The APhA Complete Review for Pharmacy

Notices

The authors, editors, and publisher have made every effort to ensure the accuracy and completeness of the information presented in this book. However, the authors, editors, and publisher cannot be held responsible for the continued currency of the information, any inadvertent errors or omissions, or the application of this information. Therefore, the authors, editors, and publisher shall have no liability to any person or entity with regard to claims, loss, or damage caused or alleged to be caused, directly or indirectly, by the use of information contained herein.

The inclusion in this book of any product in respect to which patent or trademark rights may exist shall not be deemed, and is not intended as, a grant of or authority to exercise any right or privilege protected by such patent or trademark. All such rights or trademarks are vested in the patent or trademark owner, and no other person may exercise the same without express permission, authority, or license secured from such patent or trademark owner.

The inclusion of a brand name does not mean the authors, the editors, or the publisher has any particular knowledge that the brand listed has properties different from other brands of the same product, nor should its inclusion be interpreted as an endorsement by the authors, the editors, or the publisher. Similarly, the fact that a particular brand has not been included does not indicate the product has been judged to be in any way unsatisfactory or unacceptable. Further, no official support or endorsement of this book by any federal or state agency or pharmaceutical company is intended or inferred.

NAPLEX® is a trademark of the National Association of Boards of Pharmacy® (NABP®), and NABP® in no way endorses, authorizes, or sponsors this guide.

The APhA Complete Review for Pharmacy

Sixth Edition

Dick R. Gourley, PharmD

Editor-in-Chief
Dean and Professor
University of Tennessee College of Pharmacy
Memphis, Tennessee

James C. Eoff III, PharmD

Associate Editor-in-Chief
Executive Associate Dean and Professor, Clinical Pharmacy
University of Tennessee College of Pharmacy
Memphis, Tennessee

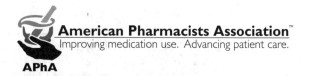
American Pharmacists Association™
Improving medication use. Advancing patient care.
APhA

Washington, D.C.

Editor: Nancy Tarleton Landis
Composition: Circle Graphics
Cover Design: Scott Neitzke, APhA Creative Services

©2009 by the American Pharmacists Association
Published by the American Pharmacists Association
1100 15th Street, NW, Suite 400
Washington, DC 20005-1707
www.pharmacist.com

APhA was founded in 1852 as the American Pharmaceutical Association.

To comment on this book via e-mail, send your message to the publisher at aphabooks@aphanet.org.

Library of Congress Cataloging-in-Publication Data

The APhA complete review for pharmacy / Dick R. Gourley, editor-in-chief;
James C. Eoff III, associate editor-in-chief. – 6th ed.
      p. ; cm.
Includes bibliographical references.
ISBN 978-1-58212-141-3
1. Pharmacy–Outlines, syllabi, etc. 2. Pharmacy–Examinations,
questions, etc. I. Gourley, D. R. (Dick R.), 1944- II. Eoff, James C.
III. American Pharmacists Association. IV. Title: Complete review for
pharmacy.
  [DNLM: 1. Pharmacy–Examination Questions. 2. Pharmaceutical
Preparations–Examination Questions. QV 18.2 A641 2009]

  RS98.A64 2009
  615.1076–dc22

                              2008053875

How to Order This Book
Online: www.pharmacist.com
By phone: 800-878-0729 (770-280-0085 from outside the United States)
VISA®, MasterCard®, and American Express® cards accepted

Contents

Katie J. Suda, PharmD
Associate Professor and Director, Drug Information
    Center
Department of Clinical Pharmacy
University of Tennessee College of Pharmacy

Anne M. Hurley, PharmD
Assistant Professor
Department of Clinical Pharmacy
University of Tennessee College of Pharmacy

Trevor McKibbin, PharmD, M.Sc., BCPS
Assistant Professor
Department of Clinical Pharmacy
University of Tennessee College of Pharmacy

Erin M. Timpe, PharmD, BCPS
Associate Professor and Director, Drug Information
Southern Illinois University, Edwardsville

Preface

It is indeed an honor to have again been asked to serve as Editor-in-Chief of *The APhA Complete Review for Pharmacy*. We are now publishing the sixth edition and sincerely appreciate the continued support of the American Pharmacists Association (APhA). The faculty of the University of Tennessee College of Pharmacy and I appreciate the confidence that APhA has demonstrated by allowing us this opportunity to assist pharmacy students in preparing for the NAPLEX® examination. This project is very important to pharmacy students across the United States, and we know they appreciate the support of APhA.

As pharmacy students prepare to take the NAPLEX® examination, it is imperative that they have available to them the most up-to-date and relevant information concerning the practice of pharmacy. The information explosion is such that information changes daily, and approximately 30 new drugs are marketed each year. The amount of information that any student in pharmacy must master is significant and doubles every two to three years.

The board examination is the culmination of at least six years of university work. It is impossible to go back to the beginning and review all aspects of pharmacy education to prepare for it. Therefore, we have developed a comprehensive review of pharmacy for students preparing to take the NAPLEX® examination.

In this new sixth edition, Chapter 38 provides a summary of all new drugs, dosage indications, and uses of medications since the last edition. The other chapters remain unchanged from the fifth edition.

This study guide has attempted to summarize the information in a user-friendly manner. Our faculty and a panel of 10 pharmacy residents believe the information included to be the most important information needed for the NAPLEX® exam. The review includes educational material (synthesizing the most salient points), key points (further delineation of the most important factors), references, and, finally, self-study questions.

This book is also an excellent review for practicing pharmacists as they continue to expand their therapeutic knowledge and for foreign graduates interested in obtaining licensure in the United States. The CD-ROM that accompanies this book contains case studies and more than 900 questions and annotated answers, and it will give students valuable practice exam experience.

It is highly recommended that any student preparing for the NAPLEX® examination review the instructions on the NABP® Web site (www.nabp.net). Students should also read the current literature in journals and review areas where they feel they have a weakness.

My thanks and appreciation go to my Associate Editor James C. Eoff III, PharmD, Executive Associate Dean of the University of Tennessee College of Pharmacy; the faculty of the University of Tennessee College of Pharmacy, who participated in preparing this comprehensive review; and Karin Ingram, Executive Assistant to the Dean, for her coordination of the preparation of the review book. I also wish to thank APhA for recognizing the need of pharmacy students for this review book. APhA's willingness to provide this for all student members who are pharmacy graduates in the United States is a true service to the profession of pharmacy.

Dick R. Gourley, PharmD
Dean and Professor
University of Tennessee College of Pharmacy
Memphis, Tennessee
December 2008

The Editors wish to thank the following contributors for the case studies and questions and answers they prepared for inclusion on the companion CD-ROM:

Mollie Cannon, PharmD

L. Paige Clement, PharmD

Amy B. Gamlin, PharmD

Tameka W. Lucas, PharmD

Kristi Nesler, PharmD

Laura Pounders, PharmD

Kristie Ramser, PharmD

Katie Wassil, PharmD

Study Guide to NAPLEX Review and Test-Taking Strategies

James C. Eoff III, PharmD
University of Tennessee College of Pharmacy

Welcome to *The APhA Complete Review for Pharmacy*. With so many different academic backgrounds, such a variety of learning experiences, and the increasing volume of information taught at U.S. colleges of pharmacy, it is impossible to cover all materials from each course you have taken while in pharmacy school. Therefore the primary purpose of *The APhA Complete Review for Pharmacy* is to provide a summary of therapeutics as well as other basic pharmaceutical principles (dosage forms, math, biopharmaceutics, kinetics, basic and parenteral compounding, among others) which will be valuable in your preparation for the NAPLEX®, and also be a resource as you enter practice.

This review book is not an exhaustive discussion of the topics presented; it utilizes an abbreviated outline format to enable you to review and organize the material in an efficient manner for easy recall and recognition. The NAPLEX® is a difficult exam, and it covers a tremendous amount of material. In recent years, the NAPLEX® has become even more relevant to professional practice, with less emphasis on the basic sciences and more emphasis on drug therapy and pharmaceutical care.

Your success in pharmacy school has been due to diligence and hard work. You should have confidence that your pharmacy education has prepared you for the NAPLEX® and you should not have anxieties about the exam. However, your self-confidence should not prevent you from being meticulous about preparation for the NAPLEX®. Realizing that approximately 10% of students fail to achieve a passing score on their first attempt at the NAPLEX®, do not take this exam lightly.

The following are helpful hints that will improve your success on this examination:

1. *Positive attitude:* You are encouraged to approach preparation for the NAPLEX® with a positive attitude. Study to learn and understand concepts, not just memorize enough facts to pass the exam. Remember that in addition to being a minimum standard required for entry into pharmacy practice, an important benefit of taking the NAPLEX® is the comprehensive review, which will make you a better pharmacy practitioner. Without the NAPLEX®, few pharmacy graduates would spend the time and effort to review the entire discipline immediately prior to completing their studies. You should be confident that you have the knowledge to pass the exam if you have prepared diligently.

2. *Plan ahead:* Do not delay your review and preparation for the NAPLEX® until the last week before your scheduled exam date. While the total amount of time varies greatly from student to student, it is recommended that you start a serious review no less than 4-6 weeks before you plan to take the exam. However, if you have limited pharmacy work experience, you should start much earlier, especially learning generic and trade names. Be conscientious about scheduling specific times to prepare for the NAPLEX® over this time period. Cramming the last few days before the NAPLEX® will potentially increase your anxiety and could also confuse you with such a large volume of material. Read one or two chapters per day 4 or 5 days per week, and review the generic and trade names daily.

3. *Generic and trade names:* The first place to begin your preparation is to learn the generic and trade names for the top 200 drugs. The importance of this basic recommendation cannot be overemphasized. Without this base, you will experience tremendous difficulty on the NAPLEX®, which is traditionally over half trade names. In addition, you will also need to learn the generic and trade names for the unique drugs, which may not be among the top 200 drugs (eg, Cogentin® & Artane®, which are used to manage the extrapyramidal side effects of psychotherapeutic agents; Tofranil®, which is used to treat enuresis; Tapazole®, which is used to treat hyperthyroidism). Most of the patient medication profiles contain numerous drugs that may be listed either by the generic or trade name. Therefore knowledge of generic and trade names is essential to identify therapeutic duplication (eg, the patient who is prescribed Corgard® who is already taking the beta-blocker propranolol). You will also be expected to determine potential causes for adverse effects, as well as screen for drug interactions and drug-disease interactions, either from drugs on the profile or the new prescriptions. In some cases drugs will be listed by their generic names and in others by their trade names.

4. **Math:** Other than generic and trade names, pharmacy math is the most important single area to review. You should practice working several examples of each type of math problem to be sure you are comfortable and confident in your ability. While some therapeutic topics may not be covered extensively, the large number of math questions on the NAPLEX® makes this a high priority. Many students struggle with math on the NAPLEX®. Therefore it is recommended that you schedule several math study sessions. The metric system is emphasized, but you must know the other systems and be able to make conversions. While the apothecary system is used infrequently, the avoirdupois system (sometimes called the "household" system) is still used (eg, prepare one pound of ointment). When apothecary or avoirdupois measures are used, you should usually convert them to metric.

5. **Competencies:** You should review the areas of emphasis defined in the NAPLEX® competency statements that are available on the NABP® website: www.nabp.net. As you review the top 200 drugs you should ask yourself the following questions:

   * What is the therapeutic category of this drug?
   * What is the mechanism of action?
   * What type of patient counseling information should be provided?
   * What are the major adverse effects (side effects and toxic effects)?
   * What is the dosage schedule (frequency)?
   * What are the major drug interactions and disease contraindications?

   These topics should also be the priority areas as you review each therapeutic class of agents.

6. **Dosage schedules:** Summary charts of the major categories of drugs are provided in each of the therapeutic chapters of this book. You will find the generic as well as trade names, along with commonly available dosage forms, dosage, and frequency of use. The frequency of use is emphasized more on the NAPLEX® than the specific dosages. The following therapeutic lists with multiple agents should also be emphasized in your studying: β-blockers, calcium channel blockers, ACE inhibitors, benzodiazepines, cephalosporins, quinolones, aminoglycosides, NSAIDs, H_2 blockers, protease inhibitors, oral antidiabetics, and statins. Be able to recognize the agents within these categories, and to know how to compare the differences within the category (eg, duration of action, dosage schedules, side effects, and distinct advantages in patients with certain diseases).

7. **Appendices:** There are also many tables that can help you recall or recognize answers for NAPLEX® questions in the appendices, such as the major drug-drug interactions, the drugs that should not be crushed, and the top 200 OTC agents. There are also other important tables to study throughout the book, such as the table of common antidotes for poisons and overdosages in the toxicology chapter. By reviewing these therapeutic agents by categories and in tables, you will increase your recall of them on the exam.

8. **Chronic and common diseases:** The NAPLEX® emphasizes the more common and chronic diseases and their therapy. While it is a good idea to have a general knowledge of the disease process, remember that the NAPLEX® is heavily weighted toward drug therapy. Therefore you should not devote the majority of your study time on the disease process (eg, etiology, pathophysiology, diagnosis, and signs and symptoms) at the expense of the therapy (including nondrug therapy). While it is helpful to review your areas of strength, you should concentrate more on your areas of weakness. The less familiar you are with a topic, the more time the topic should be given in review.

9. **Priorities:** There are several areas that should **not** be emphasized in your review: (1) the manufacturer of the specific drug (eg, Zithromax® manufactured by Pfizer); (2) chemical structures; and (3) identification or physical descriptions (eg, color, shape, etc). These areas are covered only minimally on the NAPLEX®.

10. **Review questions:** Reviewing sample exam questions is very helpful. However, to make this a more effective learning experience, study the explanations along with their answers. Do not look only at the correct answer, but look at distractors and learn why they are incorrect. Therapeutics reference texts may also be helpful in your NAPLEX® review for their more detailed information and to assist with difficult or complex material. This will also reinforce learning points about material covered in your review.

11. **Exam format:** The NAPLEX® consists of 185 multiple-choice questions in a computer adaptive format that is individualized to each candidate's level of ability. The computer adapted test system selects your next questions based on your response to previous questions, and thus each question must be answered before you can proceed. The 150 questions that have been pre-tested for validity are the basis for your evaluation. In addition, 35 questions that are being evaluated for use in future exams are distributed throughout the exam.

12. **Question format:** You should log on to the NABP® website (www.napb.net) to review the format for exam questions and the patient profiles. NABP® also offers a "pre-NAPLEX®" test for a fee, that will allow you to practice with the computerized format. This will help allay your anxiety and be especially beneficial if you are not comfortable with exams given in a computer format.

All questions have 5 choices with only *one* "best" answer. You may not continue the exam until you have answered the question. You may not skip the question and come back. Therefore you will be unable to leave any question blank. The question is superimposed at the bottom of the screen below the patient medication record. After deciding on the best answer you will:

1. Highlight the answer.
2. Request the next question.
3. Confirm that you want the next question, which will finalize your answer.

You cannot go back to change an answer after step 3.

There are two types of multiple-choice questions:

1. The traditional single-answer type as in the example below:

   The agent of choice for the initial treatment of contact dermatitis, whether irritant or allergic, is a:

   A. topical antihistamine
   B. oral antihistamine
   C. topical corticosteroid
   D. local anesthetic
   E. coal tar product

   and

2. The combined-response ("K" type) question with 1, 2, or 3 components listed, as in the example below:

   The most common side effects of isotretinoin include which of the following?

   I. Cheilitis
   II. Acute depression
   III. Decreased night vision

   A. I only
   B. II only
   C. III only
   D. I and II
   E. I, II, and III

13. **Patient medication record:** The patient medication record is usually followed by 10-15 questions. You must refer to the patient profile for many of the questions. However, some questions may be answered as presented or "stand alone." You will **not** be able to see the entire profile on the top of the screen without scrolling down to review the whole profile. You may want to write down the significant points from the profile, such as allergies, age of the patient, and preexisting diseases, on scrap paper. Note carefully if the patient has multiple diseases, and for females, look for pregnancy or nursing, or likelihood of becoming pregnant. Some prefer to read the questions prior to reviewing the profile, but you could miss an important fact like a drug allergy, a drug-disease contraindication, or an adverse effect being treated currently that resulted from a previously prescribed drug, and answer the question without all of the necessary information. Therefore always conduct a quick review of the profile prior to answering the questions.

14. **Testing center location:** If you are not familiar with the exact location of the testing center, locate it no later than the day before the exam. Arrive at the testing site at least 30 minutes prior to the scheduled time in order to be as calm as you can. You do not want to be caught in traffic or get lost trying to find the testing center and panic immediately prior to taking the exam.

15. **The night before the exam:** Do not study the night before the exam; last minute cramming will only add to your anxiety and will not improve your test score. I recommend that you

take a night off from study the evening before the exam. Go out for a relaxing dinner and/or a movie. Be sure to get to bed early, especially if you are scheduled for a morning exam, so your ability to reason, recognize, and recall information is sharp.

16. *Afternoon exam:* If your exam is scheduled in the afternoon, fatigue can dull your test-taking abilities. Be on guard against this by having a light lunch, preferably with coffee, tea, or some caffeine-containing beverage to be sure that you stay sharp for the afternoon session.

Taking the Exam

1. Read all directions carefully. Read each question a minimum of two times to determine the nature of the question and the point of asking the question. Note any modifying terms like always, all, never, most, usually, double negatives, and anything else that may change the meaning of the question. Modifiers like "always" and "never" mean what they say.

2. Read all the choices thoroughly before you answer the question. Attempt to eliminate the distractor choices or incorrect answers. Two or three answers can usually be eliminated for one reason or another, and the final choice is between two answers. The more distractors you identify and eliminate, the more you increase your probability of obtaining the best answer. Then select the *single best answer*. Your first instinct is generally the best choice. Be cautious about not reading multiple possibilities into questions; the questions are straightforward and are not designed to trick you.

3. If you are positive that you do not know the answer, eliminate any distractors and guess intelligently, making the best choice you can of the remaining answers. If you can limit your guess to two possible correct answers, your score will be much better than if you try to guess the correct answer from five possible choices. Proceeding in this fashion over the course of the exam, you can increase your success if you guess consistently. While blind guessing is not recommended, after narrowing possibilities, intelligent guessing is definitely recommended.

4. Pace yourself, but do not rush through the exam. The 4 hours, 15 minutes scheduled for the NAPLEX® is more than adequate, and the majority of students have plenty of time to complete the exam. You need to proceed at a reasonable pace and need to answer approximately 45-50 questions per hour to finish comfortably in the time available. There is a timer visible at the corner of the screen with your remaining exam time. If you notice that you have only completed 40 questions in the first hour, you should increase your speed.

5. Some of the math questions may be weighted more heavily and some will take several minutes to answer. Take the time to answer the math questions correctly. Incorrect answers may lead to additional math questions (eg, missing the first milliequivalent question could lead to more milliequivalent questions on your exam). Use the scrap paper provided for your calculations. Be sure to include units as you complete the math questions on your scrap paper.

6. It is important that you remember that you cannot return to a previous question after you have confirmed an answer. There is no need to get upset over a previous question you realize you have missed as you proceed through the exam. Do not get nervous during the exam or panic or you may lose your ability to recall or recognize common information. Remain calm and do the best you can. Best of luck with the test!

James C. Eoff III, PharmD
Executive Associate Dean and Professor
University of Tennessee College of Pharmacy
847 Monroe Avenue
Memphis, Tennessee 38163
Email: jeoff@utmem.edu

NAPLEX® is a federally registered trademark owned by the National Association of Boards of Pharmacy® (NABP®). This review course is in no way authorized or sponsored by the NABP®. Please check the NABP® website, www.nabp.net, for more complete information.

It's YOUR time to shine!

At the American Pharmacists Association (APhA), we're excited about the future of pharmacy and the arrival of our new practitioner members! We see a profession rich with innovation and future-focused perspectives on patient care that oftentimes come from our new practitioner members—**the rising stars of pharmacy!**

Most likely, you currently are or have been a member of APhA's Academy of Student Pharmacists and are acquainted with the many valuable benefits of membership in APhA: special discounts on books and products, timely news and information from our periodicals, and a variety of other programs designed to supplement your education. As you begin to practice in your chosen community and practice setting, you'll find that you need to rely on these assets more than ever.

Now that you're about to make the transition to professional practice, this is the perfect time to discover how APhA can support your career! New practitioners are welcomed into APhA through a special category of membership called the APhA New Practitioner Network (APhA-NPN). Becoming a member of APhA-NPN means you'll receive the same benefits regular members receive *plus* benefits specifically tailored to new practitioners, with modified pricing based on your graduation date! Even those in postgraduate and/or residency programs qualify for a discounted rate to help with the transition.

APhA-NPN resources cover three main areas that have proven over the years to help new pharmacists jumpstart their careers and quickly gain momentum. You'll benefit from:

- **Quality news and information resources** to help you stay on the cutting edge of trends in the profession as well as work/life balance issues.
- **Networks of like-minded professionals** to help you navigate the daily challenges of a practicing pharmacist.
- **Additional educational resources** useful for gaining new perspectives or simply fulfilling licensure requirements when the time comes.

Sound interesting? Let's take a closer look...

APhA provides quality news and information you can trust.

When you need reliable information at your fingertips to help you respond to the new demands of your career, who better to trust than the organization that has been helping tens of thousands of pharmacists meet their professional challenges for more than 150 years? APhA has a solid history of leading the profession, in part by providing periodicals containing information you can use right away or keep as a reference.

Transitions—Exclusively for pharmacist members of APhA-NPN, *Transitions* is the quarterly newsletter that provides insight on your personal and professional life, such as career advice, financial planning, maintaining work/life balance, and more. At a time when moving from one life stage to another can involve focusing on multiple priorities at once, *Transitions* can help you find ways to become acclimated to life's new events.

Pharmacy Today—Reading this monthly publication from APhA provides you with comprehensive news on new drug products and drug regimens, developments in innovative practice and medication therapy management, and trends in health care that affect pharmacists, as well as legal and regulatory updates. *Pharmacy Today* will help prepare you to meet the day-to-day challenges of your career.

Journal of the American Pharmacists Association (JAPhA)—The official peer-reviewed journal of APhA publishes research on pharmacy practice, in-depth feature articles, columns, and informed opinion. Keeping *JAPhA* on your short list of professional resources will help you stay in touch with your profession and gain new perspectives from others making great strides in improving medication use and advancing patient care. Current and past issues of *JAPhA* are available online at www.japha.org.

APhA DrugInfoLine—When you need the latest information on drug therapy developments and major therapeutic research, time is of the essence! As an APhA member, you won't have to worry because you'll have the *APhA DrugInfoLine,* which allows you to quickly and easily access "what you need to know" and "what your patients need to know" *when you need to know it.* Published monthly, *DrugInfoLine* sets the standard for offering timely clinical and drug information useful in daily practice. See the Publications link at www. pharmacist.com for current and past issues of *DrugInfoLine.*

Get involved! Stay connected! And get the support you deserve!

As you focus on becoming the best pharmacist you can be while balancing your personal life, you can easily get lost in the daily grind. But you don't want to miss out on relationships with peers! APhA makes it easy to stay connected to colleagues old and new, as well as keep up with the latest trends in pharmacy through APhA Academies, e-Communities, and social networking sites.

APhA Academies are free to members and offer an opportunity to more closely align your APhA membership with the areas of practice or research that you're most interested in pursuing. Indicating your Academy preference will enable you to receive information tailored to your interests and connect with others on issues specifically related to your practice setting. If you haven't already, consider joining one of APhA's Academies:

- APhA Academy of Pharmacy Practice and Management (APhA-APPM)
- APhA Academy of Pharmaceutical Research and Science (APhA-APRS)

APhA e-Communities are listserves that offer a quick, easy way to engage with like-minded professionals and solicit feedback on APhA and pharmacy-related issues while learning about some of the hottest areas of pharmacy. In addition, APhA has established Facebook pages and LinkedIn sites to foster networking, which is vital for healthy career growth. If you want to keep up with the movers and shakers in pharmacy, then you'll want to participate in one of the following members-only virtual communities:

- Medication Therapy Management (MTM) e-Community
- Nuclear Pharmacy e-Community
- APhA House of Delegates e-Community
- APhA and APhA-NPN Facebook and LinkedIn communities (can be accessed by visiting www.facebook.com and www.linkedin.com).

Your education is just beginning!

As your career progresses, you'll eventually need ongoing professional development and continuing education to stay on top of the latest trends and maintain licensure. Furthermore, many new practitioners take advantage of APhA's free educational opportunities as a way to *become more marketable to potential employers* by becoming more knowledgeable in their profession. APhA is the best resource for a wide variety of *quality education.* Whether you're interested in continuing education monographs, comprehensive certificate training programs, or live educational programming, you can rest assured that APhA's programs are designed to keep you on the fast track to success!

Continuing Education—Convenient, accessible, and free to members, the APhA CE Center at www. pharmacist.com offers more than 80 valuable and relevant continuing education activities. You'll also find information on state licensure requirements, instant Statements of Credit, and online personal transcript storage that automatically maintains a record of your CE.

APhA's Annual Meeting & Exposition—The nation's only education-based conference for pharmacists in all practice settings is held annually in the spring. Participants can select from numerous programs geared toward the latest drug therapies and innovations in patient-centered pharmacy practice, make or enhance professional relationships, take advantage of networking opportunities, and explore various career opportunities. In addition, there are "new practitioner only" events, including financial planning strategies workshops and several social events. APhA members benefit from discounted registration rates, and all attendees are sure to have a memorable experience. Visit www.aphameeting.org for the latest information.

Certificate Training Programs—These innovative and interactive practice-based educational programs are designed to help pharmacists develop the skills needed to become confident, successful disease state managers. Thousands of pharmacists have benefited from APhA's Certificate Training Programs. When you're ready to develop the advanced skills needed for disease management, advocate disease prevention, or assist patients with improving medication use, APhA's Certificate Training Programs are ready for you. For more information regarding programs on becoming an immunizing pharmacist, providing pharmaceutical care for patients with diabetes or dyslipidemias, providing medication therapy management, and advancing patient self-care, go to www.pharmacist.com/education.

Whether you're looking to interact with other like-minded professionals, explore additional topics in pharmacy, or keep up with the latest pharmacy news, information, and trends, be sure to visit us online at www.pharmacist.com/membership to *renew* your membership. Or, if you've never had a membership with APhA, *join today* so that you, too, can have the quality resources necessary to stay competitive with those who already enjoy being a part of APhA.

Join APhA! You'll be right at home where the rising stars of pharmacy are improving medication use and advancing patient care!

American Pharmacists Association
1100 15th Street NW, Suite 400
Washington, DC 20005-1707
800-237-2742

For additional information about APhA and the latest pharmacy news, drug information, career information, and continuing education, or to shop the APhA store, go to www.pharmacist.com, the nation's premier Web site for practicing pharmacists.

Please note—in April 2009, APhA will return to its newly renovated headquarters located at 2215 Constitution Avenue NW, Washington, DC 20037-2985.

1. Pharmacy Math

George E. Bass, PhD
Associate Professor
Director of Pharmaceutical Sciences
University of Tennessee College of Pharmacy

Contents

1. Units of Measure

Calculations in pharmacy may involve four different systems of measure: metric, apothecaries', avoirdupois, and household.

Metric System

The metric system fundamental units are the gram, the liter, and the meter. Prefixes are used extensively to express quantities much greater and much less than the fundamental units. Some of the most commonly used prefixes are provided in Table 1.

Apothecaries' System

While the metric system is the official system of measure for pharmacy today, the apothecaries' system is the traditional system and some elements might sometimes be found in prescriptions. Units of the apothecaries' system are presented in Table 2.

Avoirdupois System

The avoirdupois system measure of weight is employed in ordinary commerce. Here, the ounce corresponds to 437.5 grains. The avoirdupois grain unit is equal to the apothecaries' grain. Sixteen ounces (7000 grains) corresponds to 1 pound. Note that the avoirdupois ounce (473.5 grains) and pound (7000 grains)

Table 1.

Metric System Prefixes

mega-	one million times the base unit (10^6)
kilo-	one thousand times the base unit (10^3)
deci-	one-tenth the base unit (10^{-1})
centi-	one-hundredth the base unit (10^{-2})
milli-	one-thousandth the base unit (10^{-3})
micro-	one-millionth the base unit (10^{-6})
nano-	one billionth the base unit (10^{-9})
pico-	one-trillionth the base unit (10^{-12})

Table 2.

Apothecaries' System of Measure

Weight
- 20 grains = 1 scruple
- 3 scruples = 1 dram
- 8 drams = 1 ounce
- 12 ounces = 1 pound

Volume
- 60 minims = 1 fluidram
- 8 fluidrams = 1 fluidounce
- 16 fluidounces = 1 pint
- 2 pints = 1 quart
- 4 quarts = 1 gallon

measures are not equal to the apothecaries' ounce (480 grains) and pound (5760 grains) measures.

Household Measures

A tablespoon is equivalent to 15 mL and a teaspoon is equivalent to 5 mL.

Conversion Factors

A short list of convenient conversion factors is provided below.

Convenient Conversion Factors

1 inch = 2.54 cm
1 fluidounce = 30 milliliters
1 gram = 15.4 grains
1 kilogram = 2.20 pounds (avoir.)
1 pound (avoir.) = 454 grams
1 gallon, U.S = 3785 mL

2. Significant Figures

All measured quantities are approximations. The accuracy of a given measurement is conveyed by the number of figures that are recorded. The number of significant figures in a measurement includes the first approximate figure. The last recorded digit to the right of a measured quantity is taken to be an approximation. For example, the weight 13.24 g has four significant figures where the final digit, 4, is approximate. Calculations should be conducted so as to carry the correct numbers of significant figures.

It frequently happens in a given calculation that the different quantities in the calculation have different numbers of significant figures. When this occurs, follow the rules below.

Addition and Subtraction

When adding or subtracting decimal numbers, round all measurements to have the same number of decimal places as the least in the set. For example, 13.78 mL and 53.5 mL would be added as 13.8 + 53.5 = 67.3 mL, using and retaining only one decimal place.

Multiplication and Division

When multiplying or dividing decimal numbers, round the measurements to include the number of significant figures contained in the least accurate number. For example, 25.678 mL multiplied by 1.24 g/mL would be handled as 25.7 mL times 1.24 g/mL = 31.9 g, using and retaining three significant figures.

Handling Zero

Whether or not the digit zero is counted as a significant figure depends on where it appears in the measured number. If zero occurs at an interior position in the number (eg, as in 3052 and 2.031) it is significant. If zero occurs as the last digit to the right of the decimal (eg, 44.50), it is significant. If zero occurs as the first digit to the right of the decimal in a number that is less than 1, it is not significant. For example, in 0.078 there are only two significant figures. If zero occurs as the last digit, or digits, in a whole number (ie, no decimal is expressed), its significance is unknown without further information. For example, 3500 might have two, three, or four significant figures.

3. Ratios and Proportions

The most frequently encountered calculations in pharmacy will employ ratios and proportions. In mathematics, a ratio is the quotient of one quantity divided by another of the same kind, and a proportion is an equality between ratios. Thus a proportion involves a relationship between four quantities. You can always solve for one of these when the other three are known. If the ratio x/y is equal to the ratio a/b, one has the proportion $x/y = a/b$, and can obtain by algebraic manipulation: $x = ay/b$, etc. Such problems are frequently encountered when adjusting dosages.

One common source of error in proportion problems involves writing one of the ratios upside down, eg, writing $x/y = b/a$ when it should be $x/y = a/b$. A disciplined approach to setting up such problems can help. For example, you might follow the rule to express each ratio as the quotient of like quantities. Then, when you equate the two ratios, if the numerator of one ratio is smaller (or larger) than its denominator, the same should be true of the other ratio as well. Another source of error involves using mixed units, eg, using one number expressed in grams and the other in milligrams. To guard against this kind of error, always write the units into the equation along with the numbers. All unit expressions should cancel except those required for the quantity being solved for (dimensional analysis).

Example: If 250 mg of drug are contained in 300 mL of a preparation, what weight (x) would be contained in 1800 mL of the preparation?
Equate the ratios x:250 mg and 1800 mL:300 mL to solve for x:

$$\text{ie, } x/250 \text{ mg} = 1800 \text{ mL}/300 \text{ mL}$$
$$x = 250 \text{ mg} \times 1800 \text{ mL}/300 \text{ mL} = 1500 \text{ mg}$$

(Note that since the new volume is six times greater, the new weight should be six times greater as well.)

4. Specific Gravity and Density

At times you will be required to convert a volume measure to a weight measure or vice versa. To accomplish this, you will need to employ either the specific gravity or the density of the material. The specific gravity (SpGr) is a ratio of the weight of the material to the weight of the same volume of a standard material. For liquids, the standard material is water, which has a density of 1 g/mL. Specific gravity is unit-less. Density is the quotient of any measure of the weight of a sample of the material divided by any measure of the volume of the sample. The units must be explicitly expressed (eg, grams per milliliter, pounds per gallon, etc). When density is expressed in grams per milliliter, it is numerically equal to specific gravity. Algebraically, it is easier to work with density (d = wt/vol) than the corresponding expression for specific gravity.

Example: What is the weight of 750 mL of concentrated hydrochloric acid (SpGr = 1.20)?
From the specific gravity definition and using the volume of 750 mL,

$$\text{SpGr (HCl)} = \frac{\text{wt of 750 mL HCl}}{\text{wt of 750 mL H}_2\text{O}}$$

Rearranging and noting that the density of H_2O is 1 g/mL,

$$\text{wt of 750 mL HCl} = (\text{SpGr}) \times (\text{wt of 750 mL H}_2\text{O}) = 1.20 \times 750 \text{ g} = 900 \text{ g}$$

Alternatively, specific gravity is numerically equal to density expressed in grams per milliliter. Thus,

$$d = 1.20 = \text{wt HCl/Vol HCl};$$
$$\text{or, wt HCl} = d \times \text{vol HCl} =$$
$$1.20 \text{ g/mL} \times 750 \text{ mL} = 900 \text{ g}$$

5. Percentage Error

Associated with the fact that all measurements are approximations is the need to characterize the extent of the error involved. Percentage of error is such a quantity and is defined as:

$$\% \text{ error} = (\text{error} \times 100\%)/(\text{quantity desired})$$

The term **error** in the numerator is taken as the maximum potential error in the measurement, while the term **quantity desired** in the denominator represents the total amount measured. Percentage error may be calculated for either a weight or a volume measurement.

Example: Suppose a given quantity of material weighed 5.810 g on a prescription balance. Using a much more accurate analytical balance, the quantity was found to weigh 5.893 g. What is the percentage error for the original weighing?

$$\text{error} = 5.893 \text{ g} - 5.810 \text{ g} = 0.083 \text{ g}$$

The desired quantity is 5.810 g. Thus,

$$\% \text{ error} = 0.083 \text{ g} \times 100/5.810 = 1.4\%$$

Example: Suppose you wished to weigh out 75.0 mg of an ingredient but mistakenly weighed 65.0 mg instead. On the basis of the desired quantity, what is the percentage error?

$$\% \text{ error} = (\text{error} \times 100\%)/(\text{quantity desired})$$
$$= (10.0 \text{ mg} \times 100\%)/(75.0 \text{ mg}) = 13\%$$

6. Minimum Measurable Quantity

By regulation, weighings by a pharmacist cannot exceed a percentage error of greater than 5%. This requires that the sensitivity of the balance be known and limits the smallest quantity that can be weighed. Balance sensitivity is defined in terms of the *sensitivity requirement (SR)*, the weight that will move the indicator one marked unit on the index plate of the balance. For a class A prescription balance, SR = 6 mg. The minimum weighable quantity for a given balance can be calculated using the percentage error formula by replacing the "error" term with the SR (eg, 6 mg), the percentage error term with 5%, and the "desired quantity" term with "minimum weighable quantity." Thus, one would have:

$$\text{minimum weighable quantity} = SR \times 100/5$$

Example: What is the minimum weighable quantity for a balance that has a sensitivity requirement of 4 mg to assure an error no greater than 2%?

$$\% \text{ error} = \text{error} \times 100/\text{desired quantity}$$
$$= SR \times 100/\text{minimum weighable quantity}$$
$$\text{minimum weighable quantity} = SR \times 100/\% \text{ error}$$
$$= 4 \text{ mg} \times 100/2 = 200 \text{ mg}$$

Example: What is the sensitivity requirement (SR) for a balance with which a percentage error of 5% is obtained when weighing 120 mg?

$$\% \text{ error} = SR \times 100\%/\text{desired quantity}$$
$$SR = (\% \text{ error} \times \text{desired quantity})/100\%$$
$$= (5\% \times 120 \text{ mg})/100\% = 6 \text{ mg}$$

7. Patient-Specific Dosage Calculations

Drugs with a narrow therapeutic range often are dosed based on patient weight or body surface area. For patients with renal impairment, some drugs are dosed based on creatinine clearance.

Dosing Based on Body Weight

Weight-based dosing might involve using the patient's actual body weight (ABW), ideal body weight (IBW), or perhaps an adjusted ideal body weight that is a function of IBW and ABW. These weights are invariably expressed in kilograms.

Example: A patient weighing 180 lb is to receive 0.25 mg/kg per day amphotericin B (reconstituted and diluted to 0.100 mg/mL) by IV infusion. What volume of solution is required to deliver the daily dose?

$$\text{patient weight} = 180 \text{ lb}/2.20 = 82 \text{ kg}$$
$$\text{daily dose} = 82 \text{ kg} \times 0.25 \text{ mg/kg} = 20.5 \text{ mg}$$
$$\times \text{ mL}/1 \text{ mL} = 20.5 \text{ mg}/0.100 \text{ mg}$$
$$x = 1 \text{ mL} \times 20.5 \text{ mL}/0.100 \text{ mg} = 205 \text{ mL}$$

A commonly used equation for calculating IBW is:

$$\text{IBW} = (\text{gender factor}) + 2.3 \times (\text{each inch} > 5 \text{ ft}) \text{ kg},$$

where the gender factor for males is 50 kg and for females is 45.5 kg.

Example: The recommended adult daily dosage for patients with normal renal function for tobramycin is 3 mg/kg IBW given in three evenly divided doses. What would each injection be for a male patient who weighs 185 lb and is 5 ft 9 in. tall?

$$\text{IBW} = 50 \text{ kg} + 2.3 \times 9 \text{ kg} = 50 \text{ kg} + 21 \text{ kg} = 71 \text{ kg}$$
$$(\text{ignore ABW of 84 kg})$$
$$\text{daily dose (tid)} = 71 \text{ kg} \times 3 \text{ mg/kg}$$
$$= 213 \text{ mg (per day)}$$

Thus each injection = 213 mg/3 = 71 mg.

In the absence of other information, the usual drug doses are considered generally suitable for 70-kg individuals. Thus in the absence of more specific information, an adjusted dosage for a notably larger or smaller individual may be obtained by multiplying the usual dose by the ratio of patient weight to 70 kg (Clark's rule).

Example: If the adult dose of a drug is 100 mg and no child-specific dosing information is available, what would be the weight-adjusted dose for a child who weighs 40 kg?

$$\text{child dose} = 100 \text{ mg} \times 40 \text{ kg}/70 \text{ kg} = 57 \text{ mg}$$

Dosing Based on Body Surface Area

Dosing based on body surface area requires an estimation of the patient's body surface area, BSA, expressed in square meters (m^2). This parameter might be estimated from a nomogram using height and weight, or for adults, by using one of several equations such as:

$$\text{BSA} = [(\text{height in centimeters})(\text{weight in kilograms})/3600]^{1/2} \text{ m}^2$$

Example: What is the computed BSA for an adult who weighs 88 kg and is 5 ft 10 in. tall?

$$\text{height} = 70 \text{ in.} \times 2.54 \text{ cm/in.} = 178 \text{ cm}$$
$$\text{BSA} = [178 \text{ cm} \times 88 \text{ kg}/3600]^{1/2} \text{ m}^2 = 2.09 \text{ m}^2$$

The average adult BSA is taken to be 1.73 m^2. This value can be used to obtain an approximate child's dose given the usual dose for an adult and the child's estimated BSA.

Example: If the adult dose of a drug is 50 mg, what would be the BSA-adjusted dose for a child having an estimated BSA of 0.55 m^2?

$$\text{child dose} = 50 \text{ mg} \times 0.55 \text{ m}^2/1.73 \text{ m}^2 = 16 \text{ mg}$$

Dosing Based on Creatinine Clearance

For many drugs, the rate of elimination is dependent on kidney function. Creatinine clearance (CrCl) is a measure of the volume of blood plasma that is cleared of creatinine by kidney filtration per minute and is expressed in milliliters per minute. It can be calculated using the Cockcroft-Gault equation as a function of patient gender, age, body weight, and serum creatinine. For males:

$$\text{CrCl (mL/min)} = (140 - \text{age in years}) \times (\text{body wt in kg})/(72 \times \text{serum creatinine in mg/dL})$$

For females:

$$\text{CrCl} = 0.85 \times \text{CrCl for males}$$

Example: Calculate the creatinine clearance rate for a 76-year-old female weighing 65 kg and having a serum creatinine of 0.52 mg/dL using the Cockcroft-Gault equation.

$$\text{CrCl} = 0.85 \times (140 - 76 \text{ y}) \times 65 \text{ kg}/(72 \times 0.52 \text{ mg/dL}) = 94 \text{ mL/min}$$

Alternatively, creatinine clearance may be estimated using the Jelliffe equations. For males:

$$\text{CrCl} = [98 - 0.8 \times (\text{patient age in years} - 20)]/ \text{serum creatinine in mg/dL}]$$

For females:

$$\text{CrCl} = 0.9 \times \text{CrCl for males}$$

The normal value for creatinine clearance is taken to be 100 mL/min. It is sometimes advisable to adjust CrCl to the patient's BSA. This is calculated thus:

$$\text{adjusted CrCl} = \text{CrCl} \times \text{BSA}/1.73$$

The maintenance dose for some drugs is based on ideal body weight (IBW) and CrCl. See the chapter on pharmacokinetics, drug metabolism, and drug disposition for more detailed coverage.

8. Using Batch Preparation Formulas

The relative amounts of ingredients in a pharmaceutical product are specified in a formula. A pharmacist may be required to reduce or enlarge the formula to prepare a lesser or greater amount of product. A given formula might specify either the actual amount (weight or volume) of each ingredient for a specified total amount of product or just the relative amounts (parts) of each ingredient. In the latter case, the ingredients must all be of the same measure (eg, weight in grams).

Example: From the following formula, calculate the quantity of triethanolamine required to make 200 mL of the lotion.

Triethanolamine	10 mL
Oleic acid	25 mL
Benzyl benzoate	250 mL
Water to make	1000 mL

$$x{:}10 \text{ mL} = 200 \text{ mL}{:}1000 \text{ mL}$$
$$x = 10 \text{ mL } x \text{ } 200 \text{ mL}/1000 \text{ mL} = 2.0 \text{ mL}$$

Example: From the following formula, calculate the quantity of chlorpheniramine maleate required to make 500 g of the product.

Chlorpheniramine maleate	6 parts
Phenindamine	20 parts
Phenylpropanolamine HCl	55 parts

Note that the formula will give a total of 81 parts, which will correspond to the desired quantity of 500 g. Then,

$$x{:}500 \text{ g} = 6 \text{ parts}{:}81 \text{ parts}$$
$$x = 500 \text{ g } x \text{ } 6 \text{ parts}/81 \text{ parts} = 37 \text{ g}$$

9. Conventions in Expression of Concentration

A diversity of conventions for expressing drug concentrations is encountered in pharmacy. One must be prepared to calculate these directly from their definitions and to interconvert among them.

Percentage Strength

Percentage, strictly speaking, specifies the number of parts per 100 parts. In pharmacy, this comes in three varieties:

- Percent weight-in-weight = %(w/w) = grams of ingredient in 100 grams of product; assumed for mixtures of solids and semisolids
- Percent volume-in-volume = %(v/v) = milliliters of ingredient in 100 milliliters of product; assumed for solutions or mixtures of liquids
- Percent weight-in-volume = %(w/v) = grams of ingredient in 100 milliliters of product; assumed for solutions of solids in liquids

Example: What is the concentration in %(w/v) for a preparation containing 250 mg of drug in 50 mL of solution? Note that %(w/v) is defined as g/100 mL. So:

$$\text{concentration} = 0.250 \text{ g x } 100/50 \text{ mL} = 0.50 \text{ %(w/v)}$$

Parts (Ratio Strength)

Concentrations may be expressed in "parts" or ratio strength, when the active ingredient is highly diluted. Assumptions concerning (w/w), (v/v), and (w/v) are identical to those above for percentages.

Example: What is the concentration in %(v/v) of a solution that has a ratio strength of 1:2500 (v/v)?

$$x \text{ mL}{:}1 \text{ mL} = 100 \text{ mL}{:}2500 \text{ mL}$$
$$x = 100 \text{ mL x } 1 \text{ mL}/2500 \text{ mL} = 0.040 \text{ %(v/v)}$$

Millimoles

By definition, a 1 molar solution contains 1 gram molecular weight (1 GMW = 1 mole = weight in grams of Avogadro's number of particles) per liter of solution. The molarity expresses the number of moles per liter. The millimolarity (millimoles/liter) is 1000 times the molarity of a solution.

Example: What is the millimolar concentration of a solution consisting of 0.90 g of sodium chloride (GMW = 58.5) in 100 mL of water? The quantity of 0.9 g in 100 mL corresponds to 9.0 g in 1000 mL.

$$\text{molarity} = \text{moles}/1000 \text{ mL} = (9.0 \text{ g}/58.5 \text{ g/mole})$$
$$= 0.154$$
$$\text{millimolarity} = 1000 \times \text{molarity} = 154$$

Milliequivalents

By definition, the equivalent weight of an ion is the atomic or formula weight of the ion divided by the absolute value of its valence. Thus the equivalent weight of ferric ion, Fe^{3+} (atomic weight 55.9, valence 3) is 18.6. A milliequivalent is one-thousandth of an equivalent weight, ie, there are 1000 milliequivalent weights in 1 equivalent weight. For a molecule, the equivalent weight is obtained as the gram molecular weight (formula weight) divided by the total cation OR the total anion charge. For example, the equivalent weight of $MgCl_2$ (Mg^{2+}, atomic weight 24.3, valence +2; Cl^{1-}, atomic weight 35.5, valence –1) is $(24.3 + 2 \times 35.5)/2 = 47.7$ g. Its milliequivalent weight is 0.0477 g, or 47.7 mg. In the case of a nondissociating (nonionizing) molecule, eg, dextrose or tobramycin, the equivalent weight is equal to the formula weight.

Example: What is the concentration, in milliequivalents per liter, of a solution containing 14.9 g of potassium chloride (GMW = 74.5 g) in one liter? Note that the valence of potassium is 1+, so the equivalent wt. = molecular wt. Accordingly,

$$\text{mEq/L of KCl} = \text{mEq/L of } K^+ = \text{mEq/L of } Cl^-$$
$$= 1000 \times (14.9 \text{ g/L})/(74.5 \text{ g/Eq}) = 200 \text{ mEq/L}$$

Example: What weight of $MgSO_4$, GMW = 120, is required to prepare 1 liter of a solution that is 25.0 mEq/L in Mg^{2+}? To obtain 25.0 mEq of Mg requires 25.0 mEq of $MgSO_4$. Since the valence of Mg (and total positive charge) is 2+, the equivalent weight of $MgSO_4$ is 120/2 = 60 g. Accordingly, 60 mg corresponds to 1 mEq of $MgSO_4$. Then,

$$x:60 \text{ mg} = 25 \text{ mEq}:1 \text{ mEq}$$
$$x = 60 \text{ mg} \times 25 \text{ mEq}/1 \text{ mEq} = 1500 \text{ mg} = 1.50 \text{ g}$$

Example: How many milliequivalents of $Ca2^+$ are contained in 100 mL of a solution that is 5.0 %(w/v) in $CaCl_2$ (GMW $CaCl_2$ = 111, atomic wt. Ca^{2+} = 40, atomic wt. Cl^- = 35.5)? Note that the valence of calcium is 2+. The solution contains 5.0 g $CaCl_2$ per 100 mL. This corresponds to $(5.0 \text{ g}/111) \times 2 = 0.090$ equivalents of $CaCl_2$, as well as Ca^{2+}. Accordingly, 100 mL of the solution contains 90 mEq of Ca^{2+}.

Milliosmoles

Osmotic concentration is a measure of the total number of particles in solution and is expressed in milliosmoles (mOsm). Thus the number of milliosmoles is based on the total number of cations AND total number of anions. The milliosmolarity of a solution is the number of milliosmoles per liter of solution (mOsm/L), where

$$\text{mOsm/L} = (\text{moles/L}) \times \text{number of species}$$
$$\times 1000 \text{ moles} = \text{wt/molecular weight}$$
$$\text{number of species} = \text{number of ionic species}$$
$$\text{on complete dissociation}$$
(eg, dextrose, 1 specie; NaCl, 2 species; $MgCl_2$, 3 species, etc)

The (total) osmolarity of a solution is the sum of the osmolarities of the solute components of the solution. When calculating osmolarities, in the absence of other information, assume that salts (eg, NaCl, etc) dissociate completely (referred to as the "ideal" osmolarity). You should be aware of the distinction between the terms *milliosmolarity* (milliosmoles per liter of solution) and *milliosmolality* (milliosmoles per kilogram of solution).

Example: What is the concentration, in milliosmoles per liter, of a solution that contains 224 mg of KCl (GMW = 74.6 g) and 234 mg of NaCl (GMW = 58.5) in 500 mL? What is the number of milliosmoles per liter of K^+ alone?

$$\text{mOsm KCl/500 mL} = (0.224 \text{ g}/74.6) \times 2 \times 1000$$
$$= 6.0 \text{ for 500 mL}$$
$$\text{mOsm NaCl/500 mL} = (0.234 \text{ g}/58.5) \times 2 \times 1000$$
$$= 8.0 \text{ for 500 mL}$$
$$\text{total mOsm/L} = 2 \times (6.0 \text{ mOsm KCl} +$$
$$8.0 \text{ mOsm NaCl}) = 28.0 \text{ mOsm/L}$$
$$\text{mOsm/L of } K^+ = \text{mOsm/L of KCl}/2 = 12.0/2 = 6.0$$

Mg%; Mg/dL

Traditionally, some lab test values are reported as the number of milligrams per 100 milliliters (mg%) or equivalently, milligrams per deciliter (mg/dL).

Example: What is the %(w/v) concentration of glucose in a patient with a blood glucose reading of 230 mg/dL? Note that 1 dL = 100 mL and that 230 mg = 0.230 g. Then,

$$\text{glucose concentration} = 0.230 \text{ g}/100 \text{ mL}$$
$$= 0.230 \text{ \%(w/v)}$$

"Units" and mcg/mg

The concentrations for some drugs whose production involves incomplete isolation from natural sources might be expressed in terms of "units" of activity or micrograms per milligram (mcg/mg) as determined by a standardized bioassay.

Example: A preparation of penicillin G sodium contains 2.2 mEq of sodium (atomic wt. = 23, valence = 1+) per 1 million units of penicillin. How many milligrams of sodium are contained in an IV infusion of 5 million units? The 5 million unit dose will contain 5 x 2.2 mEq = 11.0 mEq.

$$\text{mEq weight of sodium} = 23 \text{ mg}$$
$$\text{wt. sodium} = (23 \text{ mg/mEq}) \times 11.0 \text{ mEq} = 253 \text{ mg}$$

Parts Per Million and Parts Per Billion

Very low concentrations often are expressed in terms of parts per million (ppm), the number of parts of ingredient per million parts of mixture or solution, or parts per billion (ppb), the number of parts of ingredient per billion parts of mixture or solution. Thus ppm and ppb are special cases of ratio strength concentrations.

Example: Re-express 1:25,000 in terms of parts per million.

$$x \text{ parts}:1 \text{ part} = 1{,}000{,}000 \text{ parts}:25{,}000 \text{ parts}$$
$$x = 1{,}000{,}000 \times 1/25{,}000 = 40 \text{ parts,}$$
$$\text{ie, the concentration is 40 ppm}$$

10. Dilutions and Concentrations

Simple Dilutions

In simple dilutions, a desired drug concentration is obtained by adding more solvent (or diluent) to an existing solution or mixture. Mathematically, the key feature of this process is that the initial and final amount of drug present remains unchanged. The amount of drug in any solution is proportional to the concentration times the quantity of the solution. Thus, taking the initial concentration as C_1, the initial quantity of solution as Q_1, the final concentration as C_2, and the final quantity of solution as Q_2, one has the relationship: $C_1 \times Q_1 = C_2 \times Q_2$. When provided values for any three of these variables, the fourth variable can be calculated. (Because this equation can be rearranged to $C_1/C_2 = Q_2/Q_1$, it is sometimes referred to as an "inverse proportionality.")

Example: How much water should be added to 250 mL of a solution of 0.20 %(w/v) benzalkonium chloride to make a 0.050 %(w/v) solution?

$$C_1 = 0.20 \text{ \%(w/v)} \quad Q_1 = 250 \text{ mL}$$
$$C_2 = 0.05\text{\%(w/v)} \quad Q_2 = ? \quad x = Q_2 - 250 \text{ mL}$$
$$C_1 \times Q_1 = C_2 \times Q_2$$
$$Q_2 = C_1 \times Q_1/C_2 = 0.20\% \times 250 \text{ mL}/0.050\%$$
$$= 1000 \text{ mL}$$
$$x = Q_2 - 250 \text{ mL} = 1000 \text{ mL} - 250 \text{ mL}$$
$$= 750 \text{ mL of water to be added}$$

Alcohol Solutions

The preceding treatment of dilutions assumes that solution and solvent volumes are reasonably additive. For dilutions of concentrated ethyl alcohol in water, this is not the case; a contraction in volume occurs on mixing. Consequently, you cannot extend the calculation to determine the exact volume of water to add to the initial alcohol solution. That is, the volume of water to be added cannot be obtained simply as $Q_2 - Q_1$. Rather, you can only specify that sufficient water be added to the initial concentrated alcohol solution (Q_1) to reach the specified or calculated final volume (Q_2) of the diluted alcohol solution.

Example: How much water should be added to 100 mL of 95%(v/v) ethanol to make 50%(v/v) ethanol?

$$C_1 = 95\% \quad Q_1 = 100 \text{ mL} \quad C_2 = 50\% \quad Q_2 = ?$$
$$C_1 \times Q_1 = C_2 \times Q_2$$
$$Q_2 = C_1 \times Q_1/C_2 = 95\% \times 100 \text{ mL}/50\%$$
$$= 190 \text{ mL (this is the final total volume)}$$

Thus, to the 100 mL of 95% add sufficient water to make 190 mL. This quantity will be more than 90 mL because of the contraction that occurs when concentrated alcohol is mixed with water.

Concentrated Acids

Concentrated mineral acids (hydrochloric, sulfuric, nitric, and phosphoric) are manufactured by bubbling the pure acid gas into water to produce a saturated solution. The manufacturer specifies the concentration as a %(w/w). However, when preparing diluted acids for compounding, the pharmacist must express the concentration as a %(w/v). This requires utilization of the specific gravity of the concentrated acid.

Example: What volume of 35%(w/w) concentrated HCl, specific gravity 1.20, is required to make 500 mL of 5%(w/v) solution?

First, determine the weight of HCl required for the dilute solution. Since the dilute solution is 5%(w/v), it will contain 5 g in each 100 mL, or 25 g in 500 mL.

Next, one must determine what weight, x, of the 35%(w/w) solution contains 25 g of HCl. By proportion,

$$x:100 \text{ g} = 25 \text{ g}:35 \text{ g} \quad x = 100 \text{ g} \times 25 \text{ g}/35 \text{ g}$$
$$= 71.4 \text{ g of the concentrated solution}$$

Finally, use the SpGr of the concentrated solution to convert the weight to volume. Here, recall that SpGr is numerically equal to the density when the latter is expressed in grams per milliliter. Thus, density = 1.20 g/mL = Wt/Vol. Rearranging,

$$\text{vol} = \text{wt/density} = 71.4 \text{ g}/1.20 \text{ g/mL} = 59.5 \text{ mL}$$

Triturations

Triturations (used as a noun) are simply 10%(w/w) finely powdered (triturated) mixtures of a drug in an inert substance.

Example: What weight of colchicine trituration is required to prepare 30 doses of 0.25 mg each of colchicine?

For the trituration, 10 mg of the mixture contains 1 mg of drug. Thus,

$$x \text{ mg of trituration:10 mg of trituration} =$$
$$(30 \times 0.25 \text{ mg drug}):1 \text{ mg drug}$$
$$x = 10 \text{ mg trituration} \times (30 \times 0.25 \text{ mg drug})/$$
$$1 \text{ mg drug} = 75 \text{ mg trituration}$$

Alligation Alternate

There are times when a drug concentration is required that is intermediate between those of two (or more) stock solutions (or available drug products). In this event, the alligation alternate method may be employed to quickly obtain the relative parts of each of the stock solutions needed to yield the desired concentration. If stock solutions of concentrations A% and B% (A% > B%) are to be used to make a solution of concentration C%, one sets up the diagram below to obtain the relative parts of solutions A and B.

A% (C% − B%) parts of A

C%

B% (A% − C%) parts of B

Example: In what proportion should 20%(w/v) dextrose be mixed with 5%(w/v) dextrose to obtain 15%(w/v) dextrose? How much of each is required to make 75 mL of 15%(w/v) solution?

20% 10 parts of 20%

15%

5% 5 parts of 5%

Thus, combine in the ratio of 10 parts of 20%:5 parts of 5%, ie, 2:1. Accordingly, to make 75 mL of 15% solution, mix 50 mL of 20% solution with 25 mL of 5% solution.

Alligation Medial

There may be times when one needs to know the final concentration of a solution obtained by mixing specified volumes of two or more stock solutions. In this event, the alligation medial method may be employed.

Example: What is the concentration of a solution prepared by combining 100 mL of a 10% solution, 200 mL of a 20% solution and 300 mL of a 30% solution? Proceed as illustrated below:

10%	×	100 mL	=	1000 %mL
20%	×	200 mL	=	4000 %mL
30%	×	300 mL	=	9000 %mL
		600 mL		14,000 %mL

Mixture concentration = 14,000 %mL/600 mL = 23.3%

11. Isotonic Solutions

The preparation of many solutions used in pharmacy requires attention to osmotic pressure, a colligative property that is especially relevant for membrane transport. Other colligative properties include freezing point depression and boiling point elevation. These properties are a function of the total number of particles dissolved in the solution, regardless of the identity of the particles. Here, the term "particles" corresponds to cations, anions, and neutral undissociated molecules. A solution that has the same osmotic pressure as bodily fluids (blood or tears) is said to be *isotonic* (and *isosmotic*). As points of reference, 5.0%(w/v) dextrose, a nondissociating molecule, and 0.9%(w/v) sodium chloride, a dissociating molecule, are isotonic.

Dissociating Solutes

Preparation of solutions of specific tonicities requires knowledge of the dissociation properties of the solutes involved. One must know if the solute in question dissociates, and if so, to what extent and into how many particles. For example, in weak solutions sodium chloride dissociates about 80% into two particles, yielding a solution containing Na^+ ions, Cl^- ions and undissociated NaCl molecules. A measure of the extent of dissociation is provided by the dissociation factor, i, defined as the ratio of the total number of particles following dissociation to the number of molecules prior to dissociation. For example, 100 molecules of sodium chloride (prior to dissociation) will dissociate 80% to produce 80 particles of Na^+, 80 particles of Cl^- and 20 particles of NaCl, or 180 particles in all. The dissociation factor (i) for NaCl then is 180/100 = 1.8. A nondissociating molecule (like dextrose or tobramycin) is assigned a dissociation constant of 1.0. If measured dissociation information is not available, one can assume approximately 80% dissociation for weak solutions of salts. In this event, salts (including drugs) which dissociate into 2 ions will have a dissociation factor of 1.8 (like NaCl and ephedrine hydrochloride); 3 ions (like ephedrine sulfate), 2.6; 4 ions (like sodium citrate), 3.4; and 5 ions, 4.2 (ie, 0.9 per ion).

Example: What is the dissociation factor (i) for a compound which dissociates 60% into 3 ions?

For each 100 undissolved molecules, one will obtain on dissolution:

60 x 3 = 180 particles of ions plus 40 particles of undissociated molecules for a total of 220 particles.

Thus the dissociation factor = i = 220/100 = 2.2.

Example: What is the dissociation factor for dextrose, a nondissociating compound?

For each 100 undissolved molecules, one will obtain on dissolution:

zero particles of ions and 100 particles of undissociated molecules for a total of 100 particles

Thus the dissociation factor = i = 100/100 = 1.0.

Sodium Chloride Equivalents

When preparing isotonic drug solutions, it is necessary to take into consideration the tonicity contribution of the drug. This can be accomplished by using the *sodium chloride equivalent* for the drug, defined as the number of grams of sodium chloride that would produce the same tonicity effect as 1 gram of the drug. If the value of the sodium chloride equivalent is not provided, it can be calculated using the molecular weights and dissociation factors of sodium chloride and the drug in question:

sodium chloride equivalent = (MW of NaCl) x (drug dissociation factor)/(MW of drug) x (sodium chloride dissociation factor) = (58.5)(i)/(MW of drug)(1.8)

Example: What is the sodium chloride equivalent of demecarium bromide (GMW = 717, i = 2.6)?

sodium chloride equivalent = (58.5 x 2.6)/ (717 x 1.8) = 0.12

Thus each gram of demecarium bromide is equivalent to 0.12 g of NaCl.

So how does one proceed to prepare a drug solution that must be made isotonic? Using the total volume of isotonic solution to be prepared, first calculate the hypothetical weight, x, of NaCl (alone) that would be required to make that volume of water isotonic (0.9%). Next, using the weight of drug to be incorporated in the solution and its sodium chloride equivalent, calculate the weight of NaCl, y, that would correspond to the weight of the drug. Then calculate the true weight of NaCl, z, to be added to the preparation as $z = x - y$.

Example: What weight of sodium chloride would be required to prepare 50 mL of an isotonic solution containing 500 mg of pilocarpine nitrate (sodium chloride equivalent = 0.23)?

Since isotonic saline requires 0.9 g/100 mL, 50 mL of isotonic saline will require 0.45 g, ie, $x = 0.45$ g.

The 500 mg of pilocarpine nitrate will correspond to 500 mg × 0.23 = 115 mg of NaCl, ie, $y = 0.12$ g.

Sodium chloride to add to make isotonic = $z = x - y =$ 0.45 g – 0.12 g = 0.33 g.

Example: A (fictitious) new drug, Utopical, molecular weight 175 and dissociation factor i = 3.4, is to be provided as 325 mg in 60 mL of solution made isotonic with sodium chloride. What is the required weight of sodium chloride?

Here, the sodium chloride equivalent of the drug is not given and must be calculated from the information provided.

Sodium chloride equivalent of Utopical =
(58.5 × 3.4)/(175 × 1.8) = 0.63

Since isotonic saline requires 0.9 g/100 mL, 60 mL of isotonic saline will require 0.54 g ie, $x = 0.54$ g.

The 325 mg of Utopical will correspond to 0.325 g × 0.63 = 0.20 g of sodium chloride, ie, $y = 0.20$ g.

The amount of sodium chloride to add to make isotonic = $z = (x - y) = (0.54$ g – 0.20 g) = 0.34 g.

12. Intravenous Infusion Flow Rates

The physician may specify the rate of flow of IV fluids in drops per minute, amount of drug per hour, or the duration of time of administration of the total volume of the infusion. It may then be necessary to calculate the infusion rate in per-minute or per-hour increments in order to program an infusion pump to give the medication at the correct rate.

Example: If 250 mg of a drug is added to a 500-mL D_5W bag, what should be the flow rate, in milliliters per hour, to deliver 50 mg of drug per hour?

x mL/h:500 mL/h = 50 mg/h:250 mg/h
$x = (500$ mL/h) × (50 mg/h)/(250 mg/h) = 100 mL/h

Example: If an infusion flow rate is at 100 mL/h and the infusion set delivers 15 drops/mL, what is the rate of flow in drops per minute?

15 drops/mL × 100 mL/h = 1500 drops/h
= 25 drops/min

Example: If 500 mL of an infusion is to be delivered using an IV administration set that delivers 10 drops/mL and flow rate is set at 1.25 mL per minute, how long will it take to deliver the 500 mL?

Total time of delivery = 500 mL/1.25 mL/minute =
400 minutes = 6.7 hours
(The 10 drops/mL is superfluous information.)

13. Buffers

Buffer solutions are employed to reduce pH fluctuations associated with introduction of small amounts of strong acids or bases. Typical buffer solutions are composed of a weak acid or weak base plus a salt of the acid or base. Solution pH in the presence of a buffer can be calculated using the Henderson-Hasselbalch equations.

For weak acids, $pH = pK_a + \log(\text{salt/acid})$
For weak bases, $pH = pK_w - pK_b + \log(\text{base/salt})$,
where $pK_w = 14$

Example: What is the pH of a buffer solution prepared to be 0.50 M in sodium acetate and 0.050 M in acetic acid (pK_a of acetic acid = 4.76)?

For weak acids, $pH = pK_a + \log(\text{salt/acid})$
Thus $pH = 4.76 + \log(0.50/0.050) = 4.76 + \log(10)$
$= 4.76 + 1 = 5.76$

Example: What is the pH of a buffer solution prepared to be 0.5 M in ammonia ($pK_b = 4.74$) and 0.050 M in ammonium chloride?

Ammonia forms a base in aqueous solution.
$pH = pK_w - pK_b + \log(\text{base/salt}) = 14.00 - 4.74 +$
$\log(0.50/0.05) = 14.00 - 4.74 + 1.00 = 10.26$

14. Temperature

Frequently, one must convert temperatures from Fahrenheit (F) to Centigrade (C), and conversely. The following formula can be used: $9C = 5F - 160$.

Example: A patient has an oral temperature of 100°F. What is this temperature in °C?

$$9C = 5F - 160$$
$$C = (5F - 160)/9 = (5 \times 100 - 160)/9 = 37.8$$

15. Practice Problems

1. If 100 capsules contain 340 mg of active
    ingredient, what would be the weight of active
    ingredient contained in 75 capsules?

    A. 453 mg
    B. 340 mg
    C. 255 mg
    D. 128 mg
    E. 75 mg

2. What is the weight of 500 mL of a liquid whose
    specific gravity is 1.13?

    A. 442 mg
    B. 565 g
    C. 442 g
    D. 885 mg
    E. 221 g

3. Suppose a pharmacist weighs out 325 mg of a
    substance on her class A prescription balance.
    When she subsequently checked this weight on a
    more sensitive analytical balance, she found it to
    be only 312 mg. What was the percentage error
    in the original weighing?

    A. 4%
    B. 5%
    C. 6%
    D. 10%
    E. 12%

4. What is the minimum weighable quantity for a
    maximum of 5% error using a balance with a
    sensitivity requirement of 6 mg?

    A. 80 mcg
    B. 100 mg
    C. 120 mg
    D. 150 mg
    E. 240 mg

5. A patient weighing 175 lb is to receive an initial
    daily IM dosage of procainamide HCl (500
    mg/mL vial) of 50 mg/kg (ABW) to be given in
    divided doses every 3 hours. How many
    milliliters should each injection contain?

    A. 3.98 mL
    B. 0.49 mL
    C. 8.23 mL
    D. 1.87 mL
    E. 0.99 mL

6. What is the ideal body weight of a female
    patient whose height is 5 ft 8 in.?

    A. 68 kg
    B. 64 kg
    C. 150 lb
    D. 121 lb
    E. 53 kg

7. What is the approximate BSA of an adult patient
    who weighs 154 lb and is 6 ft tall?

    A. 1.73 m^2
    B. 3.15 m^2
    C. 1.89 m^2
    D. 0.70 m^2
    E. 2.67 m^2

8. If the adult dose of a drug is 125 mg, what
    would be the dose for a child whose BSA is
    estimated to be 0.68 m^2?

    A. 485 mcg
    B. 318 mg
    C. 85 mg
    D. 49 mg
    E. 33 mg

9. What is the creatinine clearance for a 65-year-
    old female patient who weighs 50 kg and has a
    serum creatinine level of 1.3 mg/dL?

    A. 34 mL/min
    B. 40 mL/min
    C. 26 mL/min
    D. 82 mL/min
    E. 100 mL/min

10. Using the formula below, how much zinc oxide
    would be required to make 750 g of the
    mixture?

Zinc oxide	150 g
Starch	250 g
Petrolatum	550 g
Coal tar	50 g

    A. 200 g
    B. 188 g
    C. 413 g
    D. 113 g
    E. 38 g

11. Using the formula below, what weight of kaolin would be required to produce 500 g of the mixture?

Kaolin	12 parts
Magnesium oxide	3 parts
Bismuth subcarbonate	5 parts

   A. 83 g
   B. 300 g
   C. 208 g
   D. 333 g
   E. 250 g

12. How much dextrose is required to prepare 500 mL of an aqueous 10% solution?

   A. 250 mg
   B. 500 mg
   C. 10 g
   D. 25 g
   E. 50 g

13. What weight of hexachlorophene should be used in compounding 20 g of an ointment containing hexachlorophene at a concentration of 1:400?

   A. 25 mcg
   B. 50 mcg
   C. 50 mg
   D. 80 mg
   E. 5 g

14. What weight of magnesium chloride ($MgCl_2$, formula weight = 95.3) is require to prepare 200 mL of a solution which is 5.0 millimolar?

   A. 191 mg
   B. 95.3 mg
   C. 19.1 mg
   D. 477 mcg
   E. 95 g

15. What weight of magnesium chloride ($MgCl_2$, formula weight = 95.3; Mg^{2+} atomic wt. = 24.3; Cl^{1-}, atomic wt. = 35.5) is required to prepare 1000 mL of a solution which contains 5.0 mEq of magnesium?

   A. 238 mg
   B. 4.76 g
   C. 1.19 g
   D. 60.7 mg
   E. 476 mcg

16. What is the milliosmolarity (ideal) of normal saline (NaCl formula weight = 58.5)?

   A. 100 mOsm/L
   B. 154 mOsm/L
   C. 254 mOsm/L
   D. 287 mOsm/L
   E. 308 mOsm/L

17. How much water for injection should be added to 250 mL of 20% dextrose to obtain 15% dextrose?

   A. 333 mL
   B. 83 mL
   C. 250 mL
   D. 166 mL
   E. 58 mL

333-250 (handwritten)

18. What volume of a 5% dextrose solution should be mixed with 200 mL of a 20% dextrose solution to prepare 300 mL of a 15% dextrose solution?

   A. 150 mL
   B. 200 mL
   C. 100 mL
   D. 50 mL
   E. 250 mL

19. What is the final concentration obtained by mixing 200 mL of 20% dextrose with 100 mL of 5% dextrose?

   A. 10%
   B. 15%
   C. 7.5%
   D. 12.5%
   E. 17.5%

20% × 200mL = 4000 %mL
5% × 100 mL = 500 %mL
4500 %mL
300 mL
~15%

20. Magnesium chloride ($MgCl_2$) is a 3-ion electrolyte that dissociates 80% at the relevant concentration. Calculate its dissociation factor (i).

   A. 1.8
   B. 2.2
   C. 2.4
   D. 2.6
   E. 3.2

80%-100 (handwritten)

$$\frac{(80\% * 3) + 20}{100} = 2.6$$

21. Tobramycin (formula weight = 468) has a dissociation factor of 1.0. What is its sodium chloride equivalent?

A. 0.069
B. 0.0092
C. 0.117
D. 0.286
E. 0.782

(handwritten: 58.5(i)/MW ×1.8)

22. What weight of sodium chloride should be used in compounding the following prescription for ephedrine sulfate (formula weight = 429, dissociation factor = 2.6, sodium chloride equivalent = 0.23)?

Rx Ephedrine sulfate	0.25 g
Sodium chloride	qs
Purified water ad	30 mL
Make isoton. sol.	

A. 1.22 g
B. 784 mcg
C. 212 mg
D. 527 mcg
E. 429 mg

23. A patient is to receive an infusion of 2 g of lidocaine in 500 mL D_5W at a rate of 2 mg/min. What is the flow rate in milliliters per hour?

A. 2.0 mL/h
B. 6.5 mL/h
C. 15 mL/h
D. 30 mL/h
E. 150 mL/h

24. What is the pH of a buffer solution prepared with 0.05 M disodium phosphate and 0.05 M sodium acid phosphate (pK_a = 7.21)?

A. 4.55
B. 5.23
C. 6.18
D. 7.05
E. 7.21

25. Convert 104°F to centigrade.

A. 22°C
B. 34°C
C. 40°C
D. 46°C
E. 54°C

(handwritten: 9C = 5F - 160)

Answers

1. **C.**

$$x \text{ mg}:340 \text{ mg} = 75 \text{ cap}:100 \text{ cap}$$
$$x = 340 \text{ mg} \times 75 \text{ cap}/100 \text{ cap} = 255 \text{ mg}$$

2. **B.**
A specific gravity of 1.13 corresponds to a density of 1.13 g/mL.

$$\text{density} = \text{weight/volume, thus,}$$
$$\text{weight} = \text{density} \times \text{volume} = 1.13 \text{ g/mL} \times 500 \text{ mL}$$
$$= 565 \text{ g}$$

3. **A.**

$$\% \text{ error} = (\text{error} \times 100)/\text{desired quantity}$$
$$= (325 - 312) \times 100/325 = 4\%$$

4. **C.**

$$\text{minimum weighable quantity} = \text{SR} \times 100/5$$
$$= 6 \text{ mg} \times 100/5 = 120 \text{ mg}$$

5. **E.**

$$\text{daily dosage} = 50 \text{ mg/kg} \times 175 \text{ lb}/2.2 \text{ lb/kg} = 3977 \text{ mg}$$
$$\text{single IM injection} = (3977/8) \text{ mg} \times 1/500 \text{ mg/mL}$$
$$= 0.99 \text{ mL}$$

6. **B.**

$$\text{IBW} = 45.5 + 2.3 \times 8 = 64 \text{ kg}$$

7. **C.**

$$\text{wt} = 154 \text{ lb}/2.2 \text{ lb/kg} = 70 \text{ kg; ht}$$
$$= 6 \text{ ft} \times 12 \text{ in./ft} \times 2.54 \text{ cm/in.} = 183 \text{ cm}$$
$$\text{BSA} = \text{square root } [70 \times 183/3600]$$
$$= \text{square root } [3.56] = 1.89 \text{ m}^2$$

8. **D.**

$$\text{child dose} = \text{adult dose} \times \text{child BSA}/1.73$$
$$= 125 \text{ mg} \times 0.68 \text{ m}^2/1.73 \text{ m}^2 = 49 \text{ mg}$$

9. **A.**

$$\text{CrCl} = 0.85 \times (140 - 65) \times 50/(72 \times 1.3) = 34 \text{ mL/min}$$

10. **D.**
Note that the formula is designed to produce a total of 1000 g of the mixture. Then, by proportions,

x g ZnO:150 g ZnO = 750 g mix:1000 g
x = 150 g x 750 g/1000 g = 113 g

11. **B.**
Note that the formula will produce a total of 20 parts of the mixture. Then, by proportions,

x g kaolin:500 g mix = 12 parts kaolin:20 parts mix
x = 500 g x 12 parts/20 parts = 300 g

12. **E.**
Note that this will be a solution of a solid in a liquid and thus the concentration will be %(w/v).

$10\%(w/v) = x$ g dextrose x 100/500
x = 10 x 500/100 = 50 g

13. **C.**
By proportions,

x g hexachlorophene:20 g ung. = 1 part hexachlorophene:400 parts ung.
x = 20 g x 1 part/400 parts = 0.050 g = 50 mg

14. **B.**
A 1.0 molar solution will contain 95.3 g in 1000 mL. A 5.0 molar solution will contain 95.3 x 5 = 477 g in 1000 mL. A 5.0 millimolar solution will contain 477 mg in 1000 mL. Thus, 200 mL of a 5 millimolar solution will contain 477/5 = 95.3 mg in 200 mL.

15. **A.**
Because magnesium has a valence of 2, a formula weight of $MgCl_2$ will contain two equivalent weights of magnesium (and chloride for that matter). Thus, 5 equivalents of Mg is contained in 5 x 95.3/2 g = 238 g of $MgCl_2$. Accordingly, 5 milliequivalents of Mg is contained in 238 mg of $MgCl_2$.

16. **E.**
Normal saline is 0.90%(w/v), or 0.90 g/100 mL = 9.0 g/1000 mL.

mOsmolarity = (9 g/58.5) x 2 x 1000 = 308 mOsm/L

17. **B.**

C_1 = 20%, Q_1 = 250 mL, C_2 = 15%, Q_2 = ?
C_1 x Q_1 = C_2 x Q_2
Q_2 = C_1 x Q_1/C_2 = 20% x 250 mL/15% = 333 mL
added water = 333 mL – 250 mL = 83 mL

18. **C.**

20% (conc of stock A)   15 – 5 = 10 = parts of A

15% (desired conc)

5% (conc of stock B)   20 – 15 = 5 = parts of B

Relative volumes are 10:5, or 2:1. Thus, 200 mL of 20% solution (A) will require 100 mL of 5% solution (B) to produce 300 mL of 15% dextrose.

19. **B.**

20%	X	200 mL =	4000 %mL
5%	X	100 mL =	500 %mL
		300 mL	4500 %mL

Mixture concentration = 4500 %mL/300 mL = 15%.

20. **D.**
Each 100 molecules will provide:

80 Mg ions
160 Cl ions
20 undissociated molecules
260 particles total

Thus the dissociation factor = 260/100 = 2.6.

21. **A.**

sodium chloride equivalent = (58.5)(1.0)/(468)(1.8) = 0.069

22. **C.**
Since 900 mg of sodium chloride in 100 mL is isotonic,

x:900 mg = 30 mL:100 mL and
x = 900 x 30/100 = 270 mg

is the amount of NaCl alone to make 30 mL isotonic. But 1 g of ephedrine sulfate is equivalent to 0.23 g of sodium, thus

y = 0.25 g x 0.23 = 0.058 g = 58 mg of sodium chloride

Accordingly, the amount of sodium chloride to add ($z = x - y$) is (270 mg – 58 mg) = 212 mg.

23. **D.**

The bag contains 2000 mg in 500 mL, thus 4 mg/mL. A rate of 2 mg/min then corresponds to 0.5 mL/min that in turn corresponds to 30 mL/h.

24. **E.**

$$pH = pK_a + \log(\text{salt/acid}) = 7.21 + \log(0.05/0.05)$$
$$= 7.21 + \log(1) = 7.21$$

25. **C.**

$$9C = 5F - 160$$
$$9C = 5 \times 104 - 160 = 520 - 160 = 360$$
$$C = 360/9 = 40$$

16. References

Ansel HC, Stoklosa MJ. *Pharmaceutical Calculations,* 11th ed. Philadelphia: Lippincott Williams & Wilkins; 2001.

Khan MA, Reddy IK. *Pharmaceutical and Clinical Calculations,* 2nd ed. Lancaster, PA: Technomic Publishing Co; 2000.

O'Sullivan TA. *Understanding Pharmacy Calculations,* Washington: American Pharmaceutical Association; 2002.

2. Federal Pharmacy Law

Walter L. Fitzgerald, Jr, BSPharm, MS, JD
Dean, Pharmacy Education Program Development
South College
Knoxville, Tennessee

Contents

1. **Resources to Assist in Preparing for the MPJE®**

2. **The Comprehensive Drug Abuse Prevention and Control Act of 1970 and Regulations of the U.S. Drug Enforcement Administration (DEA)**

3. **The Food, Drug, and Cosmetic Act of 1938 and Regulations of the U.S. Food and Drug Administration (FDA)**

4. **The Poison Prevention Packaging Act of 1970 and Regulations of the U.S. Consumer Product Safety Commission (CPSC)**

5. **Miscellaneous Federal Laws**

Introduction

This study guide was developed for the purpose of assisting candidates for the National Association of Boards of Pharmacy® (NABP®) Multistate Pharmacy Jurisprudence Examination™ (MPJE®). It is recognized that candidates will have been exposed, through the academic pharmacy degree program, to the federal and state laws subject to inquiry on the MPJE®. Upon this recognition, this study guide is not intended to be a comprehensive collection or compilation of the text of these laws. Rather, it is a general overview of the relevant federal laws with which the candidate should be familiar.

1. Resources to Assist in Preparing for the MPJE®

Information from NABP®

NABP® offers two resources on state pharmacy law that may be beneficial to the MPJE® candidate. More about each of these resources is available on the NABP web site at *www.nabp.net*.

The first resource is the Survey of Pharmacy Law. Revised annually, the Survey contains a wealth of information regarding pharmacy and drug laws in the individual states. The Survey is provided at no cost to all final year pharmacy students, but may be purchased by others for $20.00. The latest edition is 2007 and is available exclusively on CD-ROM.

The second resource is NABPLAW® Online. This is an electronic database of the pharmacy practice act and board of pharmacy rules for each of the 50 states. There is a free NABPLAW demo, and short term access can be purchased. A 1-day subscription is available for $10.00 and a 1-week subscription is available for $50.00. Additional time periods and prices can be viewed at the NABP® web site.

Information from Electronic Databases of Federal Law

Of great assistance to the MPJE® candidate is a wealth of databases of federal law available via the Internet at no cost. The candidate is encouraged to utilize these electronic databases as necessary during the review process. One of the greatest advantages of these electronic databases is the ability, through active links contained in the databases, to quickly retrieve and review cross-references to individual sections of the laws, as well as to other relevant laws.

Because the "pharmacy law course" is taught at different times at colleges and schools of pharmacy, these electronic databases can be very beneficial. If the pharmacy law course was taught during the first professional year, the candidate may not have been exposed to changes in federal pharmacy law that occurred during the remaining years of the curriculum. Because these databases are quite current, the candidate can achieve two objectives by reviewing the federal law databases as described below. First, the candidate will be refreshed on laws studied previously in the pharmacy law course. Second, the candidate will be exposed to changes that have occurred since completing the pharmacy law course.

Accessing the Federal Food, Drug, and Cosmetic Act and the Federal Controlled Substances Act

Go to the U.S. Code Collection maintained by the Legal Information Institute of the Cornell Law School. The web site address for this collection is:

http://www.law.cornell.edu/uscode/

When the web page appears, scroll down and select Title 21. From the web page that will next appear you can access both the Federal Food, Drug, and Cosmetic Act and the Federal Controlled Substances Act.

Federal Food, Drug, and Cosmetic Act

On the web page select Chapter 9, which is titled Federal Food, Drug, and Cosmetic Act. When the next web page appears you will see all nine Subchapters that comprise the Federal Food, Drug, and Cosmetic Act. When you select a subchapter, you will then see on the next web page the individual sections of the Act contained in that subchapter, or in some cases, the individual parts contained in that subchapter. Where the subchapter contains individual parts, selecting one part leads to a web page with the individual sections of that act.

Federal Controlled Substances Act

The same web page used to access the Food, Drug, and Cosmetic Act should be used to access the Controlled Substances Act, which is located at Chapter 13 instead of Chapter 9. After selecting Chapter 13 use the same process as described immediately above.

Accessing the regulations of the U.S. Food and Drug Administration and the U.S. Drug Enforcement Administration

Go to the electronic Code of Federal Regulations (CFR) maintained by the Government Printing Office (GPO). The web site address for this collection is:

http://www.gpoaccess.gov

When the web page appears, look for the heading "GPO Access Resources by Branch" and under "Executive Resources" select "Code of Federal Regulations." When the next web page appears look for the heading "Most Current 50 Titles" and under that heading select "Browse and/or search the CFR." When the next web page appears, scroll down to Title 21, and then select the box to the right with the most current date, and then scroll down to the bottom of the web page and click "Continue." When the next web page appears, you will see a listing of the individual Parts of Title 21. Parts 1-99 through 800-1299 contain the regulations of the U.S. Food and Drug Administration (FDA). Beginning at Parts 1300-1399 you will find the regulations of the U.S. Drug Enforcement Administration (DEA).

The FDA regulations

The scope of the FDA regulations is significantly large, constituting literally thousands of pages. Rather than include the sections of FDA regulations in this guide, the MPJE® candidate should go to the GPO's CFR web site as described immediately above for review.

As to what to review, the FDA regulations governing drugs begin at Part 200, which is found on the web site at Parts 200-299. Thus the candidate should select Parts 200-299 in the column with the heading "Browse Parts." When the next web page appears, the individual parts will appear, and upon selecting any of the parts, the individual sections in that part will appear on the next web page. FDAs regulations governing drugs continue into the next set of parts, specifically, Parts 300-499. The next set of parts (500-599) contain FDAs regulations governing animal drugs, and should be reviewed. The next set of parts (600-799) concern two items, biologicals and cosmetics, and also should be reviewed. The final set of parts (800-1299) contain FDAs regulations governing medical devices, and should be reviewed.

An important note is that by use of the word "review" in the above paragraph it is not meant that the candidate should read each and every word of every FDA regulation. To do so would require an unreasonable and unnecessary time commitment. It is anticipated that the candidate can recognize whether there is a need to review the text of the section or move on to the next one. Also, from the "Competency Statements" on page 23 of the NABP® Registration Bulletin for NAPLEX® and MPJE® the candidate should be able to identify those sections that contain text not relevant to preparing for the MPJE®.

The MPJE® candidate can begin by opening Part 200 of the FDA regulations as directed above, and open the first section of Part 200. Then the candidate should recognize from the section title whether this is (1) information about which the candidate is knowledgeable and does not require review or (2) information that is not subject to inquiry on the MPJE®. In the presence of either of these, the candidate should move forward to the next section.

The DEA regulations

As with the FDA regulations, the scope of the DEA regulations is quite extensive, but fortunately is more manageable than the FDA regulations. In addition, if the candidate has worked in pharmacy practice to any degree, the DEA regulations likely will be more familiar to the candidate than the FDA regulations, since the FDA regulations are not as directly related to daily pharmacy practice as are the DEA regulations. The MPJE® candidate can review each section of the relevant DEA regulations using the process described above for the FDA regulations, beginning by opening Part 1300 and then each individual section in each part.

Information from Electronic Databases of State Law

It is anticipated that candidates for the MPJE® will have at least two resources for their study of relevant state law. The first of these is the textbook or other compilation of state law that was utilized in the pharmacy law course taught in the academic degree program. This first resource will, of course, be of value only if the candidate is taking the MPJE® and seeking licensure as a pharmacist in the same state where the candidate completed the academic degree program. The second is what is commonly referred to as the "state board of pharmacy law book." In many states, upon submission of an application for examination for licensure as a pharmacist, the applicant will be provided a copy of the state board's pharmacy law book. The candidate may also have received as a final-year pharmacy student, the *Survey of Pharmacy Law* described above in the section on resources available from NABP®.

But in addition to these resources, as with federal law, there are a number of electronic databases for accessing state law. Most directly related to preparing for the MPJE® is NABPLAW® described above in the section on resources available from NABP®. But in addition to NABPLAW® are various databases that are accessible-free of charge. The candidate should first look to his or her state's Internet homepage for resources on state law. While it is not possible to describe here for each state how to find relevant state law on the state homepage, the candidate will likely be able to successfully navigate through the state's web pages. But as an example, the candidate can search to see if the state's secretary of state has an individual homepage, and if it does, look on that homepage for a link to state agency rules and regulations, such as those of the state board of pharmacy.

Beyond the state homepage, there are legal resource web sites that the candidate can use for accessing state law, again at no cost. The following web sites may be useful to the candidate seeking additional information not only on state law, but also federal and other law:

http://www.romingerlegal.com/

http://www.findlaw.com/

http://www.law.com

http://www.alllaw.com/

http://gsulaw.gsu.edu/metaindex

Publications

At many colleges and schools of pharmacy, a textbook or other compilation of federal and state drug and pharmacy law, may have been used in the pharmacy law course. Thus the MPJE® candidate may already have a publication that covers the laws subject to inquiry on the MPJE®. If not, there are publications that may be of assistance, including the two publications listed below, that provide a practical, easy-to-understand explanation of the federal law subject to inquiry on the MPJE®. Additionally, these publications contain sample questions for the MPJE® candidate to use in gaining experience in answering questions related to federal law, as well as to obtain a measure of knowledge prior to the MPJE®.

References

Reiss, Barry S. and Hall, Gary D. *Guide to Federal Pharmacy Law*, 5th ed. Apothecary Press. Apothecary Press. Contact information: (888) 609-2665 or www.apothecarypress.com.

Strauss, Steven. *Strauss' Federal Drug Laws and Examination Review*, 5th ed. CRC Press. Contact information: (800) 272-7737 or www.crcpress.com.

2. The Comprehensive Drug Abuse Prevention and Control Act of 1970 and Regulations of the U.S. Drug Enforcement Administration (DEA)

The Comprehensive Drug Abuse Prevention and Control Act, enacted by Congress in 1970, has as its primary purpose preventing illicit manufacture, distribution, and use of controlled substances. This purpose is achieved through numerous requirements in the Act and DEA regulations.

Introduction

The Comprehensive Drug Abuse Prevention and Control Act, more commonly known as the Controlled Substances Act (CSA), establishes a "closed system" for distribution of drugs that are "controlled substances." Reference is made to a closed system because controlled substances can only be distributed by and between persons registered with the DEA. The DEA is a unit within the U.S. Department of Justice, and was established in July 1973 by an executive reorganization plan and replaced the former Bureau of Narcotics and Dangerous Drugs (BNDD). But it must be noted that the U.S. Food and Drug Administration (FDA) has also promulgated regulations that affect the distribution of controlled substances. One example is treatment programs for narcotic addicts, where the FDA regulations contain medical guidelines for a program and the DEA regulations contain requirements for dispensing and recordkeeping activities for such a program.

It is important to recognize that in 1988 Congress amended existing federal laws, including the CSA, with enactment of the Chemical Diversion and Trafficking Act. This Act establishes recordkeeping and reporting requirements for persons who manufacture, distribute, import, or export a listed precursor or essential chemical, as well as tableting and encapsulating machines. When the MPJE® candidate studies the CSA and DEA regulations, the text added as a result of this 1988 Act is generally easily recognized. For example, the DEA regulation at 21 CFR 1300.02 is entitled "definitions relating to listed chemicals." The MPJE® candidate needs to be attentive to how the CSA and DEA regulations address commercially available controlled substances versus chemicals. Finally, the CSA and DEA regulations are quite complex and technical, and have a significant effect on pharmacy practice, and thus demand thorough study by the MPJE® candidate.

Key Provisions of the CSA

Access the CSA at the web link and process listed earlier (*http://www.law.cornell.edu/uscode/*). There are 2 subchapters:

I. Control and Enforcement
II. Import and Export

The MPJE® candidate should be familiar with both subchapters, and particularly the following provisions from Subchapter I of the CSA. But in addition, the MPJE® candidate should review the sections in Subchapter II on import and export, using the web link listed above.

Subchapter I. Control and Enforcement

. . .

Part A—Introductory Provisions
§ 801. Congressional findings and declarations: controlled substances
This section sets forth the reasons why Congress enacted the CSA. The MPJE® candidate should be generally familiar with these findings and declarations.

§ 801a. Congressional findings and declarations: psychotropic substances
This section recognizes the international treaty—the Convention on Psychotropic Substances—that the U.S. entered into in 1971 and sets forth the reasons why Congress implemented the Convention. The MPJE® candidate should be generally familiar with these findings and declarations.

§ 802. Definitions
The MPJE® candidate should be familiar with all terms defined in this section of the CSA, which will aid in understanding the language of the sections that follow. Note the limitation in dispensing that results from the relationship between the definition of "dispense" and the definition of "ultimate user." Note also that some of the definitions contain important substantive content, such as the definition of a regulated transaction and its placing of "thresholds" on the retail sale of ephedrine, pseudoephedrine, and phenylpropanolamine. Finally note the definition of anabolic steroid as amended in 2004.

. . .

Part B—Authority to Control; Standards and Schedules

§ 811. Authority and criteria for classification of substances

This section gives the U.S. Attorney General the authority to add a drug to a schedule, transfer a drug between schedules, and remove a drug from a schedule. This section also contains the factors to be considered when determining whether a drug should be placed in or removed from a schedule. This section also allows for exclusion of a non-narcotic substance from a schedule if the substance may be lawfully sold, under the FDCA, without a prescription. Finally, this section provides that dextromethorphan shall not be included in any schedule by reason of enactment of the CSA unless controlled after October 27, 1970 based on the factors in this section.

§ 812. Schedules of controlled substances

This section establishes the five schedules (I-V) of controlled substances and the findings required for each schedule. The MPJE® candidate should be familiar with these findings, such as that a Schedule I controlled substance "has no currently accepted medical use in treatment."

§ 813. Treatment of controlled substance analogues

This section provides that a controlled substance analogue, to the extent intended for human use, shall be treated as a controlled substance in Schedule I.

§ 814. Removal of exemption of certain drugs

This section, among other things, allows the Attorney General to remove from exemption [see definition (39)(A)(iv) at section 802 concerning ephedrine, pseudoephedrine, and phenylpropanolamine] a drug or group of drugs that is being diverted to obtain a listed chemical for use in illicit production of controlled substances.

Part C—Registration of Manufacturers, Distributors, and Dispensers of Controlled Substances

§821. Rules and regulations

This section authorizes the U.S. Attorney General to promulgate rules and regulations and to charge reasonable fees relating to the registration and control of regulated persons and transactions.

§822. Persons required to register

This section sets forth the registration requirements for persons who handle controlled substances. The MPJE® candidate should understand who is and who is not required to obtain a registration, that a separate registration is required for separate locations, and that an inspection may be conducted prior to granting a registration.

§ 823. Registration requirements

This section provides specific detail regarding registration of practitioners, including pharmacies but not pharmacists, and the factors to be considered in determining whether to grant a registration.

§ 824. Denial, revocation, or suspension of registration

This section lists the grounds for denying, suspending, or revoking a registration. Note that a suspension or revocation may be limited to a particular schedule or schedules, and that the registration can be revoked simultaneously with initiation of proceedings (issuing an "order to show cause") if there is an imminent danger to the public health or safety.

§ 825. Labeling and packaging

This section establishes the labeling requirements for commercial containers of controlled substances.

§ 826. Production quotas for controlled substances

This section authorizes the Attorney General to determine and establish production quotas for Schedule I and II controlled substances to be manufactured each calendar year to provide for the estimated medical, scientific, research, and industrial needs of the U.S., for lawful export requirements, and for establishing and maintaining reserve stocks.

§ 827. Records and reports of registrants

This section establishes requirements for the biennial inventory (in relation to May 1, 1971) and adding any newly scheduled drug to the existing inventory. This section requires every registrant to maintain a complete and accurate record of each controlled substance received, sold, delivered or otherwise disposed of, but this section does not require a perpetual inventory. The MPJE® candidate should recognize the exceptions to the inventory requirement. Note also the recently added reporting requirements for gamma hydroxybutyric acid (GHB).

§ 828. Order forms

This section establishes the requirement that distribution of Schedule I and II controlled substances occur only pursuant to a form issued by the Attorney General (the DEA 222 Form) and also lists recordkeeping requirements for the form. As a related item, be sure to review the new DEA regulations on "electronic orders" for controlled substances.

§ 829. Prescriptions

This section sets forth the prescription requirements for each schedule of controlled substances, and notes that Schedule V controlled substances, when not dispensed pursuant to a prescription, may only be sold for a medical purpose.

§ 830. Regulation of listed chemicals and certain machines

This section establishes the recordkeeping and reporting requirements for those engaged in activities related to listed chemicals and tableting and encapsulating machines.

Part D—Offenses and Penalties
§841. Prohibited acts A

This section and the next two sections list unlawful acts and the penalties associated with these acts. It is important for the MPJE® candidate to recognize that some of the listed unlawful acts apply to all persons, while others only apply to registrants. The MPJE® candidate should recognize what acts are unlawful and generally be familiar with the associated penalties.

§ 842. Prohibited acts B

See note to section 841.

§ 843. Prohibited acts C

See note to section 841.

§ 844. Penalties for simple possession

This section makes possession, for any person or a registrant, of a controlled substance or listed chemical unlawful unless allowed under the CSA, establishes penalties for unlawful possession and defines what is meant by a "drug, narcotic, or chemical offense."

§ 844a. Civil penalty for possession of small amounts of certain controlled substances

This section provides penalties, for any person or a registrant, for unlawful possession of "personal use amounts" as specified by the U.S. Attorney General by regulation.

...

§ 846. Attempt and conspiracy

This section provides that persons who "attempt" or "conspire" to commit a controlled substance offense are subject to the same penalties as prescribed for the offense.

§ 847. Additional penalties

This section provides that any criminal penalties imposed for violation of the CSA do not preclude other civil and administrative penalties, such as monetary fines under the federal Civil Monetary Penalties Law or suspension or revocation of a DEA Certificate of Registration.

§ 848. Continuing criminal enterprise

This section defines a "continuing criminal enterprise" and imposes very severe penalties—including life imprisonment and the death penalty—for those convicted of engaging in a continuing criminal enterprise. The MPJE® candidate should also recognize that the text of this section also includes other offenses that are not a continuing criminal enterprise. For example, this section provides that any person, during the commission of, in furtherance of, or while attempting to avoid apprehension, prosecution, or service of a prison sentence for, a felony violation of the CSA who intentionally kills or counsels, commands, induces, procures, or causes the intentional killing of any federal, state, or local law enforcement officer engaged in, or on account of, the performance of such officer's official duties and such killing results, shall be sentenced to any term of imprisonment, which shall not be less than 20 years, and which may be up to life imprisonment, or may be sentenced to death.

§ 849. Transportation safety offenses

This section doubles the penalty for the first conviction, and triples the penalty for subsequent convictions, of certain controlled substance offenses in a "rest area" or "truck stop," as these terms are defined in this section.

§ 850. Information for sentencing

This section, unless provided otherwise in another federal law, establishes that no limitation be placed on the information concerning the background, character, and conduct of a person convicted of a controlled substance offense that may be received and considered for purposes of imposing an appropriate sentence.

§ 851. Proceedings to establish prior convictions

This section sets forth the process for establishing that a person has prior convictions of a controlled substance offense or offenses.

§ 852. Application of treaties and other international agreements

This section provides that no treaties and other international agreements entered into by the U.S. shall limit the provision of treatment, education, or rehabilitation as alternatives to conviction or criminal penalty for offenses involving any drug or other substance subject to a treaty or agreement.

§ 853. Criminal forfeitures

This section provides that persons convicted of controlled substance offenses shall forfeit to the U.S. all real and personal property constituting or derived from, any proceeds the person obtained, directly or indirectly, as the result of the offense; and any of the person's property used, or intended to be used, in any manner or part, to commit, or to facilitate the commission of the offense.

...

§ 854. Investment of illicit drug profits

This section makes it unlawful for a person to use or invest in certain "enterprises" as defined in this section any income derived, directly or indirectly, from a violation of the CSA punishable by imprisonment for more than one year if the person participated as a principal in the violation, and provides penalties for making such investments.

§ 855. Alternative fine

This section provides that in lieu of a fine otherwise authorized by Part D, a defendant who derives profits or other proceeds from an offense may be fined not more than twice the gross profits or other proceeds.

§ 856. Maintaining drug-involved premises

This section makes it unlawful to knowingly open or maintain any place for the purpose of manufacturing, distributing, or using any controlled substance, as well as to manage or control any building, room, or enclosure, either as an owner, lessee, agent, employee, or mortgagee, and knowingly and intentionally rent, lease, or make available for use, with or without compensation, the building, room, or enclosure for the purpose of unlawfully manufacturing, storing, distributing, or using a controlled substance, and establishes penalties for a violation.

...

§ 858. Endangering human life while illegally manufacturing controlled substance

This section provides that whoever, while unlawfully manufacturing a controlled substance, or attempting to do so, or transporting or causing to be transported materials, including chemicals, to do so, creates a substantial risk of harm to human life shall be subject to a fine and imprisonment.

§ 859. Distribution to persons under age twenty-one

This section provides enhanced penalties for first and second offenses of a person who is at least 18 years of age unlawfully distributing a controlled substance to a person under 21 years of age.

§ 860. Distribution or manufacturing in or near schools and colleges

This section provides enhanced penalties for first and second offenses of any person who is unlawfully distributing, possessing with intent to distribute, or manufacturing a controlled substance in or on, or within one thousand feet of, the real property comprising a public or private elementary, vocational, or secondary school or a public or private college, junior college, or university, or a playground, or housing facility owned by a public housing authority, or within 100 feet of a public or private youth center, public swimming pool, or video arcade facility. This section also makes it an offense for any person at least 21 years of age to knowingly and intentionally employ, hire, use, persuade, induce, entice, or coerce a person under 18 years of age to violate this section; or employ, hire, use, persuade, induce, entice, or coerce a person under 18 years of age to assist in avoiding detection or apprehension for any offense under this section by any federal, state, or local law enforcement official.

§ 861. Employment or use of persons under 18 years of age in drug operations

This section makes it unlawful for any person at least 18 years of age to knowingly and intentionally employ, hire, use, persuade, induce, entice, or coerce, a person under 18 years of age to violate any provision of the CSA; or employ, hire, use, persuade, induce, entice, or coerce, a person under 18 years of age to assist in avoiding detection or apprehension for any offense of the CSA by any federal, state, or local law enforcement official; or receive a controlled substance from a person under 18 years of age, other than an immediate family member, in violation of the CSA. This section also establishes penalties for first and subsequent violations of this section. This section also makes it unlawful to knowingly provide or distribute a controlled substance or a controlled substance analogue to a person under 18 years of age or to a pregnant person.

§ 862. Denial of federal benefits to drug traffickers and possessors

This section provides for denial of federal benefits, with differences in denial based upon whether the person is a drug trafficker or drug possessor.

§ 862a. Denial of assistance and benefits for certain drug-related convictions

This section provides for denial of federal benefits and assistance to an individual convicted under federal or state law of any offense which is classified as a felony by the law of the jurisdiction involved and which has as an element the possession, use, or distribution of a controlled substance.

§ 862b. Sanctioning for testing positive for controlled substances

This section provides that states shall not be prohibited by the federal government from testing welfare recipients for use of controlled substances nor from sanctioning welfare recipients who test positive for use of controlled substances.

§ 863. Drug paraphernalia

This section makes unlawful a number of activities with respect to drug paraphernalia, establishes penalties for violations, and defines drug paraphernalia.

§ 864. Anhydrous ammonia

This section makes it unlawful to steal anhydrous ammonia, or to transport stolen anhydrous ammonia across state lines, knowing, intending, or having reasonable cause to believe that such anhydrous ammonia will be used to manufacture a controlled substance in violation of this part.

The last two parts of Subchapter I contain a variety of sections, many of which are not of interest to the MPJE® candidate. As directed in the explanation to the study guide, the candidate should open each part, and from the titles of the sections in each part, determine those that the MPJE® candidate should review.

Subchapter II. Import and Export

This subchapter of the Controlled Substances Act contains several sections governing the importation and exportation of controlled substances, including requirements for registration of importers and exporters. These sections should be reviewed in general fashion by the MPJE® candidate.

Regulations of the U.S. Drug Enforcement Administration (DEA)

The DEA regulations may be found in Title 21 of the Code of Federal Regulations (CFR). The body of DEA regulations is divided into 17 "Parts."

The MPJE® candidate should review relevant DEA regulations on the electronic database as described in the explanation to this study guide. Following is a very basic summary of the content of each part.

Part 1300—Definitions

The DEA regulations begin at Part 1300 of Title 21 of the Code of Federal Regulations (CFR). Part 1300 has two sections, both of which contain definitions of terms related to controlled substances and to listed chemicals. Because there are many definitions, they are not included here, but as noted above for definitions contained in the CSA, the MPJE® candidate should retrieve and review all of the definitions from the following two sections of the DEA regulations. Some of these definitions are quite extensive and contain very important information for the MPJE® candidate. For example, restrictions related to the sale of ephedrine, pseudoephedrine, and phenylpropanolamine will be found in the definition of "regulated transaction" at 21 CFR 1300.02.

21 CFR 1300.01—Definitions relating to controlled substances

21 CFR 1300.02—Definitions relating to listed chemicals

Part 1301—Registration of manufacturers, distributors, and dispensers of controlled substances

Part 1301 governs the many aspects of registration with the DEA. This part includes the sections related to who is required to register, applying for registration, exemptions to registration, and allowances for importation for personal use. Also included are specific details about the DEA Certificate of Registration and the number assignment, procedure for suspension or revocation of a registration, and modification or termination of a registration. Very importantly, requirements for security, including the prohibition of employing certain individuals, are included in this part. The MPJE® candidate should study this part in detail paying particular attention to § 1301.27 and 1301.28, both added in 2005. While not included specifically here, the method for determining the legitimacy of a DEA registration number is important for the MPJE® candidate, and thus is included below.

Prior to 1 October 1985, DEA Certificate of Registration Numbers for practitioners began with the letter "A." Since that date, the DEA Certificate of Registration Numbers for practitioners begins with the letter "B." Further, a DEA Certificate of Registration Number issued to a mid-level practitioner begins with the letter "M." Following the first letter is a second letter, and this letter is the first letter of the registrant's last name. Following the two letters is a seven-digit computer-generated sequential number. The number is constructed in a way that it can be tested for verification, using the following formula.

Step 1: Determine the sum of the first, third, and fifth digits added together.
Step 2: Determine the sum of the second, fourth, and sixth digits added together, and then multiply the sum by two.
Step 3: Determine the sum of the two numbers determined in Step 1 and Step 2.
Step 4: The last digit of this third sum should be the same as the last digit of the seven-digit DEA Certificate of Registration Number.

Part 1302—Labeling and packaging requirements for controlled substances

Part 1302 contains the requirements for labeling of the "commercial container" of a controlled substance. The MPJE® candidate should be generally familiar with these requirements.

Part 1303—Quotas

Part 1303 contains the sections related to the establishment of production and procurement quotas for Schedule I and Schedule II controlled substances for the estimated medical, scientific, research and industrial needs. The MPJE® candidate should be generally familiar with the sections in this part.

Part 1304—Records and reports of registrants

Part 1304 contains the many requirements associated with recordkeeping in relation to the various aspects of handling controlled substances by practitioners, and also including narcotic treatment programs. Also included in this part are the requirements associated with inventories of controlled substances, including the "biennial inventory." The MPJE® candidate should be very familiar with the sections in this part.

Part 1305—Order forms

Part 1305 includes the sections describing the DEA Form 222 for ordering Schedule II controlled substances. Also included in this part are the details associated with the granting of a power of attorney in association with order forms. The MPJE® candidate should be very familiar with the sections in this part and be sure to review the regulations regarding electronic orders for controlled substances added in 2005.

Part 1306—Prescriptions

Part 1306 contains the sections concerning the many details of issuing, dispensing, and labeling of prescriptions for controlled substances. Also included in this part in relation to prescriptions are the requirements for electronic recordkeeping of prescription refills and for transfer of prescriptions between pharmacies. Finally, this part includes the requirements for the sale of controlled substances which are not "prescription drugs." The MPJE® candidate should be very familiar with the sections in this part and be sure to review the new regulations added in 2005 regarding prescribing of some controlled substances for narcotic treatment.

Part 1307—Miscellaneous

Part 1307 contains a few sections of interest to the MPJE® candidate. Of particular note are the sections on "distribution" by dispensers and disposal of controlled substances.

Part 1308—Schedules of controlled substances

Part 1308 describes the "Administration Controlled Substances Number" and its uses, and lists controlled substances in their respective schedules. Part 1308 also provides for "exempt" and "excluded" substances, control of immediate precursors, and emergency scheduling. The MPJE® candidate should be generally familiar with controlled substances and the schedule into which they have been placed, and those products that are exempt and excluded as described in Part 1308.

Part 1309—Registration of manufacturers, distributors, importers, and exporters of List I chemicals

Part 1309 includes several provisions related to those engaged in activities with List I chemicals. While the practice of pharmacy is not generally affected by Part 1309, the MPJE® candidate should review these sections for familiarity.

Part 1310—Records and reports of listed chemicals and certain machines

While the comment about Part 1309 immediately above also applies to some sections of Part 1310, it is noted that some sections in Part 1310 relate to ephedrine, and thus this part deserves review by the MPJE® candidate.

Part 1311—Digital certificates
Part 1311 is an entire new Part added in 2005. It governs digital certificates in association with electronic orders for controlled substances and should be studied in detail by the MPJE® candidate.

Part 1312—Importation and exportation of controlled substances
Part 1312 includes several provisions related to those engaged in importing and exporting controlled substances. While the practice of pharmacy is not generally affected by this part, the MPJE® candidate should review these sections for familiarity.

Part 1313—Importation and exportation of precursors and essential chemicals
Part 1313 includes several provisions related to those engaged in importing and exporting precursors and essential chemicals. While the practice of pharmacy is not generally affected by this part, the MPJE® candidate should review these sections for familiarity.

Part 1314—Retail sale of scheduled listed chemical products
In 2005 Congress enacted the Combat Methamphetamine Epidemic Act (CMEA) placing significant control and limitation on the sale of ephedrine, pseudoephedrine and phenylpropanolamine. In September 2006 the DEA added Part 1314 to implement CMEA. The MPJE® candidate should be very familiar with all details concerning the retail sale of these products.

. . .

Part 1316—Administrative functions, practices, and procedures
Part 1316 contains several sections that address inspections, probable cause, and other issues related to warrants, matters related to research, procedures for hearings, burden of proof, and miscellaneous other matters. The MPJE® candidate should be generally familiar with these matters.

3. The Food, Drug, and Cosmetic Act of 1938 and Regulations of the U.S. Food and Drug Administration (FDA)

The Food, Drug, and Cosmetic Act (FDCA), enacted by Congress in 1938, has as its primary purpose preventing interstate distribution of foods, drugs, cosmetics, and devices that are adulterated or misbranded. This purpose is achieved through numerous requirements in the Act and FDA regulations.

Introduction

The MPJE® candidate should be familiar with the historical development of the Food, Drug, and Cosmetic Act of 1938 (FDCA), and its predecessor, the Pure Food and Drug Act of 1906. And the candidate should also be familiar with amendments to the FDCA since 1938, including the following:

Durham-Humphrey Amendment of 1951
Kefauver-Harris Amendment of 1962
Medical Device Amendment of 1976
Orphan Drug Act of 1983
Drug Price Competition and Patent Term Restoration Act of 1984
Prescription Drug Marketing Act of 1987
Safe Medical Devices Act of 1990
Dietary Supplement Health and Education Act of 1994
Food and Drug Administration Modernization Act of 1997
Medical Device User Fee and Modernization Act of 2002
Pediatric Research Equity Act of 2003
Food and Drug Administration Amendments of 2007

Key Provisions of the FDCA

The FDCA is located at Chapter 9 of Title 21 of the United States Code. There are 9 subchapters in Chapter 9, as follows:

I.   Short Title
II. Definitions
III. Prohibited Acts and Penalties
IV. Food
V.   Drugs and Devices
VI. Cosmetics
VII. General Authority
VIII. Imports and Exports
IX. Miscellaneous

The MPJE® candidate should be particularly familiar with Subchapters II, III, V (which is divided into Subparts A through E), and VI, and particularly the following sections within the subchapters of the FDCA.

Subchapter I. Short title

...

Subchapter II. Definitions
§ 321. Definitions; generally
The MPJE® candidate should be familiar with all terms defined in this section of the FDCA, which will aid in understanding the language of the sections that follow. The candidate also should be able to distinguish between terms such as "drug," "counterfeit drug," "new drug," "device," "dietary supplement," "food," and "cosmetic."

...

Subchapter III. Prohibited acts and penalties
§ 331. Prohibited acts
The MPJE® candidate should be familiar with conduct that is prohibited by the FDCA, as set forth in this section.

§ 332. Injunction proceedings
This section provides that the U.S. district courts and all courts exercising jurisdiction in U.S. territories have jurisdiction to enjoin violations of section 331, with some exception as set forth in this section. Further, an alleged violation of an injunction or restraining order shall, upon demand of the accused, be tried before a jury.

§ 333. Penalties
The penalties for violation of the FDCA range from not very severe to very severe. The MPJE® candidate should be familiar with the penalties, and particularly those related to the prescription drug marketing violations (ie, drug samples) and distribution of human growth hormone. Notice the use of the term "knowingly," as defined in Section 321.

...

§ 334. Seizure
This section describes the process related to seizure and disposition of adulterated and misbranded foods, drugs, and cosmetics, a process with which the MPJE® candidate should be familiar.

§ 335. Hearing before report of criminal violation
This section provides that before any violation of this chapter is reported to a U.S. attorney for criminal proceedings, the person against whom the proceeding is contemplated shall be given appropriate notice and an opportunity to present his views, either orally or in writing.

§ 335a. Debarment, temporary denial of approval, and suspension
This section describes the "debarment" from submitting or assisting in the submission of applications for drug approvals of businesses and individuals based on prior misconduct related to the drug approval process. The MPJE® candidate should be able to distinguish the various characteristics of mandatory and permissive debarments.

§ 335b. Civil penalties
This section continues the matter of misconduct in the drug approval process. The MPJE® candidate should be familiar with the conduct prohibited and the associated penalties, together with the provision concerning informants.

§ 335c. Authority to withdraw approval of abbreviated drug applications
This section authorizes the withdrawal of approval of abbreviated drug applications where the approval was obtained, expedited, or otherwise facilitated through bribery, payment of an illegal gratuity, or fraud or material false statement, and further, if the manufacturer has repeatedly demonstrated a lack of ability to produce the drug for which the application was submitted in accordance with the formulations and manufacturing processes set forth in the application and has introduced, or attempted to introduce, such adulterated or misbranded drug into commerce. This section also provides procedures for withdrawals.

§ 336. Report of minor violations
This section provides that the HHS Secretary is not required to report for prosecution, or for the institution of libel or injunction proceedings, minor violations of this chapter whenever he believes that the public interest will be adequately served by a suitable written notice or warning.

§ 337. Proceedings in the name of United States; provision as to subpoenas
This section requires that legal proceedings for enforcement or restraining of violations be in the name of the U.S. However, this section also allows states to bring actions under the Act, but only upon notice being given to the HHS Secretary as set forth in this section.

Subchapter IV. Food

Although this subchapter is entitled "Food" the MPJE® candidate should review select sections of this subchapter as they contain requirements related to dietary supplements. The MPJE® candidate should review the portions addressing dietary supplements in the following sections: 341, 342, 343, 343-1, 343-2, and 350-b. In addition, the MPJE® candidate should review section 350 on vitamins and minerals.

Subchapter V. Drugs and devices
Part A—Drugs and devices
§ 351. Adulterated drugs and devices

A drug or device can be "adulterated" for several reasons, as listed in this section. The MPJE® candidate should be familiar with these reasons.

§ 352. Misbranded drugs and devices

A drug or device can be "misbranded" for several reasons, as listed in this section. The MPJE® candidate should be familiar with these reasons.

§ 353. Exemptions and consideration for certain drugs, devices, and biological products

A very key section of the FDCA, it is this section that, among other things, exempts legend drugs from the general labeling requirements of the FDCA, including when sold upon presenting a prescription. (Note the label requirement of the "Rx Only symbol" which replaces the labeling requirement of "Caution: Federal law prohibits dispensing without a prescription," a change created by the Food and Drug Administration Modernization Act of 1997.) Also included in this section are the sales restrictions imposed by the Prescription Drug Marketing Act of 1987 with respect to legend drug samples and coupons for legend drugs, together with the wholesaler licensing requirements. Finally, veterinary use drugs are addressed in this section.

§ 353a. Pharmacy compounding

This section was added to the FDCA by the Food and Drug Administration Modernization Act of 1997. However, in an April 29, 2002 opinion, the U.S. Supreme Court ruled the section unconstitutional in the case of *Thompson et al. v. Western States Medical Center et al.*, Case No. 01-344. However, it is important to realize that other sections of the FDCA also address pharmacy compounding. The MPJE® candidate should be very familiar with the federal law on pharmacy compounding. A good source for the Supreme Court opinion and other materials, particularly the FDA Compliance Policy Guidance on pharmacy compounding, is the FDA's Center for Drug Evaluation and Research at www.fda.gov/cder/pharmcomp/default.htm.

§ 354. Veterinary feed directive drugs

This section defines what is meant by a veterinary feed directive drug, and sets forth requirements in relation to use and labeling of such drugs.

§ 355. New drugs

This quite lengthy section sets forth the requirements and process for approval of a "new drug" through filing of a new drug application or abbreviated new drug application. The MPJE® candidate should be familiar with the process for approval of drugs, and note particularly in this section the definition and use of the terms "bioavailability" and "bioequivalent." The references listed in the introduction to this review provide a good overview of the drug approval process.

§ 355a. Pediatric studies of drugs

This section authorizes the HHS Secretary to request pediatric studies, which are defined in this section, from the holder of an approved application for a new or previously approved drug, where the drug may produce health benefits in the pediatric population. If the holder of the approved application completes the studies, the holder will be granted additional "market exclusivity," through extension of patent life for the periods described in this section, for the drug. Finally, this section establishes requirements relative to the conducting of pediatric studies.

§ 355b. Adverse-event reporting

This section requires that the label of a prescription drug contain a toll-free maintained by HHS to receive report of adverse events regarding drugs.

§ 355c. Research into pediatric uses for drugs and biological products

This section contains several requirements in relation to assess the safety and effectiveness of drugs and biological products in pediatric patients, and to support dosing and administration of drugs and biological products in pediatric patients.

§ 356. Fast track products

This section authorizes the HHS Secretary, at the request of the sponsor of a new drug, to facilitate the development and expedite the review of such drug if it is intended for the treatment of a serious or life-threatening condition, and it demonstrates the potential to address unmet medical needs for such a condition, which serves as the definition of a "fast track product."

§ 356-1. Accelerated approval of priority countermeasures

This section authorizes the HHS Secretary to designate a priority countermeasure as a fast track product.

§ 356a. Manufacturing changes

This section describes "manufacturing changes" and sets forth those changes that require filing of a supplemental application and those that do not.

§ 356b. Reports of postmarketing studies

This section establishes the requirements for postmarketing studies where the sponsor of a drug has entered into an agreement with the HHS Secretary to conduct such a study.

§ 356c. Discontinuance of life-saving drug

This section creates the requirement that the sole manufacturer of a drug, that has an approved application and that was not originally derived from human tissue and was replaced with recombinant product, and that is life-supporting, life-sustaining, or intended for use in the prevention of a debilitating disease or condition, notify the HHS Secretary of discontinuance of manufacture of the product at least six months prior to the discontinuance date. Reduction in the six-month notice requirement is authorized in certain circumstances, as described in this section.

. . .

§ 358. Authority to designate official names

This section authorizes the HHS Secretary to designate an official name for a drug or device, except where the official name infringes a valid trademark. It also contains a requirement that the HHS Secretary review official names in the United States Pharmacopoeia, the Homoeopathic Pharmacopoeia, and the National Formulary to determine whether revision of those names is necessary or desirable. Finally, in such reviews the HHS Secretary is required to make determinations, in relation to the designation of an official name, based upon complexity, usefulness, multiplicity, or lack of a name.

§ 359. Nonapplicability of subchapter to cosmetics

As the title of this section states, nothing in this Subchapter applies to cosmetics, unless the cosmetic is also a drug or device or component of a drug or device.

§ 360. Registration of producers of drugs or devices

This section establishes the registration and drug listing/National Drug Code requirements for drug manufacturers. The MPJE® candidate should be familiar with the National Drug Code system. And significantly, this section, at (g)(1), exempts pharmacies and certain others from the registration and drug listing requirements.

§ 360b. New animal drugs

As with drugs for human use, the MPJE® candidate should be familiar with new animal drugs under the FDCA, as described in this lengthy section.

§ 360c. Classification of devices intended for human use

The MPJE® candidate should be familiar with the FDCA provisions related to devices. This section establishes three classes of devices, as follows.

Class I   General Controls
Class II   Special Controls
Class III Premarket Approval

This section also sets forth the standards for determination of the safety and effectiveness of a device and provides for classification panel organization and operation.

§ 360d. Performance standards

This section establishes performance standards for Class II, and in some cases Class III, devices, and the procedures for establishing and recognizing the standards.

§ 360e. Premarket approval

This section establishes the requirements and procedures for an application for premarket approval of a Class III device.

§ 360f. Banned devices

This section authorizes the HHS Secretary to promulgate regulations to ban certain devices, as described in this section.

§ 360g. Judicial review

This section sets forth the procedures for judicial review of decisions of the HHS Secretary with regard to devices.

§ 360h. Notification and other remedies

This section provides that when a device presents an unreasonable risk of substantial harm and notification is necessary to eliminate the risk of harm, the HHS Secretary may issue an order to assure that adequate notification is provided in an appropriate form, by the persons and means best suited under the circumstances involved, to all health professionals who prescribe or use the device, and to any other person (including manufacturers, importers, distributors, retailers, and device users) who should properly receive such notification in order to eliminate such risk. This section also authorizes the HHS Secretary to order the manufacturer of a device to make repair, replacement, or refund in relation to the device. Finally, this section gives the HHS Secretary authority to order a recall of a device.

. . .

§ 360i. Records and reports on devices

This section requires reports, as described in the section, from device manufacturers and device user facilities, such as hospitals. It also authorizes the HHS Secretary to order a device manufacturer to adopt a method for tracking certain Class II and III devices.

§ 360j. General provisions respecting control of devices intended for human use

This section contains a variety of requirements, including provisions for custom devices, restricted devices, good manufacturing practice requirements, and exemption of devices for investigational use.

§ 360k. State and local requirements respecting devices

This section establishes the relationship between the FDCA provisions on devices and any state laws that may exist in relation to devices.

§ 360l. Postmarketing surveillance

This section authorizes the HHS Secretary to impose upon manufacturers of certain devices various postmarketing surveillance requirements related to devices.

§ 360m. Accredited persons

This section requires the HHS Secretary to establish an "accreditation program" as described in the section, for persons who review reports related to devices.

Part B—Drugs for rare diseases or conditions
§ 360aa. Recommendations for investigations of drugs for rare diseases or conditions

This section provides that a sponsor of a drug for a disease or condition which is rare may request the HHS Secretary to provide written recommendations for the nonclinical and clinical investigations that must be conducted with the drug before it may be approved for such disease or condition, or, if the drug is a biological product, before it may be licensed for such disease or condition.

§ 360bb. Designation of drugs for rare diseases or conditions

This section allows a manufacturer or sponsor of a drug to request, prior to submission of an application for approval, the HHS Secretary to designate the drug as a drug for a rare disease or condition. This section defines a "rare disease or condition" as any disease or condition that affects fewer than 200,000 persons in the U.S. or affects more than 200,000 in the U.S. and for which there is no reasonable expectation that the cost of developing and making available in the U.S. a drug for such disease or condition will be recovered from sales in the U.S. It also contains a requirement for notice to the HHS Secretary for discontinuance of production of the drug.

§ 360cc. Protection for drugs for rare diseases or conditions

This section provides that if the HHS Secretary approves an application for a drug designated for a rare disease or condition, the HHS Secretary may not approve another application for such drug for such disease or condition for a person who is not the holder of such approved application until the expiration of seven years from the date of approval, except where the holder of the approved application cannot assure the availability of sufficient quantities of the drug to meet the needs of persons with the disease or condition for which the drug was designated, or such holder provides the HHS Secretary written consent for the approval of other applications before the expiration of such seven-year period.

§ 360dd. Open protocols for investigations of drugs for rare diseases or conditions

This section provides, under certain circumstances, for the HHS Secretary to encourage the sponsor of a drug designated for a rare disease or condition to design protocols for clinical investigations of the drug that may be conducted to permit the addition to the investigations of persons with the disease or condition who need the drug to treat the disease or condition, and who cannot be satisfactorily treated by available alternative drugs.

§ 360ee. Grants and contracts for development of drugs for rare diseases and conditions

This section authorizes the HHS Secretary to make grants to and enter into contracts with public and private entities and individuals to assist in defraying the costs of qualified testing expenses incurred in connection with the development of drugs for rare diseases and conditions, defraying the costs of developing medical devices for rare diseases or conditions, and defraying the costs of developing medical foods (a food formulated to be consumed or administered enterally under the supervision of a physician) for rare diseases or conditions.

Part C—Electronic product radiation control

. . .

Part D—Dissemination of treatment information
§ 360aaa. Requirements for dissemination of treatment information on drugs or devices

This section allows a manufacturer to disseminate

written information concerning the safety, effectiveness, or benefit of a use not described in the approved labeling of a drug or device if the manufacturer meets certain requirements. Those parties to whom a manufacturer may disseminate such information are a health care practitioner; a pharmacy benefit manager; a health insurance issuer; a group health plan; and a federal or state governmental agency. Among the requirements are that the manufacturer must submit the information to the HHS Secretary at least 60 days prior to dissemination and the information must contain a prominently displayed statement that discloses very specific language as set forth in this section.

§ 360aaa-1. Information authorized to be disseminated

This section describes what information may be disseminated, such as reprints of peer-reviewed articles and reference publications, but both of which must meet standards set by this section.

§ 360aaa-2. Establishment of a list of articles and publications disseminated and a list of providers that received articles and reference publications

This section requires a manufacturer that disseminates information to biannually provide to the HHS Secretary a list containing the titles of all articles and reference publications that were disseminated, and a list of the categories of providers that received the articles and reference publications. The manufacturer must also keep records that may be used to take corrective action in relation to any information that was disseminated.

§ 360aaa-3. Requirement regarding submission of supplemental application for new use; exemption from requirement

This section generally requires that a manufacturer that disseminates information submit to the HHS Secretary a supplemental application for such use, subject to a number of conditions and exemptions as described in this section.

§ 360aaa-4. Corrective actions; cessation of dissemination

This section authorizes the HHS Secretary to take a variety of actions in relation to a manufacturer's dissemination of information, including an order that the manufacturer cease dissemination of the information, and possibly requiring the manufacturer to correct the information that was disseminated. Grounds for ordering that dissemination be ceased are set forth in the section. It also imposes a duty on manufacturers to notify the HHS Secretary of any additional knowledge of the manufacturer on clinical research or other data that relate to the safety or effectiveness of the new use.

§ 360aaa-5. Definitions

This section defines a number of terms, such as "health care practitioner" and "new use" that are essential to understanding the sections related to manufacturer dissemination of information. The MPJE® candidate should be familiar with these terms and their definitions.

§ 360aaa-6. Rules of construction

This section contains a number of what are referred to as "rules of construction." Examples from the section include that section 360aaa shall not be "construed" as prohibiting a manufacturer from disseminating information in response to an unsolicited request from a health care practitioner. The MPJE® candidate should be familiar with the content of this section.

Part E—General provisions relating to drugs and devices
§ 360bbb. Expanded access to unapproved therapies and diagnostics

This section authorizes the HHS Secretary to allow shipment of investigational drugs or investigational devices for the diagnosis, monitoring, or treatment of a serious disease or condition in emergency situations. Further, an individual patient, acting through a physician, may request from a manufacturer or distributor an investigational drug or investigational device for the diagnosis, monitoring, or treatment of a serious disease or condition if a number of conditions as set forth in this section are fulfilled.

§ 360bbb-1. Dispute resolution

This section requires the HHS Secretary to establish a procedure for a sponsor, applicant, or manufacturer to obtain a review, including by a scientific advisory panel, in situations in which there is a scientific controversy with the HHS Secretary.

§ 360bbb-2. Classification of products

This section provides that a person submitting an application for a product may submit a request to the HHS Secretary with respect to the classification of the product as a drug, biological product, device, or a combination, or with respect to the component of the Food and Drug Administration that will regulate the product. In submitting the request, the person shall recommend a classification for the product, or a component to regulate the product, as appropriate. It also provides what action the HHS Secretary shall take in response to such a request being filed.

§ 360bbb-3. Authorization for medical products for use in emergencies

This section provides for the use of unapproved drugs,

device and biological products, and the use approved drugs, devices and biological products for unapproved uses, in the event of an emergency.

Subchapter VI. Cosmetics

The MPJE® candidate should review the three sections (361 through 363) contained in this subchapter on cosmetics.

The last three subchapters of Chapter 9 contain a variety of sections, many of which are not of interest to the MPJE® candidate. As directed in the explanation to the study guide, the candidate should open each subchapter, and from the titles of the parts and sections, determine those that the MPJE® candidate should review.

Regulations of the U.S. Food and Drug Administration (FDA)

The FDA regulations may be found in Title 21 of the Code of Federal Regulations (CFR). The body of FDA regulations is divided into "Subchapters" as follows.

Subchapter A	General (21 CFR Parts 1 to 99)
Subchapter B	Food for Human Consumption (21 CFR Parts 100 to 199)
Subchapter C	Drugs: General (21 CFR 200 to 299)
Subchapter D	Drugs for Human Use (21 CFR Parts 300 to 499)
Subchapter E	Animal Drugs, Feeds, and Related Products (21 CFR Parts 500 to 599)
Subchapter F	Biologics (21 CFR Parts 600 to 699)
Subchapter G	Cosmetics (21 CFR Parts 700 to 799)
Subchapter H	Medical Devices (21 CFR Parts 800 to 899)
Subchapter I	Mammography Quality Standards Act (21 CFR Parts 900 to 999)
Subchapter J	Radiological Health (21 CFR Parts 1000 to 1099)
Subchapter K	Reserved
Subchapter L	Regulations Under Certain Other Acts (21 CFR Parts 1200 to 1299)

The MPJE® candidate should review relevant FDA regulations on the electronic database as described in the explanation to this study guide.

4. The Poison Prevention Packaging Act of 1970 and Regulations of the U.S. Consumer Product Safety Commission (CPSC)

The Poison Prevention Packaging Act (PPPA), enacted by Congress in 1970, has as its purpose preventing poisonings in children under 5 years of age. This purpose is achieved through numerous requirements in the Act and CPSC regulations.

Introduction

The Poison Prevention Packaging Act of 1970 (PPPA) establishes packaging requirements for certain household products. Included among these products are both prescription and nonprescription drug products.

Key provisions of the PPPA

The MPJE® candidate should be familiar with the packaging requirements contained in the PPPA and the regulations of the Consumer Product Safety Commission (CPSC). The PPPA is located at Chapter 39A of Title 15 of the United States Code. The MPJE® candidate should retrieve and the review the sections contained in Chapter 39A as described in the explanation to this study guide.

Regulations of the U.S. Consumer Product Safety Commission (CPSC)

The CPSC regulations may be found at Part 1700 of Title 16 of the Code of Federal Regulations (CFR). The MPJE® candidate should retrieve and the review the sections contained in Part 1700 as described in the explanation to this study guide.

5. Miscellaneous Federal Laws

Omnibus Budget Reconciliation Act of 1990

This act, more commonly referred to as OBRA '90, required the states to enact laws to require patient profiling, prospective drug utilization review, and patient counseling by pharmacies. While the federal mandate applied only to the provision of pharmacy services to Medicaid beneficiaries, the states extended application of the requirements to all pharmacy patients. While the MPJE® candidate should review state law on these requirements, the federal regulations may be found beginning at section 42 CFR 456.700.

Anti-Tampering Act of 1982

This Act makes it a federal offense to tamper with consumer products, and was passed as a result of a series of incidents of intentional contamination of Tylenol® capsules while held for sale in retail establishments. Regulatory authority resides with the Federal Bureau of Investigation, U.S. Department of Agriculture, and FDA. Regulations for specific types of products may be retrieved (as described in the explanation to this study guide) and reviewed as follows:

Over-the-counter drug products (21 CFR 211.132)
Medical devices (21 CFR 800.12)
Cosmetics (21 CFR 700.25)

Federal Law on Medicinal Use of Alcohol

Under federal law, retailers that sell alcohol are subject to an annual tax, and in order to handle any type of alcohol, a license from the U.S. Bureau of Alcohol, Tobacco, and Firearms (ATF) is required. Retailers selling take-home liquors are required to obtain a federal retail liquor dealer's stamp. In a community pharmacy, if the alcohol is sold only for medicinal purposes, a federal medicinal spirits dealer's stamp may be obtained instead of the retail liquor dealer's stamp.

Some pharmacies require much larger volumes (usually obtained in 10- or 55-gallon drums) of alcohol, and it can be purchased tax-free. However, the use of tax-free alcohol is subject to a number of federal law restrictions.

- The alcohol must be used for medicinal or scientific purposes, or patient treatment.
- The alcohol must not be sold or loaned to other pharmacies or other practitioners.
- The alcohol, whether in pure form or in combination with other substances, must not be sold to outpatients, with the exception of nonprofit clinics, so long as the patient is not charged.
- The alcohol must be kept in a secure, fire-resistant room.
- A perpetual inventory of the alcohol stock must be maintained.

For additional information, the MPJE® candidate can review the sections beginning at 27 CFR 22.1 as described in the explanation to this study guide.

3. Dosage Forms and Drug Delivery Systems

Ram I. Mahato, PhD
Associate Professor
Department of Pharmaceutical Sciences
University of Tennessee College of Pharmacy

Contents

1. Introduction

Pharmaceutical dosage forms are drug delivery systems. Some common examples are tablets, capsules, suppositories, injections, suspensions, and transdermal patches. To achieve an optimum response from any dosage form, a drug should be delivered to its site of action at a rate and concentration that both minimize its side effects and maximize its therapeutic effects. The development of safe and effective pharmaceutical dosage forms and delivery systems requires a thorough understanding of *physicochemical principles* that allow a drug to be formulated into a pharmaceutical dosage form. Design of the appropriate dosage form or delivery system depends on the:

- Physicochemical properties of the drug, such as solubility, oil-to-water partition coefficient ($K_{o/w}$), pK_a value, molecular weight, and polymorphism
- Dose of the drug
- Route of administration
- Type of drug delivery systems desired
- Pathologic condition to be treated
- Desired therapeutic effect
- Drug release from the delivery system
- Bioavailability of the drug at the absorption site
- Pharmacokinetics and pharmacodynamics of the drug

How Drug Molecules Move Across Barriers in the Body

Most drugs are absorbed from the site of their application by simple diffusion. Drug diffusion through a barrier may occur by simple molecular permeation known as *molecular diffusion* or by movement through pores and channels known as *pore-diffusion.* In pore-diffusion, drug release rate is affected by degree of crystallinity and crystal size, degree of swelling, porous structure, and tortuosity of polymers.

With passive molecular diffusion, a drug travels by *passive transport* (which does not require an external energy source) from a region of high concentration to a region of low concentration. However, other transport processes occur in the body as well. For example, *active transport* of drugs can proceed from regions of low concentration to regions of high concentration through the pumping action of one or more biologic transport systems. These active transport systems require an energy source such as an enzyme or biochemical carrier to ferry the drug across the membrane.

For passive molecular diffusion, Fick's first law of diffusion states that the amount of material (M) flowing through a unit cross-section (S) of a barrier in unit time (t), which is known as the flux (J), is proportional to the concentration gradient (dc/dx).

$$J = \frac{dM}{S \cdot dt}$$

J = flux in g/cm²s
S = cross section of barrier in cm²
dM/dt = rate of diffusion in g/s
(M = mass in grams;
    t = time in seconds)

The flux is proportional to the concentration gradient, dC/dx:

$$J = -D \frac{dC}{dx}$$

D = diffusion coefficient of a
    penetrant in cm²/s
C = concentration in g/cm³ or g/mL
x = distance in centimeters of
    movement perpendicular to the
    surface of the barrier

The diffusion coefficient, D, is a physical chemical property of the drug molecule. It is not constant and can vary with changes in concentration, temperature, pressure, solvent properties, and chemical nature of the diffusant.

Fick's first law of diffusion describes the diffusion process under the condition of steady state when the concentration gradient (dc/dx) does not change with time. Figure 1 shows the diaphragm of thickness "h" and cross-sectional area "S" which separates the two compartments of the diffusion cell. Equating both equations for flux, Fick's first law of diffusion may be written as:

$$J = \frac{dM}{S \cdot dt} = \frac{D(C_1 - C_2)}{h}$$

In which $(C_1 - C_2)/h$ approximates dC/dx. Concentrations C_1 and C_2 within the membrane can be replaced by the partition coefficient multiplied by the concentration C_d in the donor compartment or C_r in the receptor compartment. The *partition coefficient,* K, is given by $K = C_1/C_d = C_2/C_r$. Hence,

$$\frac{dM}{dt} = \frac{DSK(C_d - C_r)}{h}$$

Under sink conditions, the drug concentration in the receptor compartment is much lower than the drug concentration in the donor compartment. Therefore, $C_r \rightarrow 0$. The above equation can be simplified as:

$$\frac{dM}{dt} = \frac{DSKC_d}{h} = PSC_d$$

Figure 1.

Concentration gradient of diffusant across a diaphragm of a diffusion cell.

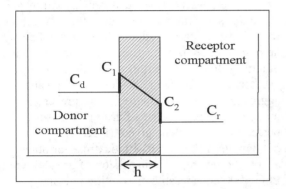

where D is the diffusion coefficient (cm^2/s), S is the surface area of the cross section of the barrier (cm^2), K is the partition coefficient, C_d is the concentration of drug in the donor compartment (g/mL), h is the barrier thickness (cm), and P is the permeability coefficient (cm/s), where P = DK/h.

Drug transport and absorption
Transport of a drug by *passive diffusion* across a membrane such as the gastrointestinal mucosa is represented by Fick's law:

$$-\frac{dM}{dt} = \frac{D_m SK}{h}(C_g - C_p)$$

where M is the amount of drug in the gut compartment at time t, D_m is drug diffusivity in intestinal membrane, S is the surface area of GI membrane available for absorption, K is the partition coefficient between the membrane and aqueous medium in the intestine, h is the thickness of the GI membrane, C_g is the drug concentration in the intestinal compartment, and C_p is the drug concentration in the plasma compartment.

Since the gut compartment usually has a high drug concentration compared to the plasma compartment, C_p may be omitted. Therefore, the above equation then becomes

$$-\frac{dM}{dt} = \frac{D_m SK \cdot C_g}{h}$$

This suggests that the rate of gastrointestinal absorption of a drug by passive diffusion depends on the surface area of the membrane available for drug absorption. The

small intestine is the major site for drug absorption due to the presence of villi and microvilli, which provide an enormous surface area for absorption.

pH-Partition Theory and Its Limitation

The pH-partition theory states that drugs are absorbed from the biological membranes by passive diffusion, depending on the fraction of the un-ionized form of the drug at the pH of the fluids close to that biological membrane. The degree of ionization of the drug depends on both the pK_a and the pH of the drug solution. The gastrointestinal tract acts as a lipophilic barrier and thus ionized drugs, compared to un-ionized ones, are more hydrophilic and have minimal membrane transport. The solution pH affects the overall partition coefficient of an ionizable substance. The pK_a of the molecule is the pH at which there is a 50:50 mixture of conjugate acid-base forms. The conjugate acid form predominates at a pH lower than the pK_a, and the conjugate base form is present at a pH higher than that of the pK_a. The extent of ionization of a drug molecule, given by the following *Henderson-Hasselbalch equations,* describes a relationship between ionized and non-ionized species of a weak electrolyte:

Weakly Acidic Drugs   **Weakly Basic Drugs**

$$pH = pK_a + \log \frac{[A^-]}{[HA]} \qquad pH = pK_a + \log \frac{[B]}{[BH^+]}$$

Where [HA] is the concentration of un-ionized acid, [A$^-$] is the concentration of ionized base, [B] is the concentration of un-ionized base, and [BH$^+$] is the concentration of ionized base.

Although pH-partition theory is useful, it often does not hold true for certain experimental observations. For example, most weak acids are well-absorbed from the small intestine, which is contrary to the prediction of the pH-partition hypothesis. Similarly, quaternary ammonium compounds are ionized at all pHs, but are readily absorbed from the GI tract. These discrepancies arise because *pH-partition theory does not take into consideration the following (this list is not exhaustive):*
- Large epithelial surface areas of small intestine compensate for ionization effects.
- Long residence time in the small intestine also compensates for ionization effects.
- Charged drugs, such as quaternary ammonium compounds and tetracyclines, may interact with opposite charged organic ions, resulting in a neutral species that is absorbable.
- Some drugs are absorbed via active transport.

The Noyes-Whitney Equation of Dissolution

The rate at which a solid drug of limited water solubility dissolves in a solvent can be determined using the *Noyes-Whitney equation:*

$$\frac{dM}{dt} = k \cdot S \cdot (C_s - C)$$

where dM/dt is the rate of dissolution (mass/time), k is the dissolution rate constant (cm/s) ($k = D/h$), S is the surface area of exposed solid (cm^2), D is the diffusion coefficient of solute in solution (cm^2/s), h is the thickness of the diffusion layer (cm), C_s is the drug solubility (g/mL), and C is the drug concentration in bulk solution at time t (g/mL).

Under *sink conditions* when C is much less than C_s, the Noyes-Whitney equation can be simplified as:

$$\boxed{\frac{dM}{dt} = k\,S\,C_s \quad \text{or} \quad \frac{dC}{dt} = \frac{kSC_s}{V}}$$

where dC/dt is the dissolution rate (conc/time) and V is the volume of the dissolution medium (mL).

Factors influencing dissolution rate

- The dissolution rate of a drug may be influenced by the physicochemical conditions in the GI tract. For example, the presence of foods that increase the viscosity of GI fluids decreases the diffusion coefficient, D, of a drug and its dissolution rate.
- The thickness of the diffusion layer, h, is influenced by the degree of agitation experienced by each drug particle in the GI tract. Hence an increase in gastric and/or intestinal motility may increase the dissolution rate of poorly soluble drugs.
- The removal rate of dissolved drugs due to absorption through the GI-blood barrier and the GI fluid volume affects drug concentration in the GI tract and thus also affects the dissolution rate.
- The dissolution rate of a weakly acidic drug in GI fluids is influenced by the drug solubility in the diffusion layer surrounding each dissolving drug particle. The pH of the diffusion layer has significant effect on the solubility of a weak electrolyte drug and its subsequent dissolution rate. The dissolution rate of a weakly acidic drug in GI fluid (pH 1-3) is relatively low because of its low solubility in the diffusion layer. If the pH in the diffusion layer could be increased, the solubility (C_s) exhibited by the weak acidic drug in this layer (and hence the dissolution rate of the drug in GI fluids) could be increased. The potassium or sodium salt form of the weakly acidic drug has a relatively high solubility at the elevated pH in the diffusion layer. Thus the dissolution of the

drug particles takes place at a faster rate.
- Particle size and the surface area of the drug have significant influence on the drug dissolution rate. An increase in the total effective surface area of drug in contact with GI fluids causes an increase in its dissolution rate. The smaller the particle size, the greater the effective surface area exhibited by a given mass of drug and the higher the dissolution rate. However, particle size reduction is not always helpful and may fail to increase the bioavailability of a drug. In case of certain hydrophobic drugs, excessive particle size reduction tends to cause re-aggregation into larger particles. To prevent the formation of aggregates, small drug particles are dispersed in polyethylene glycol (PEG), polyvinylpyrrolidone (PVP), dextrose, or other agents. For example, a dispersion of griseofulvin in PEG 4000 enhances its dissolution rate and bioavailability. Certain drugs such as penicillin G and erythromycin are unstable in gastric fluids and do not dissolve readily in them. Regarding such drugs, particle size reduction yields an increased rate of drug dissolution in gastric fluid and also increases the extent of drug degradation.
- Amorphous or noncrystalline forms of a drug may have faster dissolution rates than crystalline forms.
- Temperature also affects solubility. An increase in temperature will increase the solubility of a solid with a positive heat of solution. The solid will therefore dissolve at a more rapid rate on heating the system.
- Surface-active agents will increase the dissolution rates by lowering the interfacial tension, which allows better wetting and penetration by the solvent.

Interfacial Electrical Properties

Most dispersed substances in a solvent such as water acquire a surface electric charge by *ionization, ion adsorption,* and *ion dissolution.*

Ionization

- Surface charge arising from ionization on the particles is the function of the pH of the environment and the pK_a of the drug. Proteins acquire charge through the ionization of carboxyl and amino groups to obtain COO^- and NH_3^+ ions. Ionization of these groups, and the net molecular charge, depends on the pH of the medium. At a pH below its isoelectric point (PI), a protein molecule is positively charged, $^-NH_2 \rightarrow NH_3^+$, and at a pH above its PI, the protein is negatively charged, $-COOH \rightarrow COO^-$. At the isoelectric point of a protein, the total number of positive charges equals the total number of negative charges, and the net charge is zero. This may be represented as follows:

R-NH$_2$-COO$^-$ Alkaline solution

$\Updownarrow$

R-NH$_3^+$-COO$^-$ Isoelectric point (Zwitterion)

$\Updownarrow$

R-NH$_3^+$-COOH   Acidic solution

- Often a protein is least soluble at its isoelectric point and is readily desolvated by water-soluble salts such as ammonium sulfate.

Ion adsorption

- A net surface charge can result from the unequal adsorption of oppositely charged ions. Surfaces that are already charged usually show a tendency to adsorb counter-ions. It is possible for counter-ion adsorption to cause a reversal of charge. Surfactants strongly adsorb by hydrophobic effect and thus will determine the surface charge when adsorbed.

Ion dissolution

- Ionic substances can acquire a surface charge by virtue of unequal dissolution of the oppositely charged ions of which they are composed. For example, in a solution of silver iodide with excess [I$^-$], the silver iodide particles carry a negative charge; however, the charge is positive if excess [Ag$^+$] is present. The silver and iodide ions are referred to as *potential-determining ions* since their concentrations determine the electric potential at the particle surface.

Adsorption at solid interfaces

- Adsorption of materials at solid interfaces may take place from either an adjacent liquid or gas phase. *Adsorption* is different from *absorption,* since the process of absorption implies the penetration of an entity through the organ and tissues. The degree of adsorption depends on the chemical nature of the adsorbent (a material that is being adsorbed onto a substrate, called adsorbate), the chemical nature of the adsorbate, the surface area of the adsorbent, the temperature, and the partial pressure of the adsorbed gas. Adsorption can be physical or chemical in nature.

Physical adsorption

- Physical adsorption is rapid, nonspecific, and relatively weak. Furthermore, it is associated with van der Waals attractive forces and is reversible. Removal of the adsorbate from the adsorbent is known as *desorption.* A physically adsorbed gas may be desorbed from a solid by increasing the temperature and reducing the pressure.

Chemical adsorption

- Chemical adsorption or chemisorption is an irreversible process in which the adsorbent is attached to the adsorbate by primary chemical bonds. Chemisorption is specific, and may require an activation energy; therefore the process is slow and only a monomolecular chemisorbed layer is possible.

Factors affecting adsorption from solution

- *Solubility of adsorbate:* The extent of adsorption of a solute is inversely proportional to its solubility in the solvent from which adsorption occurs.
- *Solute concentration:* An increase in the solute concentration causes an increase in the amount of adsorption that occurs at equilibrium until a limiting value is reached.
- *Temperature:* An increase in temperature leads to decreased adsorption.
- *pH:* The influence of pH is through a change in the ionization and solubility of the adsorbate drug molecule. For many simple small molecules, adsorption increases as the ionization of the drug is suppressed, ie, the extent of adsorption reaches a maximum when the drug is completely un-ionized. For amphoteric compounds, adsorption is at a maximum at the isoelectric point. pH and solubility effects act in concert since the un-ionized form of most drugs in aqueous solution has a low solubility.
- *Surface area of adsorbent:* An increased surface area, achieved by a reduction in particle size or the use of a porous adsorbing material, increases the extent of adsorption.

Rheology

Rheology is *the study of flow properties* of liquids and deformation of solids. The flow of simple liquids can be described by viscosity, an expression of the resistance to flow; however, other complex dispersions cannot be simply expressed by viscosity.

According to *Newton's law of flow,* the rate of flow (D) is directly proportional to the applied stress (τ). That is, $\tau = \eta \cdot D$, where η is the viscosity. Fluids that obey Newton's law of flow are referred to as *Newtonian fluids* and fluids that deviate are known as *non-Newtonian fluids.* The force per unit area (F'/A) required to bring about flow is called the shearing stress (F):

$$F = \frac{F'}{A} = \eta \frac{dv}{dr}$$

where η is the viscosity, dv/dr is the rate of shear = G (s^{-1}), and F'/A units are in dynes per cm^2. For simple Newtonian fluids, a plot of the rate of shear against shearing stress gives a straight line (Figure 2A), thus η

Figure 2.

Plots of rate of shear as a function of shearing stress for (A) Newtonian, (B) plastic, (C) pseudoplastic, (D) dilatant, and (E) thixotropic flow.

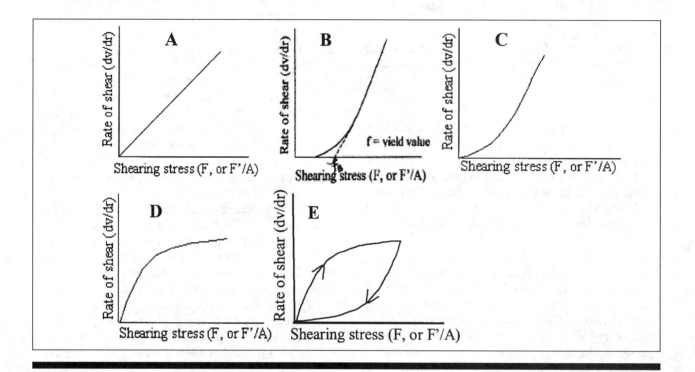

is a constant. In the case of Newtonian fluids, viscosity does not change with increasing shear rate. Various types of water and pharmaceutical dosage forms that contain a high percentage of water are examples of liquid dosage forms that have Newtonian flow properties.

Most pharmaceutical fluids (including colloidal dispersions, emulsions, and liquid suspensions) do not follow Newton's law of flow, and the viscosity of the fluid varies with the rate of shear. There are three types of non-Newtonian flow: *plastic, pseudoplastic,* and *dilatant* (Figure 2B, C, and D).

Plastic flow
Substances that undergo plastic flow are called *Bingham bodies,* which are defined as substances that exhibit a yield value (Figure 2B). Plastic flow is associated with the presence of flocculated particles in concentrated suspensions.
- Plastic flow does not begin until a shearing stress, corresponding to a *yield value,* f, is exceeded.
- The curve intersects the shearing stress axis but does not cross through the origin.
- The materials are said to be "elastic" at shear stresses below the yield value.

- Viscosity decreases with increasing shear rate at shear stress below the yield value.

Flocculated solids
Flocculated solids are light, fluffy conglomerates of adjacent particles held together by weak van der Waals forces. The yield value exists because a certain shearing stress must be exceeded in order to break up van der Waals forces. A plastic system resembles a Newtonian system at shear stresses above the yield value. Yield value, f, is an indicator of flocculation (the higher the yield value, the greater the degree of flocculation).

Pseudoplastic flow
Pseudoplastic flow is exhibited by polymers in solution. A large of number of pharmaceutical products, including natural and synthetic gums (eg, liquid dispersions of tragacanth, sodium alginate, methyl cellulose, and sodium carboxymethylcellulose) exhibit *pseudoplastic flow properties.*
- Pseudoplastic substances begin flow when a shearing stress is applied, ie, there is no yield value (it does cross the origin).

- The viscosity of a pseudoplastic substance decreases with increasing shear rate.
- With increasing shearing stress, the rate of shear increases; these materials are called *shear-thinning* systems.
- Shear thinning occurs when molecules (polymers) align themselves along their long axes and slip and slide past each other.

Dilatant flow

Certain suspensions with a high percentage of dispersed solids exhibit an increase in resistance to flow with increasing rates of shear. This type of behavior may be exhibited by dispersions containing a high percentage ($\geq$50%) of small, deflocculated particles.
- Dilatant materials *increase in volume* when sheared.
- They are also known as *shear-thickening* systems (the opposite of pseudoplastic systems).
- When the stress is removed, the dilatant system returns to its original state of fluidity.
- Viscosity increases with increasing shear rate.
- Dilatant materials may solidify under conditions of high shear.

Thixotropy

Thixotropy is a nonchemical isothermal gel-sol-gel transformation. If a thixotropic gel is sheared (by simple shaking), the weak bonds are broken and a lyophobic solution is formed. On standing the particles collide, flocculation occurs, and the gel is reformed. The advantage that thixotropic preparations have is that the particles remain in suspension during storage, but when required for use, the pastes are readily made fluid by tapping or shaking. The shearing force on the injection as it is pushed through the needle ensures that it is fluid when injected; however, the rapid resumption of the gel structure prevents excessive spreading in the tissues, and consequently a more compact depot is produced than with nonthixotropic suspensions. Thixotropy is a desirable property in liquid pharmaceutical preparations. A well-formulated thixotropic suspension will not settle out readily in the container and will become fluid upon shaking. Flow curves (rheograms) for thixotropic materials are highly dependent on the rate at which shear is increased or decreased and the length of time a sample is subjected to any one rate of shear.

Negative thixotropy

Negative thixotropy is also known as antithixotropy, which represents an increase rather than a decrease in consistency on the down-curve (an increase in thickness or resistance to flow with an increased time of shear). It may result from an increased collision frequency of dispersed particles (or polymer molecules) in suspension, which causes increased interparticle bonding with time.

Shelf-Life Stability of a Drug Product

The shelf life of a drug in a dosage form is the amount of time that the product can be stored before it becomes unfit for use because of chemical decomposition and/or physical deterioration. Shelf-life stability of a dosage form can be determined by the Arrhenius equation given below:

$$k = A \cdot e^{-Ea/RT}, \text{ which can be rewritten as}$$

$$\log k = -\frac{Ea}{2.303} \frac{1}{R}$$

$$\log \frac{k_2}{k_1} = \frac{Ea (T_2 - T_1)}{2.303 R T_2 T_1}$$

Where k_2 and k_1 are the reaction rates at the absolute temperatures T_2 and T_1, respectively, R is the gas constant (1.987 cal/Kmol), Ea is the activation energy (cal/mol), and A is the constant (based on molecular weight and molar volume of liquid).

2. Surfactants and Micelles

Surface-active agents or *surfactants* are substances that absorb to surfaces or interfaces to reduce surface or interfacial tension. They may be used as emulsifying agents, solubilizing agents, detergents, and wetting agents. Surfactants have two distinct regions in one chemical structure. One area is hydrophilic ("water-liking"); another is hydrophobic ("water-hating"). The existence of two such moieties in a molecule is known as *amphipathy* and the molecules are consequently referred to as amphipathic molecules or amphiphiles. Depending on the number and nature of the polar and nonpolar groups present, the amphiphile may be predominantly hydrophilic, lipophilic, or somewhere in between. For example, straight chain alcohols, amines, and acids are amphiphiles that change from being predominantly hydrophilic to lipophilic as the number of carbon atoms in the alkyl chain is increased. The hydrophobic portions are usually saturated or unsaturated hydrocarbon chains, or, less commonly, heterocyclic or aromatic ring systems.

Surfactants are classified according to the nature of the hydrophilic or hydrophobic groups. In addition, some surfactants possess both positively and negatively charged groups, and can exist as either anionic or cationic, depending on the pH of the solution. These surfactants are known as *ampholytic* compounds.

At low concentrations in solutions, amphiphiles exist as monomers. As the concentration is increased, aggregation occurs over a narrow concentration range. These aggregates, which may contain 50 or more monomers, are called *micelles.* Therefore, micelles are small spherical structures composed of both hydrophilic and hydrophobic regions. The concentration of monomer at which micelles are formed is called the *critical micellization concentration,* or CMC. Surface tension decreases up to the CMC, but remains constant above the CMC. The longer the hydrophobic chain or the lower the polarity of the polar group, the greater the tendency for monomers to "escape" from the water to form micelles and hence lower the CMC.

Types of Micelles

In the case of amphiphiles in water, in dilute solution (still above but close to the CMC) the micelles are considered to be spherical in shape. At higher concentrations they become more asymmetric and eventually assume *cylindrical* or *lamellar* structures. Oil-soluble surfactants have a tendency to self-associate into *"reverse micelles"* in nonpolar solvents, with their polar groups oriented away from the solvent.

Factors Affecting CMC and Micellar Size

- Structure of hydrophobic group: An increase in the hydrocarbon chain length causes a logarithmic decrease in the CMC.
- Nature of hydrophilic group: An increase in chain length increases hydrophilicity and the CMC.
- Nature of counter ions: $Cl^- < Br^- < I^-$ for cationic surfactants and $Na^+ < K^+$ for anionic surfactants
- The addition of electrolytes to ionic surfactants decreases the CMC and increases the micellar size. In contrast, micellar properties of nonionic surfactants are only minimally affected by the addition of electrolytes.
- Effect of temperature
- Alcohol: CMCs are increased by the addition of alcohols.

HLB (Hydrophile-Lipophile Balance) Systems

Griffin's method of selecting emulsifying agents is based on the balance between the hydrophilic and lipophilic portions of the emulsifying agent; this is now widely known as the hydrophile-lipophile balance (HLB) system. The higher the HLB value of an emulsifying agent, the more hydrophilic it is. The emulsifying agents with lower HLB values are less polar and more lipophilic. The Spans, ie, sorbitan esters, are lipophilic and have low HLB values (1.8-8.6); the Tweens, polyoxyethylene derivatives of the Spans, are hydrophilic and have high HLB values (9.6-16.7). Surfactants with the proper balance of hydrophilic and lipophilic affinities are effective emulsifying agents since they concentrate at the oil-water (o/w) interface. The type of an emulsion that is produced depends primarily on the property of the emulsifying agent. The HLB of an emulsifier or a combination of emulsifiers determines whether an o/w or water-oil (w/o) emulsion results. In general, o/w emulsions are formed when the HLB of the emulsifier is within the range of about 9-12; w/o emulsions are formed when the range is about 3-6. The type of emulsion is a function of the relative solubility of the supernatant. An emulsifying agent with high HLB is preferentially soluble in water and results in the formation of an o/w emulsion. The reverse situation is true with surfactants of low HLB value, which tend to form w/o emulsions.

Micellar Solubilization

Micelles can be used to increase the solubility of materials that are normally insoluble or poorly soluble in the dispersion medium used. For example, surfactants are often used to increase the solubility of poorly soluble steroids. The factors affecting micellar solubilization are: nature of surfactants, nature of solubilizates, and temperature.

3. Dispersed Systems

Dispersed systems consist of particulate matter, known as the dispersed phase, distributed throughout a continuous or dispersion medium. The particulate matter, or dispersed phase, consists of particles that range from 1 nm to 0.5 micro meter (10^{-9} m to 5×10^{-7} m). Dispersed systems are classified as follows:
- *Molecular dispersions:* <1 nm, invisible under electron microscopy (EM); examples are oxygen molecules, ions, and glucose
- *Colloidal dispersions:* 1 nm to 0.5 micro meter, visible under EM; examples are colloidal silver sols and natural and synthetic polymers
- *Coarse dispersions:* >0.5 micro meter, visible under light microscopy; examples are grains of sand, emulsions, suspensions, and red blood cells

Types of Colloidal Systems

Colloidal systems are classified as lyophilic or lyophobic. Their association is based on the interaction of the particles or molecules of the dispersed phase with the molecules of the dispersion medium.

Lyophilic or hydrophilic colloids
Systems containing colloidal particles that interact with the dispersion medium are referred to as *lyophilic colloids.* Because of their affinity for the dispersion medium, such materials form colloidal dispersions with relative ease. For example, the dissolution of acacia or gelatin in water or celluloid in amyl acetate leads to the formation of a solution. Most lyophilic colloids are polymers (eg, gelatin, acacia, povidone, albumin, rubber, and polystyrene).

Lyophobic or hydrophobic colloids
Lyophobic colloids are composed of materials that have little attraction for the dispersion medium. Lyophobic colloids are intrinsically unstable and irreversible. Hydrophobic colloids are generally composed of inorganic particles dispersed in water.

Association colloids
Association (referring to amphiphilic colloids) *colloids* are formed by the grouping or association of amphiphiles, ie, molecules that exhibit both lyophilic and lyophobic properties. At low concentrations, amphiphiles exist separately and do not form a colloid. At higher concentrations, aggregation occurs at around 50 or more monomers, which induces micelle formation. As with lyophilic colloids, formation of association colloids is spontaneous, provided that the concentration of the amphiphile in solution exceeds the CMC.

Zeta Potential and Its Effect on Colloidal Stability

Zeta (ζ) potential is defined as the difference in potential between the surface of the tightly bound layer (shear plane) and the electroneutral region of the solution. The ζ potential governs the degree of repulsion between adjacent, similarly charged, dispersed particles. If ζ potential is reduced below a certain value, the attractive forces exceed the repulsive forces, and the particles come together. This phenomenon is known as *flocculation.*

Stabilization is accomplished by providing the dispersed particles with an electric charge and a protective solvent sheath surrounding each particle to prevent mutual adherence due to collision. This second effect is significant only in the case of lyophilic colloids. Lyophilic and association colloids are thermodynamically stable and exist in a true solution so that the system constitutes a single phase. In contrast, lyophobic colloids are thermodynamically unstable, but can be stabilized by preventing aggregation/coagulation by providing the dispersed particles with an electric charge, which can prevent coagulation by repulsion of like particles.

4. Pharmaceutical Ingredients

To turn a drug substance into a pharmaceutical dosage form or a drug delivery system, pharmaceutical ingredients are required. For example, in the preparation of tablets, *diluents* or *fillers* are commonly added to increase the bulk of the formulation. *Binders* are added to promote adhesion of the powdered drug to other ingredients. *Lubricants* assist the smooth tabletting process. *Disintegrants* promote tablet break-up after administration. *Coatings* improve stability, control disintegration, or enhance appearance. Similarly, in the preparation of pharmaceutical solutions, *preservatives* are added to prevent microbial growth, *stabilizers* are added to prevent drug decomposition, and *colorants* and *flavorants* are added to ensure product appeal. Thus, for each dosage form, the pharmaceutical ingredients establish the primary features of the product and control the physicochemical properties, drug-release profiles, and bioavailability of the product. Table 1 lists some typical pharmaceutical ingredients used in different dosage forms.

Table 1

Typical Pharmaceutical Ingredients

Ingredient type	Definition	Examples
Antifungal preservative	Used in liquid and semisolid formulations to prevent growth of fungi	Benzoic acid, butylparaben, ethylparaben, sodium benzoate, sodium propionate
Antimicrobial preservative	Used in liquid and semi-solid formulations to prevent growth of microorganisms	Benzalkonium chloride, benzyl alcohol, cetylpyridinium chloride, phenyl ethyl alcohol
Antioxidant	Used to prevent oxidation	Ascorbic acid, ascorbyl palmitate, sodium ascorbate, sodium bisulfate, sodium metabisulfite
Emulsifying agent	Used to promote and maintain dispersion of finely divided droplets of a liquid in a vehicle in which it is immiscible	Acacia, cetyl alcohol, glyceryl monostearate, sorbitan monostearate
Surfactant	Used to reduce surface or interfacial tension	Polysorbate 80, sodium lauryl sulfate, sorbitan monopalmitate
Plasticizer	Used to enhance coat spread over tablets, beads, and granules	Glycerin, diethyl palmitate
Suspending agent	Used to reduce sedimentation rate of drug particles dispersed throughout a vehicle in which they are not soluble	Carbopol, hydroxymethylcellulose, hydroxypropyl cellulose, methylcellulose, tragacanth
Binder	Used to cause adhesion of powder particles in tablet granulations	Acacia, alginic acid, ethylcellulose, starch, povidone
Diluent	Used as fillers to create desired bulk, flow properties, and compression characteristics in tablet and capsule preparations	Kaolin, lactose, mannitol, cellulose, sorbitol, starch
Disintegrant	Used to promote disruption of solid mass into small particles	Microcrystalline cellulose, carboxymethylcellulose calcium, sodium alginate, sodium starch glycolate, alginic acid
Glidant	Used to improve flow properties of powder mixture	Colloidal silica, cornstarch, talc
Lubricant	Used to reduce friction during tablet compression and facilitate ejection of tablets from the die cavity	Calcium stearate, magnesium stearate, mineral oil, stearic acid, zinc stearate
Humectant	Used for prevention of dryness of ointments and creams	Glycerin, propylene glycol, sorbitol

5. Types of Commonly Used Dosage Forms

Solutions

Solutions are homogeneous mixtures of one or more solutes dispersed in a dissolving medium (solvent). Aqueous solutions containing a sugar or sugar substitute with or without added flavoring agents and drugs are classified as *syrups.* Sweetened hydroalcoholic (combinations of water and ethanol) solutions are termed *elixirs.* Hydroalcoholic solutions of aromatic materials are termed *spirits. Tinctures* are alcoholic or hydroalcoholic solutions of chemical or soluble constituents of vegetable drugs. Most tinctures are prepared by an extraction process. *Mouthwashes* are solutions used to cleanse the mouth or treat diseases of the oral membrane. *Antibacterial topical solutions* (eg, benzalkonium chloride and strong iodine) will kill bacteria when applied to the skin or mucous membrane.

Solutions intended for oral administration usually contain flavorants and colorants to make the medication more attractive and palatable to the patient. They may contain stabilizers to maintain the physicochemical stability of the drug and preservatives to prevent the growth of microorganisms in the solution. A drug dissolved in an aqueous solution is in the most bioavailable form. Since the drug is already in solution, no dissolution step is necessary before systemic absorption occurs. Solutions that are prepared to be sterile, pyrogen-free, and intended for parenteral administration are classified as *injectables.*

Some drugs, particularly certain antibiotics, have insufficient stability in aqueous solution to withstand long shelf lives. These drugs are formulated as dry powder or granule dosage forms for reconstitution with purified water immediately before dispensing to the patient. The dry powder mixture contains all of the formulation components, ie, drug, flavorant, colorant, buffers, and others, except for the solvent. Examples of dry powder mixtures intended for reconstitution to make oral solutions include cloxacillin sodium, nafcillin sodium, oxacillin sodium, and penicillin V potassium.

Sucrose is the sugar most frequently employed in syrups; in special circumstances it may be replaced in whole or in part by other sugars (eg, dextrose) or nonsugars (eg, sorbitol, glycerin, and propylene glycol). Most syrups consist of between 60 and 80% sucrose. Sucrose not only provides sweetness and viscosity to the solution; it renders the solution inherently stable (unlike dilute sucrose solutions, which are unstable).

Compared to syrups, elixirs are usually less sweet and less viscous, because they contain a lower proportion of sugar, and are consequently less effective than syrups in masking the taste of drugs. In contrast to aqueous syrups, elixirs are better able to maintain both water-soluble and alcohol-soluble components in solution due to their hydroalcoholic properties. These stable characteristics often make elixirs preferable to syrups. All elixirs contain flavoring and coloring agents to enhance their palatability and appearance. Elixirs containing over 10-12% alcohol are usually self-preserving and do not require the addition of antimicrobial agents for preservation. Alcohols precipitate tragacanth, acacia, agar, and inorganic salts from aqueous solutions; therefore such substances should either be absent from the aqueous phase or present in such low concentrations so as not to promote precipitation on standing. Examples of some commonly used elixirs include dexamethasone elixir USP, pentobarbital elixir USP, diphenhydramine HCl elixir, and digoxin elixir.

Tablets

Depending on the physicochemical properties of the drug, site and extent of drug absorption in the gastrointestinal (GI) tract, stability to heat or moisture, biocompatibility with other ingredients, solubility, and dose, the following types of tablets are commonly formulated:

- *Tablets that are swallowed whole*
- *Effervescent tablets* are dissolved in water prior to administration. In addition to the drug substance, these tablets contain sodium bicarbonate and an organic acid such as tartaric acid. These additives react in the presence of water, liberating carbon dioxide, which acts as a disintegrator and produces effervescence.
- *Chewable tablets* are used when a faster rate of dissolution and/or buccal absorption is desired. Chewable tablets consist of a mild effervescent drug complex dispersed throughout a gum base. The drug is released from the dosage form by physical disruption associated with chewing, chemical disruption caused by the interaction with the fluids in the oral cavity, and the presence of effervescent material. For example, antacid tablets should be chewed to obtain quick indigestion relief.
- *Buccal and sublingual tablets* dissolve slowly in the mouth, cheek pouch (buccal), or under the tongue (sublingual). Buccal or sublingual absorption is often desirable for drugs subject to extensive hepatic metabolism, often referred to as the *first-pass effect.* Examples are isoprenaline sulfate (bronchodilator), glyceryl trinitrate (vasodilator), nitroglycerin, and testosterone tablets. These tablets do not contain a disintegrant and are compressed lightly to produce a fairly soft tablet.

- *Controlled-release tablets* are used to improve patient compliance and to reduce side effects. Some water-soluble drugs are formulated as sustained-release tablets so that their release and dissolution is controlled over a long period. A hydrophobic matrix composed of carnauba wax and partially hydrogenated cottonseed oil were used to prepare sustained-release tablets of a highly water-soluble drug, ABT-089, a cholinergic channel modulator for the treatment of cognitive disorders. Theo-Dur® is a controlled-release tablet of theophylline and consists of two components: a matrix of compressed theophylline crystals and coated theophylline granules embedded in the matrix. In contact with fluid, theophylline diffuses slowly through the wall of the free granules, which dissolves with time. After oral administration of Theo-Dur 300-mg tablets to human subjects, serum theophylline concentrations over 1 mg/mL were maintained over 24 hours. To provide a zero-order release of ibuprofen, core-in-cup tablets were developed by compressing the mixture of ethyl cellulose and carnauba wax, followed by compression with core tablets containing ibuprofen. The combination of high- and low-viscosity grades of hydroxypropylmethylcellulose (HPMC) was used as the matrix base to prepare diclofenac sodium and zileuton sustained-release tablets. A ternary polymeric matrix system composed of protein, HPMC, and highly water-soluble drugs such as diltiazem HCl was developed by the direct compression method. Xanthan gum was used for a hydrophilic matrix for sustained-release ibuprofen tablets. Sustained-release tablets can also be prepared by formulating inert polymers like polyvinyl chloride, polyvinyl acetate, and methyl methacrylate. These polymers protect the tablet from disintegration and also reduce the dissolution rate of the drug inside the tablet. Examples of commonly used sustained-release drug delivery products are listed in Table 2.
- *Coated tablets* are used to prevent decomposition or to minimize the unpleasant taste of certain drugs. There are several types of coated tablets: film-coated, sugar-coated, gelatin-coated (gel caps), or enteric-coated tablets. Enteric coatings are resistant to gastric juices, but readily dissolve in the small intestine. These enteric coatings can protect drugs against decomposition in the acidic environment of the stomach. Commonly used polymers for enteric coating are acid-impermeable polymers, such as cellulose acetate trimellitate (CAT), hydroxypropyl methylcellulose phthalate (HPMCP), polyvinyl acetate phthalate (PVAP), cellulose acetate phthalate (CAP), and EUDRAGIT®. Aspirin has been shown to produce less gastric bleeding when formulated as enteric-coated sustained-release tablets than conventional aspirin preparations. Film-coated tablets are compressed tablets that are coated with a thin layer of a water-insoluble or water-soluble polymer, such as HPMCP, ethylcellulose, povidone, or polyethylene glycol. Abacavir is a capsule-shaped film-coated tablet containing a nucleoside reverse transcriptase inhibitor, which is a potent antiviral agent for the treatment of HIV infection.

Tablet formulation

In addition to the drug, the following materials are added to make the powder system compatible with tablet formulation by the compression or granulation methods:

- *Diluents.* A tablet should weigh at least 50 mg, and therefore, very low-dose drugs invariably require a diluent or bulking agent to bring overall tablet weight to at least 50 mg. Commonly used diluents are lactose, dicalcium phosphate, starches, microcrystalline cellulose (MCC), dextrose, sucrose, mannitol, and sodium chloride. Dicalcium phosphate absorbs less moisture than lactose and is therefore used with hygroscopic drugs such as pethidine hydrochloride.
- *Adsorbents* are substances capable of holding quantities of fluids in an apparently dry state. Oil-soluble drugs or fluid extracts can be mixed with adsorbents and then granulated and compressed into tablets. Examples are fumed silica, microcrystalline cellulose, magnesium carbonate, kaolin, and bentonite.
- *Moistening agents* are liquids that are used for wet granulation. Examples include water, industrial methylated spirits, and isopropanol.
- *Binding agents (adhesives)* bind powders together in the wet granulation process. They also help bind granules together during compression. Examples include starch, gelatin, polyvinylpyrrolidone (PVP), alginic acid derivatives, cellulose derivatives, glucose, and sucrose. Choice of binders affects the dissolution rate. For example, the tablet formulation of furosemide with PVP as the binder has a t_{50} (time required for 50% of the drug to be released during an in vitro dissolution study) of 3.65 minutes, but with starch mucilage as the binder, the t_{50} of the tablets was 117 minutes.
- *Glidants* are added to tablet formulations to improve the flow properties of the granulations. They act by reducing interparticulate friction. Commonly used glidants are fumed (colloidal) silica, starch, and talc.
- *Lubricants* have a number of functions in tablet manufacture. They prevent adherence of the tablet material to the surfaces of the punch faces and dies, reduce inter-particle friction, and facilitate the smooth ejection of the tablet from the die cavity. Many lubricants also enhance the flow properties of the granules. Commonly used lubricants are magnesium stearate, talc, stearic acid and its derivatives, PEG, paraffin, and sodium or magnesium lauryl

Table 2

Examples of Sustained-Release Drug Delivery Products

Dosage forms	Manufacturer	Active ingredients	Indications
Controlled-release tablets			
Theo-Dur	ALZA Corp.	Theophylline	Asthma
Abacavir (Ziagen®)	GlaxoWellcome Inc	Nucleoside reverse transcriptase inhibitor	HIV-1 infection
Sinemet®	Bristol Myers Squibb	Carbidopa + levodopa	Parkinson's disease
Volmax®	ALZA Corp.	Albuterol	Bronchospasm
Voltaren®	Novartis	Diclofenac sodium	Osteoarthritis and rheumatoid arthritis
Efidac 24®	ALZA Corp.	Chlorpheniramine	Allergy symptom and nasal congestion
DynaCirc® CR	ALZA Corp.	Isradipine	Hypertension
Capsules			
Dexedrine Spansules®	GlaxoSmithKline	Dextroamphetamine	Narcolepsy
Adderal XL®	Shire Pharmaceuticals	Amphetamine + dextroamphetamine	Attention-deficit/hyperactivity disorder (ADHD)
Ritalin LA®	Novartis	Methylphenidate hydrochloride	ADHD
Videx® EC	Bristol Myers Squibb	Didanosine ddL	HIV-1 infection
Aerosols			
Ventolin HFA®	GlaxoSmithKline	Albuterol sulfate	Bronchodilator
Azmacort®	Kos	Triamcinolone acetonide	Asthma
Serevent®	GlaxoSmithKline	Salmeterol	Bronchodilator
Osmotic system			
Oros® System	ALZA Corp.	Oral delivery of different drugs	
Ditropan XL®	ALZA Corp.	Oxybutynin chloride	Overreacting bladder
Covera-HS®	ALZA Corp.	Verapamil	Antihypertensive
Concerta®	ALZA Corp.	Methylphenidate HCl	Attention deficit hyperactivity disorder (ADHD)
DUROS® implant systems			
Viadur®	ALZA Corp.	Leuprolide	Prostate cancer
Inserts			
Pilocarpine Ocusert®	ALZA Corp.	Pilocarpine	Glaucoma
Lacrisert®	ALZA Corp.	Hydroxypropyl cellulose	Ophthalmic moisturizer
Progestasert®	CollaGenex	Progesterone	Contraceptive
Atridox®	ALZA Corp.	Doxycycline	Periodontal disease
Transdermal patches			
Alora®	Watson Pharma	Estradiol	Menopausal symptoms
CombiPatch™	Novartis	Estradiol/norethindrone acetate	Vasomotor symptoms associated with menopause
Androderm®	Watson Pharmaceuticals, Inc.	Testosterone	Testosterone deficiency
Nicotine transdermal system	Watson Pharmaceuticals, Inc.	Nicotine	Smoking cessation
PEGylated proteins			
PEG-Intron®	Schering Corp.	PEGylated interferon	Hepatitis C
Pegasys®	Roche	PEGylated interferon + ribavirin	Hepatitis B, hepatitis C
Liposomes			
Doxil®	Ortho Biotech	Doxorubicin HCl	Kaposi's sarcoma
DaunoXome®	NeXstar Pharmaceuticals	Daunorubicin	Kaposi's sarcoma
PLGA/PLA microspheres			
Lupron Depot®	TAP Pharmaceuticals	Luteinizing hormone-releasing hormone agonist	Prostate cancer, endometriosis
Zoladex Depot®	AstraZeneca	Goserelin acetate	Prostate cancer, endometriosis
Nutropin Depot®	Genentech	Recombinant human growth hormone	Growth deficiencies

sulfate. Among these, magnesium stearate is the most popular lubricant, as it is effective as both a die and punch lubricant. However, for many drugs, magnesium stearate is chemically incompatible (eg, aspirin) and therefore talc or stearic acid is often used. Most lubricants, with the exception of talc, are used in concentrations below 1%.

- **Disintegrating agents** are added to the tablets to promote break-up or disintegration after administration. This increases the effective surface area and promotes rapid release of the drug. Disintegrants act by either bursting open the tablet and/or by promoting the rapid ingress of water into the center of the tablet or capsule. Examples include starch, cationic exchange resins, cross-linked polyvinylpyrrolidone, celluloses, modified starches, alginic acid and alginates, magnesium aluminum silicate, and cross-linked sodium carboxymethylcellulose. Among them, starch is the most popular disintegrant, as it has a great affinity for water and swells when moistened, thus facilitating the rupture of the tablet matrix.

Disintegration, dissolution, and absorption

A solid drug product has to disintegrate into small particles and release the drug before absorption can take place. However, tablets that are intended for chewing or sustained release do not have to undergo disintegration. The various excipients for tablet formulation affect the rates of disintegration, dissolution, and absorption. Systemic absorption of most products consists of a succession of rate processes, such as:

- disintegration of the drug product and subsequent release of drug,
- dissolution of the drug in an aqueous environment, and
- absorption across cell membranes into the systemic circulation.

Rate-limiting step for absorption

In the process of tablet disintegration, dissolution, and absorption, the rate at which drug reaches the circulatory system is determined by the slowest step in the sequence. Disintegration of a tablet is usually more rapid than drug dissolution and absorption. For the drug that has poor aqueous solubility, the rate at which the drug dissolves (dissolution) is often the slowest step, and therefore exerts a rate-limiting effect on drug bioavailability. In contrast, for the drug that has a high aqueous solubility, the dissolution rate is rapid and the rate at which the drug crosses or permeates cell membranes is the slowest or rate-limiting step.

Capsules

Capsules are solid dosage forms in which the drug substance is enclosed in either a hard or soft, water-soluble container or shell of gelatin. **Coating** of capsule shell or drug particles within the capsule can affect bioavailability. There are two types of capsules: hard and soft capsules; however, hard gelatin capsules are more versatile for controlled drug delivery.

Hard gelatin capsules

A hard gelatin capsule consists of two pieces, a cap and a body, that fit one inside the other. They are produced empty and are then filled in a separate operation. Hard gelatin capsules are usually filled with powders, granules, or pellets containing the drug. After ingestion, the gelatin shell softens, swells, and begins to dissolve in the gastrointestinal tract. Encapsulated drugs are released rapidly and dispersed easily, leading to high bioavailability. Capsules are supplied in a variety of sizes, and high-speed filling machinery capable of filling ~1500 capsules per minute is available. The hard gelatin empty capsules are numbered from 000, the largest size, to 5, which is the smallest. The approximate filling capacity of capsules ranges from 6000 to 30 mg, depending on the types and bulk densities of powdered drug materials.

Formulation of hard gelatin capsules

Powder formulations for encapsulation into hard gelatin capsules require careful consideration of the filling process, such as lubricity, compactibility, and fluidity. Additives present in the capsule formulations, such as the amount and choice of fillers and lubricants, inclusion of disintegrants and surfactants, and the degree of plug compaction, can influence drug release from the capsule. Formulation factors influencing drug release and bioavailability are as follows:

- **Fillers (or diluents).** Active ingredient is mixed with a sufficient volume of a diluent, usually lactose, mannitol, starch, and dicalcium phosphate, to yield the desired amount of the drug in the capsule when the base is filled with the powder mixture.
- **Glidants.** The flow properties of the powder blend should be adequate to assure a uniform flow rate from the hopper. Glidants such as silica, starch, talc, and magnesium stearate are used to improve the fluidity. The optimal concentration of the glidant used to improve the flow of a powder mixture is generally less than 1%.
- **Lubricants** ease the ejection of plugs by reducing adhesion of powder to metal surfaces and friction between sliding surfaces in contact with the powder. Typical lubricants for capsule formulations include magnesium stearate and stearic acid.

- *Surfactants* may be included in capsule formulations to increase wetting of the powder mass and enhance drug dissolution. The most commonly used surfactants in capsule formulations are 0.1-0.5% of sodium lauryl sulfate and sodium docusate.
- *Hydrophilization.* Another approach for improving the wettability of poorly soluble drugs is to treat the drug with a hydrophilic polymer solution. Powder wettability and dissolution rate of several drugs, including hexobarbital and phenytoin, from hard gelatin capsules have been shown to be enhanced if the drug is treated with methylcellulose or hydroxyethylcellulose.

Vancomycin HCl is a highly hygroscopic antibiotic. To achieve acceptable stability, Eli Lilly has developed a hard gelatin capsule filled with a PEG 6000 matrix of vancomycin HCl, which produces plasma and urine levels of the antibiotic similar to those obtained with the solution of vancomycin HCl. Controlled-release beads and minitablets are often filled into gelatin capsules for convenient administration of an oral controlled-release dosage form. For example, sustained-release antihistamines, antitussives, and analgesics are first preformulated into extended-release microcapsules or microspheres and then placed inside a gelatin capsule. Another example is enteric-coated lipase minitablets that are placed in a gelatin capsule for more effective protection and dosing of these enzymes.

Soft gelatin capsules

Soft gelatin capsules are prepared from plasticized gelatin by a rotary die process. Soft gelatin capsules are formed, filled, and sealed in a single operation. Soft gelatin capsules may contain a nonaqueous solution, a powder, or a drug suspension, none of which solubilize the gelatin shell. In contrast to hard gelatin capsules, soft gelatin capsules contain ~30% glycerol as a plasticizer in addition to gelatin and water. The moisture uptake of soft gelatin capsules plasticized with glycerol is considerably higher than that of hard gelatin capsules. Therefore oxygen-sensitive drugs should not be inserted into soft gelatin capsules, nor should emulsions, since they are unstable and crack the shell of the capsule when the water is lost in the manufacturing process. Extreme acidic and basic pH must also be avoided, since a pH below 2.5 hydrolyzes gelatin, while a pH above 9 has a tanning effect on the gelatin. Insoluble drugs should be dispersed with an agent such as beeswax, paraffin, or ethylcellulose. Surfactants are also often added to promote wetting of the ingredients. Drugs that are commercially prepared in soft capsules include declomycin, chlortrianisene, digoxin, vitamin A, vitamin E, and chloral hydrate.

Formulation of soft gelatin capsules

Formulation of soft gelatin capsules involves liquid, rather than powder, technology. It requires careful consideration of the composition of the gelatin shell and filling materials. The composition of the soft capsule shell consists of two main ingredients: gelatin and a plasticizer. Water is used to form the capsule and other additives are often added as described below:

- *Gelatin.* Properties of gelatin shells are controlled by choice of gelatin grade and by adjusting the concentration of plasticizer in the shell.
- *Plasticizers.* The main plasticizer used for soft gelatin capsules is glycerol. Sorbitol and polypropylene glycol are also used in combination with glycerol. Compared to hard gelatin capsules and tablet film coatings, a relatively large amount (~30%) of plasticizers are added in soft gelatin capsule formulation to ensure adequate flexibility.
- *Water.* The desirable water content of the gelatin solution used to produce a soft gelatin capsule shell depends on the viscosity of gelatin used and ranges between 0.7 and 1.3 parts of water to each part of dry gelatin.
- *Other additives.* Preservatives are added to prevent mold growth in the gelatin shell. Potassium sorbate, and methyl, ethyl, and propyl hydroxybenzoate are commonly used as preservatives.

Emulsions

An *emulsion* is a thermodynamically unstable system consisting of at least two immiscible liquid phases, one of which is dispersed as globules (dispersed phase) in the other, a liquid phase (continuous phase), stabilized by the presence of an emulsifying agent. Emulsified systems range from lotions of relatively low viscosity, to ointments and creams, which are semisolid in nature.

Types of emulsions

One liquid phase in an emulsion is essentially polar (eg, aqueous), while the other is relatively nonpolar (eg, an oil).

- *Oil-in-water (o/w) emulsion:* When the oil phase is dispersed as globules throughout an aqueous continuous phase, the system is referred to as an oil-in-water (o/w) emulsion.
- *Water-in-oil (w/o) emulsion:* When the oil phase serves as the continuous phase, the emulsion is termed a water-in-oil (w/o) emulsion.
- *Multiple (w/o/w or o/w/o) emulsions:* These are emulsions whose dispersed phase contains droplets of another phase. Multiple emulsions are of interest as delayed-action drug delivery systems.
- *Microemulsions:* These consist of homogeneous transparent systems of low viscosity which contain

a high percentage of both oil and water and high concentrations of emulsifier mixture.

Microemulsions form spontaneously when the components are mixed in the appropriate ratios and are thermodynamically stable.

Externally applied emulsions may be o/w or w/o. The o/w emulsions employ the following emulsifiers: sodium lauryl sulfate, triethanolamine stearate, sodium oleate, and glyceryl monostearate. The w/o emulsions are used mainly for external applications and may contain one or several of the following emulsifiers: calcium palmitate, sorbitan esters (spans), cholesterol, and wool fats.

Interfacial free energy and emulsification

Two immiscible liquids in emulsions often fail to remain mixed due to the greater cohesive force between the molecules of each separate liquid, rather than the adhesive force between the two liquids. This leads to phase separation, which is the state of minimum surface-free energy. When one liquid is broken into small particles, the interfacial area of the globules constitutes a surface that is enormous compared with the surface area of the original liquid. The adsorption of a surfactant or other emulsifying agent at the globule interface lowers the oil-to-water or water-to-oil interfacial tension. In addition, the process of emulsification is made easier and the drug's stability may be enhanced.

Emulsifying agents

To prevent coalescence, it is necessary to introduce an emulsifying agent that forms a film around the dispersed globules. Emulsifying agents may be divided into three groups:

- **Surface-active agents.** Surfactants are adsorbed at oil-water interfaces to form **monomolecular films** and reduce interfacial tensions. Unless the interfacial tension is zero, there is a natural tendency for the oil droplets to coalesce to reduce the area of oil-water contact, but the presence of the surfactant monolayer at the surface of the droplet reduces the possibility of collisions leading to coalescence. To retain a high surface area for the dispersed phase, surface-active agents must be used to decrease the surface-free energy. Often a mixture of surfactants is used: one with hydrophilic character and the other with hydrophobic character. A hydrophilic emulsifying agent is needed for the aqueous phase, and a hydrophobic emulsifying agent is needed for the oil phase. A complex film results, which produces an excellent emulsion. Nonionic surfactants are widely used in the production of stable emulsions. They are less toxic than ionic surfactants and are less sensitive to electrolytes and pH variation. Examples include sorbitan esters, polysorbates, and others.
- **Hydrophilic colloids.** A number of hydrophilic colloids are used as emulsifying agents. These include gelatin, casein, acacia, cellulose derivatives, and alginates. These materials adsorb at the oil-water interface and form multilayer films around the dispersed droplets of oil in an o/w emulsion. Hydrated lyophilic colloids differ from surfactants since they do not cause an appreciable lowering in interfacial tension. Their action is due to the fact that multimolecular films are strong and resist coalescence. Additionally, they increase the viscosity of the dispersion medium. Hydrophilic colloids are used for formation of o/w emulsions since the films are hydrophilic. Most cellulose derivatives are not charged but can sterically stabilize the systems.
- **Finely divided solid particles** are adsorbed at the interface between two immiscible liquid phases and form a film of particles around the dispersed globules. Finely divided solid particles that are wetted to some degree by both oil and water can act as emulsifying agents. They are concentrated at the interface where they produce a film of particles around the dispersed droplets so as to prevent coalescence. Finely divided solid particles that are wetted by water form o/w emulsions; those that are wetted by oil form w/o emulsions. Examples include bentonite, magnesium hydroxide, and aluminum hydroxide.

Types of instability in emulsions

The stability of an emulsion is characterized by the absence of coalescence of the internal phase, the absence of creaming, and maintenance of elegance with respect to appearance, odor, color, and other physical properties. An emulsion becomes unstable due to creaming, breaking, coalescence, phase inversion, and some other factors.

1. **Creaming and sedimentation.** Creaming is the upward movement of dispersed droplets relative to the continuous phase, while sedimentation, the reverse process, is the downward movement of particles. These processes take place due to the density differences in the two phases and can be reversed by shaking. However, creaming is undesirable, because a creamed emulsion increases the likelihood of coalescence due to the close proximity of the globules in the cream. Factors that influence the rate of creaming are similar to those involved in the sedimentation rate of suspension particles, and are indicated by Stokes Law as follows:

$$v = \frac{d^2(\rho_s - \rho_0)g}{18\eta_o}$$

where v is the velocity of creaming, d is the globule diameter, ρ_s and ρ_0 are the densities of dispersed phase and dispersion medium, respectively, η_o is the viscosity of the dispersion medium (poise), and g is the acceleration of gravity

(981 cm/sec^2). According to this equation, the rate of creaming is decreased by:
- a reduction in the globule size,
- a decrease in the density difference between the two phases, and
- an increase in the viscosity of the continuous phase.

This may be achieved by homogenizing the emulsion to reduce the globule size and increasing the viscosity of the continuous phase by the use of thickening agents such as tragacanth or methylcellulose.

2. *Creaming, breaking, coalescence, and aggregation.* Creaming is a reversible process, whereas breaking is irreversible. When breaking occurs, simple mixing fails to resuspend the globules in a stable emulsified form, since the film surrounding the particles has been destroyed and the oil tends to coalesce. Coalescence is the process by which emulsified particles merge with each other to form large particles. The major factor preventing coalescence is the mechanical strength of the interfacial barrier. Formation of a thick interfacial film is essential for minimal coalescence. In aggregation, the dispersed droplets come together but do not fuse. Aggregation is to some extent reversible.

3. *Phase inversion.* An emulsion is said to invert when it changes from an o/w to a w/o emulsion or vice versa. Inversion can occur by the addition of an electrolyte or by changing the phase:volume ratio. For example, an o/w emulsion stabilized with sodium stearate can be inverted to a w/o emulsion by adding calcium chloride to form calcium stearate.

4. *Preservation of emulsions.* Growth of microorganisms in an emulsion can cause physical separation of the phases. Bacteria can degrade nonionic and anionic emulsifying agents and therefore preservatives must be added in adequate concentrations to the product.

Suspensions

Suspensions are dispersions of finely divided solid particles of a drug in a liquid medium in which the drug is not readily soluble. *Suspending agents* are often hydrophilic colloids (eg, cellulose derivatives, acacia, or xanthan gum) added to suspensions to increase viscosity, inhibit agglomeration, and decrease sedimentation. Highly viscous suspensions may prolong gastric emptying time, slow drug dissolution, and decrease the absorption rate. A suspension that is *thixotropic* as well as *pseudoplastic* should prove to be useful since it forms a gel on standing and becomes fluid when disturbed.

Desired characteristics of suspensions
- Suspended material should settle slowly and should readily disperse upon gentle shaking of the container.
- Particle size of the suspension should remain fairly constant.
- The suspension should pour readily and evenly from its container.

Flocculation
The large surface area of the particles is associated with a surface-free energy that makes the system thermodynamically unstable. This makes particles highly energetic and tend to regroup, resulting in the decrease in total surface area and surface-free energy. The particles in a liquid suspension, therefore, tend to *flocculate. Flocculation* is the formation of light, fluffy conglomerates held together by weak van der Waals forces. *Aggregation* occurs when crystals come together to form a compact cake (growth and fusing together of crystals in the precipitate to form a solid aggregate). *Flocculating agents* can prevent caking, whereas *deflocculating agents* increase the tendency to cake. Surfactants can reduce interfacial tension, but it cannot be made equal to zero, so suspensions of insoluble particles tend to have a positive finite interfacial tension, and particles tend to flocculate.

Forces at the surface of a particle affect the degree of flocculation and agglomeration in a suspension. *Forces of attraction* are of the London van der Waals type, whereas the *repulsive forces* arise from the interaction of the electric double layers surrounding each particle. When the repulsion energy is high, collision of the particles is opposed; the system remains deflocculated, and when sedimentation is complete, the particles form a close-packed arrangement with the smaller particles filling the voids between the larger ones. Those particles lowest in the sediment are gradually pressed together by the weight of the ones above; the energy barrier is thus overcome, allowing the particles to come into close contact with each other. To resuspend and redisperse these particles, it is necessary to overcome the high-energy barrier. Since this is not easily achieved by agitation, the particles tend to remain strongly attracted to each other and form a hard cake. When the particles are flocculated, the energy barrier is still too large to be surmounted, and so the approaching particles in the second energy minimum, which is at a distance of separation of perhaps 1000 to 2000 Å, is sufficient to form the loosely structural flocs.

Sedimentation of flocculated particles
"Flocs" tend to fall together, producing a distinct boundary between the sediment and the supernatant liquid. The liquid above the sediment is clear because

even the small particles present in the system are associated with flocs. In contrast to this are deflocculated systems with variable particle sizes; the large particles here settle more rapidly than the smaller particles, and no clear boundary is formed. The supernatant remains turbid for a longer period of time.

Flocculation or deflocculation?

Whether a suspension is flocculated or deflocculated depends on the relative magnitudes of the electrostatic forces of repulsion and the forces of attraction between the particles. Flocculated systems form loose sediments that are easily redispersible, but the sedimentation rate is usually fast. In contrast, a suspension is deflocculated when the dispersed particles remain as discrete units and will settle slowly. This prevents the entrapment of liquid within the sediment that leads to caking, which is a serious stability problem encountered in suspension formulation.

Flocculating agents

If the charge on the particle is neutralized, flocculation will occur. If a high charge density is imparted to the suspension particles, then deflocculation will be the result. To convert the suspension from a deflocculated to a flocculated state, the following flocculating agents are often used:

- *Electrolytes.* The addition of an inorganic electrolyte to an aqueous suspension will alter the zeta potential of the dispersed particles, and if this value is lowered sufficiently, then flocculation may occur. The most widely used electrolytes include sodium salts of acetates, phosphates, and citrates.
- *Surfactants.* Ionic surfactants may also cause flocculation by neutralization of the charge on each particle.
- *Polymeric flocculating agents.* Starch, alginates, cellulose derivatives, tragacanth, carbomers, and silicates are examples of polymeric flocculating agents that can be used to control the degree of flocculation. Their linear branched-chain molecules form a gel-like network within the system and become adsorbed on the surfaces of the dispersed particles, thus holding them in a flocculated state.

Formulation of suspensions

There are two ways of formulating physically stable suspensions:

- One is to use a structured vehicle to maintain deflocculated particles in suspension. However, the major disadvantage of deflocculated systems is that when the particles eventually settle, they form a compact cake.
- The other is by production of flocs, which may settle rapidly, but are easily resuspended with a minimum

of agitation. Optimum physical stability is obtained when the suspension is formulated with flocculated particles in a structured vehicle of hydrophilic colloid type.

Ointments, Creams, and Gels

Ointments, creams, and gels are semisolid preparations intended for topical applications. These semisolid formulations are designed for local or systemic drug absorption. Ointments are typically used as:

- *Emollients* to make the skin more pliable
- *Protective barriers* to prevent harmful substances from coming in contact with the skin
- *Vehicles* in which to incorporate medication

Ointment bases are classified into four general groups: (1) hydrocarbon bases, (2) absorption bases, (3) water-removable bases, and (4) water-soluble bases.

1. *Hydrocarbon (oleaginous) bases* are anhydrous and insoluble in water. They cannot absorb or contain water and are not washable in water.
    - *Petrolatum* is a good base for oil-insoluble ingredients. It forms an occlusive film on the skin and absorbs less than 5% water under normal conditions. Wax can be incorporated to stiffen the base.
    - *Synthetic esters* are used as constituents of oleaginous bases. These esters include glycerol monostearate, isopropyl myristate, isopropyl palmitate, butyl stearate, and butyl palmitate.

2. *Absorption bases* are of two types: (1) those that permit the incorporation of aqueous solutions, resulting in the formation of water-in-oil (w/o) emulsions (eg, hydrophilic petrolatum and anhydrous lanolin), and (2) those that are already w/o emulsions (emulsion bases) and thus permit the incorporation of small additional quantities of aqueous solutions (eg, lanolin and cold cream). These bases are useful as emollients although they do not provide the degree of occlusion afforded by the oleaginous bases. Absorption bases are also not easily removed from the skin with water. An aqueous solution may be first incorporated into the absorption base, and then this mixture added to the oleaginous base.

3. *Emulsion bases,* water-washable or water-removable bases commonly referred to as creams, represent the most commonly used type of ointment base. The majority of dermatologic drug products are formulated in an emulsion or cream base. Emulsion bases are washable and removed easily from skin or clothing. An emulsion base can be subdivided into three component parts, designated the oil phase, the emulsifier, and the aqueous phase. Drugs can be included in one of these phases or added to the formed emulsion. The oil

phase, also known as the internal phase, is typically made up of petrolatum and/or liquid petrolatum together with cetyl or stearyl alcohol. Types of emulsion bases include:

- *Hydrophilic ointment* is an o/w emulsion that uses sodium lauryl sulfate as an emulsifying agent. It is readily miscible with water and is removed from the skin easily. The aqueous phase of an emulsion base contains the preservative(s) that are included to control microbial growth. The preservatives in the emulsion include methylparaben, propylparaben, benzyl alcohol, sorbic acid, or quaternary ammonium compounds. The aqueous phase also contains the water-soluble components of the emulsion system, together with any additional stabilizers, antioxidants, and buffers that may be necessary for stability and pH control.
- *Cold cream* is a semisolid white w/o emulsion prepared with cetyl ester wax, white wax, mineral oil, sodium borate, and purified water. Sodium borate combines with free fatty acids present in the waxes to form sodium soaps that act as the emulsifiers. Cold cream is employed as an emollient and ointment base. Eucerin® cream is a w/o emulsion of petrolatum, mineral oil, mineral wax, wool wax, alcohol, and bronopol. It is frequently prescribed as a vehicle for delivery of lactic acid and glycerin to treat dry skin.
- *Lanolin* is a w/o emulsion that contains approximately 25% water and acts as an emollient and occlusive film on the skin, effectively preventing epidermal water loss.
- *Vanishing cream* is an o/w emulsion that contains a large percentage of water as well as a humectant (eg, glycerin or propylene glycol) that retards surface evaporation. An excess of stearic acid in the formula helps to form a thin film when the water evaporates.

4. *Water-soluble bases* may be anhydrous or may contain some water. They are washable in water and absorb water to the point of solubility. Polyethylene glycol (PEG) ointment is a blend of water-soluble PEG that forms a semisolid base. This base can solubilize water-soluble drugs and some water-insoluble drugs. It is compatible with a wide variety of drugs. This base contains 40% PEG 4000 and 60% PEG 400. Another water-soluble base is the ointment prepared with propylene glycol and ethanol, which form a clear gel when mixed with 2% hydroxypropyl cellulose. This base is a commonly used dermatologic vehicle.

Incorporation of drugs into an ointment

Drugs may be incorporated into an ointment base by levigation and fusion. Normally, drug substances are in fine powered forms before being dispersed in the vehicle. Levigation of powders into a small portion of base is facilitated by the use of a melted base or a small quantity of compatible levigation aid, such as mineral oil or glycerin. Water-soluble salts are incorporated by dissolving them in a small volume of water and incorporating the aqueous solution into a compatible base. Fusion is used when the base contains solids that have higher melting points (eg, waxes, cetyl alcohol, or glyceryl monostearate).

Suppositories

A *suppository* is a solid dosage form intended for insertion into body orifices (eg, rectum, vagina, or urethra). Once inserted, the suppository base either melts, softens, or dissolves at body temperature, distributing its medications to the tissues of the region. Suppositories are used for local or systemic effects. Rectal suppositories intended for local action are often used to relieve the pain, irritation, itching, and inflammation associated with hemorrhoids. Vaginal suppositories intended for local effects are employed mainly as contraceptives, antiseptics in feminine hygiene, and to combat invading pathogens. The suppository base has a marked influence on the release of active constituents. There are two main classes of suppository bases in use: the glyceride-type fatty bases and the water-soluble ones. The main members of water-soluble/water-miscible suppository bases are glycerinated gelatin and polyethylene glycols. Polyethylene glycol suppositories do not melt at body temperature but rather dissolve slowly in the body's fluids. Examples of rectal suppositories include Thorazine® (chlorpromazine) and Phenergan® (promethazine).

Inserts, Implants, and Devices

Inserts, implants, and *devices* are used to control drug delivery for localized or systemic drug effects. In these systems, drugs are embedded into biodegradable or nonbiodegradable materials to allow slow release of the drug. The inserts, implants, and devices are inserted into a variety of cavities (eg, vagina, buccal cavity, cul de sac of the eye, or subcutaneous tissue).

Degradable inserts consist of polyvinyl alcohol, hydroxypropylcellulose, polyvinylpyrrolidone, and hyaluronic acid. Nondegradable inserts are prepared from insoluble materials such as ethylene vinyl acetate copolymers and styrene-isoprene-styrene block copolymers. The initial use of contact lenses was for vision correction; however, they are becoming more useful as potential drug delivery devices by presoaking them in drug solutions. The use of contact lenses can simultaneously correct vision and release drug.

A number of degradable and nondegradable inserts are currently available for ophthalmic delivery. These ophthalmic inserts can be insoluble, soluble, or bioerodible. Insoluble inserts are further classified as diffusional, osmotic, and contact lens (Figure 4). Ocular inserts are no more affected by nasolacrimal drainage and tear flow than conventional dosage forms, and instead can provide slow drug release and longer residence times in the conjunctival cul-de-sac. Ocusert is an interesting device consisting of a drug reservoir (pilocarpine HCl in an alginate gel) enclosed by two release-controlling membranes made of ethylene-vinyl acetate copolymer and enclosed by a white ring, allowing positioning of the system in the eye. Pilocarpine Ocusert has demonstrated slow release of pilocarpine, which can effectively control the increased intraocular pressure in glaucoma. Other inserts (eg, medicated contact lenses, collagen shields, and minidiscs) have been shown to diminish the systemic absorption of ocularly applied drugs as a result of decreased drainage into the nasal cavity. Lacrisert is a soluble insert composed of hydroxypropylcellulose (HPC) and is useful in the treatment of dry eye syndrome. The device is placed in the lower fornix where it slowly dissolves over 6-8 hours to stabilize and thicken the tear film.

In addition to ophthalmic delivery, inserts are also used for localized delivery of drugs to various other tissues. For example, the Progestasert device is designed for implantation into the uterine cavity, where it releases 65 mg progesterone per day to provide contraception for 1 year. Similarly, Transderm® relies on the rate-limiting polymeric membranes to control drug release. Atridox is a FDA-approved product designed for controlled-release delivery of the antibiotic doxycycline for the treatment of periodontal disease. When injected into the periodontal cavity, the formulation sets, forming a drug delivery depot that delivers the antibiotic to the cavity. An implant is a drug delivery system designed to deliver a drug moiety at a desired rate over a prolonged period. Implants are available in many forms, including polymeric implants and minipumps. Diffusional and osmotic symptoms contain a reservoir that is in contact with the inner surface of a controller to which it supplies the drug. The reservoir contains a liquid, a gel, a colloid, a semisolid, a solid matrix, or a carrier containing drug. Carriers consist of hydrophilic or hydrophobic polymers.

ALZA Corporation developed ALZET® mini-osmotic pumps, which permit easy manipulation of drug release rate over a range of periods (from 1 day to 4 weeks). ALZA Corporation also developed DUROS implants for continuous therapy for up to 1 year. The nondegradable, osmotically driven system is intended to enable delivery of small drugs, peptides, proteins, and DNA for systemic or tissue-specific therapy. Viadur is a once-yearly implant for the palliative treatment of advanced prostate cancer.

One of the more commonly used devices is the oral osmotic pump, composed of a core tablet and a semipermeable coating with a 0.3- to 4-mm-diameter hole produced by a laser beam for drug exit. This system requires only osmotic pressure to be effective, but the drug release rate is dependent on the surface area, nature of the membrane, and the diameter of the hole. When the dosage form comes in contact with water, water is imbibed because of the resultant osmotic pressure of the core, and the drug is released from the orifice at a controlled rate.

Transdermal Drug Delivery Systems

Transdermal drug delivery systems (often called **transdermal patches**) deliver drugs directly through the skin and into the bloodstream. Percutaneous absorption of a drug generally results from direct penetration of the drug through the stratum corneum. Once through the stratum corneum, drug molecules may pass through the deeper epidermal tissues and into the dermis. When the drug reaches the vascularized dermal area, it becomes available for absorption into the general circulation. Among the factors influencing percutaneous absorption are the physicochemical properties of the drug, including its molecular weight, solubility, partition coefficient, nature of vehicle, and the condition of the skin. Chemical permeation enhancers and/or iontophoresis are often used to enhance the percutaneous absorption of a drug.

Figure 4.

Different types of ophthalmic inserts.

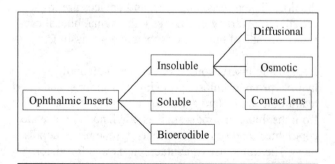

In general, patches are composed of three key compartments: a protective seal that forms the external surface and protects it from damage, a compartment that holds the medication itself and has an adhesive backing to hold the entire patch on the skin surface, and a release liner that protects the adhesive layer during storage and is removed just prior to application. Examples of transdermal patches include Estraderm® (estradiol), Nicoderm® (nicotine), Testoderm® (testosterone), Alora (estradiol), and Androderm (testosterone) .

Aerosol Products

Aerosols are pressurized dosage forms designed to deliver drugs with the aid of a liquefied or propelled gas (propellant). Aerosol products consist of a pressurizable container, a valve that allows the pressurized product to be expelled from the container when the actuator is pressed, and a dip tube that conveys the formulation from the bottom of the container to the valve assembly. Inhalation devices broadly fall into three categories: pressurized metered-dose inhalers (MDIs), nebulizers, and dry-powder inhalers (DPIs). The most commonly used inhalers on the market are MDIs. They contain active ingredient as a solution or as a suspension of fine particles in a liquefied propellant held under high pressure. MDIs use special metering valves to regulate the amount of formulation that is dispensed with each dose. Nebulizers do not require propellants and can generate large quantities of small droplets capable of penetrating into the lung. Sustained release of drugs, such as bronchodilators and corticosteroids for the treatment of asthma and chronic obstructive pulmonary diseases, involves encapsulation of the drugs in slowly degrading particles that can be inhaled. For accumulation in the alveolar zone of the lungs, which has a very large surface area, inhaled liquid or dry-powder aerosols should have particle sizes in the range of 1-5 micrometers. Inhaled drugs play a very prominent role in the treatment of asthma, because this route has significant advantages over oral or parenteral administration. Azmacort (triamcinolone acetamide), Ventolin HFA (albuterol sulfate), and Serevent (salmeterol) are examples of commercially available aerosols for the treatment of asthma.

6. Targeted Drug Delivery Systems

Targeted drug delivery systems are drug carrier systems that deliver the drug to the target or receptor site in a manner that provides maximum therapeutic activity, prevents degradation or inactivation during transit to the target sites, and protects the body from adverse reactions because of inappropriate disposition. Design of an effective delivery system requires a thorough understanding of the drug, the disease, and the target site (Figure 5). Examples include macromolecular drug carriers (protein drug carriers), particulate drug delivery systems (eg, microspheres, nanospheres, and liposomes), monoclonal antibodies, and cells. Plasma clearance kinetics, tissue distribution, metabolism, and cellular interactions of a drug can be controlled by the use of a site-specific delivery system. Targeting of drugs to specific sites in the body can be achieved by linking particulate systems or macromolecular carriers to monoclonal antibodies or to cell-specific ligands (eg, asialofetuin, glycoproteins, or immunoglobulins), or by alterations in the surface characteristics so that they are not recognized by the reticuloendothelial systems (RES).

Macromolecular Carrier Systems

Both natural and synthetic water-soluble polymers have been used as macromolecular drug carriers. The drug can be attached to the polymer chain either directly or via a spacer. Attachment of polyethylene glycol (PEG) to proteins can protect them from rapid hydrolysis or degradation within the body, and increase blood circulation time and lower the immunogenicity of proteins. PEGylated forms of interferons, PEG-Intron and PEGASYS (for treatment of hepatitis C, to reduce dosing frequency from daily injections to once-

Figure 5.

Essential components of drug delivery.

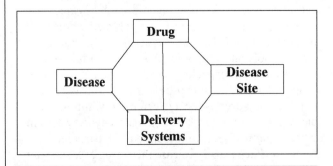

a-week injection dosing), adenosine deaminase, and L-asparaginase are currently on the market. PEGylation improves macromole solubility and stability by minimizing the uptake by the cells of the reticuloendothelial system (RES). Since PEG drug conjugates are not well absorbed from the gut, they are mainly used as injectables. The drug-polymer conjugate may also contain a receptor-specific ligand to achieve selective access to, and interaction with, the target cells.

Particulate Drug Delivery Systems

Liposomes

Liposomes are microscopic phospholipid vesicles composed of uni- or multilamellar lipid bilayers surrounding compartments. Multilamellar vesicles (MLVs) have diameters in the range of 1-5 micrometers. Sonication of MLVs results in the production of small unilamellar vesicles (SUVs) with diameters in the range of 0.02-0.08 micrometers. Large unilamellar vesicles (LUVs) can also be made by evaporation under reduced pressure, resulting in liposomes with a diameter of 0.1-1 micrometers. The bilayer-forming lipid is the essential part of the lamellar structure, while the other compounds are added to impart certain characteristics to the vesicles. Water-soluble drugs can be entrapped in liposomes by intercalation in the aqueous bilayers, while lipid-soluble drugs can be entrapped within the hydrocarbon interiors of the lipid bilayers. Liposomes can encapsulate low-molecular-weight drugs, proteins, peptides, oligonucleotides, and genes. The use of the antifungal agent amphotericin B formulated in liposomes has been approved by the FDA. Since conventional liposomes are recognized by the immune system as foreign bodies, the ALZA Corporation developed STEALTH® liposomes, which evade recognition by the immune system because of their unique polyethylene glycol coating. Doxil is a STEALTH liposome formulation of doxorubicin used for the treatment of AIDS-related Kaposi's sarcoma.

Microencapsulation

Microencapsulation is a technique that involves the encapsulation of small particles or solution of drugs in a polymer film or coat. Different methods of microencapsulation result in either microcapsules or microspheres. For example, interfacial polymerization of a monomer almost always produces microcapsules, whereas solvent evaporation may result in microspheres or microcapsules, depending on the amount of drug loading. A microcapsule is a reservoir-type system in which drug is located centrally within the particle, whereas a microsphere is a matrix-type system in which drug is dispersed throughout the particle. Microcapsules usually release their drug at a constant rate (zero-order release), whereas microspheres typically give a first-order release of drugs. Low-molecular-weight drugs, proteins, oligonucleotides, and genes can be encapsulated into microparticles to provide their sustained release at disease sites.

The most commonly used method of microencapsulation is coacervation, which involves addition of a hydrophilic substance to a colloidal drug dispersion. The hydrophilic substance, which acts as a coating material, may be selected from a variety of natural and synthetic polymers, including shellacs, waxes, gelatin, starches, cellulose acetate phthalate, and ethylcellulose, among others. Following dissolution of the coating materials, the drug inside the microcapsule is available for dissolution and absorption.

Biodegradable polylactide and its copolymers with glycolide [poly (lactic-co-glycolic acid), or PLGA] are commonly used for preparation of microparticles from which the drug can be released slowly over a period of a month or so. Microspheres can be used in a wide variety of dosage forms, including tablets, capsules, and suspensions. Lupron Depot from TAP Pharmaceuticals is a FDA-approved preparation of PLGA microspheres for sustained release of a small peptide luteinizing hormone-releasing hormone (LHRH) agonist. More recently, PLGA microspheres of recombinant human growth hormone have been developed and marked successfully by Genentech, Inc. under the trade name of Nutropin Depot.

7. Key Points

- Fick's first law of diffusion describes the diffusion process under steady-state conditions when the drug concentration gradient does not change with time.
- Drug absorption depends not only on the fraction of un-ionized form of the drug, but also on the surface area available for absorption.
- The Noyes-Whitney equation can be used for determination of the dissolution rate of a drug from its dosage form, while the Arrhenius equation can be used for the determination of the shelf life of a drug dosage form.
- Surfactants consist of hydrophilic and hydrophobic groups and can be used as emulsifying agents to reduce the interfacial tensions.
- The pharmaceutical dosage form contains the active drug ingredient in association with nondrug (usually inert) ingredients (excipients). Together they comprise the vehicle, or formulation matrix.
- Water-soluble drugs are often formulated as sustained-release tablets so that their release and dissolution rates can be controlled, while enteric-coated tablets are used to protect drugs from gastric degradation.
- Capsules are solid dosage forms with hard or soft gelatin shells that contain drugs and excipients.
- Aerosols are pressurized dosage forms designed to deliver drugs to pulmonary tissues with the aid of a liquefied or propelled gas.
- Inserts, implants, and devices allow slow release of the drug into a variety of cavities (eg, vagina, buccal cavity, cul-de-sac of the eye, and skin).
- Transdermal patches deliver drugs directly through the skin and into the bloodstream.
- The drug delivery system deals with the pharmaceutical formulation and the dynamic interactions among the drug, its formulation matrix, its container, and the physiologic milieu of the patient. These dynamic interactions are the subject of pharmaceutics.
- Macromolecular drug carriers, such as protein-polymer conjugates, and particulate delivery systems such as microspheres and liposomes, are commonly used for delivery of drugs with low molecular weight, such as peptides and proteins, to different disease targets.
- Targeted (or site-specific) drug delivery systems are used for drug delivery to the target or receptor site in a manner that provides maximum therapeutic activity, by preventing degradation during transit to the target site while avoiding delivery to nontarget sites.

8. Questions and Answers

1. Which of the following is true for Fick's first law of diffusion?

   A. It refers to the non-steady-state flow
   B. The amount of material flowing through a unit cross-section of a barrier in unit time is known as the concentration gradient
   C. Flux of material is proportional to the concentration gradient
   D. Diffusion occurs in the direction of increasing concentration
   E. All of the above

2. Which equation describes the rate of drug dissolution from a tablet?

   A. Fick's law
   B. Henderson-Hasselbalch equation
   C. Michaelis-Menten equation
   D. Noyes-Whitney equation
   E. All of the above

3. The pH of a buffer system can be calculated with

   A. the Henderson-Hasselbalch equation
   B. the Noyes-Whitney equation
   C. the Michaelis-Menten equation
   D. Yong's equation
   E. All of the above

4. Which of the following is NOT true for gas adsorption on a solid?

   A. Chemical adsorption is reversible
   B. Physical adsorption is based on weak van der Waals forces
   C. Chemical adsorption may require activation energy
   D. Chemical adsorption is specific to the substrate
   E. All of the above

5. What is bioavailability?

   A. Bioavailability is the measurement of the rate and extent of active drug that reaches the systemic circulation
   B. It is the relationship between the physical and chemical properties of a drug and its systemic absorption
   C. It is the movement of the drug into body tissues over time

D. It is dissolution of the drug in the gastrointestinal tract

E. All of the above

6. Which of the following may be used to assess the relative bioavailability of two chemically equivalent drug products in a crossover study?

   A. Dissolution test
   B. Peak concentration
   C. Time-to-peak concentration
   D. Area under the plasma level time curve
   E. All of the above

7. What condition usually increases the rate of drug dissolution for a tablet?

   A. Increase in the particle size of the drug
   B. Decrease in the surface area of the drug
   C. Use of the ionized, or salt, form of the drug
   D. Use of the free acid or free base form of the drug
   E. Use of sugar coating around the tablet

8. The characteristics of an active transport process include all of the following EXCEPT

   A. For active transport moves drug molecules against a concentration gradient
   B. For active transport follows Fick's law of diffusion
   C. For active transport is a carrier-mediated transport system
   D. For active transport requires energy
   E. For active transport of drug molecules may be saturated at high drug concentrations

9. Which of the following dosage forms may utilize surface-active agents in their formulations?

   A. Emulsions
   B. Suspensions
   C. Colloidal dosage forms
   D. Creams
   E. All of the above

10. Which of the following statements about lyophilic colloidal dispersions is true?

    A. They tend to be more sensitive to the addition of electrolytes than lyophobic systems
    B. They tend to be more viscous than lyophobic systems
    C. They can be precipitated by prolonged dialysis

D. They separate rapidly

E. All of the above

11. Which of the following is NOT true for tablet formulations?

    A. A disintegrating agent promotes granule flow
    B. Lubricants prevent adherence of granules to the punch faces of the tabletting machine
    C. Glidants promote flow of the granules
    D. Binding agents are used for adhesion of powder into granules
    E. All of the above

12. The absorption rate of a drug is most rapid when the drug is formulated as

    A. A controlled-release product
    B. A hard gelatin capsule
    C. A compressed tablet
    D. A solution
    E. A suspension

13. The passage of drug molecules from a region of high drug concentration to a region of low drug concentration is known as

    A. Active transport
    B. Simple diffusion or passive transport
    C. Pinocytosis
    D. Bioavailability
    E. Biopharmaceutics

14. Which equation is used to predict the stability of a drug product at room temperature from experiments at increased temperatures?

    A. Stokes equation
    B. Arrhenius equation
    C. Michaelis-Menten equation
    D. Fick's equation
    E. Noyes-Whitney equation

15. Choose which of the following statements is true.

    A. Flocculation is desirable for pharmaceutical suspensions
    B. The diffusion rate of molecules of a smaller particle size is less than that of a larger particle size
    C. Particle size of molecular dispersions is larger than a coarse dispersion
    D. Pseudoplastic flow is shear-thickening type and dilatant is shear-thinning type
    E. All of the above are true statements.

16. Choose which of the following statements is false.

    A. The Henderson-Hasselbalch equation describes the effect of physical parameters on the stability of pharmaceutical suspensions
    B. The passive diffusion rate of hydrophobic drugs across biological membranes is higher than that of hydrophilic compounds
    C. When the dispersed phase in an emulsion formulation is heavier than the dispersion medium, creaming can still occur.
    D. Targeted drug delivery systems deliver the drug to the target or receptor site in a manner that provides maximum therapeutic activity
    E. All of the above are false statements

17. Which of the following is an emulsifying agent?

    A. Sorbitan mono-oleate (Span 80)
    B. Polyoxyethylene sorbitan mono-oleate (Tween 80)
    C. Sodium lauryl sulfate
    D. Gum acacia
    E. All of the above

18. Which of the following surfactants is incompatible with bile salts?

    A. Polysorbate 80
    B. Potassium stearate
    C. Sodium lauryl sulfate
    D. Benzalkonium chloride
    E. All of the above

19. Which of the following statements is false?

    A. The partition coefficient is the ratio of drug solubility in n-octanol to that in water
    B. Absorption of a weak electrolyte drug does not depend on the extent to which the drug exists in its un-ionized form at the absorption site
    C. The drug dissolution rate can be determined using the Noyes-Whitney equation
    D. Amorphous forms of drug have faster dissolution rates than crystalline forms
    E. All of the above are false

20. Which of the following statements is true?

    A. Most substances acquire a surface charge by ionization, ion adsorption, and ion dissolution
    B. The term "surface tension" is used for liquid-vapor and solid-vapor tensions

    C. At the isoelectric point, the total number of positive charges is equal to the total number of negative charges
    D. All of the above are true
    E. None of the above are true

21. Agents that may be used in the enteric coating of tablets include

    A. Hydroxypropyl methylcellulose
    B. Carboxymethylcellulose
    C. Cellulose acetate phthalate
    D. All of the above
    E. None of the above

Answers

1. **C.** Fick's first law of diffusion states that the amount of material flow through a unit cross-section of a barrier in unit time, which is known as the flux, is proportional to the concentration gradient. Fick's first law of diffusion describes the diffusion process under steady-state conditions when the concentration gradient does not change with time.

2. **D.** The Noyes-Whitney equation describes the rate of drug dissolution from a tablet. Fick's first law of diffusion is similar to the Noyes-Whitney equation in that both equations describe drug movement due to a concentration gradient. The Michaelis-Menten equation involves enzyme kinetics, whereas Henderson-Hasselbalch equations are used for determination of pH of the buffer and the extent of ionization of a drug molecule.

3. **A.** The Henderson-Hasselbalch equation for a weak acid and its salt is represented as: $pH = pK_a + \log$ [salt]/[acid], where pK_a is the negative log of the dissolution constant of a weak acid, as [salt]/[acid] is the ratio of the molar concentration of salt and acid used to prepare a buffer.

4. **A.** Chemical absorption is an irreversible process, which is specific and may require activation energy, while physical adsorption is reversible and associated with van der Waals forces.

5. **A.** Bioavailability is the measurement of the rate and extent of systemic circulation of an active drug.

6. **D.** The plasma drug concentration versus time curve measures the bioavailability of a drug from a product. The peak plasma drug concentration (C_{max}) relates to the intensity of the pharmacologic response, while the time for peak plasma drug concentration (T_{max}) relates to the rate of systemic absorption.

7. **C.** The ionized, or salt, form of a drug is generally more water soluble and therefore dissolves more rapidly than the non-ionized (free acid or free base) form of the drug. According to the Noyes-Whitney equation, the dissolution rate is directly proportional to the surface area and inversely proportional to the particle size. Therefore an increase in the particle size or a decrease in the surface area slows the dissolution rate.

8. **B.** In passive transport, a drug travels from a high concentration to a low concentration, while active transport moves drug molecules against a concentration gradient and requires energy.

9. **E.** Surface-active agents facilitate emulsion formation by lowering the interfacial tension between the oil and water phases. Adsorption of surfactants on insoluble particles enables these particles to be dispersed in the form of a suspension.

10. **B.** Most lyophilic colloids are organic molecules (including gelatin and acacia), they sponta-neously form colloidal solutions, and tend to be viscous. Dispersion of lyophilic colloids is stable in the presence of electrolytes.

11. **A.** Disintegrating agents are added to the tablets to promote breakup of the tablets when placed in the aqueous environment. Lubricants are required to prevent adherence of the granules to the punch faces and dies. Binding agents are added to bind powders together in the granulation process. Glidants are added to tablet formulations to improve the flow properties of the granulations.

12. **D.** For a drug in solution, no dissolution is required before absorption. Consequently, compared with other drug formulations, a drug in aqueous solution has the highest bioavailability rate, and is often used as the reference preparation for other formulations.

13. **B.** In simple diffusion or passive transport, a drug travels from a high concentration to a low concentration, while active transport moves drug molecules against a concentration gradient and requires energy. Pinocytosis is a vesicular transport process of engulfment of small particles or fluid volumes.

14. **B.** Stability at room temperature can be predicted from accelerated testing data by the Arrhenius equation: $\log (k_2/k_1) = E_a (T_2 - T_1)/(2.303\ RT_2T_1)$, where k_2 and k_1 are the rate constants at the absolute temperatures T_2 and T_1, respectively; R is the gas constant; and E_a is the energy of activation. The Stokes equation is used to determine the sedimentation rate of a suspension, while the Noyes-Whitney equation is used to determine the dissolution rate.

15. **A.** Flocculation is the formation of light, fluffy conglomerates held together by weak van der Waals forces and is a reversible process. Pseudoplastic flow is a shear-thinning process, while dilatant is a shear-thickening type process.

16. **A.** The Henderson-Hasselbalch equation describes the relationship between ionized and non-ionized species of a weak electrolyte.

17. **E.** Surfactants such as sorbitan mono-oleate (Span 80), polyoxyethylene sorbitan mono-oleate (Tween 80), sodium lauryl sulfate, and gum acacia are surfactants used as emulsifiers.

18. **D.** Benzalkonium chloride is a cationic surfactant and can interact with bile salts.

19. **B.** According to pH partition theory, absorption of a weak electrolyte drug depends on the extent to which the drug exists in its un-ionized form at the absorption site. However, pH partition theory often does not hold true, as most weakly acidic drugs are well absorbed from the small intestine, possibly due to the large epithelial surface areas of the organ.

20. **D.** Most substances acquire a surface charge by ionization, ion adsorption, and ion dissolution. At the isoelectric point, the total number of positive charges is equal to the total number of negative charges.

21. **C.** An enteric-coated tablet has a coating that remains intact in the stomach, but dissolves in the intestine when the pH exceeds 6. Other enteric-coating materials include cellulose acetate trimellitate, polyvinyl acetate phthalate, and hydroxypropyl methylcellulose phthalate.

9. References

Ansel HC, Popovich NG, Allen LV, eds. *Pharmaceutical Dosage Forms and Drug Delivery Systems,* 6th ed. Malvern, PA: Williams & Wilkins; 1995.

Aulton ME, ed. *Pharmaceutics: The Science of Dosage Form Design.* New York: Churchill Livingstone; 1988.

Block LH, Yu ABC. Pharmaceutical principles and drug dosage forms. In: Shargel L, Mutnick AH, Souney PH, Swanson LN, eds. *Comprehensive Pharmacy Review.* New York: Lippincott Williams & Wilkins; 2001:28-77.

Block LH, Collins CC. Biopharmaceutics and drug delivery systems. In: Shargel L, Mutnick AH, Souney PH, Swanson LN, eds. *Comprehensive Pharmacy Review.* New York: Lippincott Williams & Wilkins; 2001:78-91.

Hillery AM. Advanced drug delivery and targeting: An introduction. In: Hillery AM, Lloyd AW, Swarbrick J, eds. *Drug Delivery and Targeting: For Pharmacists and Pharmaceutical Scientists.* New York: Taylor & Francis; 2001:63-82.

Martin A. *Physical Pharmacy,* 4th ed. Baltimore: Lippincott Williams & Wilkins; 1993.

Gennaro AR, Gennaro AL, eds. *Remington: The Science and Practice of Pharmacy.* Baltimore: Lippincott, Williams & Wilkins; 2000.

Mathiowitz E, Kretz MR, Bannon-Peppas L. Microencapsulation. In: *Encyclopedia of Controlled Drug Delivery.* New York: John Wiley & Sons; 1999:493-546.

Florence AT, Attwood D. *Physicochemical Principles of Pharmacy,* 3rd ed. Palgrave, NY: MacMillan; 1998

Banker GS, Rhodes CT, eds. *Modern Pharmaceutics,* 3rd ed. New York: Marcel Dekker; 1995.

Washington N, Washington C, Wilson CG. *Physiological Pharmaceutics: Barriers to Drug Absorption,* 2nd ed. New York: Taylor & Francis; 2001.

4. Compounding

Charles N. May, BSPh, MSHP
Assistant Professor, Department of Pharmaceutical Sciences
University of Tennessee College of Pharmacy

Contents

1. Introduction

Pharmacists extemporaneously compound medications to provide patients and prescribers more options for treatment and therapy than are provided by commercially available products. There are many reasons patients need individualized custom-prepared medications, and these include (1) some therapeutic agents are not commercially manufactured; (2) some therapeutic agents are not manufactured in the form or size needed; (3) some manufactured therapeutic agents contain offending ingredients such as dyes, preservatives, fillers, and binders, among others; (4) some manufactured therapeutic agents contain offending flavors, fragrances, or colors; and (5) some patients do not fit into the standard categories that manufactured products treat. In addition, from time to time commercially manufactured products are unavailable for a variety of reasons, such as (1) drug recalls, (2) the manufacturing facility is closed down, (3) strikes or disasters, (4) the product is no longer commercially profitable, or (5) for other corporate reasons the manufacturer no longer supplies the product. There are several segments of the population that are not properly served by pharmaceutical manufacturers and these include pediatric patients, geriatric patients, veterinary patients, and patients with rare and/or very complicated disease states. Prescribers and pharmacists working very closely with patients improve the quality of life for those patients as no other practice can do.

2. Philosophy of Compounding

- Extemporaneous per patient
- Fulfills needs for unique dosage forms and sizes
- Works as part of a three-member team: the patient, the pharmacist, and the prescriber, to satisfy a patient's unique needs that cannot be satisfied by commercially available products
- Follows-up with patient and/or prescriber to determine if the compounded preparation needs further adjustment or refinement to completely satisfy the patient's needs

3. Compounding versus Manufacturing

Compounding

- Patient-specific in conjunction with the prescriber
- Regulated by the state board of pharmacy
- Compounded preparations are not advertised.
- Compounded preparations have "beyond-use dates."
- Compounded preparations are not prepared in advance except in the case of documented usage or demand.
- Compounded preparations have no NDC number.

Manufacturing

- Products are subject to an approved NDA.
- Products are subject to FDA-approved labeling.
- Products are manufactured in FDA-approved plants in accordance with Good Manufacturing Practices.
- Products may be advertised.
- Products carry an expiration date.
- Products carry an NDC number.
- Regulated by the FDA.

4. Guidelines for Compounding

The following are published guidelines pharmacists utilize in designing and carrying out their compounding activities. Pharmacists' compounding practices are regulated by the laws of the state board of pharmacy of the state in which the pharmacist practices.

Allen Jr LV. Extemporaneous prescription compounding: Chapter 98. *Remington: The Science and Practice of Pharmacy,* 20th ed. Baltimore: Lippincott Williams & Wilkins; 2000:1706-1715.

Compliance Policy Guide, Compliance Policy Guidance for FDA Staff and Industry, Chapter 4, Sub Chapter 460, Sec. 460.200. Pharmacy Compounding, Washington: U.S. Food and Drug Administration; June, 2002.

Good Compounding Practices Applicable to State Licensed Pharmacies. Park Ridge, IL: The National Association of Boards of Pharmacy; 1993.

Good Compounding Practices: Chapter 1075. *U.S. Pharmacopeia 28/National Formulary 23,* Rockville, MD: U.S. Pharmacopeial Convention, Inc.; 2005:2620-2624.

Pharmaceutical Calculations in Prescription Compounding: Chapter 1160. *U.S. Pharmacopeia 28/National Formulary 23,* Rockville, MD: U.S Pharmacopeial Convention, Inc.; 2005:2712-2721.

Pharmaceutical Compounding–Nonsterile Preparations: Chapter 795. *U.S. Pharmacopeia 28/National Formulary 23,* Rockville, MD: U.S. Pharmacopeial Convention, Inc.; 2005:2457-2460.

5. Requirements

Pharmacy

Space
- Appropriate amount: a dedicated area is ideal.
- Properly arranged and maintained: ingredients and equipment close at hand
- Controlled atmosphere: limited traffic flow, air flow away from operator
- Separate areas for sterile and nonsterile compounding
- Source of potable water and purified water: sink readily available
- Constructed of materials that are nonporous and seamless as possible: a well lit space with bright fixtures, walls, and floors give a clean, professional appearance

Equipment
- Appropriate measuring devices: eg, graduated cylinders, pharmacy graduates, pipettes, etc
- Appropriate balances for weighing: eg, electronic balance or class A prescription balance
- Appropriate mixing devices: eg, Wedgwood, porcelain, and glass mortars and pestles, blenders, etc
- Appropriate counters and shelves: sufficient countertop space must be available so compounding will not be cramped and shelving must be sufficient and appropriately located so ingredients can be convenient and properly stored.
- Appropriate processing equipment: eg, hot plates and magnetic stirrers, ointment mills, electronic mortar and pestle, tablet pulverizers, etc
- Appropriate safety equipment: eg, rubber gloves, face masks, hair covers, etc, for personnel; devices that gently exhaust the air from the work area to keep the air free of contamination with ingredients; and containment areas in which to work when personnel are working with light, fine, fluffy ingredients or ingredients that are irritating or foul-smelling
- Appropriate packaging equipment: eg, capsule filling machines, tube sealing equipment, calibrated measuring and filling devices, etc
- Appropriate computer equipment: eg, for processing labels, profiles, formulas, and maintaining required records regarding ingredients

Other

Formulas
Ingredient classification and quality
- USP/NF (United States Pharmacopeia/National Formulary) (ingredients meet official standards and are suitable for human use)
- FCC (Food Chemicals Codex) (Food Grade)
- ACS (American Chemical Society) (Reagent Grade)
- AR (Analytical Reagent) (High Purity)
- CP (Chemically Pure) (Uncertain Quality)
- Tech (Technical) (Industrial Quality)

Supplies
- These include weigh boats, weighing paper (parchment and glassine), filter paper, ointment paper, spatulas (stainless steel and hard rubber), stirring rods (glass and polypropylene), rubber scrapers, beakers, flasks, funnels, casseroles, and containers of all types and sizes to properly package all the unique dosage forms and sizes patients require. These also include all sizes of prescription bottles, powder jars, capsule vials, and ointment jars as well as ointment tubes, troche molds, plastic suppository molds, powder paper boxes, suppository boxes, "ride-up" tubes, etc.

Records
- An exact record of each compounded prescription must be made and maintained. A chronological record of each day's compounding activity should be made and kept for future reference and use.

Policies and procedures including
- Standard Operating Procedures (SOPs)
- Material Safety Data Sheets (MSDSs)
- Certificates of Analysis (COAs)
- Quality Assurance Checks, etc

The Pharmacist

- *Interest:* a distinct interest in being creative, solving difficult patient problems, working closely with prescribers and patients, and formulating and compounding special customized medications is very important.
- *Education:* the emphasis on compounding varies among the colleges of pharmacy. Even graduates of programs that require students to compound a wide variety of formulations may find they need more training.
- *Training:* additional training is often obtained through CE courses, seminars, professional development programs, or professional associations.
- *Experience:* experience in compounding is perhaps the key to how effective a pharmacist can be in creating special formulations that make a significant difference in a patient's life when everything else up to that point has failed.
- Experience enables the pharmacist to suggest to the prescriber a therapeutic agent in a unique dosage form that has a better chance of solving the patient's problem. Conversely, a pharmacist with less-than-

optimal experience and interest may compound a medication that is not effective, and thereby not satisfy the patient's need, and perhaps even undermine the prescriber's confidence in all compounded medications. Pharmacists who compound must be certain they possess the appropriate requisites for the level of compounding they perform.

- *Compounding support:* compounding pharmacists should join professional organizations that support compounding such as the International Academy of Compounding Pharmacists; they should subscribe to journals that focus on compounding such as the *International Journal of Pharmaceutical Compounding,* the *U.S. Pharmacist,* etc; and they should utilize the professional resources of the companies that fulfill their compounding needs.

Professional considerations
- Is there a commercially available product in the exact dosage, size, form, and package required?
- Is there an alternative product that will completely satisfy the patient's needs?
- Can I do the required pharmaceutical calculations to make and package the product?

Quality Control Requirements

- Accurate calculations
- Accurate weights
- Accurate measurements
- Proper processing techniques
- Proper packaging
- Proper records
- Proper labeling including "beyond-use date"

Beyond-use dates
- Pharmacists assign beyond-use dates to compounded preparations to provide patients guidance in the proper use of the preparation.
- The goal is to provide a beyond-use date that will allow the patient enough time to fully utilize the amount of preparation dispensed, but not enough time to allow the preparation to degrade and/or lose potency or be stored for future use.
- If the pharmacist does not have a reference on stability of the specific dosage form or if experience with it is insufficient, the USP guidelines are followed.

6. Compounded Preparations

Solutions

- *Definition:* chemically and physically homogenous mixtures of two or more substances
- *Types:* syrups, elixirs, aromatic waters, tinctures, spirits, nonaqueous, etc
- *Properties:* hypertonic, isotonic, hypotonic, osmolar, osmolal, etc
- Stability is enhanced by adjusting pH or adding preservatives, antioxidants, etc.
- Rate of dissolution is enhanced by stirring, heat, particle size reduction, etc.
- Beyond-use dates: aqueous solutions have short beyond-use dates.
- Testing: organoleptic, pH, etc

An example of an isotonic **aqueous** solution:

Ephedrine sulfate	1%
Sodium chloride	qs
Purified water qs ad	30 mL
M.Ft. isotonic solution	

Steps in compounding:
1. Calculate the required quantity of each ingredient (NaCl equivalent of ephedrine sulfate is 0.2).
2. Accurately weigh or measure each ingredient.
3. Dissolve the solid ingredients in about 25 mL of purified water.
4. Add sufficient purified water to measure 30 mL.

The following is an example of a **nonaqueous** solution:

Urea	10 g
Salicylic acid	5 g
Coal tar solution	5 mL
Propylene glycol qs ad	100 mL

Steps in compounding:
1. Accurately weigh or measure each ingredient.
2. Dissolve the urea and salicylic acid in about 75 mL of propylene glycol.
3. Add the coal tar solution and mix well.
4. Add sufficient propylene glycol to measure 100 mL

Note: If using a mechanical stirrer, it may take significant time to dissolve the urea and salicylic acid.

Suspensions

- *Definition:* a two-phased system containing a finely divided solid in a vehicle

- **Requirement:** drug is uniformly dispersed throughout vehicle.
- **Suspending agents** are typically used in a concentration of 0.5-6%.

Categories of suspending agents
* Natural hydrocolloids: acacia, alginic acid, gelatin, guar gum, sodium alginate, tragacanth, xanthan gum
* Semisynthetic hydrocolloids: ethylcellulose, methylcellulose, sodium carboxymethylcellulose
* Synthetic hydrocolloids: carbomers (carbopol), poloxamers (pluronic), polyvinyl alcohol, polyvinylpyrolidone
* Clays: bentonite, magnesium aluminum silicate (veegum)

- The vehicle has enough viscosity to keep drug particles suspended separately.
- Active ingredient is insoluble in vehicle

Tip: Wet insoluble powder with vehicle-miscible liquid.

- Advantage: a suspension allows the preparation of a liquid form of an insoluble drug.
- Stability is enhanced by adding a preservative.
- Testing: organoleptic

An example of an oral suspension:

Progesterone, micronized	1.2 g
Glycerin	3 mL
Methylcellulose 2 % soln	30 mL
Flavored syrup qs ad	60 mL

Steps in compounding:
1. Accurately weigh or measure each ingredient.
2. In a glass mortar, wet the progesterone with the glycerin, making a thick paste.
3. Slowly add the methylcellulose solution while triturating.
4. When mixed thoroughly, pour into a graduate.
5. Add small amounts of syrup in mortar, mix, and add to graduate until the desired volume is reached.

Emulsions

- **Definition:** a two-phase system of two immiscible liquids, one of which is dispersed throughout the other as small droplets
- **Components:** a dispersion medium or external or continuous phase, an internal or discontinuous or dispersed phase, and an emulsifying agent
- **Type:** oil-in-water (o/w) or water-in-oil (w/o), based on which is the internal and which is the external phase

Emulsifying agents
* Natural gums: acacia, agar, chondrus, pectin, tragacanth
* Hydrophilic/lipophilic agents: the esters of sorbitan
  - Lipophilic: trade names Arlacel® and Span™
  - Hydrophilic: trade names Myrj™ and Tween™

- A lower hydrophilic-lipophilic balance (HLB) value favors a w/o emulsion; a higher HLB value favors an o/w emulsion.
- Agents with an HLB value of 1 through 9 are considered to be lipophilic; agents with an HLB value of 10 and above are considered to be hydrophilic.
- Other agents include bentonite, cholesterol, gelatin, lecithin, methylcellulose, soaps of fatty acids, sodium docusate, sodium lauryl sulfate, and triethanolamine.
- Equipment: mortar and pestle, homogenizers, colloid mill, mechanical mixers, agitators, ultrasonic vibrators, etc
- Solid ingredients should be dissolved before they are incorporated into the emulsion, or if a sizeable quantity is added, a levigating or wetting agent may be needed.
- Flavors should be incorporated into the external phase.
- Preservatives should be added in the aqueous phase; may also be added to the oily phase if needed.
- Stability: either cream or crack (coalesce)
- The Continental or dry gum method of preparing an emulsion nucleus involves using the oil:water:dry gum emulsifier in a 4:2:1 ratio.
- Advantages of an emulsion as a vehicle: to mask taste, improve palatability, increase absorption, and enhance bioavailability

An example of preparing an emulsion by the Continental or dry gum or 4-2-1 method:

Cod liver oil	50 mL
Acacia	12.5 g
Syrup	10 mL
Flavor oil	0.4 mL
Purified water, qs ad	100 mL

Steps in compounding:
1. Accurately weigh or measure each ingredient.
2. Place the cod liver oil in a dry mortar.
3. Add the acacia and give it a very quick mix.

4. Add 25 mL of purified water and immediately triturate rapidly to form the thick, white, homogenous emulsion nucleus.
5. Add the flavor and mix thoroughly.
6. Add the syrup and mix thoroughly.
7. Add sufficient purified water to measure 100 mL.

Capsules

- *Definition:* a dosage form incorporating ingredients into a shell called a capsule
- *Procedure:* triturate powders to reduce particle size, mix powders by geometric dilution, incorporate diluent by geometric dilution, calculate total weight to fit a certain size capsule, clean the outside of the filled capsules.
- *Advantages:* mask unpleasant taste; mix ingredients that could not be mixed in other vehicles; alter the release rate of ingredients; incorporate several ingredients into one dosage form; provide an accurate dosage size for liquids, semisolids, and powders; provide a dosage form that is easier to swallow and more acceptable to the patient.
- Method of filling: hand punch from powder on pill tile; use capsule filling machine
- Sizing: determining the size of capsule to use for your dosage size involves assessing the density /fluffiness of your powder, comparing it to known weights of various reference powders with published capsule size capacities, then actually weighing your capsule; if the requested dosage doesn't fill a specific size capsule, a filler should be added to fill the capsule.

An example of an altered-release capsule:

Progesterone, micronized	25 mg
Methocel E4M®	50%
Lactose, qs ad	
M.Ft. capsules	dtd #15

Steps in compounding:
1. Select capsule size and calculate the required quantity of each ingredient.
2. Accurately weigh each ingredient.
3. If necessary, reduce particle size and mix thoroughly.
4. Fill capsules.
5. Weigh capsules, calculate average weight, and determine percentage of error.

Tablet Triturates (Sublingual or Molded Tablets)

- *Definition:* a small tablet made in a mold and intended for sublingual administration, usually weighing about 30-250 mg
- *Advantages:* rapidly dissolves under the tongue, rapidly absorbed, avoids first pass through liver, provides rapid therapeutic response
- *Components:* active ingredient and base, which may consist of lactose, sucrose, dextrose, mannitol, etc
- *Formulation:* based on the size of the mold cavities, mix the active ingredient with the base, which often consists of 4 parts lactose and 1 part sucrose. Thoroughly triturate powders and mix by geometric dilution, then moisten with a solution containing 4 parts alcohol and 1 part purified water until the powder mixture is adhesive. Press into mold.

Tip: Tablets may be flavored and colored by adding flavor and color to the wetting solution.

An example of a tablet triturate:

Testosterone	3 mg
Base, qs ad	
M.Ft. tabs	

Steps in compounding:
1. The base may consist of a 1:4 mixture of sucrose and lactose.
2. The wetting solution may consist of a 1:4 mixture of water and alcohol.
3. Based on the size mold you will use and the number of tablets it makes, calculate the required quantity of each ingredient.
4. Accurately weigh or measure each ingredient.
5. Reduce particle size and mix ingredients by geometric dilution.
6. In a glass mortar gradually moisten the powder mixture until it becomes adhesive.
   Note: Drop the wetting solution onto the powder a few drops at a time and triturate after each addition until powder becomes moist and adhesive.
7. Press moist powder evenly into all holes in the tablet triturate mold plate.
8. Place the mold plate on the base plate and press down until the tablets rest on top of the pegs.
9. Let tablets air dry.
10. Very gently remove dried tablets from pegs.

Troches, Lozenges, and Lollipops (Suckers)

- *Definition:* solid dosage forms intended to be slowly dissolved in the mouth for local or systemic effects

- **Formulation:** active ingredient and base that may consist of sugar and other carbohydrates that produce a hard candy troche, or the polyethylene glycols with other ingredients that produce a softer troche, or a glycerin-gelatin combination that produces a chewable troche
- Formulations made in a sucker mold complete with sticks are called lollipops or suckers.
- Formulations must be calculated to fit the size mold that will be utilized.
- Flavors and colors are added just before the molds are filled.
- **Advantages:** easy to administer, convenient for patients who cannot swallow oral dosage forms, maintain a constant level of drug in the oral cavity and throat, pleasant taste

An example of a troche:

Gelatin	4.68 g
Glycerin	16.70 mL
Purified water	2.30 mL
Acacia	0.50 g
Bentonite	0.50 g
Benzocaine	0.30 g
Citric acid	0.66 g
Saccharin sodium	0.17 g
Flavor and color	qs

Steps in compounding:
1. Based on the size of the mold to be used and the number of troches to be made, calculate the required quantity of each ingredient.
2. Accurately weigh or measure each ingredient.
3. Heat the glycerin in a boiling water bath for several minutes.
4. Add the water and heat for a few more minutes.
5. While stirring, VERY SLOWLY add the gelatin. **Note:** Gelatin must be lump-free; the mixture must be homogenous.
6. Triturate and thoroughly mix the powders.
7. Add the powders to the warm liquid and mix thoroughly.
8. Add flavor and color, mix, pour into the mold, and let cool.

Transdermal Gels

- **Definition:** gels that move medications through the skin in quantities sufficient to produce a therapeutic effect

Components
  * Active ingredient(s)

  * Gelling agents: the carbomers (eg, Carbopol 934P®), methylcellulose, the poloxamers (eg, Pluronic F-127®), sodium carboxymethylcellulose, etc
  * Wetting/levigating agents: propylene glycol, glycerin, etc
  * Penetration-enhancing agents: water, alcohol, lecithin, dimethyl sulfoxide, isopropyl myristate, isopropyl palmitate, propylene glycol, polyethylene glycol, etc
  * Suspending/dispersing agents: bentonite, silica gel, etc

- **Advantages:** convenient, effective, has great acceptability to patients, and avoids problems other dosage forms have such as GI irritation from oral dosages, pain from injections, and undesirability of suppositories
- **Formulation:** use proper techniques for creating the gel, adjust the pH for carbomer gels, respect the temperature for poloxamer gels, use small amounts of nonaqueous solvents, and if possible keep electrolyte ingredients to a minimum.

Tip: Do not use transdermal gels for the systemic use of antibiotics, and do not try to get large molecules such as proteins through the skin via transdermal gels.

An example of a transdermal gel using carbomer as the base:

Ketoprofen	5%
Carbomer 934P	2%
Alcohol	qs
Trolamine	2 mL
Purified water, qs ad	30 mL

Steps in compounding:
1. Calculate the required quantity of each ingredient.
2. Accurately weigh or measure each ingredient.
3. Triturate the carbomer 934P in a glass mortar.
4. While triturating, gradually add about 18 mL of purified water.
5. Be sure the carbomer and water are thoroughly mixed and the mixture is homogenous.
6. Dissolve the ketoprofen in about 10 mL of alcohol.
7. While triturating, add this to the carbomer/water mixture and mix thoroughly.
8. If necessary, add purified water to make about 28 mL and pour into the ointment jar.
9. Add trolamine and stir quickly with a stirring rod until the gel is thoroughly formed.

Note: A trade name for carbomer 934P is Carbopol 934P®.

An example of a transdermal gel using organogel (PLO) as the base:

Ketoprofen	5%
Propylene glycol	10%
Lecithin isopropyl palmitate liq.	20%
Poloxamer 407 20% gel qs ad	100 mL

Steps in compounding:
1. Calculate the required quantity of each ingredient.
2. Accurately weigh or measure each ingredient.
3. In a glass mortar triturate the ketoprofen with the propylene glycol.
4. Make a smooth uniform paste.
5. Add the lecithin isopropyl palmitate liquid and mix well.
6. Add sufficient poloxamer 407 20% gel to measure 100 mL.
7. Triturate until a high-quality gel is produced.
8. Package in a light-resistant container.

Note: The lecithin isopropyl palmitate liquid and the poloxamer 407 20% gel should be prepared ahead of time so they are ready for use.

The lecithin isopropyl palmitate liquid may be prepared as follows:

Soy lecithin, granular	10 g
Isopropyl palmitate	10 g
Sorbic acid	0.2 g

1. Accurately weigh or measure each ingredient.
2. Add the soy lecithin granules and the sorbic acid to the isopropyl palmitate, mix well, and allow to set overnight at room temperature.
3. The next morning, very gently stir to assure complete mixing.

Note: Isopropyl myristate may be used in place of isopropyl palmitate.

The poloxamer 407 20% gel may be prepared as follows:

Poloxamer 407	20 g
Potassium sorbate	0.2 g
Purified water, qs ad	100 mL

1. Accurately weigh or measure each ingredient.
2. Add the poloxamer 407 and the potassium sorbate to a portion of the purified water, mix well and add purified water to make 100 mL.
3. Mix thoroughly, ensuring that the poloxamer 407 is completely wet.

4. Allow to set overnight in the refrigerator.
5. The next morning, stir slowly to be sure mixing is complete.
6. Store in the refrigerator.

Note: A trade name for poloxamer 407 is Pluronic F-127®.

Suppositories

- **Definition:** solid dosage forms for insertion into the rectum, vagina, or urethra to provide localized therapy or systemic therapy
- **Sizes:** rectal, approx. 2 g; vaginal, 3-5 g; urethral, 2 g female, 4 g male (urethral suppositories formerly called bougies)
- **Formulation:** usually made by fusion with either a fatty or water-miscible base (can also be hand molded or made by compression)
- Usually made in a metal or plastic mold
- The active ingredients in powder form should be triturated (comminuted) to reduce particle size and should be levigated with a levigating or wetting agent before incorporation into the melted base.
- The melted formulation should be poured continuously into the mold to prevent layering.
- Calculations: the capacity in grams of the suppository mold must be known to determine the quantity of base needed (if this capacity is not known, the capacity must be determined by filling the mold with the suppository base and weighing the resulting suppositories). The space in the suppository occupied by the active ingredient(s) must calculated using the density factor of each active ingredient (if the density factor is not known, it can be calculated by making a suppository containing a known amount of the active ingredient).
- Advantages: delivers medication for local or systemic effects (the systemically absorbed medication avoids the first pass through the liver); delivers medication systemically when patients cannot take it orally or by injection

An example of a rectal suppository:

Progesterone, micronized	25 mg
Polyethylene glycol base	qs
M.Ft. supp	dtd #12

Steps in compounding:
Use the following formula for the polyethylene glycol base:

Polyethylene glycol 300	50%
Polyethylene glycol 6000	50%

1. Based on the size of the mold, calculate the required amount of each ingredient.
2. Accurately weigh or measure each ingredient.
3. Carefully heat the PEG 6000 until it melts.
4. Add the PEG 300 and mix well.
5. Very slowly add the micronized progesterone and mix thoroughly.
6. Pour the mixture into the suppository mold.

Note: When using the plastic molds (shells), the liquid mixture must not be too hot.

Powders

- **Definition:** fine particles that result from the comminution of dry substances; particle sizes are usually determined by the size sieve they will pass through, and may be described as very coarse, coarse, moderately coarse, fine, and very fine.
- Mixtures of powders should have the same or similar sized particles and mixing should be accomplished by geometric dilution.
- **Preparation:** comminution is the process of reducing particle size in powders and is accomplished manually by trituration, levigation, and/or pulverization by intervention, and mechanically by grinders and various types of mills.
- **Uses:** powders taken by mouth may provide systemic effects. Powders are applied topically for local effects. Powders that contain mucoadhesive ingredients, when insufflated into body cavities, will adhere to moist body surfaces.
- **Advantages:** since they are dry, they often have greater stability and they may not react with ingredients with which they are otherwise incompatible (except explosive mixtures). Once in the GI tract they are ready to be absorbed, and they tend to have longer beyond-use dates.

An example of a powder for external use:

Calamine	
Zinc oxide, aa	8%
Red mercuric oxide	1%
Magnesium oxide, heavy, qs ad	60 g
M.Ft. powder	

Steps in compounding:
1. Calculate the required amount of each ingredient.
2. Accurately weigh each ingredient.
3. Thoroughly mix the powders by geometric dilution.
4. If using a mortar and pestle, use a porcelain mortar and begin with the ingredient having the smallest weight.

5. Use the "spread test" to determine when the mixture is totally homogenous.

Powder Papers (Charts)

- **Definition:** powders or mixtures of powders enfolded in papers containing one dose each and dispensed in an appropriate box or container
- **Preparation:** powders are finely subdivided (comminuted), mixed by geometric dilution, and the appropriate sized dose is placed on a powder paper and properly folded. The appropriate sized dose can be obtained by weighing. An alternate method is to place all the powder on a pill tile and "blocking and dividing" the powder into the proper number of doses, placing one dose on each powder paper.
- **Advantages:** for patients who cannot swallow, those who have difficulty swallowing certain tablets or capsules, and for those who have indwelling nasogastric tubes, powder papers provide an ideal dosage form. Several medications can be given as one dose. The medication is in powder form and ready to be absorbed once in the gastrointestinal tract. For patients who have many medications to take each day, they may be combined into a smaller number of powder papers. Powder papers have longer beyond-use dates than many other compounded dosage forms.

An example of a powder paper (chart):

Aspirin	3.5 grains
Acetaminophen	2.5 grains
Caffeine	0.5 grains
M.Ft. chart	dtd #12

Steps in compounding:
1. Calculate the required quantity of each ingredient.
2. Accurately weigh each ingredient.
3. Triturate each ingredient separately to reduce particle size.
4. Thoroughly mix the ingredients by geometric dilution.
5. Weigh the correct amount for each chart on a separate paper.
6. Properly fold each paper and place in powder box.

Ointments and Creams

- **Definition:** semisolid dosage forms for external application
- Properties are typically characteristic of the base selected (eg, white petrolatum, hydrophilic petrolatum, cold cream, hydrophilic ointment, polyethyl-

ene glycol ointment). Ointments and creams protect the skin and mucous membranes, moisturize the skin, and provide a vehicle for various types of medications.

Types and classifications of ointment bases

Oleaginous/hydrocarbon ointment bases

Characteristics	*Examples*
Occlusive	White petrolatum
Greasy	White ointment
Emollient	Vegetable shortening
Not water washable	
Will not absorb water	
Insoluble in water	

Absorption ointment bases

Characteristics	*Examples*
Occlusive	Hydrophilic petrolatum
Greasy	Lanolin, USP (anhydrous)
Emollient	Aquaphor®
Not water washable	Aquabase®
Can absorb water	
Insoluble in water	

Emulsion, water/oil ointment bases

Characteristics	*Examples*
Occlusive	Cold cream
Greasy	Rose water ointment
Emollient	Eucerin®
Not water washable	Hydrous lanolin
Will absorb water	Hydrocream
Insoluble in water	Nivea®

Emulsion, oil/water ointment bases

Characteristics	*Examples*
Nonocclusive	Hydrophilic ointment
Nongreasy	Acid mantle cream
Water washable	Cetaphil®
Will absorb water	Dermabase®
Insoluble in water	Keri® lotion
	Lubriderm®
	Neobase®
	Unibase®
	Vanishing cream
	Velvachol®

Water soluble ointment bases

Characteristics	*Examples*
Nonocclusive	Polyethylene glycol ointment
Nongreasy	Polybase®
Water washable	
Will absorb water	
Water soluble	

- *Preparation:* typically by fusion or levigation; powders should be comminuted to fine particles; some powders may be dissolved.
- If using the fusion method, only enough heat should be used to melt the ingredient having the highest melting point.
- If using the levigation method, an ointment slab and metal spatula usually work well. Levigating agents should be carefully selected considering both the ingredient(s) to be incorporated and the base. The following list shows commonly used levigating agents grouped by type and matched with the appropriate group of ointment base classifications:

Aqueous agents	*Ointment base classifications*
Glycerin	Oil-in-water emulsion
Propylene glycol	Water soluble
Polyethylene glycol 400	Water washable

Oily agents	*Ointment base classifications*
Mineral oil	Oleaginous/hydrocarbon
Castor oil	Absorption
Cottonseed oil	Water-in-oil emulsion

Note: Other agents may be useful for certain preparations such as Tween 80® for incorporating coal tar. Castor oil is useful for incorporating ichthammol and peru balsam.

- Uses: an effective dosage form for treating skin and mucous membranes; on occasion an ointment or cream will move sufficient quantities of medication through the skin to produce a systemic effect; some formulations provide effective protection for the skin and mucous membranes.
- Packaging: typically ointments and creams are packaged in ointment jars. The tube is often an ideal alternative package because it protects the product until it is squeezed out and used.

An example of a nongreasy ointment:

Benzoyl peroxide	10%
Sulfur	1%
Polyethylene glycol base qs ad	30 g

Steps in compounding:

1. Calculate the required quantity of each ingredient.
   Note: Benzoyl peroxide, hydrous, USP contains about 26% water.
   Note: The polyethylene glycol base consists of:
   Polyethylene glycol 400   65%
   Polyethylene glycol 3350   35%

2. Accurately weigh or measure each ingredient.
3. Triturate each powder to a fine particle size.
4. Melt the polyethylene glycol 3350 and remove from heat source.
5. Add the polyethylene glycol 400 and mix thoroughly.
6. Add the powders and mix thoroughly.
7. Before the preparation begins to harden, stir thoroughly and pour into ointment jar.

An example of a greasy ointment:

Salicylic acid	3%
White petrolatum, qs ad	30 g

Steps in compounding:
1. Calculate the required quantity of each ingredient.
2. Accurately weigh each ingredient.
3. Triturate the salicylic acid to reduce particle size.
4. Levigate with a small quantity of mineral oil.
5. By geometric dilution, incorporate the levigated salicylic acid into the white petrolatum.

The following is an example of a cream:

Almond oil	56 g
White wax	12 g
Light mineral oil	10 g
Cetyl esters wax	2.5 g
Sodium borate	0.5 g
Purified water	19 g
Total	100 g

M.Ft. cream, S.A.

Steps in compounding:
1. Accurately weigh or measure each ingredient.
2. Melt the white wax.
3. Add the cetyl esters wax, almond oil, and light mineral oil.
4. Bring to a temperature of 70°C.
5. Dissolve the sodium borate in the purified water.
6. Bring to a temperature of 70°C.
7. With both liquids at 70°C, mix and stir.
8. Stir until the cream is completely formed.
9. Package in a tube or jar.

Sticks

- **Definition:** a topical dosage form made in the shape of a rod or stick or variation thereof and packaged in a container that allows it to be advanced upward as it is used/consumed
- **Advantages:** an effective, convenient method of applying a topical agent exactly in the location

desired; can deliver a variety of agents, including those that are therapeutic, protective, and cosmetic; very portable
- **Preparation:** select a semisolid vehicle from a variety of polyethylene glycols, waxes, and oils that will produce the consistency desired. Triturate solid ingredients and wet them with an appropriate wetting/levigating agent and add them along with any liquid ingredients to the melted vehicle. Mix thoroughly. Pour into an appropriate "ride-up" container.

Tip: Sticks can usually be considered a stable dosage form and assigned a corresponding beyond-use date.

An example of a stick:

Menthol	1%
Camphor	0.5%
Phenol	0.25%
Flavor	qs
Color	qs
Polyethylene glycol 400	7 g
Polyethylene glycol 4500	3 g

Steps in compounding:
1. Calculate the required quantity of each ingredient.
2. Accurately weigh or measure each ingredient.
3. Melt the polyethylene glycol 4500.
4. Remove from heat source.
5. Add the polyethylene glycol 400 and mix thoroughly.
6. Mix the menthol, camphor, and phenol together; they will liquefy, forming a eutectic mixture.
7. Add the eutectic mixture and the other ingredients and mix thoroughly.
8. Pour into a "ride-up" lip balm tube and let cool.

7. Key Points

- Each extemporaneously compounded prescription is for a specific patient.
- Three parties are involved in extemporaneous compounding: the prescriber, the patient, and the pharmacist.
- A thorough knowledge of pharmacy math is required for extemporaneous compounding of prescriptions.
- The sensitivity of the pharmacy balance must be determined and the minimum weighable quantity calculated for that particular balance.
- All weighing and measuring must be accurate; avoid errors of 5% or more.
- Once an ingredient is removed from the stock container, it may not be returned to the stock container.
- Trituration is utilized to reduce the particle size of powders so a greater surface area will be available, to uniformly mix powders using geometric dilution, and to dissolve solutes in solvents.
- Levigation is the process of mixing or triturating a powder with a liquid in which it is insoluble to reduce particle size and aid in incorporating it into the ointment base.
- The pharmacist must choose a levigating agent that is miscible with the ointment base.
- Mineral oil is an appropriate levigating agent for a hydrophobic ointment base such as white petrolatum.
- Up to 5% of levigating agent is usually sufficient unless the amount of powder is large.
- Heat should be used sparingly in compounding, using only enough heat to melt ingredients, effect solution, enhance a reaction, etc—never any extra.
- Use of a water bath normally prevents overheating ingredients when compounding.
- Care must be taken to never lose or waste any ingredients in the preparation process since this can alter the concentration of active ingredients in the finished preparation and produce a sub-potent or super-potent preparation.
- To promote accuracy in the compounding process, place all unused stock containers on the left side of the work station; as each one is used, place it on the right side.
- The dry gum (or Continental) method of preparing an emulsion uses the oil, purified water, and gum (eg, acacia) in a ratio of 4:2:1, respectively.
- The extemporaneously compounded preparation has no NDC number.

8. Questions and Answers

1. When water is an ingredient in a nonsterile compounded preparation and the type of water is not specified, the pharmacist is correct to use

   A. tap water
   B. potable water
   C. purified water
   D. water for injection
   E. sterile water for injection

2. When alcohol is an ingredient in a nonsterile compounded preparation and the type and percent alcohol is not specified, the pharmacist is correct to use

   A. ethyl alcohol 100%
   B. ethyl alcohol 95%
   C. ethyl alcohol 70%
   D. ethyl alcohol 50%
   E. isopropyl alcohol 70%

3. Ingredients that soften the skin and make it more flexible when applied topically are called

   A. keratolytics
   B. emollients
   C. rubefacients
   D. counterirritants
   E. astringents

4. To increase the stability of potassium iodide oral solution (SSKI), _____ may be used as an antioxidant to prevent the release of free iodine.

   A. sodium alginate
   B. sodium borate
   C. sodium glycinate
   D. sodium succinate
   E. sodium thiosulfate

5. In preparing diluted hydrochloric acid, a temperature change is noted. The reaction is called *heat generated*

   A. hypothermic
   B. hyperthermic
   C. endothermic
   D. exothermic
   E. isothermic

6. Ingredients that tend to tighten or shrink tissues when applied topically are called

A. astringents
B. emollients
C. keratolytic agents
D. occlusive agents
E. suspending agents

7. A solution expressed as 35% w/w has the following:

A. 35 mg of solute dissolved in 100 mL of solution
B. 35 g of solute dissolved in 100 g of solvent
C. 35 mg of solute dissolved in 100 g of solvent
D. 35 g of solute dissolved in 100 g of solution
E. 35 mL of solute dissolved in 100 mL of solution

8. When dissolving potassium iodide in purified water, a temperature change is noted. The reaction is called   *gets cold*

A. hypothermic
B. hyperthermic
C. endothermic
D. exothermic
E. isothermic

9. A solution expressed as 35% w/v has the following:

A. 35 mg of solute dissolved in 100 mL of solvent
B. 35 g of solute dissolved in 100 mL of solution
C. 35 mg of solute dissolved in 100 mL of solution
D. 35 g of solute dissolved in 100 mL of solvent
E. 35 mL of solute dissolved in 100 g of solution

10. Hydrophilic ointment, USP is an o/w type of ointment base, therefore it possesses the property of being

A. emollient
B. greasy
C. occlusive
D. water washable
E. anhydrous

11. When compounding an emulsion that contains a flavoring agent, the flavoring agent should be in

A. the continuous (external) phase
B. the discontinuous (internal) phase
C. the aqueous phase

D. the oil phase
E. the emulsifier

The next four questions pertain to the following compounded prescription.

Mineral oil	60 mL
Acacia	qs
Syrup	12 mL
Flavor	qs
Purified water, qs ad	120 mL

M.Ft. emulsion using dry gum method

12. Mineral oil is in the

I. internal phase
II. external phase
III. discontinuous phase

A. I only
B. II only
C. I and III only
D. II and III only
E. I, II, and III

13. Acacia is the

A. primary active ingredient
B. preservative
C. emulsifying agent
D. wetting agent
E. coloring agent

14. How much acacia is needed for this preparation?

A. 5 g
B. 10 g
C. 15 g
D. 30 g
E. 35 g

15. How much purified water is needed to make the initial emulsion?

A. 5 mL
B. 10 mL
C. 15 mL
D. 30 mL
E. 48 mL

16. When cocoa butter is used as a suppository base, its melting point can pose a problem. To overcome this problem, the compounding pharmacist can replace _____ of the cocoa butter with white wax.

A. 5%
B. 10%
C. 15%
D. 20-25%
E. 30%

17. When cocoa butter is used as a suppository base, its melting point can pose a problem. To overcome this problem, the compounding pharmacist can replace _____ of the cocoa butter with cetyl esters wax.

    A. 5%
    B. 10%
    C. 15%
    D. 20-25%
    E. 30%

18. Hydrophilic petrolatum, USP is used as an ointment base. It possesses the characteristic(s) of being

    I.   emollient
    II. occlusive
    III. greasy

    A. I only
    B. II only
    C. I and III only
    D. II and III only
    E. I, II, and III

19. When lime water and olive oil are processed together to form an emulsion, a reaction occurs that produces the emulsifying agent

    A. Lime oil
    B. Lime oxide
    C. Calcium oxide
    D. Calcium oleate
    E. Olive oxide

20. The advantage(s) of sublingual tablets as a dosage form is/are

    I.   quick absorption into the bloodstream
    II. rapid onset of action
    III. avoids the first pass through the liver

    A. I only
    B. II only
    C. I and III only
    D. II and III only
    E. I, II, and III

Compounded Rx

Camphor	1%
Menthol	1%
Thymol	0.5%
White petrolatum, qs ad	30 g
M.Ft. oint	

21. To prepare this compounded prescription, the pharmacist should

    A. dissolve the camphor, menthol, and thymol in alcohol and incorporate into the white petrolatum by geometric dilution
    B. dissolve the camphor, menthol, and thymol in glycerin and incorporate into the white petrolatum by geometric dilution
    C. dissolve the camphor, menthol, and thymol in propylene glycol and incorporate into the white petrolatum
    D. form a eutectic mixture and incorporate it into the white petrolatum by geometric dilution
    E. alter the formula to avoid incompatibilities

22. The advantage(s) of capsules as a dosage form is/are

    I.   provides an accurate dose
    II. masks unpleasant tastes
    III. provides an immediate therapeutic response

    A. I only
    B. II only
    C. I and II only
    D. II and III only
    E. I, II, and III

Compounded Rx

| Salicylic acid | 5% |
| White petrolatum, qs ad | 30 g |

23. The pharmacist has on hand 2% salicylic acid ointment to use in preparing this prescription. When using it, the pharmacist should

    A. weigh 0.5 g of salicylic acid powder and qs to 30 g with 2% salicylic acid ointment, incorporating the salicylic acid powder by geometric dilution
    B. weigh 0.5 g of salicylic acid powder, levigate it with 5 mL of alcohol and qs to 30 g with 2% salicylic acid ointment, incorporating the salicylic acid by geometric dilution

C. weigh 1.5 g of salicylic acid powder, levigate it with 6 mL of mineral oil and qs to 30 g with 2% salicylic acid ointment, incorporating the salicylic acid by geometric dilution

D. weigh 1.5 g of salicylic acid powder and qs to 30 g with 2% salicylic acid ointment, incorporating the salicylic acid powder by geometric dilution

E. weigh 1 g of salicylic acid powder, levigate it with 4.5 mL of mineral oil (SpGr 0.89) and incorporate it into 25 g of 2% salicylic acid ointment by geometric dilution

24. The advantage(s) of a transdermal gel as a dosage form is/are

I. convenience of administration/application
II. quick therapeutic response
III. patient acceptance

A. I only
B. II only
C. I and II only
D. II and III only
E. I, II, and III

25. One gram of iodine is soluble in 3000 mL of water. In Lugol's solution (strong iodine solution) 1 g of iodine is dissolved in 20 mL of solution. Lugol's solution contains 5% iodine and 10% potassium iodide. The phenomenon by which the KI increases the solubility of iodine is known as

A. alligation
B. coalescence
C. comminution
D. complexation
E. diffusion

Answers

1. C. For nonsterile compounding, the USP specifies that purified water be used.

2. B. When type or percentage of alcohol is not specified, alcohol, USP is used and it is 95% ethyl alcohol.

3. B. Ingredients that make the skin soft and pliable when applied locally are called emollients.

4. E. Sodium thiosulfate is the antioxidant that prevents the iodide ion from oxidizing to form free iodine.

5. D. When diluted hydrochloric acid is prepared, heat is generated and the reaction is called exothermic.

6. A. Ingredients that shrink or tighten the skin when applied locally are called astringents.

7. D. W/w means weight in weight, consequently 35 g of solute must be contained in 100 g of solution to have a 35% w/w solution.

8. C. When potassium iodide is dissolved in purified water, the solution becomes distinctively cold and the reaction is called endothermic.

9. B. W/v means weight in volume, consequently 35 g of solute must be contained in 100 mL of solution to have a 35% w/v solution.

10. D. Hydrophilic ointment is water washable, but does not possess the other properties listed.

11. A. For the flavoring agent to be tasted, it must be in the external or continuous phase.

12. C. Mineral oil is in the internal or discontinuous phase and should not be tasted.

13. C. Acacia is the emulsifying agent forming an oil-in-water emulsion.

14. C. Using the 4:2:1 ratio, the 1 part or 15 g is the acacia.

15. D. Using the 4:2:1 ratio, the 2 parts or 30 mL is the water for the initial emulsion.

16. A. Five percent cocoa butter replaced by white wax will overcome the low melting point problem.

17. D. Twenty to twenty-five percent cocoa butter replaced by cetyl esters wax will overcome the low melting point problem.

18. E. Hydrophilic petrolatum is greasy, occlusive, and emollient.

19. D. The lime water is calcium hydroxide solution and the olive oil contains oleic acid. The two react together to form calcium oleate, which is

the emulsifying agent that forms a water-in-oil emulsion.

20. **E.** All three items are advantages of sublingual tablets as dosage forms.

21. **D.** The camphor, menthol, and thymol are three ingredients which when mixed together will liquefy, forming what is called a eutectic mixture. This liquid mixture is then gradually incorporated into the white petrolatum by geometric dilution.

22. **C.** Capsules do not provide an immediate therapeutic response; the other two choices are correct.

23. **E.** Your compounded preparation must contain 1.5 g of salicylic acid. Twenty-five grams of your 2% ointment contains 500 mg. You must weigh out 1 g of salicylic acid powder. The remaining ingredients must not contain any salicylic acid. The remaining weight can be made up with the levigating agent or a combination of the levigating agent and white petrolatum.

24. **E.** All three choices are correct.

25. **D.** In solution KI ionizes into potassium and the iodide ion. The iodide ion complexes with elemental iodine to form the soluble I^3 complex.

9. References

The following are references that should be available in the compounding pharmacy to provide assistance as the pharmacist formulates the variety of dosage forms of customized medications patients require.

Allen Jr LV. *The Art, Science and Technology of Pharmaceutical Compounding,* 2nd ed. Washington: American Pharmaceutical Association; 2002.

Ansel HC, Allen Jr LV, Popovich NG. *Ansel's Pharmaceutical Dosage Forms and Drug Delivery Systems,* 8th ed. Baltimore: Lippincott Williams & Wilkins; 2005.

Ansel HC, Stoklosa MJ. *Pharmaceutical Calculations,* 11th ed. Baltimore: Lippincott Williams & Wilkins; 2001.

Bodavari S, ed. *The Merck Index,* 13th ed. Whitehouse Station, NJ: Merck & Co.; 2001.

Gennaro AR, ed. *Remington: The Science and Practice of Pharmacy,* 20th ed. Baltimore: Lippincott Williams & Wilkins; 2000.

Parfitt K, ed. *Martindale: The Complete Drug Reference,* 32nd ed. London: Pharmaceutical Press; 1999.

Shrewsbury R. *Applied Pharmaceutics in Contemporary Compounding,* Englewood, CO: Morton Publishing; 2001.

Thompson JE. *A Practical Guide to Contemporary Pharmacy Practice,* Baltimore: Williams & Wilkins; 1998.

Trissel LA. *Stability of Compounded Formulations,* 2nd ed. Washington: American Pharmaceutical Association; 2000.

U.S. Pharmacopeia 28/National Formulary 23. Rockville, MD: U.S. Pharmacopeial Convention, Inc.; 2005.

5. Sterile Products

Laura A. Thoma, PharmD
Associate Professor,
Department of Pharmaceutical Sciences
Director, Parenteral Medications Lab
University of Tennessee College of Pharmacy

Contents

1. Parenteral Products

- Parenteral products are products that are administered by injection and therefore bypass the gastrointestinal (GI) tract. Parenteral products must be sterile and free of pyrogens and particulate matter. Drugs that are destroyed, inactivated in the GI tract, or poorly absorbed can be given by a parenteral route. Parenteral routes of administration may also be used when the patient being treated is uncooperative, unconscious, or unable to swallow. This route is also used when rapid drug absorption is essential, such as in emergency situations.

Parenteral Routes of Administration

Intravenous route
- An intravenous (IV) medication is administered directly into the vein. The IV route gives a rapid effect with a predictable response. The IV route is used for irritating medications because the medication is rapidly diluted. This route does not have as much volume restriction as other parenteral routes.
- A *bolus* is injected into the vein over a short period of time. A bolus is used to administer a relatively small volume and is often written as "IV push" (IVP).
- An *infusion* refers to the introduction of larger volumes of solution given over a longer period of time. A continuous infusion is used to administer a large volume of solution at a constant rate. Intermittent infusions are used to administer a relatively small volume of solution over a specified amount of time at specific intervals.

Intramuscular route
- An intramuscular medication (IM) is injected deep into a large muscle mass, such as the upper arm, thigh, or buttocks. The medication is absorbed from the muscle tissue, acting more quickly than when given by the oral route, but not as quickly as a medication given by the IV route. Up to 2 mL may be administered intramuscularly as a solution or suspension given in the upper arm, and 5 mL may be given in the gluteal medial muscle of each buttock. A sustained-release–type action can be achieved with certain drugs that have low solubility as they are released from muscle tissue at a slow rate. IM injections are often painful, and reversing adverse effects from medications given by this route is very difficult. Antibiotics are often given by this route.

Subcutaneous route
- Subcutaneous (SC or SQ) injections of solution or suspension are given beneath the surface of the skin. Medications administered by this route are not absorbed as well and have a slower onset of action than medications given by the IV or IM route. The volume of solution or suspension that can be injected subcutaneously is 2 mL or less. Drugs often given by this route include epinephrine, insulin, heparin, and vaccines.

Intradermal route
- An intradermal (ID) injection is injected into the top layer of the skin. The injection is not as deep as a SC injection. Medications used for diagnostic purposes such as a tuberculin (TB) test or an allergy test are often administered by this route. The volume of solution that can be administered intradermally is limited to 0.1 mL. The onset of action and the rate of absorption of medication from this route is slow.

Intra-arterial route
- An intra-arterial injection is injected directly into an artery. It delivers a high drug concentration to the target site with little dilution by the circulation. Generally, this route is used only for radiopaque materials and some antineoplastic agents.

Other routes
- *Intracardiac:* an injection directly into the heart
- *Intra-articular:* administration by injection into a joint space; corticosteroids are often administered by this route for the treatment of arthritis.
- *Intrathecal:* injection into the lumbar intraspinal fluid sacs; local anesthetics are frequently administered via this route during surgical procedures. Preservative-free drugs should be used for intrathecal administration.

2. Definitions for Sterile Product Compounding

admixture: when parenteral dosage forms are combined for administration as a single entity

aseptic processing: when product components, containers, and closures, and the product itself, are sterilized separately and then brought together and assembled in an aseptic environment; the primary objective of aseptic processing is to create a product that is sterile.

aseptic technique: carrying out a procedure or procedures under controlled conditions in a manner that will minimize the chance of contamination; contaminants can be introduced from the environment, equipment and supplies, or personnel (see ISO Classification, below).

controlled area (buffer area): the area the laminar flow workbench is in

critical site: any opening or surface that can provide a pathway between the sterile product and the environment

hypertonic: a solution that contains a higher concentration of dissolved substances than the red blood cell, which causes the red blood cell to shrink

hypotonic: a solution that contains a lower concentration of dissolved substances than the red blood cell, causing the red blood cell to swell and possibly burst

isotonic: a solution that is isotonic has an osmotic pressure close to that of body fluids. This minimizes patient discomfort and damage to red blood cells. Dextrose 5% in water and sodium chloride 0.9% solutions are approximately isotonic.

sterilizing filter: a filter which, when challenged with the microorganism *Brevundimonas diminuta*, at a minimum concentration of 10^7 organisms per cm^2 of filter surface, will produce a sterile effluent; a sterilizing filter has a pore size rating of 0.2 or 0.22 micron.

tonicity: refers to osmotic pressure exerted by a solution from the solutes or dissolved solids present.

validation: establishing documented evidence that provides a high degree of assurance that a specific process will consistently produce a product meeting predetermined specifications and quality attributes

International Organization of Standardization (ISO) Classification

- The International Organization of Standardization (ISO) Classification of Particulate Matter in Room Air is the new standard for clean rooms and associated environments. Limits are expressed in particles 0.5 micron and larger per cubic meter, compared to the limits from Federal Standard 209E, which are in particles 0.5 micron and larger per cubic foot (1 cubic meter = 35.31 cubic feet.)

ISO 5 area

- The air in the area has a count of no more than 3520 particles 0.5 micron or larger per cubic meter of air. This is equivalent to the class 100 area, in which the air in the area has a count of no more than 100 particles that are 0.5 micron or larger per cubic foot of air. This is the quality of air required for sterile product preparation.

ISO 7 area

- The air in the area has a count of no more than 352,000 particles 0.5 micron or larger per cubic meter. This is equivalent to a class 10,000 area, in which the air in the area has a count of no more than 10,000 particles that are 0.5 micron or larger per cubic foot of air.

ISO 8 area

- The air in the area has a count of no more than 3,520,000 particles 0.5 micron or larger per cubic meter. This is equivalent to a class 100,000 area, in which the air in the area has a count of no more than 100,000 particles that are 0.5 micron or larger per cubic foot of air.

3. Sterile Product Preparation Area

Horizontal Laminar Flow Workbench (HLFW)

- The horizontal laminar flow workbench works by drawing air in through the pre-filter. The prefiltered air is pressurized in the plenum for consistent distribution of air to the HEPA (high-efficiency particulate air) filter (Figure 1).
- The pre-filter protects the HEPA filter from prematurely clogging. Pre-filters should be checked regularly and changed as needed. A record of these checks and changes of the pre-filter must be kept.
- The plenum of the hood is the space between the pre-filter and the HEPA filter. Air is pressurized here and distributed over the HEPA filter.
- *Laminar flow* is defined as air in a confined space moving with uniform velocity along parallel lines. Inside the laminar flow workbench is an ISO 5 area (Class 100 area).

Vertical Laminar Flow Workbench (VLFW)

- The vertical laminar flow workbench (VLFW) works just like a HLFW in that the air is drawn in through the pre-filter, and pressurized in the plenum to distribute it over the HEPA filter. However, the air is blown down from the top of the workstation onto the work surface, not across it (Figure 2).

Figure 1.

Horizontal laminar flow workbench.

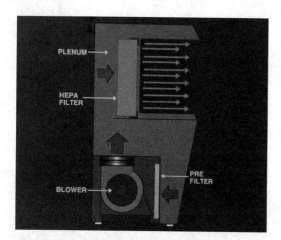

Illustration courtesy of the University of Tennessee Parenteral Medications Lab.

Figure 2.

Vertical laminar flow workbench.

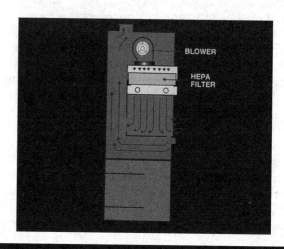

Illustration courtesy of the University of Tennessee Parenteral Medications Lab.

- Working in vertical laminar flow (VLF) requires different techniques than working in horizontal laminar flow (HLF). In VLF, the hands of the operator or any object must not be above an object in the hood. In HLF, the hands of the operator or any object must not be in back of another object. The hands of the operator must never come between the HEPA filter and the object.

The High-Efficiency Particulate Air (HEPA) Filter

- The HEPA filter consists of a bank of filter media separated by corrugated pleats of aluminum. These pleats act as baffles to direct the air into laminar sheets. The HEPA filter is 99.97% efficient at removing particles 0.3 micron and larger.

Certification of the HEPA filter
- The velocity of air from the HEPA filter is checked with a velometer or hot wire anemometer. ISO 14644 recommends that the average air velocity should be >0.2 m/s.

Integrity of the HEPA filter (DOP test)
- The integrity of the HEPA filter is checked by introducing a high concentration of aerosolized Emery 3004 (a synthetic hydrocarbon) upstream of the filter on a continuous basis, while monitoring the penetration on the downstream side of the HEPA filter.

- The aerosol has an average particle size of 0.3 micron. An aerosol photometer is used to check for leaks by passing the wand slowly over the filter and the gasket. None of the surfaces should yield greater than 0.01% of the upstream smoke concentration. Any value greater than 0.01% indicates that a serious leak is present and it must be sealed. All repaired areas must be retested for compliance. At one time DOP (dioctyl phthalate) was used to generate the aerosol. However, since DOP is a carcinogen, Emery 3004 is now used. An electronic particle counter cannot be used to certify the integrity of the HEPA filter. The particle counter is used to determine room classification.

Buffer Area (Controlled Area)

- The laminar flow workstation is the most clean area and has an ISO 5 (class 100) area inside the LFW. It must be located in a controlled environment, away from excess traffic, doors, air vents, or anything that could produce air currents greater than the velocity of the airflow from the HEPA filter. Air currents greater than the velocity of the airflow from the HEPA filter may introduce contaminants into the hood. It is very easy to overcome air flowing at 90 feet per minute.
- The buffer area should be enclosed from other pharmacy operations. Floors, walls, ceiling, shelving, counters, and cabinets of the controlled area must be of nonshedding, smooth, and nonporous material to allow for easy cleaning and disinfecting. All surfaces should be resistant to sanitizing agents. Cracks, crevices, and seams should be avoided, as should ledges or other places that could collect dust. The floor of the buffer area should be smooth and seamless with coved edges up the wall.
- The walls of the buffer area can be sealed panels, or if drywall, painted with epoxy paint, which is nonshedding. The corner of the ceiling and the walls should be sealed to avoid cracks. A solid ceiling may be painted with epoxy paint, or nonshedding washable ceiling tiles that are caulked into place may be used.
- Light fixtures should be mounted flush with the ceiling and sealed. Anything that penetrates the ceiling or walls should be sealed.
- Air entering the room should be fresh, HEPA filtered, and air-conditioned, and the room must be maintained in positive pressure in relation to the adjoining rooms or corridors (air flow should be out from the room, not into it). There should be at least 10 air changes per hour.
- People entering the buffer area should be properly scrubbed and gowned. Access to the buffer area should be restricted only to qualified personnel.

Controlling the traffic in the buffer area is a critical factor in keeping the area clean. Only items required to compound should be brought into the buffer room. These items must be cleaned and sanitized before being taken into the buffer area. Items may be stored in the buffer room for a limited time. However, try and keep the number of items stored in the buffer room to a minimum. All equipment used in the buffer room should remain in the room except for calibration or repair.

- These items should not be in the buffer room (controlled area): Refrigerators and freezers should be kept out of the buffer area, as they can harbor many organisms. Sinks or floor drains should not be in the buffer area for the same reason. If you have a sink or floor drain in the buffer area, disinfectants must be poured down the drain on a regular basis. Computers and printers should be located outside of the buffer area since they generate many particles. Cardboard boxes should also not be stored in the buffer area. However, vials stored in laminated cardboard may be stored in the buffer area.

Preparation of Operators

- The operator must be properly scrubbed before entering the controlled area. This is critical to the maintenance of asepsis. The greatest source of contamination in a clean room is the people in the area. A seated or standing person without movement releases an average of 100,000 particles greater than 0.3 micron in diameter per minute. A person standing up with full body movement releases an average of 2,000,000, particles, and if moving at a slow walk can release an average of 5,000.000 particles per minute greater than 0.3 micron in diameter. The garb is designed to help contain the particles that are being shed.
- The operator should scrub from elbows to hands for an appropriate length of time using an antimicrobial skin cleanser. After scrubbing, the operator should don a hair cover, shoe covers, and a clean knee-length nonshedding gown and sterile latex gloves. Once the gloves are out of the package they are no longer sterile. Frequent rinsing with sterile 70% isopropyl alcohol is essential to keep the gloves sanitized. Before working in the hood the operator should put on a facemask. All facial hair must be covered at all times.

Validation of the Operator

- A *media fill* or *media transfer* is when media is used instead of the drug product, and all the normal compounding manipulations are done. Usually the medium used is soybean casein digest, which is also called trypticase soy broth (TSB). This medium will support the growth of many organisms, including some fungi and mold. A media fill can be used to check an operator's aseptic technique or to validate a compounding process.

- Initially, before an operator can compound low- or medium-risk sterile injectable products he or she must successfully complete one media fill. This means no growth in any of the units. The media fill should closely simulate the most challenging or stressful conditions encountered during the compounding of low-risk and medium-risk products. The operator should perform a revalidation at a minimum of once a year by completing one media fill. Ideally, the media fills should be designed to mimic techniques the operator will use during a normal day. Validation for high-risk compounding focuses on making sure the process, along with the operator, is capable of producing a sterile product with all its purported quality attributes. Revalidation must be done on at least a semi-annual basis. An example of a high-risk operation is the compounding of a sterile product from nonsterile drug powder. All media fills should take place in an ISO 5 environment and must be completed without interruption.

4. Working in the Laminar Flow Workbench

- Items not in a protective overwrap should be wiped with a lint-free wipe soaked with sterile 70% isopropyl alcohol (IPA) before being placed in the hood. Check containers for cracks, tears, and particles. Items in a protective overwrap, such as syringes and bags, should be taken from the overwrap at the edge of the hood (within the first 6 inches of the hood), and placed in the hood with the injection port facing the HEPA filter. The overwrap should not be placed in the hood, as this would introduce particles and organisms into the hood.
- When working in the HLFW, supplies should be arranged to the left or right of the critical work area. The critical site must be in uninterrupted laminar airflow at all times. The operator must be careful not to place an object or hand in between the HEPA filter and the critical site. To do so would interrupt the airflow to the critical site and potentially cause particles to be washed from the hand or object onto the critical site.
- All work done in the HLFW must be done at least 6 inches inside the hood. The laminar air flow is blowing toward the operator. The body acts as a barrier to the laminar airflow, causing it to pass around the person and create backflow. This turbulence can cause room air to be carried into the front of the hood.
- Items placed in the HFLW disturb the laminar flow. The laminar airflow is disturbed downstream of the item for approximately three times the diameter of the object. If the item is placed next to the sidewall of the hood, the airflow is disturbed approximately six times the diameter of the object. Air downstream from the nonsterile objects also becomes contaminated with particles. For these reasons, it is very important that a direct path exists between the HEPA filter and the area where the manipulations will occur.
- With the VLFH, supplies in the hood should be placed so that the operator may work without placing a hand or object above the critical site. It is possible to place many more items in the VLFH and still work without compromising the laminar flow. It must be kept in mind that within 1 inch of the work surface is turbulent air. The air is coming from the HEPA filter and striking the work surface. It then has to change directions and move horizontally across the work surface. All work in the VLFW should be done at least 1 inch above the work surface.

• When compounding sterile products it is important that all movements into and out of the hood be minimized, to decrease the risk of carrying contaminants into the critical site. This can be achieved by introducing all items needed for the aseptic manipulation into the work area at one time, by dropping discarded items over the edge of the hood, or leaving the items within the first 6 inches until the manipulations are complete.

5. Needles, Syringes, Ampuls, and Vials

The Syringe

• The basic parts of the syringe are the barrel, plunger, collar, the rubber tip of the plunger, and the tip of the syringe. The syringes are sterile, pyrogen-free, and packaged either in paper or in a rigid plastic container. It is important that the syringe packages be inspected to make sure the wrap is intact to ensure that the syringe is still sterile. Syringes have either a Luer-Lok tip, in which the needle is screwed tightly onto the threaded tip, or a slip tip, in which case the needle is held on by friction (Figure 3). Syringes are supplied with and without needles attached, and are available in a variety of sizes. Some syringes are packaged with a protective tip on them to keep the syringe sterile until the needle is attached. Other syringes do not have the protective tip, so care must be taken not to lay the syringe down under the hood until the needle has been attached.

• There are calibration marks on the barrel of the syringe. These marks are accurate to one-half the interval marked on the syringe. The critical sites on the syringe are the tip of the syringe and the ribs of the plunger. This is because the ribs of the plunger go back inside the syringe upon injection of the fluid from the syringe and could potentially contaminate the syringe.

Figure 3.

Types of syringes.

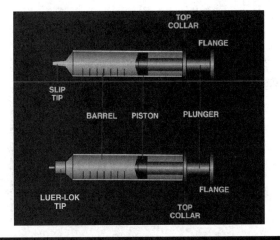

Illustration courtesy of the University of Tennessee Parenteral Medications Lab.

The Needle

- The basic parts of a needle include the hub, needle shaft, bevel, bevel heel, and the tip of the needle (Figure 4).
- Needles are sterile and come wrapped in plastic with a twist-off top or wrapped in paper. This wrap must be inspected for integrity before using the needle. The gauge of the needle refers to the outer diameter of the needle. The larger the number, the smaller the bore of the needle. The smallest is 27 gauge and the largest is 13 gauge. The length of the needle is measured in inches, and the most common lengths are 1-1$\frac{1}{2}$ inches.
- The critical sites on the needle are the hub of the needle, the needle shaft, and the tip of the needle.

Ampuls

- Ampuls are single-dose containers. Once ampuls are broken, they are an open-system container, and air can pass freely in and out of the ampul. Any solution taken from an ampul must be filtered with a 5-micron filter needle, because glass particles fall into the ampul when it is broken. Before breaking the ampul, the neck of the ampul should be wiped with a sterile alcohol prep pad.

Vials

- A vial is a molded glass or plastic container with a rubber closure secured in place with an aluminum seal. They may contain sterile solutions, dry-filled powders, lyophilized drugs, or may be an empty evacuated container. Vials may be single-dose or multiple-dose containers.
- A single-dose container usually contains no preservative system to prevent the growth of microorganisms if they are accidentally introduced into the container. The proposed revision of UPS <797> states that a single-dose vial punctured in an environment worse than ISO class 5 air shall be used within 1 hour. Currently, single-dose vials continuously exposed to ISO class 5 air may be used up to 6 hours after initial needle puncture. When the vial is first used, it should be labeled with the date, time, and initials of the person using the vial so the length of time the vial has been in the hood can be determined.
- A multi-dose vial contains preservatives, and these vials can be entered more than once. The pharmaceutical manufacturer has done studies to prove the preservative system will remain effective and the closure will reseal after penetration by the needle. Therefore the beyond-use date for opened or entered multiple-dose containers is 28 days, unless otherwise specified by the manufacturer.

Figure 4.

Needle.

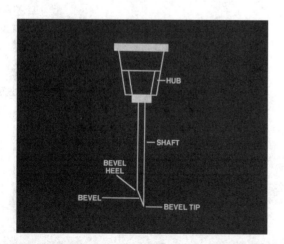

Illustration courtesy of the University of Tennessee Parenteral Medications Lab.

6. Biological Safety Cabinets

• A class II biological safety cabinet (BSC) should be used to prepare cytotoxic and other hazardous drugs. All BSCs are vertical flow hoods, but not all vertical flow hoods are BSCs. There are four different types of class II BSCs. The most often used is a class II type A cabinet, which has approximately 70% of the air recirculated and 30% of the air exhausted through a HEPA filter into the room. Intake of the make-up air is through the front grill of the workbench.

Preparation of Cytotoxic Drugs

• When working with cytotoxic drugs it is imperative that positive pressure is not allowed to build up in the vial. It is recommended that some type of air venting device be used, such as a Chemo Dispensing Pin®. The 0.2-micron hydrophobic filter on this device allows air to pass in and out of the vial, but prevents the passage of aerosolized drug (Figure 5). If this type of device is not available, care must be taken to keep the vial at negative pressure to prevent spewing of drug into the BSC.

• When preparing cytotoxic drugs it is recommended that the operator wear a nonshedding and nonabsorptive gown with a closed front and elastic or knit cuffs. Sterile gloves should be worn, and the operator should double-glove. The first set of gloves should be put under the cuff of the gown and the second pair should be pulled up over the cuff of the gown.

• When compounding, syringes and IV sets with Luer-Lok fittings should be used. Use a large enough syringe so the plunger does not separate from the barrel of the syringe when filled with solution. When possible, attach IV sets and prime them before adding the hazardous drug. Wipe the outside of the bag or bottle to remove any inadvertent contamination. The use of nonshedding plastic-backed absorbent pads is also conducive to keeping the BSC as clean as possible.

Figure 5.

Chemo Dispensing Pin.

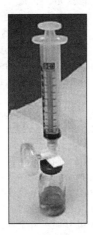

Illustration courtesy of the University of Tennessee Parenteral Medications Lab.

7. Overview of Standards of Practice Related to Sterile Products

American Society of Health-System Pharmacists (ASHP)

- The ASHP published the Technical Assistance Bulletin on Quality Assurance for Pharmacy-Prepared Sterile Products in September 1993. This document has been revised and is now called the ASHP Guidelines on Quality Assurance for Pharmacy-Prepared Sterile Products.
- This document groups sterile products into three risk levels based on the risk to the patient posed by the compounded product. Level I products have the least risk and level III products have the greatest risk for the patient. Some factors can increase the risk of microbial contamination of the product, such as increased complexity of compounding steps, lengthy exposure of the critical site, increased storage time, and the temperature of the prepared injectable product. The document provides a method to match quality assurance/quality control (QA/QC) activities with the potential risk of the product to the patient. Information is provided on QA/QC activities that should be in place.
- For risk levels I and II the product is prepared using sterile equipment, ingredients, solutions, and sterile contact surfaces for the final product.

A level I product exhibits a, b, and c, below:
a. Stored at room temperature and administered within 28 hours, or refrigerated under USP conditions for ≤7 days, or frozen for ≤30 days prior to complete administration to a patient over a period not to exceed 24 hours
b. A product prepared for one patient that is unpreserved or a batch product compounded for multiple patients that contains a preservative
c. A product prepared by closed-system aseptic transfer of sterile product to sterile final container

If the compounded product exhibits a, b, or c, below, it is considered a level II product:
a. Stored beyond 7 days in the refrigerator or greater than 30 days in the freezer, or administered beyond 28 hours from preparation time at room temperature
b. Sterile batch preparation made without preservatives, intended for use by more than one patient
c. Product compounded by combining multiple sterile ingredients, obtained from a licensed manufacturer using closed-system aseptic transfer, before subdivision into multiple units to be dispensed to patients

Any compounded parenteral product that exhibits a or b, below, is a level III product:
a. Sterile products made from nonsterile ingredients or using nonsterile components or equipment
b. Prepared by combining multiple ingredients, sterile or nonsterile, by using open-system transfer or open reservoir before terminal sterilization or subdivision into multiple dispensing units

The United States Pharmacopeia 28/ National Formulary 23

- Chapter <797>, Pharmaceutical Compounding–Sterile Preparations in USP 28/NF 23, became official January 2004. This change of chapter number from <1206> to <797> is very important. Chapters numbered <1> to <999> contain general requirements. Chapters numbered <1000> to <1999> are informational only. Chapter <797> has three risk levels of compounded sterile products. The risk levels are determined based on the potential for the introduction of microorganisms, spores, and endotoxins into the product. The potential of contaminating the product with chemical and physical contaminants is evaluated. The chapter covers such topics as validation of sterilization and of the aseptic process, environmental control and monitoring, end-product testing, bacterial endotoxins, training, and a quality assurance program.

Compounding is classified as low-risk when all of the following conditions prevail:
1. Commercially available sterile products, components, and devices are used in compounding within an ISO class 5 or better air quality
2. Compounding involves few aseptic manipulations.
3. Closed-system transfers are used. Withdrawal from an open ampul is classified as a closed system.
4. In the absence of passing a sterility test the storage periods cannot exceed the following time periods before administration:
    a. stored for not more than 48 hours at controlled room temperature
    b. stored for not more than 14 days at a cold temperature of 2-8°C
    c. stored for not more than 45 days in solid frozen state at −20°C or colder

Medium-risk compounds are compounded under low-risk conditions and one or more of the following conditions exist:

1. Compounding involves pooling of additives for the administration to either multiple patients or to one patient on multiple occasions.
2. Compounding involves complex manipulations other than a single volume transfer.
3. The compounding process requires a long time to complete dissolution or homogeneous mixing.
4. The finished product does not contain a bacteriostatic substance and is administered over several days.
5. In the absence of passing a sterility test the storage periods cannot exceed the following time periods before administration:
   a. exposed for not more than 30 hours at controlled room temperature
   b. stored for not more than 7 days at a cold temperature
   c. stored for not more than 45 days in a solid frozen state at –20°C or colder

High-risk level compounds are compounded under any of the following conditions. They are either contaminated or at high risk to become contaminated with infectious microorganisms:

1. A sterile product compounded from nonsterile ingredients
2. Sterile ingredients or components are exposed to air quality inferior to ISO class 5; this includes storage in environments inferior to ISO class 5 of opened or partially used packages of manufactured sterile products with no antimicrobial preservative system.
3. Nonsterile preparations are exposed for at least 6 hours before being sterilized.
4. No examination of labeling and documentation from suppliers or direct determination that the chemical purity and content strength of ingredients meet their original or compendia specification
5. In the absence of passing a sterility test the storage periods cannot exceed the following time periods before administration:
   a. stored for not more than 24 hours at controlled room temperature
   b. stored for not more than 3 days at a cold temperature
   c. stored for not more than 45 days in solid frozen state at –20°C or colder

8. Sterilization Methods

Filtration

- Filtration works by a combination of sieving, adsorption, and entrapment. When deciding which filter to use to sterilize the product, care must be taken to choose the correct filter. Membrane filters generally are compatible with most pharmaceutical solutions, but interactions do occur. This is often due to sorption or leaching. Sorption is the binding of drug or other formulation components to the filter. This can occur with peptide or protein formulations. There are filters that have little or no affinity for peptides or proteins. Leaching is the extracting of components of the filter into the solution. Often surfactants are added to the filter to make it hydrophilic, and these may leach into the product. Large-molecular-weight peptides may be affected by filtration. The passage through a filter with a small pore size may cause shear stress and alter the three-dimensional structure of the peptide. Filters may also be affected by solvents in the parenteral formulation. All filter manufacturers have compatibility data on their membrane type and are a great source of information when choosing a membrane.

Choosing a Filter

- Choose the appropriate size and configuration of filtration device that will accommodate the volume being filtered to permit complete filtration without clogging of the membrane. A 25-mm syringe disk filter should filter no more than 100 mL of solution. If the solution you are filtering has a heavy particulate load, a 5-micron filter should be used before the 0.2-micron filter to decrease the particulate load to the 0.2-micron filter. The filter membrane and housing must be physically and chemically compatible with the product to be filtered and capable of withstanding the temperature, pressures, and hydrostatic stress imposed on the system.
- A pharmacy may rely on the certificate of quality provided by the vendor. Certification should include microbial retention testing with *Brevundimonas diminuta* at a minimum concentration of 10^7 organisms per cm^2, as well as testing for membrane and housing integrity, nonpyrogenicity, and extractables.

Hydrophobic and Hydrophilic Filters

- *Hydrophilic membranes* wet spontaneously with water. They are used for filtration of aqueous solutions and aqueous solutions containing water-miscible solvents. *Hydrophobic filters* do not wet spontaneously with water. They are used for filtering gases and solvents.

Filter Integrity

- A sterilizing filter assembly should be tested for integrity after filtration has occurred. The *bubble point* is a simple, nondestructive check of the integrity of the filtration assembly, including the filter membrane. The test is based on the fact that liquid is held in the capillary structure of the membrane by surface tension. The minimum pressure required to force the liquid out of the capillary space is a measure of the largest pores in the membrane.
- A bubble point test is performed by wetting the filter with water, increasing the pressure of air upstream of the filter, and watching for air bubbles downstream, to indicate passage of air through the filter capillaries. The typical water bubble point pressure of a sterilizing filter with a pore size rating of 0.2 micron is >50 pounds per square inch gauge (psig). As pore size decreases, the bubble point increases. Keep in mind that the bubble point given on the certificate of quality from the filter manufacturer is usually the water bubble point. Many drug formulations have a lower surface tension than water and will have a lower bubble point. Bubble points are also often given for 70% IPA and water. If you have a hydrophobic filter, you should use the alcohol test.
- After filtration of your solution, and before checking the integrity of the filter membrane, the filter should be flushed with water to wash the product off the membrane as much as possible. Then the integrity test may be performed.

Heat Sterilization

Moist-heat sterilization (autoclave)
- Moist-heat sterilization is one of the most widely used methods of sterilization. Saturation of steam at high pressure is the foundation for the effectiveness of moist heat sterilization. When steam makes contact with a cooler object, it condenses and loses latent heat to the object. The amount of energy released is ~524 kcal/g at 121°C. Most sterilization cycles are at 121°C at 15 psig for a minimum of 15 minutes. Moist heat sterilization is quicker and does not require as high a temperature as dry heat.

Dry-heat sterilization
- Dry-heat sterilization is usually done as a batch process in an oven designed for sterilization. It is designed to provide heated filtered air that is evenly distributed throughout the chamber by a blower. The oven is equipped with a system to control the temperature and exposure period. Dry-heat sterilization requires higher temperatures and longer exposure times than moist-heat sterilization. Typical sterilization cycles are 120-180 minutes at 160°C or 90-120 minutes at 170°C. Dry heat is also used to depyrogenate equipment.

9. Stability

- Each compounded sterile product must have a label that specifies the product's storage requirements and the expiration date. Stability refers to physical, chemical, and microbial stability. Any product that is not meant for immediate use should be refrigerated at a temperature no higher than 4°C, as this is the temperature that will inhibit microbial growth. If the sterile product is intended for multi-day administration, the infusion should be started as soon as possible after preparation. There are several good references available on drug stability, such as *Trissel's Handbook on Injectable Drugs*. When compounding sterile products for home use, there is often a need to push the envelope on expiration dating. When setting the expiration date, consideration must be given to the concentration of the product, the temperature at which the product will be administered, and the duration of administration. For example, if the product will be in an implantable infusion device where it will be exposed to body temperature for several days, the stability data referenced must take into account the increased temperature and the increase in concentration that is required for this dosing regimen. The most accurate way to determine stability is to do a product-specific experiment.
- *Instability* usually refers to chemical reactions that are incessant, irreversible, and result in distinctly different chemical entities. These new chemical entities can be both therapeutically inactive and possibly exhibit greater toxicity.
- *Incompatibility* usually refers to physicochemical phenomena such as concentration-dependent precipitation and acid-base reactions that occur when one drug is mixed with others to produce a product unsuitable for administration to the patient. An incompatibility could cause the patient not to receive the full therapeutic effect, or toxic decomposition products could form. A precipitated incompatibility may irritate the vein or cause occlusion of vessels.
- There are three categories of incompatibilities: *therapeutic incompatibility, physical incompatibility,* and *chemical incompatibility.*

Therapeutic Incompatibility

- This results when two or more drugs administered at the same time result in undesirable antagonistic or synergistic pharmacologic action.

Physical Incompatibility

- This is the combination of two or more drugs in solution, resulting in a change in the appearance of the solution, a change in color, formation of turbidity or a precipitate, or the evolution of a gas. Physical incompatibilities are related to solubility changes or container interactions rather than to molecular change to the drug entity itself.

Six major areas of concern about physical incompatibility:

1. *The compatibility or incompatibility of two or more drugs mixed in the same syringe.*
   For example, preoperative medications: a combination of a narcotic, an analgesic, an antiemetic, and an anticholinergic; these drugs are mixed in the same syringe to save the patient from multiple IM injections.

2. *The compatibility of two or more drugs given through the same IV administration line.*
   This is common in intensive care units where patients are on a number of IV meds and could also be fluid restricted.
   An example: dopamine HCl 800 mg in 500 mL D_5W. The nurse wants to push 2 amps of sodium bicarbonate through the IV line.
   pH of dopamine: 3.0-4.5
   pH of $NaHCO_3$: ~8
   If this is done a color change occurs due to decomposition of the product. The pH of the bicarb is too high for dopamine stability.

3. *Compatibility of two or more drugs placed in the same bottle or bag of IV fluid.*
   KCl, the most common additive, is a neutral salt composed of monovalent ions which are not likely to produce compatibility problems. Therefore, if a drug is compatible in NS, it is probably compatible in KCl.

- Parenteral nutrition solutions can be especially difficult. The number of components, the long duration of contact time, and exposure to ambient temperature and light enhance the potential for an adverse compatibility interaction to occur. The interaction of Ca and PO_4 to form $CaPO_4$, which appears as fine white particles that create a milky solution, is a problem.

   Ways to decrease the risk of injury:
   a. Calculate the solubility of the added calcium from the volume at the time when calcium is added. Flush the line between addition of any potentially incompatible components.
   b. Add the calcium before the lipid emulsion, so if a precipitate forms, the lipid will not obscure its presence.

c. Periodically agitate the admixture and check for precipitates. Train patients and caregivers to visually inspect for signs of precipitation and to stop the infusion if precipitation is noted.

- The following factors enhance formation of precipitate of calcium and phosphate:
    * High concentrations of calcium and phosphate
    * Increases in solution pH
    * Decreases in amino acid concentrations
    * Increases in temperature
    * Addition of calcium before phosphate
    * Lengthy time delay or slow infusion rates
    * Use of the chloride salt of calcium
- Do not exceed 15 mEq of calcium with up to 15 mL PO$_4$ per 1000 mL of solution.

4. *Compatibility of the additive with the composition of the IV container itself.*
    Nitroglycerin readily migrates into many plastics, especially PVC. Insulin adsorbs to both glass and plastic containers, IV tubing, and filters.

5. *Compatibility of the additive with the additional equipment used to prepare or administer the IV admixture.*
    Cisplatin interacts with aluminum by forming a black precipitate when coming in contact with it.

6. *Stability of the drug after admixture.*
    Ampicillin sodium is stable for 72 hours refrigerated and 24 hours at room temperature in normal saline. However, if it is added to D$_5$W, it is stable for only 4 hours refrigerated and 2 hours at room temperature.

Other potential sources of physical incompatibilities
Concentration
- A drug will remain in aqueous solution as long as its concentration is less than its saturation solubility.

Cosolvent system
- Drugs that are poorly water soluble are often formulated using water-miscible cosolvents. Examples of water-miscible cosolvents include ethanol, propylene glycol, and polyethylene glycol. Dilution of drugs that are in a cosolvent system often causes precipitation of the drug. A good example is diazepam injection. Dilution of the drug results in precipitation in some concentrations, but sufficient dilution to a point below diazepam's saturation solubility results in a physically stable admixture.

pH
- The greatest single factor in causing an incompatibility is a change in acid-base environment. Solubility of drugs that are weak acids or bases is a direct function of solution pH. The drug's dissocia-

tion constant and pH control the portion of drug in its ionized form and the solubility of the un-ionized form. A drug that is a weak acid may be formulated at a pH sufficient to yield the desired solubility. Sodium salts of barbiturates, phenytoin, and methotrexate are formulated at high pH values to achieve adequate solubility.
- Sodium salts of weak acids precipitate as free acids when added to IV fluids having an acidic pH. If the pH of these drugs is lowered, the drug's solubility at the final pH may be exceeded, resulting in possible precipitation. Drugs that are salts of weak bases may precipitate in an alkaline solution.

Ionic interactions
- Large organic anions and cations may also form precipitates. An example of this is the precipitation that occurs when heparin (anionic) and aminoglycoside antibiotics (cationic) are mixed. These heparin salts of the cationic drug are relatively insoluble in water.

Sorption phenomena
- The intact drug is lost from the solution by adsorption to the surface or absorption into the matrix of container material, administration set, or filter.
- Adsorption to the surface can result from interactions of functional groups within the drug's molecule to binding sites on the surfaces.
- Absorption of lipid-soluble drug into the matrix of plastic containers and administration sets, especially those made from polyvinyl chloride (PVC), does occur. The substantial amount of phthalate plasticizer used to make the PVC bag pliable and flexible allows the lipid-soluble drugs to diffuse from the solution into the plasticizer in the plastic matrix. Plastics such as polyethylene and polypropylene, which contain little or no phthalate plasticizer, do not readily absorb lipid-soluble drug into the polymer core. Leaching of the phthalate plasticizer into the solution may also occur, especially if surface-active agents or a large amount of organic cosolvent is present in the formulation.

Chemical Incompatibility

- Chemical incompatibilities are interactions resulting in molecular changes or rearrangements to different chemical entities. Most chemical interactions are not visibly observable.

Chemical degradation pathways
- *Hydrolysis* is a common mode of chemical decomposition. Water attacks labile bonds in dissolved drug molecules. Functional groups labile to hydrolysis are carboxylic acid and phosphate esters, amides, lactams, and imines.

- *Oxidation* is an electron loss, causing a positive increase in valence. Many drugs are in the reduced form and oxygen creates stability problems. Steroids, epinephrine, and tricyclic compounds are sensitive to oxygen. To control the stability problem, oxygen can be excluded, pH can be adjusted, and chelating agents or antioxidants can be added.
- *Reduction* is when an electron is gained, causing a decrease in valence and the addition of halogen or hydrogen to the double bond. β-Lactam antibiotics can produce reducing aldehydes upon hydrolysis.
- *Photolysis* is the catalysis by light of degradation reactions such as oxidation or hydrolysis. Examples of drugs that are light sensitive are amphotericin B, furosemide, and sodium nitroprusside. The reaction rate depends on the intensity and wavelength of light. Sodium nitroprusside in D_5W has a faint brownish cast, but exposure to light causes deterioration, which is evident by a change to a blue color due to the reduction of the ferric to ferrous ion.
- *Extreme pH* can be a catalysis of drug degradation. Drug reaction rates are generally less at intermediate pH values than at high or low ranges. Many times a buffer system is used to ensure the maintenance of the proper pH.
- *Effects of temperature.* Usually, but not always, an elevation in temperature may increase reaction rates.
- *An increase in drug concentration* will usually increase the degradation rate exponentially. Again, this rule does not always apply. Some drugs appear to have a lower rate of decomposition at high concentration. An example of this is the reduced hydrolysis of nafcillin in the presence of aminophylline. Greater buffer concentration at higher nafcillin concentrations protects the drug from aminophylline's high pH and slows the hydrolysis.
- *Expiration dates and removal of IV bag overwrap.* The overwrap protects against evaporation of the solution, desiccation of the container, drug oxidation, and photochemical inactivation of the drug. Substantial moisture loss may occur, increasing drug concentration. With ready-to-use dopamine or dobutamine injections, removal of the overwrap can allow oxygen to enter the container, reducing drug stability. After removal of the overwrap the expiration date should be changed at once.

10. Sterile Products Compounded from Nonsterile Drugs

- When compounding a sterile drug product from a nonsterile component, several concerns arise: how to sterilize the drug and/or the container and closure; and how to ensure the drug and components are sterile. All sterilization processes must be validated, whether it is terminal sterilization of the product in the final container or aseptic processing of the product. End-product testing must be done on all high-risk-level compounded sterile products (CSPs) if they are prepared in groups of more than 25 single-dose packages, or in multiple-dose vials for administration to multiple patients and are for administration by injection into the vascular or central nervous system. High-risk-level CSPs that are exposed longer than 12 hours to temperatures of 2-8°C and longer than 6 hours at warmer than 8° before sterilization must also undergo end product testing. Besides visual inspection for particulate matter and compounding accuracy checks, end-product testing for the high-risk products meeting the above criteria must include the sterility test and the bacterial endotoxin test. The product should not be dispensed from the pharmacy until the results of the bacterial endotoxin test are known. Because the USP sterility test takes 14 days, the sterile product is usually dispensed before the results are known. However, a method must be in place to track the product in case it does not meet the requirement of the sterility test.

Sterility Testing

- There are two methods of sterility testing: direct inoculation and membrane filtration. The USP states that when possible, membrane filtration should be performed, and two culture media are required: fluid thioglycollate medium (FTM) and trypticase soy broth (TSB), also called soybean casein digest medium.

Media suitability test

- Before beginning the test it must be confirmed that the medium being used is sterile, and it will support the growth of microorganisms.

Sterility

- Confirm the sterility of each sterilized batch of medium by incubating a portion of the batch at the specified incubation temperature (TSB 20-25°C, FTM 30-35°C) for 14 days, or by incubating uninoculated containers as negative controls during a sterility test procedure. When purchasing a new batch of sterile media from a vendor, it is advisable to incubate a portion for several days to make sure it did not become contaminated during shipment.

Growth promotion test (GP)

- Each lot of ready-prepared medium and each batch of dehydrated medium bearing the manufacturer's lot number must be tested for its growth-promoting qualities. Separately inoculate, in duplicate, containers of each medium with fewer than 100 viable microorganisms of each of the strains listed below. If visual evidence of growth appears in all inoculated media containers within 3 days of incubation in the case of bacteria and 5 days of incubation in the case of fungi, the test media is satisfactory. The test may be conducted simultaneously with testing of the media for sterility.
- The organisms to be used for the growth promotion test of fluid thioglycollate media are *Staphylococcus aureus* (*Bacillus subtilis* may be used instead), *Pseudomonas aeruginosa* (*Micrococcus luteus* may be used instead), and *Clostridium sporogenes* (*Bacteroides vulgatus* may be used instead). The test organisms for soybean casein digest media are *Bacillus subtilis*, *Candida albicans,* and *Aspergillus niger.* Soybean casein digest media is incubated at 20-25°C, and fluid thioglycollate media is incubated at 30-35°C, both under aerobic conditions.

Validation test bacteriostasis/fungistasis test (B&F)

- The B&F must be done on each product to determine if the product itself will inhibit the growth of microorganisms. This test only needs to be done one time for each product tested. The organisms used are the same as for growth promotion. The test uses two sets of containers. One set is inoculated with the drug product and microorganisms. The other set is inoculated with just the microorganisms. Both sets will be incubated at the appropriate temperature for no more than 5 days. The same amount of growth should be seen in both sets.

Number of articles to test

- Below is the minimum number of articles to be tested in relation to the number of articles in the batch:
  - * For up to 100 articles, test 10% or 4 articles, whichever is greater.
  - * For more than 100 but not more than 500 articles, test 10 articles.

Interpretation of results

No growth

- At days 3, 5, 7, and 14, examine the media visually for growth. If no microbial growth is seen, the article complies with the test for sterility. No growth does not prove that all units in the lot are sterile.

Growth observed

- When microbial growth is observed and confirmed microscopically, the article does not meet the requirements of the test for sterility. If there is no doubt that the microbial growth can be ascribed to faulty aseptic techniques or materials used in conducting the testing procedure, the test is invalid and must be repeated.
- An investigation must take place, and the organism must be identified down to the species. All records must be reviewed, including all employee training procedures and records, aseptic gowning practices, equipment maintenance records, component sterilization data, and environmental monitoring data.

Visual inspection

- Every unit compounded in the pharmacy should be subjected to a physical inspection against a white background and a black background.
- Any container whose contents show evidence of contamination with visible foreign material must be rejected.

Pyrogens

- An endotoxin is a type of pyrogen. A pyrogen is a substance that produces fever.
- Gram-negative bacteria produce more potent endotoxins than gram-positive bacteria and fungi. The lipopolysaccharide (LPS) portion of the cell wall causes the pyrogenic response. The LPS can be sloughed off and the bacteria do not have to be living for the LPS to be pyrogenic.
- Some of the effects caused by pyrogens in the body are an increase in body temperature, chills, cutaneous vasoconstriction, a decrease in respiration, an increase in arterial blood pressure, nausea and malaise, and severe diarrhea.
- The official endotoxin limits are 5 endotoxin units (EU)/kg per hour or 350 EU/total body per hour for drugs and biologicals. Drugs for intrathecal use have a much lower endotoxin limit of 0.2 EU/kg.
- Water is the number one source of pyrogens. This is because *Pseudomonas,* a gram-negative bacterium, grows readily in water. Other sources of endotoxins or pyrogens are raw material, equipment, processing, and human contamination. It is very important to use good quality raw materials, and request a certificate of analysis with each lot of material when compounding. Endotoxins can be destroyed by dry heat. Three to five hours at 200°C will depyrogenate glass vials and beakers. The endotoxin concentration can be reduced by rinsing with sterile water for injection. When compounding a sterile product from a nonsterile product, any equipment that can withstand the heat of 200°C should be depyrogenated. If an article is depyrogenated it is also sterile. Endotoxins are not

completely removed by filtration, and steam sterilization only reduces endotoxin levels by a small amount.

Pyrogen test (rabbit test)

- The pyrogen test is designed to limit, to an acceptable level, the patient's risk of febrile reaction in the patient to the administration, by injection, of the product concerned. The test involves measuring the rise in the temperature of rabbits following the intravenous injection of a test solution, and is designed for products that can be tolerated by the test rabbit in a dose, not to exceed 10 mL/kg, injected intravenously within a period of no more than 10 minutes.
- The rabbit test has several limitations. It is an invivo method, it is expensive and time-consuming, and it is not a very sensitive test. Drugs that have pyretic side effects, or that are antipyretics, cannot be tested by the rabbit test. The test is not quantitative, and the pyrogenic response is dose-dependent, not concentration-dependent.

Bacterial endotoxin test (limulus amebocyte lysate test; LAL)

- The bacterial endotoxin test (BET) provides a method for estimating the concentration of bacterial endotoxins that may be present in, or on the sample of, the article to which the test is applied using LAL reagent. The blood cells of the horseshoe crab are sensitive to endotoxin and form a gel in its presence. LAL reagent is made from the lysate of amebocytes from the horseshoe crab.
- There are two types of techniques for this test. The gel-clot technique, which is based on the formation of the gel, and the photometric technique, which is based on either the development of turbidity or the development of color in the test sample.
- The routine gel-clot test requires 0.1 mL of test sample to be mixed with 0.1 mL of LAL reagent. This mixture is incubated for 1 hour at 37°C. A positive reaction is confirmed by formation of a firm gel that remains intact when the tube is slowly inverted 180 degrees.
- The BET is 5-50 times more sensitive, more simple and rapid, and less expensive than the pyrogen test. However, the clotting enzyme is heat sensitive, pH sensitive, and chemically related to trypsin. It is only dependable for detection of pyrogens originating from gram-negative bacteria. Also, some drugs can inhibit the reaction, while other drugs can enhance the reaction. The BET does not determine the fever-producing potential of the bacterial endotoxins.
- The photometric technique requires the establishment of a standard regression curve. The endotoxin content of the test material is determined by interpolation from the curve. The test can either be an endpoint determination, with the reading made immediately at the end of the incubation period, or a kinetic test, in which the absorbance is measured throughout the reaction period.

11. Key Points

- A sterilizing filter (0.2 micron) is required to filter sterilize a drug product. The filter must be integrity tested before the product may be released. The test is often referred to as the "bubble point test."
- The HEPA (high-efficiency particulate air) filter is 99.97% efficient at filtering out particles 0.3 microns and larger. Certification of the HEPA filter involves testing the velocity of airflow from the filter and the integrity of the filter.
- The air in an ISO class 5 area has no more than 3520 particles 0.5 microns and larger per cubic meter of air. The laminar flow workbench provides an ISO class 5 area.
- The critical site is any opening or pathway between the product and the environment. The larger the critical site and the longer it is exposed to the environment, the greater the risk of contamination of the product.
- The bacterial endotoxin test is designed to detect the level of bacterial endotoxin from gram-negative organisms in the drug product. All bacterial endotoxins are pyrogens, but not all pyrogens are bacterial endotoxins.
- The sterility test and the bacterial endotoxin test should be done on all high-risk-level compounded sterile products intended for administration by injection into the vascular or central nervous system that are prepared in groups of more than 25 identical individual single-dose packages, or in multiple-dose vials for administration to multiple patients. The bacterial endotoxin test must be done before the product can be dispensed.
- Any pharmacist preparing sterile products must have training in aseptic technique. One way to validate aseptic technique is by performing media fills. The growth media most often used is trypticase soy broth, also called soybean casein digest in the USP.
- The laminar airflow in a horizontal laminar flow workbench (HLFW) flows toward the operator. The pharmacist must never put his or her hands in back of an object, between the HEPA filter and the critical site.
- The laminar airflow in a vertical laminar flow workbench (VLFW) flows down onto the work surface.
- A biological safety cabinet should always be used for preparing cytotoxic drugs. All biological safety cabinets have vertical laminar flow.
- The hot air oven is used to depyrogenate items used in compounding.
- Moist-heat sterilization is a common way to sterilize equipment used in the compounding process. Only items that can be moistened by steam can be sterilized by autoclaving.

12. Questions and Answers

1. A high-risk-level compounded sterile product which will be administered by intravascular injection and is prepared in a lot size of 30 single-dose vials must undergo all of these tests except one before release to a patient. Choose the test that does not have to be completed before release of the product.

    A. Bacterial endotoxin test
    B. Visual inspection
    C. Sterility test
    D. Verification of the sterilizing filter integrity
    E. LAL test

2. Choose the correct answer concerning certification of a laminar flow workbench.

    A. The particles introduced into the plenum of the hood must be approximately 0.5 micron in size
    B. Air flow from the HEPA filter must be 120 fpm
    C. A leak of 0.01% of the upstream smoke concentration through the filter is considered a serious leak
    D. A total particle counter can be used to check the integrity of the HEPA filter
    E. If a HEPA filter leaks it cannot be patched but must be replaced

3. Please choose the correct answer. The bacterial endotoxin test is used to determine:

    A. the amount of pyrogens
    B. the level of pyrogens from gram-negative bacteria
    C. the fever-producing potential of bacterial endotoxins from gram-negative bacteria
    D. the level of bacterial endotoxin from gram-positive bacteria
    E. the amount of live bacteria present in the drug solution

4. Please choose the correct answer concerning USP media transfers.

    A. An operator must successfully complete one media fill before compounding any sterile products
    B. An operator who passes a written exam may compound sterile products until the chief pharmacist gets time to watch their aseptic

technique

C. An operator who has successfully completed a media fill must requalify semi-annually if they are preparing low-risk-level products

D. Once an operator successfully completes one media fill for high-risk compounding, they need to revalidate quarterly by completing one media fill

E. Fluid thioglycollate media is used for media transfers

5. Choose the correct answer. When transferring product into the controlled area:

A. bottles, bags, and syringes must be removed from brown cardboard boxes before being brought into the buffer area

B. vials stored in laminated cardboard may not be brought into the controlled area

C. stainless steel carts may be used to transfer items into the controlled area directly from the storage area

D. large-volume parenteral bags of IV solution must be removed from their protective overwrap before being brought into the controlled area

E. the refrigerator should be placed next to the laminar flow hood for easy access

6. Choose the correct answer concerning a vertical laminar flow hood.

A. A VLFH is always a biological safety cabinet

B. In vertical laminar flow the hands of the operator must not be behind an object

C. A VLFH has turbulent airflow within 1 inch of the work surface

D. A VLFH has the laminar flow air blowing at the operator

E. The operator works in a vertical flow hood and a horizontal flow hood in the same manner

7. Certain factors may increase the risk of microbial contamination of a sterile product. Please choose the item that would not be a risk factor.

A. Very complex compounding steps

B. Lengthy exposure of a critical site during compounding

C. Using appropriate aseptic technique

D. Batch compounding for multiple patients without preservatives

E. Preparing a sterile product from nonsterile powders

8. Choose the true statement concerning the ASHP risk levels of compounded sterile products.

A. Products intended for administration over 3 days would be classified as risk level I

B. A sterile product that is stored in the refrigerator for 6 days would be classified as a risk level II product

C. A sterile product that is unpreserved and compounded for one patient is classified as a risk level II product

D. An intrathecal injection compounded from nonsterile powder would be classified as a risk level III product

E. A batch of unpreserved product prepared for multiple patients is at risk level I

9. Choose the correct statement.

A. When working in a horizontal laminar flow workbench, arrange items in the hood such that when working, one's hand never is between the HEPA filter and an object

B. When working in a horizontal laminar flow workbench, vials that are not being used should be stacked up along the side of the hood to increase workspace in the hood

C. 70% isopropyl alcohol is used to sterilize the laminar flow workbench before each shift

D. An object placed in the HLFW disturbs the airflow downstream of the object equal to two times the diameter of the object

E. Syringes and IV bags are placed in the hood in their protective overwrap

10. Operators in the buffer area must be properly gowned. Choose the correct statement.

A. Operators gown because they shed particles and the nonshedding gowns keep the operator sterile

B. Sterile gloves are used so that if the operator accidentally touches a critical site during compounding of the sterile product it will not become contaminated

C. Frequent sanitization with sterile 70% isopropyl alcohol is essential in order to keep your hands sterile during the compounding process

D. Nonshedding garb and sterile gloves help to contain the particles shed from the operator

E. Operators must gown before working at the laminar flow workbench, but not before entering the buffer area

11. Concerning placement of items in the laminar flow workstation and working in the laminar flow workstation, choose the correct answer.

    A. Items should be placed in a horizontal flow hood to the right or left of the work area
    B. Items in a vertical laminar flow hood should be placed so that when working in the hood your hand never goes over the top of a critical site
    C. An object placed in a horizontal flow hood disturbs the airflow three times the diameter of the object downstream of the object
    D. When working in a horizontal laminar flow workstation, all work must be done at least 6 inches inside the hood
    E. All of the above are correct

12. Which parts of the syringe are considered critical sites?

    I.   The ribs of the plunger
    II. The collar of the syringe
    III. The tip of the syringe

    A. I only
    B. II only
    C. I and III only
    D. II and III only
    E. I, II, and III

13. Which parts of the needle are considered critical sites?

    I.   The hub
    II. The needle shaft
    III. The bevel and bevel tip of the needle

    A. I only
    B. II only
    C. I and III only
    D. II and III only
    E. I, II, and III

14. Which of the following statements are true concerning ampuls?

    I.   Ampuls are single-dose containers
    II. Ampuls must have the neck wiped with a sterile alcohol pad before breaking
    III. Ampuls can be left in the hood and used for several days once opened

    A. II only
    B. I and III only

C. I and II only
D. I, II, and III

15. When working with cytotoxic agents, several steps are taken to protect the operator. Which of the statements below are true?

    I.   Preparation of cytotoxic drugs must occur in a biological safety cabinet
    II. Syringes with Luer-lok tips should be used when compounding cytotoxic sterile products
    III. It is very important that positive pressure is not allowed to build up inside the vial when working with cytotoxic drugs

    A. I only
    B. II only
    C. I and III only
    D. II and III only
    E. I, II, and III

16. Choose the correct statement.

    A. Filter integrity testing of the filter membrane is done to determine at what pressure the filter will break
    B. The manufacturer of the filter membrane determines the bubble point of the membrane; this value is always the same, no matter what solution has been filtered
    C. As the pore size of the filter membrane decreases, the pressure at which the air can be pushed from the largest pore increases
    D. The bubble point test is a destructive test
    E. It is not necessary to perform the bubble point test if there is a certificate of quality from the filter manufacturer

17. When choosing a sterilizing filter there are several items that must be considered. Choose the correct statement.

    A. The volume of product to be filtered
    B. The compatibility of the membrane with the product to be filtered
    C. Whether the solution to be filtered is hydrophobic or hydrophilic
    D. The compatibility of the filter housing with the product to be filtered
    E. All of the above statements are correct

18. Please choose the correct statement concerning the USP sterility test.

    A. The validation test must be done on each product to determine if the article to be tested adversely affects the reliability of the test

B. The growth promotion test does not require that the test organisms listed in the USP be used

C. After inoculation the media must be incubated for 14 days or less at the appropriate temperature

D. No growth on the sterility test proves that the aseptically-produced product is sterile

E. Trypticase soy broth is incubated at 30-35°C and fluid thioglycollate is incubated at 20-25°C

19. Choose the correct answer from the following statements.

   A. Gram-negative bacteria must be alive to cause a pyrogenic response

   B. The lipopolysaccharide portion of the cell wall of gram-negative bacteria causes the causes the pyrogenic response

   C. Endotoxin can be removed by a 0.2-micron filter

   D. Steam sterilization will depyrogenate the object just as well as the hot air oven

   E. An article that is depyrogenated is not necessarily sterile

20. Choose the correct answer from the following statements.

   A. The rabbit test and the LAL test are the same test

   B. LAL reagent will determine the fever-producing potential of the pyrogens

   C. There are two types of techniques for the bacterial endotoxin test: the gel clot technique and the photometric technique

   D. The drug product being tested has no effect on the test

   E. All drug products may be tested by the rabbit test

21. Choose the correct statement.

   A. The rabbit test is the most sensitive test because it can detect pyrogens from all sources

   B. The rabbit test is an *in-vitro* test

   C. Some drugs may inhibit the formation of a gel in the bacterial endotoxin test

   D. No drug will enhance the formation of the gel in the bacterial endotoxin test

   E. The pyrogen test is a quantitative test

22. Please choose the correct statement. The plenum in a laminar flow workbench is:

   A. where the air is prefiltered

   B. the area where air is pressurized for distribution over the HEPA filter

   C. the area where compounding takes place

   D. an area that serves no purpose

   E. an area directly above the HEPA filter in a horizontal laminar flow hood

23. Calcium and phosphate can interact to form a precipitate in parenteral nutrition solutions. Listed below are some situations that could enhance precipitate formation. Please choose the one that would ***not***.

   A. High concentration of calcium and phosphate

   B. Increase in solution pH

   C. Decrease in temperature

   D. The use of the chloride salt of calcium

   E. A slow infusion rate

24. Listed below are some potential sources of physical or chemical incompatibilities. Please choose the one that is ***not***.

   A. Dilution of a drug in a cosolvent system into an aqueous system

   B. Addition of a drug solution with a high pH into a solution with a low pH

   C. Adsorption of a lipid-soluble drug into the matrix of a polypropylene container

   D. A photosensitive drug such as sodium nitroprusside in 5% dextrose in water exposed to light

   E. Leaching of phthalate plasticizer into the solution from a polyvinyl chloride container

Answers

1. **C.** The bacterial endotoxin test, LAL, visual inspection test, and bubble point test should all be completed before the product is dispensed. Because the sterility test takes 14 days, the product may be dispensed before the results are known. However, a system to recall the product must be in place in case the product does not meet the requirement of the test.

2. **C.** Any leak greater than 0.01% of upstream smoke concentration is a serious leak. The HEPA filter can be patched. The smoke particles are 0.3 micron in size. The air flow from the HEPA filter should be 90 fpm plus or minus 20%. A total particle counter is used to classify the environment, not certify the integrity of the HEPA filter.

3. **B.** The BET determines the level of bacterial endotoxin only from gram-negative bacteria. The BET cannot determine fever-producing potential of the endotoxins. The gram-negative bacteria do not have to be alive for the endotoxin to produce an effect.

4. **A.** The operator must successfully complete one media fill before compounding a sterile product. Once validated for low- or medium-risk compounding the operator must revalidate annually. For high-risk compounding the operator must revalidate semi-annually. Passing only a written exam does not allow the operator to compound a sterile product. Trypticase soy broth is the medium most often used in media fills.

5. **A.** Cardboard must be kept out of the buffer area. Vials in laminated cardboard may be stored in the buffer area. No items should be brought into the buffer area without being sanitized. Large-volume parenteral bags should be removed from their overwrap just before being used. The refrigerator should not be in the buffer room. It is a source of contamination.

6. **C.** There are several types of vertical laminar flow hoods, of which the biological safety cabinet is one. The operator must never work over the top of items in the hood, and all work should be done at least 1 inch above the work surface.

7. **C.** Using good aseptic technique is one way to ensure a good product.

8. **D.** Any sterile product that is made from nonsterile ingredients is a risk level III product. A product that is at room temperature for longer than 28 hours is a risk level II product. A batch of unpreserved product intended for use by one patient is a risk level I product. If this batch is intended for multiple patients it is a risk level II product.

9. **A.** In HLF, never put your hand behind an object, whereas in VLF, never put your hand above an object. A vial disturbs the laminar air flow three times the diameter of the object when in HLF. If the vial is next to the side wall, the air flow is disturbed six times the diameter of the object. Syringes and IV bags should be taken from their overwrap at the edge of the hood.

10. **D.** Operators in the buffer area should wear clean nonshedding gowns and gloves to help contain the particles that they shed. The sterile gloves that are worn are not sterile once they are out of the package. Proper aseptic technique must always be used.

11. **E.** All of the following are true statements concerning placement of items in the laminar flow workstation and working in the laminar flow workstation: A. Items should be placed in a horizontal flow hood to the right or left of the work area. B. Items in a vertical laminar flow hood should be placed so that when working in the hood one's hand never goes over the top of a critical site. C. An object placed in a horizontal flow hood disturbs the airflow three times the diameter of the object downstream of the object. D. When working in a horizontal laminar flow workstation all work must be done at least 6 inches inside the hood.

12. **C.** The ribs of the plunger and the tip of the syringe are considered critical sites of the syringe.

13. **E.** The hub, the needle shaft, the bevel, and bevel tip of the needle are all considered critical sites.

14. **C.** Once an ampul is opened it must be used immediately.

15. **E.** When working with cytotoxic agents the following steps are taken to protect the operator: 1. Preparation must occur in a biological safety cabinet. 2. Syringes with Luer-lok tips should be used. 3. Positive pressure is not allowed to build up inside the vial.

16. **C.** The bubble point test is not a destructive test, and the value is dependent on the solution being filtered. When filter sterilizing a product, the bubble point test must be done before the product may be dispensed.

17. **E.** All of the statements are correct.

18. **A.** The validation (B&F) must be completed one time for each product. The growth promotion organisms listed in the USP are used for the validation test and for the growth promotion test.

19. **B.** Endotoxin will pass through a 0.2-micron filter. Steam sterilization will not depyrogenate an article. Bacteria do not have to be alive to be pyrogenic.

20. **C.** The pyrogen test is also known as the rabbit test, which determines the fever-producing potential of the pyrogens. The bacterial endotoxin test is also known as the LAL test. The drug product can inhibit or enhance the gel formation in the BET test.

21. **C.** The pyrogen (rabbit) test, is an in-vivo test, and is not as sensitive as the BET test. It is not a quantitative test.

22. **B.** The plenum is the area behind the HEPA filter in an HFLW that allows air to be pressurized for even distribution over the filter.

23. **C.** An increase in temperature could enhance precipitate formation.

24. **C.** Absorption of lipid-soluble drug into the matrix of polyvinyl chloride containers does occur. Polypropylene and polyethylene contain little or no phthalate plasticizer.

13. References

Akers MJ. *Parenteral Quality Control.* New York: Marcel Dekker; 1994.

American Society of Health-System Pharmacists. ASHP Guidelines on Quality Assurance for Pharmacy-Prepared Sterile Products. *Am J Hosp Pharm* 2000;57:1150-1169.

Anderson RA. The status of environmental control. Practical approaches to the safe handling of anticancer products. Proceedings of a Symposium in Mayaguez, Puerto Rico, November 2-5, 1983.

Bacterial endotoxin test. In: *United States Pharmacopeia,* 28th rev.: national formulary, 23rd ed. Rockville, MD: United States Pharmacopeial Conventions; 2005:2264-2267.

Buchanan C, McKinnon B, Scheckelhoff D, Schneider P. *Principles of Sterile Product Preparation.* Bethesda, MD: American Society of Health-System Pharmacists; 2002:50.

Commission, Federal Supply Service, General Services Administration. Federal Standard 209e. Clean room and work station requirements, controlled environments. Washington: U.S. Government Printing Office; 1992.

McKinnon B, Avis K. Membrane filtration of pharmaceutical solutions. *Am J Hosp Pharm* 1993;50:1021-1036.

Pyrogen test. In: *United States Pharmacopeia,* 28th rev.: national formulary, 23rd ed. Rockville, MD: United States Pharmacopeial Convention; 2005:2289-2290.

Sterile drug products for home use. In: *Pharmaceutical Compounding—Sterile Preparations,* 28th rev: national formulary, 23rd ed. Rockville, MD: United States Pharmacopeial Convention; 2005:2461-2477.

Sterility tests. In: *United States Pharmacopeia,* 28th rev: national formulary, 23rd ed. Rockville, MD: United States Pharmacopeial Convention; 2005:2251-2256.

Trissel LA. *Handbook on Injectable Drugs,* 11th ed. Bethesda, MD: American Society of Health-System Pharmacists; 2001.

6. Pharmacokinetics, Drug Metabolism, and Drug Disposition

Charles R. Yates, PharmD, PhD
Associate Professor
Department of Pharmaceutical Sciences

Bernd Meibohm, PhD, FCP
Associate Professor
Department of Pharmaceutical Sciences
University of Tennessee College of Pharmacy

Contents

1. Pharmacokinetics

Pharmacokinetics is the science of a drug's fate in the body. A drug's therapeutic potential is intimately linked to its pharmacokinetic profile. For example, a drug's pharmacologic response may be severely diminished as a result of poor absorption and/or rapid elimination from the body. The most important factors contributing to drug disposition include absorption, distribution, metabolism, and excretion (ADME).

Absorption

The rate and extent of drug absorption is referred to as bioavailability. The fraction of drug absorbed (f_a), an important determinant of the extent of bioavailability, is affected not only by its physicochemical properties, but also by physiologic barriers at the site of absorption. For example, intestinal expression of the drug efflux transporter P-glycoprotein is known to limit oral drug absorption.

Distribution

Many drugs circulate in the body and are bound to plasma proteins (eg, human serum albumin). The fraction of drug not bound to protein (f_{up}) is responsible for the pharmacologic effect. A drug may also bind significantly to tissue proteins resulting in a small unbound fraction of drug in the tissue (f_{ut}). Drugs with a large f_{up}:f_{ut} ratio have a large volume of distribution, whereas drugs with a small f_{up}:f_{ut} ratio are largely confined to the vascular space. Volume of distribution is directly related to half-life ($t_{1/2}$), the time required to eliminate half the drug from the body.

Metabolism

Approximately 50% of drugs undergo some form of hepatic metabolism. The cytochrome P450 (CYP450) family of drug metabolizing enzymes is primarily responsible for drug inactivation in the liver. Hepatic clearance is dependent on liver blood flow and the extraction ratio. The hepatic extraction ratio can be used to estimate the fraction of drug escaping first-pass metabolism (F*), an important determinant of oral bioavailability. Intestinal inactivation of drugs by CYP450 enzymes in the gut is responsible for reduced F of a number of drugs.

Excretion

The primary purpose of hepatic metabolism is to increase a drug's water solubility to facilitate its renal elimination. The kidneys also serve as the primary eliminating organ for drugs that do not undergo hepatic metabolism. Renal clearance comprises three main physiologic processes: glomerular filtration, reabsorption, and secretion. Filtration clearance is the product of f_{up} and glomerular filtration rate (a physiologic parameter that diminishes with age). Renal reabsorption is a predominantly passive process dependent upon physicochemical drug properties and urine drug concentration and pH, whereas secretion is an active process facilitated by various transport mechanisms. The net of filtration, reabsorption, and secretion determine a drug's total renal clearance.

Variability in drug response can be partially explained by inter-individual differences in drug pharmacokinetics. Thus a thorough understanding of the physiologic processes affecting drug disposition is essential to drug individualization and optimization.

2. Absorption and Disposition

Drug Input

Drugs are administered to the body by one of two routes, intravascular or extravascular. For intravascular administration, drugs are usually administered via intravenous infusion (continuous, short-term, or bolus). The concentration C is given by the following expressions:

IV bolus

$$C = \frac{Dose}{V} * e^{-K*t}$$

$\frac{dC}{dt}$ (Rate of change in plasma concentration) = Rate of drug elimination (output rate)

K = Elimination rate constant = CL/V

Clearance = Dose/AUC

IV infusion

For drugs that are administered extravascularly (PO, IM, and SC) and act systemically, absorption must occur.

First-order absorption

$$C = \frac{k_a * F * Dose}{V * (k_a - K)} * \left(e^{-K*t} - e^{-k_a * t} \right)$$

k_a = First-order rate constant for drug absorption
Absorption half-life = $0.693/k_a$
K = First-order rate constant for drug elimination (CL/V)
CL = F * Dose/AUC
Oral clearance = CL/F = Dose/AUC
F = bioavailability; fraction of drug absorbed

3. Bioavailability

Bioavailability refers to the rate and extent of absorption. The extent of absorption can be expressed as absolute or relative bioavailability.

Absolute Bioavailability

This is the fraction (or percentage) of a dose administered nonintravenously (or extravascularly) that is systemically available (compared to an intravenous dose). If given orally, absolute bioavailability (F) is:

$$F = \frac{D_{IV}}{D_{PO}} * \frac{AUC_{PO}}{AUC_{IV}}$$

Relative Bioavailability

This is the fraction of a dose administered as a test formulation that is systemically available as compared to a reference formulation:

$$F = \frac{AUC_{test\ formulation}}{AUC_{reference}} * \frac{D_{reference}}{D_{test\ formulation}}$$

Determinants of the Plasma Concentration-Time Curve After an Extravascular Dose

Four pharmacokinetic parameters determine the plasma concentration-time profile after an extravascular dose: k_a, F, CL, and V.

$$\frac{dC}{dt} = (\text{Rate in}) - (\text{Rate out})$$

$$\frac{dC}{dt} = (\text{Rate of drug absorption}) - (\text{Rate of drug elimination})$$

$$\frac{dC}{dt} = \frac{k_a * F * Dose}{V} - K * C$$

Time to peak (t_{max})
The maximum plasma concentration occurs when dC/dt = 0.

The equation below can be derived to determine the factors that affect t_{max}.

$$t_{max} = \frac{\ln \left(\frac{k_a}{K} \right)}{k_a - K}$$

Maximum plasma concentration (C_{max})

The maximum plasma concentration occurs at t_{max}. The following equation for C_{max} can be used to determine which factors affect C_{max}.

$$C_{max} = \frac{k_a * F * Dose}{V * (k_a - K)} * \left(e^{-K * t_{max}} - e^{-k_a * t_{max}} \right)$$

Area under the plasma concentration-time curve (AUC)

$$AUC = \frac{F * Dose}{CL} = \frac{F * Dose}{V * K}$$

Terminal half-life ($t_{1/2}$)

$$t_{1/2} = \frac{0.693 * V}{CL}$$

4. Constant Rate Regimens

Introduction

For many drugs to be therapeutically effective, drug concentrations of a certain level have to be maintained at the site of action for a prolonged period of time (eg, β-lactam antibiotics and antiarrhythmic medications), while for others, alternating plasma concentrations are more preferable (eg, aminoglycoside antibiotics like gentamicin).

To continuously maintain drug concentrations in a certain therapeutic range over a prolonged period of time, two basic approaches to administer the drug can be applied:

1. Drug administration at a constant input rate
2. Sequential administration of discrete single doses (multiple dosing)

Drug Administration as Constant Rate Regimens

At any time during the infusion, the rate of change in drug concentration is the difference between the input rate (infusion rate R_0 / volume of distribution V) and the output rate (elimination rate constant K * concentration C):

$$\text{Rate of change} = \text{Input rate} - \text{Output rate}$$

In concentrations:

$$\frac{dC}{dt} = \frac{R_0}{V} - K * C$$

In amounts:

$$V * \frac{dC}{dt} = R_0 - CL * C$$

R_0 = Infusion rate (in amount/time [eg, mg/h])
V = Volume of distribution
CL = Clearance
K = First-order rate constant for drug elimination (CL/V)
As

$$\frac{dC}{dt} = 0 \qquad \frac{R_0}{V} = K * C_{ss} \quad \text{or} \quad R_0 = CL * C_{ss}$$

Hence, the steady-state concentration C_{ss} is only determined by the infusion rate R_0 and the clearance CL.

Drug concentration at steady-state:

$$C_{ss} = \frac{R_0}{CL}$$

Drug concentration before steady-state:

$$C = \frac{R_0}{CL} * \left(1 - e^{-K*t}\right)$$

Time to Reach Steady-State

For therapeutic purposes, it is often of critical importance to know how long it will take after initiation of an infusion to finally reach the targeted steady-state concentration C_{ss}.

Concentration during an infusion:

before steady-state $\quad C = \dfrac{R_0}{CL} * \left(1 - e^{-K*t}\right)$

steady-state $\quad C_{ss} = \dfrac{R_0}{CL}$

the fraction of steady-state f is then

$$f = \frac{C}{C_{ss}} = \left(1 - e^{-K*t}\right)$$

After a duration of infusion of:
1 $t_{1/2} \rightarrow$ 50% of steady-state is reached
2 $t_{1/2} \rightarrow$ 75% of steady-state is reached
3 $t_{1/2} \rightarrow$ 87.5% of steady-state is reached
3.3 $t_{1/2} \rightarrow$ 90% of steady-state is reached
4 $t_{1/2} \rightarrow$ 93.8% of steady-state is reached
5 $t_{1/2} \rightarrow$ 96.9% of steady-state is reached

The following conclusions can be drawn:
1. The approach to the steady-state concentration C_{ss} is exponential in nature and is controlled by the elimination process (elimination rate constant K), **not** the infusion rate R_0.
2. Only the value of the steady-state concentration C_{ss} is controlled by the infusion rate R_0 (and of course by the clearance CL).
3. Assuming for clinical purposes that a concentration of >95% of steady-state is therapeutically equivalent to the final steady-state concentration C_{ss}, it takes approximately **five elimination half-lives $t_{1/2}$** to reach steady-state after initiation of an infusion.

Concentration-Time Profiles Postinfusion

The postinfusion plasma concentration cannot be distinguished from readings following administration of an intravenous bolus dose. As the drug input has been discontinued, the rate of change in drug concentration is only determined by the output rate. If the drug follows one-compartment characteristics, then the plasma concentration profile can be described by

$$C = C * e^{-K*t_{pi}}$$

where C = concentration at the end of the infusion, and t_{pi} = time postinfusion (ie, time after the infusion has stopped).

Thus, a general expression can be used to calculate the plasma concentration during and after a constant rate infusion:

$$C = \frac{R_0}{CL} * \left(1 - e^{-K*t}\right) * e^{-K*t_{pi}}$$

where t = is the elapsed time after the beginning of the infusion
t_{pi} = the postinfusion time, ie, the difference between the duration of the infusion (infusion time T_{inf}) and t: $t_{pi} = t - T_{inf}$
For describing concentrations during the infusion, t_{pi} is set to zero.
For describing concentrations postinfusion, t is set to T_{inf}.

Four different cases can be distinguished:
1. *During the infusion, but before steady-state is reached:*

$$t = t, t_{pi} = 0 \Rightarrow \quad C = \frac{R_0}{CL} * \left(1 - e^{-K*t}\right)$$

2. *During the infusion at steady-state:*

$$t \rightarrow \infty, t_{pi} = 0 \Rightarrow \quad C = \frac{R_0}{CL}$$

3. *After cessation of the infusion before steady-state:*

$$t = T_{inf}, t_{pi} = t - T_{inf} \Rightarrow C = \frac{R_0}{CL} * \left(1 - e^{-K*T_{inf}}\right) * e^{-K*(t - T_{inf})}$$

4. *After cessation of the infusion at steady-state:*

$$t \rightarrow \infty, t_{pi} = t - T_{inf} \Rightarrow C = \frac{R_0}{CL} * e^{-K*(t - T_{inf})}$$

Determination of Pharmacokinetic Parameters

- The elimination rate constant K, and the elimination half-life $t_{1/2}$ can be determined from:
  a) the terminal slope after the infusion has been stopped
  b) the time to reach half of C_{ss}
  c) the slope of the relationship of ln $(C_{ss} - C)$ versus t, based on

$$C = C_{ss} * \left(1 - e^{-K*t}\right)$$

and the resulting $\ln \left(C_{ss} - C\right) = \ln C_{ss} - K * t$

- The clearance CL can be determined from the relationship:

$$CL = \frac{R_0}{C_{ss}}$$

- The volume of distribution can be determined from the relationship:

$$V = \frac{CL}{K}$$

Loading Dose and Maintenance Dose

- The loading dose (LD) is supposed to immediately (t = 0) reach the desired target concentration C_{target}. It is administered as an IV bolus injection, or more frequently as a short-term infusion.
- The maintenance dose (MD) is intended to sustain C_{target}. It is administered as a constant rate infusion.

Loading dose (LD)
Target concentration calculated for a drug with one-compartment characteristics:

$$C_{target} = \frac{LD}{V} \rightarrow LD = C_{target} * V$$

Maintenance dose (MD)
The maintenance dose is the infusion rate necessary to sustain the target concentration:

$$C_{target} = \frac{MD}{CL} \rightarrow MD = R_0 = C_{target} * CL$$

5. Multiple Dosing

Introduction

Continuous drug concentrations for prolonged therapy can be maintained either by drug administration at a constant input rate or by sequential administration of discrete single doses. The latter is the more frequently used approach and can be applied to extravascular as well as intravascular routes of administration.

Multiple dose regimens are defined by two components, the **dose D** that is administered at each dosing occasion, and the **dosing interval τ,** the time period between the administration of two subsequent doses. Dose and dosing interval can be summarized in the **dosing rate DR:**

$$DR = \frac{D}{\tau}$$

Concentration-Time Profiles During Multiple Dosing

The **multiple dose function MDF** can be used for calculating drug concentrations before steady-state (during a multiple dose regimen) has been reached:

$$MDF = \frac{1 - e^{-n*K*\tau}}{1 - e^{-K*\tau}}$$

where K is the respective rate constant of the drug, τ the dosing interval, and n the number of the dose.

Once steady-state has been reached, n approaches infinity and the MDF simplifies to the **accumulation factor AF:**

$$AF = \frac{1}{1 - e^{-K*\tau}}$$

Multiple Dosing Regimens: Instantaneous Input (IV Bolus)

For an IV bolus multiple dose regimen, the concentrations during the first dosing interval, the nth dosing interval, and at steady-state are described by the following relationships:

Dose number	Equation	Maximum or peak concentration	Minimum or trough concentration at the end of the dosing interval
1	$C = \dfrac{D}{V} * e^{-K*t}$	$C_{1,max} = \dfrac{D}{V}$	$C_{1,min} = \dfrac{D}{V} * e^{-K*\tau}$
n	$C = \dfrac{D}{V} * e^{-K*t} * \dfrac{1 - e^{-n*K*\tau}}{1 - e^{-K*\tau}}$	$C_{n,max} = \dfrac{D}{V} * \dfrac{1 - e^{-n*K*\tau}}{1 - e^{-K*\tau}}$	$C_{n,min} = \dfrac{D}{V} * e^{-K*\tau} * \dfrac{1 - e^{-n*K*\tau}}{1 - e^{-K*\tau}}$
Steady-state	$C = \dfrac{D}{V} * \dfrac{e^{-K*t}}{1 - e^{-K*\tau}}$	$C_{ss,max} = \dfrac{D}{V} * \dfrac{1}{1 - e^{-K*\tau}}$	$C_{ss,min} = \dfrac{D}{V} * \dfrac{e^{-K*\tau}}{1 - e^{-K*\tau}}$

The peak and trough concentrations at steady-state can thus be expressed as the peak and trough after the first dose multiplied by the accumulation factor AF:

$$C_{ss,max} = \frac{C_{1,max}}{1 - e^{-K*\tau}}$$

$$C_{ss,min} = \frac{C_{1,min}}{1 - e^{-K*\tau}} = \frac{C_{1,max} * e^{-K*\tau}}{1 - e^{-K*\tau}}$$

Average Steady-State Concentration

By definition, the average drug input rate is equal to the average drug output rate at steady-state. While the average input rate is the drug amount entering the systemic circulation per dosing interval, the average output rate is equal to the product of clearance CL and the average plasma concentration within one dosing interval $C_{ss,av}$:

$$\frac{D}{\tau} = CL * C_{ss,av}$$

Thus, the average steady-state concentration $C_{ss,av}$ during multiple dosing is only determined by the dose, the dosing interval τ (or both together as dosing rate DR = D/τ) and the clearance CL:

$$C_{ss,av} = \frac{D}{\tau * CL}$$

The area under the curve resulting from administration of a single dose AUC_{single} is equal to the area under the curve during one dosing interval at steady-state AUC_{ss}, if the same dose is given per dosing interval τ:

$$C_{ss,av} = \frac{AUC_{ss}}{\tau} = \frac{D}{\tau * CL} = \frac{AUC_{single}}{\tau}$$

Thus:

$$AUC_{single} = AUC_{ss}$$

Extent of Accumulation

The extent of accumulation during multiple dosing at steady-state is determined by the dosing interval τ and the half-life of the drug $t_{1/2}$ (or the elimination rate constant K):

$$AF = \frac{1}{1 - e^{-k*\tau}}$$

Thus, the extent of accumulation is not only dependent on the pharmacokinetic properties of a drug, but also on the multiple dosing regimen chosen.

$$Fluctuation = \frac{C_{ss,max} - C_{ss,min}}{C_{ss,min}}$$

Fluctuation

The degree of fluctuation between peak and trough concentrations during one dosing interval, ie, $C_{ss,max}$ and $C_{ss,min}$, is determined by the relationship between elimination half-life $t_{1/2}$ and dosing interval τ.

Multiple Dosing Regimens: First-Order Input (Oral Dosing)

The average steady-state concentration $C_{ss,av}$ is now determined by the bioavailable fraction F of the dose

(D) administered per dosing interval τ and the clearance (CL):

$$C_{ss,av} = \frac{F * D}{\tau * CL}$$

As the concentration-time profile after a single oral dose is given by

$$C = \frac{F * D * k_a}{V * (k_a - K)} * \left(e^{-K*t} - e^{-k_a*t}\right),$$

the concentration at any time within a dosing interval during multiple dosing at steady-state is determined by

$$C = \frac{F * D * k_a}{V * (k_a - K)} * \left(\frac{e^{-K*\tau}}{1 - e^{-K*\tau}} - \frac{e^{-k_a*t}}{1 - e^{-k_a*\tau}}\right)$$

Thus, the trough concentration is readily available assuming that the absorption is completed:

$$C_{ss,min} = \frac{F * D * k_a}{V * (k_a - K)} * \left(\frac{e^{-K*\tau}}{1 - e^{-K*\tau}}\right)$$

The peak concentration is assessable via the time-to-peak t_{max}, which is dependent on the rate of absorption and has to be determined via:

$$t_{max} = \frac{\ln\left(\frac{k_a * (1 - e^{-k_e*\tau})}{K * (1 - e^{-K*\tau})}\right)}{(k_a - K)}$$

6. Volumes of Distribution and Protein Binding

Introduction

Drug distribution means the reversible transfer of drug from one location to another within the body.

Once a drug has entered the vascular system, it becomes distributed throughout the various tissues and body fluids. However, most drugs do not distribute uniformly and in a similar manner throughout the body. This is reflected by the difference in their volumes of distribution. Thus in the following, we will focus on the factors and processes determining the rate and extent of distribution and the resulting consequences for pharmacotherapy.

Factors affecting distribution:
• Binding to blood or tissue elements
• Blood flow (ie, the delivery of drug to the tissues)
• Ability to cross biomembranes
• Physicochemical properties of the drug (lipophilicity and extent of ionization) that determine partitioning into tissues

Protein Binding

The fraction unbound in plasma varies widely among drugs. Drugs are classified as
• Highly protein bound:
  $f_{up} \leq 0.1$ ($\leq 10\%$ unbound, $\geq 90\%$ bound)
• Moderately protein bound:
  $f_{up} = 0.1\text{-}0.4$ (10-40% unbound, 60-90% bound)
• Low protein binding:
  $f_{up} \geq 0.4$ ($\geq 40\%$ unbound, $\leq 60\%$ bound)

Factors Determining the Degree of Protein Binding

The reversible binding of a drug to proteins obeys the law of mass action,

$$[\text{Drug}] + [\text{Protein}] \underset{k_2}{\overset{k_1}{\rightleftharpoons}} [\text{Drug-Protein-Complex}]$$

where the expressions in brackets represent the molar concentrations of the components. k_1 and k_2 are rate constants for the forward and reverse reactions, respectively. The equilibrium association constant K_a is defined as k_1/k_2.

This results in the following relationship for the fraction unbound:

$$f_{up} = \cfrac{1}{1 + \cfrac{N}{(1/K_a) + C_u}}$$

where N is the number of available binding sites and C_u is the unbound concentration.

Binding Proteins

Human plasma contains over 60 proteins. Of these, three proteins account for the binding of most drugs. *Albumin,* which comprises approximately 60% of total plasma protein, fully accounts for the plasma binding of most anionic drugs and many endogenous anions (high-capacity, low-affinity binding site). Many cationic and neutral drugs bind appreciably to *α₁-acid glycoprotein (AAG)* (high-affinity, low-capacity binding site) and/or *lipoproteins* in addition to albumin. Other proteins, such as transcortin, thyroid-binding globulin, and certain antibodies have specific affinities for a small number of drugs.

Volumes of Distribution

Volume of distribution at steady-state V_{ss}

The volume of distribution at steady-state is by definition the sum of the pharmacokinetic volumes of distribution for the different pharmacokinetic compartments. Theoretically:

$$V_{ss} = V_p + \frac{f_u}{f_{u,t}} * V_t$$

where V_p is the volume of plasma (3 L) and V_t is the volume of tissue water (total body water minus plasma volume: 42 − 3 = 39 L based on a "standard" person). f_{up} and f_{ut} are the fraction unbound for the drug in plasma and tissue, respectively.

The relationship for V_{ss} shows that the extent of distribution is (besides physicochemical properties of the drug) largely determined by the differences in protein binding in plasma and tissue, respectively:

$$V_{ss} = 3\,L + \frac{f_u}{f_{u,t}} * 39\,L$$

Unbound steady-state concentrations

The average steady-state concentration during a multiple dose regimen or during a constant rate infusion is determined by

$$C_{ss} = \frac{Dose\ rate}{CL} = \frac{Dose\ rate}{f_{up} * CL_u}$$

The free steady-state concentration $C_{ss,u}$ is given by

$$C_{ss,u} = f_{up} * C_{ss}$$

Thus, the unbound steady-state concentration $C_{ss,u}$ is determined by

$$\frac{C_{ss,u}}{f_{up}} = \frac{Dose\ rate}{f_{up} * CL_u} \Rightarrow C_{ss,u} = \frac{Dose\ rate}{CL}$$

7. Elimination and Clearance Concepts

Clearance (CL) is defined as the irreversible removal of drug from the body by an organ of elimination. Since the units of CL are flow per time (eg, mL/min or L/h), CL is often defined as the volume of blood irreversibly cleared of drug per unit of time.

CL by the eliminating organ (CL_{organ}) is defined as the product of (blood flow to the organ) and (the extraction ratio of that organ).

$$CL_{organ} = Q * ER$$
Organ clearance = Blood flow * Extraction ratio

Individual organ clearances are additive. For the majority of drugs we use clinically, the liver is the major, and sometimes only, site of metabolism; the kidneys are the major site of excretion for drugs and metabolites. Thus the equation for total clearance can be written to include renal clearance (CL_R) and hepatic clearance (CL_H):

$$CL = CL_R + CL_H$$

The fraction of drug excreted unchanged by the kidneys (f_e) tells us what fraction of the drug we administered will be excreted into the urine.

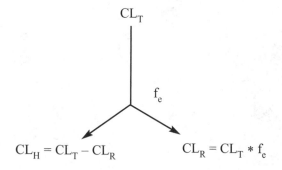

$$CL_T$$

$$f_e$$

$$CL_H = CL_T - CL_R \qquad CL_R = CL_T * f_e$$

8. Renal Clearance

Drugs may undergo three processes in the kidney, two of which act to remove drug from the body—filtration and secretion—while the other acts to return the drug to the body—reabsorption. Thus we may express renal clearance of a drug as:

$$CL_R = [CL_{filtration} + CL_{secretion}] * (1 - f_{reabsorbed})$$

Calculating Filtration Clearance of Creatinine (CL_{cr})

Normal serum concentrations of creatinine are:
0.8-1.3 mg/dL for men
0.6-1.0 mg/dL for women

Creatinine is a useful marker of renal function since it is an endogenous by-product of muscle breakdown. Creatinine is eliminated by the kidney at a rate approximately equal to the glomerular filtration rate (GFR). A number of formulas have been developed that allow us to estimate creatinine clearance (CL_{cr}) from serum creatinine concentrations. The most widely used clinically is the *Cockcroft-Gault equation:*

$$CL_{cr} = \frac{(140 - age) * IBW}{S_{cr} * 72}$$

(multiply result by 0.85 if patient is female)
where S_{cr} is the serum creatinine concentration in milligrams per deciliter, and IBW is the ideal body weight.

$$IBW_{males} (kg) = 50 + (2.3 * \text{height in inches} >5 \text{ ft})$$
$$IBW_{females} (kg) = 45.5 + (2.3 * \text{height in inches} >5 \text{ ft})$$

Secretion Clearance

Drug in blood may also be secreted into the kidney tubule. This occurs *against* a concentration gradient (concentration of drug in the kidney tubule is very high because of water reabsorption) and therefore is *an active process.*

Cellular processes (eg, presence of active transporters) exist to facilitate tubular secretion. The two most well characterized include transporters responsible for the secretion of *basic* (cationic) and *acidic* (anionic) drugs.

Reabsorption

Passive reabsorption of many drugs also occurs in the kidneys. Since reabsorption is a passive process (ie, diffusion), reabsorption will depend on the physicochemical properties of the drug (eg, molecular weight, polarity, and pK_a).

$$\text{Weak bases: } B + H \leftrightarrow BH^+$$

Low urine pH = **more ionized, less reabsorption**
High urine pH = **less ionized, more reabsorption**

Thus, only weak bases with pK_a between 6 and 12 show changes in the extent of reabsorption (and thus CL_R) with changes in urine pH.

$$\text{Weak acids: } HA \leftrightarrow A^- + H^+$$

Low urine pH = **less ionized, more reabsorption**
High urine pH = **more ionized, less reabsorption**

Thus, only weak acids with pK_a in the range of 3-7.5 show changes in the extent of reabsorption (and thus CL_R) with changes in urine pH.

All drugs that are not bound to plasma proteins are filtered, therefore filtration clearance is:

$$CL_{filtration} = f_{up} * GFR = f_{up} * 125 \text{ mL/min}$$

Some drugs are secreted or reabsorbed, or both. We can determine the net process a drug undergoes by calculating the excretion ratio (E_{ratio}):

$$E_{ratio} = \frac{CL_R}{CL_{filtration}} = \frac{CL_R}{f_{up} * 125 \text{ mL/min}}$$

9. Hepatic Clearance

Relation of Hepatic Extraction Ratio and Bioavailability

The fraction of drug escaping first-pass metabolism (F*) can be described in terms of the hepatic extraction ratio (ER).

$$F^* = 1 - ER$$

The overall oral bioavailability (F) of a drug is dependent on the fraction absorbed (f_a), the fraction escaping metabolism in the intestinal wall (f_g), and the fraction escaping hepatic first-pass metabolism (F*).

$$F = f_a * f_g * F^*$$

Venous Equilibrium Model for Hepatic Clearance

The venous equilibrium model relates hepatic extraction ratio (ER) to f_{up}, intrinsic clearance (CL_{int}), and liver blood flow (Q) as follows (from Wilkinson et al, 1975):

$$ER = \frac{f_{up} * CL_{int}}{Q + f_{up} * CL_{int}}$$

and (remembering that $CL_H = Q_H * ER_H$),

$$CL_H = \frac{Q * f_{up} * CL_{int}}{Q + f_{up} * CL_{int}}$$

The fraction of drug escaping hepatic first-pass metabolism using the venous equilibrium model.

$$F^* = \frac{Q}{Q + f_{up} * CL_{int}}$$

Drugs undergoing hepatic metabolism can be broadly divided into three categories:
1. Low-extraction drugs: ER <0.3 and thus F* >0.7
2. Intermediate-extraction drugs: 0.3 < ER < 0.7 and thus 0.3 < F* < 0.7
3. High-extraction drugs: ER >0.7 and thus F* <0.3

Determinants of Hepatic Clearance

The determinants of hepatic extraction ratio, hepatic clearance, and the fraction escaping hepatic first-pass metabolism are Q, f_{up}, and CL_{int}.
1.   Liver blood flow (Q)

2. Protein binding (f_{up})

    ER < f_{up}. For some drugs, hepatic clearance is limited or restricted to the unbound or free drug. This is known as **restrictive clearance**. Because clearance is limited to unbound drug, changes in protein binding will alter the concentration of drug that is available for elimination.

    ER > f_{up}. Some drugs defy this principle such that the hepatic extraction ratio (ER) is greater than the fraction of drug unbound in plasma (f_{up}). When this occurs, it suggests that drug clearance is not restricted to unbound drug. Drugs behaving in this manner are said to undergo **nonrestrictive clearance**. Because nonrestrictive clearance is not limited to the fraction unbound in plasma, changes in protein binding will not alter the concentration of drug that is available for elimination (ie, all drug is available for elimination regardless of whether it is bound or unbound).

3. Intrinsic clearance (CL_{int})

    Intrinsic clearance (CL_{int}) is defined as the intrinsic ability of the hepatic enzymes to eliminate drug when there are no limitations due to blood flow or protein binding.

    CL_{int} is a measure of the capacity and affinity of drug-metabolizing enzymes (eg, cytochrome P450s) for the drug. The determinants of CL_{int} can be explained using the Michaelis-Menten equation:

    $$v = \frac{V_{max} * C_u}{K_m + C_u} \text{ and } CL_u = \frac{V_{max}}{K_m + C_u}$$

    where v is the rate of drug metabolism (amount/time), V_{max} is the maximal rate of metabolism for a given metabolic pathway (amount/time), K_m is the concentration of the drug at which the rate of metabolism is half-maximal (amount/volume), and C_u is the unbound drug concentration (amount/volume).

    Physiologically, V_{max} describes the quantity (capacity) of a drug-metabolizing enzyme to metabolize drug. K_m describes the interaction between the drug-metabolizing enzyme and the drug.

Factors that affect CL_{int}

a. **Enzyme induction:** this refers to an increased number (capacity) of drug-metabolizing enzymes, which results in an increase in clearance. An increased number (capacity) of drug-metabolizing enzymes results in an increase in V_{max} and Cl_{int}.

b. **Enzyme inhibitors:** this is competitive inhibition of the drug-metabolizing enzyme by another drug. The apparent K_m is increased in this situation (ie, a higher concentration of drug will be required to achieve a half-maximal rate of metabolism). Increase in apparent K_m results in a decrease in CL_{int}.

An extensive list of potential CYP450 inducers and inhibitors can be found at: www.drug-interactions.com

10. Clinical Examples

Clinical Example #1

A patient (age 55, weight 73 kg) was started on a multiple dose regimen with gentamicin 80 mg q8h given as an IV short-term infusion over 30 minutes. As his infection was serious, it was decided to set the target for a peak concentration of 10 mg/L and a trough concentration of 1 mg/L. Three blood samples were drawn 30 minutes prior to the third dose, and 30 minutes and 7 hours after the end of the infusion of the third dose, respectively. The measured plasma concentrations were 1.73, 5.96, and 1.80 mg/L, respectively.

Optimize the gentamicin dosing regimen based on the individual pharmacokinetic parameters of the patient to achieve the therapeutically-targeted concentrations.

Step 1: Calculate the elimination rate constant K

$$K = \frac{\ln\left(\frac{C^*_{max}}{C^*_{min}}\right)}{t} = \frac{\ln\left(\frac{5.96}{1.80}\right)}{(8-1-0.5)\text{h}} = 0.184 \text{ h}^{-1}$$

Step 2: Calculate volume of distribution V

$$C_{max} = \frac{C^*_{max}}{e^{-K*t}} = \frac{5.96 \text{ mg/L}}{e^{-0.184 \text{ h}^{-1}*0.5 \text{ h}}} = 6.53 \text{ mg/L}$$

$$C_{min} = C^*_{min} * e^{-K*t^*} = 1.73 \text{ mg/L} * e^{-0.184 \text{ h}^{-1}*0.5 \text{ h}} = 1.58 \text{ mg/L}$$

$$V = \frac{R_0}{K} * \frac{1-e^{-K*T_{inf}}}{C_{max} - C_{min} * e^{-K*T_{inf}}} =$$

$$\frac{80 \text{ mg}}{0.184 \text{ h}^{-1} * 0.5 \text{ h}} * \frac{1-e^{-0.184 \text{ h}^{-1}*0.5 \text{ h}}}{6.53 \text{ mg/L} - 1.58 * e^{-0.184 \text{ h}^{-1}*0.5 \text{ h}}} = 15.0 \text{ L}$$

Step 3: Calculate recommended dosing interval τ

$$\tau = \frac{\ln\left(\frac{C_{ss,max(desired)}}{C_{ss,min(desired)}}\right)}{K} + T_{inf} \quad \frac{\ln\left(\frac{10}{1}\right)}{0.184 \text{ h}^{-1}} + 0.5\text{ h} = 13.0 \text{ h}$$

Practically reasonable, recommended dosing interval: 12 hours

Step 4: Calculate recommended dose D

$$D = C_{ss,max(desired)} * K * V * T_{inf} * \frac{1-e^{-K*\tau}}{1-e^{-K*T_{inf}}}$$

$$D = 10 \text{ mg/L} * 0.184 \text{ h}^{-1} * 15 \text{ L} * 0.5 \text{ h} * \frac{1-e^{-0.184 \text{ h}^{-1}*12 \text{ h}}}{1-e^{-0.184 \text{ h}^{-1}*0.5 \text{ h}}}$$

$$= 139.7 \text{ mg}$$

Recommended dosing regimen:
140 mg every 12 hours

Step 5: Check expected peak $C_{ss,max}$ and trough $C_{ss,min}$

$$C_{ss,max} = \frac{R_0}{K*V} * \frac{1-e^{-K*T_{inf}}}{1-e^{-K*\tau}} * \frac{140 \text{ mg}}{0.184 \text{ h}^{-1} * 15 \text{ L} * 0.5 \text{ h}} *$$

$$\frac{1-e^{-0.184 \text{ h}^{-1}*0.5 \text{ h}}}{1-e^{-0.184 \text{ h}^{-1}*12 \text{ h}}} = 10.0 \text{ mg/L}$$

$$C_{ss,min} = C_{ss,max} * e^{-K*(\tau - T_{inf})} = 10.0 \text{ mg/L} * e^{-0.184 \text{ h}^{-1}*(12 \text{ h}-0.5 \text{ h})}$$

$$= 1.21 \text{ mg/L}$$

Clinical Example #2

A 70-year-old white male who weighs 95 pounds and is 5 feet tall has a serum creatinine of 1.1 mg/dL. He is admitted to the hospital complaining of shortness of breath; he denies chest pain. Digoxin is prescribed for him. You are asked to design a dosage regimen using tablets for him to achieve and maintain a $C_{target,ss}$ of 1 ng/mL. The PK parameters for digoxin are as follows: CL = 2.7 mL/min/kg (TBW) ; f_e = 0.68; V_{ss} = 6.7 L/kg (IBW); F of tablet = 0.75.

1. Estimate CL, CL_{cr}, RF, and CL* (clearance in this renally impaired patient) of digoxin in this patient.
    IBW = 45.5 kg; TBW = 43 kg
    Therefore, use TBW for all calculations.

    CL for a normal 43-kg patient = 116 mL/min

    CL_{cr} and RF are:

    $$CL_{cr} = \frac{(140-70)*43}{1.1*72} = 38 \text{ mL/min}$$

    $$RF = \frac{38 \text{ mL/min}}{125 \text{ mL/min}} = 0.304$$

2. Estimate CL, clearance of digoxin, in this patient with renal impairment.

    CL* = 116 mL/min * [1 − .68 * (1− .304)] = 61.1 mL/min

3. Calculate dose rate.

$$\text{Dose rate} = \frac{1 \text{ ng/mL} * 61.1 \text{ mL/min}}{0.75} = 81.5 \text{ ng/min}$$

4. Determine dosing interval τ^*: estimate half-life of digoxin.

$$\tau^*_{1/2} = \frac{\mathbf{0.693 * V_{ss}}}{\mathbf{CL^*}}$$

V_{ss} (V_d) for digoxin from PK tables is 6.7 L/kg, or 289 L in this patient. Thus,

$$\tau^*_{1/2} = \frac{0.693 * 289 \text{ L}}{0.061 \text{ L/min}} = 3283 \text{ minutes} \cong 55 \text{ hours}$$

We normally administer digoxin every 24 hours ($\tau = 24$ h); we could administer 0.25 mg every 48 hours ($\tau = 48$ h). However, I would not change the dosing interval here because dosing every 24 hours is very convenient, and the resultant peak:trough ratio would be lower with a $\tau = 24$ compared to a $\tau = 48$ hours.

Clinical Example #3

A.M. is a 6'0", 195-pound, 61-year-old white male with a diagnosis of pneumonia. His serum creatinine is 2.3 mg/dL. Design a dosage regimen of gentamicin to achieve C_{peak} and C_{trough} values of 8 and 1 mg/L, respectively. $V_d = 0.2$ L/kg IBW

1. CL of gentamicin and f_e in normal adults.
   CL of gentamicin is 85 mL/min and $f_e = 1.0$

2. Degree of renal impairment.

$$CL = CL_{cr} = \frac{(140 - 61) * 77.6}{2.3(72)}$$

$$RF = \frac{37 \text{ mL/min}}{125 \text{ mL/min}} = .296$$

3. CL of gentamicin in this patient.

$CL^* = 85 \text{ mL/min} * [1 - 1 (1 - .296)] = 25.2 \text{ mL/min} = 1.5 \text{ L/h}$

4. Elimination rate constant in this patient.

$$k = \frac{CL}{V_{ss}} = \frac{1.5 \text{ L/h}}{0.2 \text{ L/kg} * 77.6 \text{ kg}} = 0.097 \text{ h}^{-1}$$

5. Infusion rate and dosing interval.

$$\tau = \frac{\ln\left(\frac{C_{ss,max(desired)}}{C_{ss,min(desired)}}\right)}{K} + T_{inf} = \frac{\ln\left(\frac{8 \text{ mg/L}}{1 \text{ mg/L}}\right)}{0.097 \text{ h}^{-1}} + 0.5 \text{ h} = 22 \text{ h} \cong 24 \text{ h}$$

$$D = C_{ss,max} * K * V * T_{inf} * \frac{1 - e^{-K*\tau}}{1 - e^{-K*T_{inf}}} = 8 \text{ mg/L} * .097 \text{ h}^{-1}$$

$$* (.2 * 77.6) * 0.5 * \frac{1 - e^{-.097 \text{ h}^{-1} *24}}{1 - e^{-.097 \text{ h}^{-1} *0.5}} = 115 \text{ mg} \cong 120 \text{ mg}$$

Clinical Example #4

Patient D.M. is a 50-year-old white male (74.1 kg) who is being treated with phenytoin ($V_d = 0.6$ L/kg), 300 mg/d (using the capsule formulation) for seizure control. He has been taking phenytoin for 2 weeks. He experienced a seizure on day 14 of treatment. His blood level was 5.2 mg/L. His dose rate was increased to 400 mg/d of the capsule formulation. Three weeks later his level was 11.8 mg/L.

Phenytoin capsules and parenteral solution = sodium phenytoin
Phenytoin tablets and suspension = phenytoin acid
100 mg phenytoin sodium = 92 mg phenytoin acid

1. The V_{max} (mg phenytoin per day) for phenytoin in patient D.M. is:
   a. 491
   b. 499
   c. 542
   d. 590
   e. 614

Since D.M. is using capsules, we need to multiply the R_{in} by 0.92.

DR (mg/day)	C_{ss} (mg/L)	DR/C_{ss} (L/day)
300 * 0.92 = 276	5.2	53.08
400 * 0.92 = 368	11.8	31.19

$$\mathbf{DR = V_{max} - \left(\frac{DR}{C_{ss}}\right) * K_m}$$

$\mathbf{Y = intercept + X * (- slope)}$ Plot DR vs DR/C_{ss}.

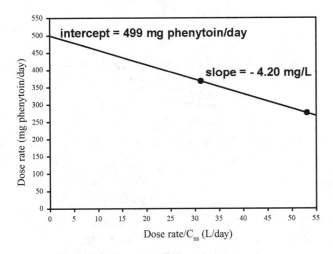

Y-intercept = V_{max} = 499 mg phenytoin/day,
slope = $-K_m$ = -4.20 mg/L, therefore, K_m = 4.2 mg/L

2. What dosage regimen is recommended to achieve an average steady-state phenytoin concentration of 15 mg/L in patient D.M. using the capsule formulation?
   a. 100 mg q6h
   b. 100 mg q8h
   c. 200 mg q6h
   d. 200 mg q8h

$$DR = CL * C_{ss,target} = \frac{V_{max} * C_{ss, target}}{K_m + C_{ss,target}} = \frac{499 \text{ mg/d} * 15 \text{ mg/L}}{4.2 \text{ mg/L} + 15 \text{ mg/L}}$$

$$= 390 \text{ mg phenytoin/d}$$

390 mg/d phenytoin = 424 mg/d sodium phenytoin. Give 400 mg Dilantin Kapseals® in three or four divided doses (eg, 100 mg q6h).

3. Estimate the time required to achieve steady-state levels of phenytoin in patient D.M. if he were changed to a dosage regimen of a 100 mg capsule q6h.
   a. 1 day
   b. 5 days
   c. 9 days
   d. 13 days
   e. 17 days

$$t_{90} = \frac{K_m * V_{ss}}{(V_{max} - DR)^2} * (2.3 * V_{max} - 0.9 * DR)$$

$$t_{90} = \frac{4.2 \text{ mg phenytoin/L} * 0.6 \text{ L/kg} * 74.1 \text{ kg}}{(499 \text{ mg phenytoin/d} - 368 \text{ mg phenytoin/d})^2}$$

$$* (2.3 * 499 \text{ mg phenytoin/d} - 0.9 * 368 \text{ mg phenytoin/d})$$

$$t_{90} = 8.9 \text{ days}$$

About 9 days to reach 90% of new steady state plasma concentration

4. In this patient, calculate the loading dose of phenytoin that would be needed to achieve a phenytoin blood level of 12 mg/L (assume that blood levels of phenytoin = 0 at the time of administration of the LD).
   a. 491 mg
   b. 535 mg
   c. 580 mg
   d. 603 mg

$LD = C_{ss,target} * V_{ss}$ = 12 mg phenytoin/L * 0.6 L/kg * 74.1 kg = 534 mg of phenytoin = 580 mg of phenytoin sodium (parenteral)

Clinical Example #5

In order to treat her asthma exacerbation, L.Y. (55 kg, 68 years of age) has received a continuous infusion of aminophylline (infusion rate 0.45 mg/kg/h) for 5 days. This morning, she suffers from theophylline toxicity indicated by tachycardia, headache, and dizziness. A blood sample is drawn and the theophylline plasma concentration is 24.3 mg/L. The therapeutic range is 10-20 mg/L, and the population average of the volume of distribution is 0.5 L/kg.

1. What is the theophylline clearance in this patient under the assumption that steady-state had already been reached at the time the blood sample was obtained?
   a. 0.81 L/h
   b. 0.95 L/h
   c. 1.35 L/h
   d. 2.15 L/h
   e. 2.80 L/h

$$CL = \frac{R_0}{C_{ss}} = \frac{0.45 \text{ mg/kg/h} * 0.8 * 55 \text{ kg}}{24.3 \text{ mg/L}} = 0.81 \text{ L/h}$$

2. To what aminophylline infusion rate should the infusion be reduced to achieve a steady-state concentration in the middle of the therapeutic range, ie, 15 mg/L?

a. 0.17 mg/kg/h
b. 0.18 mg/kg/h
c. 0.20 mg/kg/h
d. 0.22 mg/kg/h
e. 0.28 mg/kg/h

$MD = C_{target} * CL = 15$ mg/L $* 0.81$ L/h
$\qquad = 12.15$ mg/h theophylline
$\qquad = 15.2$ mg/h aminophylline
BW 55 kg: MD = 0.28 mg/kg/h

3. Approximately how long does it take to achieve the new steady-state after the infusion rate has been changed?
   a. 26 h
   b. 68 h
   c. 118 h
   d. 156 h
   e. 192 h

Estimated V = 55 kg $* 0.5$ L/kg = 27.5 L

$$t_{1/2} = \frac{\ln 2}{K} = \frac{\ln 2 * V}{CL} = \frac{0.693 * 27.5 \text{ L}}{0.81 \text{ L/h}} = 23.5 \text{ h}$$

Time to new steady-state is approximately
$5 \; t_{1/2} = 118$ hours

4. The pharmacist suggests that the new target concentration can be achieved faster if the first infusion with the higher infusion rate is completely stopped and the second infusion with the lower infusion rate is not initiated until the plasma concentration has decreased to 15 mg/L, the target concentration. Calculate the period of time the therapy has to pause (ie, the time one waits after cessation of the first infusion before the second infusion is started).
   a. 14.7 h
   b. 16.4 h
   c. 20.7 h
   d. 36.1 h
   e. 55.1 h

$$C_{target} = C_{ss,old} * e^{-K * t_{pause}}$$

$$t_{pause} = \frac{\ln\left(\dfrac{C_{target}}{C_{ss,old}}\right)}{-K} = \frac{\ln\left(\dfrac{15 \text{ mg/L}}{24.3 \text{ mg/L}}\right) * 27.5 \text{ L}}{-0.81 \text{ L/h}} = 16.4 \text{ h}$$

11. Key Points

- The clearance CL can be determined from the relationship

$$CL = \frac{DR}{C_{ss,avg}} \quad \text{or} \quad CL = \frac{D}{AUC}$$

- The volume of distribution can be determined from the relationship

$$V = \frac{CL}{K}$$

- The average steady-state concentration $C_{ss,av}$ during multiple dosing is only determined by the dose, the dosing interval τ (or both together as dosing rate DR $= D/\tau$), and the clearance CL:

$$C_{ss,av} = \frac{D}{\tau * CL}$$

- The area under the curve resulting from administration of a single dose AUC_{single} is equal to the area under the curve during one dosing interval at steady-state AUC_{ss}, if the same dose is given per dosing interval τ.

$$C_{ss,av} = \frac{AUC_{ss}}{\tau} = \frac{D}{\tau * CL} = \frac{AUC_{single}}{\tau}$$

- The volume of distribution at steady-state is by definition the sum of the pharmacokinetic volumes of distribution for the different pharmacokinetic compartments. It is the theoretical:

$$V_{ss} = V_p + \frac{f_u}{f_{u,t}} * V_t$$

where V_p is the volume of plasma (3 L), V_t is the volume of tissue water (total body water minus plasma volume: $42 - 3 = 39$ L, based on a "standard" person). f_{up} and f_{ut} are the fraction unbound for the drug in plasma and tissue, respectively.

- Clearance (CL) is defined as the irreversible removal of drug from the body by an organ of elimination. Since the units of CL are flow per time (eg, milliliters per minute or liters per hour), CL is often defined as the volume of blood irreversibly cleared of drug per unit of time.

- The venous equilibrium model can be simplified for drugs with low ER (<0.3) and high ER (>0.7). For low-ER drugs, $CL_H = f_{up} * CL_{int}$. For high-ER drugs, $CL_H = Q$.

$$CL_H = \frac{Q * f_{up} * CL_{int}}{Q + f_{up} * CL_{int}}$$

- The absolute bioavailability is the fraction (or percentage) of a dose administered non-intravenously (or extravascularly) that is systemically available as compared to an intravenous dose. The overall oral bioavailability (F) of a drug is dependent on the fraction absorbed (f_a), the fraction escaping metabolism in the intestinal wall (f_g), and the fraction escaping hepatic first-pass metabolism (F*).

- Drugs may undergo three processes in the kidney. Two of these act to remove drug from the body: filtration and secretion. The other, reabsorption, acts to return the drug to the body. We can determine the net process a drug undergoes by calculating the excretion ratio (E_{ratio}) using total renal clearance (CL_R) and filtration clearance (CL_F):

$$E_{ratio} = \frac{CL_R}{CL_F} = \frac{CL_R}{f_{up} * 125 \text{ mL/min}}$$

12. Questions and Answers

1. A pediatric patient receives immunosuppressive therapy with oral cyclosporine solution. His concentration-adjusted dosing regimen is 85 mg every 12 hours. Due to a recent change in his insurance coverage, he needs to be switched from the drug product he is currently using to a generic solution dosage form of cyclosporine that is covered by his insurance. The bioavailability of the dosage form he previously used is 43%, and the bioavailability of the generic dosage form is 28%. What is the appropriate dosage regimen for the generic dosage form in order to maintain the same systemic exposure as obtained from the previously used dosage form?

   A. 25 mg every 12 hours
   B. 55 mg every 12 hours
   C. 184 mg every 12 hours
   D. 130 mg every 12 hours
   E. 305 mg every 12 hours

2. A drug is administered via continuous infusion at a rate of 60 mg/h, resulting in a steady-state plasma concentration of 5 mcg/mL. If the plasma concentration is intended to be doubled to 10 mcg/mL, the infusion rate must be

   A. left the same
   B. increased by 30 mg/h
   C. increased by 60 mg/h
   D. increased by 120 mg/h
   E. decreased by 30 mg/h

3. Jonathan R. (72 kg, 23 years of age) has been admitted to the emergency department with acute asthma symptoms. He shall be started on a continuous infusion of aminophylline with a target theophylline concentration of 12 mg/L (therapeutic range 10-20 mg/L). To achieve the target concentration more rapidly, an additional loading dose shall be administered as a short-term infusion over 30 minutes. The population mean values for clearance and volume of distribution of theophylline are 2.7 L/h and 34 L, respectively. What aminophylline loading and maintenance dose should be given? (Select practical and useful doses and remember that aminophylline contains 80% theophylline.)

3a. Loading dose:
   A. 400 mg
   B. 450 mg

C. 500 mg
D. 550 mg
E. 600 mg

3b. Maintenance dose:
    A. 35 mg/h
    B. 40 mg/h
    C. 45 mg/h
    D. 50 mg/h
    E. 55 mg/h

4. Lidocaine shall be given as a constant rate infusion for the treatment of ventricular arrhythmia. A plasma concentration of 3 mcg/mL was decided as the therapeutic target concentration. The concentration of the infusion solution is 20 mg/mL lidocaine. The average volume of distribution of lidocaine is 90 L, the elimination half-life is 1.1 hours. What infusion rate (in milliliters per minute) has to be set on the infusion pump in order to achieve the desired target concentration?

    A. 5 mL/h
    B. 8.5 mL/h
    C. 14 mL/h
    D. 23.5 mL/h
    E. 194 mL/h

5. After termination of an intravenous constant rate infusion, the plasma concentration of a drug declines monoexponentially ($C = C * e^{-k * t}$). Concentrations measured at 2 hours and 12 hours after the end of the infusion are 12.9 mcg/mL and 6.0 mcg/mL, respectively. Calculate the initial concentration at the end of the infusion, and predict the concentration 24 hours after termination of the infusion.

    A. 13.5 and 2.9 mcg/mL
    B. 16.5 and 3.8 mcg/mL
    C. 16.5 and 1.3 mcg/mL
    D. 15 and 2.4 mcg/mL
    E. 15 and 1.3 mcg/mL

6. Margaret Q. (100 kg, 26 years of age) presents to the emergency department with acute symptoms of asthma. She recently started smoking again and has been taking oral theophylline for several years. The immediate determination of her theophylline plasma concentration results in a level of 4 mg/L. Theophylline population pharmacokinetic parameters: CL 0.04 L/h/kg, V 0.5 L/kg
Therapeutic range: 10-20 mg/L. The appropriate intravenous loading dose of aminophylline for

Margaret to achieve a target concentration of 12 mg/L is:

    A. 300 mg
    B. 400 mg
    C. 500 mg
    D. 600 mg
    E. 750 mg

7. For a drug product in clinical drug development, an oral dosing regimen needs to be established for a phase III study that maintains an average steady-state concentration of 50 ng/mL. In single-dose studies, an oral dose of 80 mg resulted in an AUC of 962 ng/h/mL and an elimination half-life of 10.3 hours. What dosing regimen should be used?

    A. 35 mg every 12 hours
    B. 50 mg every 12 hours
    C. 72 mg every 12 hours
    D. 95 mg every 12 hours
    E. 125 mg every 12 hours

8. Mary D. (47 years of age, 68 kg) has recently received her first 0.25-mg dose of digoxin. Plasma digoxin concentrations 12 and 24 hours following oral administration of this dose are 0.72 and 0.33 mcg/L, respectively. The therapeutic plasma concentration range is 0.8-2.0 mcg/L. Predict Mary's digoxin trough concentration at steady state, assuming that oral digoxin therapy is continued at a dose rate of 0.25 mg once daily.

    A. 0.62 mcg/L
    B. 0.93 mcg/L
    C. 1.32 mcg/L
    D. 1.57 mcg/L
    E. 1.95 mcg/L

9. The population average values for the clearance and volume of distribution of nifedipine have been reported as 0.41 L/h/kg and 1.2 L/kg. What would be the maximum dosing interval you can use for a multiple-dose regimen with an immediate-release oral dosage form of nifedipine if peak-to-trough fluctuation should not exceed 100%?

    A. 2 hours
    B. 4 hours
    C. 6 hours
    D. 8 hours
    E. 12 hours

10. Beth R. (63 years of age, 58 kg) is suffering from symptomatic ventricular arrhythmia. She will be started on an oral multiple-dose regimen with the antiarrhythmic mexiletine. The population average values of mexiletine for clearance and volume of distribution are CL = 0.5 L/h/kg and V = 6 L/kg, respectively. Although a therapeutic range of 0.5-2.0 mg/L has been described, it is recommended to avoid large peak-to-trough fluctuations. The available oral dosage forms are 150-, 200-, and 250-mg capsules with an oral bioavailability of F = 0.9. Design an appropriate and practically reasonable oral dosing regimen that keeps the plasma concentrations at an average concentration of approximately 1 mg/L, with a peak-to-trough fluctuation of 100% (ie, with concentrations within the limits of 0.75 and 1.5 mg/L).

A. 150 mg q6h
B. 200 mg q6h
C. 200 mg q8h
D. 250 mg q8h
E. 375 mg q12h

11. Edgar W. (20 years old, 58 kg) is receiving 80 mg of gentamicin as an IV infusion over a 30-minute period q8h. Two plasma samples are obtained to monitor serum gentamicin concentrations as follows: one sample 30 minutes after the end of the short-term infusion and one sample 30 minutes before the administration of the next dose. The serum gentamicin concentrations at these times are 4.9 and 1.7 mg/L, respectively. Assume steady state. Develop a practically reasonable dosing regimen that will produce peak-and-trough concentrations of approximately 8 and 1 mg/L, respectively.

A. 120 mg q8h
B. 160 mg q8h
C. 140 mg q12h
D. 180 mg q12h
E. 280 mg q24h

12. A patient who is receiving chronic phenytoin therapy is hospitalized for an elective surgical procedure. On admission labs, it is noted that the patient has a phenytoin concentration of 8 mcg/mL (therapeutic range: 10-20 mcg/mL) and an albumin concentration of 3.0 g/dL. Phenytoin: F = 0.2-0.9, CL variable, <1% excreted unchanged in the urine, 88-93% bound to plasma proteins (primarily albumin).

Based on this information, and the therapeutic range of phenytoin, you would recommend that the physician

A. decrease the dose of phenytoin, because high-E drugs (eg, phenytoin) exhibit increased unbound concentrations with increases in fraction unbound in the plasma
B. increase the dose rate of phenytoin, because low-E drugs (eg, phenytoin) exhibit increased CL with increases in fraction unbound in the plasma
C. not change the dose rate of phenytoin because low-E drugs (eg, phenytoin) do not exhibit changes in unbound concentrations with increases in fraction unbound in the plasma
D. not change the dose rate of phenytoin because low-E drugs (eg, phenytoin) exhibit equal and offsetting changes in CL and F with increases in fraction unbound in plasma

13. The conditions that indicate the possibility of renal clearance of a weakly acidic drug being sensitive to changes in urine pH are that

I. it is secreted and not reabsorbed
II. it has a pK_a value of 5.0
III. it has a small volume of distribution
IV. all of the drug is excreted unchanged by the kidneys (ie, $f_e = 1$)

A. Only item I is correct
B. Only item II is correct
C. Only item III is correct
D. Items II and III are correct
E. Items II and IV are correct

14. A young man (age 28 years, 73 kg, creatinine clearance 124 mL/min) receives a single 200-mg oral dose of an antibiotic. The following pharmacokinetic parameters of the antibiotic are reported in the literature: F: 90%; V_d: 0.31 L/kg; $t_{1/2}$: 2.1 h; f_{up}: 0.77. 67% of the antibiotic's absorbed dose is excreted unchanged in the urine. Determine the renal clearance of the antibiotic. What is the probable mechanism for renal clearance of this drug?

A. 84 mL/min; glomerular filtration and tubular reabsorption
B. 98 mL/min; glomerular filtration and tubular reabsorption
C. 112 mL/min; glomerular filtration
D. 167 mL/min; glomerular filtration and tubular reabsorption

E. 236 mL/min; glomerular filtration and tubular secretion

15a. The pharmacokinetic parameters for captopril in healthy adults are
Clearance: 800 mL/min; $f_e = 0.5$; V_{ss}: 0.81 L/kg
Plasma protein binding: 75%
Captopril is a weakly basic drug used in the treatment of hypertension. Assume a glomerular filtration rate of 125 mL/min. The mechanism(s) for renal clearance of captopril is:

A. Filtration only
B. Reabsorption only
C. Secretion only
D. Filtration and net secretion
E. Filtration and net reabsorption

15b. When cimetidine (a highly lipid-soluble weak base that is highly secreted in the renal proximal tubules) and captopril are co-administered, the renal clearance of captopril is reduced to approximately 125 mL/min. What is the most likely mechanism to account for this reduction in renal clearance?

A. Cimetidine reduces the filtration clearance of captopril
B. Cimetidine enhances the reabsorption of captopril
C. Cimetidine increases the unbound fraction of captopril
D. Cimetidine blocks the renal secretion of captopril

16. One of the most severe drug interactions is that between digoxin and quinidine. Administration of quinidine to patients taking digoxin results in a two- to threefold increase in digoxin C_{ss} and AUC after oral and intravenous administration of digoxin. Digoxin and quinidine are substrates for the multidrug-resistance transporter P-glyco-protein. Based on the following pharmacokinetic data for digoxin, what is the most likely mecha-nism to explain this drug/drug interaction?
CL: 125 mL/min; V_{ss}: 1.2 L/kg (IBW)
f_e: >0.99; f_{up}: 0.25

A. Quinidine reduces the digoxin fraction escaping first-pass metabolism
B. Quinidine inhibits renal secretion of digoxin by blocking P-glycoprotein
C. Quinidine decreases the digoxin fraction reabsorbed in the kidney tubule
D. Quinidine reduces the fraction of digoxin absorbed

17. The drug transporter P-glycoprotein (Pgp) is involved in numerous processes in drug disposition. Pgp activity is directly responsible for the following processes:

I. Glomerular filtration
II. Transport of drug from hepatocytes into the bile
III. Transport of drug from the small intestine into the systemic circulation (ie, bloodstream)
IV. Degradation of drug in the lumen of the duodenum
V. Maintenance of the integrity of the blood-brain barrier by transport of drug out of the brain

A. Only V
B. II and V
C. II and III
D. I, II, and V
E. All of the above

18. A 59-year-old white female is hospitalized for a ruptured duodenal diverticulum. She is 5' 6", weighs 65 kg, and has a serum creatinine of 1.5 mg/dL. Design a dosage regimen to achieve C_{peak} and C_{trough} values of 8 and 0.5 mg/L, respectively, with an infusion time of 30 minutes. Assume V_d of gentamicin of 0.2 L/kg IBW in this patient. The typical population value of CL for gentamicin is 85 mL/min/70 kg. Which of the following dosage regimens would you recommend for this patient?

A. 100 mg q8h
B. 100 mg q18h
C. 100 mg q24h
D. 160 mg q12h
E. 160 mg q24h

19. J.D. is a 47-year-old white male who has been prescribed codeine for lower back pain. The pharmacist dispensing the medication remembers reading a study in which patients who took codeine with grapefruit juice experienced an enhanced analgesic effect. The study found that grapefruit juice enhanced oral bioavailability (F) of codeine. Interestingly, there was no effect on codeine hepatic clearance or volume of distribution. Thus the pharmacist counseled the patient not to take his codeine with grapefruit juice. Based on the pharma-cokinetic data for codeine listed below, what is the most likely explanation for the enhanced oral bioavailability (F) of codeine?
CL: 1350 mL/min; f_e: 0.10; V_{ss}: 3.3 L/kg
Plasma protein binding: 35%

A. Grapefruit juice increases the absorption (f_a) of codeine

B. Grapefruit juice decreases the fraction escaping first-pass metabolism (F*)

C. Grapefruit juice increases renal secretion of codeine

D. Grapefruit juice increases the fraction escaping first-pass metabolism (F*)

20. The pharmacokinetic parameters for codeine in healthy adults are:
Oral F: 50%; f_e <0.01; V_{ss}: 2.6 L/kg
Plasma protein binding: 7%
Codeine is well absorbed ($f_a = 1$, $f_g = 0.8$). You may assume that hepatic blood flow in a 70-kg adult is 1350 mL/min. The hepatic clearance of codeine is:

A. 851 mL/min
B. 1350 mL/min
C. 500 mL/min
D. 675 mL/min

Answers

1. **D.** The systemic exposure or average steady-state concentration for an oral dosing regimen is given by

$$C_{ss,av} = \frac{F * DR}{CL}$$

where DR is the dose rate and F the oral bioavailability of the respective dosing regimens.
If $C_{ss,av}$ should be maintained constant, it follows that

$$C_{ss,av} = \frac{F_1 * DR_1}{CL} = \frac{F_2 * DR_2}{CL} \quad \text{or} \quad F_1 * DR = F_2 * DR$$

where the subscript denotes the different dosing regimens. Thus DR_2, the dose rate for the generic dosage form, can be calculated as

$$DR_2 = \frac{F_1 * DR_1}{F_2} = \frac{43\% * 85 \text{ mg}/12 \text{ h}}{28\%} = 130.5 \text{ mg}/12 \text{ h}$$

2. **C.** Steady-state plasma concentration of a constant rate infusion is directly proportional to the infusion rate R_0 via

$$C_{ss} = \frac{R_0}{CL}$$

Thus R_0 has to be doubled from 60 mg/h to 120 mg/h in order to increase C_{ss} from 5 to 10 mcg/mL, ie, an increase of the infusion rate by 60 mg/h.

3a. **C.** Give 500 mg for the loading dose.

3b. **B.** Give 40 mg/h for the maintenance dose.

The loading dose (LD) and the maintenance dose (MD) can be calculated from the target concentration and volume of distribution or clearance:

LD = C_{target} * V = 12 mg/L * 34 L
  = 408 mg theophylline
  = 510 mg aminophylline

MD = C_{target} * CL = 12 mg/L * 2.7 L/h
  = 32.4 mg/h theophylline
  = 40.5 mg/h aminophylline

4. **B.** The infusion rate R_0 or maintenance dose MD needed to achieve and maintain a steady-state concentration of 3 mcg/mL is given by

$$MD = R_0 = C_{ss} * CL = C_{ss} * V * \frac{0.693}{t_{1/2}}$$

$$= 3 \text{ mcg/mL} * 90 \text{ L} * \frac{0.693}{1.1 \text{ h}} = 170 \text{ mg/h}$$

The infusion pump setting can then be calculated as

$$Infusion\ volume/time = \frac{170 \text{ mg/h}}{20 \text{ mg/mL}} = 8.5 \text{ mL/h}$$

5. **D.** The first step is to calculate the elimination rate constant k from the measured plasma concentrations:

$$k = \frac{\ln\left(\dfrac{C_{12\,h}}{C_{2\,h}}\right)}{12 \text{ h} - 2 \text{ h}} = \frac{\ln\left(\dfrac{12.9 \text{ mcg/mL}}{6.0 \text{ mcg/L}}\right)}{12 \text{ h} - 2 \text{ h}} = 0.077 \text{ h}^{-1}$$

The initial concentration C_0 at the end of the infusion can then be back-extrapolated by solving the following relationship for C_0:

$$C = C_0 * e^{-k * t}$$

$$C_0 = \frac{12.9 \text{ mcg/mL}}{e^{-0.077 \text{ h}^{-1} * 2 \text{ h}}} = 15 \text{ mcg/mL}$$

The concentration 24 hours after termination of the infusion can be predicted by

$$C_{24\,h} = 15 \text{ mcg/mL} * e^{-0.077 \text{ h}^{-1} * 24 \text{ h}} = 2.4 \text{ mcg/mL}$$

6. **C.** The loading dose can be determined based on the target concentration to be achieved and the volume of distribution. The predose level of 4 mg/L needs to be subtracted from the target concentration, since the loading dose only has to

account for the concentration difference. The calculated theophylline dose needs to be converted to aminophylline:

$$LD = (C_{target} - C_{predose}) * V_d = (12 - 4) \text{ mg/L} * 0.5 \text{ L/kg} * 100 \text{ kg} = 400 \text{ mg theophylline}$$

A loading dose of 400 mg theophylline is equivalent to 500 mg aminophylline.

7. **B.** The maintenance dose MD required to achieve an average steady-state concentration of 50 ng/mL for an oral dosing regimen is given by

$$MD = C_{ss,av} * CL/F$$

The oral clearance CL/F can be determined from the relationship between dose and area under the plasma concentration-time curve AUC:

$$CL/F = \frac{D}{AUC}$$

Thus the required MD can be calculated as

$$MD = C_{ss,av} * \frac{D}{AUC} = 50 \text{ ng/mL} * \frac{80 \text{ mg}}{962 \text{ ng/h/mL}} = 4.16 \text{ mg/h}$$

This corresponds to a dosing regimen of 50 mg (4.16 mg/h x 12 h) given every 12 hours.

8. **D.** Since trough concentrations after the first dose are known (0.33 mcg/L), trough concentrations during multiple doses at steady state can be predicted by multiplying the trough after the first dose with the accumulation factor:

$$C_{ss,min} = C_{ss,1} * \frac{1}{e^{-k*\tau}}$$

The dosing interval τ is 24 hours, and k can be calculated from

$$k = \frac{\ln\left(\frac{C_1}{C_2}\right)}{t} = \frac{\ln\left(\frac{0.72}{0.33}\right)}{(24 - 12) \text{ h}} = 0.065 \text{ h}^{-1}$$

Thus,

$$C_{ss,min} = 0.33 \text{ mcg/L} * \frac{1}{e^{-0.065 \text{ h}^{-1}*24 \text{ h}}} = 1.57 \text{ mc/L}$$

9. **A.** For immediate-release formulations, upper limits for peak concentrations ($C_{ss,max}$) and lower limits for trough concentrations ($C_{ss,min}$) can be estimated by assuming immediate drug absorption. If fluctuation is equal to 100%, $C_{ss,min}$ is exactly one-half of $C_{ss,max}$. This is the case when the dosing interval τ is equal to the elimination half-life $t_{1/2}$ of the drug. A

population average half-life for nifedipine can be calculated as

$$k = \frac{CL}{V} = \frac{0.41 \text{ L/h/kg}}{1.21 \text{ L/kg}} = 0.34 \text{ h}^{-1}$$

$$t_{1/2} = \frac{0.693}{0.34 \text{ h}^{-1}} = \frac{0.41 \text{ L/h/kg}}{1.21 \text{ L/kg}} = 2.03 \text{ h}$$

Thus τ has to be smaller than 2.03 hours in order to avoid peak-to-trough fluctuation exceeding 100%.

10. **D.** Calculate the necessary dose rate DR to maintain $C_{ss,avg} = 1$ mg/L:

$$DR_{necessary} = \frac{D}{\tau} = \frac{C_{ss,av} * CL}{F} = \frac{1 \text{ mg/L} * 0.5 \text{ L/h/kg} * 58 \text{ g}}{0.90}$$
$$= 32.22 \text{ mg/h} = 773.3 \text{ mg/d}$$

Determine the maximum dosing interval:

$$\tau_{max} = \frac{\ln\left(\frac{C_{ss,max}}{C_{ss,min}}\right)}{K} = \frac{\ln\left(\frac{C_{ss,max}}{C_{ss,min}}\right) * V}{CL} = \frac{\ln\left(\frac{1.5}{0.75}\right) * 6 \text{ L/kg}}{0.5 \text{ L/h/kg}}$$
$$= 8.3 \text{ h}$$

Reasonable and practical dosing interval: 8 hours

$$D = DR_{necessary} * \tau = 32.22 \text{ mg/h} * 8 \text{ h} = 257.8 \text{ mg}$$

Recommended dosing regimen: 250 mg every 8 hours

11. **C.** Calculate the elimination rate constant k:

$$k = \frac{\ln\left(\frac{C_1}{C_2}\right)}{t} = \frac{\ln\left(\frac{4.9}{1.7}\right)}{6.5 \text{ h}} = 0.163 \text{ h}^{-1}$$

Calculate volume of distribution assuming steady state:

$$C_{ss,max} = \frac{C_{measured\ peak}}{e^{-k*t}} = \frac{4.9 \text{ mg/L}}{e^{-0.163 \text{ h}^{-1}*0.5 \text{ h}}} = 5.32 \text{ mg/L}$$

$$C_{ss,min} = C_{measured\ trough} * e^{-k*t} = 1.7 \text{ mg/L} * e^{-0.163 \text{ h}^{-1}*0.5 \text{ h}}$$
$$= 1.57 \text{ mg/h}$$

$$V = \frac{R_0}{k} * \frac{1 - e^{-k*T_{inf}}}{C_{max} - C_{min} * e^{-k*T_{inf}}} = \frac{80 \text{ mg}}{0.163 \text{ h}^{-1} * 0.5 \text{ h}} *$$

$$\frac{1 - e^{-0.163 \text{ h}^{-1}*0.5 \text{ h}}}{5.32 \text{ mg/h} - 1.57 \text{ mg/h} * e^{-0.163 \text{ h}^{-1}*0.5 \text{ h}}} = 19.8 \text{ L}$$

Calculate the recommended dosing interval:

$$\tau = \frac{\ln\left(\dfrac{C_{ss,\max(desired)}}{C_{ss,\min(desired)}}\right)}{k} + T_{inf} = \frac{\ln\left(\dfrac{8}{1}\right)}{0.163 \text{ h}} + .5 \text{ h} = 13.3 \text{ h}$$

Recommend dosing interval: 12 hours
Calculate recommended dose:

$$D = C_{ss,\max(desired)} * K * V * T_{inf} * \frac{1 - e^{-K*\tau}}{1 - e^{-K*T_{inf}}} =$$

$$= 8 \text{ mg/L} * 0.163 \text{ h}^{-1} * 19.8 \text{ L} * 0.5 \text{ h} * \frac{1 - e^{-0.163 \text{ h}^{-1}*12 \text{ h}}}{1 - e^{-0.163 \text{ h}^{-1}*0.5 \text{ h}}}$$

$D = 142$ mg
Recommended dosing regimen: 140 mg
every 12 hours

12. **C.** Phenytoin has to be a low-extraction drug since its bioavailability is as high as 90%. The large range in F is due to variability in the absorption of the drug. You know it is not high E because if it was, you could never get an F of 90%. Assume ER <0.1, f_{up} = 0.07 to 0.12. You should assume that all low-extraction drugs are restrictively cleared. Normal albumin range: 3.5-5 g/dL. Thus the patient probably has increased f_{up} because of decreased albumin. f_{up} (based on the equation below) would be 0.14 (slightly elevated).

$$f_{up} = \frac{1}{1 + 2.1 * albumin}$$

It is a low-E drug, therefore CL is dependent on f_{up} and CL_{int}. Increased f_{up} would lead to increased CL and decreased total plasma concentrations (thus C_{peak} of 8, which is below the therapeutic range). However, unbound concentrations would be predicted to be normal (therapeutic) even though total concentration is low. You would not recommend an increase in the patient's phenytoin dose, as it may result in toxic concentrations. If available from the hospital's lab, it may be reasonable to obtain a free phenytoin plasma concentration to document therapeutic concentrations.

13. **B.** Only item II is correct.

Item I is incorrect. No pH sensitivity in CL_R is expected unless the drug is reabsorbed (ie, E_{ratio} <<1).

Item II is possible. Weakly acidic drugs with pK_a values between 3 and 7.5 can be highly un-

ionized in the range of urine pH (5-8) and thus undergo significant reabsorption if the un-ionized form is nonpolar.

Item III is incorrect. CL and V have nothing to do with a drug's likelihood of being affected by changes in urine pH.

Item IV is also incorrect. The fraction excreted unchanged tells us nothing about the mechanisms of renal elimination. However, it is important to note that for drugs with high f_e values that are susceptible to changes in urine pH, large changes in the PK of the drug (ie, CL_R) may be observed.

14. **A.** The antibiotic's total clearance can be determined from the reported Vd and $t_{1/2}$:

$$CL = Vd * \frac{\ln 2}{t_{1/2}} = 0.31 \text{ L/kg} * 73 \text{ kg} * \frac{0.693}{2.1 \text{ h}} = 7.47 \text{ L/h}$$

Renal clearance CL_R is then given by total clearance and the fraction excreted fe:

$$CL_R = f_e * CL = 0.67 * 7.47 \text{ L/h} = 5.00 \text{ L/h} = 83.3 \text{ mL/min}$$

The predominant renal clearance mechanism can be estimated by determining the E_{ratio}:

$$E_{ratio} = \frac{CL_R}{f_{up} * GFR} = \frac{83.3 \text{ mL/min}}{0.77 * 124 \text{ mL/min}} = 0.87$$

The E_{ratio} <1 indicates that glomerular filtration and net reabsorption are the probable renal clearance mechanisms.

15a. **D.** The excretion ratio for captopril is significantly greater than 1, indicating that captopril undergoes filtration and net secretion.

$$CL_R = CL_T * f_e$$

$$CL_R = 800 \text{ mL/min} * 0.5 = 400 \text{ mL/min}$$

$$E_{ratio} = \frac{CL_R}{f_{up} * GFR} = \frac{400 \text{ mL/min}}{0.25 * 125 \text{ mL/min}}$$

$$= 12.8 = \text{filtration and net secretion}$$

15b. **D.** The most likely mechanism to account for this reduction in renal clearance is that the cimetidine blocks the renal secretion of captopril.

16. **B.** Digoxin undergoes net secretion via active transport processes (eg, P-glycoprotein). Quinidine is a potent inhibitor of P-glycoprotein. Therefore, P-glycoprotein inhibition by

quinidine results in a reduced renal clearance of digoxin.

$$CL_R = CL_T * f_e$$

$$CL_R = 125 \text{ mL/min} * 1.0 = 125 \text{ mL/min}$$

$$E_{ratio} = \frac{CL_R}{f_{up} * GFR} = \frac{125 \text{ mL/min}}{0.25 * 125 \text{ mL/min}}$$

$$= 4.0 = \text{filtration and net secretion}$$

17. **B.** The drug transporter P-glycoprotein (Pgp) is directly responsible for the transport of drug from hepatocytes into the bile and maintenance of the integrity of the blood-brain barrier by transport of drug out of the brain.

18. **C.** Calculation of CL: IBW = 59.3 kg

$$CL_{cr} = \frac{(140 - \text{age}) * IBW}{72 * S_{cr}} \quad \frac{(140 - 59) * 59.3}{72 * 1.5}$$

$$* 0.85 = 37.8 \text{ mL/min}$$

RF = 37.8/125 = 0.30. CL of gentamicin is 85 mL/min/70 kg TBW (1.2 mL/min/kg). CL of gentamicin in this patient if she did not have renal impairment would be:

CL = 1.21 mL/min/kg * 65 kg = 79 mL/min

$$CL^* = CL * [1 - f_e * (1 - RF)]$$
$$= 79 * [1 - 1 * (1 - 0.30)]$$
$$= 23.7 \text{ mL/min}$$
$$= 1.42 \text{ L/h}$$

$$K^* = \frac{CL^*}{V_{ss}} = \frac{1.42 \text{ L/h}}{0.2 \text{ L/kg} * 59.3 \text{ kg}} = 0.12 \text{ h}^{-1}$$

Calculate the dosing interval (τ) that you would recommend:

$$\tau = \frac{\ln\left(\frac{8}{0.5}\right)}{0.12 \text{ h}^{-1}} + 0.5 \text{ h} = 23.1 \text{ h}$$

Calculate the dose of gentamicin that will maintain C_{peak} and C_{trough} of 8 and 0.5 mg/L, respectively:

$$\text{Dose} = C_{ss,max} * K * V * t_{inf} * \frac{1 - e^{-K*\tau}}{1 - e^{-K*t_{inf}}}$$

$$\text{Dose} = 8 \text{ mg/L} * 0.12 \text{ h}^{-1} * 11.86 \text{ L} * 0.5 \text{ h} * \frac{1 - e^{-0.12*24}}{1 - e^{-0.12*0.5}}$$
$$= 92.3 \text{ mg}$$

Administration of 100 mg of gentamicin infused over 30 minutes given every 24 hours will provide C_{peak} and C_{trough} of approximately 8 and 0.5 mg/L, respectively.

19. **A.**

$$CL_H = 1350 * 0.9 = 1215 \text{ mL/min}$$

$$ER = \frac{1215 \text{ mL/min}}{1350 \text{ mL/min}} \approx 1$$

$$F = f_a * f_g * F^*$$

No effect on CL_H. No effect on F^*.

20. **C.**

$$F = f_a * f_g * F^*$$

$$F = \frac{F}{fa * fg} = \frac{0.5}{1 * 0.8} = 0.63$$

$$ER = 1 - F^* = 1 - 0.63 = 0.37$$

$$CL_H = Q * ER = 1350 \text{ mL/min} * 0.37$$
$$= 500 \text{ mL/min}$$

13. References

Atkinson A, Daniels C, Dedrick R, Grudzinskas C, Markey S. *Principles of Clinical Pharmacology.* San Diego, CA: Academic Press; 2001.

Ensom MH, Davis GA, Cropp CD, Ensom RJ. Clinical pharmacokinetics in the 21st century. Does the evidence support definitive outcomes? *Clin Pharmacokinet.* 1998;34:265-279.

Levy RH, Bauer LA. Basic pharmacokinetics. *Ther Drug Monit.* 1986;8:47-58.

Meibohm B, Derendorf H. Basic concepts of pharmacokinetic/pharmacodynamic (PK/PD) modelling. *Int J Clin Pharmacol Ther.* 1997;35:401-413.

Rolan PE. Plasma protein binding displacement interactions—why are they still regarded as clinically important? *Br J Clin Pharmacol.* 1994;37:125-128.

Rowland M, Tozer T. *Clinical Pharmacokinetics.* 3rd ed. Media, PA: Williams & Wilkins; 1995.

Saitoh A, Jinbayashi H, Saitoh AK, et al. Parameter estimation and dosage adjustment in the treatment with vancomycin of methicillin-resistant *Staphylococcus aureus* ocular infections. *Ophthalmologica.* 1997;211:232-235.

Sawchuck RJ, Zaske DE, Cipolle RJ, Wargin WA, Strate RG. Kinetic model for gentamicin dosing with the use of individual patient parameters. *Clin Pharmacol Ther.* 1977;21:362-369.

Tod MM, Padoin C, Petitjean O. Individualising aminoglycoside dosage regimens after therapeutic drug monitoring: simple or complex pharmacokinetic methods? *Clin Pharmacokinet.* 2001;40:803-814.

Wilkinson GR, Shand DG. Commentary: a physiological approach to hepatic drug clearance. *Clin Pharmacol Ther.* 1975;18:377-390.

7. Biotechnology and Pharmacogenomics

P. David Rogers, PharmD, PhD
Associate Professor
Department of Clinical Pharmacy
University of Tennessee College of Pharmacy

Contents

1. Introduction to Biotechnology and Pharmacogenomics

Since the discovery of the DNA double helix half a century ago, man has made significant use of biotechnology for the improvement of human health (Table 1). Accompanying these advances are a number of biological products with therapeutic applications. With the arrival of the post-genomic era, the field of pharmacogenomics has emerged and shows great promise to revolutionize the way in which pharmacy and medicine is practiced. This chapter highlights key concepts relevant to the practicing pharmacist in the areas of biotechnology and pharmacogenomics.

Biotechnology has revolutionized the pharmaceutical industry by imparting the ability to mass produce safe and pure versions of chemicals produced naturally in the body. A multitude of disease states have been impacted by therapeutic agents derived through biotechnology, including AIDS, anemia, cancer, cystic fibrosis, congestive heart failure, diabetes, hemophilia, hepatitis B and C, growth hormone deficiency, and multiple sclerosis, to name a few.

Biotechnology is defined by the United States Food and Drug Administration as "the use of recombinant

Table 1

Milestones in Biotechnology

Event	Year
Identification of DNA as the genetic material	1940
Discovery of DNA double helix by James Watson and Francis Crick	1953
Elucidation of the genetic code (64 nucleic acid triplets, or codons, encode 20 amino acids)	1961
Cloning of DNA and the production of the first recombinant DNA derived protein	1973
Introduction of monoclonal antibodies	1975
Production of the first human protein (somatostatin) from recombinant DNA technology	1977
Cloning of the human insulin gene	1978
Human insulin derived from recombinant DNA technology licensed in the U.S.	1982
Conception of the polymerase chain reaction (PCR) for amplification of DNA	1983
Initiation of the Human Genome Project	1990
Sequencing of the human genome	2001

DNA (or RNA) technology; direct DNA transfer technology; nucleic acid amplification technology; hybridoma technology; cell fusion; molecular modification of cellular receptors; or the application of cells, tissues, or their components such that their potential biological activity has been modified."

Key Terms

antibody (immunoglobulin): a protein produced by β-lymphocytes in response to antigen molecules determined to be non-self. Antibodies recognize and bind to antigens, resulting in their inactivation or opsonization for phagocytosis or complement-mediated destruction. A number of immunoglobulin (Ig) G products have been developed for therapeutic use in various immune disorders.

antigen: a molecule that elicits an antibody-mediated immune response.

bioinformatics: the application of computer sciences and information technology to the management and analysis of biological information.

biotherapy: any treatment involving the administration of a microorganism or other biologic material.

clotting factor (blood factor): chemical blood constituents that interact to cause blood coagulation.

combinatorial chemistry: a drug development strategy that utilizes nucleic acids and amino acids in various combinations to synthesize vast libraries of oligonucleotide or peptide compounds for high-throughput lead compound screening.

cytokine: an extracellular signaling protein that mediates communication between cells.

DNA (deoxyribonucleic acid): a polynucleotide molecule consisting of covalently linked nucleic acids. DNA serves as the genetic material.

enzyme: a protein that catalyzes a chemical reaction.

gene: a region of DNA that encodes a specific RNA or protein responsible for a specific hereditary characteristic.

gene therapy: therapeutic technologies that directly target human genes responsible for disease.

genome: the complete set of genetic information for a given organism.

genomics: the scientific discipline of mapping, sequencing, and analyzing genomes. It encompasses structural genomics, functional genomics, and pharmacogenomics.

hormone: a chemical substance that imparts specific cellular effects that is transmitted by the bloodstream to cells distant from its physiologic source.

hybridoma: a cell line generated by the fusion of antibody-producing β-lymphocytes with lymphocyte tumor cells for the production of monoclonal antibodies.

interferon: a member of a group of cytokines that prevents viral replication and slows the growth and replication of cancer cells.

interleukin: a member of a group of cytokines involved in orchestration and regulation of the immune response.

liposome: a microscopic, sphere-like lipid droplet that functions as a therapeutic carrier.

monoclonal antibody: an antibody derived from a hybridoma cell line.

pharmacogenomics: the scientific discipline of using genome-wide approaches to understand the inherited basis of differences between individuals in the response to drugs. This is an expansion of the field of pharmacogenetics, which traditionally considered such inherited differences on a gene-by-gene basis.

plasmid: a small, circular, extrachromosomal DNA molecule capable of replication independent of that of the genome.

polymerase chain reaction (PCR): a molecular biologic technique for amplification of specific DNA molecules.

protein: a functional product of a specific gene consisting of amino acids linked together through peptide bonds in a specific sequence.

proteomics: the scientific field of the study of sequencing and analyzing the expression, modification, and function of proteins on a genome-wide or global scale.

recombinant DNA (rDNA) technology: the application of DNA molecules derived by joining two DNA molecules from different sources.

restriction endonucleases: an enzyme capable of cleaving a DNA molecule in a site-specific manner.

ribozymes: RNA molecules with intrinsic enzymatic activity.

RNA (ribonucleic acid): a polynucleotide molecule consisting of covalently linked ribonucleic acids. Messenger RNA serves as the template for protein synthesis. Transfer RNA serves as the adaptor molecules between amino acids and mRNA during protein synthesis. Ribosomal RNA serves as a component of the ribosome and participates in protein synthesis.

small molecule chemistry: the field of drug development focusing on small organic nucleotide or peptide-based molecules derived through either combinatorial chemistry or rational drug design.

single nucleotide polymorphism: common DNA sequence variations among individuals involving a single nucleotide substitution.

vaccine: a preparation of antigenic material administered to stimulate the development of antibodies conferring active immunity against a particular pathogen or disease.

Biological Products

There are many FDA-approved biological products currently on the market, including blood factors, cytokines, enzymes, growth factors, hormones, interferons, monoclonal antibodies, and vaccines. A list of such biological products is provided in Table 2.

Gene Expression and Protein Synthesis

Proteins are the major macromolecular component of the cell and are responsible for conducting most of a cell's biological activity. Proteins consist of a linear polymer of amino acids linked together in a specific sequence. This specific sequence is responsible for a protein's structure and function. The initial code for the synthesis of a given protein is stored in a gene on a sequence of DNA that is part of a chromosome within the nucleus of a cell.

- The central dogma of molecular biology is that DNA encodes RNA, which in turn encodes protein.
- A given amino acid within a protein is encoded by a triplet of nucleic acid base pairs within the gene encoding the protein. This triplet is called a *codon.*
- There are 64 codons encoding 20 different amino acids as dictated by the genetic code.

Table 2

Approved Biological Products

Generic name	Brand name (manufacturer)	Indications
Blood factors		
Factor VII	NovoSeven (Novo Nordisk)	Hemophilia
Factor VIII	Bioclate, Recombinate, Advate (Baxter)	Hemophilia A
	Kogenate, Helixate (Bayer)	
	ReFacto (Genetics Institute)	
Factor IX	BeneFIX (Genetics Institute)	Hemophilia B
Cytokines		
Aldesleukin (IL-2)	Proleukin (Chiron)	Metastatic renal cell carcinoma and melanoma
Denileukin diftitox	Ontak (Ligand)	Cutaneous T-cell lymphoma
Interferon alfacon-1	Infergen (InterMune)	Hepatitis C
Interferon alfa-n1	Wellferon (GlaxoSK)	Chronic hepatitis C
Interferon alfa-2a	Roferon-A (Roche)	Hairy cell leukemia; AIDS-related Kaposi's sarcoma; CML
Interferon alfa-2b	Intron-A (Schering)	Hairy cell leukemia; AIDS-related Kaposi's sarcoma; chronic hepatitis B and C; condylomata acuminata; malignant melanoma
Interferon alfa-n3	Alferon-N (InterMune)	Condylomata acuminata
Interferon beta-1b	Betaseron (Berlex)	Acute relapsing-remitting multiple sclerosis
Interferon beta-1a	Avonex (Biogen); Rebif (Serono)	Acute relapsing-remitting multiple sclerosis
Interferon gamma-1b	Actimmune (InterMune)	Chronic granulomatous disease; osteoporosis
Oprelvekin (IL-11)	Neumega (Genetics Institute)	Thrombocytopenia from chemotherapy
Enzymes		
Agalsidase beta	Fabrazyme (Genzyme)	Fabry disease
Alteplase	Activase (Genentech)	Acute myocardial infarction; pulmonary embolism; stroke
Bivalirudin	Angiomax (Medicines Co.)	Coronary angioplasty (PTCA); unstable angina
Dornase alfa	Pulmozyme (Genentech)	Respiratory complication from cystic fibrosis
Eptifibatide	Integrelin (Millennium)	Acute coronary syndromes; angioplasties
Imiglucerase	Cerezyme (Genzyme)	Type 1 Gaucher's disease
Laronidase	Aldurazyme (Biomarin)	Mucopolysaccharidosis
Lepirudin	Refludan (Berlex)	Heparin-induced thrombocytopenia
Rasburicase	Elitek (Sanofi-Synthelabo)	Elevated plasma uric acid in pediatric malignancy
Reteplase	Retavase (Centocor/J&J)	Acute myocardial infarction
Tenecteplase	TNKase (Genentech)	Acute myocardial infarction
Tirobifan	Aggrastat (Merck)	Acute coronary syndromes
Growth factors		
Becaplermin (PDGF)	Regranex (Ortho-McNeil)	Diabetic foot ulcer
Darbepoetin alfa	Aranesp (Amgen)	Anemia associated with end-stage renal disease and chronic renal insufficiency
Epoetin alfa	EPOGEN (Amgen); Procrit (Ortho Biotech)	Anemia due to chronic renal disease; zidovudine-induced anemia; anemia due to chemotherapy; surgery patients
Filgrastim	Neupogen (Amgen)	Neutropenia due to myelosuppressive chemotherapy; myeloid reconstitution after BMT; severe chronic neutropenia; peripheral blood progenitor cell transplant; induction and consolidation therapy in AML
Pegfilgrastim	Neulasta (Amgen)	Febrile neutropenia due to myelosuppressive chemotherapy
Palifermin	Kepivance (Amgen)	Oral mucositis
Sargramostim	Leukine (Berlex)	Myeloid reconstitution after BMT; BMT failure; adjunct to chemotherapy in AML; peripheral blood progenitor cell transplant
Hormones		
Choriogonadotropin alfa	Ovidrel (Serono)	Fertility
Follitropin alpha	Gonal-F (Serono)	Ovulatory failure
Follitropin beta	Follistim (Organon)	Ovulatory failure

(continued)

Table 2

BIOTECHNOLOGY AND PHARMACOGENOMICS 137

Approved Biological Products (continued)

Generic name	Brand name (manufacturer)	Indications
Hormones (cont.)		
Human insulin	Humulin ; Humalog (Eli Lilly); Novolin (Novo Nordisk); Lantus (Aventis)	Insulin-dependent diabetes mellitus
Human growth hormone	Protopin , Nutropin (Genentech)	Growth hormone deficiency in pediatric patients
	Humatrope (Eli Lilly)	Growth retardation in chronic renal disease
	Saizen , Serostim (Serono)	AIDS wasting
	Norditropin (Novo Nordisk)	Turner's syndrome
	Genotropin (Pharmacia); Biotropin (Sol Source Technologies)	Growth hormone deficiency in adults
Ganirelix	Antagon (Organon)	LH surge during fertility therapy
Glucagon	GlucaGen (Novo Nordisk)	Hypoglycemia
Growth hormone-releasing hormone	Geref (Serono)	GH deficiency in pediatric patients
Thyrotropin	Thyrogen (Genzyme)	Thyroid cancer
Monoclonal antibodies		
Abciximab	ReoPro (Centocor)	Prevention of blood clots post PCI; unstable angina prior to PCI
Adalimumab	Humira (Abbott)	Acute rheumatoid arthritis
Alemtuzumab	Campath (Berlex)	Chronic lymphocytic leukemia
Basiliximab	Simulect (Novartis)	Acute organ transplant rejection
Bevacizumab	Avastin (Genentech)	Colorectal cancer
Cetuximab	Erbitux (ImClone Systems)	Colorectal cancer
Daclizumab	Zenapax (Roche)	Kidney transplant, acute rejection
Efalizumab	Raptiva (Genentech)	Psoriasis
Gemtuzumab (ozogamicin)	Mylotarg (Wyeth/PDL) Zevalin (IDEC)	Acute myeloid leukemia (CD33+)
Ibritumomab (tiuxetan)	Remicade (Centocor)	B-cell non-Hodgkin's lymphoma
Infliximab	Xolair (Genentech)	Crohn's disease; rheumatoid arthritis
Omalizumab	Synagis (MedImmune)	Asthma
Palivizumab	Rituxan (IDEC/Genentech)	Prevention of RSV and fatal pneumonia in pediatrics
Rituximab	Bexxar (Corixa)	Low-grade non-Hodgkin's lymphoma
Tositumomab	Herceptin (Genentech/PDL)	CD20+ non-Hodgkin's lymphoma
Trastuzumab		Metastatic breast cancer (Her 2 Neu+)
Vaccines		
Haemophilus b/ hepatitis B	Comvax (Merck)	Prevention of *H influenzae* and hepatitis B
Hepatitis B vaccine	Engerix-B (GlaxoSK); Recombivax HB (Merck)	Prevention of hepatitis B
Others		
Anakinra	Kineret (Amgen)	Rheumatoid arthritis
BCNU-polymer	Gliadel (Guilford)	Recurrent glioblastoma multiforme
Daunorubicin-liposomal	DaunoXome (Gilead)	Kaposi's sarcoma
Doxorubicin-liposomal	DOXIL (Alza)	Kaposi's sarcoma; ovarian cancer
Drotrecogin alfa	Xigris (Eli Lilly)	Sepsis
Etanercept	Enbrel (Amgen)	Rheumatoid arthritis; psoriatic arthritis
Fomivirsen	Vitravene (Isis)	CMV retinitis
Glatiramer	Copaxone (Teva)	Relapsing multiple sclerosis
Lipid-based amphotericin B	Abelcet (Elan); Amphotec (Sequus); AmBisome (Fujisawa/Gilead)	Aspergillosis, cryptococcal meningitis in HIV, systemic fungal infections
Nesiritide	Natrecor (Scios/Innovex)	Congestive heart failure

AIDS, acquired immunodeficiency syndrome; AML, acute myelogenous leukemia; BMT, bone marrow transplant; CML, chronic myelogenous leukemia; CMV, cytomegalovirus; GH, growth hormone; HIV, human immunodeficiency virus; IL, interleukin; LH, luteinizing hormone; PDGF, platelet-derived growth factor, PCI, percutaneous coronary intervention; PTCA, percutaneous transluminal coronary angioplasty.

- An overview of transcription, translation, and post-translational modification is shown in Figure 1.

Recombinant DNA Technology

- Recombinant DNA (rDNA) technology uses several molecular biological tools to insert a desired DNA fragment with a specific purpose in proximity to other DNA fragments within a DNA molecule. Most often, a gene encoding a desired protein is isolated through screening the genomic library or by utilization of the viral enzyme reverse transcriptase to generate cDNA from the mRNA transcript of the gene.

Enzymes called restriction endonucleases allow the cleavage of DNA in the plasmid at very specific locations. The gene is then ligated into a vector such as a plasmid for gene cloning or to control the expression of the encoded protein.

- An **expression vector** is a plasmid designed to allow inducible expression of the inserted gene within a host cell (such as the bacterium *Escherichia coli* or the yeast *Saccharomyces cerevisiae*). This mechanism permits production of large quantities of the desired protein. The protein must then be isolated and purified for further use. Such techniques, used on an industrial scale, mass-produce therapeutically

Figure 1.

Gene expression: The synthesis of proteins.

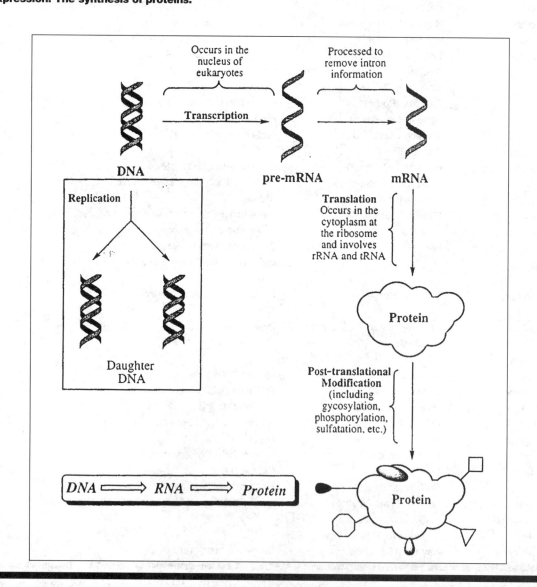

useful biological products such as cytokines, enzymes, hormones, blood factors, and vaccines (Figure 2).

- Cytokines (ie, molecules secreted by cells) orchestrate the immune response and activate immune cells such as lymphocytes, monocytes, macrophages, and neutrophils. Therapeutically useful recombinant cytokines include interferons, interleukins, and colony-stimulating factors. Examples of these include interferon beta-1b (Betaseron), which is used to treat acute relapsing-remitting multiple sclerosis; aldesleukin (IL-2) (Proleukin), which aids in the management of metastatic renal cell carcinoma and melanoma; and oprelvekin (IL-11) (Neumega), which treats thrombocytopenia caused by chemotherapy.

Figure 2.

Summary of typical rDNA production of a protein from either genomic DNA or cDNA.

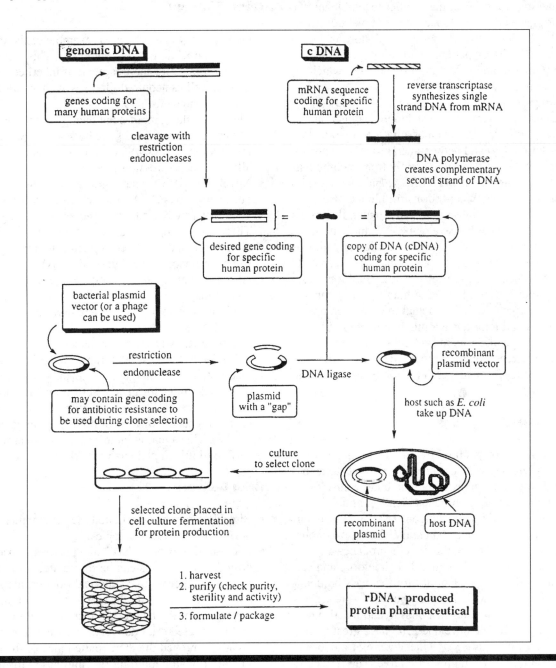

Reprinted by permission of Sindelar, 2002.

- An enzyme is a protein that catalyzes a specific chemical reaction. A number of different enzymes with therapeutic use have been produced using recombinant DNA technology. Alteplase (Activase), for example, treats acute myocardial infarction, pulmonary embolism, and stroke. Dornase alfa (Pulmozyme) treats respiratory complications that develop in cystic fibrosis. Eptifibatide (Integrelin) is used to treat acute coronary syndromes.

- Hormones, chemical substances transmitted via the bloodstream, are designed to impart specific cellular effects to cells distant from their physiologic source. Since the introduction and success of recombinant human insulin in 1982, many other recombinant hormones have been developed; for example, human growth hormone, which treats growth hormone deficiency in pediatric patients, and follitropin alpha and beta (Gonal-F and Follistim, respectively), which are used to remedy ovulatory failure.

- Clotting or blood factors are chemical blood constituents that interact to cause blood coagulation. Patients suffering from hemophilia A (due to factor VIII deficiency) and hemophilia B (due to factor IX deficiency) have benefited greatly from recombinant DNA technology. Factors VIII, IX, and factor VII are available in recombinant forms for clinical use.

- Vaccines, preparations of antigenic material administered to stimulate the development of antibodies, confer active immunity against a particular pathogen or disease. Vaccine development has also benefited from advances in rDNA technology. Traditional vaccine production used killed or nonvirulent organisms, microbial toxins, or actual microbial components to elicit long-term immune protection. Safer and more specific vaccine antigens have been devised as recombinant proteins. This technology has led to the very successful recombinant hepatitis B vaccine.

Monoclonal Antibodies

- Antibodies, proteins produced by the immune system's β-lymphocytes, use specific methods to recognize foreign molecules within the body. Subsets of β-lymphocyte clones produce identical antibodies that recognize the same antigen. These identical antibodies are said to be *monoclonal.* Fusing β-lymphocytes with lymphocyte tumor cells produces a hybridoma. This fused cell type is immortal and can be cultured in large quantities for the mass production of a given monoclonal antibody.

- Monoclonal antibodies that bind to and inactivate their targets can be developed and have great therapeutic utility (Figure 3). Nomenclature of monoclonal antibodies is highly structured. The first component of the name is product-specific. The second

component indicates its therapeutic use: *ci* denotes cardiovascular use; *li* for use in inflammation; and *tu* for use in cancer. The third component indicates the type of monoclonal antibody: *mo* for murine; *xi* for chimeric; and *zu* for humanized. The fourth component, *mab*, represents "monoclonal antibody." An example of a monoclonal antibody used clinically is abciximab (ReoPro), which prevents blood clots post-PTCA and prevents unstable angina prior to PTCA. Another example, infliximab (Remicade), is used to treat Crohn's disease and rheumatoid arthritis.

Gene Therapy

- Gene therapy is an excellent example of the therapeutic application of biotechnology. This technology holds promise for the treatment of inherited disorders as well as acquired illnesses such as infectious diseases and cancer.

- The molecular goal of gene therapy is to repair or correct a dysfunctional gene by selectively introducing recombinant DNA into cells or tissues, thereby allowing the expression of a functional gene product.

- Novel drug delivery strategies must be used to introduce exogenous DNA into the cell to treat retroviruses, lentiviruses, and adeno-associated virus. These novel drug delivery strategies have applications for nonviral delivery systems as well (eg, liposomes or uncomplexed plasmid DNA).

- Alternative approaches using ribozymes (eg, RNA repair) may prove effective. The enzymatic activity of these RNA molecules can be used to repair defective mRNAs.

- Chimeric RNA/DNA oligonucleotides make use of the cell's "DNA mismatch repair apparatus" to correct mutations at the genomic level. Antisense oligonucleotides for gene inactivation have proved clinically useful. Fomivirsen (Vitravene), one such agent, targets the mRNA of human cytomegalovirus (CMV). This agent is indicated for the treatment of CMV retinitis in patients with AIDS.

Drug Delivery

- Biotechnology has facilitated the development of novel drug delivery strategies.

- The use of liposomes has had a positive impact on drug delivery. Drugs can be formulated into liposomes, ie, microscopic spherical lipid droplets. The outer membrane of the liposome fuses with the membrane of the target cell, thereby facilitating highly targeted drug delivery. Such technology has greatly improved the therapeutic index of the antifungal drug amphotericin B. Lipid-based formulations now allow greater quantities of the drug to be

Figure 3.

Production of monoclonal antibodies.

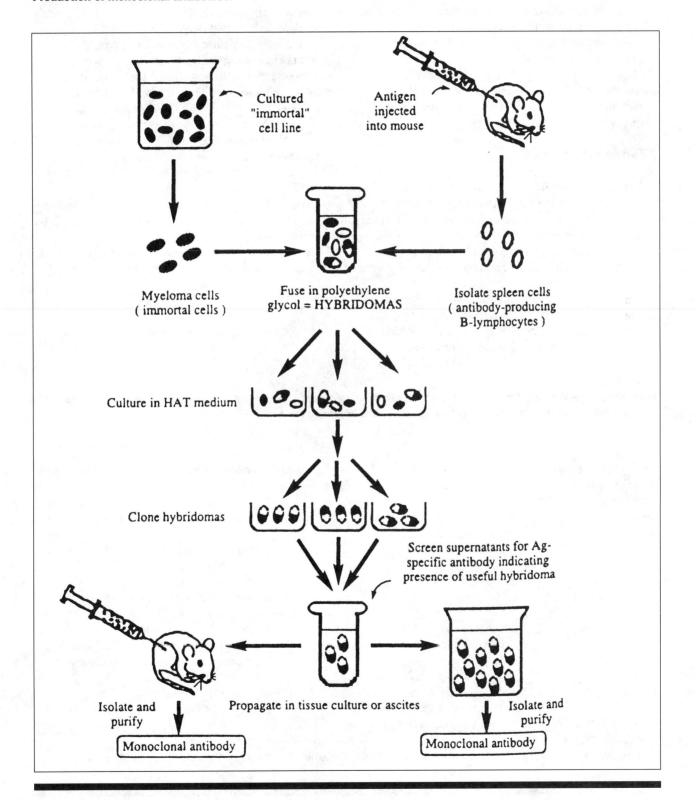

delivered with substantially less toxicity to the patient.

- Another promising approach is the use of immuno-toxins. These delivery agents combine a monoclonal antibody with a toxin such as an anticancer or antimicrobial agent, thereby allowing targeted drug delivery with minimal toxicity.
- Another novel strategy is the use of pegylation, ie, the addition of polyethylene glycol to therapeutic proteins to minimize the deleterious immune response to an individual protein.

Pharmacogenomics

- **Pharmacogenomics** is the scientific discipline of using genome-wide approaches to understand the inherited basis of differences between individuals in the response to drugs. This is an expansion of the field of pharmacogenetics, which traditionally considered such inherited differences on a gene-by-gene basis.
- Genetic differences in drug metabolism, drug disposition, and drug targets have a large impact on efficacy and toxicity. Comprehension of the relationships between specific genetic factors and drug response can be used to predict drug response and optimize drug therapy in any given individual.
- Of particular significance are single nucleotide polymorphisms (SNPs). SNPs are differences in a single nucleotide base that occur at a significant frequency (usually >5%) within the population. An SNP may or may not promote change in the encoded amino acid of a codon. It may change the encoded amino acid, but yield no change in the function of the encoded protein. When an SNP causes amino acid substitution, a phenotypic difference that carries clinical relevance may result. Even when the SNP results in no change in the encoded amino acid, it may be associated with a phenotypic change, thereby serving as a predictive marker of that change.
- Examples of significant genetic polymorphisms that can influence drug response are shown in Tables 3 and 4.
- Examples of significant genetic polymorphisms in drug-metabolizing enzymes are shown in Tables 5 and 6.

Table 3

Genetic Polymorphisms in Drug Target Genes That Can Influence Drug Response[1]

Gene or gene product	Medication	Drug effect associated with polymorphism
Angiotensin-converting enzyme (ACE)	ACE inhibitors (eg, enalapril)	Renoprotective effects; blood pressure reduction; reduction in left ventricular mass; endothelial function
	Fluvastatin	Lipid changes (reductions in low-density lipoprotein cholesterol and apolipoprotein B); progression or regression in coronary atherosclerosis
Arachidonate 5-lipoxygenase	Leukotriene inhibitors	Improvement of FEV_1
β_2-Adrenergic receptor	β_2-Agonists	Bronchodilatation; susceptibility to agonist-induced desensitization; cardiovascular effects
Bradykinin B_2 receptor	ACE inhibitors	ACE inhibitor–induced cough
Dopamine receptors (D_2, D_3, D_4)	Antipsychotics (eg, haloperidol, clozapine)	Antipsychotic response (D_2, D_3, D_4); antipsychotic-induced tardive dyskinesia (D_3); antipsychotic-induced acute akathisia (D_3)
Estrogen receptor-α	Conjugated estrogens	Increase in bone mineral density
	Hormone replacement therapy	Increase in high-density lipoprotein cholesterol
Glycoprotein IIIa subunit of glycoprotein IIb/IIIa	Aspirin or glycoprotein IIb/IIIa inhibitors	Antiplatelet effect
Serotonin (5-hydroxytryptamine transporter)	Antidepressants (eg, clomipramine, fluoxetine, paroxetine)	Serotonin neurotransmission; antidepressant response

FEV_1, forced expiratory volume in 1 second.

[1]The examples shown are illustrative and not representative of all published studies.

Reprinted by permission from Evans et al, 2003.

Table 4

Genetic Polymorphisms in Disease-Modifying or Treatment-Modifying Genes That Can Influence Drug Response[1]

Gene or gene product	Disease or response association	Medication	Influence of polymorphism on drug effect or toxicity
Adducin	Hypertension	Diuretics	Myocardial infarction or strokes
Apolipoprotein E (APOE)	Progression of atherosclerosis; ischemic cardiovascular events	Statins (eg, simvastatin)	Enhanced survival
	Alzheimer's disease	Tacrine	Clinical improvement
Human leukocyte antigen (HLA)	Toxicity	Abacavir	Hypersensitivity reaction
Cholesterol ester transfer protein (CETP)	Progression of atherosclerosis	Statins (eg, pravastatin)	Slowing of progression of atherosclerosis
Ion channels (HERG, KvLQT1, Mink, MiRP1)	Congenital long-QT syndrome	Erythromycin; terfenadine; cisapride; clarithro-mycin; quinidine	Increased risk of drug-induced torsade de pointes
Methylguanine methyltransferase (MGMT)	Glioma	Carmustine	Response of glioma to carmustine
Parkin	Parkinson's disease	Levodopa	Clinical improvement and levodopa-induced dyskinesias
Prothrombin and factor V	Deep-vein thrombosis and cerebral-vein thrombosis	Oral contraceptives	Increased risk of deep-vein thrombosis and cerebral-vein thrombosis with oral contraceptives
Stromelysin-1	Atherosclerosis progression	Statins (eg, pravastatin)	Reduction in cardiovascular events by pravastatin (death, myocardial infarction, stroke, angina, and others); reduction in risk of repeated angioplasty

[1]The examples shown are illustrative and not representative of all published studies.
Reproduced with permission from Evans et al, 2003.

Table 5

Pharmacogenomics of Phase I Drug Metabolism[1]

Drug-metabolizing enzyme	Frequency of variant poor-metabolism phenotype	Representative drugs metabolized	Effect of polymorphism
Cytochrome P-450 2D6 (CYP2D6)	6.8% in Sweden	Debrisoquin	Enhanced drug effect
	1% in China	Sparteine	Enhanced drug effect
		Nortriptyline	Enhanced drug effect
		Codeine	Decreased drug effect
Cytochrome P-450 2C9 (CYP2C9)	Approximately 3% in England (those homozygous for the *2 and *3 alleles)	Warfarin	Enhanced drug effect
		Phenytoin	Enhanced drug effect
Cytochrome P-450 2C19 (CYP2C19)	2.7% among white Americans 3.3% in Sweden 14.6% in China 18% in Japan	Omeprazole	Enhanced drug effect
Dihydropyrimidine dehydrogenase	Approximately 1% of population is heterozygous	Fluorouracil	Enhanced drug effect
Butyrylcholinesterase (pseudocholinesterase)	Approximately 1 in 3500 Europeans	Succinylcholine	Enhanced drug effect

[1]Examples of genetically polymorphic phase I enzymes that catalyze drug metabolism are listed, including selected examples of drugs that have clinically relevant variations in their effect.
Reproduced with permission from Weinshilboum, 2003.

Table 6

Pharmacogenetics of Phase II Drug Metabolism[1]

Drug-metabolizing enzyme	Frequency of variant poor-metabolism phenotype	Representative drugs metabolized	Effect of polymorphism
N-Acetyltransferase 2	52% among white Americans	Isoniazid	Enhanced drug effect
	17% of Japanese	Hydralazine	Enhanced drug effect
Uridine diphosphate-glucuronosyltransferase 1A1 (TATA box polymorphism)	10.9% among whites	Procainamide	Enhanced drug effect
	4% of Chinese	Irinotecan	Enhanced drug effect
	1% of Japanese	Bilirubin	Gilbert's syndrome
Thiopurine S-methyltransferase	Approximately 1 in 300 whites	Mercaptopurine	Enhanced drug effect (toxicity)
	Approximately 1 in 2500 Asians	Azathioprine	Enhanced drug effect (toxicity)
Catechol O-methyltransferase	Approximately 25% of whites	Levodopa	Enhanced drug effect

[1]Examples of genetically polymorphic phase II (conjugating) enzymes that catalyze drug metabolism are listed, including selected examples of drugs that have clinically relevant variations in their effects.
Reproduced with permission from Weinshilboum, 2003.

2. Key Points

- Biotechnology, as defined by the United States Food and Drug Administration, is "the use of recombinant DNA (or RNA) technology; direct DNA transfer technology; nucleic acid amplification technology; hybridoma technology; cell fusion; molecular modification of cellular receptors; or the application of cells, tissues, or their components such that their potential biological activity has been modified."
- The central dogma of molecular biology is that DNA encodes RNA, which in turn encodes protein.
- Recombinant DNA (rDNA) technology makes use of several molecular biological tools that allow for the placement of a desired DNA fragment in proximity to other DNA fragments within a DNA molecule for a specific purpose.
- Cytokines are molecules secreted by cells that orchestrate the immune response. They activate immune cells such as lymphocytes, monocytes, macrophages, and neutrophils.
- An enzyme is a protein that catalyzes a specific chemical reaction.
- Hormones are chemical substances transmitted by the bloodstream to cells distant from their physiologic source that impart specific cellular effects.
- Clotting or blood factors are chemical blood constituents that interact to cause blood coagulation.
- Vaccines are preparations of antigenic material administered to stimulate the development of antibodies for the purpose of conferring active immunity against a particular pathogen or disease.
- Subsets of β-lymphocyte clones produce identical antibodies that recognize the same antigen. These identical antibodies are said to be monoclonal. Fusing β-lymphocytes with lymphocyte tumor cells produces a hybridoma that can be cultured in large quantities for the mass production of a given monoclonal antibody.
- Gene therapy, an application of biotechnology, has great potential therapeutic benefit.
- Biotechnology has facilitated the development of novel drug delivery strategies, including liposomal technology, immunotoxins, and pegylation.
- Pharmacogenomics is the scientific discipline of using genome-wide approaches to understand the inherited basis of differences between individual responses to drugs.
- Single nucleotide polymorphisms (SNPs) are differences in a single nucleotide base occurring at a significant frequency (usually >5%) within the population. They may result in no change in the encoded amino acid of a codon or a change in the encoded amino acid with no change in the function of the encoded protein. However, when the amino acid substitution due to a SNP results in a phenotypic difference, it may carry clinical relevance.

3. Questions and Answers

1. The process whereby the ribosome in the cytoplasm reads mRNA codons and matches them with the appropriate tRNAs (which in turn carry amino acids responsible for protein synthesis) is referred to as

   A. transcription
   B. translation
   C. transformation
   D. transfection
   E. transduction

2. How many nucleotide triplets (or codons) exist for the encoding of the 20 possible amino acids specified by the genetic code?

   A. 4
   B. 12
   C. 20
   D. 61
   E. 64

3. A plasmid designed to allow for the expression of an inserted gene within a host cell for the production of the specified protein is referred to as which of the following?

   A. Cloning vector
   B. Expression vector
   C. Transcription factor
   D. Translation initiation factor
   E. Transposable genetic element

4. An example of a recombinant DNA-generated cytokine used for the management of acute relapsing-remitting multiple sclerosis is which of the following?

   A. Interferon beta-1b (Betaseron)
   B. Aldesleukin (IL-2) (Proleukin)
   C. Eptifibatide (Integrelin)
   D. Bivalirudin (Angiomax)
   E. Abciximab (ReoPro)

5. Alteplase (Activase) is a recombinant DNA protein of which of the following types?

   A. Hormone
   B. Enzyme
   C. Clotting factor
   D. Chemokine
   E. Cytokine

6. Which of the following biological agents is indicated for treatment of ovulatory failure?

   A. Ganirelix (Antagon)
   B. Glucagon (Glucagen)
   C. Follitropin alpha (Gonal-F)
   D. Eptifibatide (Integrelin)
   E. Thyrotropin (Thyrogen)

7. Which of the following recombinant blood factors is available in recombinant form for clinical therapeutic use?

   A. Factor III
   B. Factor V
   C. Factor VI
   D. Factor VII
   E. Factor X

8. Recombinant DNA technology has led to the development of vaccines for which of the following diseases?

   A. Hepatitis B
   B. Hepatitis A
   C. *Haemophilus influenzae* type B infection
   D. Malaria
   E. AIDS

9. As dictated by the nomenclature for monoclonal antibodies, which of the following is a chimeric monoclonal antibody therapeutically used for inflammatory disease?

   A. Abciximab
   B. Infliximab
   C. Palivizumab
   D. Rituximab
   E. Trastuzumab

10. The repair or correction of a dysfunctional gene by selectively introducing recombinant DNA into cells or tissues (ultimately leading to the expression of a functional gene product) best describes which of the following?

    A. Monoclonal antibody therapy
    B. Gene therapy
    C. Antiviral therapy
    D. Cell therapy
    E. Recombinant DNA therapy

11. Fomivirsen (Vitravene) is an example of which of the following biological products?

A. A liposomal formulation
B. An antisense oligonucleotide
C. An siRNA molecule
D. A recombinant DNA-produced protein
E. A monoclonal antibody

12. The use of liposomal technology has favorably impacted the therapeutic index of which of the following drugs?

    A. Cyclosporine
    B. Itraconazole
    C. Amphotericin B
    D. Cisplatin
    E. Propofol

13. The scientific discipline of using genome-wide approaches to understand the inherited basis of differences between individuals in the response to drugs best describes which of the following?

    A. Pharmacogenomics
    B. Functional genomics
    C. Comparative genomics
    D. Pharmacodynamics
    E. Molecular genetics

14. A single nucleotide polymorphism (SNP) always results in a change in which of the following?

    A. The nucleotide sequence in the genome
    B. The nucleotide sequence of a codon
    C. The encoded amino acid of the codon
    D. The encoded amino acid of the codon, with no change in function of the encoded protein
    E. The encoded amino acid of the codon, with a clinically relevant change in the function of the encoded protein

15. "The use of recombinant DNA (or RNA) technology; direct DNA transfer technology; nucleic acid amplification technology; hybridoma technology; cell fusion; molecular modification of cellular receptors; or the application of cells, tissues, or their components such that their potential biological activity has been modified" best describes which of the following?

    A. Biology
    B. Biotechnology
    C. Biotherapy

D. Bioinformatics
E. Nanotechnology

16. A drug discovery strategy that utilizes nucleic acids and amino acids in various combinations to synthesize vast libraries of oligonucleotide or peptide compounds for high throughput lead compound screening is which of the following?

    A. Whole cell screening
    B. Natural product screening
    C. Gene therapy
    D. Combinatorial chemistry
    E. rDNA technology

17. The application of computer sciences and information technology to the management and analysis of biological information best defines which of the following?

    A. Biometrics
    B. Biotherapy
    C. Bioinformatics
    D. Biostatistics
    E. Biotechnology

18. Which of the following best outlines the central dogma of molecular biology?

    A. RNA→DNA→Protein
    B. DNA→RNA→Protein
    C. Protein→RNA→DNA
    D. DNA→Protein→RNA
    E. Protein→DNA→RNA

19. Which of the following biotechnology agents is indicated for treating anemia caused by chronic renal disease?

    A. Epoetin alfa
    B. Becaplermin
    C. Filgrastim
    D. Alemtuzumab
    E. Sargramostim

20. Which of the following products is indicated for prevention of blood clots post PTCA?

    A. Abciximab
    B. Basiliximab
    C. Infliximab
    D. Trastuzumab
    E. Becaplermin

Answers

1. **B.** Transcription is the process by which RNA polymerase copies a strand of DNA into complementary RNA. Transformation refers to the alteration of the heritable properties of a eukaryotic cell. Transfection is the introduction of foreign DNA into a eukaryotic cell. Transduction can refer to the transfer of DNA from one bacterium to another via a bacteriophage.

2. **D.** There is degeneracy in the genetic code. Some amino acids may be encoded by as many as six codons, whereas others may be encoded by only one. Of the 64 possible codons, three are stop codons (UAA, UGA, and UAG).

3. **B.** A cloning vector is used to carry a fragment of DNA into a cell for cloning. A transcription factor is a protein that regulates transcription in eukaryotic cells. A translation initiation factor, as its name implies, is involved in the initiation of translation. A transposable genetic element, or transposon, is a portion of DNA that can move from one part of the genome to another.

4. **A.** Aldesleukin (IL-2) (Proleukin) is a recombinant cytokine indicated for the treatment of metastatic renal cell carcinoma and melanoma. Eptifibatide (Integrelin) is a recombinant enzyme indicated for treatment of acute coronary syndromes. Bivalirudin (Angiomax) is an enzyme indicated for use in coronary angioplasty and unstable angina. Abciximab (ReoPro) is a monoclonal antibody indicated for prevention of blood clots post-PTCA and unstable angina prior to PTCA.

5. **B.** Alteplase (Activase) is a recombinant DNA protein of the enzyme type.

6. **C.** Ganirelix (Antagon) is a recombinant hormone indicated for the treatment of LH surge during fertility therapy. Glucagon (Glucagen) is a recombinant hormone indicated for treatment of hypoglycemia. Eptifibatide (Integrelin) is a recombinant enzyme indicated for the treatment of acute coronary syndromes. Thyrotropin (Thyrogen) is a recombinant hormone indicated for the treatment of thyroid cancer.

7. **D.** The other factors listed are not clinically available in recombinant form.

8. **A.** While promising, this technology has not yet yielded vaccines for hepatitis A, malaria, AIDS, or infections caused by *H influenzae* type B.

9. **B.** Nomenclature of monoclonal antibodies is highly structured. The first component of the name is product specific, the second component indicates its therapeutic use (*ci* for cardiovascular, *li* for inflammation, *tu* for cancer), the third component indicates the type of monoclonal antibody (*mo* for murine, *xi* for chimeric, *zu* for humanized), and the fourth component (*mab*) represents "monoclonal antibody."

10. **B.** The repair or correction of a dysfunctional gene by selectively introducing recombinant DNA into cells or tissues, ultimately leading to the expression of a functional gene product, is called gene therapy.

11. **B.** Fomivirsen (Vitravene) is the first product based on this technology to come to market.

12. **C.** Formulation of this antifungal agent as a liposomal preparation (Ambisome) has significantly reduced the nephrotoxicity and other adverse effects associated with this drug.

13. **A.** The scientific discipline of using genome-wide approaches to understand the inherited basis of differences between individuals in the response to drugs best describes pharmacogenomics.

14. **A.** An SNP may occur outside of an open reading frame (coding region), it may induce a mutation where no change in encoded amino acid occurs, and it may or may not cause a functional change in an encoded protein.

15. **B.** "The use of recombinant DNA (or RNA) technology; direct DNA transfer technology; nucleic acid amplification technology; hybridoma technology; cell fusion; molecular modification of cellular receptors; or the application of cells, tissues, or their components such that their potential biological activity has been modified" best describes biotechnology.

16. **D.** A drug discovery strategy that utilizes nucleic acids and amino acids in various combinations

to synthesize vast libraries of oligonucleotide or peptide compounds for high throughput lead compound screening is called combinatorial chemistry.

17. **C.** The application of computer sciences and information technology to the management and analysis of biological information best defines bioinformatics.

18. **B.** DNA is transcribed into mRNA, which is translated ultimately to protein.

19. **A.** Becaplermin is indicated for the management of diabetic foot ulcers. Filgrastim is indicated for treatment of neutropenia. Alemtuzumab is indicated for treatment of chronic lymphocytic leukemia. Sargramostim is indicated for myeloid reconstitution after BMT, BMT failure, as an adjunct to chemotherapy in AML, and in peripheral blood progenitor cell transplant.

20. **A.** Basiliximab is indicated for management of acute organ transplant rejection. Infliximab is indicated for the treatment of Crohn's disease and rheumatoid arthritis. Trastuzumab is indicated for management of metastatic breast cancer. Becaplermin is indicated for the treatment of diabetic foot ulcers.

4. References

Adams VR, Karlix JL. Monoclonal antibodies. In: *Concepts in Immunology and Immunotherapeutics,* 3rd ed. Bethesda, MD: American Society of Health-System Pharmacists' Production Office; 1997:269-299.

Alberts B, Bray D, Lewis J, et al, eds. *Molecular Biology of the Cell,* 3rd ed. New York: Garland Publishing; 1994.

Carrico JM. Human Genome Project and pharmacogenomics—implications for pharmacy. *J Am Pharm Assoc.* 2000;40:115-116.

Evans WE, McLeod HL. Pharmacogenomics—drug disposition, drug targets, and side effects. *N Engl J Med.* 2003;348:538-549.

Glick BR, Pasternak JJ, eds. *Molecular Biotechnology: Principles & Applications of Recombinant DNA,* 2nd ed. Washington: ASM Press; 1998.

Hollinger P, Hoogenboom H. Antibodies come back from the brink. *Nature Biotech.* 1998;16:1015-1016.

Regan JW. Biotechnology and drug discovery. In: Delgado JN, Remers WA, eds. *Textbook of Organic Medicinal and Pharmaceutical Chemistry,* 10th ed. Philadelphia: Lippincott-Raven; 1998:139-152.

Rogers CS, Sullenger BA, George AL Jr. Gene therapy. In: Hardman JG, Limbird LE, eds. *Goodman & Gilman's The Pharmacological Basis of Therapeutics,* 10th ed. New York: McGraw-Hill; 2001:81-112.

Sindelar RD. Pharmaceutical biotechnology. In: Williams DA, Lemke TL, eds. *Foye's Principles of Medicinal Chemistry,* 5th ed. Philadelphia: Lippincott Williams & Wilkins; 2002:982-1015.

U.S. Food and Drug Administration (FDA). Center for Biologics Evaluation and Research webpage: http://www.fda.gov/cber

U.S. Food and Drug Administration (FDA). Center for Drug Evaluation and Research webpage: http://www.fda.gov/cder/

Vaughan TJ, Osbourn JK, Tempest PR. Human antibodies by design. *Nature Biotech.* 1998;16:535-539.

Weinshilboum R. Inheritance and drug response. *N Engl J Med.* 2003;348:529-537.

8. Hypertension

L. Brian Cross, PharmD, CDE
Assistant Professor
Department of Clinical Pharmacy
University of Tennessee College of Pharmacy

Contents

1. Disease Overview

- Hypertension is defined as a systolic blood pressure >140 mm Hg, a diastolic blood pressure >90 mm Hg, or any patient requiring antihypertensive therapy.
- 65 million Americans are affected by hypertension.
  - * Approximately 3 of every 4 hypertensive Americans are not well controlled (Table 1).
- Increased incidence with increasing age
- Its onset is most commonly in third to fifth decades of life; lifetime risk of hypertension is 90% for those surviving to an age of 80 years.
- Prevalence differs by ethnic group, socioeconomic group, and by geographical region (Table 2).

Classification

- Classification of hypertension is based on the Seventh Report of the Joint National Committee on Detection, Evaluation, and Treatment of High Blood Pressure (JNC-VII) (Table 3).

Clinical Presentation and Complications

Cardiovascular effects
- Left ventricular hypertrophy (LVH)
- Congestive heart failure (CHF)
- Peripheral arterial disease
- Angina pectoris
- Myocardial infarction
- Sudden death

Renal effects
- Nephropathy
- Renal failure
- Requirements for dialysis

Cerebrovascular effects
- Transient ischemic attacks (TIAs)
- Stroke

Ophthalmologic effects
- Retinal hemorrhage
- Retinopathy
- Blindness

Pathophysiology and Etiology

- Blood pressure = (stroke volume x heart rate) x peripheral resistance (Figure 1)

Table 1

Trends in Awareness, Treatment, and Control of High Blood Pressure in Adults Ages 18-74

	NATIONAL HEALTH AND NUTRITION EXAMINATION SURVEY, PERCENT			
	II (1976–80)	III (PHASE 1) 1988–91	III (PHASE 2) 1991–94	1999–2000
Awareness	51	73	68	70
Treatment	31	55	54	59
Control[†]	10	29	27	34

[†]SBP <140 mm Hg and DBP <90 mm Hg.

High blood pressure is systolic blood pressure (SBP) ≥140 mm Hg or diastolic blood pressure (DBP) ≥90 mm Hg or taking antihypertensive medication.

Sources: Unpublished data for 1999-2000 computed by M. Woltz, National Heart, Lung, and Blood Institute.

Adapted from JNC-7 Express. Source: National Heart, Lung, and Blood Institute.

Sympathetic nervous system activation
Central activation
1. Presynaptic α_2 stimulation is a negative feedback mechanism, leading to decreased norepinephrine release.
2. Presynaptic β stimulation leads to increased norepinephrine release.

Peripheral activation
1. β_1 Stimulation leads to increased heart rate and contractility, causing increased cardiac output.
2. β_2 Stimulation leads to arterial vasodilation.
   - * β Stimulation also causes increased renin release, causing increased angiotensin II production.
3. α_1 Stimulation leads to arterial and venous vasoconstriction.

Renin-angiotensin-aldosterone system
- Decreased renal perfusion pressure causes increases in renin levels.

Table 2

Prevalence of Hypertension by Ethnic Group for Adults Aged 20-74

	Male	Female
Caucasians	24%	19%
African-Americans	35%	34%
Mexican-Americans	25%	22%
Asian-Americans	13%	13%

Figure 1.

Sympathetic nervous system activation.

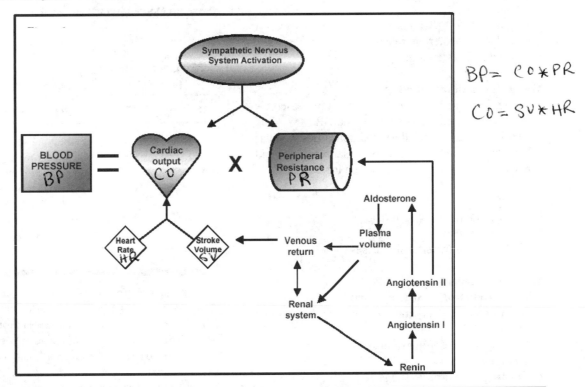

$$BP = CO * PR$$
$$CO = SV * HR$$

Table 3

Classification and Management of Blood Pressure for Adults

BP CLASSIFICATION	SBP* mmHg	DBP* mmHg	LIFESTYLE MODIFICATION	INITIAL DRUG THERAPY	
				WITHOUT COMPELLING INDICATION	WITH COMPELLING INDICATIONS (SEE TABLE 8)
NORMAL	<120	and <80	Encourage	No antihypertensive drug indicated.	Drug(s) for compelling indications.‡
PREHYPERTENSION	120–139	or 80–89	Yes		
STAGE 1 HYPERTENSION	140–159	or 90–99	Yes	Thiazide-type diuretics for most. May consider ACEI, ARB, BB, CCB, or combination.	Drug(s) for the compelling indications.‡ Other antihypertensive drugs (diuretics, ACEI, ARB, BB, CCB) as needed.
STAGE 2 HYPERTENSION	≥160	or ≥100	Yes	Two-drug combination for most† (usually thiazide-type diuretic and ACEI or ARB or BB or CCB).	

*Treatment determined by highest BP category.

†Initial combined therapy should be used cautiously in those at risk for orthostatic hypotension.

‡Treat patients with chronic kidney disease or diabetes to BP goal of <130/80 mm Hg.

ACEI, angiotensin-converting enzyme inhibitor; ARB, angiotensin receptor blocker; BB, β-blocker; CCB, calcium channel blocker; DBP, diastolic blood pressure; SBP, systolic blood pressure

Adapted from JNC-7 Express. Source: National Heart, Lung, and Blood Institute.

- Renin reacts with angiotensinogen to produce angiotensin I (AT-I).
- Angiotensin converting enzyme (ACE) causes AT-I to become AT-II.
- Angiotensin II (AT-II) is a potent vasoconstrictor and stimulates aldosterone release, which increases sodium and fluid retention.

Water and sodium retention
- Acute: increased fluid volume causes increased cardiac output, which causes increased BP.
- Chronic: excess intracellular sodium causes vascular hypertrophy, which increases vascular resistance and response to vasoconstriction, which increases BP.

Etiology
Primary (essential) hypertension
- Unknown cause
- 85-95% of all hypertension cases

Secondary hypertension
- *Renovascular disease* (suggested by increased blood urea nitrogen [BUN] and creatinine, and abdominal bruits)
- *Primary aldosteronism* (suggested by unprovoked hypokalemia)
- *Cushing's syndrome* (suggested by unprovoked hypokalemia and truncal obesity with purple striae)
- *Pheochromocytoma* (suggested by increased urinary catecholamine excretion [ie, vanillylmandelic acid and metanephrine] accompanied by headache, palpitations, and perspiration)
- *Aortic coarctation* (suggested by delayed or absent femoral pulses and decreased blood pressure in the lower extremities)

- *Drug-induced*
  * Steroids and estrogens (including oral contraceptives)
  * Alcohol
  * Cocaine
  * Cyclosporine and tacrolimus
  * Sympathomimetics
  * Erythropoietin
  * Licorice (in chewing tobacco)
  * Monoamine oxidase (MAO) inhibitors
  * Tricyclic antidepressants
  * NSAIDs

Diagnostic Criteria

- Diagnosis and treatment begin with proper blood pressure measurement, assessment, and follow-up planning (Table 4):
1. Patient should avoid smoking or caffeine for 30 minutes prior to BP measurement.

Table 4

Recommendations for Follow-Up Based on Initial Blood Pressure Measurements for Adults

Initial blood pressure (mm Hg)[1]		Recommended follow-up[2]
Systolic	**Diastolic**	
<130	<85	Recheck in 2 years
130-139	85-89	Recheck in 1 year[3]
140-159	90-99	Confirm within 2 months[3]
160-179	100-109	Evaluate or refer to source of care within 1 month
≥180	≥110	Evaluate or refer to source of care immediately or within 1 week depending on clinical situation

[1]If systolic and diastolic readings are different, follow recommendations for shorter time follow-up (eg, 160/86 mm Hg should be evaluated or referred to source of care within 1 month).
[2]Modify the scheduling of follow-up according to reliable information about past blood pressure measurements, other cardiovascular risk factors, or target organ disease.
[3]Provide advice about lifestyle modifications.
Adapted from JNC-7 Express. Source: National Heart, Lung, and Blood Institute.

2. Patient should be resting for 5 minutes before measuring BP.
3. Position arm (brachial artery) at heart level.
4. Uncover arm; do not put cuff over clothes.
5. Determine proper size cuff:

Upper arm circumference	*Cuff size required*
16-22.5 cm	pediatric cuff
22.6-30 cm	regular adult cuff
30.1-37.5 cm	large adult cuff
37.6-43.7 cm	thigh cuff

6. Position cuff 1 inch above antecubital crease.
7. Ask patient about previous readings.
8. Place stethoscope over brachial artery (medial to the center).
9. Inflate cuff rapidly to approximately 30 mm Hg above previous readings.
10. Deflate cuff slowly.
11. Remember to deflate cuff completely when done.
12. Wait 1-2 minutes before repeating.
13. Take pressure in both arms.
14. If orthostatic hypotension is suspected, take BP sitting, standing, and supine.

15. Two readings separated by at least 2 minutes should be averaged.
16. If readings differ by >5 mm Hg, additional readings should be taken.

Treatment Principles and Goals

Goals of therapy (Figure 2A and B)
- Reduce end-organ damage
- Minimize or control other risk factors for cardiovascular disease
- Maintain blood pressure, with minimal side effects, at or below the level appropriate for the patient's risk:
  * 140/90 with uncomplicated hypertension
  * 140/90 with target organ damage or CV disease
  * <130/80 with diabetes and chronic kidney disease
  * <125/75 with proteinuria >1 g/24 h

Monitoring and Evaluation

Goals of initial evaluation of patients with hypertension (Table 5)
- Identify known causes of high blood pressure.
- Assess presence or absence of target organ damage and CV disease, extent of the disease, and the response to therapies (Figure 3).
- Identify other CV risk factors or concomitant disorders that may affect prognosis and guide therapy (Figure 3).

Initial evaluation
History
- Duration and levels of elevated blood pressure
- History or symptoms of CHD, heart failure, cerebrovascular disease, pulmonary vascular disease, diabetes mellitus, renal disease, dyslipidemia
- Family history of hypertension, premature CHD, stroke, diabetes, dyslipidemias, or renal disease
- Symptoms suggesting the cause of hypertension
- Recent weight changes, physical activity levels, smoking or other tobacco use
- Dietary assessment: intake of sodium, alcohol, saturated fat, and caffeine
- Complete medication history including prescription, over-the-counter, and herbal/natural products that may increase blood pressure or decrease effectiveness of antihypertensive agents
- Results and adverse effects of previous antihypertensive therapy
- Psychosocial/environmental factors that may influence hypertension control

Examination
- Two or more blood pressure measurements separated by at least 2 minutes
- Measurement of height, weight, and waist circumference
- Funduscopic exam for hypertensive retinopathy
- Exam of neck for carotid bruits, distended veins, or an enlarged thyroid gland

Table 5

Identifiable Causes, Diagnostic Tests, and Clinical Findings for Secondary Hypertension

Cause/diagnosis	Diagnostic test (clinical finding)
Chronic kidney disease	Estimated GFR (abdominal or flank mass for polycystic kidney disease)
Coarctation of the aorta	CT angiography (delayed or absent femoral pulse)
Cushing's syndrome and other glucocorticoid excess states including chronic steroid therapy	History/dexamethasone suppression test (truncal obesity, moon facies, buffalo hump, abdominal striae, hirsutism)
Drug-induced or drug-related	History; drug screening
Pheochromocytoma	24-hour urinary metanephrine and normetanephrine (headache, palpitations, sweating)
Primary aldosteronism and other mineralocorticoid excess states	24-hour urinary aldosterone level or specific measurements of other mineralocorticoids (hypokalemia)
Renovascular hypertension	Doppler flow study; magnetic resonance angiography (abdominal bruit)
Sleep apnea	Sleep study with oxygen saturation (obesity, snoring, tired during waketime)
Thyroid/parathyroid disease	TSH; serum PTH (goiter; hypercalcemia)

CT, computed tomography; GFR, glomerular filtration rate; PTH, parathyroid hormone; TSH, thyroid-stimulating hormone.

Figure 2A.

Algorithm for the treatment of hypertension.

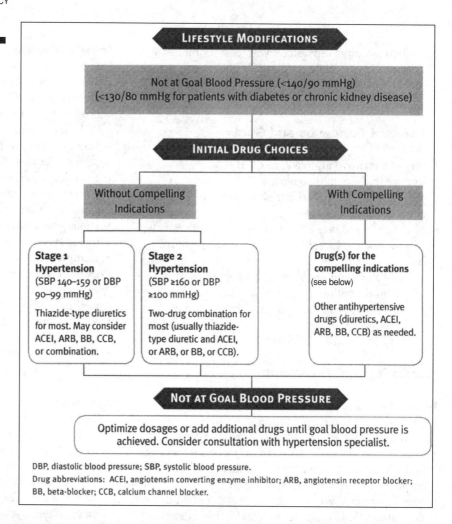

LIFESTYLE MODIFICATIONS

Not at Goal Blood Pressure (<140/90 mmHg)
(<130/80 mmHg for patients with diabetes or chronic kidney disease)

INITIAL DRUG CHOICES

Without Compelling Indications

With Compelling Indications

Stage 1 Hypertension
(SBP 140–159 or DBP 90–99 mmHg)

Thiazide-type diuretics for most. May consider ACEI, ARB, BB, CCB, or combination.

Stage 2 Hypertension
(SBP ≥160 or DBP ≥100 mmHg)

Two-drug combination for most (usually thiazide-type diuretic and ACEI, or ARB, or BB, or CCB).

Drug(s) for the compelling indications (see below)

Other antihypertensive drugs (diuretics, ACEI, ARB, BB, CCB) as needed.

NOT AT GOAL BLOOD PRESSURE

Optimize dosages or add additional drugs until goal blood pressure is achieved. Consider consultation with hypertension specialist.

DBP, diastolic blood pressure; SBP, systolic blood pressure.
Drug abbreviations: ACEI, angiotensin converting enzyme inhibitor; ARB, angiotensin receptor blocker; BB, beta-blocker; CCB, calcium channel blocker.

Figure 2B.

Clinical trial and guideline basis for compelling indications for individual drug classes.

COMPELLING INDICATION*	RECOMMENDED DRUGS†						CLINICAL TRIAL BASIS‡
	DIURETIC	BB	ACEI	ARB	CCB	ALDO ANT	
Heart failure	•	•	•	•		•	ACC/AHA Heart Failure Guideline, MERIT-HF, COPERNICUS, CIBIS, SOLVD, AIRE, TRACE, ValHEFT, RALES
Postmyocardial infarction		•	•			•	ACC/AHA Post-MI Guideline, BHAT, SAVE, Capricorn, EPHESUS
High coronary disease risk	•	•	•		•		ALLHAT, HOPE, ANBP2, LIFE, CONVINCE
Diabetes	•	•	•	•	•		NKF-ADA Guideline, UKPDS, ALLHAT
Chronic kidney disease			•	•			NKF Guideline, Captopril Trial, RENAAL, IDNT, REIN, AASK
Recurrent stroke prevention	•		•				PROGRESS

* Compelling indications for antihypertensive drugs are based on benefits from outcome studies or existing clinical guidelines; the compelling indication is managed in parallel with the BP.

† Drug abbreviations: ACEI, angiotensin converting enzyme inhibitor; ARB, angiotensin receptor blocker; Aldo ANT, aldosterone antagonist; BB, beta-blocker; CCB, calcium channel blocker.

‡ Conditions for which clinical trials demonstrate benefit of specific classes of antihypertensive drugs.

Figure 2A and B adapted from JNC-7 Express. Source: National Heart, Lung, and Blood Institute.

Figure 3.

Cardiovascular risk factors.

Major risk factors
Hypertension[1]
Cigarette smoking
Obesity[1] (body mass index ≥30 kg/m^2)
Physical inactivity
Dyslipidemia[1]
Diabetes mellitus[1]
Microalbuminuria or estimated GFR <60 mL/min
Age (>55 for men, >65 for women)
Family history of premature cardiovascular disease
  (men under age 55, women under 45)

Target organ damage
Heart
  • Left ventricular hypertrophy
  • Angina or prior myocardial infarction
  • Prior coronary revascularization
  • Heart failure
Brain
  • Stroke or transient ischemic attack
Chronic kidney disease
Peripheral arterial disease
Retinopathy

GFR, glomerular filtration rate.
[1]Components of the metabolic syndrome.
Adapted from JNC-7 Express. Source: National Heart, Lung, and Blood Institute.

• Exam of heart for abnormalities in rate and rhythm, increased size, precordial heave, clicks, murmurs, and third and fourth heart sounds
• Exam of lungs for rales and evidence of bronchospasm
• Exam of abdomen for bruits, enlarged kidneys, masses, and abnormal aortic pulsation
• Exam of extremities for decreased or absent peripheral arterial pulsations, bruits, and edema
• Neurologic assessment

Laboratory
Routine tests
• Urinalysis
• Complete blood cell count
• Blood chemistries (sodium, potassium, creatinine, BUN, glucose)
• Fasting lipid profile (total cholesterol, triglycerides, HDL, LDL)
• ECG

Optional tests
• Creatinine clearance
• Microalbuminuria
• 24-Hour urinary protein
• Blood calcium
• Uric acid
• Glycosylated hemoglobin
• Thyroid-stimulating hormone
• Limited echocardiography
• Ankle-brachial index (ABI)
• Plasma renin activity/urinary sodium determination

Follow-up evaluation
• Follow-up evaluation includes any of the previous exams completed during the initial evaluation as required to monitor both response to and possible adverse effects from prescribed antihypertensive therapies, in addition to assessment of any new symptoms of target organ damage and the assessment of patient adherence to therapy (Figure 4).

Figure 4.

General guidelines to improve patient adherence to antihypertensive therapy.

• Be aware of signs of patient nonadherence to antihypertensive therapy.
• Establish the goal of therapy: to reduce blood pressure to nonhypertensive levels with minimal or no adverse effects.
• Educate patients about the disease, and involve them and their families in its treatment. Have them measure blood pressure at home.
• Maintain contact with patients; consider telecommunication.
• Keep care inexpensive and simple.
• Encourage lifestyle modifications.
• Integrate pill-taking into routine activities of daily living.
• Prescribe medications according to pharmacologic principles, favoring long-acting formulations.
• Be willing to stop unsuccessful therapy and try a different approach.
• Anticipate adverse effects, and adjust therapy to prevent, minimize, or ameliorate side effects.
• Continue to add effective and tolerated drugs, stepwise, in sufficient doses to achieve the goal of therapy.
• Encourage a positive attitude about achieving therapeutic goals.
• Consider using nurse case management.

Adapted from JNC-7 Express. Source: National Heart, Lung, and Blood Institute.

2. Nondrug Therapy

- Lifestyle modifications are recommended to improve both blood pressure and overall cardiovascular health (Figure 5).
- Research has shown that diets rich in fruits, vegetables, and low-fat dairy foods, and with reduced saturated and total fats, significantly lower blood pressure (Figures 6 and 7).

Figure 5.

Lifestyle modifications to manage hypertension.

MODIFICATION	RECOMMENDATION	APPROXIMATE SBP REDUCTION (RANGE)
Weight reduction	Maintain normal body weight (body mass index 18.5–24.9 kg/m^2).	5–20 mmHg/10 kg weight loss
Adopt DASH eating plan	Consume a diet rich in fruits, vegetables, and lowfat dairy products with a reduced content of saturated and total fat.	8–14 mmHg
Dietary sodium reduction	Reduce dietary sodium intake to no more than 100 mmol per day (2.4 g sodium or 6 g sodium chloride).	2–8 mmHg
Physical activity	Engage in regular aerobic physical activity such as brisk walking (at least 30 min per day, most days of the week).	4–9 mmHg
Moderation of alcohol consumption	Limit consumption to no more than 2 drinks (1 oz or 30 mL ethanol; e.g., 24 oz beer, 10 oz wine, or 3 oz 80-proof whiskey) per day in most men and to no more than 1 drink per day in women and lighter weight persons.	2–4 mmHg[30]

DASH, Dietary Approaches to Stop Hypertension.

For overall cardiovascular risk reduction, stop smoking.

The effects of implementing these modifications are dose and time dependent, and could be greater for some individuals.

Adapted from JNC-7 Express. Source: National Heart, Lung, and Blood Institute.

Figure 6.

━━

Dietary suggestions for hypertensive patients.

Food group	Daily servings	Serving sizes	Examples and notes	Significance of each food group to the DASH diet pattern
Grains and grain products	7-8	1 slice bread; $^1/_2$ c. dry cereal; $^1/_2$ c. cooked rice, pasta, or cereal	Whole wheat bread, english muffins, pita bread, bagel, cereals, grits, oatmeal	Major sources of energy and fiber
Vegetables	4-5	1 c. raw leafy vegetable; $^1/_2$ c. cooked vegetable; 6 oz. vegetable juice	Tomatoes, potatoes, carrots, peas, squash, broccoli, turnip greens, collards, kale, spinach, artichokes, beans, sweet potatoes	Rich sources of potassium, magnesium, and fiber
Fruits	4-5	6 oz. fruit juice; 1 medium fruit; $^1/_4$ c. dried fruit; $^1/_4$ c. fresh, frozen or canned fruit	Apricots, bananas, dates, grapes, oranges, orange juice, grapefruit, grapefruit juice, mangoes, melons, peaches, pineapple, prunes, raisins, strawberries, tangerines	Important sources of potassium, magnesium, and fiber
Low-fat or nonfat dairy foods	2-3	8 oz. milk; 1 c. yogurt; 1.5 oz. cheese	Skim or 1% milk, skim or low-fat buttermilk, nonfat or low-fat yogurt, part-skim mozzarella cheese, nonfat cheese	Major sources of calcium and protein
Meats, poultry, and fish	2 or less	3 oz. cooked meats, poultry, or fish	Select only lean; trim away visible fats; broil, roast, or boil, instead of frying; remove skin from poultry	Rich sources of protein and magnesium
Nuts, seeds, and legumes	4-5 per week	1.5 oz. or $^1/_3$ c. nuts; $^1/_2$ oz. or 2 T. seeds; $^1/_2$ c. cooked legumes	Almonds, filberts, mixed nuts, peanuts, walnuts, sunflower seeds, kidney beans, lentils	Rich sources of energy, magnesium, potassium, protein, and fiber

━━

Adapted from JNC-7 Express. Source: National Heart, Lung, and Blood Institute.

DASH, Dietary Approaches to Stop Hypertension.

Figure 7.

The DASH diet sample menu based on 2000 calories/day.

Food	Amount	Servings provided
Breakfast		
Orange juice	6 oz.	1 fruit
1% Lowfat milk	8 oz. (1 c.)	1 dairy
Cornflakes (with 1 t. sugar)	1 c.	2 grains
Banana	1 medium	1 fruit
Whole wheat bread (with 1 T. jelly)	1 slice	1 grain
Soft margarine	1 t.	1 fat
Lunch		
Chicken salad	$^3/_4$ c.	1 poultry
Pita bread	$^1/_2$ large	1 grain
Raw vegetable medley:		
Carrot and celery sticks	3-4 sticks each	
Radishes	2	1 vegetable
Loose-leaf lettuce	2 leaves	
Part-skim mozzarella cheese	1.5 slice (1.5 oz.)	1 dairy
1% lowfat milk	8 oz. (1 c.)	1 dairy
Fruit cocktail in light syrup	$^1/_2$ c.	1 fruit
Dinner		
Herbed baked cod	3 oz.	1 fish
Scallion rice	1 c.	2 grains
Steamed broccoli	$^1/_2$ c.	1 vegetable
Stewed tomatoes	$^1/_2$ c.	1 vegetable
Spinach salad:		
Raw spinach	$^1/_2$ c.	
Cherry tomatoes	2	1 vegetable
Cucumber	2 slices	
Light Italian salad dressing	1 T.	$^1/_2$ fat
Whole wheat dinner roll	1 small	1 grain
Soft margarine	1 t.	1 fat
Melon balls	$^1/_2$ c.	1 fruit
Snacks		
Dried apricots	1 oz. ($^1/_4$ c.)	1 fruit
Minipretzels	1 oz. ($^3/_4$ c.)	1 grain
Mixed nuts	1.5 oz. ($^1/_3$ c.)	1 nuts
Diet ginger ale	12 oz.	0

Total number of servings in 2000-calorie-per-day menu

Food group	Servings
Grains	= 8
Vegetables	= 4
Fruits	= 5
Dairy foods	= 3
Meats, poultry, and fish	= 2
Nuts, seeds, and legumes	= 1
Fats and oils	= 2.5

Tips on eating the DASH way

- Start small. Make gradual changes in your eating habits.
- Center your meal around carbohydrates, such as pasta, rice, beans, or vegetables.
- Treat meat as one part of the whole meal, instead of the focus.
- Use fruits or low-fat, low-calorie foods such as sugar-free gelatin for desserts and snacks.

REMEMBER! If you use the DASH diet to help prevent or control high blood pressure, make it part of a lifestyle that includes choosing foods lower in salt and sodium, keeping a healthy weight, being physically active, and if you drink alcohol, doing so in moderation.

Adapted from JNC-7 Express. Source: National Heart, Lung, and Blood Institute.
DASH, Dietary Approaches to Stop Hypertension.

3. Drug Therapy

- All patient factors (severity of blood pressure elevation, presence of target organ damage, and presence of CV disease or other risk factors) must be considered when initiating therapy.

Initial Therapy

- Candidates for therapy (Figure 2A and 2B)
- Use of lifestyle modifications should continue to be stressed to patients after the decision to initiate drug therapy has been made (Figure 5) to further decrease the risk of complications from cardiovascular disease.
- Prehypertension represents a new classification in JNC-VII (Table 3) and represents a significant risk for future development of stage 1 hypertension. Lifestyle modifications should be stressed for this classification, and medication therapy should only be used for patients with compelling indications.
- β-Blockers and diuretics are considered the initial agents for treatment of hypertension by JNC-VI unless compelling indications for the use of other medication classes exist or the patient has comorbid conditions that would suggest the use of classes other than β-blockers and diuretics (Figure 2A and 2B and Table 6).
- Recent data suggest that angiotensin-converting enzyme inhibitors (ACEIs), calcium channel blockers (CCBs), and possibly angiotensin II receptor blockers (ARBs) might also be considered as initial agents for treatment of hypertension.
- For patients who are 20/10 mm Hg greater than their goal blood pressure, 2-drug combination therapy (one drug a diuretic) should be strongly considered.
- If a patient requires a second agent for treatment of hypertension, it is strongly recommended to be a diuretic if one is not chosen as the initial agent.
- All causes for inadequate response should be addressed before additional agents are added to a patient's antihypertensive regimen (Figure 8).
- Vasodilators, α_1-receptor antagonists, α_2-receptor agonists, and postganglionic adrenergic neuron blockers should be avoided as initial agents for hypertension.

Diuretics

Thiazide and thiazide-like diuretics (Table 7)
Mechanism of action
- Direct arteriole dilation
- Reduction of total fluid volume through the inhibition of sodium reabsorption in the distal tubules, which causes increased excretion of sodium, water, potassium, and hydrogen
- Increase the effectiveness of other antihypertensive agents by preventing re-expansion of plasma volume
- Significant decrease in efficacy in renal failure (serum creatinine >2 mg/dL or GFR <30 mL/min)

Adverse drug events (Table 7)

Patient instructions and counseling
- Can be taken with food or milk
- Take early in the day to avoid nocturia.
- Patients may become more sensitive to sunlight; consider using sunscreen with SPF >15.
- May increase blood glucose in diabetics
- Report problems with muscle cramps that may indicate decreased potassium level.

Drug-drug and drug-disease interactions
- Steroids: cause salt retention and antagonize thiazide action
- NSAIDs: blunt thiazide response
- Class IA or III antiarrhythmics (that prolong the QT interval) may cause torsades de pointes with diuretic-induced hypokalemia.
- Probenecid and lithium: block thiazide effects by interfering with thiazide excretion into the urine
- Lithium: thiazides decrease lithium renal clearance and increase risk of lithium toxicity

Parameters to monitor
- Blood pressure
- Weight
- Serum electrolytes and uric acid
- BUN and creatinine
- Cholesterol levels

Loop diuretics (Table 7)
Mechanism of action
- Reduction of total fluid volume through the inhibition of sodium and chloride reabsorption in the ascending loop of Henle, which causes increased excretion of water, sodium, chloride, magnesium, and calcium
- Are more effective than thiazides in patients with renal failure (serum creatinine >2 mg/dL or GFR <30 mL/min)
- Diuretics are also available in combination with other drugs (Table 8).

Adverse drug events (Table 7)

Patient instructions and counseling
- Can be taken with food or milk
- Take early in the day to avoid nocturia.

Table 6

Considerations for Individualizing Antihypertensive Drug Therapy[1]

Indication	Drug therapy
Compelling indications unless contraindicated	
Diabetes mellitus (type 1) with proteinuria	ACEI
Heart failure	ACEI, diuretics
Isolated systolic hypertension (older patients)	Diuretics (preferred), calcium antagonists (long-acting DHP)
Myocardial infarction	β-Blockers (non ISA), ACEI (with systolic dysfunction)
May have favorable effects on comorbid conditions[2]	
Angina	β-Blockers, calcium antagonists
Atrial tachycardia and fibrillation	β-Blockers, calcium antagonists (non-DHP)
Cyclosporine-induced hypertension (caution with the dose of cyclosporine)	Calcium antagonists
Diabetes mellitus (types 1 and 2) with proteinuria	ACEI (preferred), calcium antagonists
Diabetes mellitus (type 2)	Low-dose diuretics
Dyslipidemia	α-Blockers
Essential tremor	β-Blockers (non-CS)
Heart failure	Carvedilol, losartan potassium
Hyperthyroidism	β-Blockers
Migraine	β-Blockers (non-CS), calcium antagonists (non-DHP)
Myocardial infarction	Diltiazem hydrochloride, verapamil hydrochloride
Osteoporosis	Thiazides
Preoperative hypertension	β-Blockers
Prostatism (benign prostatic hyperplasia)	α-Blockers
Renal insufficiency (use caution in renovascular hypertension and if creatinine ≥265.2 micromole/L [3 mg/dL])	ACEI
May have unfavorable effects on comorbid conditions[2,3]	
Bronchospastic disease	β-Blockers[4]
Depression	β-Blockers, central α-agonist, reserpine[4]
Diabetes mellitus (types 1 and 2)	β-Blockers, high-dose diuretics
Dyslipidemia	β-Blockers (non-ISA), diuretics (high-dose)
Gout	Diuretics
Second- or third-degree heart block	β-Blockers,[4] calcium antagonists (non-DHP)[4]
Heart failure	β-Blockers (except carvedilol), calcium antagonists (except amlodipine besylate, felodipine)
Liver disease	Labetalol hydrochloride, methyldopa[4]
Peripheral vascular disease	β-Blockers
Pregnancy	ACEI,[4] angiotensin II receptor blockers[4]
Renal insufficiency	Potassium-sparing agents
Renovascular disease	ACEI, angiotensin II receptor blockers

ACEI, angiotensin-converting enzyme inhibitors; DHP, dihydropyridine; ISA, intrinsic sympathomimetic activity; non-CS, noncardioselective.

[1]For initial drug therapy recommendations, see Tables 7-15.

[2]Conditions and drugs are listed in alphabetical order.

[3]These drugs may be used with special monitoring unless contraindicated.

[4]Contraindicated.

Adapted from JNC-7 Express. Source: National Heart, Lung, and Blood Institute.

Figure 8.

<hr>

Causes of inadequate responsiveness to therapy.

<hr>

Pseudoresistance
"White-coat hypertension" or office elevations
Pseudohypertension in older patients
Use of regular cuff on a very obese arm

Nonadherence to therapy

Volume overload
Excess salt intake
Progressive renal damage (nephrosclerosis)
Fluid retention from reduction of blood pressure
Inadequate diuretic therapy

Drug-related causes
Doses too low
Wrong type of diuretic
Inappropriate combinations
Rapid inactivation (eg, hydralazine)
Drug actions and interactions
  Sympathomimetics
  Nasal decongestants
  Appetite suppressants
  Cocaine and other illicit drugs
  Caffeine
  Oral contraceptives
  Adrenal steroids
  Licorice (as may be found in chewing tobacco)
  Cyclosporine, tacrolimus
  Erythropoietin
  Antidepressants
  Nonsteroidal anti-inflammatory drugs

Associated conditions
Smoking
Increasing obesity
Sleep apnea
Insulin resistance/hyperinsulinemia
Ethanol intake of more than 1 oz. (30 mL) per day
Anxiety-induced hyperventilation or panic attacks
Chronic pain
Intense vasoconstriction (arteritis)
Organic brain syndrome (eg, memory deficit)

Identifiable causes of hypertension

<hr>

Adapted from JNC-7 Express. Source: National Heart, Lung, and Blood Institute.

- May become more sensitive to sunlight; consider using sunscreen with SPF >15
- May increase blood glucose in diabetics
- Report problems with muscle cramps that may indicate decreased potassium level.
- Rise slowly from a lying or sitting position.

Drug-drug and drug-disease interactions
- Aminoglycosides: combined with loop diuretics can precipitate ototoxicity
- NSAIDs: blunt diuretic response
- Class IA or III antiarrhythmics (that prolong the QT interval) may cause torsades de pointes with diuretic-induced hypokalemia.
- Probenecid: blocks loop diuretic effects by interfering with excretion into the urine

Parameters to monitor
- Weight
- Serum electrolytes
- BUN and creatinine
- Uric acid
- Hearing (in high doses)

Potassium-sparing diuretics (Table 7)
Mechanism of action
- Interferes with potassium/sodium exchange in the distal tubule; decreases calcium excretion, increases magnesium loss

Adverse drug events (Table 7)

Patient instructions and counseling
- Take early in day to avoid nocturia.
- Take after meals.
- Avoid excessive ingestion of foods high in potassium and use of salt substitutes.
- May increase blood glucose in diabetics.
- Report problems with muscle cramps that may indicate decreased potassium levels.
- Sexual dysfunction

Drug-drug and drug-disease interactions
- ACE inhibitors: may increase risk of hyperkalemia
- Indomethacin: combination with triamterene can cause decrease in renal function
- Cimetidine: increases bioavailability and decreases clearance of triamterene

Parameters to monitor
- Weight
- Serum electrolytes (especially potassium)
- BUN and creatinine

Table 7

Thiazide Diuretics, Thiazide-Like Diuretics, Loop Diuretics, Potassium-Sparing Agents, and Aldosterone-Receptor Blocker

Drug	Trade name	Usual dose range, total mg/d (frequency per day)	Adverse events and comments[1]
Thiazide diuretics			
Bendroflumethiazide	Naturetin	2.5-5 (1)	**Short-term:** increased cholesterol and glucose
Benzthiazide	Aquatag , Exna	12.5-50 (1)	**Biochemical:** decreased potassium, sodium, and
Chlorothiazide	Diuril	125-500 (1)	magnesium; increased uric acid and calcium
Chlorthalidone	Hygroton , Hylidone	12.5-25 (1)	**Rare:** blood dyscrasias, photosensitivity, pancreatitis,
Hydrochlorothiazide	HydroDIURIL , Microzide	12.5-50 (1)	hyponatremia, sulfonamide-type immune reactions
	Saluron , Diucardin		**Other:** impotence, fatigue, headache, rash, vertigo
Hydroflumethiazide		25-50 (1)	
Methyclothiazide	Renese	2.5-5 (1)	
Polythiazide	Metahydrin , Naqua	2-4 (1)	
Trichlormethiazide		2-4 (1)	
Thiazide-like diuretics	Mykrox		
Metolazone	Zaroxolyn	2.5-10 (1)	(Less or no hypercholesterolemia compared to other
Metolazone	Lozol	2.5-5 (1)	thiazides; decreased microalbuminuria in diabetes)
Indapamide		2.5-5 (1)	
Loop diuretics	Bumex		
Bumetanide	Lasix	0.5-2 (2)	Ototoxicity at high doses
Furosemide	Demadex	20-80 (2)	(Short duration, no hypercalcemia)
Torsemide		2.5-10 (1)	(Short duration, no hypercalcemia)
Potassium-sparing agents[2]	Midamor		
Amiloride	Dyrenium	5-10 (1-2)	Hyperkalemia
Triamterene		50-100 (1-2)	(Avoid with history of kidney stones or hepatic disease)
Aldosterone-receptor blocker	Aldactone		
Spironolactone		25-50 (1-2)	

[1]Side effects listed are for the class of drugs except where noted for individual drugs (in parentheses).
[2]See Table 8 for combination products.
Adapted from JNC-7 Express. Source: National Heart, Lung, and Blood Institute.

Adrenergic Inhibitors

Postganglionic adrenergic neuron blockers (Table 9)
- *This medication class is best avoided unless necessary to treat refractory hypertension unresponsive to all other agents, as they are poorly tolerated.*

Mechanism of action
- Causes presynaptic inhibition of the release of neurotransmitter from peripheral neurons by agonistic

activity on the α receptor and depletion of neurotransmitter through competitive uptake into the neurosecretory vesicles.

Adverse drug events (Table 9)

Patient instructions and counseling
- Report symptoms of dizziness or hypotension.
- Don't take OTC cold products without first asking the doctor or pharmacist.

Table 8

Combination Drugs for Hypertension

Combination Type*	Fixed-Dose Combination, mg†	Trade Name
ACEIs and CCBs	Amlodipine/benazepril hydrochloride (2.5/10, 5/10, 5/20, 10/20)	Lotrel
	Enalapril maleate/felodipine (5/5)	Lexxel
	Trandolapril/verapamil (2/180, 1/240, 2/240, 4/240)	Tarka
ACEIs and diuretics	Benazepril/hydrochlorothiazide (5/6.25, 10/12.5, 20/12.5, 20/25)	Lotensin HCT
	Captopril/hydrochlorothiazide (25/15, 25/25, 50/15, 50/25)	Capozide
	Enalapril maleate/hydrochlorothiazide (5/12.5, 10/25)	Vaseretic
	Lisinopril/hydrochlorothiazide (10/12.5, 20/12.5, 20/25)	Prinzide , _Zestoretic_
	Moexipril HCl/hydrochlorothiazide (7.5/12.5, 15/25)	Uniretic
	Quinapril HCl/hydrochlorothiazide (10/12.5, 20/12.5, 20/25)	Accuretic
ARBs and diuretics	Candesartan cilexetil/hydrochlorothiazide (16/12.5, 32/12.5)	Atacand HCT
	Eprosartan mesylate/hydrochlorothiazide (600/12.5, 600/25)	Teveten/HCT
	Irbesartan/hydrochlorothiazide (150/12.5, 300/12.5)	Avalide
	Losartan potassium/hydrochlorothiazide (50/12.5, 100/25)	Hyzaar
	Telmisartan/hydrochlorothiazide (40/12.5, 80/12.5)	Micardis/HCT
	Valsartan/hydrochlorothiazide (80/12.5, 160/12.5)	Diovan/HCT
BBs and diuretics	Atenolol/chlorthalidone (50/25, 100/25)	Tenoretic
	Bisoprolol fumarate/hydrochlorothiazide (2.5/6.25, 5/6.25, 10/6.25)	Ziac
	Propranolol LA/hydrochlorothiazide (40/25, 80/25)	Inderide
	Metoprolol tartrate/hydrochlorothiazide (50/25, 100/25)	Lopressor HCT
	Nadolol/bendrofluthiazide (40/5, 80/5)	Corzide
	Timolol maleate/hydrochlorothiazide (10/25)	Timolide
Centrally acting drug and diuretic	Methyldopa/hydrochlorothiazide (250/15, 250/25, 500/30, 500/50)	Aldoril
	Reserpine/chlorothiazide (0.125/250, 0.25/500)	Diupres
	Reserpine/hydrochlorothiazide (0.125/25, 0.125/50)	Hydropres
Diuretic and diuretic	Amiloride HCl/hydrochlorothiazide (5/50)	Moduretic
	Spironolactone/hydrochlorothiazide (25/25, 50/50)	Aldactazide
	Triamterene/hydrochlorothiazide (37.5/25, 50/25, 75/50)	Dyazide, Maxzide

*Abbreviations: ACEI, angiotensin-converting enzyme inhibitor; ARB, angiotensin receptor blocker; BB, β-blocker; CCB, calcium channel blocker.
†Some drug combinations are available in multiple fixed doses. Each drug dose is reported in milligrams.
Adapted from JNC-7 Express. Source: National Heart, Lung, and Blood Institute.

- Rise slowly from a lying or sitting position.
- Report new fluid retention.
- Sexual dysfunction

Drug-drug and drug-disease interactions
- OTC sympathomimetics: may potentiate an acute hypertensive effect
- Tricyclic antidepressants/chlorpromazine: antagonize therapeutic effects of guanethidine
- Pheochromocytoma is a contraindication to this class of medications.

- Should be avoided in patients with CHF, angina, and cerebrovascular disease

Parameters to monitor
- History of depression (reserpine)
- Sleep disturbances, drowsiness, lethargy (reserpine)
- Symptoms of peptic ulcer (reserpine)

Table 9

Postganglionic Adrenergic Neuron Blockers

Drug	Trade name	Usual dose range, total mg/d (frequency per day)	Adverse events and comments
Guanadrel	Hylorel	10-75 (2)	Postural hypotension, diarrhea
Guanethidine monosulfate	Ismelin	10-150 (1)	Postural hypotension, diarrhea
Reserpine[1]	Serpasil	0.05-0.25 (1)	Nasal congestion, sedation, depression, activation of peptic ulcer, dizziness, lethargy, memory impairment, sleep disturbances, weight gain

[1] Also acts centrally.

Adapted from JNC-7 Express. Source: National Heart, Lung, and Blood Institute.

Centrally active α-agonists (Table 10)
Mechanism of action
- Causes decreased sympathetic outflow to the cardio-vascular system by agonistic activity on central α_2 receptors

Stimulate α_2

Patient instructions and counseling
- Report symptoms of dizziness or hypotension
- Sedation precautions
- Fever and flu-like symptoms may represent hepatic dysfunction (methyldopa).
- Report new fluid retention
- Sexual dysfunction

Drug-drug and drug-disease interactions
- Use cautiously with other sedating medications.
- Use cautiously in patients with angina, recent MI, CVA, and hepatic or renal disease (guanabenz and guanfacine).

Parameters to monitor
- CBC, positive Coombs' test in 25%, less than 1% develop hemolytic anemia (methyldopa)

Table 10

Centrally Active α₂ Agonists

Drug	Trade name	Usual dose range, total mg/d (frequency per day)	Adverse events and comments[1]
Clonidine HCl[2]	Catapres	0.1-0.8 (2)	Sedation, dry mouth, bradycardia, withdrawal hypertension, orthostatic hypotension, depression, impotence, sleep disturbances (More withdrawal)
Guanabenz acetate	Wytensin	8-32 (2)	
Guanfacine HCl	Tenex	1-3 (1)	(Less withdrawal)
Methyldopa	Aldomet	250-1000 (2)	(Hepatic and "autoimmune" disorders)

[1] Side effects listed are for the class of drugs except where noted for individual drugs (in parentheses).

[2] Also available as a once-weekly transdermal patch.

Adapted from JNC-7 Express. Source: National Heart, Lung, and Blood Institute.

- Sleep disturbances, drowsiness, dry mouth
- Symptoms of depression
- Impotence
- Pulse
- Rebound hypertension

Peripherally acting α-adrenergic blockers (Table 11)

Mechanism of action

- Blocks peripheral α_1 postsynaptic receptors, which causes vasodilation of both arteries and veins (indirect vasodilators)
- Causes less reflex tachycardia than direct vasodilators (hydralazine/minoxidil)

Adverse drug events (Table 11)

Patient instructions and counseling

- Take first dose of no more than 1 mg of any agent and take at bedtime.
- Rise slowly from a lying or sitting position.
- May cause dizziness
- Priapism

Drug-drug and drug-disease interactions

- NSAIDs: decreased antihypertensive effects of α_1 blockers
- Increased antihypertensive effects with diuretics and β-blockers

Parameters to monitor

- Blood pressure and pulse
- Peripheral edema

β-Blockers (Table 12)

Mechanism of action

- Competitively blocks response to β-adrenergic stimulation:
  * Blocked secretion of renin
  * Decreased cardiac contractility, thereby decreases cardiac output
  * Decreased central sympathetic output
  * Decreased heart rate, thereby decreasing cardiac output

↓ CO ↓ HR
↓ SNS

Adverse drug events (Table 12)

Patient instructions and counseling

- Report symptoms of dizziness or hypotension.
- Sedation precautions (with lipid-soluble compounds)
- Abrupt withdrawal of the drug should be avoided.
- Sexual dysfunction

Drug-drug and drug-disease interactions

- Use with caution in patients with diabetes.
- Use with caution in patients with Raynaud's phenomenon or peripheral vascular disease.
- Sulfonylureas: β-blockers may decrease effectiveness of sulfonylureas.
- Nondihydropyridines: may increase effect/toxicity of β-blockers

Parameters to monitor

- ECG
- Rebound hypertension
- Cholesterol levels
- Pulse (apical and radial)
- Glucose levels

Table 11

Peripherally Acting α_1 Blockers

antagonist

Drug	Trade name	Usual dose range, total mg/d (frequency per day)	Adverse events and comments
Doxazosin mesylate	Cardura	1-16 (1)	Postural hypotension, syncopal episode with first dose, postural hypotension, diarrhea, weight gain, peripheral edema, dry mouth, urinary urgency, constipation, priapism, nausea, dizziness, headache, palpitations, and sweating; no effects on glucose or cholesterol
Prazosin HCl	Minipress	2-20 (2-3)	
Terazosin HCl	Hytrin	1-20 (1-2)	

Reprinted with permission from JNC-VI.

Table 12

β-Blockers and Combination α- and β-Blockers

Generic name (trade name)	Lipid solubility/primary (secondary) routes of elimination	Usual dose range, total mg/d (frequency per day)	Adverse events and comments[3]
β-Blockers			
Acebutolol (Sectral)[1,2]	low/H (R)	200-800 (1)	Bronchospasm, bradycardia, heart failure, may mask insulin-induced hypoglycemia; *less serious*: impaired peripheral circulation, insomnia, fatigue, decreased exercise tolerance, hypertriglyceridemia (except agents with intrinsic sympathomimetic activity)
Atenolol (Tenormin)[1]	low/R (H)	25-100 (1)	
Betaxolol (Kerlone)[1]	low/H (R)	5-20 (1)	
Bisoprolol fumarate (Zebeta)[1]	low/R (H)	2.5-10 (1)	
Carteolol HCl (Cartrol)[2]	low/R	2.5-10 (1)	
Metoprolol tartrate[1] (Lopressor)	moderate/H (R)	50-100 (2)	
Metoprolol succinate[1] (Toprol-XL)	moderate/H (R)	50-100 (1)	
Nadolol (Corgard)	low/R	40-120 (1)	
Penbutolol sulfate (Levatol)[2]	high/H (R)	10-20 (1)	
Pindolol (Visken)[2]	moderate/H (R)	10-60 (2)	
Propranolol HCl (Inderal)	high/H	40-160 (2)	
(Inderal LA)		60-180 (1)	
Timolol maleate (Blocadren)	low-moderate/H (R)	20-40 (2)	
			Postural hypotension, bronchospasm
Combined α- and β-blockers			
Carvedilol (Coreg)	moderate/bile into feces	12.5-50 (2)	
Labetalol (Normodyne, Trandate)	moderate/R (H)	200-800 (2)	

H, hepatic; R, renal.

[1]Cardioselective.

[2]Intrinsic sympathomimetic activity.

[3]Side effects listed are for the class of drugs except where noted for individual drugs (in parentheses).

Reprinted with permission from JNC-VI.

[handwritten: except sweat + hunger]

Direct Vasodilators

- *This medication class is best avoided (second-line agents) unless necessary to treat refractory hypertension unresponsive to all other agents.*
- *These agents should NOT be used alone secondary to increases in plasma renin activity, cardiac output, and heart rate, and should therefore be used only when β-blockers and diuretics are part of the antihypertensive regimen.*

Mechanism of action
- These agents cause direct relaxation of peripheral arterial smooth muscle and thereby significantly decrease peripheral resistance.

Adverse drug events (Table 13)

Patient instructions and counseling
- Report symptoms of dizziness or hypotension.
- Hirsutism (minoxidil)

Table 13

Direct Vasodilators

Drug	Trade name	Usual dose range, total mg/d (frequency per day)	Adverse events and comments[1]
			Headaches, fluid retention, tachycardia, peripheral neuropathy, postural hypotension
Hydralazine HCl	Apresoline	25-100 (2)	(Lupus syndrome)
Minoxidil	Loniten	2.5-80 (1-2)	(Hirsutism)

[1]Side effects listed are for the class of drugs except where noted for individual drugs (in parentheses).
Adapted from JNC-7 Express. Source: National Heart, Lung, and Blood Institute.

- Report any new symptoms of fatigue, malaise, low-grade fever, and joint aches.
- Report rapid weight gain (>5 lb), unusual swelling, and pulse increases of >20 beats/min above normal.
- Rise slowly from a lying or sitting position.

Drug-drug and drug-disease interactions
- Use with caution in patients with pulmonary hypertension.
- Use with caution in patients with significant renal failure or CHF.
- Use with caution in patients with CAD or a recent MI.

Parameters to monitor
- Weight (fluid status)
- Blood pressure and pulse
- CBC with ANA (hydralazine)

Calcium Antagonists

- Low-renin hypertensive, black, and elderly patients respond well to this class of medications.

Mechanism of action
- Inhibit the influx of calcium ions through slow channels in vascular smooth muscle and cause relaxation of both coronary and peripheral arteries
- Sinoatrial (SA) and atrioventricular (AV) nodal depression and decrease in myocardial contractility (nondihydropyridines)

Adverse drug events (Table 14)

Patient instructions and counseling
- Report symptoms of dizziness or hypotension.
- Constipation (verapamil)

- Report any new symptoms of shortness of breath, fatigue, or increased swelling of the extremities.
- Rise slowly from a lying or sitting position.

Drug-drug and drug-disease interactions
- Use with caution in patients on β-blockers (nondihydropyridines) which may increase CHF and bradycardia; this combination can also cause conduction abnormalities to the AV node.
- Use with extreme caution in patients with conduction disturbances in the SA or AV nodes.
- Grapefruit juice may increase the levels of some dihydropyridines.

Parameters to monitor
- ECG
- Peripheral edema   *gingival hyperplasia*
- Blood pressure and pulse
- Bowel habits
- Symptoms of conduction disturbances

Angiotensin-Converting Enzyme Inhibitors (ACEIs) and Angiotensin II Receptor Blockers (ARBs)

- Ethnic differences in the response to these classes of medications exist. These agents are relatively ineffective as monotherapy in black patients. However, the addition of diuretic therapy has been shown to sensitize black patients to these agents to obtain similar responses as in non-black patients.

Mechanism of action
ACEIs
- Inhibit the conversion of angiotensin I to angiotensin II (a potent vasoconstrictor; see Figure 1)

Table 14

Calcium Antagonists

Drug	Trade name	Usual dose range, total mg/d (frequency per day)	Adverse events and comments[1]
Nondihydropyridines			
Diltiazem HCl	Cardizem SR , Cardizem CD ,	180-420 (1)	Conduction defects, worsening of systolic
	Dilacor XR , Tiazac	120-360 (1)	dysfunction, gingival hyperplasia
Verapamil immediate-release	Calan , Isoptin	80-320 (2)	(Nausea, headache)
Verapamil long-acting	Calan SR , Isoptin SR	120-360 (1-2)	(Constipation)
Verapamil—Coer	Covera HS , Verelan PM	120-360 (1)	
Dihydropyridines —dipines			Edema of the ankle, flushing, headache, gingival
Amlodipine besylate	Norvasc	2.5-10 (1)	hyperplasia
Felodipine	Plendil	2.5-20 (1)	
Isradipine	DynaCirc	2.5-10 (2)	
	DynaCirc CR	5-20 (1)	
Nicardipine	Cardene SR	60-120 (1)	
Nifedipine	Procardia XL , Adalat CC	30-60 (1)	
Nisoldipine	Sular	10-40 (1)	

[1]Side effects listed are for the class of drugs except where noted for individual drugs (in parentheses).
Adapted from JNC-7 Express. Source: National Heart, Lung, and Blood Institute.

- Indirectly inhibit fluid volume increases by inhibiting angiotensin II–stimulated release of aldosterone

ARBs
- Inhibit the binding of angiotensin II to the angiotensin II receptor, thereby inhibiting the vasoconstrictive properties of angiotensin II as well its ability to stimulate release of aldosterone
- Currently considered as alternative therapy in patients not able to tolerate ACEIs due to cough

Adverse drug events (Table 15)

Patient instructions and counseling
- Report symptoms of dizziness or hypotension.
- Symptoms of swelling of the lips, mouth, or face should be considered an emergency, and the patient should immediately report to a doctor's office or emergency department.
- Report new rashes (especially with captopril).
- Do not use salt substitutes containing potassium, and do not take OTC potassium supplements.
- Rise slowly from a lying or sitting position.

Drug-drug and drug-disease interactions
- NSAIDs will decrease the effectiveness of ACEIs and ARBs.
- Potassium-sparing diuretics, potassium supplements, and salt substitutes will increase the risk of hyperkalemia when used in combination with ACEIs and ARBs.
- ACEIs and ARBs should be avoided in patients with bilateral renal artery stenosis or stenosis in a single kidney.
- ACEIs and ARBs should be avoided in pregnant patients.

Parameters to monitor
- Serum electrolytes (especially creatinine and potassium)
- Symptoms of angioedema
- Blood pressure
- Symptoms of hypotension
- CBC (especially with captopril and enalapril) for neutropenia, which is more common in patients with preexisting renal impairment
- Cough
- Urinary proteins

Table 15

Angiotensin-Converting Enzyme Inhibitors (ACEIs) and Angiotensin II Receptor Blockers (ARBs)

Drug	Trade name	Usual dose range, total mg/d (frequency per day)	Adverse events and comments
ACEIs – pril			
Benazepril HCl	Lotensin	10-40 (1-2)	**Common:** cough
Captopril	Capoten	25-100 (2-3)	**Rare:** angioedema, hyperkalemia, rash, loss of
Enalapril maleate	Vasotec	2.5-40 (1-2)	taste, leukopenia
Fosinopril	Monopril	10-40 (1-2)	**Other:** vertigo; headache; fatigue; first-dose
Lisinopril	Prinivil , Zestril	10-40 (1)	hypotension; minor GI disturbances; acute
Moexipril	Univasc	7.5-30 (1)	renal insufficiency in patients with
Perindopril	Aceon	4-8 (1-2)	predisposing factors such as renal stenosis
Quinapril HCl	Accupril	10-40 (1-2)	and coadministration with thiazide diuretics;
Ramipril	Altace	1.25-20 (1)	proteinuria (especially in patients with history
Trandolapril	Mavik	1-4 (1)	of renal disease)
ARBs			
Candesartan – sartans	Atacand	8-32 (1)	Angioedema, hyperkalemia
Eprosartan	Teveten	400-800 (1-2)	
Irbesartan	Avapro	150-300 (1)	
Losartan	Cozaar	25-100 (1-2)	
Olmesartan	Benicar	20 (1)	
Telmisartan	Micardis	40-80 (1)	
Valsartan	Diovan	80-320 (1)	

Reprinted with permission from JNC-VI.

4. Hypertensive Urgencies and Emergencies

- The classification of hypertensive urgencies and emergencies is determined by the presence or absence of acute target organ damage, not by blood pressure, and determines the appropriate treatment approach.
- The relative rise and rate of increase in blood pressure is more important than the actual blood pressure.

Hypertensive Emergencies

- Acute elevations of blood pressure (>180 mm Hg systolic or >120 mm Hg diastolic) with the presence of acute or ongoing target organ damage constitutes a hypertensive emergency (Table 16).
- This requires immediate lowering of blood pressure to prevent or minimize target organ damage.

Treatment (Table 17)
- Initial goal: reduce mean arterial pressure (MAP) by no more than 25% within minutes to hours; reach 160/100 mm Hg within 2-6 hours.

- Measure BP every 5-10 minutes until goal MAP is reached and life-threatening target organ damage resolves.
- Maintain goal BP for 1-2 days, and further reduce BP toward normal over several weeks.
- Excessive falls in BP may precipitate renal, cerebral, or coronary ischemia.
- IV agents are preferred due to the ability to titrate dosages based on BP response; however, specific agents should be chosen based on patient findings (Table 18).

Hypertensive Urgencies

- These are accelerated, malignant, or perioperative elevations in blood pressure in the absence of new or progressive target organ damage; therefore immediate lowering of BP is not required.

Treatment (Table 19)
- There is no agent of choice; medications should be selected based on patient characteristics.
- Oral therapy is preferred.
- Onset of action should be in 15-30 minutes, and peak effects seen in 2-3 hours.

Table 16

Clinical Findings of Target Organ Damage

Target organ damage:
  Hypertensive encephalopathy
  Intracranial hemorrhage
  Unstable angina
  Acute myocardial infarction
  Acute left ventricular failure with pulmonary edema
  Dissecting aortic aneurysm
  Eclampsia

Clinical findings:
  Funduscopic: papilledema, hemorrhage, exudates
  Neurologic: somnolence, confusion, seizures, coma, visual deficits
  or blindness
  Cardiac: S_4 gallop, ischemic changes on ECG, chest x-ray
  consistent with pulmonary edema, chest pain
  Renal: oliguria, progressive azotemia, hematuria, proteinuria
  Other: dyspnea

Reprinted with permission from JNC-VI.

- Check BP every 15-30 minutes to ensure response.
- Use of immediate-release nifedipine is inappropriate to lower blood pressure in patients with hypertensive urgencies.

5. Key Points

- Hypertension is defined as a systolic blood pressure >140 mm Hg, a diastolic blood pressure >90 mm Hg, or any patient requiring antihypertensive therapy.
- Prehypertension (120-139/80-89 mm Hg) represents a new classification in JNC-VII that significantly increases the risk of developing stage 1 hypertension. Lifestyle modifications should be stressed for this classification, and medication therapy should only be used for patients with compelling indications.
- Secondary causes of hypertension include: renovascular disease, primary aldosteronism, Cushing's syndrome, pheochromocytoma, aortic coarctation, and drugs (steroids/estrogens, alcohol, cocaine, cyclosporine/tacrolimus, sympathomimetics, erythropoietin, licorice, MAO inhibitors, TCA antidepressants, NSAIDs).
- Recommended lifestyle modifications both to improve blood pressure and overall cardiovascular health include: lose weight; limit alcohol intake; increase aerobic physical activity; reduce sodium intake; maintain adequate dietary intake of potassium, magnesium, and calcium; stop smoking; and reduce dietary cholesterol and saturated fat intake.
- Diuretics are considered by JNC-VII to be the initial agent for treatment of hypertension in most patients unless compelling indications for the use of other medication classes exist or the patient has comorbid conditions that would suggest the use of classes other than diuretics.
- JNC-VII considers angiotensin-converting enzyme inhibitors (ACEIs), angiotensin II receptor blockers (ARBs), β-blockers (BBs), and calcium channel blockers (CCBs) equivalent choices as initial therapy for hypertension.
- Vasodilators, α_1-receptor antagonists, α_2-receptor agonists, and postganglionic adrenergic neuron blockers should be avoided as initial agents for hypertension.
- Antihypertensive drug therapy should be individualized, and there are classifications of recommendations from JNC-VII based on the level of evidence, which include: compelling indication unless contraindicated, may have favorable effects on comorbid conditions, and may have unfavorable effects on comorbid conditions.
- The classification and treatment of hypertensive urgencies and emergencies is determined by the presence or absence of acute target organ damage and not on blood pressure.

Table 17

Parenteral Drugs for Treatment of Hypertensive Emergencies[1]

Drug	Dose[2]	Onset of action	Duration of action	Adverse effects[3]	Special indications
Vasodilators					
Sodium nitroprusside	0.25-10 mcg/kg per min as IV infusion[4] (maximal dose for 10 min only)	Immediate	1-2 min	Nausea, vomiting, muscle twitching, sweating, thiocyanate and cyanide intoxication	Most hypertensive emergencies; caution with high intracranial pressure or azotemia
Nicardipine hydrochloride	5-15 mg/h IV	5-10 min	1-4 h	Tachycardia, headache, flushing, local phlebitis	Most hypertensive emergencies except acute heart failure; caution with coronary ischemia
Fenoldopam mesylate	0.1-0.3 mcg/kg per min IV infusion	<5 min	30 min	Tachycardia, headache, nausea, flushing	
Nitroglycerin	5-100 mcg/min as IV infusion[4]	2-5 min	3-5 min	Headache, vomiting, methemoglobinemia, tolerance with prolonged use	Coronary ischemia
Enalaprilat	1.25-5 mg every 6 h IV	15-30 min	6 h	Precipitous fall in pressure in high-renin states; response variable	Acute left ventricular failure; avoid in acute myocardial infarction
Hydralazine hydrochloride	10-20 mg IV; 10-50 mg IM	10-20 min; 20-30 min	3-8 h	Tachycardia, flushing, headache, vomiting, aggravation of angina	Eclampsia
Diazoxide	50-100 mg IV bolus repeated, or 15-30 mg/min infusion	2-4 min	6-12 h	Nausea, flushing, tachycardia, chest pain	Now obsolete; when no intensive monitoring available
Adrenergic inhibitors					
Labetalol hydrochloride	20-80 mg IV bolus every 10 min; 0.5-2.0 mg/min IV infusion	5-10 min	3-6 h	Vomiting, scalp tingling, burning in throat, dizziness, nausea, heart block, orthostatic hypotension	Most hypertensive emergencies except acute heart failure
Esmolol hydrochloride	250-500 mcg/kg/min for 1 min, then 50-100 mcg/kg/min for 4 min; may repeat sequence	1-2 min	10-20 min	Hypotension, nausea	Aortic dissection, perioperative
Phentolamine	5-15 mg IV	1-2 min	3-10 min	Tachycardia, flushing, headache	Catecholamine excess

[1]These doses may vary from this in the *Physicians' Desk Reference* (51st ed.).
[2]IV indicates intravenous; IM, intramuscular.
[3]Hypotension may occur with all agents.
[4]Requires special delivery system.
Reprinted with permission from JNC-VI.

- All causes for inadequate response should be addressed before additional agents are added to a patient's antihypertensive regimen (ie, pseudo-resistance, nonadherence, volume overload, drug-related causes, associated conditions, and secondary causes of hypertension).

Table 18

Selected Agents for Specific Hypertensive Emergencies

Emergency	Recommended therapy	Comments
Encephalopathy	Labetalol; nicardipine; nitroprusside	*Avoid:* methyldopa (sedation); diazoxide (reduces cerebral blood flow); reserpine (sedation); hydralazine (increases intracranial pressure)
Myocardial infarction (MI)/ unstable angina	Nitroglycerin; esmolol	Reduce BP until pain is relieved, use in conjunction with conventional therapy for MI/angina *Avoid:* Diazoxide and hydralazine (increases oxygen demand); dihydropyridines (may worsen angina); nitroprusside (coronary steal)
Congestive heart failure	Nitroprusside; nitroglycerin; enalaprilat	*Avoid:* labetalol, esmolol, other β-blockers (reduces cardiac output)
Subarachnoid hemorrhage, intracerebral hemorrhage, stroke	Nitroprusside	BP reduction is controversial as it may cause hypoperfusion; generally recommended for severe hypertension (systolic >220 or diastolic >120 mm Hg)
Dissecting aortic aneurysm	Trimethaphan; esmolol; nitroprusside	*Avoid:* diazoxide and hydralazine (increase shear force)
Pheochromocytoma, cocaine overdose	Phentolamine; labetalol	Anecdotal reports of increased BP with labetalol; unopposed β blockade may worsen crisis
Renal insufficiency	Nitroprusside; calcium channel blocker; labetalol	Monitor cyanide and thiocyanate levels
Postoperative hypertension	Nitroprusside; nicardipine; labetalol	

Table 19

Agents Used to Treat Hypertensive Urgencies

Drug	Dose	Onset	Duration	Adverse effects
Captopril	25 mg, repeat in 1-2 hours as needed	5-15 minutes	4-6 hours	Hypotension, acute renal failure, angioedema
Clonidine	0.1-0.2 mg, repeat in 1-2 hours as needed (up to 0.6 mg)	5-15 minutes	6-12 hours	Hypotension, drowsiness, sedation, dry mouth
Labetalol	100-400 mg, repeat in 2-3 hours as needed	15-30 minutes	4-6 hours	Hypotension, heart block, bronchoconstriction

6. Questions and Answers

1. All of the following agents are suitable as initial therapy for the treatment of uncomplicated hypertension according to the Seventh Report of the Joint National Committee on Detection, Evaluation, and Treatment of High Blood Pressure (JNC-VII) EXCEPT

   A. hydrochlorothiazide *HCTZ,*
   B. chlorthalidone *Hygrotin*
   C. indapamide *Lozol*
   D. hydralazine *Apresoline*
   E. atenolol *Tenormin*

2. Hyperkalemia is a possible adverse effect of all the following medications EXCEPT

   A. trandolapril *Mavik*
   B. Teveten *Eprosartan*
   C. doxazosin *Cardura*
   D. amiloride *Midamor*
   E. captopril *Capoten*

3. A 48-year-old patient presents with a new diagnosis of hypertension. The patient is also noted to have congestive heart failure (CHF) with an ejection fraction of 28%. Which agent would be an appropriate choice as initial therapy in this patient based on JNC-VII?

   A. Clonidine *Catapress*
   B. Guanethidine *Ismelin* *PG-neur block*
   C. Diltiazem *Cartia, Cardizem*
   D. Perindopril *Aceon*
   E. Nisoldipine *Sular*

4. A 62-year-old patient with a history of hypertension and gout presents to begin pharmacotherapy for hypertension. Which agent is the most appropriate choice as initial therapy based on JNC-VII?

   A. Chlorothiazide *Diuril*
   B. Torsemide *Demadex*
   C. Tenormin *Atenolol*
   D. Chlorthalidone *Hygroton*
   E. Metolazone *Mykrox, Zaroxolyn*

5. All of the following medications can cause bradycardia EXCEPT

   A. terazosin - *Hytrin*
   B. verapamil - *Calan, Verelan*
   C. diltiazem - *Cartia, Cartizem*
   D. Ziac® *Bisoprolol / HCTZ*
   E. clonidine *Catapress*

6. A patient requires a cardioselective β-blocker in their outpatient medication regimen after recent discharge from the hospital with a new myocardial infarction. You suggest:

   A. Labetalol *Normodyne*
   B. Esmolol *brevibloc*
   C. Propranolol *Inderal*
   D. Atenolol *Tenormin*
   F. Carvedilol *Coreg*

7. A patient presents to your ambulatory clinic with a blood pressure of 210/125 mm Hg. Past medical history is significant for type 2 diabetes, CHF, and renal insufficiency. Which of the following would cause the patient to be classified as a hypertensive emergency?

   A. Blood glucose levels >300 mg/dL, which increase the patient's risk for acute renal failure
   B. A serum creatinine of 3 mg/dL
   C. Nausea, vomiting, and diarrhea for 3 days
   D. S_4 gallop and a chest x-ray consistent with pulmonary edema
   E. Polyuria combined with polydipsia

8. What are the treatment goals for the patient with hypertensive emergency described in the Question 7?

   A. Systolic pressure should be reduced to 120 mm Hg within the first hour of treatment to reduce the risk of further end organ damage
   B. Diastolic pressure should be reduced to 80 mm Hg within the first hour of treatment to reduce the risk of further end organ damage
   C. Reduce blood pressure to 160/100 mm Hg in the first 2-6 hours of therapy
   D. Reduce mean arterial pressure by at least 50% within the first minutes to hours of therapy
   E. Reduce blood pressure to no lower than 180/110 mm Hg in the first hour, as excessive falls in blood pressure may precipitate coronary ischemia

9. What would be the recommended treatment for the patient with hypertensive emergency in Question 7?

    A. Clonidine orally 0.1-0.2 mg, repeat in 1-2 hours as needed (up to 0.6 mg)
    B. Labetalol orally 100-400 mg, repeat in 2-3 hours as needed
    C. Nifedipine sublingually 10 mg, repeat in 0.5-1 hours as needed (up to 60 mg)
    D. Labetalol intravenously 20- to 80-mg bolus, followed by 0.5-2 mg/min infusion
    E. Enalaprilat intravenously 1.25-5 mg every 6 hours

10. Which of the following antihypertensive agents can cause first-dose syncope, palpitations, peripheral edema, and priapism?

    A. Hydralazine
    B. Nitroprusside
    C. Prazosin
    D. Verapamil
    E. Moexipril

11. Which of the following antihypertensive agents is most likely to cause lupus syndrome, postural hypotension, and peripheral neuropathy?

    A. Atenolol
    B. Hydralazine
    C. Guanfacine
    D. Mibefradil
    E. Nitroprusside

12. Which of the following medications is not associated with drug-induced hypertension?

    A. Prednisone
    B. Indomethacin
    C. Rosiglitazone
    D. Cocaine
    E. Cyclosporine

13. What is the best recommendation for antihypertensive medication in a patient who has atrial fibrillation, CAD with angina, and hyperthyroidism?

    A. Minoxidil
    B. Betaxolol
    C. Telmisartan
    D. Nicardipine
    E. Amiloride

14. What antihypertensive agent should not be used in a patient with essential hypertension and a history of depression with suicidal ideation?

    A. Captopril
    B. Prazosin
    C. Metolazone
    D. Reserpine
    E. Amlodipine

15. All of the following are secondary causes of hypertension EXCEPT

    A. renovascular disease
    B. pheochromocytoma
    C. systemic lupus erythematosus
    D. primary aldosteronism
    E. aortic coarctation

Answer Questions 16-20 based on the patient medication profile provided on the next page.

    A. I only is correct
    B. III only is correct
    C. I and II are both correct
    D. II and III are both correct
    E. I, II, and III are correct

16. Possible complications that the patient is at risk of developing secondary to uncontrolled hypertension include:

    I.   Hyperaldosteronism
    II. Myocardial infarction
    III. Blindness

17. Education regarding lifestyle modification issues in this patient should include:

    I.   Limit smoking to $1/2$ pack per day and alcohol intake to no more than 2 drinks per day
    II. Maintain adequate intake of dietary magnesium, calcium, and sodium
    III. Increase aerobic physical activity, lose weight, and limit dietary saturated fat and cholesterol

18. Possible reasons for the patient's blood pressure being uncontrolled include:

    I.   Use of NSAIDs causes decreased effectiveness of ACE inhibitor therapy
    II. Possible problems with adherence to antihypertensive therapy
    III. Lack of blood pressure response to ACE inhibitor therapy, which should not be used in combination with diuretics in an African-American patient

---

DATE: 04/12/03

PATIENT MEDICATION PROFILE

PATIENT'S NAME _____Buddy Manwich_____

ADDRESS _____61 Heavenly Highway_____

Phone No. _____555-8181_____

Date of Birth _____4/14/44_____

Known diseases: _DM (15 yrs), HTN (20 yrs),_

Obstructive Sleep Apnea (5yrs), Osteoarthritis

Allergies/Sensitivities__NKDA_____

NOTES: __+ tobacco – 1 ½ ppd,_____

_____4-5 cups of coffee / day_____

_____ETOH - 2 drinks / week_____

Race: _____African American_____

Ht: __5'11"_____

Wt: __248 lbs_____

OTC use: Aleve, Actron

DATE	RX#	MEDICATION/ STRENGTH	ROUTE	QUANTITY	REGIMEN	REFILLS	PHARMACIST	PRESCRIBER
1/15/03	001	Glipizide 5mg	PO	30	1 qd	5	BCE	NTE
1/15/03	002	Lisinopril 5mg	PO	30	1 qd	5	BCE	NTE
1/15/03	003	Hydrodiuril 12.5mg	PO	30	1 qd	5	BBC	NPR
1/20/03	004	Ibuprofen 800mg	PO	90	1 tid	5	REM	FTD
2/11/03	001-RF	Glipizide 5mg	PO	30	1 qd	4	BCE	NTE
2/11/03	003-RF	Hydrodiuril 12.5mg	PO	30	1 qd	4	BBC	NPR
2/11/03	004-RF	Ibuprofen 800mg	PO	90	1 tid	4	REM	FTD
3/13/03	001-RF	Glipizide 5mg	PO	30	1 qd	3	BCE	NTE
3/13/03	002-RF	Lisinopril 5mg	PO	30	1 qd	3	BCE	NTE
3/13/03	004-RF	Ibuprofen 800mg	PO	90	1 tid	3	REM	FTD

19. The appropriate initial antihypertensive agent in this patient could be

I. benazepril
II. terazosin
III. minoxidil

20. If the patient is not able to tolerate lisinopril due to adverse effects such as cough, an appropriate alternative agent would be

I. telmisartan
II. labetalol
III. guanabcnz

Answers

1. **D.** Appropriate choices for initial agents in the treatment of uncomplicated hypertension include β-blockers and diuretics. Hydralazine is a direct vasodilator, which would never be considered a first-line agent in the treatment of hypertension.

2. **C.** Hyperkalemia is a possible side effect with angiotensin-converting enzyme inhibitors, angiotensin II receptor antagonists, and potassium-sparing diuretics. Doxazosin is a peripherally acting α_1 blocker, which does not cause hyperkalemia.

3. **D.** For patients who have hypertension and congestive heart failure, JNC-VII recommends the use of ACE inhibitors, diuretics, β-blockers, and aldosterone antagonists (see Table 6). The only listed ACE inhibitor is perindopril.

4. **C.** For patients who have hypertension and gout, JNC-VI recommends not using diuretic therapy, which increases the risk of gouty attacks (see Table 6). The only medication listed that is not a diuretic is atenolol, which is a β-blocker.

5. **A.** Verapamil and diltiazem are nondihydropyridine calcium channel blockers; Ziac (bisoprolol/hydrochlorothiazide) is a β-blocker; and clonidine is a centrally acting α_2 agonist, and all these have negative inotropic effects on the myocardium. Terazosin is a peripherally acting α_1 blocker, which does not cause bradycardia.

6. **D.** Labetalol, propranolol, and carvedilol are all nonselective β-blockers. Esmolol is a cardio-selective agent only available in injectable form, and therefore would not be for outpatient use. Atenolol is a cardioselective β-blocker that is available as an oral tablet, and therefore can be used for outpatient dosing.

7. **D.** The classification of hypertensive urgencies and emergencies is determined by the presence or absence of acute target organ damage and not by the actual blood pressure measurement. Presence of an S_4 gallop and a chest x-ray consistent with pulmonary edema suggests acute left ventricular failure with pulmonary edema, which represents defined target organ damage, which means this patient should be classified as a hypertensive emergency.

8. **C.** According to JNC-VII, the initial goal of blood pressure lowering in patients with hypertensive emergencies is a drop in mean arterial pressure (MAP) of no more than 25% within minutes to hours, and to 160/100 mm Hg within 2-6 hours.

9. **E.** In a patient with CHF and a hypertensive emergency, recommended treatments include nitroglycerin, nitroprusside, and enalaprilat (Table 18). Clonidine and labetalol (PO) are incorrect choices because the patient requires IV therapy. Nifedipine SL is not indicated for immediate reduction of blood pressure. Labetalol IV is not an appropriate choice in this patient with CHF, as it could decrease cardiac output.

10. **C.** Possible side effects of peripherally acting α_1 blockers (prazosin) include first-dose syncope, palpitations, peripheral edema, and priapism (Table 11).

11. **B.** Possible side effects of direct vasodilators (hydralazine) include postural hypotension and peripheral neuropathy. However, lupus syndrome is unique to hydralazine and does not occur with minoxidil (Table 13).

12. **C.** All agents listed are possible causes of drug-induced hypertension through multiple mechanisms except rosiglitazone (Figure 8).

13. **B.** The diagnoses of atrial fibrillation, CAD with angina, and hyperthyroidism are all considered comorbid conditions with hypertension in which the use of β-blockers may have favorable effects.

14. **D.** Because of its possible increased risk of depression, reserpine should not be used in patients in whom the risk for depression and/or suicide already exists.

15. **C.** All listed diseases are possible causes of secondary hypertension through various mechanisms, except systemic lupus erythematosus.

16. **D.** Uncontrolled hypertension causes multiple organ system problems, including cardiovascular (CHF, MI, PAD), ophthalmologic (retinopathy, blindness), cerebrovascular (TIA, CVA), and renovascular (nephropathy, renal failure, dialysis). Therefore this patient is at risk for MI and blindness, not hyperaldosteronism.

17. **B.** Lifestyle modification issues to be considered in hypertensive patients include weight loss; limit of alcohol intake; increased aerobic activity; reduced sodium intake; maintenance of adequate dietary potassium, calcium, and magnesium intake; and smoking cessation.

18. **C.** Possible causes for inadequate responsiveness to therapy are listed in Figure 8.

19. **A.** In patients with hypertension and comorbid conditions of CHF and diabetes, the initial agent should be an ACE inhibitor (Table 6).

20. **A.** In patients who cannot tolerate ACE inhibitor therapy secondary to the adverse effect of cough, angiotensin II receptor antagonists are considered good alternative agents.

7. References

Carter BL, Saseen JL. Hypertension. In: DiPiro JT, ed. *Pharmacotherapy: A Pathophysiologic Approach.* New York: McGraw-Hill; 2002:157-183.

The Seventh Report of the Joint National Committee on Prevention, Detection, Evaluation and Treatment of High Blood Pressure (JNC VII), *Hypertension.* 2003;42:1206-1252.

Joint National Committee on Prevention, Detection, Evaluation, and Treatment of High Blood Pressure (JNC-7) Express. NIH Pub. No. 03-5233, May 2003. Available at http://www.nhlbi.gov/guidelines/hypertension/express.pdf

9. Heart Failure

Robert B. Parker, PharmD
Professor, Department of Clinical Pharmacy
University of Tennessee College of Pharmacy

Contents

1. Overview

Heart failure is a clinical syndrome resulting from a variety of cardiac disorders that impair the ability of the ventricle to fill with or eject blood. This in turn results in the heart being unable to pump blood at a sufficient rate to meet the metabolic demands of the body.

- Nearly 5 million people in the U.S. have heart failure, with 550,000 new patients diagnosed each year.
- It is the only major cardiovascular disease that is increasing in prevalence.
- Approximately 300,000 patients die from heart failure each year. At the time of heart failure diagnosis, the 5-year mortality rate is nearly 50%.
- A large majority of patients are elderly; approximately 10% of individuals over the age of 75 have heart failure.
- Heart failure is the most common hospital discharge diagnosis for Medicare patients. More Medicare dollars are spent for diagnosis and treatment of heart failure than for any other disorder.

Classification

- The New York Heart Association Functional Classification has been widely used for many years. It primarily reflects the severity of symptoms based on a subjective assessment by the provider. A patient's functional class can change frequently over a short period due to changes in medications, diet, or intercurrent illnesses. This classification scheme does not recognize preventive measures or the progressive nature of heart failure.
  - * *Functional class I* includes patients with cardiac disease but without limitations of physical activity. Ordinary physical activity does not cause undue fatigue, dyspnea, or palpitations.
  - * *Functional class II* includes patients with cardiac disease that results in slight limitations of physical activity. Ordinary physical activity results in fatigue, palpitations, dyspnea, or angina.
  - * *Functional class III* includes patients with cardiac disease that results in marked limitation of physical activity. Although patients are comfortable at rest, less than ordinary activity will lead to symptoms.
  - * *Functional class IV* includes patients with cardiac disease that results in an inability to carry on physical activity without discomfort. Symptoms of heart failure are present even at rest. With any physical activity increased discomfort is experienced.

- The most recent guidelines for evaluation and management of heart failure from the American College of Cardiology (ACC)/American Heart Association (AHA) recommend an additional classification scheme that emphasizes both the evolution and progression of the disease. It more objectively identifies patients within the course of the disease and links to treatments that are appropriate for each stage.
  - * *Stage A* includes patients at high risk of developing heart failure because of the presence of conditions that are strongly associated with heart failure. These patients have no known cardiac abnormalities and no heart failure signs or symptoms. Examples include patients with hypertension, coronary artery disease, and diabetes mellitus.
  - * *Stage B* includes patients who have developed structural heart disease that is strongly associated with the development of heart failure but who have never shown signs or symptoms of heart failure. Some examples include previous myocardial infarction, left ventricular hypertrophy, and/or impaired left ventricular function.
  - * *Stage C* includes patients who have current or prior symptoms of heart failure associated with underlying structural heart disease. Examples include patients with dyspnea or fatigue due to left ventricular systolic dysfunction and asymptomatic patients who are undergoing treatment for prior symptoms of heart failure. Most patients with heart failure are in this stage.
  - * *Stage D* includes patients with advanced structural heart disease and marked symptoms of heart failure at rest despite maximal medical therapy and who require specialized interventions. Examples include patients who are frequently hospitalized for heart failure and cannot be safely discharged from the hospital, patients in the hospital awaiting heart transplantation, and patients supported with a mechanical circulatory assist device.

Advanced or decompensated heart failure
- Patients with advanced heart failure have persistent limiting symptoms despite therapy with drugs of proven efficacy. Decompensated heart failure is defined as an exacerbation of previously stable symptoms (usually due to volume overload and/or hypoperfusion) and frequently requires hospitalization for acute treatment.
- Causes include medication and dietary noncompliance, atrial fibrillation, myocardial ischemia, and progression of heart failure.
- Assignment to one of four hemodynamic profiles assists in determining approach to therapy.

* Warm and dry: adequate perfusion (ie, cardiac output) and no signs or symptoms of volume overload
* Warm and wet: adequate perfusion but signs or symptoms of volume overload
* Cold and dry: inadequate perfusion and no signs or symptoms of volume overload
* Cold and wet: inadequate perfusion and signs or symptoms of volume overload
* Most patients (about 70%) present with the warm and wet classification.

Clinical Presentation

* The primary manifestations of heart failure are dyspnea and fatigue that may limit exercise tolerance, and fluid retention that may lead to pulmonary and peripheral edema. Both abnormalities can limit a patient's functional capacity and quality of life, but do not necessarily occur at the same time. Some patients may have marked exercise intolerance but little evidence of fluid retention, whereas others have prominent edema with few symptoms of dyspnea or fatigue.
* Other symptoms may include paroxysmal nocturnal dyspnea, orthopnea, tachypnea, cough, ascites, and nocturia.
* Other signs include jugular venous distension, hepatojugular reflux, hepatomegaly, bibasilar rales, pleural effusion, tachycardia, pallor, and S_3 gallop.
* Symptoms in advanced heart failure are similar but may be more severe.

Pathophysiology

* Heart failure can result from any disorder (see below) that impairs the heart's systolic (ie, pumping ability) or diastolic (impaired cardiac relaxation) function. Many patients have manifestations of both abnormalities. In either case, a decrease in cardiac output is the initiating event in heart failure. The reduction in cardiac output results in activation of a number of compensatory mechanisms that attempt to maintain an adequate cardiac output.
* The beneficial effects of ACE inhibitors (ACEIs), β-blockers, and aldosterone antagonists on reducing mortality and slowing heart failure progression resulted in the neurohormonal model of heart failure pathophysiology.
  * The decrease in cardiac output leads to activation of systems that release a number of neurohormones including angiotensin II, norepinephrine, aldosterone, proinflammatory cytokines, and vasopressin. These neurohormones can increase renal sodium and water retention, vasoconstriction, tachycardia, and ventricular hypertrophy and remodeling.
  * Activation of the compensatory systems results in a systemic disorder that is not just confined to the heart, whose progression is largely mediated by these neurohormones.

Specific Causes of Heart Failure

* Coronary artery disease is the cause of heart failure in about 65% of patients with left ventricular systolic dysfunction. Other causes include nonischemic cardiomyopathy (eg, due to hypertension, thyroid disease, or valvular disease). Most of these patients have a reduced left ventricular ejection fraction (usually <40%).
* Approximately 20%-50% of patients with heart failure have preserved (normal) left ventricular systolic function and their heart failure is secondary to diastolic dysfunction. This is most often seen in elderly patients.
* A number of drugs can precipitate or worsen heart failure.

Drugs with negative inotropic effects
  * Antiarrhythmics: disopyramide, flecainide, propafenone
  * β-Blockers
  * Calcium channel blockers: verapamil and diltiazem
  * Oral antifungals: itraconazole and terbinafine
* Cardiotoxic drugs
  * Doxorubicin
  * Daunorubicin
  * Cyclophosphamide
  * Alcohol
* Sodium and water retention
  * NSAIDs (including the COX-2 inhibitors) also can attenuate the efficacy and increase the toxicity of diuretics and ACEIs.
  * Glucocorticoids
  * Rosiglitazone and pioglitazone

Diagnostic Criteria

* There is no single diagnostic test for heart failure; it is a clinical diagnosis based on history, signs and symptoms, and physical examination.

* A rapid bedside assay for B-type natriuretic peptide (BNP) is often used in acute care settings (eg, emergency departments) as an aid in the diagnosis of suspected heart failure. BNP is synthesized and released from the ventricles in response to pressure or volume overload. BNP counteracts the increased sympathetic nervous and renin-angiotensin-

aldosterone system activity by increasing diuresis, renal sodium excretion, and vasodilation. The degree of elevation of BNP correlates with prognosis. The test is useful to differentiate between heart failure exacerbations and other causes of dyspnea (eg, COPD, asthma, or infection). Patients with dyspnea secondary to heart failure will have elevated plasma BNP concentrations.

- The echocardiogram is one of the most useful diagnostic tests in patients with heart failure.
- Patients with a left ventricular ejection fraction <40% are generally considered to have systolic dysfunction.
- Note that in general there is a poor correlation between the ejection fraction and symptoms.

Treatment Principles and Goals of Therapy

- Goals of therapy are to improve the patient's quality of life, reduce symptoms, reduce hospitalizations for heart failure exacerbations, slow progression of the disease, and improve survival.
- ACC/AHA guidelines for heart failure treatment according to stage are shown in Figure 1. Therapy in stages A and B is primarily targeted toward prevention of heart failure development, whereas stages C and D focus on treatment of patients with symptomatic heart failure.
- An algorithm for treatment of patients with advanced or decompensated heart failure is shown in Figure 2.

2. Drug Therapy of Heart Failure

- The following section on drug therapy focuses on treatment of stage C heart failure patients (ie, patients with left ventricular dysfunction with current or prior symptoms). This is also commonly referred to as outpatient treatment of patients with heart failure. These patients should be routinely managed with a combination of three drugs: a diuretic, an ACE inhibitor or an angiotensin receptor blocker (ARB), and a β-blocker. Drug therapies that can be considered in selected patients include digoxin, aldosterone antagonists, and hydralazine/isosorbide dinitrate.

Loop Diuretics

- Most heart failure patients require use of the more potent loop diuretics versus thiazide diuretics (Table 1).

Mechanism of action
- Reduce the sodium retention associated with heart failure by inhibiting reabsorption of sodium and chloride in the loop of Henle

Patient instructions and counseling
- Patients allergic to sulfa-containing medications may also be allergic to these medications.
- Take once a day in the morning, or if taking twice daily, take in the morning and afternoon.
- Can cause frequent urination
- Patients should weigh themselves daily (best in the morning after urinating). Patients who gain more than 1 pound per day for several consecutive days or 3-5 pounds in a week should contact their health care provider.
- Report muscle cramps, dizziness, excessive thirst, weakness, or confusion, as these may be signs of overdiuresis.
- Photosensitivity: patients should use sunscreen and/or avoid sun exposure.

Adverse drug events
- Electrolyte depletion: hypokalemia and hypomagnesemia
- Hypotension
- Renal insufficiency

Drug-drug and drug-disease interactions
- Furosemide bioavailability and its diuretic effect are decreased by food and it should be taken on an empty stomach. Food does not affect torsemide absorption.

Figure 1.

American College of Cardiology/American Heart Association stages of heart failure and recommended therapy by stage.

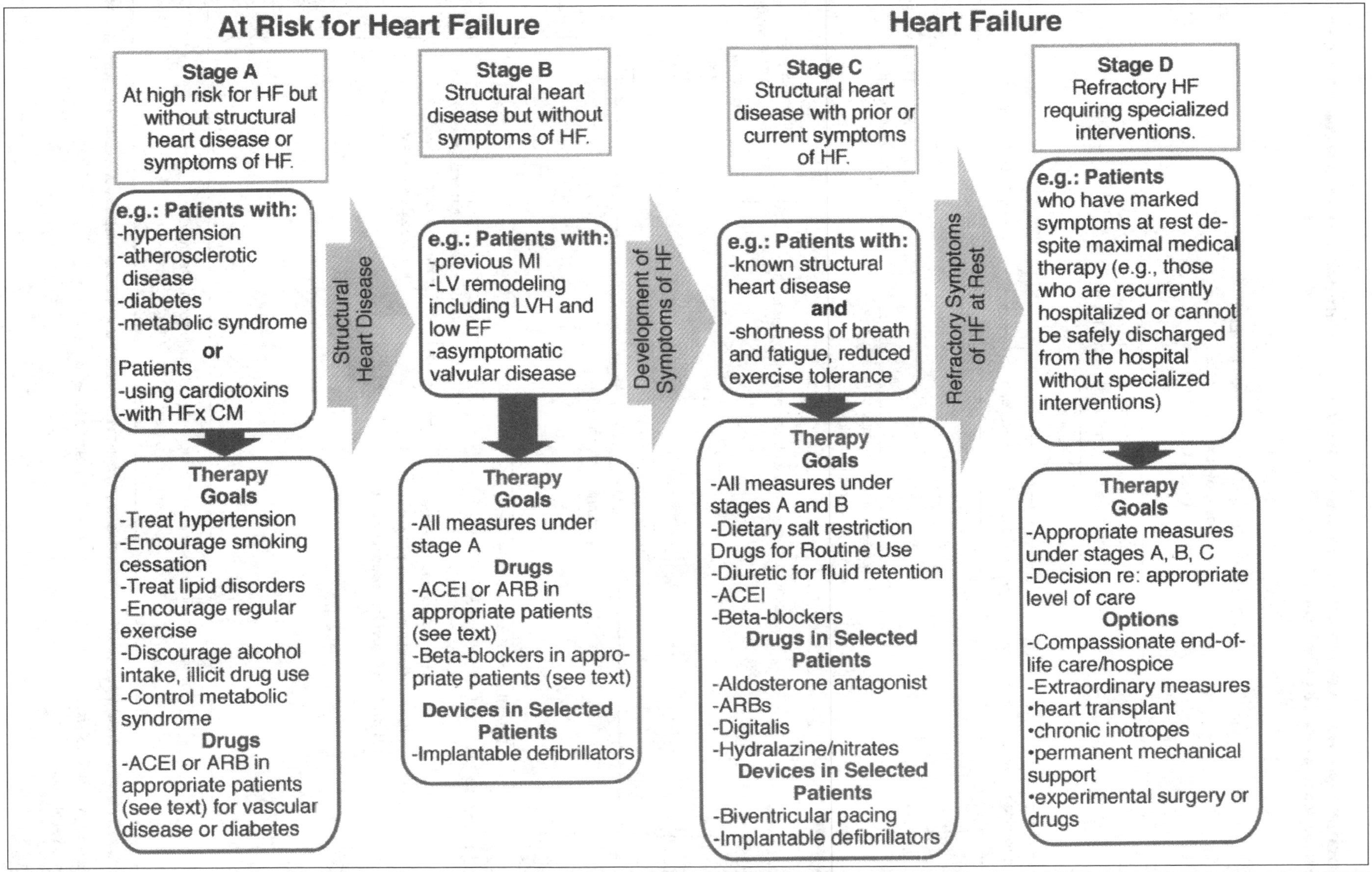

Heart Failure

At Risk for Heart Failure

Stage A
At high risk for HF but without structural heart disease or symptoms of HF.

e.g.: Patients with:
-hypertension
-atherosclerotic disease
-diabetes
-metabolic syndrome
or
Patients
-using cardiotoxins
-with HFx CM

Therapy Goals
-Treat hypertension
-Encourage smoking cessation
-Treat lipid disorders
-Encourage regular exercise
-Discourage alcohol intake, illicit drug use
-Control metabolic syndrome
Drugs
-ACEI or ARB in appropriate patients (see text) for vascular disease or diabetes

Structural Heart Disease →

Stage B
Structural heart disease but without symptoms of HF.

e.g.: Patients with:
-previous MI
-LV remodeling including LVH and low EF
-asymptomatic valvular disease

Therapy Goals
-All measures under stage A
Drugs
-ACEI or ARB in appropriate patients (see text)
-Beta-blockers in appropriate patients (see text)
Devices in Selected Patients
-Implantable defibrillators

Development of Symptoms of HF →

Stage C
Structural heart disease with prior or current symptoms of HF.

e.g.: Patients with:
-known structural heart disease
and
-shortness of breath and fatigue, reduced exercise tolerance

Therapy Goals
-All measures under stages A and B
-Dietary salt restriction
Drugs for Routine Use
-Diuretic for fluid retention
-ACEI
-Beta-blockers
Drugs in Selected Patients
-Aldosterone antagonist
-ARBs
-Digitalis
-Hydralazine/nitrates
Devices in Selected Patients
-Biventricular pacing
-Implantable defibrillators

Refractory Symptoms of HF at Rest →

Stage D
Refractory HF requiring specialized interventions.

e.g.: Patients
who have marked symptoms at rest despite maximal medical therapy (e.g., those who are recurrently hospitalized or cannot be safely discharged from the hospital without specialized interventions)

Therapy Goals
-Appropriate measures under stages A, B, C
-Decision re: appropriate level of care
Options
-Compassionate end-of-life care/hospice
-Extraordinary measures
•heart transplant
•chronic inotropes
•permanent mechanical support
•experimental surgery or drugs

Source: Hunt SA, Abraham WT, Chin MH, et al. ACC/AHA 2005 guideline update for the diagnosis and management of chronic heart failure in the adult: a report of the American College of Cardiology/American Heart Association Task Force on Practice Guidelines (Writing Committee to update the 2001 guidelines for the evaluation and management of heart failure).

Figure 2.

Advanced or decompensated heart failure.

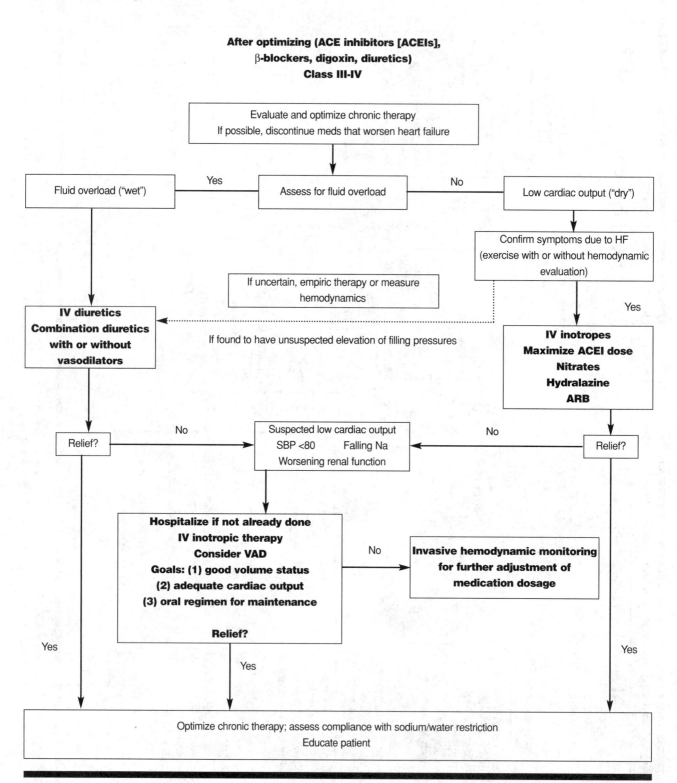

After optimizing (ACE inhibitors [ACEIs],
β-blockers, digoxin, diuretics)
Class III-IV

ARB, angiotensin receptor blocker; SPB, systolic blood pressure; VAD, ventricular assist device.
From Johnson et al, 2002.

Table 1

Loop Diuretics

Generic name (trade name)	Dosage form	Dosage range and frequency
Furosemide (Lasix®)	Oral tablet	20-160 mg qd-bid
Bumetanide (Bumex®)	Oral tablet	0.5-5 mg qd-bid
Torsemide (Demadex®)	Oral tablet	10-100 mg qd-bid

- The absorption of oral furosemide is significantly slowed in patients with decompensated heart failure, resulting in decreased diuretic response. Therefore, these individuals will usually require the use of IV furosemide.
- NSAIDs may diminish the diuretic effect.
- Potassium supplementation may not be required in patients also receiving ACE inhibitors, ARBs, and/or aldosterone antagonists.

Parameters to monitor
- Serum sodium, potassium, magnesium, creatinine, and BUN
- Patient weight: loss of 0.5-1.0 kg daily is desired until the patient achieves their dry weight.
- Urine output
- Blood pressure
- Improvement in heart failure symptoms: dyspnea, peripheral edema

Kinetics
- Bioavailability of torsemide is less variable than that of furosemide and is not affected by food.

Angiotensin-Converting Enzyme Inhibitors (ACEIs)

- These are the cornerstone of therapy in heart failure patients (Table 2). Clinical trials in over 7000 patients consistently demonstrate that ACEIs alleviate symptoms, improve clinical status and quality of life, and improve mortality. Current guidelines recommend that all patients with heart failure due to left ventricular systolic dysfunction should receive an ACEI unless contraindicated.

Mechanism of action
- They interfere with the renin-angiotensin system by inhibiting angiotensin-converting enzyme that is responsible for the conversion of angiotensin I to the potent vasoconstrictor angiotensin II. This results in

Table 2

Angiotensin-Converting Enzyme Inhibitors

Generic name (trade name)	Dosage form	Dosage range and frequency
Captopril (Capoten®)	Oral tablet	6.25-50 mg tid
Enalapril (Vasotec®)	Oral tablet	2.5-20 mg bid
Fosinopril (Monopril®)	Oral tablet	5-40 mg qd
Lisinopril (Zestril®, Prinivil®)	Oral tablet	2.5-40 mg qd
Quinapril (Accupril®)	Oral tablet	10-40 mg bid
Ramipril (Altace®)	Oral capsule	2.5-5 mg bid
Trandolapril (Mavik®)	Oral tablet	0.5-4 mg qd

a decrease in plasma angiotensin II and aldosterone concentrations, thus reducing the adverse effects of these neurohormones. Inhibition of angiotensin-converting enzyme also prevents the breakdown of the endogenous vasodilator bradykinin.
- They improve hemodynamics by increasing cardiac output and reducing left ventricular filling pressures, systemic vascular resistance, blood pressure, and heart rate.
- They improve heart failure symptoms and reduce hospitalizations for heart failure.
- They reduce mortality by 20%-30% and slow the progression of heart failure.

Patient instructions and counseling
- Patients that are pregnant or breast-feeding should not take ACEIs. If they become pregnant while taking an ACEI, they should contact their physician immediately.
- Captopril should be taken on an empty stomach, 1 hour before or 2 hours after meals.
- Use salt substitutes that contain potassium cautiously.
- Call your doctor immediately if you experience swelling of the face, eyes, lips, tongue, arms, or legs, or if you have difficulty breathing or swallowing.
- May cause cough

Adverse drug events
- Hypotension
- Dizziness
- Renal insufficiency
- Cough
- Angioedema
- Hyperkalemia
- Rash
- Taste disturbances

Drug-drug and drug-disease interactions

- NSAIDs (including the COX-2 inhibitors) can increase the risk of renal insufficiency and attenuate the beneficial hemodynamic effects of ACEIs.
- Use potassium supplements or potassium-sparing diuretics with caution in patients receiving ACEIs.
- Cyclosporine and tacrolimus may increase the risk of nephrotoxicity and hyperkalemia.
- Diuretics increase the risk of hypotension.

Parameters to monitor

- Blood pressure
- Renal function (ie, serum BUN and creatinine)
- Serum potassium
- Heart failure symptoms
- Dose: therapy should be initiated at low doses followed by gradual increases if lower doses are well tolerated.

Other

- Pregnancy category C (first trimester) and D (second and third trimesters); ACEIs can cause fetal and neonatal morbidity and death when administered to pregnant women.

Angiotensin Receptor Blockers (ARBs)

- ACEIs remain the drugs of choice for inhibiting the renin-angiotensin-aldosterone system in patients with chronic heart failure. Recent clinical trials confirm the efficacy and safety of candesartan and valsartan in the treatment of heart failure. Whether other ARBs are equally effective is unknown. Current guidelines recommend the use of candesartan or valsartan in patients that are intolerant to ACEIs—both of these agents are approved for use in patients with heart failure. Intolerance is most often due to cough or angioedema, although caution is advised when used in patients that have angioedema secondary to an ACEI. Note that ARBs are just as likely as ACEIs to cause impaired renal function, hyperkalemia, or hypotension. (Table 3)

Mechanism of action

- Interfere with the renin-angiotensin system by blocking the angiotensin-1 receptor thus attenuating the detrimental effects of this hormone.
- Unlike ACEIs, the ARBs do not affect the kinin system and thus are not associated with cough.
- Reduce hospitalizations and improve survival.

Patient instructions and counseling

- Patients that are pregnant or breast-feeding should not take ARBs. If they become pregnant while taking an ARB, they should contact their physician immediately.
- Use salt substitutes that contain potassium cautiously.
- Dizziness or light-headedness may occur, especially in patients taking diuretics.

Adverse drug events

- Hypotension
- Dizziness
- Renal insufficiency
- Hyperkalemia

Drug-drug and drug-disease interactions

- Use potassium supplements or potassium-sparing diuretics with caution in patients receiving ARBs.
- Diuretics: increase risk of hypotension

Parameters to monitor

- Blood pressure
- Renal function (ie, serum BUN and creatinine)
- Serum potassium
- Heart failure symptoms
- Dose: therapy should be initiated at low doses followed by gradual increases if lower doses are well tolerated.

Other

- Pregnancy category C (first trimester) and D (second and third trimesters). Can cause fetal and neonatal morbidity and death when administered to pregnant women.

Table 3

Angiotensin Receptor Blockers (ARBs)

Generic name (trade name)	Dosage form	Dosage range and frequency
Candesartan (Atacand®)	Oral tablet	4-32 mg qd
Valsartan (Diovan®)	Oral tablet	20-160 mg bid

Beta-Blockers

- Because of their negative inotropic effects, β-blockers were classically considered to be contraindicated in patients with heart failure. However, by inhibiting the deleterious effects of long-term activation of the sympathetic nervous system in heart failure, these agents have been repeatedly shown to provide hemodynamic, symptomatic, and survival benefits. Metoprolol succinate (extended-release metoprolol), bisoprolol, and carvedilol have all been shown to be effective and one of these three agents should be used for the treatment of heart failure (Table 4).

Mechanism of action

- Blockade of β-receptors by these agents antagonizes the increase in sympathetic nervous system activity that is one of the important mechanisms responsible for progression of heart failure. Bisoprolol and metoprolol succinate are β_1-selective agents, whereas carvedilol blocks β_1-, β_2-, and α_1-receptors. It remains uncertain whether these differences in pharmacologic actions have any important effects on outcomes in patients with heart failure.
- Treatment with β-blockers reduces symptoms, improves the clinical status, and decreases the risk of death and hospitalization.
- β-Blockers should be used in all patients with stable heart failure due to left ventricular systolic dysfunction unless they have a contraindication or have been shown not to tolerate them.
- In general, β-blockers should be used in combination with ACEIs and diuretics.

Patient instructions and counseling

- May cause fluid retention or worsening of heart failure with initiation of therapy or an increase in dose. Report any cases of body or leg swelling or increased shortness of breath. Patients should weigh themselves daily and if they gain more than 1 pound per day for several consecutive days or 3-5 pounds in a week, they should contact their health care provider.
- Fatigue or weakness may occur in the first few weeks of treatment, but will usually resolve spontaneously.
- Report any cases of dizziness, lightheadedness, or blurred vision. These may be caused by blood pressure being too low or from bradycardia or heart block.
- Take carvedilol with food.
- It is important not to miss doses or abruptly stop taking these medications.
- If patients have diabetes, β-blockers may cause their blood sugar to rise and mask the signs of hypoglycemia except for sweating.

Adverse drug events

- The adverse events listed below are the most common observed in heart failure patients receiving β-blockers. For other adverse effects of β-blockers, see the chapters on hypertension and ischemic heart disease.
  * Fluid retention and worsening heart failure
  * Fatigue
  * Bradycardia and heart block
  * Hypotension
  * Abrupt withdrawal can lead to hypertension, tachycardia, or myocardial ischemia.

Drug-drug and drug-disease interactions

- Amiodarone and calcium channel blockers (verapamil and diltiazem): increased risk of bradycardia, heart block, hypotension
- Quinidine, fluoxetine, paroxetine, and other inhibitors of cytochrome P450 2D6: inhibit hepatic metabolism of metoprolol and carvedilol and may result in increased plasma concentrations and enhanced effects.
- Ophthalmic β-blockers increase risk of bradycardia, heart block, and hypotension.
- May cause bronchoconstriction in patients with asthma or COPD
- Should not use in patients with symptomatic bradycardia or heart block unless a pacemaker is present
- May worsen blood glucose control in diabetics and mask the signs of hypoglycemia

Parameters to monitor

- Blood pressure and heart rate
- Heart failure symptoms
- Weigh daily

Table 4

Beta-Blockers

Generic name (trade name)	Dosage form	Dosage range and frequency
Bisoprolol (Zebeta®)	Oral tablet	1.25-10 mg qd-bid
Carvedilol (Coreg®)	Oral tablet	3.125-50 mg bid
Metoprolol succinate extended-release (Toprol-XL®)	Oral tablet	12.5-200 mg qd

Kinetics

- Bisoprolol is eliminated about 50% by the kidneys, so dosage adjustment may be required in patients with renal insufficiency.
- Both metoprolol and carvedilol are metabolized by the liver.

Other

- Patients must be stable (ie, minimal evidence of fluid overload or volume retention) before β-blocker treatment is initiated.
- Treatment should be initiated with low doses and titrated slowly upward until the target dose is reached. Doses are usually increased no more frequently than every 2 weeks with close monitoring of symptoms required during this titration period.
- Fluid accumulation during dose titration can usually be managed by adjusting diuretic doses.
- Staggering the schedule of other heart failure medications that lower blood pressure (eg, ACEIs and diuretics) may help reduce risk of hypotension.
- A recent study comparing the effects of carvedilol with immediate-release metoprolol (metoprolol tartrate) in patients with heart failure found that survival was improved in patients receiving carvedilol. Whether carvedilol is superior to extended-release metoprolol (Toprol-XL, metoprolol succinate) is unknown. Therefore these results strongly argue that only β-blockers proven to improve survival (carvedilol, metoprolol succinate, and bisoprolol) should be used in these patients.

Aldosterone Antagonists

- Elevated plasma aldosterone plays an important detrimental role in the pathophysiology and progression of heart failure. Although short-term treatment with ACEIs or ARBs lowers circulating aldosterone concentrations, this suppression is not sustained with long-term therapy. In low doses, the aldosterone antagonists spironolactone and eplerenone reduce the risk of death and hospitalization in patients with moderate to severe heart failure. Current guidelines recommend the addition of aldosterone antagonists in patients with moderately severe to severe symptoms of heart failure and reduced left ventricular ejection fraction that can be closely monitored for renal function and serum potassium (Table 5).

Mechanism of action

- Antagonism of aldosterone results in reduced renal potassium excretion.

Patient instructions and counseling

- Avoid potassium-containing salt substitutes.
- Call physician immediately for muscle weakness or cramps; numbness or tingling in hands, feet, or lips; or slow or irregular heartbeat
- Spironolactone may cause swollen or painful breasts in men

Adverse drug events

- Hyperkalemia
- Gynecomastia (only with spironolactone)
- Irregular menses

Drug-drug and drug-disease interactions

- ACE inhibitors, ARBs, NSAIDs increase risk of hyperkalemia.
- Spironolactone can increase digoxin plasma concentrations
- Potassium supplements
- Patients with diabetes as well as the elderly are at increased risk of hyperkalemia
- Erythromycin, clarithroymycin, verapamil, ketoconazole, fluconazole, itraconazole, and other inhibitors of cytochrome P450 3A4: inhibit hepatic metabolism of eplerenone and may result in increased plasma concentrations and enhanced effects.

Parameters to monitor

- Serum creatinine: should be <2.5 mg/dL in men or < 2.0 mg/dL in women before therapy is initiated
- Serum potassium: should be <5.0 mEq/L before therapy is initiated. Potassium should be evaluated in three days and one week after therapy is started and at least monthly for the first 3 months of therapy.

Table 5

Aldosterone Antagonists

Generic name (trade name)	Dosage form	Dosage range and frequency
Spironolactone (Aldactone®)	Oral tablet	25-50 mg qd or qod
Eplerenone (Inspra®)	Oral tablet	25-50 mg qd

Digoxin

- Unlike ACEIs or β-blockers, digoxin does not improve mortality, but does appear to produce symptomatic benefits (Table 6).

Mechanism of action
- Inhibits the Na^+-K^+-ATPase pump, which results in an increase in intracellular calcium, that in turn causes a positive inotropic effect.

- Recent evidence indicates that digoxin reduces sympathetic outflow from the central nervous system, thus blunting the excessive sympathetic activation that occurs in heart failure. These effects occur at low plasma concentrations where little positive inotropic effect is seen.

Patient instructions and counseling
- The patient should report to the health care provider if any of the following occur:
  * Dizziness, lightheadedness, fatigue
  * Changes in vision (blurred or yellow vision)
  * Irregular heartbeat
  * Loss of appetite
  * Nausea, vomiting, or diarrhea

Adverse drug events
- Major adverse effects involve three systems:
  * Cardiovascular: cardiac arrhythmias, bradycardia, and heart block
  * Gastrointestinal: anorexia, abdominal pain, nausea, and vomiting
  * Neurological: visual disturbances, disorientation, confusion, fatigue
- Toxicity is more commonly associated with serum digoxin concentrations >2 ng/mL but may occur at lower levels if patients have hypokalemia, hypomagnesemia, and in the elderly.

Drug-drug and drug-disease interactions
- Drugs that increase serum digoxin concentrations:
  * Quinidine, verapamil, amiodarone: the dose of digoxin should be decreased by 50% if these medications are added
  * Propafenone
  * Flecainide
  * Macrolide antibiotics: erythromycin and clarithromycin
  * Itraconazole, ketoconazole
  * Spironolactone
  * Cyclosporine
- Drugs that decrease serum digoxin concentrations:
  * Antacids
  * Cholestyramine, colestipol
  * Kaolin-pectin
  * Metoclopramide
- Diuretics: increase the risk of digoxin toxicity in the presence of hypokalemia or hypomagnesemia
- Digoxin clearance is reduced in patients with renal insufficiency (see section on kinetics).

Parameters to monitor
- Digoxin serum concentration
  * There is little relationship between serum digoxin concentration and therapeutic effects in heart failure.
  * Current guidelines suggest a target range of 0.5-1.0 ng/mL.
- Heart rate
- Serum potassium and magnesium
- Renal function: serum BUN and creatinine
- Heart failure symptoms

Kinetics (Table 7)
- Approximately 60%-80% of the dose is eliminated unchanged in the kidney. Dosage adjustment is

---

Table 6

Digoxin

Generic name (trade name)	Dosage form	Dosage range and frequency
Digoxin (Lanoxin®)	Oral tablet, IV, elixir	0.125-0.25 mg qd
Digoxin (Lanoxicaps®)	Oral capsule	0.1-0.2 mg qd

Table 7

Digoxin Pharmacokinetics

Oral bioavailability	
Tablets	0.5-0.9 (average 0.65)
Elixir	0.75-0.85 (average 0.80)
Capsules	0.9-1.0 (average 0.95)

Elimination half-life	
Normal renal function	36 hours
Anuric patients	5 days
Volume of disribution	7 L/kg
Fraction excreted unchanged in urine	0.65-0.70

required in patients with renal insufficiency.
- Lower doses (0.125 mg daily or every other day) should be used in the elderly or patients with a low lean body mass.
- No loading dose is needed in the treatment of heart failure.
- Because of the long distribution phase after either oral or intravenous digoxin administration, blood samples for determination of serum digoxin concentrations should be collected at least 6 and preferably 12 hours or more after the last dose.

Hydralazine-Isosorbide Dinitrate

- These were initially combined because of complementary hemodynamic actions. An early clinical trial reported reduced mortality compared to placebo with this combination. A comparison with an ACEI showed that the ACEI was superior to hydralazine-isosorbide dinitrate. Adverse effects with the combination are common (primarily headache and gastrointestinal complaints), and result in many patients discontinuing therapy. Current guidelines indicate this combination can be considered a therapeutic option in patients who cannot be given an ACEI or an ARB due to drug intolerance, hypotension, or renal insufficiency.
- A recent clinical trial found that the combination of hydralazine-isosorbide dinitrate, when added to standard background therapy (ACEIs or ARBs, β-blockers, diuretics, digoxin), reduced mortality by 40% compared to placebo in African-Americans with heart failure. Whether these benefits are specific for African-Americans remains to be determined. The current heart failure treatment guidelines indicate that the addition of hydralazine and a nitrate is reasonable in patients with persistent heart failure symptoms despite therapy with ACEIs and β-blockers.

- A fixed-dose combination product is now available (BiDil®)

3. Drug Therapy of Advanced or Decompensated Heart Failure

- Patients with advanced or decompensated heart failure are usually admitted to the hospital for aggressive treatment with IV diuretics, vasodilators, or positive inotropic drugs. Treatment goals are to reduce volume overload and improve cardiac output. The approach to treatment is dictated by the patient's hemodynamic profile.

Warm and dry
- No specific therapy is needed.

Warm and wet
- The goal is to reduce volume overload and minimize congestive symptoms.
- IV loop diuretics are often used. For patients unresponsive to loop diuretics, addition of supplemental thiazide diuretics (eg, metolazone) may be helpful.
- Addition of IV vasodilators (nitroglycerin, nitroprusside, and nesiritide) can also reduce symptoms.
- Inotropic therapy is usually not necessary.

Cold and dry
- May be clinically stable and often do not present with acute symptoms
- Need to rule out volume depletion from overdiuresis as the cause of decreased cardiac output
- Gradual introduction of β-blockers may be helpful.

Cold and wet
- Improve cardiac output first (ie, before removing excess volume).
- Cardiac output can be increased by IV vasodilators and/or inotropes.
- The relative roles of vasodilators and inotropes are this patient population is controversial.

Vasodilators
- See Table 8.

Inotropes
- See Table 9.

Table 8

Vasodilators

Generic name (trade name)	Mechanism of action	Dose[1]	Adverse effects and comments
Nitroprusside (Nipride®)	Arterial and venous dilator	Initial dose 0.1-0.25 mcg/kg per min and titrate to response	Hypotension, headache, tachycardia, cyanide and thiocyanate toxicity, myocardial ischemia
Nitroglycerin (Nitro-Bid®, Nitrostat®)	Venous dilator but also an arterial dilator at higher doses	Initial dose 5-10 mcg/min and titrate to response	Hypotension, headache, tachycardia, tolerance to hemodynamic effects
Nesiritide (Natrecor®)	B-type natriuretic peptide that increases diuresis and is an arterial and venous dilator	Initially 2 mcg/kg bolus followed by 0.01 mcg/kg per min infusion; can increase to 0.03 mcg/kg per min	Hypotension, headache when used in combination with diuretics

[1]All are given by continuous IV infusion.

Table 9

Inotropes

Generic name (trade name)	Mechanism of action	Dose[1]	Adverse effects and comments
Dopamine (Intropin®)	Dose-dependent agonist of dopamine and β and α₁ receptors	0-3 mcg/kg per min: stimulates dopamine receptors (may improve urine output) 3-10 mcg/kg per min: stimulates β_1 and β_2 receptors to increase cardiac output >10 mcg/kg per min: stimulates α_1 receptors to increase blood pressure	Increases heart rate, contractility, myocardial oxygen demand, myocardial ischemia, arrhythmias, and systemic vascular resistance; should only be used in patients with marked systemic hypotension or cardiogenic shock
Dobutamine (Dobutrex®)	β_1- and β_2-receptor agonist and weak α_1 agonist; increases cardiac output and vasodilates	2.5-20 mcg/kg per min	Increases heart rate, contractility, myocardial oxygen demand, myocardial ischemia, arrhythmias; not useful to increase blood pressure in hypotensive patients
Milrinone (Primacor®)	Inhibits phosphodiesterase III, resulting in positive inotropic and vasodilating effects	50 mcg/kg loading dose over 10 min, followed by 0.375 mcg/kg per min; can titrate to 0.75 mcg/kg per min based on response	Arrhythmias, hypotension, headache; alternative to patients not responding to dobutamine or dopamine; may be useful in patients receiving β-blockers since its positive inotropic effects are not mediated by β receptors; adjust dose in patients with renal insufficiency; preferred over amrinone because of decreased risk of thrombocytopenia

[1]All are given by continuous IV infusion.

4. Nondrug Therapy

Intra-aortic balloon pump

Left ventricular assist devices

Biventricular pacing

Implantable cardioverter-defibrillator (ICD)

Cardiac transplantation

5. Key Points

- Heart failure is a clinical syndrome caused by the inability of the heart to pump sufficient blood to meet the needs of the body.
- Although there are many causes of heart failure, the most common are coronary artery disease and hypertension.
- A number of compensatory mechanisms are activated to help maintain adequate cardiac output, and activation of these systems is responsible for heart failure symptoms and contributes to disease progression. Medications that improve patient outcomes antagonize these compensatory mechanisms.
- Drugs that can precipitate or worsen heart failure should be avoided (eg, NSAIDs, verapamil, diltiazem).
- All patients with stage C (symptomatic) heart failure should be treated with diuretics, ACEIs, and β-blockers.
- The goal of treatment with diuretics is to eliminate signs of fluid retention, thus minimizing symptoms.
- ACEIs are an integral part of heart failure pharmacotherapy. They improve survival and slow disease progression. ARBs are the preferred alternative for patients intolerant to ACEIs.
- β-Blockers are recommended for all patients with systolic dysfunction and mild to moderate symptoms. They improve survival, decrease hospitalizations, and slow disease progression. The agents with proven benefits are bisoprolol, carvedilol, and metoprolol extended-release. They should be started at low doses with slow upward titration to the target dose.
- Digoxin does not improve survival in patients with heart failure but does provide symptomatic benefits. The goal plasma concentration is 0.5-1.0 ng/mL.
- Spironolactone and eplerenone improve survival in patients with moderate to severe heart failure.
- Patients with advanced or decompensated heart failure often require hospitalization and aggressive therapy with IV diuretics, vasodilators, and positive inotropic drugs.

6. Questions and Answers

1. Which of the following combinations represents optimal pharmacotherapy of heart failure?

   A. Furosemide, clonidine, hydrochlorothiazide, and propranolol
   B. Furosemide, lisinopril, and carvedilol
   C. Carvedilol, verapamil, amlodipine, and nesiritide
   D. Diltiazem, hydrochlorothiazide, digoxin, and furosemide
   E. Dobutamine, milrinone, furosemide, and nitroglycerin

2. Which of the following mechanisms most likely contributes to the benefits of β-blockers in the treatment of heart failure?

   A. Stimulation of β_2 receptors
   B. Increased heart rate and decreased blood pressure
   C. Increased plasma norepinephrine
   D. Blockade of increased sympathetic nervous system activity
   E. Blockade of angiotensin II receptors

3. Appropriate monitoring parameters for enalapril therapy of heart failure include

   I. serum creatinine
   II. serum potassium
   III. serum calcium

   A. I only
   B. III only
   C. I and II only
   D. II and III only
   E. I, II, and III

4. Patients taking eplerenone for heart failure should avoid taking

   A. potassium supplements
   B. ACEIs
   C. β-blockers
   D. Furosemide
   E. calcium supplements

5. All of the following are adverse effects of digoxin EXCEPT

   A. nausea
   B. anorexia
   C. confusion
   D. arrhythmias
   E. acute renal failure

6. Heart failure may be exacerbated by which of the following medications?

   I. Naproxen
   II. Glipizide
   III. Simvastatin

   A. I only
   B. III only
   C. I and II only
   D. II and III only
   E. I, II, and III

7. Cough is an adverse effect associated with which of the following medications?

   A. Enalapril
   B. Valsartan
   C. Carvedilol
   D. Torsemide
   E. Eplerenone

8. Which of the following ACEIs has the shortest duration of action?

   A. Ramipril
   B. Captopril
   C. Lisinopril
   D. Monopril
   E. Fosinopril

9. Candesartan can be used for treating heart failure in patients intolerant to

   A. Milrinone
   B. Torsemide
   C. Enalapril
   D. Metoprolol
   E. Bisoprolol

10. A significant interaction can occur if digoxin is administered with

    A. Clarithromycin
    B. Fosinopril
    C. Glyburide
    D. Pravastatin
    E. Warfarin

11. All of the following medications can cause bradycardia EXCEPT

   A. Carvedilol
   B. Amiodarone
   C. Digoxin
   D. Verapamil
   E. Dobutamine

12. Which of the following is contraindicated in patients with a history of lisinopril-induced angioedema?

   A. Captopril
   B. Bumetanide
   C. Spironolactone
   D. Milrinone
   E. Aspirin

13. Nesiritide would be indicated in

   A. patients with asymptomatic left ventricular dysfunction.
   B. patients with acute decompensated heart failure not responsive to IV diuretics.
   C. patients with stage B heart failure.
   D. patients with type 2 diabetes.
   E. patients intolerant to digoxin.

14. All of the following are true about the use of furosemide in heart failure EXCEPT:

   A. The drug reduces mortality and slows heart failure progression.
   B. Hypokalemia is a common adverse effect.
   C. Response can be evaluated by monitoring patient weight.
   D. Oral absorption is slowed in patients with advanced or decompensated heart failure.
   E. The bioavailability is reduced by food.

15. Which of the following is an important consideration when using β-blockers for treating heart failure?

   A. They are only effective in post-MI patients.
   B. All β-blockers are equally effective for the treatment of heart failure.
   C. Therapy should be initiated at the target dose.
   D. Patients with fluid overload are the optimal candidates for initiating therapy.
   E. Therapy should be initiated at low doses and titrated upward slowly.

16. The dose of which of the following medications should be reduced in patients with renal insufficiency?

   A. Metoprolol
   B. Carvedilol
   C. Digoxin
   D. Nitroglycerin
   E. Dobutamine

17. The plasma concentration of digoxin is NOT affected by

   A. renal function
   B. Amiodarone
   C. Quinidine
   D. Metoprolol
   E. Bismuth subsalicylate

18. Which of the following β-blockers also blocks α_1 receptors and is effective for treating heart failure?

   A. Metoprolol
   B. Carvedilol
   C. Bisoprolol
   D. Propranolol
   E. Atenolol

19. Patients with heart failure who experience fluid retention after β-blocker initiation should have

   A. the β-blocker dose increased.
   B. the digoxin dose increased.
   C. the β-blocker discontinued.
   D. their ACEI discontinued.
   E. adjustment of their diuretic dose.

20. Which of the following agents should be used in patients with advanced or decompensated heart failure and hypotension?

   A. Dopamine
   B. Milrinone
   C. Nitroprusside
   D. Dobutamine
   E. Hydralazine

Use Patient Profile #1 to answer Questions 21 and 22.

21. Which of the following medications should be added to Mr. Johnson's regimen?

    A. Lisinopril and metoprolol
    B. Valsartan and prazosin
    C. Torsemide and amlodipine
    D. Verapamil and gemfibrozil
    E. Clonidine and hydrochlorothiazide

22. Mr. Johnson's serum potassium level of 2.0 mEq/L (normal 4.0-5.0 mEq/L) could

    A. increase the risk of lanoxin toxicity
    B. be treated by increasing the dose of Lasix
    C. be considered a side effect of therapy with EC aspirin
    D. be caused by an interaction between Zocor and Lanoxin
    E. increase his blood pressure

Patient Profile #1

Patient Name	William Johnson		
Age	64	Height	5'11"
Sex	Male	Weight	185 lbs
Allergies	NKA		

DIAGNOSIS
Myocardial infarction 1999
Hypertension
Heart failure
Hyperlipidemia

LABORATORY AND DIAGNOSTIC TESTS
Echocardiogram in 12/02 showed LV ejection fraction 30%
Blood pressure on 4/1/03: 145/90 mm Hg
Heart rate on 4/1/03: 88 bpm
Lipid profile on 4/1/03:
Total cholesterol 160 mg/dL
LDL cholesterol 95 mg/dL
HDL cholesterol 50 mg/dL
Triglycerides 100 mg/dL
Serum potassium 2.0 mg/dL

MEDICATION RECORD

Date	Rx #	Physician	Drug/Strength	Quantity	Sig	Refills
4/1	1000	Smith	Lanoxin 0.125 mg	90	1 tab qd	2
4/1	1001	Smith	Lasix 40 mg	60	1 tab q AM	3
4/1	1002	Smith	KCl 20 mEq	90	1 tab q AM	1
4/1	1003	Smith	Zocor® 40 mg	90	1 tab qhs	3
4/1	1004	Smith	EC aspirin 325 mg	90	1 tab q AM	2

Use Hospital Inpatient Profile #2 to answer Questions 23 and 24.

23. Based on her profile, the recent worsening of Mrs. Jones's heart failure is most likely related to

A. zestril
B. ibuprofen
C. subtherapeutic serum digoxin concentration.
D. furosemide
E. drug interaction between zestril and furosemide.

24. Toprol-XL is an agent that

A. is contraindicated in heart failure.
B. blocks β_1, β_2, and α_1 receptors.
C. blocks only β_1 receptors.
D. should not be used in combination with Zestril.
E. increases the serum digoxin concentration.

Answers

1. **B.** Furosemide, lisinopril (an ACEI), and carvedilol (a β-blocker) in combination should routinely be used in patients with heart failure.

2. **D.** Activation of the sympathetic nervous system plays an important role in the initiation and progression of heart failure. The benefits of β-blockers are thought to be due to blockade of this increased activity of the sympathetic nervous system.

3. **C.** Enalapril, as well as other ACEIs, can cause renal insufficiency and an increase in serum potassium. Thus serum creatinine and potassium should be monitored.

4. **A.** Use of eplerenone is associated with renal potassium retention. Concomitant use of potassium supplements significantly increases the risk of hyperkalemia.

Hospital Inpatient Profile #2

Patient Name	Ellen Smith		
Age	71	Height	5'4"
Sex	Female	Weight	150 lbs
Allergies	NKA		

DIAGNOSIS   Heart failure exacerbation with 20-lb weight gain over last 3-4 weeks
Hypertension
Osteoarthritis

LABORATORY AND DIAGNOSTIC TESTS
Echocardiogram in 2/03 showed LV ejection fraction 25%
Blood pressure on 4/1/03: 130/85 mm Hg
Heart rate on 4/1/03: 80 bpm
Serum digoxin concentration on 4/1/03: 0.8 ng/mL

MEDICATION RECORD

Date	Rx #	Physician	Drug/Strength	Quantity	Sig	Refills
2/1	100	Jones	Lanoxin 0.125 mg	90	1 tab qd	2
3/1	101	Jones	Furosemide 80 mg	60	1 tab q AM	3
1/1	102	Jones	Zestril 20 mEq	90	1 tab q AM	1
1/1	103	Jones	Toprol-XL 50 mg	90	1 tab qd	3
3/1	1004	Nelson	Ibuprofen 600 mg	90	1 tab qid with food	3

5. **E.** Nausea, anorexia, confusion, and arrhythmias are all common signs and symptoms of digoxin toxicity. Digoxin does not affect renal function.

6. **A.** Naproxen, an NSAID, can worsen heart failure by increasing renal sodium and water retention and by attenuating the efficacy and enhancing the toxicity of ACEIs and diuretics. Neither glipizide or simvastatin affect heart failure.

7. **A.** Cough is a frequently encountered adverse effect of ACEIs.

8. **B.** Captopril must be given three times daily in patients with heart failure. The other agents can be given once daily.

9. **C.** The angiotensin receptor blocker candesartan is an alternative agent for patients intolerant to ACEIs.

10. **A.** The macrolide antibiotic clarithromycin is associated with a 50%-100% increase in serum digoxin concentrations.

11. **E.** Dobutamine is a β-receptor agonist and is associated with an increase in heart rate. The other choices all slow heart rate through various mechanisms.

12. **A.** Lisinopril is an ACEI and angioedema is a known adverse effect of all agents in this class. Thus captopril, which is also an ACEI, should not be used in this situation.

13. **B.** Nesiritide is only indicated for use in patients with severe or decompensated heart failure. It can only be given intravenously.

14. **A.** Although furosemide plays an important role in patients with heart failure by interfering with sodium and water retention, they only provide symptomatic benefit. Neither furosemide nor other diuretics improve survival or affect heart failure progression.

15. **E.** When used in heart failure, β-blocker therapy should be started at low doses and gradually titrated upward to the target dose that was established in clinical trials to improve survival. Starting at the target dose or initiating treatment in patients with fluid overload increases the risk of worsening heart failure. Only carvedilol, bisoprolol, and metoprolol extended-release are proven to be effective in heart failure.

16. **C.** Only digoxin is eliminated by the kidneys.

17. **D.** Renal insufficiency reduces digoxin clearance and results in increased plasma concentrations. Amiodarone and quinidine both increase digoxin concentrations by 50%-100%. Bisumth subsalicylate can reduce digoxin concentrations by binding it in the gut, thus reducing absorption.

18. **B.** Only carvedilol blocks α_1 receptors and has been shown to be effective in patients with heart failure.

19. **E.** Some patients with heart failure may experience increases in fluid retention after initiation of β-blocker therapy. This can usually be best managed by adjustment of the diuretic dose and close monitoring of patient weight.

20. **A.** Dopamine is a β- and α-receptor agonist and is useful in patients with severe heart failure and hypotension. The other agents listed all have vasodilatory effects and are not useful for increasing blood pressure.

21. **A.** An ACEI and β-blocker are indicated in this patient with heart failure to improve survival and slow disease progression.

22. **A.** Hypokalemia increases the risk of digoxin toxicity.

23. **B.** The addition of the NSAID ibuprofen ~3-4 weeks before admission is the likely cause of this episode of decompensated heart failure. NSAIDs can increase sodium and water retention and negate the effects of diuretics and ACEIs.

24. **C.** Toprol-XL (metoprolol succinate) is a cardioselective β-blocker. It blocks only the β_1 receptor at usual therapeutic doses.

7. References

Brater DC. Diuretic therapy. *N Engl J Med.* 1998;339:387-395.

Cohn JN, Tognoni G, for the Valsartan Heart Failure Trial Investigators. A randomized trial of the angiotensin receptor blocker valsartan in chronic heart failure. *N Engl J Med.* 2001;345:1667-1675.

Effect of metoprolol CR/XL in chronic heart failure: Metoprolol CR/XL Randomised Intervention Trial in Congestive Heart Failure (MERIT-HF). *Lancet.* 1999;353:2001-2007.

Flather MD, Yusuf S, Kober L, et al. for the ACE-Inhibitor Myocardial Infarction Collaborative Group. Long term ACE-inhibitor therapy in patients with heart failure or left-ventricular dysfunction: A systematic overview of data from individual patients. *Lancet.* 2000;355:1575-1581.

Hunt SA, Abraham WT, Chin MH, et al. ACC/AHA 2005 guideline update for the diagnosis and management of chronic heart failure in the adult: a report of the American College of Cardiology/American Heart Association Task Force on Practice Guidelines (Writing Committee to update the 2001 guidelines for the evaluation and management of heart failure). American College of Cardiology Web Site. Available at http://www.acc.org/clinical/guidelines/failure//index.pdf

Parker RB, Patterson JH, Johnson JA. Heart failure. In: DiPiro JT, Talbert RL, Yee GC, et al, eds. *Pharmacotherapy: A Pathophysiologic Approach.* 6th Ed. New York, NY: McGraw-Hill; 2005:219-260.

Nohria A, Lewis E, Stevenson LW. Medical management of advanced heart failure. *JAMA.* 2002;287:628-640.

Packer M, Bristow MR, Cohn JN, et al. The effect of carvedilol on morbidity and mortality in patients with chronic heart failure. U.S. Carvedilol Heart Failure Study Group. *N Engl J Med.* 1996;334:1349-1355.

Pitt B, Zannad F, Remme WJ, et al. The effect of spironolactone on morbidity and mortality in patients with severe heart failure. Randomized Aldactone Evaluation Study Investigators. *N Engl J Med.* 1999;341:709-717.

Reuning RH, Geraets DR, Rocci ML, Vlasses PH. Digoxin. In: Evans WE, Schentag JJ, Jusko WJ, eds. *Applied Pharmacokinetics: Principles of Therapeutic Drug Monitoring.* Spokane, WA: Applied Therapeutics, Inc.; 1992:20-1 to 20-48.

The Digitalis Investigation Group. The effect of digoxin on mortality and morbidity in patients with heart failure. *N Engl J Med.* 1997;336:525-533.

Taylor AL, Ziesche S, Yancy C, et al. Combination of isosorbide dinitrate and hydralazine in blacks with heart failure. *N Engl J Med.* 2004;351:2049-2057.

Poole-Wilson PA, Swedberg K, Cleland JGF, et al. Comparison of carvedilol and metoprolol on clinical outcomes in patients with chronic heart failure in the Carvedilol Or Metoprolol European Trial (COMET): randomised controlled trial. *Lancet.* 2003;362:7-13.

Pfeffer MA, Swedberg K, Granger CB, et al. Effects of candesartan on mortality and morbidity in patients with chronic heart failure: the CHARM-Overall programme. *Lancet.* 2003;362:759-766.

Pitt B, Remme W, Zannad F, et al. Eplerenone, a selective aldosterone blocker, in patients with left ventricular dysfunction after myocardial infarction. *N Engl J Med.* 2003;348:1309-1321.

10. Cardiac Arrhythmias

Robert B. Parker, PharmD
Professor, Department of Clinical Pharmacy
University of Tennessee College of Pharmacy

Contents

1. Cardiac Arrhythmias

- Cardiac arrhythmias are abnormal heart rhythms resulting from alterations in impulse formation and/or conduction.

Electrophysiology

Impulse generation (automaticity) and conduction
- Initiation and propagation of the electrical impulse in cardiac cells is dependent on regulation of the action potential.
- Conduction velocity is determined by regulation of action potential, specifically the slope of phase 0 depolarization (Figure 1 and Table 1).
- The *absolute refractory period* is the time during which cardiac cells cannot conduct or propagate an action potential (Figure 1 and Table 1).
- The *relative refractory period* is the time during which cardiac cells may conduct and propagate action potentials secondary to strong electrical stimuli.

Normal conduction system
- The sinoatrial (SA) node, located in the right atrium, initiates an impulse, which:
  * Stimulates the left atrium and atrioventricular (AV) node, which
  * Stimulates the left and right bundle branches via the bundle of His, which then
  * Stimulates Purkinje fibers and causes ventricular contraction.

Mechanisms of Arrhythmia

- Cardiac arrhythmias arise secondary to disorders of:
  * Automaticity (impulse generation)
  * Latent pacemaker (non-SA node pacemaker)

Figure 1.

Action potential for atrial and ventricular tissue.

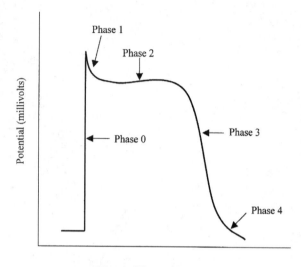

Time (milliseconds)

  * Triggered automaticity (early or late after-depolarizations)
  * Reentry
  * Impulse conduction
  * Automaticity and impulse conduction

Clinical Manifestations

Symptoms
- Except for ventricular tachycardia (VT) and ventricular fibrillation (VF), the patient may be asymptomatic. VT may be asymptomatic, but it can also

Table 1

Phases of Atrial and Ventricular Tissue Action Potential

Phase	Process	Ion flow	Corresponding ECG
0	Depolarization	Na^+ fast channel opens, Na^+ enters cell	Atrial: P wave; ventricular: QRS
1	Initial repolarization	Na^+ channel closes; passive Cl^- influx	
2	Prolongs depolarized state	Predominantly Ca^{2+} enters cell	ST segment
3	Repolarization	Rapid efflux of K^+ out of cell	T wave, QT interval
4	Repolarization	Na^+ leaks into cell, K^+ pumped out of cell	

result in hypotension, syncope, or death. VF produces no cardiac output and is the cause of most cases of sudden cardiac death.

- Symptoms generally related to poor cardiac output include dizziness, syncope, chest pain, fatigue, confusion, and exacerbation of heart failure.
- Patients with tachyarrhythmias may report palpitations.
- With atrial fibrillation/flutter, patients may also experience signs and symptoms of transient ischemic attack (TIA) or stroke.

Signs

- Electrocardiogram (ECG) abnormalities
- Ventricular rate can be assessed by documenting the heart rate from the radial artery or carotid palpation.

Diagnostic Criteria and Therapy According to Arrhythmia Classification

Arrhythmias are defined by:
- Anatomic location
    * Supraventricular: these arise from abnormalities in the SA node, atrial tissue, the AV node, or bundle of His.
    * Ventricular: these arrhythmias originate from below the bundle of His.
- Ventricular rate
    * Bradycardia: heart rate <60 bpm
    * Tachycardia: heart rate >100 bpm

Supraventricular Arrhythmias

Bradyarrhythmias
Sinus bradycardia
Diagnostic criteria and characteristics
    * HR <60 bpm; otherwise normal ECG

Mechanism of arrhythmia
    * Decreased SA node automaticity

Clinical etiology
    * Acute myocardial infarction, hypothyroidism, drug-induced (β-blockers, digoxin, calcium channel blockers [diltiazem, verapamil], clonidine, amiodarone, and cholinergic agents), hyperkalemia

Treatment goals
    * Restore normal sinus rhythm if the patient is clinically symptomatic.

Drug and nondrug therapy
    * Intermittent symptomatic episodes: atropine 0.5-1 mg IV repeated up to maximum dose of 3 mg

    * For persistent episodes or if atropine nonresponsive: place transvenous or transcutaneous pacemaker.

Atrioventricular (AV) block
Diagnostic criteria and characteristics
    * First-degree: prolonged PR interval >0.20 seconds, 1:1 atrioventricular conduction
    * Second-degree Mobitz type I: gradual prolongation of PR interval followed by P wave without ventricular conduction
    * Second-degree Mobitz type II: constant PR interval with intermittent P wave without ventricular contraction; often widened QRS complex
    * Third-degree: HR 30-60 bpm; no temporal relation between atrial and ventricular contraction; ventricular contraction initiated by AV junction or ventricular tissue.

Mechanism of arrhythmia
    * Prolonged conduction

Clinical etiology
    * AV nodal disease, acute myocardial infarction, myocarditis, increased vagal tone, drug-induced (β-blockers, digoxin, calcium channel blockers [diltiazem and verapamil], clonidine, amiodarone, cholinergic agents), hyperkalemia

Treatment goals
    * Restore sinus rhythm if the patient is symptomatic.

Drug and nondrug therapy
    * If the cause is reversible, treat with a temporary pacemaker or intermittent atropine; if chronic, implant a permanent pacemaker.

Tachyarrhythmias
Atrial fibrillation and atrial flutter
Diagnostic criteria and characteristics
    * Fibrillation: no P waves, irregularly irregular QRS pattern
    * Flutter: sawtooth P-wave pattern; regular QRS pattern

Mechanism of arrhythmia
    * Enhanced automaticity and reentrant circuits

Clinical etiology
    * Rheumatic heart disease, heart failure, hypertension, ischemic heart disease, pericarditis, cardiomyopathy, mitral valve prolapse, cardiac surgery, infection, alcohol abuse, hyperthyroidism, chronic obstructive pulmonary dis-

ease, pulmonary embolism, idiopathic (lone atrial fibrillation)

   * The risk of developing atrial fibrillation increases with age.
   * Complications: stroke, heart failure exacerbation

Specific treatment goals for atrial fibrillation (Figure 2)

• Control ventricular rate
   * Digoxin (slow-onset, poor control in hyper-adrenergic-induced AF)
   * β-Blockers (esmolol, metoprolol, propranolol, others)

Figure 2.

Treatment algorithm for atrial fibrillation.

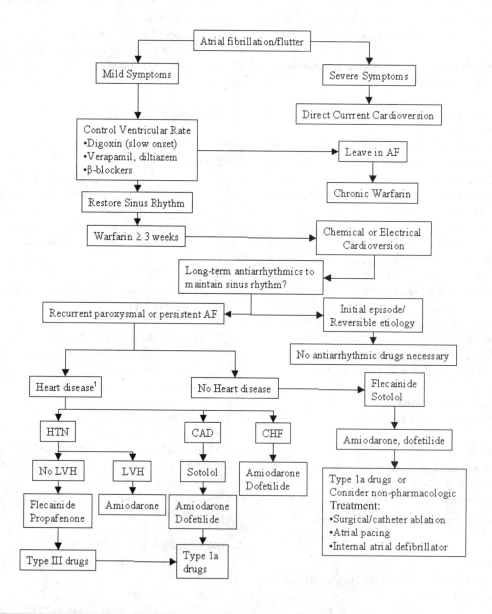

[1]Most patients with heart disease who receive antiarrhythmic drugs to maintain sinus rhythm should also receive chronic warfarin therapy titrated to an INR of 2-3.

CAD, coronary artery disease; CHF, congestive heart failure; HTN, hypertension; LVH, left ventricular hypertrophy.

* Calcium channel blockers (diltiazem, verapamil)
* Digoxin, calcium channel blockers, and β-blockers do not restore sinus rhythm.

Restore and maintain sinus rhythm

* Restoration of sinus rhythm is usually accomplished by electrical cardioversion or administration of antiarrhythmic drugs.
* An important area of controversy centers on whether chronic antiarrhythmic drug therapy should be administered to maintain sinus rhythm after cardioversion (rhythm control approach) or whether patients should simply be treated with agents to control ventricular response and anticoagulants to prevent thromboembolic stroke (rate control approach).
* Historically, antiarrhythmic drugs were frequently used to restore and maintain sinus rhythm in patients with atrial fibrillation (rhythm control approach). With chronic therapy, antiarrhythmic drugs approximately double the chances of a patient remaining in sinus rhythm. However, this approach exposes patients to the large number of adverse effects associated with antiarrhythmic drugs. The rationale for this approach includes the possibility of fewer symptoms, lower risk of stroke, improved quality of life, and reduced mortality. However, these benefits had never been proven in large clinical trials.
* The alternative approach, so called "rate control," involves using drugs to control the ventricular response and chronic anticoagulation, usually with warfarin, for stroke prevention.
* The rate control and rhythm control approaches have recently been compared and the studies demonstrate no advantage for rhythm control over the rate control approach. Regardless of the approach, adequate anticoagulation is needed to prevent stroke.
* Chronic antiarrhythmic therapy is usually reserved for patients with recurrent, symptomatic episodes.

Prevent thromboembolism

* Pharmacologic or direct-current (DC) cardioversion: if atrial fibrillation is present for >48 hours, anticoagulate with warfarin (INR 2-3) for 3-4 weeks prior to cardioversion unless transesophageal echocardiography (TEE) rules out atrial thrombus.
* Postcardioversion, continue anticoagulation for at least 4 weeks.
* Risk factors for nonvalvular atrial fibrillation thromboembolism:

  • Previous stroke or TIA
  • Hypertension
  • Congestive heart failure
  • Diabetes mellitus
  • Age >75 years

Recommended antithrombotic therapy

* ***Aspirin 325 mg daily:***
  Age <65 years and no risk factors
  Age <65 years and coronary artery disease but no risk factors (risk factors: see above)
  Age 65-75 years and no risk factors (warfarin is an acceptable alternative in this group)
* ***Warfarin (INR 2-3):***
  Age ≥75
  Any age and presence of risk factors for thromboembolism

Warfarin (Coumadin®)

Dosage forms

• Tablets:
  * 1 mg (pink), 2 mg (lavender), 2.5 mg (green), 3 mg (tan), 4 mg (blue), 5 mg (peach), 6 mg (teal), 7.5 mg (yellow), 10 mg (white)
• Injections (intravenous):
  * 5 mg powder for reconstitution (2 mg/mL)

Mechanism of action

• Inhibits vitamin K epoxide-reductase and vitamin K reductase, preventing the conversion of vitamin K-epoxide to vitamin K; ultimately inhibits formation of vitamin K–dependent coagulation factors II, VII, IX, and X, as well as proteins C and S.

Pharmacokinetics

Absorption

• Bioavailability 80-100% following oral administration
• Absorbed in the upper gastrointestinal tract
• Food/enteral feedings may decrease rate and extent of absorption.

Distribution

• 99.0-99.5% protein bound, primarily to albumin

Metabolism and elimination

• Metabolized in the liver via cytochrome P450 (CYP450) 2C9 (S-(–)-enantiomer) and mixed function CYP450 enzymes to inactive metabolites. Genetic differences in the *CYP2C9* gene may significantly affect the activity of this enzyme, thus affecting the dose of warfarin needed for adequate anticoagulation.
• Low extraction pharmacokinetic characteristics
• Clearance decreases with increasing age

- Half-life: R-(+)-enantiomer, 45 hours; S-(−)-enantiomer, 33 hours

Pharmacodynamics

- The S-isomer is approximately 2-5 times more potent than the R-isomer in inhibiting vitamin K reductase.
- Its pharmacodynamic effect (change in INR) is an indirect effect of the decreased formation of the vitamin K–dependent coagulation factors II, VII, IX, and X. The long half-lives of these factors results in delayed onset of action and delayed response to dosage changes.

Adverse effects

- Bleeding, roughly proportional to the degree of anticoagulation
- Skin necrosis related to depletion of or deficiency of protein C; usually occurs within 10 days of warfarin initiation; the incidence is low.
- Purple-toe syndrome: usually occurs 3-8 weeks after warfarin initiation; the incidence is low.

Some common drug interactions

- Medications decreasing warfarin anticoagulant response:
  * Rifampin
  * Barbiturates
  * Carbamazepine
  * Phenytoin (chronic therapy)
  * Cholestyramine
  * Griseofulvin
  * Nafcillin
- Medications increasing warfarin anticoagulant response:
  * Amiodarone
  * Propafenone
  * Cimetidine
  * Clofibrate
  * Omeprazole (R-enantiomer)
  * Erythromycin, clarithromycin
  * Metronidazole
  * Trimethoprim-sulfamethoxazole
  * Phenytoin (acute therapy)
  * Allopurinol
  * Phenylbutazone
  * Azole antifungal agents
  * Ciprofloxacin
  * Sulfinpyrazone
  * Acetaminophen

Dosing management

- Once-daily dose of 1-10 mg orally; patient response is highly variable.
- Management of elevated INR (Table 2)

Monitoring

- The standard for assessing the degree of anticoagulation is the International Normalized Ratio (INR)

Table 2

Management of Elevated International Normalized Ratio

INR	Significant bleeding	Recommendations
<5.0 but above therapeutic range	No	Lower dose or omit single dose and restart at lower dose
>5.0 and <9.0	No	Omit 1-2 doses, resume at lower dose when the INR is in the therapeutic range; alternatively, omit dose and give 1-2.5 mg vitamin K orally (2-4 mg if urgent surgery is required); restart warfarin at lower dose when the INR is therapeutic or clinically appropriate
>9.0	No	Hold warfarin and give 5-10 mg vitamin K orally; resume warfarin at lower dose when the INR is therapeutic
Serious bleeding at any elevation of INR	Yes	Hold warfarin; give 10 mg vitamin K IV via slow infusion[1]; supplement with fresh frozen plasma or prothrombin complex concentrate if necessary; repeat vitamin K 10 mg IV q12h if necessary
Life-threatening bleeding at any elevation of INR	Yes, life-threatening	Hold warfarin; give prothrombin complex concentrate with vitamin K 10 mg via IV slow infusion[1]; repeat as necessary

[1]Infused over at least 10 minutes.

- INR = (observed prothrombin ratio)^{ISI}, where ISI is the International Standardized Index, which corrects for variability in thromboplastin sensitivity
- Initially the INR is monitored every 1-2 days until the desired INR is achieved and has stabilized at a given dose. Periodic INR monitoring (ie, monthly) is recommended thereafter unless dosage changes are made.

Paroxysmal supraventricular tachycardia (PSVT)
Diagnostic criteria and characteristics
- PSVT: rate 160-240 bpm that is abrupt in onset and termination with regular QRS interval; 1:1 AV conduction

Mechanism of arrhythmia
- Reentry

Clinical etiology
- Idiopathic, fever, drug-induced (sympathomimetics, anticholinergics, β-agonists)

Treatment goals (Figure 3)
- Acute: terminate reentry circuit by prolonging refractoriness and slowing conduction
- Chronic: prevent or minimize the number and severity of episodes

Acute nonpharmacologic therapy
- Vagal maneuvers may terminate PSVT: carotid massage and Valsalva maneuver (most common), squat-

Figure 3.

Treatment algorithm for paroxysmal supraventricular tachycardia.

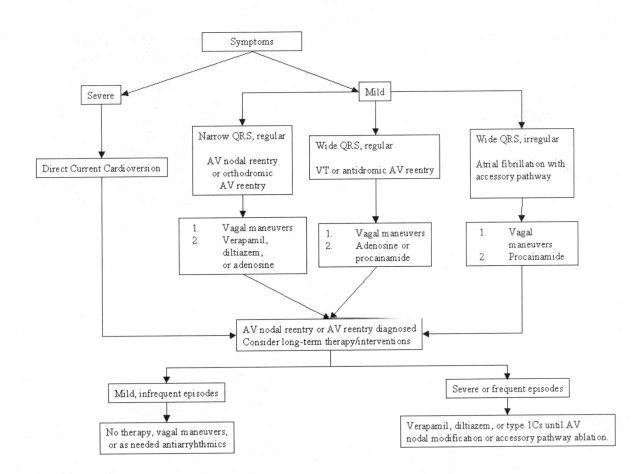

Reproduced with permission from Bauman et al, 2002.

ting, deep breathing, coughing, inducing eyeball pressure, and diving reflex (less common)

Ventricular Arrhythmias

Major classifications and diagnostic criteria
Ventricular tachycardia (VT)
- Three or more consecutive premature ventricular contractions (PVCs) at rate >100 bpm; wide QRS interval (>0.12 seconds), usually regular pattern
- Nonsustained VT (NSVT): episode lasting <30 seconds
- Sustained VT: episode lasting >30 seconds

Ventricular fibrillation
- Absence of organized cardiac electrical or mechanical activity, no recognizable P waves, QRS complexes, or T waves on the ECG; rapidly results in no effective cardiac output, blood pressure, or pulse

Mechanism of arrhythmia
- Reentry

Clinical etiology
- Acute myocardial infarction, electrolyte disturbances, catecholamines, drug-induced

Treatment goals
- Restore sinus rhythm
- Prevent/minimize recurrences

2. Drug and Nondrug Therapy

Nonsustained Ventricular Tachycardia

- Patients with heart disease and ejection fraction ≥30%
    * If asymptomatic, no drug therapy is warranted
    * If symptomatic (palpitations), β-blocker and other therapy to reduce the risk of recurrent cardiovascular events (eg, aspirin, ACE inhibitors, statins)
- Patients with heart disease and ejection fraction <30%
    * Recent studies indicate these patients are at increased risk for sudden cardiac death (usually from ventricular fibrillation). Use of an implantable cardioverter defibrillator (ICD) improves survival in this group, whereas amiodarone does not affect survival.
    * Unless contraindicated, these patients should also receive standard background therapy which includes aspirin, ACE inhibitors, β-blockers, statins, and aldosterone antagonists.

Sustained Ventricular Tachycardia or Ventricular Fibrillation (Postresuscitation)

- If it occurs within 24-48 hours of myocardial infarction or due to other reversible causes, no antiarrhythmic drug therapy is needed except β-blockers.
- If not secondary to myocardial infarction or other reversible cause, ICD placement is recommended.
- Antiarrhythmic drugs (ie, amiodarone) may still be required to decrease the number of defibrillator discharges, increase patient comfort, and prolong battery life.
- Amiodarone can be considered if the patient refuses ICD placement.

Torsades de Pointes

- QRS complexes that appear to twist around an axis; associated with prolonged QT interval

Clinical etiology
- Genetic abnormalities in cardiac potassium channels
- Acquired
    * Hypokalemia, hypomagnesemia
    * Myocardial ischemia or infarction
    * Subarachnoid hemorrhage
    * Hypothyroidism
    * Myocarditis or cardiomyopathy
    * Arsenic poisoning

* Drug-induced (known association with torsades de pointes)
  * Antiarrhythmics: quinidine, procainamide, disopyramide, sotalol, ibutilide, dofetilide, amiodarone
  * Antipsychotics: chlorpromazine, haloperidol, droperidol, mesoridazine, thioridazine, pimozide, quetiapine, risperidone, ziprasidone
  * Antidepressants: amitriptyline, desipramine, doxepin, imipramine, nortriptyline
  * Antibiotics: erythromycin, clarithromycin, sparfloxacin, gatifloxacin, moxifloxacin, pentamidine, trimethoprim-sulfamethoxazole

Treatment
* Stop the offending drug if possible.
* Administer direct current cardioversion for hemodynamically unstable patients.
* Administer magnesium sulfate 2 g over 1 minute IV.
* Use a pacemaker or isoproterenol infusion to increase heart rate.
* Correct hypokalemia or hypomagnesemia.

Drug therapy (Tables 3, 4, and 5)
* Antiarrhythmic drugs terminate or minimize arrhythmias via:
  * Decreasing automaticity of abnormal pacemaker tissues
  * Altering conduction characteristics of reentry
    * Increasing refractory period
  * Eliminating premature impulses that trigger reentry

Table 3

Effects of Antiarrhythmic Drugs on Cardiac Electrophysiology

Drug class	Ion block	Conduction	Refractory period	Automaticity
Ia	Sodium	↓	↑	↓
Ib	Sodium	0/↓	↓	↓
Ic	Sodium	↓↓	↑	↓
II	Calcium	↓	↑	↓
III	Potassium	0	↑↑	0
IV	Calcium	↓	↑	↓

Sotalol also possesses β-blocking activity.
Amiodarone also possesses sodium and calcium channel blockade.

Patient counseling
* Take medication as prescribed. If a dose is missed, have the patient take the dose as soon as it is remembered, unless it is close to the next scheduled dose. In this case, the patient should skip the missed dose and continue the regular regimen; do not double doses.
* Many drug interactions are possible; patients should inform health care providers of medications prescribed prior to starting new medications, including over-the-counter medications (Table 6).
* Periodic ECG and laboratory assessments may be required to minimize or prevent adverse effects.
* Patients should be educated that complete remission of their arrhythmia is unlikely. However, symptomatic arrhythmias that have increased in frequency or severity should be reported to the physician immediately.
* Patients with atrial fibrillation/flutter should be educated about the importance of antithrombotic therapy as well as the signs and symptoms of stroke. Patients with symptoms including sudden onset of slurred speech, facial drooping, or muscle weakness should seek emergent care.
* Antiarrhythmic drugs that are administered as extended-release formulations should not be crushed, opened, or chewed. Advise patients to swallow the dose whole.

Drug-specific information
Amiodarone
* The FDA now requires that a medication guide be distributed directly to each patient to whom amiodarone is dispensed.
* Visual disturbances are rare but should be reported immediately to the physician.
* Difficulty breathing, shortness of breath, wheezing, or persistent cough should be reported immediately to the physician.
* Nausea or vomiting, passing brown or dark-colored urine, feeling more tired than usual, skin or whites of the eyes turning yellow, or stomach pain should be reported immediately to the physician.
* Cardiac symptoms such as pounding heart, skipping a beat, or very rapid or slow heartbeats, as well as lightheadedness or feeling faint should be reported immediately to the physician.
* Periodic laboratory tests to evaluate thyroid function, liver function, and pulmonary function, as well as diagnostic tests such as chest x-ray, ECG, and eye exams may be necessary to assess and prevent adverse events (Table 7).
* May cause skin photosensitivity. Patients should be advised to wear protective clothing and sunscreen when exposed to sunlight or ultraviolet light.

Table 4

Antiarrhythmic Drug Availability and Standard Dosing Regimens

Generic name (trade name)	Dosage forms	Loading dose	Maintenance dose
Class Ia			
Quinidine gluconate (Quinaglute Dura-Tabs, Duraquin, Quinalan, Quinatime)	324-mg tablets		328-648 mg PO tid
	80-mg/mL inj	IV: not recommended	
Quinidine sulfate (Quinidex Extentabs, Cin-Quin, Quinora)	200-, 300-mg tablets	PO: 200 mg q 2-3 h for 5-8 doses (sulfate salt only)	200-400 mg PO qid
Quinidine polygalacturate (Cardioquin)	275-mg tablets		275 mg PO bid-tid
Procainamide (Procanbid, Pronestyl)	IR: 250-, 375-, 500-mg capsules/tablets	IV: 15-18 mg/kg at 20-50 mg/min	IV: 1-6 mg/min
	SR: 250-, 500-, 750-, 1000-mg tablets		PO: up to 50 mg/kg divided q3-6h for immediate release; divided q6h for sustained release
	100- and 500-mg/mL inj		
Disopyramide (Norpace, Norpace CR)	100-, 150-mg capsules		150-300 mg q6h
	100-, 150-mg capsules		300-600 mg q12h
Moricizine (Ethmozine)	200-, 250-, 300-mg tablets		200-300 mg q8h
Class Ib			
Lidocaine	10 mg/mL (5 mL and 10 mL)	IV: 100 mg repeat up to 2 times	IV: 1-4 mg/min
	20 mg/mL (5 mL)		
	IV infusion: 2 (500 mL), 4 (250, 500, 1000 mL), 8 (250, 500 mL) mg/mL in D$_5$W		
Tocainide (Tonocard)	400-, 600-mg tablets		400-600 mg q8h
Mexiletine (Mexitil)	150-, 200-, 250-mg capsules		100-300 mg q8h
Class Ic			
Flecainide (Tambocor)	50-, 100-, 150-mg tablets		50-200 mg q12h
Propafenone (Rythmol)	150-, 225-, 300-mg tablets		150-300 mg q8h
Class II: β-blockers			
Metoprolol (Lopressor, Toprol XL)	50-, 100-mg tablets	IV: 2.5-5 mg up to 3 doses	25-450 mg PO daily
	25-, 50-, 100-, 200-mg tablets; 1-mg/mL injection		
Propranolol (Inderal, Inderal LA)	10-, 20-, 40-, 60-, 80-mg tablets	IV: 0.15 mg/kg	PO: 80-240 mg daily
	60-, 80-, 120-, 160-mg capsules	IV: 0.5 mg/kg	
	20-, 40-mg/mL oral solution		
	1-mg/mL (5 mL) injection		
Esmolol (Brevibloc)	10- and 250-mg/mL injection	0.5 mg/kg/min x 1 min	IV: 0.05-0.2 mg/kg/min
Class III			
Bretylium (Bretylol)	50 mg/mL (10 and 20 mL) for injection		IV: 1-4 mg/min
	In D$_5$W 2 mg/mL (250 mL), 4 mg/mL (250, 500 mL)		
Amiodarone (Cordarone)	200-, 400-mg tablets	800-1600 mg/d in divided doses x 2-4 weeks	PO: 100-400 mg qd
	50-mg/mL IV solution	IV (VT/VF): 150 mg/10 min or 900 mg in 500 mL D$_5$W at 1 mg/min x 6 h	IV: 0.5 mg/min
		IV (cardiac arrest): 300 mg	

(continued)

Table 4

Antiarrhythmic Drug Availability and Standard Dosing Regimens (continued)

Generic name (trade name)	Dosage forms	Loading dose	Maintenance dose
Sotalol (Betapace, Betapace AF)	80-, 120-, 160-, 240-mg tablets		80-320 mg q12h N/A
Ibutilide (Corvert)	0.1-mg/mL (10 mL) injection	1.0 mg IV over 10 min; repeat x 1 if needed	
Dofetilide (Tikosyn)	125-, 250-, 500-mcg capsules		CrCl >60 mL/min = 500 mcg bid; 40-60 mL/min = 250 mcg bid; 20-39 mL/min = 125 mcg bid; <20 mL/min = not recommended
Class IV: calcium channel blockers			
Verapamil (Calan, Calan SR, Isoptin SR, Covera-HS, Verelan, Verelan-PM)	40-, 80-, 120-mg tablets 120-, 180-, 240-mg tablets 180-, 240-mg tablets 120-, 180-, 240-, 360-mg capsules 100-, 200-, 300-mg capsules	2.5-10 mg IV over 2 min	PO: 120-360 mg/d IV: 5-15 mg/h Calan: tid-qid Calan SR, Isoptin SR, Covera-HS, Verelan: qd
Diltiazem (Cardizem, Cardizem CD, Cardizem Monovial, Cardizem Lyo-Ject, Cardizem SR, Cartia XT, Dilacor XR, Diltia XT, Tiazac)	30-, 60-, 190-, 120-mg tablets; 25-mg/mL injection 120-, 180-, 240-, 300-, 360-mg capsules 100-mg/mL injection 25-mg injection 60-, 90-, 120-mg capsules 120-, 180-, 240-, 300-mg capsules 120-, 180-, 240-mg tablets 120-, 180-, 240-, 300-mg capsules	20 mg IV over 2 min	IV: 5-15 mg/h; PO: 120-360 mg/d Cardizem: qid Cardizem SR: bid Cardizem CD, Dilacor XR, Tiazac: qd
Miscellaneous			
Atropine	0.1-, 0.3-, 0.4-, 0.5-, 0.8-, 1.0-mg/mL injection	0.5-1.0 mg q 5 min up to 3 mg total	
Adenosine (Adenocard)	3-mg/mL injection	IV and PO: 0.25 mg q 2 h up to 1.5 mg	Initial dose: 6 mg IV bolus; if necessary, can be followed by 12 mg q 2 min as IV bolus; flush IV line after each administration
Digoxin (Lanoxin)	125-, 250-, 500-mcg tablets 50-mcg/mL elixir 100-, 250-mcg/mL injection		IV and PO: 0.125-0.375 mg qd
Digoxin (Lanoxicaps)	50-, 100-, 200-mcg capsules		

- Prolonged use may cause blue-gray skin discoloration.
- Tell your doctor and pharmacist about all the other medicines you take including prescription and non-prescription medicine, vitamins, and herbal supplements.
- Frequent administration with grapefruit juice may increase oral absorption. Encourage patients to drink

Table 5

Pharmacokinetics of Antiarrhythmic Drugs

Drug	Bioavailability (%)	Protein binding (%)	Primary route of elimination	Substrate for	Inhibitor of	Half-life	Therapeutic range (mg/L)
Quinidine	70-80	80-90	Hepatic	CYP 3A4	CYP 2D6, CYP 3A4, P-gp	5-9 h	2-6
Procainamide	75-95	10-20	Hepatic/renal	NAT		2.5-5.0 h	4-15
Disopyramide	70-95	50-80	Hepatic/renal	CYP 3A4		4-8 h	2-6
Moricizine	34-38	92-95	Hepatic			1-6 h	
Lidocaine	20-40	65-75	Hepatic	CYP 3A4, CYP 2B6, CYP 1A2	CYP 1A2	60-180 min	1.5-5.0
Tocainide	90-95	10-30	Hepatic			12-15 h	4-10
Mexiletine	80-95	60-75	Hepatic	CYP 2D6, CYP 1A2	CYP 1A2	6-12 h	0.8-2.0
Flecainide	90-95	35-45	Hepatic/renal	CYP 2D6	CYP 2D6	13-20 h	0.3-2.5
Propafenone	11-39	85-95	Hepatic	CYP 2D6, CYP 1A2, CYP 3A4	CYP 2D6	12-32 h	
Bretylium	15-20	0	Renal	CYP 3A4		5-10 h	0.5-2.0
Amiodarone	22-88	95-99	Hepatic	CYP 3A4	CYP 1A2, CYP 2C9, CYP 2D6, CYP 3A4, P-gp	15-100 d	1.0-2.5
Sotalol	90-95	30-40	Renal			12-20 h	
Ibutilide		40	Hepatic			6	
Dofetilide	>90	60-70	Renal	CYP 3A4		8-10 h	
Digoxin	60-85 (90-100 for lanicaps)	20-30	Renal	P-gp		34-44	0.5-2.2 ng/mL
Diltiazem	35-50	70-85	Hepatic	CYP 3A4	CYP 3A4, P-gp	4-10 h	>0.05
Verapamil	20-40	95-99	Hepatic	CYP 3A4, CYP 1A2	CYP 3A4, P-gp	4-12 h	>0.05

CYP, cytochrome P450 isoenzyme; P-gp, P-glycoprotein.

water with amiodarone or separate grapefruit juice consumption by at least 2 hours.

β-Blockers (including sotalol)
- Patients with asthma and chronic obstructive pulmonary disease should be advised that β-blockers may worsen their symptoms of airway disease. Advise patients to notify physician immediately if this occurs.
- Patients with diabetes should be advised that β-blockers may mask symptoms of hypoglycemia.
- Patients should avoid abrupt withdrawal of β-blocker therapy. If withdrawal of β-blocker therapy is desired, the patient should contact the physician for the dosage tapering regimen, if necessary.

Digoxin
- Refer to "Heart Failure" chapter.

Warfarin
- Warfarin should be avoided at any time during pregnancy.
- To determine the correct dosage, your physician may need to check your blood regularly.
- Encourage patients to maintain consistency in their diet. Abrupt changes, particularly in the intake of green leafy vegetables, may alter the effectiveness of warfarin.
- Minor cuts may take longer to stop bleeding. If a cut or injury fails to stop bleeding, contact your health care provider.
- Excessive alcohol intake may alter the effectiveness of this medication.
- Tell your doctor and pharmacist about all the other medicines you take including prescription and non-prescription medicine, vitamins, and herbal supplements.

Table 6

Antiarrhythmic Drug Interactions and Significant Adverse Effects

Drug	Effect of disease/drugs on antiarrhythmic drug concentrations	Effect of antiarrhythmic on other drug concentrations	Common or severe adverse effects
Quinidine	*Elevated:* cimetidine, amiodarone, verapamil, diltiazem, ketoconazole, urine alkalinization; *reduced:* enzyme inducers	*Elevated:* warfarin, digoxin, β-blockers, disopyramide, procainamide, propafenone, mexiletine, flecainide	QTc prolongation, torsades de pointes, diarrhea
Procainamide	*Elevated:* cimetidine, trimethoprim, amiodarone		Lupus-like syndrome, QTc prolongation, torsades de pointes, hypotension, dizziness, blurred vision, GI distress
Disopyramide	*Reduced:* enzyme inducers; *elevated:* erythromycin, protease inhibitors, cimetidine		Anticholinergic side effects, decreased cardiac contractility, heart failure, QTc prolongation, torsades de pointes, hypoglycemia
Moricizine	*Elevated:* cimetidine	*Elevated:* theophylline	Dizziness, nausea, paresthesias, proarrhythmia
Lidocaine	*Increased:* with decreased cardiac output		CNS toxicity: paresthesias, dizziness, confusion, nausea and vomiting, seizures
Tocainide	*Decreased:* cimetidine, enzyme inducers		GI distress; CNS: dizziness, paresthesias, confusion, seizures; pulmonary fibrosis/pneumonitis; agranulocytosis
Mexiletine	*Reduced:* enzyme inducers; elevated: quinidine, amiodarone, ritonavir	*Elevated:* theophylline	GI distress; CNS: tremor, dizziness, confusion, vertigo, nystagmus, diplopia; hypotension, sinus bradycardia, AV block
Flecainide	*Elevated:* cimetidine, amiodarone	*Elevated:* digoxin	Proarrhythmia, prolonged PR interval and QRS complex; dizziness, blurred vision, heart failure
Propafenone	*Reduced:* enzyme inducers; elevated: cimetidine, quinidine	*Elevated:* warfarin, digoxin, cyclosporine, theophylline	Metallic/bitter taste; CNS: dizziness, paresthesias, fatigue; GI distress; heart failure, liver injury, agranulocytosis
Bretylium			Adrenergic blocking effects: initial hypertension followed by hypotension; GI distress; hyperthermia
Amiodarone[1]		*Elevated:* quinidine, procainamide, warfarin, digoxin, phenytoin, cyclosporine, lovastatin, simvastatin	IV: phlebitis; general: corneal microdeposits, photophobia, increased liver enzymes, photosensitivity, blue-gray skin discoloration, pulmonary fibrosis, hyper- and hypothyroidism, polyneuropathy
Sotalol			β-blocking effects: bradycardia, fatigue, dyspnea, bronchospasm, heart failure; QTc prolongation, torsades de pointes
Ibutilide			QTc prolongation, torsades de pointes
Dofetilide	*Elevated:* verapamil, cimetidine, ketoconazole, trimethoprim, megestrol, prochlorperazine		QTc prolongation, torsades de pointes
Digoxin	*Elevated:* quinidine, amiodarone, verapamil, diltiazem		
Diltiazem	*Elevated:* cimetidine	*Elevated:* cyclosporine, carbamazepine, digoxin	Hypotension, bradycardia, heart failure
Verapamil	*Reduced:* rifampin, phenobarbital	*Elevated:* theophylline, digoxin, carbamazepine, cyclosporine	Hypotension, bradycardia, heart failure, constipation

[1]See Table 7.

Table 7

Suggested Monitoring Guidelines for Amiodarone

Test	Baseline	3 Months	6 Months	12 Months
Electrocardiogram	•	•	•	•
Pulmonary function tests	•	Routine monitoring controversial; may repeat tests if patient becomes symptomatic		
Ophthalmologic examination	•	Periodic exam recommended		
Chest x-ray	•	•	•	•
Thyroid function tests	•		•	•
Liver enzymes	•		•	•

3. Key Points

- All antiarrhythmic drugs are proarrhythmic.
- Cardiac arrhythmias range from benign to lethal.
- Antiarrhythmic drug therapy should be individualized to patient response while minimizing adverse effects.
- Most antiarrhythmic drugs are hepatically eliminated and are associated with significant drug interactions.
- Nonpharmacologic therapy is an important treatment modality, particularly for life-threatening ventricular tachycardia and ventricular fibrillation.
- Treatment of atrial fibrillation should always include an assessment of antithrombotic therapy.
- Direct current cardioversion is typically the treatment of choice for severely symptomatic arrhythmias.
- Anticoagulant response to warfarin therapy is influenced by numerous factors, including diet, drug interactions, and disease.
- The treatment of excessive anticoagulation secondary to warfarin should be based on the INR, the presence of active bleeding, and the risk of recurrent thromboembolism.
- Patient education and appropriate monitoring are important aspects of successful therapy while minimizing adverse effects.

4. Questions and Answers

1. Which of the following is (are) an adverse effect(s) of orally administered amiodarone?

   I. Gastrointestinal upset
   II. Pulmonary fibrosis
   III. Phlebitis

   A. I only
   B. III only
   C. I and II only
   D. II and III only
   E. I, II, and III

2. Which of the following antiarrhythmic agent's mechanism of action is primarily the result of sodium ion transport blockade?

   A. Quinidine
   B. Ibutilide
   C. Sotalol
   D. Verapamil
   E. Diltiazem

3. First-degree atrioventricular heart block can be categorized as a disorder of

   I. automaticity
   II. reentry
   III. conduction

   A. I only
   B. III only
   C. I and II only
   D. II and III only
   E. I, II, and III

4. Each of the following can be symptoms of atrial fibrillation except

   A. dizziness
   B. palpitations
   C. angina
   D. hypertension
   E. sudden-onset slurred speech

5. Each of the following are recommended monitoring tools for patients requiring chronic amiodarone therapy except

   A. electrocardiogram
   B. coagulation tests
   C. thyroid function tests
   D. liver function tests
   E. chest x-ray

6. For the treatment of persistent atrial fibrillation, each of the following patients should receive chronic warfarin therapy with a target INR 2.0-3.0 except for

   A. patients with heart failure
   B. patients ≥65 years old with hypertension
   C. a 50-year-old male with no risk factors for thromboembolism
   D. a 77-year-old female with diabetes
   E. a 63-year-old male who has had a previous stroke

7. Patients with which type of arrhythmia should be educated on performing vagal maneuvers to restore sinus rhythm?

   A. Paroxysmal supraventricular tachycardia
   B. Torsades de pointes
   C. Atrial flutter
   D. Sinus bradycardia
   E. Ventricular fibrillation

8. In the absence of an acute myocardial infarction, what is the treatment of choice for resuscitated patients with sustained ventricular tachycardia?

   A. β-Blocker
   B. Amiodarone
   C. No antiarrhythmic therapy
   D. Digoxin
   E. Implantable cardioverter defibrillator (ICD)

9. Which of the following medications is (are) associated with torsades de pointes?

   I. Dofetilide
   II. Droperidol
   III. Erythromycin

   A. I only
   B. III only
   C. I and II only
   D. II and III only
   E. I, II, and III

10. Which of the following would result in the greatest risk of lidocaine toxicity?

    A. Rifampin
    B. Cimetidine
    C. Amiodarone
    D. Heart failure
    E. Bradycardia

11. What is the recommended dosage regimen for dofetilide in a patient with a calculated creatinine clearance of 30 mL/min?

    A. Dofetilide therapy not recommended
    B. 125 mcg PO bid
    C. 125 mg PO bid
    D. 500 mcg PO bid
    E. 500 mg PO bid

12. Quinidine is metabolized by and inhibits the metabolism of which cytochrome P450 enzymes, respectively?

    A. CYP 3A4 and CYP 2D6
    B. CYP 2D6 and CYP 3A4
    C. P-gp and CYP 2D6
    D. P-gp and CYP 3A4
    E. CYP 1A2 and CYP 3A4

13. Which of the following antiarrhythmic agents does not increase digoxin concentrations when used concomitantly?

    A. Quinidine
    B. Lidocaine
    C. Amiodarone
    D. Diltiazem
    E. Verapamil

14. J.S. is a 66-year-old male with a past medical history of congestive heart failure and hypertension for which he is receiving lisinopril 10 mg PO qd, digoxin 0.25 mg PO qd, and spironolactone 25 mg PO qd at home. J.S. now presents to the emergency room with a 1-week history of intermittent palpitations and dizziness. A stat ECG reveals atrial fibrillation with a

ventricular rate of 130 bpm. The decision is made to attempt to restore normal sinus rhythm. Which of the following represents the best therapeutic approach to cardioverting this patient?

    A. Perform transesophageal echocardiography; if no thrombus is present, cardiovert; no need for anticoagulation

    B. Perform transesophageal echocardiography; if no thrombus is present, cardiovert; anticoagulate for at least 4 weeks post-cardioversion

    C. Anticoagulate for 4 weeks prior to cardioversion; discontinue anticoagulation post-cardioversion

    D. Anticoagulate for 2 weeks prior to cardioversion; continue anticoagulation for at least 4 weeks post-cardioversion

    E. Direct current cardiovert immediately

15. After the initial successful cardioversion, J.S. continues to have recurrent atrial fibrillation episodes. Chronic therapy to maintain sinus rhythm is to be initiated. Which of the following antiarrhythmic drugs would be the best choice to maintain sinus rhythm?

    A. Flecainide
    B. Amiodarone
    C. Sotalol
    D. Ibutilide
    E. Esmolol

16. In a patient with mildly symptomatic paroxysmal supraventricular tachycardia, verapamil should be used for which rhythm(s)?

  I. Narrow QRS complex, regular interval
  II. Wide QRS complex, regular interval
  III. Wide QRS complex, irregular interval

    A. I only
    B. III only
    C. I and II only
    D. II and III only
    E. I, II, and III

17. R.J. is a 53-year-old male with a past medical history of coronary artery disease and hypertension. He presents to his doctor complaining of short (about 10 seconds in duration), intermittent palpitations during the last 2 days. Tests rule out an acute myocardial infarction and an echocardiogram shows a left ventricular ejection fraction of 52%. The patient is sent home with a Holter monitor to identify

any arrhythmias. The Holter monitor reveals episodes of ventricular tachycardia. What is the most appropriate intervention for R.J.?

    A. No therapy
    B. Place an implantable cardioverter defibrillator (ICD)
    C. Start amiodarone
    D. Start a β-blocker
    E. Direct current cardioversion

18. Treatment of torsades de pointes may include all of the following except

    A. discontinue any drugs associated with prolonged QT interval
    B. isoproterenol infusion
    C. adenosine
    D. magnesium sulfate
    E. atrial/ventricular pacing

19. Which of the following antiarrhythmic agents has anticholinergic properties?

    A. Sotalol
    B. Amiodarone
    C. Lidocaine
    D. Disopyramide
    E. Propafenone

20. Which of the following is not a characteristic of atrial fibrillation?

    A. No discernable P waves
    B. Ventricular rate 100-130 bpm
    C. Regular QRS pattern
    D. Narrow QRS complex
    E. Chaotic atrial contractions

21. Which of the following would be the best choice for ventricular rate control in atrial fibrillation secondary to hyperthyroidism?

    A. Adenosine
    B. Digoxin
    C. Verapamil
    D. Propranolol
    E. Atropine

22. A dose-limiting adverse effect of sotalol is

    A. bradycardia
    B. polyneuropathy
    C. metallic taste
    D. agranulocytosis
    E. lupus-like syndrome

23. Which of the following is not available in both intravenous and oral dosage forms?

    A. Procainamide
    B. Amiodarone
    C. Verapamil
    D. Digoxin
    E. Ibutilide

24. Warfarin dosage adjustment should be considered for the following drugs, except for

    A. amiodarone
    B. sotalol
    C. quinidine
    D. propafenone
    E. diltiazem

Answers

1. **C.** Gastrointestinal upset is common, particularly with larger oral doses (ie, during the loading dose phase), and pulmonary fibrosis occurs during prolonged therapy. Phlebitis would only be expected to occur during intravenous amiodarone infusion, particularly through a peripheral intravenous line. To decrease risk of phlebitis, a central line is preferred.

2. **A.** Quinidine blocks sodium entry into the cardiac cell, slowing depolarization. Ibutilide and sotalol act primarily by blocking potassium transport, whereas verapamil and diltiazem inhibit the calcium channel.

3. **B.** Atrioventricular heart block is caused by slowed conduction through the atrioventricular node.

4. **D.** Due to loss of functional atrial contraction and rapid ventricular rate (producing palpitations), cardiac output may decrease, resulting in decreased perfusion of major organs, particularly the brain (dizziness, confusion, etc) and heart (angina and heart failure exacerbation). Depending on the vascular tone, blood pressure may remain stable or fall as a direct result of decreased cardiac output; however, hypertension would not be expected. Patients with atrial fibrillation are at increased risk of thrombosis, particularly stroke, secondary to pooling of blood in the left atrium and subsequent thrombus formation.

5. **B.** See Table 7 for recommended monitoring parameters and schedule. Coagulation tests are not routinely recommended for patients receiving amiodarone therapy. Coagulation tests may be required if a patient develops severe hepatotoxicity secondary to amiodarone or simply requires concomitant warfarin therapy for atrial fibrillation.

6. **C.** Patients under age 65 with no thromboembolic risk factors are at low risk of stroke and should be treated with aspirin 325 mg/day rather than warfarin.

7. **A.** Vagal maneuvers are effective nonpharmacologic therapy for PSVT since the reentry impulse circuit exists in the atrioventricular node. Although vagal maneuvers will slow the rate in atrial fibrillation/flutter, it will not terminate the arrhythmia since the reentry circuit is in the atrial tissue. Vagal maneuvers will have no effect on ventricular arrhythmia since the impulse arises from below the AV node.

8. **E.** Based on the results of several clinical trials, implantable cardioverter defibrillator (ICD) treatment has a significant mortality benefit over antiarrhythmic drug therapy alone. Antiarrhythmic therapy may be considered if the patient refuses surgical placement of the ICD or to decrease the number of discharges from the ICD if recurrences are frequent.

9. **E.**

10. **D.** Lidocaine is nearly 100% metabolized in the liver. Lidocaine metabolism is dependent upon liver blood flow rather than enzymatic activity (ie, high extraction ratio). Therefore, poor cardiac output secondary to congestive heart failure may decrease lidocaine delivery to the liver for metabolism. Bradycardia typically does not decrease cardiac output secondary to a compensatory increase in left ventricular stroke volume.

11. **B.** Dofetilide is renally eliminated and therefore must be adjusted to decrease the significant risk of torsades de pointes.

12. **A.**

13. **B.**

14.　**B.** Since the patient appears to have been in atrial fibrillation for 1 week by history, there is a significant risk of thromboembolism during conversion to sinus rhythm. Proper treatment would require at least 3-4 weeks of anti-coagulation (warfarin INR 2-3) prior to cardio-version, followed by at least 4 weeks of anti-coagulation post-cardioversion. Alternatively, a transesophageal echocardiogram can be used to rule out an atrial thrombus, allowing immediate cardioversion. Since the atria will require time to recover normal contractile activity, anti-coagulation will be required for at least 4 weeks post-conversion.

15.　**B.** Since the patient has heart failure, the results of the CAST trials indicate the avoidance of class Ic agents due to increased risk of death. Sotalol may worsen heart failure. Ibutilide is indicated for chemical conversion only, not for maintenance of sinus rhythm. Esmolol will only control the ventricular rate but will have no effect on maintaining sinus rhythm.

16.　**A.** A wide QRS complex signifies conduction via an accessory pathway other than the AV node. Since calcium channel blockers prolong conduction in the AV node and not in the accessory pathways, administration of these agents will block the AV node and force impulses to be conducted via the accessory pathways, which have shorter refractory periods. Consequently, the ventricular response will significantly increase.

17.　**D.** According to the patient's presentation, he has nonsustained ventricular tachycardia, since the duration of each event is less than 30 seconds. Since he is symptomatic and has no heart failure, the treatment of choice is β-blocker therapy.

18.　**C.** Adenosine is typically only used to terminate paroxysmal supraventricular tachycardia. Dis-continuation of drugs that prolong the QT interval is essential to terminate torsades de pointes and prevent recurrences. Treatment should consist of intravenous magnesium sulfate and electrical pacing. An isoproterenol infusion can be used while waiting for electrical pacing.

19.　**D.**

20.　**C.** Atrial fibrillation represents chaotic atrial activity resulting in no identifiable P wave. Since atrial fibrillation originates above the AV node, the QRS complex is narrow and the ventricular rate is typically >100 bpm.

21.　**D.** β-Blockers are the preferred rate-controlling agent for hyperthyroidism since they inhibit the adrenergic response and decrease thyroid hormone conversion (especially propranolol). Digoxin is not as effective in controlling the ventricular rate related to an hyperadrenergic state (hyperthyroidism).

22.　**A.** Sotalol possesses significant β-blocking activity and therefore the patient may experience adverse effects similar to traditional β-blockers.

23.　**E.**

24.　**B.** Warfarin is metabolized via multiple cytochrome P450 isoenzymes, including CYP 2C9, CYP 1A2, and CYP 3A4. Amiodarone inhibits CYP 2C9, CYP 1A2, and CYP 3A4, quinidine via unknown mechanisms, propafenone via CYP 1A2 and CYP 3A4, and diltiazem via CYP 3A4. Sotalol is primarily renally eliminated and does not result in cytochrome P450–mediated drug interactions.

5. References

ACC/AHA/ESC guidelines for the management of patients with atrial fibrillation: executive summary. *Circulation.* 2001;104:2118-2150.

Ansell J, Hirsh J, Poller L, et al. The pharmacology and management of the vitamin K antagonists. *Chest.* 2004;126:204s-233s.

Bauman JL, Schoen MD. Arrhythmias. In: Dipiro JT, Talbert RL, Yee GC, et al, eds. *Pharmacotherapy: A Pathophysiologic Approach,* 5th ed. New York: McGraw-Hill; 2002:273-303.

Blomstrom-Lundqvist C, Scheinman MM, Aliot EM, et al. ACC/AHA/ESC guidelines for the management of patients with supraventricular arrhythmias—executive summary. *J Am Coll Cardiol.* 2003;42:1493-531.

Echt DS, Liebson PR, Mitchell LB, et al. Mortality and morbidity in patients receiving encainide, flecainide, or placebo. *N Engl J Med.* 1991;324:781-788.

Harder S, Thurmann P. Clinically important drug interactions with anticoagulants: an update. *Clin Pharmacokinet.* 1996;30:416-444.

Josephson M, Wellens HJ. Implantable defibrillators and sudden cardiac death. *Circulation.* 2004;2685-2691.

Klein AL, Grimm RA, Murray RD, et al. Use of transesophageal echocardiography to guide cardioversion in patients with atrial fibrillation. *N Engl J Med.* 2001;344:1411-1420.

McNamara RL, Tamariz LJ, Segal JB, Bass EB. Management of atrial fibrillation: Review of the evidence for the role of pharmacologic therapy, electrical cardioversion, and echocardiography. *Ann Intern Med.* 2003;139:1018-1033.

Ommen SR, Odell JA, Stanton MS. Atrial arrhythmias after cardiothoracic surgery. *N Engl J Med.* 1997;336:1429-1434.

Singer DE, Albers GW, Dalen JE, et al. Antithrombotic therapy in atrial fibrillation. *Chest.* 2004;126:429S-456S.

The Antiarrhythmics Versus Implantable Defibrillators (AVID) Investigators. A comparison of antiarrhythmic-drug therapy with implantable defibrillators in patients resuscitated from near fatal ventricular arrhythmias. *N Engl J Med.* 1997;337:1576-1583.

The Atrial Fibrillation Follow-up Investigation of Rhythm Management (AFFIRM) Investigators. A comparison of rate control and rhythm control in patients with atrial fibrillation. *N Engl J Med.* 2002;347:1825-1833.

Trujillo TC, Nolan PE. Antiarrhythmic agents: drug interactions of clinical significance. *Drug Safety.* 2000;23:509-512.

11. Ischemic Heart Disease

Carrie S. Oliphant, PharmD, BCPS
Assistant Professor, Department of Clinical Pharmacy
University of Tennessee College of Pharmacy

Shannon Finks, PharmD, BCPS
Assistant Clinical Professor, Department of Clinical Pharmacy
University of Tennessee College of Pharmacy

Kelly C. Rogers, PharmD
Associate Professor, Department of Clinical Pharmacy
University of Tennessee College of Pharmacy

Contents

1. Introduction

Definitions

Ischemia
- Lack of oxygen from inadequate perfusion due to an imbalance between oxygen supply and demand

Ischemic heart disease (IHD)
- Disease caused most frequently by atherosclerosis
- May present as silent ischemia, chest pain (at rest or on exertion), or myocardial infarction (MI)

Angina
- Syndrome described as discomfort or pain in the chest, arm, shoulder, back, or jaw
- Frequently worsened by physical exertion or emotional stress and usually relieved by sublingual (SL) nitroglycerin (NTG)
- Patients with angina usually have coronary artery disease (CAD) in at least one large epicardial artery.

Atypical angina
- Transient pain or discomfort lacking one or more of the criteria of classic angina
- More common presentation for women

Acute coronary syndrome (ACS)
- ACS encompasses the following:
  * Unstable angina (UA)
  * Non ST-segment myocardial infarction (NSTEMI)
  * ST-segment myocardial infarction (STEMI)

Coronary artery disease (CAD)
- Chronic disorder that typically cycles in and out of the clinically defined phases of ACS and asymptomatic, stable, or progressive angina

Percutaneous coronary intervention (PCI)
- Procedure to reopen a partially or completely occluded coronary vessel to restore blood flow

Coronary artery bypass graft (CABG)
- Surgical procedure in which a vein is harvested from the leg and attached to the heart as a new coronary vessel in order to bypass a diseased vessel

Epidemiology of IHD

- Leading cause of death in the U.S.
- Causes more deaths than the next five leading causes combined (cancer, chronic lower respiratory diseases, accidents, diabetes mellitus, influenza and pneumonia)
- Approximately 61 million Americans have some type of cardiovascular (CV) disease, which includes high blood pressure, coronary heart disease (CHD), heart failure, stroke, and congenital defects.
- Approximately 950,000 Americans die of CV disease per year; nearly 2600/day.
- Every 34 seconds an American will die of heart disease or stroke.
- Approximately every 26 seconds an American will suffer a coronary event and every minute someone will die from one.
- In 2002, there were 4,648,000 visits to emergency departments and 80,092,000 physician office visits with a primary diagnosis of CV disease.
- In 2005, the estimated direct and indirect cost of CV disease is $393.5 billion.
- CHD, which includes AMI, angina, atherosclerotic CVD, and all forms of chronic ischemic heart disease, is the single largest killer of American men and women. CHD caused 1 of every 5 deaths in the U.S. in 2002.
- In 2005, an estimated 700,000 people will have a new coronary attack. About 500,000 will have a recurrent attack and approximately 175,000 silent attacks occur per year.

2. Normal Physiology versus Pathophysiology

Normal Physiology

- The arterioles change their resistance and dilate as needed to enable the heart to receive a fixed amount of O_2.
- In response to physical exertion, an increase in blood pressure (BP), or an increase in myocardial oxygen demand (MVO_2), the arterioles dilate to maintain O_2 supply to the heart.
- *Note:* In atherosclerosis, plaque narrows the conductance vessel causing the arterioles to dilate under normal or resting conditions to prevent ischemia. With stress or exercise, the vasodilator response is minimal, which causes ischemia and angina.

Pathophysiology

Determinants of MVO_2
- Heart rate (HR)
    * Tachycardia will increase MVO_2.
- Contractility
    * Increases will increase MVO_2.
- Myocardial wall tension
    * Dependent on ventricular volume and pressure
    * Increased pressure or enlargement of the ventricle will increase systolic wall force and increase MVO_2.

Determinants of Myocardial Oxygen Supply and Flow

- Limits of flow: thrombi, spasm, congenital abnormalities, severe anemia, and severe ventricular hypertrophy due to hypertension (HTN) or aortic stenosis (abnormally high oxygen demands)
- Autoregulation of coronary blood flow
    * Adenosine, a potent vasodilator, is released from myocardial cells in response to decreased O_2 supply (ie, occlusion), increased sympathetic activity (exercise, mental stress, exposure to cold), increased BP, and increased HR, which leads to increased MVO_2.
- Normal arteries respond to increased demand with increased blood flow and some vasodilation of the large epicardial vessels.
    * Note: Atherosclerotic vessels lose this vasodilator response and develop constriction.
- Vascular endothelium
    * Protective surface of the artery wall
    * Promotes smooth muscle relaxation and inhibits thrombogenesis

* If damaged, the endothelium produces nitric oxide (NO) which produces vasodilation similar to the therapeutic effects of nitroglycerin (NTG).
* Loss of the vascular endothelium due to primary transcutaneous coronary angioplasty (PTCA), cigarettes, oxidized LDL, HTN, or atherosclerosis results in loss of NO and the defense mechanism.
- Diastole
    * Normally, the distribution of blood flow between the epicardial and endocardial layers is equal during the period when coronary artery filling occurs.
    * In atherosclerosis, there is a reduction in subendocardial blood flow.
- Coronary vasospasm
    * Reduces blood flow, thereby causing ischemia in areas of atherosclerotic plaques
- Atherosclerosis
    * Most common cause of myocardial ischemia
    * Decrease in the lumen of coronary arteries due to stenosis leads to reduced myocardial perfusion and subsequent ischemia.
    * Segmental atherosclerotic narrowing is most commonly caused by a plaque, which can fissure, hemorrhage, and cause thrombosis, which then worsens the obstruction, reduces blood flow further, and leads to ACS.

3. Diagnostic Procedures

- History and physical examination
- Laboratory work-up (Table 1)
- Resting ECG

Exercise Tolerance Test (ETT, Treadmill)

Drugs that can interfere with test
- Digoxin causes abnormal exercise-induced ST depression in ~30% of healthy patients.
- β-Blockers and vasodilators alter hemodynamic response to BP.
    * Hold 4-5 half-lives before ETT
    * Withdraw β-blockers gradually to avoid precipitating an attack.
- Nitrates can attenuate angina.
- Flecainide may cause exercise-induced ventricular tachycardia.

Stress Imaging

Thallium treadmill (exercise thallium test)

Pharmacologic stress imaging
- Drugs "do the exercise" by increasing MVO_2.

Dobutamine
- High doses up to 40 mcg/kg/min cause positive inotropic and chronotropic effects which increase cardiac demand as a result of positive inotropic and chronotropic effects and lead to ischemia.
- Commonly used with ECHO. Side effects (SE) include nausea, anxiety, tremor, arrhythmias, angina, and headache.

Dipyridamole and adenosine
- Induce coronary vasodilation; used in conjunction with myocardial perfusion scintigraphy

- Dipyridamole SEs occur in up to 50% of patients: angina, headache, nausea, dizziness, flushing, and severe bronchospasm in patients with COPD or asthma.
- Adenosine SEs occur in up to 80% of patients: chest pain, headache, flushing, shortness of breath (SOB), first-degree AV block, and severe bronchospasm in patients with COPD or asthma.

Drug interactions
- Xanthines (theophylline, caffeine) are adenosine receptor antagonists that attenuate the effects of adenosine and dipyridamole.
- β-Blockers interact with dobutamine, but the interaction can be overcome by increasing the dose of dobutamine.

Cardiac Catheterization (Cath, Angiography)

- A catheter is inserted into the femoral artery and guided to the heart.
- Radiocontrast dye is injected directly into the coronary arteries.
- The dye shows which arteries are involved and the extent of occlusion.
- Complications
    * Allergic reaction to iodine in the dye
    * Dye is nephrotoxic.
    * Arterial bleeding from access site, stroke, MI, death (rare)

Table 1

Pertinent Laboratory Tests in Ischemic Heart Disease

Complete blood cell count (CBC) with platelet count
Serial creatine kinase-myocardial bound (CK-MB) and troponin levels
   (enzyme markers specific for myocardial necrosis)
Activated partial thromboplastin time (aPTT)
Prothrombin time (PT) and international normalized ratio (INR)
Fasting lipid panel (FLP) within 24 hours of admission

4. Chronic Stable Angina, Prinzmetal's (or Variant) Angina, and Silent Ischemia

Clinical Presentation

Chronic stable angina
- Symptoms are caused by decreased O_2 supply due to reduced flow.
- Considered stable if symptoms have been occurring for several weeks without worsening (Table 2)

Prinzmetal's or variant angina (uncommon)
- Usually due to spasm without increased MVO_2
- Most patients have severe atherosclerosis.
- Characterized by recurrent, prolonged attacks of severe ischemia
- Patients are often between 30 and 40 years old.
- Pain usually occurs at rest or awakens the patient from sleep.
- Electrocardiogram (ECG) shows ST segment elevation, which returns to baseline when the patient is given NTG.

Silent ischemia
- Ischemia in the absence of symptoms.
- ~75% of ischemic episodes in patients with stable angina are undetected.
- ECG shows ST segment changes and there is elevation or depression during activity, but patient experiences no symptoms.
- Occurs in ~20-30% of post-MI patients
- 50% of patients with stable angina have silent ischemia; common in diabetics

Table 2

Characteristics of Stable Angina

1. Pain located over sternum and may radiate to left shoulder or arm, jaw, back, right arm, or neck
2. Description of symptoms: pressure or heavy weight on chest, burning, tightness, deep, squeezing, aching, vise-like, suffocating, crushing
3. Duration of 0.5-30 minutes
4. Precipitating factors: exercise, cold weather, postprandial, emotional stress, sexual activity
5. Pain relief: sublingual (SL) nitroglycerin or rest

Pharmacologic Management

Chronic stable angina
Goals of therapy:
- Prevent MI and death
- Reduce symptoms of angina and occurrence of ischemia to improve quality of life

Agents
Antiplatelets
- Aspirin decreases the incidence of MI, adverse CV events, and sudden death.
- Clopidogrel (Plavix®) has a greater antithrombotic effect than ticlopidine (Ticlid®) and has fewer SEs.
- **Note:** Ticlopidine has not been shown to reduce CV events in stable angina.
- Indications for therapy (Table 3)

Table 3

Antiplatelet Use in Stable Angina

- Aspirin (75-325 mg qd) in all patients with acute and chronic IHD (with or without symptoms) in the absence of contraindications
- Clopidogrel is chosen when aspirin is absolutely contraindicated
- Ticlopidine is not recommended due to poor side-effect profile
- The combination of clopidogrel plus aspirin is not indicated in patients with stable disease not undergoing PCI

Anti-ischemic therapy
- β-Blockers (BBs)
- Effects on MVO_2
  - * Inhibit catecholamine effects, thereby decreasing MVO_2
  - * Decrease HR (negative chronotrope-decreases conduction through the AV node)
  - * Decreases contractility (negative inotrope-decreases force of contraction)
  - * Reduces BP
- Effects on oxygen supply
  - * No direct improvement on oxygen supply
  - * Increases diastolic perfusion time (coronary arteries fill during diastole) due to decreased HR, which may enhance left ventricle (LV) perfusion
  - * Ventricular relaxation causes increased subendocardial blood flow.
  - * Unopposed alpha stimulation may lead to coronary vasoconstriction.
- Dosing
  - * Start low, go slow.
  - * Titrate to resting HR of 50-60 bpm, maximal exercise HR ≤100.

* Avoid abrupt withdrawal, which can precipitate more severe ischemic episodes and MI. Taper over 2 days.
* Basis of selection of BBs
    * Cardioselectivity to decrease adverse effects; lose cardioselectivity at higher doses
    * The intrinsic sympathomimetic activity (ISA) with acebutolol, carteolol, penbutolol, and pindolol may not be as effective because the reduction in HR would be minimal; therefore, there is a small reduction in MVO_2. BBs with ISA are generally reserved for patients with low resting HR who experience angina with exercise.
    * Lipophilicity is associated with more central nervous system (CNS) SEs.
    * Preferred in young patients who are hypertensive, post-MI, with high resting HR, fixed angina threshold, and mild heart failure (HF)
* Indications for therapy (Table 4)

Nitrates (endothelium-independent vasodilators)
* Effects on MVO_2
    * Peripheral vasodilation leads to decreased blood return to the heart (preload) which leads to decreased LV volume, decreased wall stress, and decreased O_2 demand.
    * Arterial vasodilation leads to decreased peripheral resistance (afterload), decreased systolic BP (SBP), and decreased O_2 demand.
    * Nitrates can cause a reflex increase in sympathetic activity, which may increase HR/contractility and lead to an increase in O_2 demand in some patients. This can be overcome with the use of a BB.

* Effects on O_2 supply
    * Dilation of large epicardial coronary arteries and collateral vessels in areas with or without stenosis leads to increased O_2 supply.

* Indications for therapy (Table 5)

Calcium channel blockers (CCBs)
* Effects on MVO_2
    * Primarily by decreasing systemic vascular resistance and arterial BP by vasodilation of systemic arteries
    * Decreased contractility and O_2 requirement (all CCBs exert varying degrees of negative inotropic effects): verapamil > diltiazem > nifedipine
    * Verapamil and diltiazem promote additional decreases in MVO_2 by decreasing conduction through the AV node, thereby decreased HR.
* Effects on O_2 supply
    * Increased diastolic perfusion time due to decreased HR which may enhance LV perfusion
    * Decreased coronary vascular resistance and increased coronary blood flow by vasodilation of coronary arteries
    * Coronary vasodilation at sites of stenosis
    * Prevents/relieves vasospastic angina by dilation of the epicardial coronary arteries
* Indications for therapy (Table 6)

Combination therapy
BBs and nitrates
* BBs can potentially increase LV volume and left venticular end-diastolic pressure.

Table 4

β-Blocker Use in Stable Angina

* First-line therapy if not contraindicated in patients with prior MI
* Initial therapy if not contraindicated in patients without prior MI
* More effective than nitrates and calcium channel blockers (CCBs) in silent ischemia
* Effective as monotherapy and in combination with nitrates and/or CCBs
* Avoid in Prinzmetal's angina
* Improves symptoms 80% of the time
* All BBs are effective, but not all are FDA-indicated

Table 5

Nitrate Use in Stable Angina

* Sublingual nitroglycerin or NTG spray for the immediate relief of angina
* Long-acting nitrates as initial therapy to reduce symptoms if BBs are contraindicated
* Long-acting nitrates in combination with BBs when initial treatment with BBs is ineffective
* Long-acting nitrates as a substitute for BBs if BBs cause unacceptable side effects
* In patients with CAD or other vascular disease
* Preferred agents in treatment of Prinzmetal's/vasospastic angina
* Improves exercise tolerance
* In combination with BBs or CCBs, nitrates produce greater effects

Table 6

Calcium Channel Blocker Use in Stable Angina

- Initial therapy for reduction of symptoms when BBs are contraindicated
- In combination with BBs when initial treatment with BBs is not successful
- As a substitute for BBs if initial treatment with BBs causes unacceptable side effects
- Slow-release/long-acting dihydropyridines and nondihydropyridines are effective in stable angina
- Avoid short-acting dihydropyridines
- Newer-generation dihydropyridines such as amlodipine or felodipine can be used safely in patients with depressed LV systolic function

---

    * Nitrates attenuate this effect.
- Nitrates increase sympathetic tone and may cause a reflex tachycardia.
    * BBs attenuate this response.

BBs and CCBs
- BBs and long-acting diydropyridine CCBs are usually efficacious and well-tolerated.
- CCBs, especially the dihydropyridines, increase sympathetic tone and may cause reflex tachycardia.
    * BBs attenuate this effect.
- BBs and nondihydropyridine CCBs should be used together cautiously as the combination can lead to excessive bradycardia or AV block. The combination can also precipitate symptoms of HF.

ACE-inhibitors (ACEIs)
- Potential CV protective effects:
    * Reduce the incidence of MI, CV death, and stroke in patients at high risk for vascular disease (data from the Heart Outcomes Prevention Evaluation [HOPE] trial).
- Controversy exists as to whether all ACEIs are equally effective or if "tissue ACEIs" provide better protection.
- Based on a recent clinical trial, low-risk patients with stable CAD and normal or slightly reduced left ventricular function may not benefit from ACEI therapy as greatly as a high-risk patient.
- Indications for therapy (Table 7)

Lipid-lowering therapy
- Clinical trials have proved that lipid-lowering therapy should be recommended in patients with established CAD, including chronic stable angina,

Table 7

Angiotensin-Converting Enzyme Inhibitor Use in Stable Angina

- In all patients with CAD (by angiography or previous MI) who also have diabetes mellitus (DM) and/or left ventricular dysfunction
- In patients with CAD or other vascular disease
- In all patients with DM who do not have contraindications due to severe renal disease

---

even if only mild-moderate elevations of LDL cholesterol are present.
- Indications for therapy (Table 8)

Table 8

Low Density Lipoprotein–Lowering Therapy in Stable Angina

- In patients with documented or suspected CAD or CHD risk equivalents and LDL ≥100 mg/dL: target LDL <100 mg/dL
- In high-risk patients: target LDL <70 mg/dL may be appropriate

---

Prinzmetal's or variant angina
- BBs have no role in management and may increase painful episodes.
- BBs may induce coronary vasoconstriction and prolong ischemia.
- Nitrates are often used for acute attacks.
- CCBs may be more effective, may be dosed less frequently, and have fewer SEs than nitrates.
- Nifedipine, diltiazem, or verapamil are all equally effective as single agents.
- Nitrates can be added if there is no response to CCB.
- Combination therapy with nifedipine + diltiazem and nifedipine + verapamil have been reported to be useful.
- Dose titration is recommended to obtain efficacy without unacceptable SEs.
- Treat acute attacks and provide prophylactic treatment for 6-12 months.

Silent ischemia
- Goal is to decrease the number of episodes, both symptomatic and asymptomatic

- Initial step is to modify risk factors for IHD (smoking, hypercholesterolemia, hypertension)
- BBs have shown improvement in patients with ischemic episodes and are preferred in patients post-MI.
- CCBs are somewhat less effective than BBs.

5. Unstable Angina/Non-ST-Segment Elevation Myocardial Infarction (UA/STEMI)

Pathophysiology

- The process of ischemic syndromes involves two essential events:
    * Disruption of an atherosclerotic plaque
    * Formation of a platelet-rich thrombus
- The clinical manifestation depends on the extent and duration of the thrombotic occlusion.
- In UA/NSTEMI the thrombus does not completely occlude the vessel.
- Pathogenesis and clinical presentations of UA and NSTEMI are similar but differ in severity.

Presentation

- Central/substernal or crushing chest pain that can radiate to the neck, jaws, back, shoulders, and arm(s).
- Patients may present with diaphoresis, nausea, vomiting, arm tingling, weakness, shortness of breath, or syncope.
- Pain may be similar to typical angina except that the occurrences are more severe, may occur at rest, and may be caused by less exertion than typical angina.
- May be incorrectly interpreted as dyspepsia or indigestion
- Pain is not relieved by NTG.
- May evolve into STEMI without treatment.

Diagnosis

- Chest pain persisting longer than 5 minutes that is unrelieved by NTG
- Cardiac enzymes and ECG changes (Table 9)

Table 9

Cardiac Enzymes and Electrocardiographic Changes: UA versus NSTEMI

	UA	NSTEMI
Cardiac enzymes	Negative	Positive
ECG changes: ST-segment, T-wave changes	If present, are transient	Always present

Goals of Therapy

- Complete restoration of blood flow to the myocardium
- Prevent MI, arrhythmias, and ischemia

Pharmacologic Management of UA/NSTEMI

Morphine, oxygen, nitrates, and aspirin (MONA)
- Indications for therapy (Table 10)

Anti-ischemic therapy
β-Adrenergic blockade
- Preference is for an agent without ISA
- Agents with β_1 selectivity are preferred in patients with bronchoconstrictive disease.
- No evidence that one agent is superior to another
- Initial choices include metoprolol, atenolol, and propranolol.
- Indications for therapy (Table 11)

Nitrates (see MONA, Table 10)

Calcium channel blockers (CCBs)
- There is no mortality benefit from the use of CCBs,

Table 11

β-Blocker Use in UA/NSTEMI

- All patients without contraindications
- In patients with continued chest pain, the first dose should be given IV

therefore they are not recommended as first-line therapy.
- Indications for therapy (Table 12)

Angiotensin-converting enyzme inhibitors
- Indications for therapy (Table 13)

Antiplatelet therapy

Aspirin (see MONA, Table 10)

Table 10

Morphine, Oxygen, Nitrates, and Aspirin (MONA) Therapy

Morphine	**Rationale:** vasodilatory properties on both arterial and venous sides, therefore decreases both preload and afterload. Pain relief decreases tachycardia, along with decrease in preload and afterload; all work to decrease myocardial O_2 demand **Dosing:** increments of 2-4 mg IV every 5-15 minutes until pain relief **Adverse effects:** nausea, vomiting, hypotension, sedation, and respiratory depression **Cautions and contraindications:** produces a vagotonic effect that may be contraindicated in patients with bradycardia. Watch closely for hypotension, respiratory depression, and allergic reactions.
Meperidine	Can be used in patients who are intolerant to morphine. Has vagolytic effects, so it is the analgesic of choice in patients who are bradycardic; 25-75 mg IV
Oxygen	Supplemental O_2 2-4 L/min by nasal cannula is recommended to correct and avoid hypoxia, particularly within the first 2-3 hours. More aggressive ventilatory support should be considered and given as needed.
Nitroglycerin (NTG)	• All patients should receive NTG as a sublingual tablet or spray, followed by IV administration as needed for the relief of ischemia. • Long-acting nitrates (oral, transdermal) should be used as secondary prevention in patients who do not tolerate BBs and CCBs. These nitrates can be used in patients who have continual chest pain despite the use of BBs and CCBs.
Aspirin (ASA)	• Aspirin 160-325 mg should be given at the onset of chest pain unless contraindicated. Chew and swallow the first dose. • Daily dose of 75-325 mg for life • Clopidogrel may be substituted if true aspirin allergy is present or if the patient is unresponsive to ASA.

Table 12

Calcium Channel Blocker Use in UA/NSTEMI

- In patients with contraindications to BBs, a nondihydropyridine CCB (verapamil, diltiazem) should be used in the absence of severe LV dysfunction or other contraindication
- Oral long-acting CCBs provide additional control of anginal symptoms in patients who are already receiving BBs and nitrates
- Avoid short-acting dihydropyridines

Thienopyridines (ie, clopidogrel [Plavix] and ticlopidine [Ticlid])
   * Inhibition of platelet aggregation is irreversible and takes 2-5 days to achieve full effect. Often clopidogrel or ticlopidine is given in a loading dose for a more rapid effect (within 2 hours).
   * Clopidogrel is the preferred agent in this class.
   * Ticlopidine is rarely used as a result of severe toxicities.
   * The mechanism of platelet aggregation for clopidogrel and ASA differ; therefore, their effects are additive.
- Indications for therapy (clopidogrel) (Table 14)

Glycoprotein IIb/IIIa receptor inhibitors (GPIs)
   Agents
- Abciximab (ReoPro®)
- Eptifibatide (Integrilin®)
- Tirofiban (Aggrastat®)

   Uses
- All of the agents can be used as adjunctive therapy in patients undergoing PCI.

Table 13

Angiotensin-Converting Enzyme Inhibitor Use in UA/NSTEMI

- Not indicated for the immediate treatment of UA/NSTEMI
- Recommended in patients with HF, DM, patients with high-risk CAD and in patients with persistent hypertension not controlled by the use of BBs or nitrates
- Based on the results from the HOPE trial, which showed a mortality reduction when ramipril was used in patients with vascular disease and no history of HF, may consider in all patients without contraindications

Table 14

Clopidogrel Use in UA/NSTEMI

- Alternative for patients who are allergic to ASA or who have a gastrointestinal intolerance to ASA
- Clopidogrel should be combined with ASA in patients undergoing stent implantation for at least 1-6 months depending on type of stent used and possibly up to one year.
- Clopidogrel should be combined with ASA in patients without a planned PCI procedure for up to 9 months

- Eptifibatide and tirofiban can also be used in patients who will be managed medically. Medical management can be used in patients who refuse a PCI procedure or in patients who are at high risk of complications related to a PCI procedure.
- In combination with heparin and ASA, eptifibatide and abciximab have been shown to reduce the incidence of combined death, MI, and recurrent ischemia in patients with UA/NSTEMI who undergo PCI.
- Indications for therapy (Table 15)

Anticoagulant therapy
Unfractionated heparin (UFH)
- Indications for therapy (Table 16)

Low molecular weight heparin (LMWH)
- Agents
   * Enoxaparin (Lovenox®)
   * Dalteparin (Fragmin®)
- Differ from UFH in size and affinity for thrombin
- Advantages of LMWH over UFH include: better bioavailability, a more predictable response, ease of

Table 15

Glycoprotein IIb/IIIa Receptor Inhibitor Use in UA/NSTEMI

- In addition to heparin, ASA and clopidogrel should be given to all patients with a planned PCI procedure. The GPI can be given during the interventional procedure just before stent deployment or angioplasty
- Eptifibatide or tirofiban should be given in combination with ASA and LMWH/UFH to patients with ACS who will not undergo a PCI procedure

Table 16

Heparin Use in UA/NSTEMI

- Heparin or LMWH should be given to all patients in combination with ASA and clopidogrel
- Heparin is continued for a total of 24-48 hours or until a PCI procedure is completed
- In patients with a planned CABG within 24 hours, heparin use is preferred to LMWH

Table 17

Low Molecular Weight Heparin (LMWH) Use in UA/NSTEMI

- LMWH or heparin in combination with aspirin and clopidogrel should be given to all patients
- Enoxaparin may be superior to heparin in patients with UA/NSTEMI

administration, fewer SEs, and no recommended routine monitoring.
- A total of four clinical trials have compared UFH to LMWH for the treatment of UA/NSTEMI. Two of the trials showed superiority of enoxaparin over UFH. The remaining two trials with dalteparin showed equivalence to UFH.
- Indications for therapy (Table 17)

Lipid-lowering therapy
- Indications for therapy (Table 18)

Table 18

LDL-Lowering Therapy in UA/STEMI

- In patients with documented or suspected CAD or CHD risk equivalents and LDL ≥100 mg/dL: target LDL <100 mg/dL
- In high-risk patients: target LDL <70 mg/dL may be appropriate

6. Acute Myocardial Infarction (ST-Segment Elevation MI or STEMI)

Pathophysiology

- More than 85% of all MIs occur by thrombus formation precipitated by atherosclerotic plaque rupture.
- Aggregated platelets after plaque rupture can serve as a substrate for thrombus propagation, leading to formation of an occlusive thrombus.
- This complete occlusion results in abrupt and persistent ischemia that clinically manifests as ST-segment elevation MI. Left untreated, occlusion of the coronary arteries can lead to sudden cardiac death.

STEMI vs UA/ NSTEMI (Table 19)

Location
- Patients with RV wall infarction should be managed similarly to LV infarction with the exception that NTG, diuretics, and other preload reducing agents should be avoided in RV wall MIs because these patients are dependent on preload.
- RV MI may require volume loading with IV fluids to maintain preload and cardiac output.

Table 19

STEMI versus UA/NSTEMI

STEMI	NSTEMI
Totally occlusive thrombus	Platelet-rich thrombi, which do not completely block coronary blood flow
More extensive damage	Smaller, less extensive damage
Results in an injury that affects the entire thickness of the myocardial wall	NSTEMI involves only the subendocardial myocardium
Occlusion persists long enough to compromise myocardial function and leads to myocardial necrosis	Unstable angina is ischemia; NSTEMI may still result in necrosis, but not to the extent of STEMI
ST-segment elevation on ECG	ST depression or no ST elevation on ECG
Lytic therapy or primary reperfusion is a main treatment strategy	Antiplatelet agents such as GPIs are used to target platelet-rich thrombus

- Symptoms differ from a LV wall MI in that an RV wall MI can cause hypotension, elevated jugular venous pressure, and cardiogenic shock because of inadequate filling of the LV.

Ventricular remodeling
- Can occur as a result of myocardial necrosis and may continue for months following MI.
- Leads to activation of the neurohormonal and renin-angiotensin systems that will ultimately affect ventricular shape, size, and function
- Precipitates chronic changes in ventricular volume, ventricular dilation, hypertrophy, and eventually heart failure (HF)
- ACEIs and BBs reduce the progression of ventricular remodeling. Carvedilol may reverse ventricular remodeling.

Prognosis

Mortality
- The highest risk of death from MI is generally within the first 48 hours.
- Anterior MIs usually involve a larger area of the myocardium than do inferior MIs, and thereby have a higher mortality.
- An important prognostic factor following MI is LV function, as HF is one of the most serious complications of MI.
- Large anterior wall MIs, LV dysfunction, and complex ventricular ectopy carry the highest mortality rate post-MI.
- Early identification and risk stratification can reduce mortality following MI.

Predictors of death
- High troponin concentration correlates with higher death rates in STEMI and NSTEMI.
- Predictors of death within 30 days post-MI include: age >70 years, HTN, atrial fibrillation (afib), tachycardia, large infarct size, previous MI, and female gender.
- Lower-risk patients include those younger than 71 years of age with an LV ejection fraction (EF) ≥40%.
- Patients who continue to have frequent ventricular arrhythmias following MI are at a high risk of sudden cardiac death.

Presentation

- Symptoms similar to UA/NSTEMI
- Atypical presentation is common in women, elderly, and in those with DM.

Diagnosis (Table 20)

Table 20

Criteria for the Diagnosis of Myocardial Infarction
(Two of these three must be met)

Chest pain	Generally lasting for >30 minutes
ECG changes	ST-segment elevation of 0.1 mV in two limb leads or 0.1-0.2 mV elevation in at least two precordial leads
Cardiac isoenzymes	Troponin T or I elevation
	CK-MB elevations

Goals of Therapy in Acute MI

- Limit infarct size
- Reverse myocardial ischemia and thereby salvage myocardium
- Minimize complications.
- Reduce mortality.
- Strict glucose control

Pharmacologic Management of STEMI

Morphine, oxygen, nitrates, aspirin (refer to Table 10 in UA/NSTEMI section)

Nitrates
- Indications for therapy (Table 21)

Table 21

Nitrate Use in STEMI

- Nitrates may be used for the first 24 hours in all patients with MI who do not have hypotension, bradycardia, or tachycardia. Nitrates salvage ischemic myocardium by relaxation of vascular smooth muscle in veins, arteries, and arterioles.
- Insignificant reductions in mortality beyond 48 hours. Use is reserved for those patients with large AMIs, persistent chest discomfort, HF, HTN, or persistent pulmonary congestion.
- Cautions and contraindications: carefully titrate in patients with inferior wall MI because of its frequent association with RV infarction. Such patients are especially dependent on adequate RV preload to maintain cardiac output and can experience profound hypotension during nitrate administration.

Reperfusion therapy

Primary PTCA (see section 7 for more information)

- Intervention designed to reopen a partially or completely occluded coronary artery to reestablish blood flow
- Goal is time to balloon <90 minutes.
- Mechanical reperfusion (PTCA such as balloon angioplasty and coronary stenting) has been shown to be more successful than fibrinolysis.
- In patients who receive a stent, clopidogrel therapy should be added to the regimen as in UA/NSTEMI.

Fibrinolytic therapy (also known as thrombolytic therapy)

- Improves myocardial O_2 supply, limits infarct size, and decreases mortality
- Controversy exists in regard to one lytic agent's superiority over another.
- A door-to-needle time <30 minutes is an important goal.
- Signs of successful reperfusion include relief of CP, resolution of ST-segment changes, and reperfusion arrhythmias, usually ventricular in nature.
- Fibrinolytic therapy is unsuccessful in approximately 22-30% of patients.
- Indications for therapy (Table 22)

Heparin therapy

- Indications for therapy (Table 23)

LMWH

- Indications for therapy (Table 24)

Table 23

Heparin Use in STEMI

- Adjunct with fibrinolytics for the prevention of recurrent coronary thrombosis.
- Combination of UFH with streptokinase (SK) is less clear because it is a nonspecific fibrinolytic. UFH may increase the risk of bleeding because of SK's long half-life.
- Patients at high risk for systemic emboli (large or anterior MI, afib, previous emboli, or known LV thrombus) should have UFH held for 6 hours (postthrombolytic) and aPTT monitoring begun at that time. After 48 hours a change to SC heparin, warfarin or ASA alone should be considered.
- IV UFH or LMWH or dalteparin 120 units/kg SC bid in patients at high risk for systemic emboli
- Can use SC UFH (7500 units bid x 7 days or until the patient is fully ambulatory) or LMWH in all patients not treated with a thrombolytic (who have no contraindications to UFH).
- Consider SC UFH or LMWH for DVT prophylaxis.

β-Adrenergic blockade (BB)

- Early BB use post-MI reduces infarct size, CV mortality, reinfarction rate, and nonfatal cardiac arrests, and increases probability of long-term survival.
- Late administration of a BB (at least 24 hours after MI) improves left ventricular diastolic filling and reduces risk of recurrent MI and death
- Indications for therapy (Table 25)

Table 22

Use of Fibrinolytic Therapy in STEMI

- ST-segment elevation >1 mm in two or more contiguous leads or Left Bundle Branch Block (obscuring ST observational changes)
- Presentation within 12 hours or less of symptom onset
- Patient has no contraindications to fibrinolytic therapy and has indications for therapy
- In patients age >75 years may be useful and appropriate
- Can be used in STEMI when time to therapy is 12-24 hours if chest pain is ongoing
- Should not be used if the time to therapy is >24 hours, and the ischemic pain is resolved
- Should not be used for ST depression

Table 24

LMWH Use in STEMI

- Can be used as an alternative to UFH for patients </5 years of age without significant renal dysfunction (men: SCr >2.5 mg/dl; women: SCr >2 mg/dl) who are receiving fibrinolytic therapy. Enoxaparin (30 mg IV bolus, 1 mg/kg SC q12h until discharge) + tenecteplase (full dose) is the most studied regimen in this population.
- Should not be used in patients >75 years of age or in patients <75 years of age with renal dysfunction
- LMWH or IV UFH in patients at high risk for systemic emboli
- Patients not treated with a thrombolytic without contraindications can be treated with SC or IV UFH or LMWH (enoxaparin 1 mg/kg SC bid or dalteparin 120 units/kg SC bid) for at least 48 hours.
- Consider LMWH or SC UFH for DVT prophylaxis.

Table 25

β-Blocker Use in STEMI

Early therapy: BBs should be given to all patients with acute MI who can be treated within 12 hours of MI, regardless of administration of concomitant thrombolytic therapy. IV or PO treatment should be started as soon as possible in all patients within 12-24 hours after onset of symptoms.

Late therapy: BBs should be given to all patients without a clear contraindication to BB therapy. Treatment should begin within a few days of the event (if not initiated early) and be continued indefinitely.

Glycoprotein IIb/IIIa Inhibitors (GPIs)

- The role of platelet GPI in STEMI is rapidly evolving, and trials to date in combination with full- and half-dose fibrinolytic agents have shown a more complete reperfusion at the price of higher bleeding rates, especially in elderly patients.
- Abciximab reduces the incidence of combined death, MI, and recurrent ischemia in patients with STEMI.

Inhibition of the renin-angiotensin-aldosterone (RAA) system (ACEIs, angiotensin receptor blockers [ARBs], and aldosterone inhibitors)

- Primary goal is to limit postinfarction LV dilatation and hypertrophy so that pump function is preserved or improved. ACEIs attenuate the remodeling process and thereby slow the progression to HF post-MI.
- Benefits of ACEIs are clearly most pronounced in patients with evidence of ventricular dysfunction (either objective evidence such as LVEF ≤40% or subjective evidence such as HF symptoms).
- Marked benefit of ACEIs in other high-risk patients (previous MI, HF, and anterior MI without thrombolytic therapy)
- Recent studies of ACEI therapy suggest acute treatment should be given to patients considered at higher risk due to a history of HTN, DM, or previous MI, and should be continued indefinitely.
- An ARB can be used for those patients who are intolerant of an ACEI and have either clinical or radiological signs of heart failure and an LVEF of ≤40%.
- The combination of an ACEI and an ARB may be considered in patients with persistent heart failure. Due to results from clinical trials when this combination is considered, candesartan is the preferred ARB.
- Aldosterone blockade (eplerenone, spironolactone)

Table 26

ACEI, ARB, and Aldosterone Blocker Use Post-STEMI

- Patients within the first 24 hours of a suspected MI or with clinical HF without contraindications should receive an ACEI.
- All other patients without contraindications should receive an ACEI within the first 24 hours.
- ACEIs remain the first choice for inhibition of the RAAS system in the long-term management of patients post-STEMI.
- IV ACEIs should not be given to patients within the first 24 hours of STEMI because of the risk of hypotension.
- ARBs should be given to those patients who are intolerant of an ACEI. Valsartan and candesartan are the only ARBs that have established efficacy for this indication.
- Long-term aldosterone blockade should be prescribed for post-STEMI patients without contraindications with an LVEF ≤40%, and having either symptomatic heart failure or diabetes.

should be prescribed post-STEMI in those patients already on an ACEI with an LVEF ≤40% and having either symptomatic heart failure or diabetes.
- Aldosterone blockers should be avoided in patients with renal dysfunction (SCr ≥2.5 mg/dL in men or ≥2.0 in women) or hyperkalemia (potassium >5 mEq/L).
- Less is known about the combination of an aldosterone blocker and an ARB and the triple combination of an ACEI, ARB, and aldosterone blocker.
- Indications for therapy (Table 26)

Lipid lowering

- Indications for therapy (see Table 18 in UA/STEMI section)

Calcium channel blockers (CCBs)

- Indications for therapy (Table 27)

Warfarin

- Indications for therapy (Table 28)

Treatment of ventricular fibrillation (VF) post-MI

- The risk of VF is at highest during the first 4 hours post-MI and then declines sharply.
- Prophylactic antiarrhythmic use has been shown to increase all-cause mortality when used to prevent VF. The use of lidocaine for VF prophylaxis is not recommended.
- Amiodarone may be utilized if patients experience VF or hemodynamically compromising ventricular tachycardia following MI.

Table 27

Calcium Channel Blockers Post-STEMI

- Verapamil or diltiazem only with continuing ischemia when BB use is either contraindicated or used at maximum dose with nitrates.
- Verapamil or diltiazem should not be used in patients with systolic dysfunction, AV block, or bradycardia.

Table 28

Warfarin Use Post-STEMI

- The indications for long-term anticoagulation with warfarin are evolving yet remain controversial.
- Recommended in patients with indications for anticoagulation (ie, LV thrombus, atrial fibrillation, extensive wall motion abnormalities, etc)
- Patients over age 75 have not been adequately studied in secondary prevention trials post-STEMI. Warfarin is not recommended in these patients unless a clear indication for anticoagulation exists.
- Clopidogrel is preferred in patients who cannot tolerate aspirin for secondary prevention unless a clear indication for warfarin exists.

7. Revascularization

Percutaneous Coronary Intervention (PCI)

Procedures
- Procedure types include: balloon angioplasty (PTCA), coronary stenting, and ablative technologies (laser, atherectomy).
- Primary PCI is a very effective method for re-establishing coronary perfusion and is suitable for at least 90% of patients.
- Primary PCI should be performed as quickly as possible with the goal of a medical contact-to-balloon or door-to-balloon time of 90 minutes or less.
- Primary PCI is favored over fibrinolytic therapy because PCI-treated patients experience lower short-term mortality rates, fewer nonfatal reinfarctions and hemorrhagic strokes than those treated with fibrinolytic therapy.
- Facilitated PCI refers to a strategy of planned immediate PCI after an initial pharmacologic regimen such as full-dose fibrinolytics, GPIs, or another pharmacologic regimen.
- Potential complications of invasive PCI include problems with arterial access site, technical complications, acute vessel closure, restenosis, and acute renal failure secondary to nephrotoxic dye.

Drug eluting stents (DES)
- Restenosis is the loss of 50% or more of the diameter of the in-stent lumen at the site of an initially successful intervention; it usually occurs within the first 3-6 months after PTCA.
- DES were introduced in 2003, and have the principal advantage of reducing in-stent thrombosis and restenosis over bare metal stents (BMS).
- Sirolimus and paclitaxel are two options of pharmacologic agents that are embedded in the steel stent with release modulated by a polymeric coating so the agent is released over a period of time.
- Clopidogrel in combination with aspirin is used to reduce in-stent thrombosis, and is used for at least 1 month with BMS, 3 months for sirolimus-coated, and 6 months for paclitaxel-coated stents.

Anticoagulation during PCI
- Mandatory, as the vessel manipulation during PCI is inherently thrombogenic.

Possible agents
- UFH is currently the mainstay of therapy.
- Bivalirudin: studies have shown that this direct thrombin inhibitor may be as effective as heparin but with less bleeding.

- LMWHs have been utilized in varying doses during PCI; however, there is no consensus on their use during PCI.

Glycoprotein inhibitors (GPIIb/IIIa inhibitors)
- Although similar effects have been noted with each of the GPIs, the timing of PCI should be determined before an agent is selected.
- Use abciximab or eptifibatide if PCI is anticipated soon after presentation (<4 hours), reserving tirofiban for patients treated medically during the first 48 hours.
- Abciximab should not be used for patients who are conservatively managed without plans for PCI.

Coronary artery bypass graft surgery (CABG)
- Indicated in patients with multivessel disease with LV dysfunction or significant disease of a major coronary vessel

8. Primary Prevention: Risk Factor Modification

Background

- The majority of the causes of cardiovascular disease are known and modifiable.
- Risk factor screening should begin at age 20 with the hope that all adults know the levels and significance of risk factors as routinely assessed by their primary care provider.

Nonmodifiable Risk Factors

Age
- Men >45; women >55 (or those who had an early hysterectomy regardless of age)

Race
- Higher risk in African-American males and females compared to Caucasian males and females

Family history
- Father or brother with a coronary event before age 55
- Mother or sister with a coronary event before age 65

Modifiable Risk Factors

- Smoking
- Hypertension
- Hyperlipidemia
- Hyperhomocysteinemia
- Diabetes
- Metabolic syndrome
- Obesity
- Physical inactivity
- Alcohol consumption

Pharmacologic Therapy

Aspirin
- The Seventh ACCP Consensus Conference on Antithrombotic Therapy (Chest Guidelines) recommends that ASA (80-325 mg/day) be considered for individuals >50 years old who have at least one major risk factor for CAD and who are free of contraindications.
- The ACC/AHA recommends doses of 75-162 mg/day in persons at higher risk of CVD (especially those with a 10-year risk of CHD >10%).
- The American Diabetes Association recommends ASA therapy to prevent CV events in most patients

with DM who are >40 years of age and have no contraindications to ASA.

- The recommendation for aspirin use for primary prevention is stronger in men than in women.

Angiotensin-converting enzyme inhibitors (ACEIs)

- In the HOPE trial, ramipril demonstrated effectiveness in reducing the risk of MI, stroke, and death from cardiovascular causes in patents at high risk of a major cardiovascular event. ACEIs may be used as protective agents.
- EUROPA similarly showed perindopril to be beneficial in patients with evidence of coronary heart disease but without heart failure, and has led to the increased use of ACEIs in patients with vascular disease but without heart failure or LV dysfunction.
- Results from PEACE suggest that low-risk patients with CAD, who are receiving maximal therapy with β-blockers, aspirin, and lipid-lowering therapies, do not gain additional benefit from the addition of trandolapril 4 mg daily.
- Chronic ACEI therapy may be most beneficial in high-risk patients (uncontrolled hyperlipidemia, hypertension, smoking, proteinuria, vascular disease).

Lipid lowering

- Consider in all patients at risk for a coronary event.

Antioxidants

- There is no consistent evidence with vitamin E or other antioxidant therapy to recommend its use for primary prevention of heart disease.

Nonpharmacologic Therapy for IHD

Smoking cessation

- One of the most important risk-modifying behaviors
- Evidence suggests that the best adherence to a cessation program combines pharmacotherapy with behavioral modification.
- A wide range of smoking cessation aids (prescription and nonprescription) products are available.
- Nicotine replacement alone is not an effective management strategy for smoking cessation. Nicotine combined with bupropion has been the most successful.

Diet

- Diets low in saturated fat and high in fruits, vegetables, whole grains, and fiber are associated with a reduced risk of CVD.
- Omega-3 fatty acids: the AHA Dietary Guidelines recommends inclusion of at least two servings of fish per week (particularly fatty fish).
- Food sources high in alpha-linolenic acid (eg, soy-

bean, canola, walnut, and flaxseed oil and walnuts and flaxseeds) are also recommended.

Exercise

- Regular aerobic physical activity increases a person's capacity for exercise. Exercise plays a role in both primary and secondary prevention of cardiovascular disease.
- Current guidelines from the CDC and NIH recommend that Americans should accumulate at least 30 minutes of moderate-intensity physical activity on most, preferably all, days of the week to prevent risk of chronic disease in the future.
- The Institute of Medicine recommends 60 minutes of physical activity per day.

Weight loss

- Weight loss can reduce blood pressure, lower blood glucose levels, and improve blood lipid abnormalities.
- A goal of 5-10% of body weight loss is associated with decreased morbidity and mortality.
- Pharmacotherapy used for weight loss should be reserved for those with a BMI >30, or in those with BMI >25 with other risk factors for comorbid diseases.

Alcohol consumption

- Lowest CV mortality occurs in those who consume 1 or 2 drinks per day. People with no alcohol consumption have higher total mortality than those drinking 1 to 2 drinks per day.
- In the absence of alcohol-related illnesses, 1 to 2 drinks per day in males and 1 alcoholic drink per day in females may be considered for high-risk patients.
- A drink equivalent amounts to a 12-ounce bottle of beer, a 4-ounce glass of wine, or a 1.5-ounce shot of 80-proof spirits.
- A general increase in alcohol consumption at the population level is not recommended.

9. Pharmacology

Anti-Ischemic Drug Therapy

β-Blockers (see hypertension chapter)

Nitrates
Mechanism of action
- Organic nitrates are prodrugs that must be transformed to exert pharmacological effect.
- NTG leads to denitration of the nitrate, liberation of nitric oxide (NO), guanylyl cyclase stimulation, the conversion of guanosine triphosphate to cGMP, and vasodilation.
- NO also reduces platelet adhesion and aggregation and affects endothelial function and vascular growth.

Properties
- Oral: Isosorbide dinitrate (ISDN) and NTG undergo extensive first-pass metabolism when given orally. Mononitrate does not; it is completely bioavailable.
- IV: Achieves highest concentrations; usually used for only 24 hours to avoid developing tolerance
- SL tablet/spray for immediate-release
    * Spray does not degrade when exposed to air like tablets.
    * Half-life: 1-5 minutes regardless of route

Doses (Table 29)

Monitoring parameters
- Blood pressure, heart rate

Adverse drug reactions (Table 30)

Table 29

Pharmacologic Properties and Doses of Nitrates

Drug	Route	Onset (min)	Duration of action	Dose
Nitroglycerin sublingual tablet (Nitrostat®, Nitroquick®)	Sublingual	1-3	30-60 min	0.2-0.6 mg every 5 minutes. Seek emergency treatment if chest pain is unrelieved after 1 dose
Nitroglycerin spray (Nitrolingual®)	Translingual	2	30-60 min	0.4 mg every 5 minutes. Seek emergency treatment if chest pain unrelieved after 1 spray
Nitroglycerin transmucosal tablets (Nitroguard®)	Buccal	1-2	3-5 h	Insert 1 tablet into cheek every 3-5 h
Nitroglycerin ointment (Nitrobid®, Nitrol®)	Topical	30-60	2-12 h	1-2 inches every 8 h up to 4-5 inches every 4 h
Nitroglycerin transdermal patches (Nitro-dur®, Transderm Nitro®, Nitrek®, Nitrodisc®, Deponit®, Minitran®)	Topical	30-60	Up to 24 h	Starting dose: 0.2-0.4 mg/h. Apply and allow patch to stay in place for 12 h. Remove the patch after 12 h to allow for a nitrate-free interval
Nitroglycerin sustained-release tablets/capsules (Nitrong®, Nitroglyn®, Nitro-Time®)	Oral	20-45	3-8 h	Starting dose: 2.5 mg tid-qid. Increase the dose by 2.5 mg two to four times daily to reach effective dose
Nitroglycerin intravenous (Tridil®, Nitro-Bid IV®)	IV	1-2	3-5 min	Starting dose: 5 mcg/min. Titrate to response
Isosorbide mononitrate (Ismo®, Monoket®)	Oral	30-60	No data	20 mg bid (given 7 hours apart). May need to start with 5 mg bid for low-weight patients
Isosorbide mononitrate, extended-release (Imdur®, Isotrate ER®)	Oral	30-60	No data	Starting dose: 30-60 mg qd. Maximum dose: 240 mg qd
Isosorbide dinitrate (Isordil Titradose®, Sorbitrate®)	Oral	20-40	4-6 h	Starting dose: 5-20 mg q6h. Maintenance dose: 10-40 mg q6h
Isosorbide dinitrate, sustained-release tablets/capsules (Isordil Tembids®, Dilatrate-SR®)	Oral	Up to 4 h	6-8 h	Initial dose: 40 mg q8h. Maintenance dose: 40-80 mg q8-12 h

Table 30

Nitrate Adverse Reactions

Tolerance	Tolerance to the vasodilatory effects can develop if dosing does not allow for a nitrate-free interval (10-12 h)
CNS	Headache (up to 50%), dizziness, anxiety, nervousness
CV	Hypotension, tachycardia, palpitations, syncope
GI	Nausea, vomiting, dyspepsia
Dermatologic	Rash, dermatitis
Other	Blurred vision, muscle twitching, perspiration, edema, arthralgia

Drug-drug interactions (Table 31)

Drug-disease interactions
- Glaucoma
    * Intraocular pressure may increase.
    * Use with caution in patients with glaucoma.
- Hypertrophic obstructive cardiomyopathy
- Severe aortic stenosis
    * Can cause hypotension and syncope

Contraindications
- Sildenafil and vardenafil: use within 24 hours
- Tadalafil: use within 48 hours
- Hypersensitivity to nitrates

Table 31

Nitrate Drug-Drug Interactions

Interacting medication	Effect
Sildenafil (Viagra®), vardenafil (Levitra®), tadalafil (Cialis®)	Significant reduction of systolic and diastolic blood pressure. Do not give sildenafil or vardenafil within 24 hours of nitrate use. Do not give tadalafil within 48 hours of nitrate use.
Calcium channel blockers	Marked symptomatic hypotension may occur
Alcohol	Severe hypotension may occur

Patient instructions/counseling
- Avoid alcohol consumption.
- May cause dizziness; use caution when driving or engaging in hazardous activities until drug effect is known.
- When standing from a sitting position, rise slowly to avoid an abrupt drop in blood pressure.
- Notify physician of acute headache, dizziness, or blurred vision.
- Sublingual tablets
    * Keep tablets in their original container.
    * Dissolve tablet under the tongue. Lack of tingling does not indicate a lack of potency.
    * Take one tablet at the first sign of chest pain. If chest pain is unrelieved, seek emergency medical attention.
- Translingual spray
    * Spray under tongue or onto tongue.
    * Hold spray nozzle as close to the mouth as possible and spray medicine onto or under the tongue.
    * Do not inhale the spray or use near heat, open flame, or while smoking.
    * Close mouth immediately after spraying
    * Avoid eating, drinking, or smoking for 5-10 minutes.
    * If the pain does not go away after 1 spray, seek emergency medical attention.
- Transmucosal tablets
    * Place between cheek and gum. Do not chew tablet; allow to dissolve over a 3- to 5-hour period.
    * Touching the tablet with the tongue or hot liquids may increase release of the medication.
- Ointment
    * Measure the correct amount using the papers provided with the product.
    * Use papers for the application, not fingers.
    * Apply to the chest or back.
- Transdermal patches
    * Tear the wrapper open carefully. Never cut the wrapper or patch with scissors. Do not use any patch that has been cut by accident.
    * Apply to a hairless area and rotate sites to avoid irritation. Be sure to remove the old patch before applying a new one.
    * Do not put the patch over burns, cuts, or irritated skin.
    * Remove the patch approximately 12-14 hours after placing it on every day. This prevents tolerance to the beneficial effects of NTG.
    * Used patches may still contain residual medication; use caution when disposing around children and pets.

* Store the patches at room temperature in a closed container, away from heat, moisture, and direct light. Do not refrigerate.
* Sustained-release tablets
    * Take at the same time each day as directed.
    * Do not chew or crush tablets/capsules.

Inhibition of the renin-angiotensin-aldosterone (RAA) system

Angiotensin-converting enzyme Inhibitors (see heart failure chapter)

Angiotensin receptor blockers (see heart failure chapter)

Aldosterone blockers (see heart failure chapter)

Calcium channel blockers (see hypertension chapter)

Antiplatelet Drug Therapy

Aspirin
Mechanism of action
* Blocks prostaglandin synthesis, which prevents the formation of thromboxane A_2

Dose
* At the onset of chest pain: 160-325 mg chewed and swallowed
* Maintenance dose: 75-325 mg for life
* Monitoring parameters: signs of bleeding, renal function, tinnitus

Adverse drug reactions (Table 32)

Table 32

Aspirin Adverse Reactions

CV	Hypotension, edema, tachycardia
CNS	Fatigue, nervousness, dizziness
Dermatologic	Rash, urticaria, angioedema
GI	Nausea, vomiting, dyspepsia, gastrointestinal ulceration, gastric erosion, duodenal ulcers
Hematologic	Bleeding, anemia
Otic	Hearing loss, tinnitus
Renal	Renal impairment, increased serum creatinine, proteinuria
Respiratory	Asthma, bronchospasm, dyspnea, tachypnea, respiratory alkalosis

Drug-drug interactions
* Clopidogrel, GPI, UFH, LMWH, NSAIDs, and warfarin may all increase the risk of bleeding if used in combination with ASA.

Drug-disease interactions
* PUD
* Other active bleeding
    * May cause gastric ulceration
    * Recommend enteric-coated tablet

Patient instructions/counseling
* Avoid additional over-the-counter (OTC) products containing ASA, NSAIDs, or salicylate ingredients without the direction of a physician.
    * Patients who have received a stent will need the combination of clopidogrel and aspirin.
* Notify physician of dark, tarry stools, persistent stomach pain, difficulty breathing, unusual bruising or bleeding, or skin rash.
* Do not crush an enteric-coated product.

Thienopyridines
Mechanism of action
* Blocks adenosine diphosphate (ADP)-mediated activation of platelets by selectively and irreversibly blocking ADP activation of the glycoprotein IIb/IIIa complex

Dose
Clopidogrel
* Loading dose: 300-600 mg PO
* Maintenance dose
    * 75 mg daily combined with aspirin for up to 9 months in patients who did not undergo cardiac cath
    * 75 mg daily combined with aspirin for at least 1 month with BMS, 3 months for sirolimus-coated, and 6 months for paclitaxel-coated stents and possibly continued for up to one year.
    * 75 mg daily for life in patients with aspirin allergy
Ticlopidine
* Loading dose: 500 mg PO
* Maintenance dose: 250 mg bid
* Monitoring parameters
    * Clopidogrel: signs of bleeding
    * Ticlopidine: CBC with differential every 2 weeks for the first 3 months of therapy; liver function tests periodically; signs of bleeding
    * Discontinue ticlopidine if the absolute neutrophil count drops to <1200 or platelet count drops to <80,000.

Adverse drug reactions (Table 33)

Table 33

Thienopyridine Adverse Reactions

Clopidogrel	Chest pain, headache, dizziness, abdominal pain, vomiting, diarrhea, arthralgia, back pain, upper respiratory infections, flu-like symptoms; <1% blood dyscrasias, bleeding, rash
Ticlopidine	Rash, nausea, dyspepsia, diarrhea; 2.4% neutropenia; <1% blood dyscrasias, thrombotic thrombocytopenic purpura (TTP), bleeding

Table 34

Thienopyridine Drug-Drug Interactions

Interacting medication	Effect
ASA, GPI, UFH, LMWH, NSAIDs, warfarin	Combination may increase the risk of bleeding
CYP450-2C9 substrates (phenytoin, fluvastatin, NSAIDs, losartan, irbesartan, valsartan)	May have increased serum levels

Drug-drug interactions (Table 34)

Drug-disease interactions
• PUD or other active bleeding

Contraindications
• Hypersensitivity to an individual product
• Active bleeding (eg, PUD or intracranial hemorrhage)
• Severe liver disease
• Ticlopidine: neutropenia, thrombocytopenia

Patient instructions/counseling
• Combination with ASA is necessary in patients receiving stents
• Avoid additional ASA, salicylates, and NSAID products unless under the direction of a physician
• Notify physician for unusual bleeding or bruising, blood in the urine, stool, or emesis; skin rash or yellowing of the skin or eyes.
• Do not stop taking without discussing with physician.

Glycoprotein IIb/IIIa receptor inhibitors (GPI)
Mechanism of action
• Blockade of the GP receptor prevents fibrinogen bind-

Table 35

Pharmacologic Properties of the Glycoprotein IIb/IIIa Receptor Inhibitors

Drug	Chemical nature	Duration of effect	Renal elimination	Renal dosing adjustment
Abciximab (ReoPro®)	Antibody	>12 h. Note: action can be reversed by a platelet infusion	No	No
Eptifibatide (Integrilin®)	Nonpeptide	4-8 h	Yes	Yes
Tirofiban (Aggrastat®)	Peptide fragment	4 h	Yes	Yes

ing, thus inhibiting platelet aggregation; the receptor is the final common pathway for platelet aggregation.

Properties of individual agents (Table 35)

Indications and dose (Table 36)

Monitoring parameters
• Hematocrit/hemoglobin, platelet count, PT/aPTT, activated clotting time (ACT) with PCI

Adverse drug reactions
• Bleeding, thrombocytopenia, allergic reaction from repeated exposure (abciximab)

Drug-drug interactions
• ASA, clopidogrel, UFH, LMWH, NSAIDs and warfarin may increase the risk of bleeding if used in combination with GPI

Drug-disease interactions
• PUD or other active bleeding

Contraindications
• Active bleeding
• Platelet count <100,000
• History of intracranial hemorrhage, neoplasms, AV malformations, or aneurysm
• History of stroke within the past 30 days or any history of hemorrhage stroke
• Severe hypertension (BP >180/110 mm Hg)

Table 36

Indications and Doses of the Glycoprotein IIb/IIIa Receptor Inhibitors

Drug	Indication	Dose
Abciximab (ReoPro)	Adjunct to PCI or when PCI is planned within 24 hours	0.25 mg/kg IV bolus, 0.125 mg/kg infusion continued for 12 hours postprocedure; maximum length of infusion: 18-24 h
Eptifibatide (Integrilin)	Adjunct to PCI	180 mcg/kg IV bolus x 2, 10 minutes apart; 2 mcg/kg/min infusion (SCr >2 mg/dL or CrCl <50 mL/min; 1 mcg/kg/min) started after the 1st bolus and continued for 18-24 h postprocedure
	Patients with ACS managed with or without PCI	180 mcg/kg IV bolus, 2 mcg/kg/min infusion (SCr >2 mg/dL or CrCl <50 mL/kg; 1 mcg/kg/min) continued for 18-24 h postprocedure; maximum length of infusion: 96 hours
Tirofiban (Aggrastat)	Adjunct to PCI	0.4 mcg/kg IV bolus over 30 minutes, 0.1 mcg/kg/min infusion for 72 h; minimum infusion time: 48 h
		OR
	Patients with ACS managed with or without PCI	10 mcg/kg IV bolus over 3 minutes followed by 0.15 mcg/kg/min infusion for 36 h 0.4 mcg/kg IV bolus over 30 minutes, 0.1 mcg/kg/min infusion for 72 h *Note:* If CrCl <30 mL/min, bolus and infusion are reduced by 50%

- Major surgery within the past 6 weeks
- SCr >4 mg/dL or dialysis dependent (eptifibatide only)

Anticoagulants

Heparin
Mechanism of action
- Enhances the action of antithrombin III, thereby inactivating thrombin and preventing the conversion of fibrinogen to fibrin

Dose
- UA/NSTEMI: 60-70 units/kg (maximum 5000 units) IV bolus, 12-15 units/kg/h (maximum 1000 units/h) infusion titrated to an aPTT 1.5-2 times control
- STEMI (in combination with tPA, rPA or tenecteplase):
    * 60 units/kg (maximum 4000 units) IV bolus, 12 units/kg/h (maximum 1000 units/h) infusion
    * Titrate to an aPTT of 1.5-2 times control for 48 hours.

Monitoring parameters
- aPTT, PT, platelet count, hemoglobin/hematocrit, signs of bleeding, ACT (w/PCI)

Adverse drug reactions
- Bleeding, thrombocytopenia, hemorrhage, epistaxis, allergic reactions, osteoporosis.
- Protamine can be used to reverse the effects of heparin. Dose: 1 mg of protamine neutralizes 100 units of heparin.

Drug-drug interactions
- ASA, clopidogrel, GPI, NSAIDs, and warfarin may increase the risk of bleeding if used in combination with UFH.
- LMWH: combination may increase the risk of bleeding and has been reported to cause death.

Drug-disease interaction
- PUD or other active bleeding

Contraindications
- History of heparin-induced thrombocytopenia (HIT)
- Severe thrombocytopenia
- Active bleeding
- Suspected intracranial hemorrhage

Low molecular weight heparin (LMWH)
Mechanism of action
- Same mechanism as heparin; stronger inhibitor of thrombin (factor Xa)

Properties (Table 37)

Dose
- Enoxaparin (Lovenox): 1 mg/kg SC q12h (CrCl <30 mL/min: 1 mg/kg SC q24h)
- Dalteparin (Fragmin): 120 IU/kg q12h (maximum 10,000 IU q12h)

Monitoring parameters
- Platelet count, hemoglobin/hematocrit, anti-Xa levels, signs of bleeding
- *Note:* It is not necessary to monitor aPTT, PT.

Table 37

Properties of Low Molecular Weight Heparin versus Unfractionated Heparin

Drug	Half-life	MW (daltons)	Anti-Xa: Anti-IIa	Renal elimination
Enoxaparin	4.5 h	4500	2.7:1	Yes
Dalteparin	3-5 h	5000	2.0:1	Yes
UFH	1 h	15,000	1:1	No

Adverse drug reactions
• Bleeding, thrombocytopenia, hemorrhage, epistaxis

Drug-drug interactions
• ASA, clopidogrel, GPI, NSAIDs, and warfarin may increase the risk of bleeding if used in combination with LMWH.
• UFH: combination may increase the risk of bleeding and has been reported to cause death.

Drug-disease interactions
• PUD or any active bleeding.

Warnings
• Patients with recent or anticipated epidural or spinal anesthesia are at risk of hematoma and subsequent paralysis.

Contraindications
• Severe thrombocytopenia
• Active bleeding
• Suspected intracranial hemorrhage

Thrombolytic Therapy

Mechanism of action
• Acts either directly or indirectly to activate or convert plasminogen to plasmin to lyse a formed clot; the conversion of plasminogen to plasmin activates the body's natural thrombolytic/fibrinolytic system, which lyses the clot and releases fibrin degradation products.

Dose (Table 38)

Monitoring parameters
• CBC, ECG, aPTT, signs of bleeding, signs of reperfusion

Adverse drug reactions
• Bleeding, intracranial hemorrhage (<1%), stroke (<2%), epistaxis

Drug-drug interactions
• ASA, clopidogrel, GPI, UFH, LMWH, NSAIDs and warfarin may increase the risk of bleeding if used in combination with thrombolytics.

Table 38

Thrombolytic Doses

Drug	Dose
Streptokinase (SK, Streptase®)	1.5 million units in 50 mL of normal saline or D₅W given over 60 minutes
Tissue plasminogen activator (tPA, Alteplase®)	15-mg IV bolus, followed by 0.75-mg/kg IV infusion over 30 minutes (not to exceed 50 mg); then 0.5-mg/kg IV infusion over 1 hour (not to exceed 35 mg)
Reteplase (rPA, Retevase®)	10 U IVP over 2 minutes, followed in 30 minutes by a repeat 10-U IV bolus over 10 minutes
Tenecteplase (TNK, TNKase®)	<60 kg give 30-mg IV bolus; 60-69.9 kg give 35-mg IV bolus; 70-79.9 kg give 40-mg IV bolus; 80-89.9 kg give 45-mg IV bolus; >90 kg give 50-mg IV bolus; *Note:* Each bolus is given over 5 seconds

Contraindications (Table 39)

Table 39

Contraindications and Cautions for Fibrinolytic Use

Contraindications:
1. Any prior intracranial hemorrhage.
2. Known structural cerebrovascular lesion.
3. Ischemic stroke within 3 months; except acute ischemic stroke within 3 hours
4. Known intracranial neoplasm (primary or metastatic)
5. Active internal bleeding or bleeding diathesis (does not include menses)
6. Suspected aortic dissection
7. Significant closed head or facial trauma within 3 months

Relative contraindications:
1. Severe uncontrolled hypertension (BP >180/110 mm Hg)
2. History of prior ischemic stroke greater than 3 months, dementia, or known intracerebral pathology not covered in contraindications
3. Current use of anticoagulants in therapeutic doses (INR >2-3)
4. Traumatic or prolonged (>10 min) CPR or major surgery (<3 wk)
5. Noncompressible vascular punctures
6. Recent (within 2-4 weeks) internal bleeding
7. For streptokinase: prior exposure (especially within 5 d-2 y) or prior allergic reaction
8. Pregnancy
9. Active peptic ulcer
10. History of chronic severe hypertension

10. Key Points

- Angina is a syndrome described as discomfort or pain in the chest, arm, shoulder, back, or jaw. Angina is frequently worsened by physical exertion or emotional stress and is usually relieved by sublingual nitroglycerin (NTG). Patients with angina usually have coronary artery disease (CAD).
- Anginal symptoms are caused by a decrease in O_2 supply due to reduced flow.
- The goals for treating stable angina are to prevent death, reduce symptoms, and improve quality of life.
- Aspirin has been shown to decrease the incidence of MI, adverse CV events, and sudden death in patients with coronary artery disease.
- β-Blockers are first-line therapy for treatment of angina in patients with or without a history of MI if there are no contraindications.
- Patients prescribed nitrates for treatment of angina need to be counseled on their appropriate use.
- Upon hospital presentation with UA/NSTEMI/ STEMI, initial therapy for all patients is MONA (morphine, oxygen, nitroglycerin, and aspirin). If there are no contraindications, all patients should be given aspirin therapy for life.
- The first-line anti-ischemic therapy for the treatment of UA/NSTEMI is a β-blocker. If chest pain continues or a β-blocker is contraindicated, a calcium channel blocker or long-acting nitrate should be considered, in that order.
- In addition to aspirin therapy for life, clopidogrel should be administered to all patients who undergo stent replacement for at least 1 month after BMS, 3 months for sirolimus-coated, and 6 months for paclitaxel-coated stents and may be continued up to one year. Long-term treatment with clopidogrel may be beneficial in patients with established vascular disease. Clopidogrel should be withheld for 5-7 days prior to surgery to reduce the risk of major bleeding.
- Any of the available GP IIb/IIIa agents should be considered in patients undergoing a PCI procedure. In patients without a planned PCI, eptifibatide or tirofiban can be used for medical treatment.
- All patients presenting with UA/NSTEMI should receive anticoagulation with UFH or LMWH.
- STEMI differs from UA/NSTEMI in that there is a totally occlusive clot that causes damage across the entire thickness of the myocardial wall. The damage to the heart is more extensive with STEMI and ECG changes differ.
- Primary reperfusion (either percutaneous coronary intervention or fibrinolytic therapy) is the main treatment strategy for STEMI.
- Ventricular remodeling (post-MI) resulting after myocardial damage can be slowed and possibly reversed by using long-term ACE inhibition and β-blockade.
- Secondary prevention of MI should include aspirin, β-blockers, ACE inhibitors, and statin therapy (to achieve an LDL goal of <100 mg/dL; <70 mg/dL in high-risk patients) in all patients who have no contraindications.
- Aldosterone blockade should be considered post-STEMI in patients with an LVEF ≤40% and either symptomatic heart failure or diabetes.

11. Questions and Answers

Mr. Smith is a 66-year-old white male who presented to his local physician with complaints of chest pain. He described the pain as sharp, aching, and non-radiating. The pain, which he has had for the past few weeks, has occurred mainly during his daily walk and is usually relieved when he stops to rest.

PMH: HTN, PUD, asthma, CAD
FH: Father died of a stroke at 86; mother age 82 with DM, HF; sister died of MI at 52
SH: Smokes 1 ppd x 40 years; drinks alcohol socially 1-2 times a week
Meds: Proventil MDI 2 puffs prn
        Flovent 44 mcg 2 puffs bid
        Prilosec 20 mg qd
        Aspirin 75 mg qd
        HCTZ 25 mg qd
VS: BP 148/92; HR 82; RR 18; Ht 72"; Wt 200 lbs
Labs: (fasting) total cholesterol 226 mg/dL, TG 110 mg/dL, HDL 38 mg/dL, LDL 166 mg/dL, Chem 12-WNL
ECG: Normal (patient currently pain-free)
Cath 6 years ago: Minimal two-vessel disease.

1. How would you classify Mr. Smith's chest pain?

    A. Unstable angina
    B. Stable angina
    C. Variant angina
    D. Silent Ischemia
    E. NSTEMI

2. Considering Mr. Smith's situation, which of the following would be the most appropriate therapeutic intervention?

    A. SL NTG prn
    B. Propranolol
    C. Tirofiban
    D. Verapamil and SL NTG prn
    E. Atenolol, amlodipine and SL NTG

3. What additional medication should be considered for Mr. Smith?

    A. Ticlopidine
    B. Atorvastatin
    C. Clopidogrel
    D. Eptifibatide
    E. Reteplase

4. Which of the following effects on myocardial oxygen demand do β-blockers NOT cause?

    A. Decrease HR
    B. Decrease BP
    C. Decrease contractility
    D. Peripheral vasodilation
    E. Decrease conduction through the AV node

5. Which of the following statements is true regarding the use of calcium channel blockers in IHD?

    A. Amlodipine and felodipine reduce MVO_2 by decreasing conduction through the AV node
    B. They should be used as first-line therapy in patients with stable angina
    C. Newer-generation dihydropyridines like nifedipine immediate-release are safe in the treatment of IHD
    D. Can use in combination with β-blockers to attenuate the effect of increased sympathetic tone that some dihydropyridines may cause
    E. The combination of verapamil and metoprolol in a patient with reduced LV systolic function is safe and well-tolerated by most patients

6. Which of the following counseling points should be made to a patient being prescribed SL NTG?

    I.   Take at the same time each day as directed
    II. Keep tablets in their original container
    III. Take at the first sign of chest pain; if chest pain is unrelieved, seek emergency medical attention

    A. III only
    B. I, II, and III
    C. I and III only
    D. I and II only
    E. II and III only

7. Which of the following are not considered potential cardiovascular benefits of ACE inhibitors in IHD?

    A. Reduce the incidence of MI
    B. Reduce the incidence of CV death and stroke in patients at high risk for vascular disease
    C. Agents with high tissue ACE inhibition have been proven to be superior and provide better protection
    D. ACE inhibitors should be used in all stable angina patients with known CAD who also have diabetes
    E. ACE inhibitors have shown greater benefit post-MI in higher-risk patients

8. Which of the following drugs do not appear to interact with an exercise tolerance test (ETT)?

   A. Nitrates
   B. Digoxin
   C. Atenolol
   D. Flecainide
   E. Clopidogrel

9. Ideal properties for a β-blocker in the treatment of UA/NSTEMI include all of the following, EXCEPT

   A. available in both IV and PO forms
   B. low lipophilicity
   C. has intrinsic sympathomimetic activity (ISA)
   D. does not have ISA
   E. cardioselectivity

10. Nitrates decrease oxygen demand via the following mechanism(s):

   I. Peripheral vasodilation
   II. Arterial vasodilation
   III. Decreasing contractility

   A. I only
   B. II only
   C. I and II only
   D. II and III only
   E. I, II, and III

11. The possible benefits of LMWH over UFH include all of the following EXCEPT

   A. predictable response
   B. ease of administration
   C. no recommended routine monitoring
   D. stronger affinity for thrombin
   E. no renal adjustment necessary

12. Which of the following β-blocker has ISA activity?

   A. Tenormin
   B. Sectral
   C. Inderal
   D. Lopressor
   E. Coreg

13. Which of the following medications is contraindicated within 24 hours of a nitrate?

   A. Metoprolol
   B. Quinapril
   C. Verapamil

   D. Sildenafil
   E. Felodipine

14. The preferred narcotic to relieve chest pain after the use of SL NTG is:

   A. meperidine
   B. oxycodone
   C. morphine
   D. hydromorphone
   E. fentanyl

Questions 15 and 16 refer to this case:
J.O. is a 54-year-old male who presents to the hospital with crushing substernal chest pain and radiation to his left arm. Past medical history is significant for HTN, COPD, and gout. J.O. has a history of smoking x 30 years and occasionally consumes alcohol. Vital signs on admission include BP 170/85; Pulse 72; RR 18; Temp 97. Before admission the patient was taking enteric coated aspirin 81 mg qd; Combivent inhaler two puffs qid; Tiazac 240 mg qd; allopurinol 300-mg qd.

Allergies: sulfa
Lab/diagnostic tests:
1. ECG: ST-segment depression, T-wave changes
2. Troponin: T-positive x 3
3. Ejection fraction: <35%
4. LDL: 135 mg/dL

Diagnosis:
1. NSTEMI
2. Heart Failure

15. What is the preferred β-blocker for this patient?

   A. Propranolol
   B. Carvedilol
   C. Labetalol
   D. Atenolol
   E. Nadolol

16. All of the following therapies should be considered in this patient, EXCEPT

   A. reteplase
   B. clopidogrel
   C. enalapril
   D. simvastatin
   E. eptifibatide

Questions #17-18 refer to this case:

S.D. is a 56-year-old female who presents to the local ER complaining of crushing, substernal CP x 3 hours, which has been unrelieved by SL NTG. PMH is pertinent for HTN, T2DM, hypercholesterolemia, and metabolic syndrome. Heart rate and rhythm are regular and no S$_3$ or S$_4$ sounds are present. Vital signs include BP 184/119, HR 100, and RR 32/min. S.D.'s ECG shows ST-segment elevation >1 mm in leads II, III, and aVF. She is immediately admitted to the chest pain center and started on oxygen.

17. Which of the following criteria for the diagnosis of MI are present in S.D.?

    A. Chest pain symptoms relieved by SL NTG
    B. ST-segment elevation >1 mm in two or more noncontiguous leads
    C. Chest pain symptoms with ECG changes that are consistent with myocardial ischemia or necrosis
    D. S.D. does not meet the criteria for MI based on the above presentation, because myocardial enzymes have not been evaluated
    E. Since S.D. has negative enzymes, MI is ruled out

18. Which of the following agents should be administered to S.D.?

    A. tPA 100 mg IV over 90 minutes
    B. IV magnesium
    C. Prophylactic lidocaine
    D. Metoprolol 5 mg IV
    E. Cardizem 240 mg

19. What medications should a patient who is post-MI with preserved LVEF receive as discharge therapy?

    A. Aspirin, Plavix, Cardizem, and simvastatin
    B. Aspirin, metoprolol, enalapril, atorvastatin, and SL NTG
    C. Plavix, metoprolol, enalapril, and simvastatin
    D. Morphine, aspirin, SL NTG, and Lovenox
    E. Morphine, IV NTG, aspirin, and oxygen

20. The anticoagulant effect of unfractionated heparin requires the binding to which plasma co-factor?

    A. Thrombospondin
    B. Antithrombin III
    C. Plasminogen
    D. Factor XIIa
    E. Factors II, VII, IX, and X

S.P. is a 45-year-old marathon runner. He presents to the emergency department with complaints of chest pain during his morning run. His father died of a myocardial infarction at age 48. His past medical history is positive for angina, hyperlipidemia, and hypertension. His current medications include aspirin, pravastatin, nifedipine, and clonidine. His electrocardiogram is consistent with acute ischemia. His HR is 52/min and BP is 170/100. CBC and Chem-7 are within normal limits.

21. All of the following interventions are appropriate for S.P. EXCEPT

    A. enoxaparin 1 mg/kg SC bid
    B. IV metoprolol followed by PO metoprolol
    C. nitroglycerin SL prn and IV drip titrated to pain and blood pressure
    D. continue aspirin
    E. morphine if NTG does not control the pain

22. Which one of the following agents is not indicated in the setting of STEMI when pharmacologic reperfusion is the planned strategy?

    A. Eptifibatide
    B. LMWH
    C. Aspirin
    D. tPA
    E. Metoprolol

23. Which of the following agents would not be administered at the same time as heparin?

    A. tPA
    B. Reteplase
    C. Eptifibatide
    D. TNKase
    E. Streptokinase

24. Which of the following statements about the GPIs is NOT true?

    A. Abciximab, eptifibatide, and tirofiban are all administered as a bolus followed by a continuous infusion
    B. It is possible to experience an allergic reaction after repeat exposure of abciximab
    C. Eptifibatide, tirofiban, and abciximab can all be reversed by a platelet infusion
    D. Tirofiban and eptifibatide are renally eliminated; therefore, dosage adjustment is required for patients with renal dysfunction
    E. Abciximab, eptifibatide, and tirofiban are all indicated as adjuncts to PCI

Answers

1. **B.** Angina is considered stable if symptoms have been occurring for several weeks without worsening, it lasts <30 minutes, and is relieved by rest or SL NTG.

2. **D.** This regimen will help control his angina without β_2-blocking effects in this asthmatic patient, as well as lower his BP. SL NTG will be useful for acute attacks. **A** is not the best answer, as this patient also needs a medication to lower his BP. **B** is incorrect, as propranolol is not β_1-selective and could worsen his asthma. **C** is incorrect, as GP IIb/IIIa inhibitors are not indicated in stable angina. **E** is incorrect; combination therapy is not recommended as first-line therapy and should only be considered when initial treatment with a β-blocker is not successful.

3. **B.** Mr. Smith has an elevated LDL with known heart disease and he needs to be treated to a goal LDL of <100 mg/dL (consider LDL <70 mg/dL). **A** and **C** are incorrect; these antiplatelet agents are not indicated for treating stable angina unless a patient cannot tolerate aspirin. **D** and **E** are incorrect, as glycoprotein IIb/IIIa inhibitors and thrombolytics are not indicated in stable angina.

4. **D.** β-Blockers do not cause peripheral vasodilation like nitrates or calcium channel blockers.

5. **D.** The increased sympathetic tone caused by some dihydropyridines can lead to a reflex tachycardia, which would be detrimental in an IHD patient. Therefore, using a β-blocker to block this effect would be desirable. **A** is incorrect; the dihydropyridines do not decrease conduction through the AV node like verapamil or diltiazem. **B** is incorrect; CCBs are not indicated as first-line therapy unless a patient has a contraindication to a β-blocker. **E** is incorrect, as both verapamil and metoprolol can lead to worsening systolic function, and used in combination would be unsafe.

6. **E.** SL NTG should be kept in the original amber bottle, as exposure to light or extreme temperatures will cause it to lose potency. III is correct and patients should be counseled to take 1 tablet and seek medical attention if chest pain is not relieved. I is incorrect; SL NTG is used on a prn basis and should not be taken at the same time each day.

7. **C.** It has not been proven that so-called "tissue" ACE inhibitors are better than other ACE inhibitors.

8. **E.** Clopidogrel, or Plavix, does not have any pharmacologic interaction with an ETT. Digoxin can cause an abnormal exercise-induced ST depression in ~30% of healthy patients. β-Blockers and vasodilators can alter hemodynamic response to BP and should be withdrawn gradually 4-5 half-lives before ETT. Nitrates can attenuate angina and flecainide may cause exercise-induced ventricular tachycardia.

9. **C.** It has ISA. β-Blockers with ISA reduce heart rate to a lesser degree than non-ISA β-blockers, thus producing a smaller decrease in oxygen demand. Ideally, a β-blocker used for the treatment of UA/NSTEMI would be available in IV and PO formulations. In addition, it would have β_1-receptor selectivity, no ISA, and low lipophilicity.

10. **C.** Nitrates are vasodilators acting on both arteries and in the periphery, thereby decreasing preload and afterload. As far as anti-ischemic therapy, only β-blockers and nondihydropyridine calcium channel blockers reduce contractility.

11. **E.** Renal adjustment is necessary with LMWH. UFH does not require dosage adjustment in renal patients and is preferred to LMWH in patients with a CrCl <30 mL/min. LMWH does appear to have advantages over UFH in ease of administration, its affinity to thrombin (stronger than UFH), its more predictable response, and the fact that it does not require monitoring.

12. **B.** β-Blockers with ISA activity include Sectral (acebutolol), Cartrol (carteolol), Levatol (penbutolol), and Visken (pindolol). Tenormin (atenolol), Inderal (propranolol), Lopressor (metoprolol), and Coreg (carvedilol) do not have ISA activity.

13. **D.** Sildenafil. Viagra (sildenafil) use is contraindicated within 24 hours of a nitrate. Likewise, if sildenafil has been used within 24 hours, a nitrate cannot be used. β-Blockers (metoprolol), ACE inhibitors (quinapril), and calcium channel blockers (verapamil, felodipine) can be safely combined with nitrates.

14. **C.** Morphine. Morphine has vasodilator properties, thereby decreasing both preload and afterload, which decreases oxygen demand. In addition, morphine lowers heart rate by relieving pain and anxiety. If a true morphine allergy exists, meperidine may be used as an alternate agent. Oxycodone, hydromorphone, and fentanyl are not recommended for the treatment of anginal pain.

15. **D.** Atenolol. With the patient's history of COPD, a β-blocker with $β_1$-receptor selectivity is preferred. The only agent with $β_1$-selectivity in this list is atenolol. All of the remaining agents are nonselective.

16. **A.** Reteplase. Reteplase is a thrombolytic agent, which does not have a role in the treatment of NSTEMI. Thrombolytic therapy is indicated for the treatment of STEMI. Clopidogrel and GPI (eptifibatide) should be considered in all patients with NSTEMI with or without PCI. Eptifibatide and tirofiban can be used in patients who are medically managed; abciximab is reserved for patients with a scheduled PCI procedure. Lipid-lowering therapy with an HMG-CoA reductase inhibitor (eg, simvastatin) should be initiated in this patient due to his LDL level of >130 mg/dL. This patient has a clear indication for an ACE inhibitor (enalapril) due to his EF of <40%.

17. **C.** A is incorrect, as chest pain unrelieved by NTG is a diagnostic criterion for MI, but two criteria must be present before the diagnosis can be made. B is incorrect because ST-segment elevation >1 mm must be found in two or more contiguous leads. S.D. has both CP symptoms and ECG changes that are consistent with myocardial infarction. C is correct because she meets two of the three criteria for diagnosing MI. S.D. does not have positive enzymes, which would meet the third diagnostic criteria. D is incorrect because positive enzymes do not have to be present for the diagnosis of MI to be made (as in the case with S.D.).

18. **D.** One of the relative contraindications to fibrinolytic therapy is severe uncontrolled hypertension (BP >180/110 mm Hg). **A** is not appropriate in this patient with BP of 184/119 mm Hg. Routine use of magnesium post-MI is not recommended and should only be reserved for patients with hypomagnesemia. No labs were given for S.D., so answer **B** is not appropriate at

this time. Prophylactic lidocaine has been shown to increase all-cause mortality, and is not recommended in the early management of STEMI for prevention of VF. Therefore, **C** is incorrect. β-Blockers reduce the incidence of ventricular arrhythmias, recurrent ischemia, reinfarction, infarct size, and mortality in patients with STEMI. Since S.D. does not have any contraindications to β-blockade, **D** is the correct choice. **E**, calcium channel blockers, do not have a role in STEMI when a β-blocker can be given.

19. **B.** ACE inhibitors, β-blockers, aspirin, statin therapy, and SL NTG should be given to all patients without contraindications post-MI. Plavix can be combined with aspirin, and can be continued for 1 to 9 months. All of the answers including Plavix are incorrect, however, because **A** omits β-blockade, and **C** omits aspirin therapy. Calcium channel blockers can be given if a patient has contraindications to β-blockade, but it is not recommended as first-line treatment. Answers **D** and **E** are incorrect because ACE inhibition and β-blockade are omitted. Answer **E** would be a correct choice for the immediate treatment of someone who presents with STEMI, but not as discharge medications.

20. **B.** Heparin's anticoagulant effect requires binding to antithrombin (previously antithrombin III), and that binding converts antithrombin from a slow, progressive thrombin inhibitor to a very rapid inhibitor of thrombin and factor Xa.

21. **B.** One of the contraindications to β-blockade is a HR <55 bpm. Since S.P. has a HR of 52 bpm at this time, the only inappropriate therapy out of the above choices would be **B**. Enoxaparin, NTG, morphine, and aspirin are all therapies that should be continued.

22. **A.** GP IIb/IIIa inhibition is still controversial in the setting of STEMI, especially when a fibrinolytic agent is administered. The role of platelet GPI in STEMI is rapidly evolving, and trials to date in combination with full- and half-dose fibrinolytic agents have shown a more complete reperfusion at the price of higher bleeding rates. At this point, there is no formal recommendation on using eptifibatide or another GPI in STEMI.

23. **E.** A GPI should be administered with heparin, and therefore **C** is not the correct answer. Combination of UFH with streptokinase (SK) is less desirable because it is a nonspecific fibrinolytic, and UFH may increase the risk of bleeding because of SK's long half-life. Therefore, answer **E** is the correct choice. Heparin should be administered for at least 48 hours with the other lytic choices to reduce risk of reocclusion.

24. **C.** The only GPI that is reversed by a platelet infusion is abciximab. All of the remaining selections are true statements. All of the available GPI agents are administered as a bolus and infusion. **A**, abciximab, is a monoclonal antibody; therefore it is possible to develop an allergic reaction upon rechallenge. There are only two GPIs that are renally eliminated: eptifibatide and tirofiban. All of the agents are indicated as adjunct to PCI, so **E** is true.

12. References

American Heart Association. Heart Disease and Stroke Statistics—2005 Update. Dallas, TX: American Heart Association; 2005.

Antman EM, Anbe DT, Armstrong PW, et al. ACC/AHA guidelines for the management of patients with ST-elevation myocardial infarction: a report of the American College of Cardiology/American Heart Association Task Force on Practice Guidelines (Committee to revise the 1999 guidelines for the management of patients with acute myocardial infarction). 2004. Available at www.acc.org/clinical/guidelines/stemi/index.pdf.

Aspirin therapy in diabetes. *Diabetes Care.* 2004;27: 72S-73S.

Braunwald E, Antman EM, Beasley JW, et al. ACC/AHA 2002 guideline update for the management of patients with unstable angina and non-ST-segment elevation myocardial infarction. A report of the American College of Cardiology/American Heart Association Task Force on Practice Guidelines (Committee on the Management of Patients with Unstable Angina). *Circulation.* 2002;106:1893-1900. Available at: http://www.acc.org/clinical/guidelines/unstable/incorporated/index.htm

Dagenais GR, Yusuf S, Bourassa MG, et al. Effects of Ramipril on Coronary Events in High-risk persons. Results from the Heart Outcomes Prevention Evaluation Study. *Circulation.* 2001;104:522-526.

Deepak LB, Fox KA, Hacke W, et al. Clopidogrel and aspirin versus aspirin alone for the prevention of atherothrombotic events. *N Engl J Med.* 2006;354: 1706-1717.

Ginnons RJ, Abrams J, Chatterjee K, et al. ACC/AHA 2002 guideline update for the management of patients with chronic stable angina: A report of the American College of Cardiology/American Heart Association Task Force on Practice Guidelines (Committee to Update the 1999 Guidelines for the Management of Patients with Chronic Stable Angina), 2002. Available at: http://www.acc.org/clinical/guidelines/stable/stable.pdf.

Grundy SM, Cleeman JI, Berz NB, et al. Implications of recent clinical trials for the national cholesterol education program adult treatment panel III guidelines. *Circulation.* 2004;110:227-239.

Hirsh J, Anand S, Halperin JL. Guide to anticoagulant therapy: heparin. A statement for healthcare professionals from the American Heart Association. *Circulation.* 2001;103:2994-3018.

Malinow MR, Bostom AG, Krauss RM. Homocysteine, diet, and cardiovascular diseases. *Circulation.* 1999;99:178-182.

Mehta SR, Yusuf S, Peter RJ, et al. Effects of pretreatment with clopidogrel and aspirin followed by long-term therapy in patients undergoing percutaneous coronary intervention: the PCI-CURE study. *Lancet.* 2001;358:527-533.

Meister FL, Stringer KA, Spinler SA, et al. Thrombolytic therapy for acute myocardial infarction. *Pharmacotherapy.* 1998;18:686-698.

Ridker PM, Cook NR, Lee I-M, et al. A randomized trial of low-dose aspirin in the primary prevention of cardiovascular disease in women. *N Engl J Med.* 2005;352:1293-1304.

Smith SC, Blair SN, Bonow RO, et al. AHA/ACC Guidelines for Preventing Heart Attack and Death in Patients with Atherosclerotic Cardiovascular Disease: 2001 Update. *Circulation.* 2001;104:1577-1579.

Steinhubl SR, Berger PB, Mann JT, et al. Early and sustained dual oral antiplatelet therapy following percutaneous coronary intervention. A randomized controlled trial. *JAMA.* 2002;288:2411-2420.

Stringer KA, Lopez LM. Acute myocardial infarction. In: DiPiro JT, Talbert RL, Hayes PE, et al, eds. *Pharmacotherapy: A Pathophysiologic Approach,* 3rd ed. Norwalk, CT: Appleton & Lange; 1997:295-322.

Summary of the Second Report of the National Cholesterol Education Program (NCEP). Expert Panel on Detection, Evaluation, and Treatment of High Blood Cholesterol in Adults (Adult Treatment Panel III). *JAMA.* 2001;285:2486-2497.

Talbert RL. Ischemic heart disease. In: DiPiro JT, Talbert RL, Yee GC, Martzke GR, et al, eds. *Pharmacotherapy: A Pathophysiologic Approach,* 5th ed. New York: McGraw-Hill; 2002:219-250.

The EURopean trial On reduction of cardiac events with Perindopril in stable coronary Artery disease investigators. Efficacy of perindopril in reduction of cardiovascular events among patients with stable coronary artery disease: randomized, double-blind, placebo-controlled, multicenter trial (the EUROPA study). *Lancet.* 2003;362:782-788.

The PEACE trial investigators. Angiotensin-converting enzyme inhibition in stable coronary artery disease. *N Engl J Med.* 2004;351:2058-2068.

The Seventh ACCP Consensus Conference on Antithrombotic Therapy. *Chest.* 2004;126:163S-703S.

Wong GC, Giugliano RP, Antman EM. Use of low-molecular-weight heparins in the management of acute coronary artery syndromes and percutaneous coronary intervention. *JAMA.* 2003;289:331-342.

12. Hyperlipidemia

Lawrence Brown, PharmD, PhD
Assistant Professor
Department of Pharmaceutical Sciences
University of Tennessee College of Pharmacy

Contents

1. Hyperlipidemia

- **Hyperlipidemia** is an elevation in the blood concentration of a lipid such as cholesterol or triglyceride (in the form of lipoprotein).
- **Dyslipidemia** refers to any lipid disorder.
- **Lipids** include cholesterol, triglycerides (TG), and phospholipids.
- Lipoproteins: apolipoproteins + cholesterol + triglyceride + phospholipids
- Major lipoproteins are chylomicrons, very-low density lipoproteins (VLDL), intermediate-density lipoproteins (IDL), low-density lipoproteins (LDL), high-density lipoproteins (HDL), and lipoprotein (a).
- Apolipoproteins: structural components of lipoproteins
- Friederwald equation: formula used to calculate LDL:

$$LDL = \text{total cholesterol} - (HDL + TG/5)$$

Classification of Lipids

- Total cholesterol, LDL, HDL, and triglycerides are measured in mg/dL.
- ATP III: Adult Treatment Panel III recommendations from the National Cholesterol Education Program [NCEP] are shown in Table 1.

Clinical Presentation

- Hyperlipidemia can cause atherosclerosis, atheroma formation, atherothrombosis, and the subsequent consequences of these disease processes:
  - * Coronary artery disease (angina and myocardial infarction)
  - * Cerebrovascular disease (TIA and/or stroke)
  - * Peripheral arterial disease (intermittent claudication)
  - * A state of elevated lipids alone generally promotes no symptoms except in some familial lipid disorders, in which there may be cutaneous manifestations of lipid deposition (eg, tendon xanthomas, planar xanthomas, xanthelasmas, and eye manifestations [corneal arcus]).

Pathophysiology of Atherosclerosis

- Progressive, systemic disease starting early in life
  - * Atheroma lesions, called fatty streaks, develop in the arterial vascular walls and result from the accumulation of cholesterol within vessel walls.

Table 1

Classification of Lipids

LDL cholesterol: primary target of therapy

<100	Optimal
100-129	Near optimal/above optimal
130-159	Borderline high
160-189	High
≥190	Very high

Total cholesterol

<200	Desirable
200-239	Borderline high
≥240	High

HDL cholesterol

<40	Low
≥60	High

Triglycerides: secondary target of therapy after LDL

<150	Normal
150-199	Borderline high
200-499	High
>500	Very high

- * Atheroma lesions may lead to occlusion by thrombus or embolus formation.
- * LDL cholesterol accumulates below the intimal surface of the artery. General guideline: the higher the cholesterol elevation in the blood, the more LDL migrates into the artery.
- * Endothelial dysfunction occurs, and this increases LDL cholesterol's permeability.
- * LDL becomes oxidized and recruits monocytes.
- * Monocytes are transformed into macrophages and ingest the oxidized LDL.
- * This process results in lipid-filled cells called foam cells.
- * Foam cells are the initial lesion of atherosclerosis. Growth factors are produced by macrophages.
- * Other processes are also occurring (eg, additional endothelial cell injury and inflammatory responses that can further accelerate the development of plaque).
- * Elevated cholesterol and hyperlipidemia enhance this process.
- * Plaque may continue to develop, may become stable, or it may rupture.

* Plaque rupture exposes atherogenic materials in the lesion to blood.
* Platelets are activated and a clot may form.
* Partial occlusion or obstruction can result in angina; complete occlusion results in myocardial infarction.
* Other vascular beds promote similar outcomes.

Diagnostic Criteria

• Lipid disorders (dyslipidemias) are classified as familial or secondary.
  * Familial disorders usually are caused by a defect in lipid metabolism.
    • Categorized into the hypercholesterolemias and the combined hyperlipidemias
    • Assessment of fasting lipid panels provides diagnostic information and classification of lipid disorders.
    • Familial hypercholesterolemia (FH): LDL = 250-450 mg/dL
    • Familial defective apolipoprotein B-100
    • Polygenic hypercholesterolemia is the most common form (LDL = 160-250 mg/dL)
  * Combined hyperlipidemias:
    • Familial combined hyperlipidemia (FCH): (LDL = 160-250 mg/dL and triglycerides = 200-800 mg/dL)
    • Familial hyperapobetalipoproteinemia
    • Hypoalphalipoproteinemia
    • Dysbetalipoproteinemia
    • Elevated Lp(a)
• These disorders are characterized by variations in the amounts of LDL, IDL, VLDL, and HDL.
• The most common secondary causes of lipid disorders:
  * Diabetes mellitus
  * Hypothyroidism
  * Renal failure
  * Obstructive liver disease
  * Drugs such as β-blockers, thiazide diuretics, oral contraceptives, oral estrogens, glucocorticosteroids, and cyclosporinc
• Risk factors are used to assess the potential for an individual to develop coronary heart disease (CHD) or another equivalent atherosclerotic process over the next 10 years. The Framingham Global Risk Score is calculated to provide this information. The major nonlipid risk factors for CHD are counted and used to assess the 10-year risk of developing CHD.
• Major nonlipid risk factors for CHD:
  * Cigarette smoking
  * Hypertension (BP ≥140/90 mm Hg or on antihypertensive medication)
  * Low HDL cholesterol (<40 mg/dL)
  * Family history of premature CHD (CHD in a male first-degree relative aged <55 years and CHD in a female first-degree relative aged <65 years)
  * Age (men ≥45 years; women ≥55 years)
• HDL ≥60 mg/dL counts as a negative risk factor and acts to remove one of the other risk factors from the total count.

Treatment Principles

• Treatment and target lipid goals are based on the estimation of risk for coronary heart disease using the Framingham Global Risk Score.
• If a patient has a form of clinical CHD, such as angina, myocardial infarction, stroke, or transient ischemic attack, he or she is considered to be at high risk for another ischemic event within the next 10 years.
• Those at highest risk require the most aggressive therapy (ie, drug therapy and achieving the lowest possible LDL level). The major nonlipid risk factors above are used in the risk analysis for those individuals who do not have CHD or a CHD risk equivalent. Table 2 identifies risk categories, lipid goals, and risk of event.
• Treatment consists of lifestyle changes, ie, therapeutic lifestyle changes (TLC), which are discussed in the nonpharmacologic and pharmacotherapy sections of this chapter.
• Algorithm for drug therapy in primary prevention (<20% risk):
  * Initiate LDL-lowering drug therapy (statins, niacin, resin) for 6 weeks. If LDL goal is not met, intensify LDL-lowering therapy (higher dose or combination) for 6 weeks. If LDL goal is still not achieved, intensify drug therapy or

Table 2

Risk Categories, Lipid Goals, and Risk of Event

Risk category	LDL goal	Risk of event
CHD and CHD risk equivalent[1]	<100 mg/dL	>20% over 10 years
Multiple risk factors (2+)	<130 mg/dL	10-20% over 10 years
0-1 Risk factor	<160 mg/dL	<10% over 10 years

[1]CHD risk equivalent = clinical CHD, symptomatic carotid artery disease, peripheral arterial disease, abdominal aortic aneurysm, and diabetes.

refer to a lipid specialist for 4-6 months. Monitor response and adherence.
- Drug therapy in secondary prevention (>20% risk):
  * The most aggressive treatment is required.
  * A large LDL reduction requires a statin and possibly a statin in combination with another agent. Follow the same algorithm as outlined in primary prevention above.

Monitoring (Clinical Evaluation)

- Screening: The National Cholesterol Education Program (NCEP) Adult Treatment Panel III (ATP III) recommends that starting at age 20, adults receive a fasting lipid profile (FLP). If this is normal, then repeat in 5 years.
- Children do not need to be screened without the presence of significant family history or other reasons to test the lipids.

Monitoring

- The main tool is fasting lipid profile (FLP).
  * Baseline FLP is done before drug or dietary interventions.
  * After therapeutic lifestyle changes and/or drug therapy is started, monitor every 6 weeks times two initially, again in 4-6 months, and then periodically thereafter (usually annually). Results of FLP will show the effects of lifestyle and drug therapy interventions and help direct changes in therapy.

2. Drug Therapy

- See Tables 3, 4, and 5 for details on dosing, efficacy, and drug combinations.

Statins
- Conduct baseline liver function tests (LFTs) and creatine kinase (CK) before therapy is initiated. LFTs should be repeated again in 4-6 weeks, at 3 months, and then periodically (usually annually).
- Creatine kinase needs to be monitored only if the patient has suspected muscle damage.
- Assess effectiveness at 6 weeks.

Resins
- Determine baseline FLP to screen for hypertriglyceridemia.
  * If TG >200 mg/dL, use with caution.
  * Contraindicated if TG >400 mg/dL
- Assess effectiveness at 6 weeks.

Nicotinic acid
- Determine baseline fasting glucose, LFTs, and serum uric acid levels before initiating therapy.
- Repeat these tests 4-6 weeks after each dose level is reached.
- Sustained-release niacin requires monthly LFT readings while dosage is titrated; subsequent LFT readings should occur every 12 weeks for the first year and then periodically.
- Diabetics require routine fasting glucose tests.
- Monitor serum uric acid after the highest dose level is achieved in those with a history of hyperuricemia or gout.
- Assess effectiveness at 6 weeks.

Fibric acids
- Determine baseline fasting lipid panel (total cholesterol, HDL, LDL, and TG) before therapy and again at 3 and 6 months.
- Monitor changes in triglycerides at 3 months and assess effectiveness.

Cholesterol inhibitors
- Determine baseline lipid panel.
- Assess effectiveness at 6 weeks.

Mechanism of Action

HMG-CoA reductase inhibitors (statins)
- Competitively inhibit HMG-CoA reductase, which is the enzyme responsible for conversion of HMG-CoA to mevalonate.
- Mevalonate is an early precursor and a rate-limiting step in cholesterol synthesis. This reduction in liver

Table 3

Drug Products and Dosage

Generic name (trade name)	Dosage range and schedule	Dosage form and strength
Statins		
Atorvastatin (Lipitor)	10-80 mg/d qhs	10-, 20-, 40-, 80-mg tablet
Fluvastatin (Lescol)	20-80 mg/d qhs	20- and 40-mg capsule; 80-mg XL tablet
Lovastatin (Mevacor)	20-80 mg/d qhs	10-, 20-, 40-mg tablet
Lovastatin extended-release (Altoprev)	10-60 mg/d qhs	10-, 20-, 40-, 60-mg tablet
Pravastatin (Pravachol)	20-80 mg/d qhs	10-, 20-, 40-, 80-mg tablet
Simvastatin (Zocor)	20-80 mg/d qhs	5-, 10-, 20-, 40-, 80-mg tablet
Rosuvastatin (Crestor)	5-40 mg/d hs	5-, 10-, 20-, 40-mg tablet
Bile acid sequestrants		
Cholestyramine (Questran)	4-16 g/d divided	Powder
Colestipol (Colestid)	5-20 g/d divided	Powder/tablet
Colesevelam (WelChol)	2.6-3.8 g/d (once or bid)	625-mg tablet
Nicotinic acid		
Immediate release (Niacor)	1.5-3 g/d (divided tid)	500-mg tablet
Sustained release (Slo-Niacin)	1-2 g/d qhs	250-, 500-, 750-mg tablet
Extended release (Niaspan)	1-2 g/d qhs	500-, 750-, 1000-mg tablet
Fibric acids		
Gemfibrozil (Lopid)	600 mg before meals bid	600-mg tablet
Fenofibrate (Tricor)	48-145 mg/d	48-, 145-mg tablet
Cholesterol inhibitors		10-mg tablet
Ezetimibe (Zetia)	10 mg/d	
Combinations		
Aspirin + pravastatin (Pravigard PAC)	81/20-325/80 mg qhs	81/20-, 81/40-, 81/80-mg tablets
		325/20-, 325/40, 325/80-mg tablets
		(Note: Aspirin tablets and pravastatin tablets are separate tablets within the PAC)
Ezetimibe + simvastatin (Vytorin)	10/10-10/80 mg qhs	10/10-, 10/20-, 10/40-, 10/80-mg tablet
Lovastatin + Niaspan (Advicor)	20/500-40/2000 mg/d	20/500-, 20/750-, 20/1000-mg tablets

[Handwritten margin notes: SE ↑ BS ↑ LFT ↑ Uric Acid]

cholesterol synthesis results in upregulation of liver LDL receptors and increased clearance of LDL and VLDL particles in the blood. These actions induce a decrease in total cholesterol and LDL cholesterol, promote a slight increase in HDL cholesterol, and affect a modest decrease in triglycerides.

Bile acid sequestrants (BAS or resins)
- Nonabsorbable anion exchange resins exchange chloride ions for bile acids and other anions in the intestine.

- This inhibits enterohepatic recycling, which results in bile excretion and a decrease in the cholesterol pool in the liver.
- LDL receptors are upregulated, increased LDL is cleared, and LDL is lowered.

Niacin
- Reduces LDL cholesterol and triglycerides, increases HDL
- May decrease VLDL synthesis, thereby leading to decreased LDL cholesterol and triglycerides
- Niacin may inhibit metabolism of apolipoprotein A-I, which increases HDL cholesterol.

Table 4

Efficacy of Drugs Used to Treat Hyperlipidemia

Drug class	Lipid/lipoprotein effect
Statins	LDL ↓18-55%
	HDL ↑5-15%
	TG ↓7-30%
Resins	LDL ↓15-30%
	HDL ↑3-5%
	TG (no change)
Nicotinic acid	LDL ↓5-25%
	HDL ↑15-35%
	TG ↓20-50%
Fibric acids	LDL ↓5-20%
	HDL ↑10-20%
	TG ↓20-50%
Cholesterol inhibitors	LDL ↓17%
	HDL ↓1.3%
	TG ↓6%

Fibric acids (fibrates)
- Reduce triglycerides by reduction of apolipoproteins B, C-III, and E
- Increase HDL by increasing apolipoproteins A-I and A-II

Cholesterol inhibitors (ezetimibe)
- Selectively inhibit intestinal absorption of dietary and biliary cholesterol at the brush border of the small intestine, which results in a decrease in the

Table 5

Pharmacotherapeutic Options for Treatment of Hyperlipidemia

Lipid target	Pharmacotherapy
LDL	Statin most potent and effective for large LDL reductions
	Niacin and resins effective for moderate LDL reductions
	Combination of statin + niacin; statin + ezetimibe; statin + resin
LDL + TG	Statin + niacin or statin + fibric acid
TG	Fibric acid or niacin

absorption of cholesterol and a decrease in cholesterol in the blood.

Patient Instructions and Counseling

Statins
- Usually administered in the evening because most hepatic cholesterol production occurs during the night.
- Lovastatin conventional tablets should be given with the evening meal since absorption is better with food; however, the extended-release lovastatin products should be taken at bedtime.
- The lovastatin + Niaspan combination product should be taken at bedtime with a low-fat snack.
- Non-extended release statins can be dosed once daily.
- Other regular dosage forms should be divided as the doses are raised above 40 mg/d.
- Atorvastatin may be given any time of the day because of its longer half-life.
- Rosuvastatin dosage adjustment is required in patients with severe renal impairment. Plasma concentrations of rosuvastatin increased to a clinically significant extent (about 3-fold) in patients with severe renal impairment (CL_{CR}<30 mL/min/1.73m^2) compared with healthy subjects (CL_{CR}>80 mL/min/1.73m^2). Dosage adjustment is also required in patients with liver disease.
- Monitor LFTs and muscle toxicity as described above.

Bile acid sequestrants (resins)
- Cholestyramine and colestipol: start with 1 dose daily with the largest meal. May be increased (after the patient adjusts to the resin) to two doses daily with the largest meals or divided between breakfast and dinner.
- Titrate doses slowly to avoid gastrointestinal side effects.
- Powered doses can be mixed with food such as soup, oatmeal, nonfat yogurt, applesauce, etc. The mixture can also be chilled overnight to improve palatability.
- Do not use carbonated beverages to mix, as this promotes increased air swallowing.
- Drinking through a straw may also help.
- Patients who suffer constipation with the resins may mix them with psyllium; however, this mixture should be ingested immediately after mixing in order to prevent a gel from forming.
- Counsel the patient to rinse the glass to ensure ingestion of all resin.
- Colesevelam is a tablet formulation, which may be easier for some patients to self-administer. However, the tablets are large, and some patients may not be able to swallow them.
- Monitor for adherence and gastrointestinal side effects for all resins.

Nicotinic acid (niacin)

- Immediate-release (IR) niacin should be started at a low dose and slowly titrated upward:
  - * Start with 100 mg tid and adjust upward the second week to 200 mg tid; the next week increase to 350 mg tid; the following week raise to 500 mg tid. When 1500 mg/d is reached and maintained for 4 weeks, assess effectiveness before increasing the dose.
  - * If further titration is needed, go to 750 mg tid and assess effectiveness after 4 weeks before increasing. Maximum dose is 1000 mg tid.
  - * Aspirin 325 mg or ibuprofen 200 mg must be given 30 minutes before the morning dose to minimize flushing and itching.
  - * Caution patients to avoid hot beverages and hot showers so as not to exacerbate the flushing effect.
- Extended-release formulation (ER) should be taken at bedtime (500 mg) and titrated weekly to a maximum of 1500 mg/d. Aspirin should be taken 30 minutes before the dose.
- Sustained-release formulations are started at 250 mg bid and increased at weekly intervals to a maximum of 2000 mg/d. Aspirin should be given 30 minutes before the dose.
- Monitor for adherence and side effects. The titration schedule for some patients may have to be gradual due to flushing and itching.

Fibric acids (fibrates)

- Gemfibrozil should be taken twice daily 30 minutes before meals.
- Tricor can be taken with or without food once daily.
- Reduce dose in renal insufficiency and monitor for muscle toxicity, especially when used in combination with statins and niacin.

Cholesterol inhibitors

- Dosed once daily without regard to food
- Can be taken simultaneously in combination with statins

Adverse Drug Events

HMG-CoA reductase inhibitors (statins)

- Myopathy due to muscle damage
- Myalgia from muscle soreness or tenderness
- Myositis occurs in 0.2% of patients

myalgia + ↑creatine kinase
(3-10 times upper limit of normal)

- Rhabdomyolysis occurs rarely, but can cause acute renal failure. Stop drug immediately.

severe myositis + creatine kinase
10 x upper limit of normal,
↑serum creatinine and urine myoglobin

- Elevated liver enzymes occur in 0.1-2.3% of patients. Obtain baseline LFTs, repeat at 4-6 weeks, again at 6 months, and yearly thereafter.
- Flu-like symptoms and headache
- Mild GI complaints
- Absolute contraindication in active or chronic liver disease
- Relative contraindication in combination with certain drugs (see drug interactions)

Bile acid sequestrants (resins)

- Gastrointestinal distress
- Palatability problems with the resin slurry
- Constipation that increases with dose and in the elderly
- Decreased absorption of other drugs:
  - * Dose other drugs 1 hour before or 4 hours after resin.
- An absolute contraindication is dysbetalipoproteinemia (highly elevated VLDL) and TG >400 mg/dL.
- Relative contraindication when TG >200 mg/dL

Nicotinic acid (niacin)

- Flushing is common. Pretreat with aspirin (325 mg) 30 minutes before the first niacin dose of the day.
- Hyperglycemia risk; use with caution in diabetics.
- Hyperuricemia (or gout)
  - * Upper GI distress
  - * Hepatotoxicity
  - * Absolute contraindication in chronic liver disease and severe gout
  - * Relative contraindication in diabetes, hyperuricemia, or severe gout

Fibric acids (fibrates)

- Dyspepsia
- Gallstones
- Myopathy increases when combined with statins.
- Absolutely contraindicated in severe renal or severe hepatic disease

Cholesterol inhibitors

- Elevated liver enzymes (same as placebo)
- GI distress (less than with resins)
- Absolutely contraindicated in moderate to severe hepatic disease

Drug-Drug and Drug-Disease Interactions

HMG-CoA reductase inhibitors (statins)
- CYP450 mixed function oxidase enzymes metabolize statins, and drugs that inhibit this process can cause increases in statin concentrations, thus predisposing to myopathy and liver toxicity.
  - * Common CYP450 3A4 inhibitors include amiodarone, clarithromycin, cyclosporine, danazol, delavirdine, diltiazem, erythromycin, fluoxetine, fluvoxamine, grapefruit juice, indinavir, itraconazole, ketoconazole, miconazole, nefazodone, nelfinavir, nicardipine, nifedipine, pimozide, propoxyphene, quinidine, ritonavir, saquinavir, sildenafil, tacrolimus, tamoxifen, testosterone, troleandomycin, verapamil, and zafirlukast.
  - * Pravastatin is not metabolized by the CYP450 system; therefore, these drug-drug interactions are avoided.
- Absolute contraindication in active or chronic liver disease

Bile acid sequestrants (resins)
- Avoid concomitant use with all other drugs, especially warfarin, digoxin, levothyroxine, tetracycline, fat-soluble vitamins, and minerals.
- Always separate other drugs by 1 hour before use and 4 hours after.
- Colesevelam does not appear to have these drug and nutrient interactions.
- Absolute contraindication in dysbetalipoproteinemia

Nicotinic acid (niacin)
- Use caution in combination with resins.
- Combination therapy with statins and gemfibrozil may cause an increased risk of myopathy.
- Absolute contraindications in chronic liver disease and severe gout

Fibric acids (fibrates)
- Highly protein-bound and metabolized by the CYP450 3A4 enzyme system
- Increased warfarin effect
- Cyclosporine may increase gemfibrozil concentrations.
- Fenofibrate may have less interaction potential with warfarin and cyclosporine.
- BAS (resins) decrease fibrate absorption.
  - * Combinations with statins and niacin may increase the risk of myopathy.
  - * Absolute contraindications are severe renal disease and severe liver disease.

Cholesterol inhibitors
- Cyclosporine may increase ezetimibe concentrations.
- Combination with a resin may decrease absorption.

- Combination with a fibric acid may predispose to gallbladder disease.
- Absolute contraindication in moderate to severe hepatic disease

Landmark Clinical Trials with Statins

Primary prevention trials
West of Scotland Study (WOSCOPS)
- This trial with pravastatin showed decreased coronary morbidity and mortality in hypercholesterolemic men with no clinical evidence of coronary heart disease (CHD).

Air Force/Texas Coronary Atherosclerosis Prevention Study (AFCAPS/TexCAPS)
- This trial with lovastatin showed reduced incidence of first acute major coronary events in patients who did not have CHD but did have normal to mildly elevated total cholesterol and LDL with low HDL.

Secondary prevention trials
Scandinavian Simvastatin Survival Study (4S)
- This trial with simvastatin showed decreased cardiac morbidity and mortality in patients with CHD and elevated cholesterol.

Cholesterol and Current Events Study (CARE)
- This trial with pravastatin showed reduced incidence of myocardial infarction (MI), death from CHD, stroke, and need for revascularization procedures in patients with recent MI and normal cholesterol levels.

Long-term Intervention with Pravastatin in Ischemic Disease Study (LIPID)
- This trial with pravastatin showed reduced mortality and incidence of MI and stroke in patients with CHD and a broad range of cholesterol.

Heart Protection Study (HPS)
- This trial with simvastatin is the largest single cholesterol trial (as of 2002) in patients at high-risk of CHD (prior MI, diabetes, or hypertension) and LDL >135 mg/dL. Antioxidants studied included vitamins E and C and beta-carotene. Simvastatin therapy showed a reduced incidence of CHD regardless of age (also elderly) or pre-existing condition. There was not a threshold for LDL at 100 mg/dL (ie, benefits extended below this level). In addition, there was no cardiovascular protective effect from vitamins E and C and beta-carotene.

3. Nondrug Therapy

- Nonpharmacologic therapy focuses on therapeutic lifestyle changes (TLC), which incorporate dietary changes, physical activity, and weight reduction.
    * "Heart healthy" nutrition is the foundation for any therapeutic interventions.

General Therapeutic Lifestyle Change (TLC) Recommendations

- Decrease the amount of high-fat foods consumed (especially foods high in saturated fat).
- Decrease intake of high-cholesterol foods.
- Replace saturated fats with monounsaturated fats and fish oils.
- Use foods high in complex carbohydrates (fiber, starch, fruits, vegetables).
- Strive for and maintain an acceptable weight.
- Patients should be instructed on how to read a nutrition label.
- Recommended nutrient makeup of the TLC diet is shown in Table 6.

Algorithm for Therapeutic Lifestyle Changes

- Begin lifestyle therapies and continue for 6 weeks. Evaluate LDL response, and if the LDL goal is not achieved, intensify LDL-lowering therapy (diet + weight management + physical activity) for 6 more weeks. Evaluate LDL response, and if LDL goal is not achieved, consider adding drug therapy (if not already added). Monitor adherence to TLC every 4-6 months.

Other Nonpharmacologic Therapies

- Soluble fiber and plant sterols/stanols can help lower LDL.
- Viscous or soluble fiber such as psyllium or pectin in the amount of 5-10 g/d, or other sources of fiber such as vegetables, fruits, and whole grains can reduce LDL by up to 8%.
- Fish oils
    * Active ingredient is omega-3 fatty acid
    * Can reduce triglycerides as much as 30-60%
    * Can be added when niacin or fibrates do not control triglycerides
- Antioxidant and vitamin therapy
    * Recent clinical trials have shown that the antioxidants, vitamins A, C, E, and beta-carotene are not protective for cardiovascular disease.
- Alcohol
    * Light to moderate alcohol use (1 drink per day for women, 2 drinks per day for men) has been associated with reductions in coronary heart disease rates. The benefit may be potentially due to a rise in HDL.
    * Use of alcohol should not be encouraged as a means of lowering cholesterol.
    * Excessive alcohol can cause elevations of triglycerides.
- Alternative therapies
    * Herbal therapies have not been systematically studied in hyperlipidemia and should not be recommended for treatment of hyperlipidemia or other lipid disorders.

Table 6

Nutrient Makeup of the TLC Diet

Nutrient	Recommended Intake
Saturated fat	<7% of total calories
Polyunsaturated fat	Up to 10% of total calories
Monounsaturated fat	Up to 20% of total calories
Total fat	25-35% of total calories
Carbohydrate	50-60% of total calories
Fiber	20-30 g/d
Protein	About 15% of total calories
Cholesterol	<200 mg/d
Total calories	Individualize to balance energy intake and expenditure to maintain desirable weight and/or prevent weight gain

4. Key Points

- Hyperlipidemia is the elevation of the blood concentration of a lipid such as cholesterol or triglyceride (in the form of lipoprotein).
- There are four major classifications of lipids: total cholesterol, low-density lipoproteins (LDL), high-density lipoproteins (HDL), and triglycerides.
- The process of atherosclerosis begins with atheroma lesions in the arterial vascular walls resulting from the accumulation of cholesterol within vessel walls.
- Polygenic hypercholesterolemia (LDL = 160-250 mg/dL) is the most common form of familial dyslipidemia.
- Major nonlipid risk factors for coronary heart disease (CHD) are cigarette smoking, hypertension, family history of premature CHD, and age (men over 45 years, women over 55 years).
- Persons with a history of CHD such as angina, MI, stroke, or transient ischemic attack are considered at highest risk of having another ischemic event in the next 10 years and require the most aggressive therapy and the lowest target LDL goal (<100 mg/dL).
- Monitoring for drug therapy of hyperlipidemia includes laboratory monitoring for adverse effects (eg, liver function tests, uric acid, and creatine kinase) and fasting lipid profiles (FLPs) for effectiveness.
- The mechanism of action of statin agents to treat hyperlipidemia is to competitively inhibit HMG-CoA reductase, which is the enzyme responsible for conversion of HMG-CoA to mevalonate, which is an early precursor and a rate-limiting step in cholesterol synthesis.
- The statins are usually administered in the evening because most hepatic cholesterol production occurs during the night, except for atorvastatin, which has a longer half-life than the other agents in this class.
- The only class of agents to control hyperlipidemias that is not contraindicated in patients with active or chronic liver disease is the bile acid sequestrant (resin) type.
- Pravastatin is not metabolized by the CYP450 enzyme system and thus avoids most of the drug interactions with the other statin agents.
- Advicor should not be substituted for equivalent doses of immediate-release (crystalline) niacin. For patients switching from immediate-release niacin to extended-release niacin, therapy with the latter should be initiated with low doses (ie, 500 mg once daily at bedtime) and the dose should then be titrated to the desired therapeutic response.
- The bile acid sequestrants (resins) may decrease the absorption of warfarin, digoxin, levothyroxine, tetracycline, fat-soluble vitamins, and minerals.
- The new formulation of Tricor can be taken with or without food once daily.
- Therapeutic lifestyle changes (TLC) that incorporate dietary changes, increased physical activity, and weight reduction, are the first recommended therapy for hyperlipidemia for 6-12 weeks prior to addition of drug therapy.

5. Questions and Answers

Case Presentation: Medication Profile—Community

H.L. is a 50-year-old man who comes to your pharmacy for cholesterol and medication monitoring. His medical history is notable for stage 1 hypertension, recent-onset type 2 diabetes, and hypercholesterolemia. Family history is noncontributory. Social history indicates he neither smokes nor uses alcohol. He has no known allergies. His medication history reveals that he occasionally takes acetaminophen for headaches and no other OTC medications or herbal products. Current medications include hydrochlorothiazide 25 mg/d (for 4 years) and a new prescription today for atorvastatin 10 mg/d. Your physical assessment reveals the following:

BP 144/90 mm Hg, pulse 70 and regular, weight 185 lb, height 5'9"
FLP today reveals total cholesterol = 250 mg/dL, HDL = 40 mg/dL, and triglycerides = 145 mg/dL.

Answer Questions 1-5 using the above case.

1. What is H.L.'s LDL cholesterol?

   A. 130 mg/dL
   B. 153 mg/dL
   C. 162 mg/dL
   D. 178 mg/dL
   E. 181 mg/dL

   $$LDL = TC - \left(HDL + \frac{TG}{5}\right)$$
   $$250 - \left(40 + \frac{145}{5}\right)$$
   $$40 \quad 29$$
   $$250 - 69$$

2. What is H.L.'s LDL goal?

   A. <100 mg/dL
   B. 130-160 mg/dL
   C. 160-189 mg/dL
   D. <200 mg/dL
   E. >40 mg/dL

3. H.L. is started on TLC and atorvastatin because of his high LDL. When should you assess the effectiveness of therapy?

   A. 12 weeks
   B. 6 months
   C. 3 weeks
   D. 6 weeks
   E. Annually

4. H.L. is most likely to have which of the following?

   A. Familial hypercholesterolemia
   B. Polygenic hypercholesterolemia
   C. Familial combined hyperlipidemia
   D. Elevated triglycerides
   E. Isolated low HDL

5. H.L. returns for reassessment at the appropriate time. His FLP shows that his LDL is now 100 mg/dL. What is your recommendation?

   A. Stop the statin since you have achieved optimal LDL
   B. Increase statin dose
   C. Intensify TLC
   D. Add gemfibrozil
   E. Add cholestyramine

6. The National Cholesterol Education Program (NCEP) Expert Panel identifies which of the following as a positive risk factor for coronary heart disease (CHD)?

   A. Hypertension
   B. Low HDL (<40 mg/dL)
   C. Family history of premature CHD
   D. Current cigarette smoking
   E. All of the above

7. Which of the following is NOT a secondary cause of hyperlipidemia?

   A. High LDL
   B. Hypothyroidism
   C. Diabetes
   D. Renal disease
   E. β-Blockers

8. Cholesterol biosynthesis can be decreased by which of the following?

   A. Statins
   B. Oat bran
   C. Bile acid sequestrants (resins)
   D. Ezetimibe
   E. Aspirin

9. Choose the medication with the greatest effect on raising HDL.

   A. Lovastatin
   B. Pravastatin

C. Gemfibrozil
D. Niaspan
E. Colesevelam

10. Choose the drug class with the most potent lowering effect on LDL.

   A. Nicotinic acid
   B. Fibric acids
   C. Bile acid sequestrants (resins)
   D. Cholesterol inhibitors
   E. HMG-CoA reductase inhibitors

11. The initial lesion in the development of atherosclerosis is

   A. development of foam cells
   B. increase in HDL reverse transport
   C. rupture of a vulnerable plaque
   D. clot formation in the artery lumen
   E. development of a thin cap over the lipid pool

12. Choose the correct statement.

   A. Diabetes is an absolute contraindication to the use of nicotinic acid.
   B. Aspirin is dosed three times per day in order to prevent flushing from niacin.
   C. Gemfibrozil may reduce triglycerides by as much as 50%.
   D. Colesevelam has similar patient tolerability problems as cholestyramine.
   E. Ezetimibe frequently causes muscle toxicity.

13. Hyperlipidemia refers to

   A. elevation of apolipoproteins
   B. hypercholesterolemia
   C. high levels of white blood cells
   D. increased ingestion of protein
   E. endothelial dysfunction

14. Which of the following indicates an optimal LDL?

   A. >190 mg/dL
   B. <40 mg/dL
   C. >60 mg/dL
   D. <100 mg/dL
   E. <150 mg/dL

15. Polygenic hypercholesterolemia is characterized by which of the following?

   A. LDL = 150-450 mg/dL
   B. LDL = 160-250 mg/dL
   C. Triglycerides >400 mg/dL
   D. HDL = 50 mg/dL
   E. LDL = 160-250 mg/dL + triglycerides >400 mg/dL

16. Identify a baseline laboratory test required before statin treatment.

   A. White blood cell count
   B. Complete blood cell count
   C. Liver function test
   D. Serum creatinine
   E. Creatinine clearance

17. The major troublesome side effect in nicotinic acid therapy is:

   A. Diarrhea
   B. Vomiting
   C. Hair growth
   D. Flushing
   E. Dizziness

18. Which of the following medications has the following warning: "For patients switching from immediate-release niacin, therapy with this drug should be in initiated with a low dose and then titrated to the desired therapeutic response"?

   A. Pravigard
   B. Vytorin
   C. Advicor *Niaspan + Lovastatin*
   D. Atorvastatin
   E. Ezetimibe

19. Identify the drug interaction that involves the CYP450 system.

   A. Ezetimibe + niacin
   B. Colestipol + simvastatin
   C. Gemfibrozil + cholestyramine
   D. Fenofibrate + ezetimibe
   E. Lovastatin + itraconazole

20. A TLC diet could include

   A. antioxidant therapy such as vitamin E
   B. <7% of total calories from saturated fat
   C. 150-250 g/d of fiber
   D. 2-4 drinks of alcohol per day
   E. assessing the effectiveness of TLC at 12-week intervals

Answers

1. **E.** Use the Friederwald equation to calculate LDL.

   $$LDL = TC - (HDL + TG/5)$$

2. **A.** H.L. has type 2 diabetes that is a CHD risk equivalent, therefore he is at highest risk for an event in the future and his LDL goal should be optimal or <100 mg/dL.

3. **D.** Both TLC and drug therapy measures should be assessed at 6-week intervals.

4. **B.** H.L.'s LDL is 181 mg/dL, which falls into the range for polygenic hypercholesterolemia (160-250 mg/dL) and he does not have elevated triglycerides or low HDL.

5. **C.** Since H.L.'s LDL is still slightly above optimal; intensify TLC. That is, continue to decrease saturated fat in the diet and to intensify weight reduction and physical activity. If after the next assessment in 6 weeks the LDL is still above 100 mg/dL, options would be to increase the statin dose (double it), or add another agent such as niacin or ezetimibe.

6. **E.** All of the answers are positive risk factors for CHD as defined by the NCEP ATP III. The remaining positive risk factors are gender and age (ie, males 45 and over and females 55 and over).

7. **A.** Causes of hyperlipidemia must be ruled out. The common secondary causes are renal failure, hypothyroidism, obstructive liver disease, diabetes, and drugs such as β-blockers, thiazide diuretics, oral contraceptives, oral estrogens, glucocorticoids, and cyclosporine.

8. **A.** Statins competitively inhibit HMG-CoA reductase, which is the enzyme responsible for converting HMG-CoA to mevalonate. Inhibition of mevalonate reduces cholesterol synthesis.

9. **D.** Nicotinic acid (Niaspan) has the most efficacy in raising HDL compared to other therapies. HDL may be raised 15-35%.

10. **E.** Statins (HMG-CoA reductase inhibitors) have the most efficacy in lowering LDL. LDL may be lowered 18-55%.

11. **A.** Foam cells represent the initial lesion of atherosclerosis and develop as a result of the ingestion of oxidized LDL by macrophages in the subintimal space of the artery.

12. **C.** Diabetes is a relative contraindication to the use of nicotinic acid. Aspirin is dosed once daily, before the first nicotinic acid dose of the day. Gemfibrozil can reduce TGs 20-50%. Colesevelam is a tablet and avoids most of the palatability problems of other resins. Ezetimibe does not cause muscle toxicity.

13. **B.** Hyperlipidemia is defined as an elevation of a lipid in the blood. The lipid can be cholesterol or triglyceride in the form of a lipoprotein.

14. **D.** Level <100 = optimal; 100-129 = near optimal/above optimal; 130-159 = borderline high; 160-189 = high; ≥190 = very high

15. **B.** Polygenic hypercholesterolemia is the most common cause of mild to moderately elevated LDL (LDL = 160-250 mg/dL).

16. **C.** Baseline tests before statin use include liver function tests (LFTs) and creatine kinase (CK).

17. **D.** The most common side effect is flushing, which may occur in many patients. To decrease flushing intensity, aspirin 325 mg should be taken 30 minutes prior to the first dose of nicotinic acid. Itching may also occur with flushing.

18. **C.** Advicor (Niaspan + lovastatin) contains Niaspan, which is not dose-equivalent to immediate-release niacin or modified-release (sustained-release or time-release) niacin preparations.

19. **E.** Lovastatin is metabolized by CYP450 3A4 enzymes, and itraconazole will inhibit this enzyme system. Inhibition causes lovastatin blood and tissue concentrations to rise, thus predisposing to potential muscle or liver toxicity.

20. **B.** TLC diet includes <7% saturated fat, 20-30 g/d fiber, avoidance of alcohol, and assessment at 6 weeks. Vitamin E is not recommended for cardiovascular risk reduction.

6. References

ACC/AHA/NHLBI Clinical Advisory on the Use and Safety of Statins. *J Am Coll Cardiol.* 2002;40:568-573.

Beaird SL. HMG-CoA reductase inhibitors: assessing differences in drug interactions and safety profiles. *J Am Pharm Assoc.* 2000;40:6337-6344.

Downs JR, Clearfield M, Weis S, et al. Primary prevention of acute coronary events with lovastatin in men and women with average cholesterol levels: results of AFCAPS/TexCAPS. Air Force/Texas Coronary Atherosclerosis Prevention Study. *JAMA.* 1998;279:1615-1622.

Executive Summary of the Third Report of the National Cholesterol Education Program (NCEP) Expert Panel on Detection, Evaluation, and Treatment of High Blood Cholesterol in Adults (Adult Treatment Panel III). *JAMA.* 2001;285:2486-2497.

Heart Protection Study Collaborative Group. *Lancet.* 2002;360:7-22.

Knopp RH. Drug treatment of lipid disorders. *N Engl J Med.* 1999;341:498-511.

McKenney JM, Hawkins DW, eds. *Handbook on the Management of Lipid Disorders.* Springfield, New Jersey: Scientific Therapeutics Information/National Pharmacy Cardiovascular Council; 2001.

Scandinavian Simvastatin Survival Study Group. Randomized trial of cholesterol lowering in 4444 patients with coronary heart disease: The Scandinavian Simvastatin Survival Study (4S). *Lancet.* 1994;344:1383-1389.

Sudhop T, Lutjohann D, Kodal A, et al. Inhibition of intestinal cholesterol absorption by ezetimibe in humans. *Circulation.* 2002;106:1943-1948.

The Long-Term Intervention with Pravastatin in Ischaemic Disease (LIPID) Study Group. *N Engl J Med.* 1998;338:1349-1357.

Talbert RL. Hyperlipidemia. In: DiPiro JT, Talbert RL, Yee GC, et al, eds. *Pharmacotherapy: A Pathophysiologic Approach,* 5th ed. New York: McGraw-Hill; 2002.

West of Scotland Coronary Prevention Study Group. Influence of pravastatin and plasma levels on clinical events in the West of Scotland Coronary Prevention Study (WOSCOPS). *Circulation.* 1998;97:1440-1445.

Wolf MI, Vartnian SF, Ross JL, et al. Safety and effectiveness of Niaspan when added sequentially to a statin for treatment of dyslipidemia. *Am J Cardiol.* 2001;87:476-479.

13. Diabetes Mellitus

Joni Foard, PharmD, CDE
Assistant Professor
Department of Pharmacy
University of Tennessee College of Pharmacy

L. Brian Cross, PharmD, CDE
Associate Professor
Department of Pharmacy
University of Tennessee College of Pharmacy

Contents

1. Overview

Diabetes mellitus (DM) is a group of chronic metabolic diseases due to defects in insulin secretion and/or action, which result in hyperglycemia; abnormal metabolism of carbohydrates, fats, and proteins; and long-term macrovascular and microvascular complications.

- Affects 20.8 million people or ~7% of the population
  - *14.6 million diagnosed
  - *6.2 million undiagnosed
- Sixth leading cause of death
- Risk of death is two times that of people without diabetes of similar age

Classification

Type 1 diabetes
- Previously called insulin-dependent diabetes mellitus (IDDM) or juvenile-onset diabetes
- Requires exogenous insulin for survival
- 5%-10% of all diagnosed cases

Type 2 diabetes
- Previously called non-insulin dependent diabetes mellitus (NIDDM) or adult-onset diabetes
- 90%-95% of all diagnosed cases

Gestational diabetes mellitus (GDM)
- Glucose intolerance with onset or first recognition during pregnancy (second and third trimesters)
- Approximately 4%-7% of pregnancies in American women; >200,000 annually
- Up to 50% later develop type 2 diabetes; 5%-10% of those diagnosed in the postpartum period.
- Primary fetal complication of concern: macrosomia

Other types (secondary DM)
- Due to genetic defects of β-cell function (eg, maturity onset diabetes of youth [MODY]), surgery, drugs, malnutrition, infections, and other illnesses
- 1%-5% of all diagnosed cases

Prediabetes
- Plasma glucose levels are higher than normal but lower than those diagnostic for diabetes
- Formerly characterized as IFG (impaired fasting glucose) and IGT (impaired glucose tolerance)

- Risk factor for future diabetes and cardiovascular disease

Clinical Presentation

- Classic signs and symptoms include polydipsia, polyuria, and polyphagia
- Other common findings include fatigue, blurred vision, and frequent infections
- Type 1: rapid onset; unexplained weight loss; potentially ketonuric or in ketoacidosis
  - * May experience a "honeymoon" period, a phase of erratic insulin secretion lasting months to a year during destruction of β-cells
- Type 2: progressive onset; asymptomatic or mild classic signs and symptoms; 80% are obese or have history of obesity; may present with microvascular and macrovascular chronic complications

Pathophysiology and Etiology

Type 1 DM
- β-Cell destruction leading to absolute insulin deficiency
- Subgroups:
  - * Immune mediated
- Strong HLA (human leukocyte antigen) association indicates genetic predisposition
- Related to environmental factors; stimulus (eg, virus) triggers immunologic process
  - * Idiopathic: no evidence of autoimmunity or other known etiology
- Prone to ketoacidosis
- Peak onset occurs at the time of puberty but may occur at any age

Type 2 DM
- Insulin resistance and progressive β-cell dysfunction
- Strong genetic predisposition
- Associated with environmental factors such as excessive calorie intake, decreased activity, weight gain and obesity
- Insulin resistance may be present years before the onset of diabetes
- Initially normal glucose levels are maintained by increased insulin secretion by β-cells
- Increasing insulin resistance or a failure of β-cells to maintain insulin secretion leads to glucose intolerance and development of diabetes
- Insulin resistance is influenced by age, ethnicity, physical activity, medications, and weight

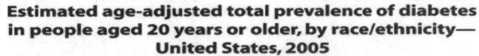

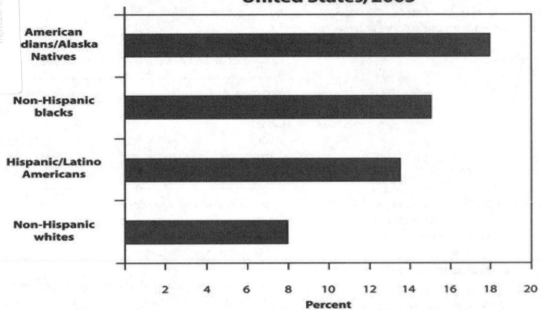

Estimated age-adjusted total prevalence of diabetes in people aged 20 years or older, by race/ethnicity— United States, 2005

Source: *For American Indians/Alaska Natives, the estimate of total prevalence was calculated using the estimate of diagnosed diabetes from the 2003 outpatient database of the Indian Health Service and the estimate of undiagnosed diabetes from the 1999-2002 National Health and Nutrition Examination Survey. For the other groups, 1999-2002 NHANES estimates of total prevalence (both diagnosed and undiagnosed) were projected to year 2006.*

* Graph and information obtained from CDC (Center for Disease Control and Prevention) website at http://www.cdc.gov/diabetes/pubs/estimates05.htm#prev4 on December 1, 2006.

- Usually diagnosed in adulthood but can occur at any age
- The incidence of type 2 diabetes is higher among certain ethnic populations (Figure 1)

Diagnostic Criteria

Type 1 and type 2 DM (Table 1)

- Diagnosis can be made based on a fasting plasma glucose (FPG), a random plasma glucose, or an oral glucose tolerance test (OGTT)
- Diagnosis must be confirmed on a subsequent day using any of the three methods
- FPG is the test of choice due to simplicity, accuracy and reproducibility
- Abnormal results not meeting criteria outlined in Table 1 are classified as prediabetes
    * impaired fasting glucose (IFG) = FPG ≥100 mg/dL and ≤126 mg/dL
- * Impaired glucose tolerance (IGT) = 2-hour OGTT plasma glucose ≥140 mg/dL and <200 mg/dL

- Serum C peptide level: diagnostic for functioning of β-cells and may be used for classification

Gestational diabetes mellitus

- OGTT is preferred screening test in pregnancy
- For average-risk patients test at 24-28 weeks of gestation
- For high-risk patients (marked obesity, personal history of GDM, glycosuria, or strong family history of DM) perform risk assessment at first prenatal visit and test as soon as possible; if negative at initial screenings, retest between 24 and 28 weeks of gestation
- In average- or high-risk patients use one of two approaches:
    * One-step approach: diagnostic 75-g or 100-g OGTT
    * Two-step approach: 1-hour 50-mg glucose challenge test followed by diagnostic OGTT if 1-hour level ≥140 mg/dL

Table 1

Criteria for the Diagnosis of Diabetes Mellitus[1]

Symptoms of diabetes and a casual plasma glucose ≥ 200 mg/dL (11.1 mmol/L). Casual is defined as any time of day without regard to time since last meal. The classic symptoms of diabetes include polyuria, polydipsia, and unexplained weight loss.

OR

FPG ≥126 mg/dL (7.0 mmol/L). Fasting is defined as no caloric intake for at least 8 h.

OR

2-h plasma glucose ≥200 mg/dL (11.1 mmol/L) during an OGTT. The test should be performed as described by the World Health Organization, using a glucose load containing the equivalent of 75 g anhydrous glucose dissolved in water.

[1]In the absence of unequivocal hyperglycemia with acute metabolic decompensation, criteria should be confirmed by repeat testing on a different day.
Report of the Expert Committee on the Diagnosis and Classification of Diabetes Mellitus. Copyright 1997 American Diabetes Association from Diabetes Care, Vol. 20, 1997; 1183-1197. Reprinted with permission from The American Diabetes Association.

Table 2

Summary of Recommendations for Adults with Diabetes

Glycemic control	
A_{1C}	<7.0%
Preprandial capillary plasma glucose	90–130 mg/dL
Peak postprandial capillary plasma glucose†	<180 mg/dL
Blood pressure	<130/80 mmHg
Lipids‡	
LDL	<100 mg/dL
Triglycerides	<150 mg/dL
HDL	>40 mg/dL§

Key concepts in setting glycemic goals:

A_{1C} is the primary target for glycemic control

Goals should be individualized

Certain populations (children, pregnant women, and elderly) require special considerations

More stringent glycemic goals (ie, a normal A_{1C}, <6%) may further reduce complications at the cost of increased risk of hypoglycemia

Less intensive glycemic goals may be indicated in patients with severe or frequent hypoglycemia

Postprandial glucose may be targeted if A_{1C} goals are not met despite reaching preprandial glucose goals

* Referenced to a nondiabetic range of 4.0–6.0% using a DCCT-based assay.
† Postprandial glucose measurements should be made 1–2 h after the beginning of the meal, generally peak levels in patients with diabetes.
‡ Current NCEP/ATP III guidelines suggest that in patients with triglycerides ≥ 200 mg/dL, the "non-HDL cholesterol" (total cholesterol minus HDL) be utilized. The goal is 130 mg/dL.
§ For women, it has been suggested that the HDL goal be increased by 10 mg/dL.
Adapted from *Standards of Medical Care in Diabetes* – 2007.
Source: American Diabetes Association

- Diagnostic criteria with 100-g glucose load—fasting: 95 mg/dL; 1-hour: 180 mg/dL; 2-hour: 155 mg/dL; 3-hour: 140 mg/dL
- Diagnostic criteria with 75-g glucose load—fasting: 95 mg/dL; 1-hour: 180 mg/dL; 2-hour: 155 mg/dL
- Diagnosis positive if two glucose values meet or exceed those listed for 100-mg or 75-g load
- FPG >126 mg/dL or casual PG >200 mg/dL confirmed on subsequent day precludes the need for glucose challenge
- At least 6 weeks postpartum re-evaluation and reclassification should be conducted

Treatment Principles and Goals

- Achieve and maintain glycemic control (Table 2)
- Attain recommended blood pressure and lipid goals (Table 2)
- Lifestyle modifications to promote general health and achieve weight management goals
- Prevent or slow progression of chronic complications
- Prevent or resolve acute complications
- Achieve an acceptable quality of life and satisfaction with care

Prevention of complications

- Smoking cessation
- Aspirin/antiplatelet therapy
    * Use as secondary prevention with a history of CVD
    * Use as primary prevention if >40 years of age or have additional risk factors (family history of CVD, hypertension, smoking, dyslipidemia, or albuminuria)
    * Aspirin 75-162 mg/d
- Immunization
    * Annual influenza vaccine if 6 months of age or older and no contraindications
    * At least one lifetime pneumococcal vaccine for adults with no contraindications
    * One-time pneumococcal revaccination if >64 years of age, previously immunized at <65 and vaccine administered >5 years ago
- Foot care: self-inspection daily; visual inspection at each office visit, and annual comprehensive exam
- Skin inspection and care daily
- Dental care: annual examination
- Eye care: annual dilated eye examination

Complications of diabetes

Chronic complications

- Coronary atherosclerosis: death rate is 2 to 4 times higher than adults without diabetes
- Cerebrovascular atherosclerosis: risk of stroke is 2 to 4 times higher among people with diabetes
- Peripheral vascular disease: pain due to intermittent claudication; insufficient circulation impairs healing, increases risk of gangrene and amputation

Microvascular disease

- Retinopathy
    * Leading cause of new cases of blindness in adults 20-74
    * May develop without symptoms; annual dilated eye examination recommended for detection
    * Treatment includes glycemic and blood pressure control, laser photocoagulation
- Nephropathy
    * Occurs in 20%-40% of diabetics and is the leading cause of end-stage renal disease (ESRD)
    * May develop without symptoms; detection relies on laboratory screening which should be done annually
    * Random spot collection of the albumin-to-creatinine ratio is the easiest screening to perform; a value of >30 mg/g is considered abnormal
    * Serum creatinine should be measured at least annually for the estimation of glomerular filtration rate (GFR)
    * Treatment includes glycemic and blood pressure control; ACE inhibitors or ARBs should be used except during pregnancy.
- Polyneuropathy
    * Sensorimotor nervous system dysfunction; pain and diminished sensation with progression from lower to upper extremities; poor detection of trauma, which increases risk for ulcers and infection, particularly in lower extremities and feet
- Autonomic neuropathy
    * Gastrointestinal: gastroparesis, constipation, diarrhea
    * Genitourinary: neurogenic bladder and sexual dysfunction in men
    * Cardiovascular: orthostatic hypotension, resting tachycardia

- Diabetic foot problems
  - * DM accounts for >60% of nontraumatic amputations in the U.S.
  - * Prevention, early detection with regular foot exams, and prompt treatment of lesions are essential to avoid complications

Acute complications

- Hypoglycemia
  - * Plasma glucose <70 mg/dL
  - * Glucose (15-20 g) is the preferred treatment
  - * Other forms of carbohydrate that contain glucose can be used
  - * Treatment effects should be seen in 15 minutes
  - * Symptoms can range from mild (tremor, palpitations, sweating) to severe (unresponsiveness, unconsciousness, or convulsions)
  - * Severe hypoglycemia may require assistance from another individual for treatment with glucagon or IV glucose

- Diabetic ketoacidosis (DKA)
  - * Medical emergency in type 1 diabetes due to absolute or relative insulin deficiency
  - * Omission of insulin, major stress, infection or trauma may precipitate DKA
  - * Characterized by glucose >250 mg/dL, elevated ketones, arterial pH <7.2, plasma bicarbonate <15 mEq/l
  - * Ketone bodies are formed in excess due to fatty acid metabolism in the liver, leading to ketonuria and ketonemia and ultimately diabetic ketoacidosis.
  - * Kussmaul respirations (deep and rapid); attempt to compensate for metabolic acidosis
  - * Requires prompt intervention with insulin, fluids and electrolytes to prevent coma and death

- Hyperosmolar hyperglycemic state (HHS)
  - * Also known as hyperglycemic hyperosmolar nonketotic coma (HHNC)
  - * Complication of type 2 diabetes
  - * Elevated plasma glucose (typically >500 mg/dL), dehydration, and hyperosmolality in the absence of significant ketoacidosis

- * May be triggered by infection or other stressors such as stroke or myocardial infarction
- * Treatment includes fluid and electrolyte replacement and treatment with insulin

2. Drug Therapy

Oral Medications for the Treatment of Diabetes Mellitus

SECRETAGOGUES

Mechanism of Action: Primary mechanism is to cause a reduction in blood glucose by stimulating the release of insulin from the pancreas. This may in turn cause a decrease in hepatic gluconeogenesis and a slight decrease in insulin resistance at the muscle level. Effectiveness is dependent on pancreatic beta-cell function.

Clinical/Counseling Considerations:
- Should be taken before meals (sulfonylureas [QD-BID], meglitinides [before each meal])
- Causes 1-2 kg weight gain
- + risk of hypoglycemia (sulfonylureas > meglitinides)
- Typically not indicated during pregnancy, breastfeeding, or in children
- Carry fast-acting oral carbohydrate for emergency use
- Wear medical identification
- Store drug in a cool, dry place (not the bathroom or kitchen)

A_{1c} Reduction: 1%-2% (sulfonylureas)
0.5%-2% (meglitinides)

Monthly Cost: generically available / ~$75-$200 (meglitinides)

Cautions / Contraindications:
- Caution in elderly (do NOT use chlorpropamide)
- Caution in renal and hepatic insufficiency (glipizide & glimepiride safer)
- Avoid in pts with significant alcohol use
- Drug interactions (worse with 1st generation sulfonylureas) may cause ↑ risk of hypoglycemia: anticoagulants, fluconazole, salicylates, gemfibrozil, sulfonamides, tricyclic antidepressants, digoxin
- Contraindicated in patients with DKA, severe infection, surgery, or trauma
- SIADH, disulfiram-like reaction with ETOH, and sun-sensitivity reactions more common in 1st vs. 2nd generation sulfonylureas

SULFONYLUREAS

FIRST-GENERATION

NAME (generic/brand/strength)	DAILY DOSE	DURATION OF ACTION	COMMENTS
Acetohexamide (*Dymelor*®) 250, 500 mg	250 – 1500 mg	up to 16 hours	Active metabolite excreted by kidney
Chlorpropamide (*Diabinese*®) 100, 250 mg	100 – 500 mg	up to 72 hours	Contraindicated in renal insufficiency
Tolazamide (*Tolinase*®) 100, 250, 500 mg	100 – 1000 mg	up to 10 hours	
Tolbutamide (*Orinase*®) 250, 500 mg	500 – 3000 mg QD - BID	up to 10 hours	

SECOND-GENERATION

NAME (generic/brand/strength)	DAILY DOSE	DURATION OF ACTION	COMMENTS
Glipizide (*Glucotrol*®, *Glucotrol XL*®) 5, 10 mg	5-40 mg QD-BID / 5-20 mg QD (XL)	up to 20 hours	Given with or without meal; do not cut XL tab
Glyburide (*DiaBeta*®, *Micronase*®) 1.25, 2.5, 5 mg	1.25-20 mg QD-BID	up to 24 hours	3mg *Glynase*® = 5mg Glyburide
Glyburide micronized (*Glynase*®) 1.5, 3, 4.5, 6mg	1.5-12 mg QD	up to 24 hours	
Glimepiride (*Amaryl*®) 1, 2, 4 mg	1-8 mg QD	24 hours	Begin with 1 mg in renal insufficiency

(Continued)

SULFONYLUREAS (cont.)

MEGLITINIDES / PHENYLALANINES

NAME (generic/brand/strength)	DAILY DOSE	DURATION OF ACTION	COMMENTS
Repaglinide (*Prandin* ®) 0.5, 1, 2 mg	0.5-4 mg before each meal MAX DOSE = 16 mg/day	Peak effect: ~ 1 hour Duration: ~ 2-3 hours	skip dose if meal skipped; do not give in combination with sulfonylureas
Nateglinide (*Starlix* ®) 60, 120 mg	60-120 mg before each meal	Peak effect: ~ 1 hour Duration: ~ 4 hours	EFFICACY: *Prandin* ® > *Starlix* ®

BIGUANIDES

Mechanism of Action: Primary mechanism is seen through decreased hepatic gluconeogenesis, as well as improved glucose utilization and uptake in peripheral tissues and decreased intestinal absorption of glucose.

Clinical Considerations:
- Considered first choice to begin in newly diagnosed DM patients unless contraindicated
- Minimal risk of hypoglycemia unless combined with secretagogues or insulin
- May decrease weight up to 5 kg
- ↓ triglycerides, ↓ LDL, ↔/↑ HDL
- GI symptoms (nausea, vomiting, bloating, flatulence, anorexia, and diarrhea) are the most common adverse effects
  - ➢ Take doses with or after meals to reduce GI symptoms
  - ➢ GI symptoms are transient and improve in most patients over time
  - ➢ Titrate the dose up slowly to minimize GI symptoms
- 500 mg QD with the largest meal X 1 week, then ↑ to
- 500 mg BID with the 2 largest meals X 1 week, then ↑ to
- 1 gm [two 500 mg tabs] with largest meal & 500 mg with the 2nd largest meal X 1 week, then ↑ to
- 1 gm BID with the 2 largest meals of the day
  - ➢ Interferes with vitamin B_{12} absorption
- May require as much as 8 weeks of therapy before assessing effectiveness
- Generally not indicated during pregnancy or breastfeeding
- Indicated for the treatment of type 2 DM in children 10 years and older
- May decrease the progression to diabetes from IGT & IFG (prediabetes)
- +CV benefits when used in obese patients with DM

A_{1c} Reduction: 1%-2%

Monthly Cost: generically available

Cautions / Contraindications:
- Most cautions & contraindications are related to their ability to ↑ the risk of lactic acidosis with metformin
  - ➢ CONTRAINDICATIONS:
    - Renal Insufficiency (SCr ≥1.4 females; SCr ≥1.5 males)
    - Hepatic dysfunction
    - Excessive alcohol use (binge or chronic use >2 drinks per day or at one sitting)
    - May be contraindicated in CHF (NYHA III & IV)
  - ➢ CAUTIONS:
    - Should be held in situations of increased risk for lactic acidosis, including acute MI, CHF exacerbation, severe respiratory disease, shock, septicemia
    - Should be held X 48 hours after iodinated contrast media and major surgeries

NAME (generic/brand/strength)	DAILY DOSE	DURATION OF ACTION	COMMENTS
Metformin (*Glucophage* ®) 500, 850, 1000 mg	1000-2550 mg (adult) up to 2000 mg (10 yo +)	≥ 24 hours	
Metformin extended release (*Glucophage XR* ®) 500, 750 mg (*Glumetza* ®) 500, 1000 mg	2000 mg QPM; may take 1gm BID if QD dosing causes GI symptoms		DO NOT cut, crush, or chew

NAME (generic/brand/strength)	DAILY DOSE	DURATION OF ACTION	COMMENTS
Rosiglitazone (*Avandia*®) 2, 4, 8 mg	4-8 mg QD OR 2-4 mg BID	24 hours	May be more effective when given BID
Pioglitazone (*Actos*®) 15, 30, 45 mg	30-45 mg QD	24 hours	

THIAZOLADINEDIONES (GLITAZONES/TZDs)
Mechanism of Action:
- Agonists of the PPAR$_\gamma$ (peroxisome proliferators-activated receptor-$_\gamma$) receptor which, when stimulated, improves peripheral muscle and adipose tissue insulin sensitivity as well as suppresses hepatic glucose output.

Clinical Considerations:
- Minimal risk of hypoglycemia unless combined with secretagogues or insulin
- May cause a 5 kg weight gain, more if combined with secretagogues or insulin
- ↓ triglycerides (PIO > ROSI), ↑ HDL (PIO = ROSI), ↑ LDL (ROSI) / ↔LDL (PIO)
- Dosed QD, though ROSI may be slightly more effective when dosed BID
- May require as much as 16 weeks of therapy before assessing effectiveness
- Generally not indicated during breastfeeding or pregnancy
- May decrease the progression to diabetes from IGT & IFG (prediabetes)
- Edema may best be treated by aldosterone antagonists
- Not FDA-indicated for treatment of type 2 DM in children, though has been used
- May be helpful in Non-Alcoholic Fatty Liver Disease (NAFLD)
- Generally not indicated during pregnancy or breastfeeding

A$_{1c}$ Reduction: 1%-2%

Monthly Cost: ~ $120-$200

Cautions/Contraindications:
- Edema – with PO therapies (~5%), with insulin (~15%) – this may occur in patients with NO history of heart problems [may be dose related]. Recommendation: D/C therapy if significant problem of edema, decrease dose if minor problem of edema → consider further cardiac workup.
- Recent black box warning added for CHF (PIO & ROSI)
- Hepatotoxicity – incidence = ~ 0.2% of ALT > 3X ULN for both agents. Recommendation: LFT's every other month for 1st 12 months, periodically thereafter. If ALT >2.5 ULN, don't start; if ALT = 1-2.5 ULN, monitor closely; if ALT 3X ULN, D/C medication.
- May cause resumption of ovulation in anovulatory women
- ↓ oral contraceptive effectiveness

NAME (generic/brand/strength)	DAILY DOSE	DURATION OF ACTION	COMMENTS
Acarbose (*Precose* ®) 50, 100 mg	25-100 mg TID	1-3 hours	MAX DOSE: <60 kg = 50 mg TID >60 kg = 100 mg TID
Miglitol (*Glyset* ®) 25, 50, 100 mg	25-100 mg TID	1-3 hours	

ALPHA-GLUCOSIDASE INHIBITORS

Mechanism of Action: Causes delay in the digestion of carbohydrates into simple sugars, and their subsequent absorption in the small intestine.

Clinical Considerations:
- Minimal risk of hypoglycemia unless combined with secretagogues or insulin
- Minimal effect on weight, possible ↓ weight secondary to side effects
- Main target of therapy should be post-prandial hyperglycemia
- GI symptoms (flatulence, GI upset, abdominal pain, diarrhea, bloating) are the most common side effects. These tend to dissipate over time with continued treatment. Dosing must be individualized and slowly titrated up as tolerated:
  - ➢ 25 mg QD X 1 week, then
  - ➢ 25 mg BID X 1 week, then
  - ➢ 25 mg TID X 1 week, then
  - ➢ continued increased dose as tolerated up to 50 mg TID
- Diet considerations: pt should be counseled to ↑ complex carbohydrate intake and ↓ intake of simple sugars
- Treatment of hypoglycemia:
  - ➢ should use milk (lactose) or fruit juice (fructose), NOT SUCROSE
  - ➢ any carbohydrate can be used if >2-3 hours since last dose of alpha-glucosidase inhibitor agent
- Generally not indicated during pregnancy, breastfeeding or in children
- Drug Interactions: ↓ bioavailability of digoxin, propranolol, and ranitidine.

A$_{1c}$ Reduction: 0.5%-1%

Monthly Cost: ~ $75-$100

Cautions/Contraindications:
- Avoid use in patients with GI disorders: ulcerative colitis, Crohn's disease, possible bowel obstruction, short bowel syndrome.
- Avoid use in patients with SCr >2 mg/dL (acarbose) or CrCl of ≤ 25mL/min (both agents)
- Possible increased LFTs (acarbose) – dose related (>300mg/day) and weight (of patient) related. [Avoid use in patients with cirrhosis.]

DIPEPTIDYL PEPTIDASE– 4 (DPP-4) INHIBITORS

Mechanism of Action: Inhibits the degradation of endogenous glucagon-like peptide-1 (GLP-1) and glucose-dependent insulinotropic polypeptide (GIP), which in turn causes: 1) increased insulin production in a glucose-dependent fashion, 2) decreased production of glucagon, and 3) improved beta-cell functioning.

Clinical Considerations:
- Minimal risk of hypoglycemia unless combined with secretagogues or insulin
- Minimal/no effect on weight
- Can be used either as monotherapy or in combination with metformin or thiazoladinediones, and possibly insulin

- Only drug class impacting the GLP-1 system dosed orally
- Generally, very well tolerated with the most common side effects including nasopharyngitis and upper respiratory tract infections
- Secondary to newness of the drug, no significant long-term outcome data is yet available

A_{1c} **Reduction:** 0.6%-1.2%

Monthly Cost: ~ $150

Cautions / Contraindications:
- Dose should be adjusted for renal insufficiency
- May cause adverse immunologic reactions through T-cell inhibition
- Should not be used in patients with DKA or type 1 DM

COMBINATION ORAL AGENTS FOR DIABETES MELLITUS (See write-up of individual agents for details)

NAME (generic/brand/strength)	DAILY DOSE	DURATION OF ACTION	COMMENTS
Sitagliptin (*Januvia* ®) 25, 50, 100 mg	100 mg QD	24 hours	CrCl 30-50: 50 mg QD CrCl <30: 25 mg QD

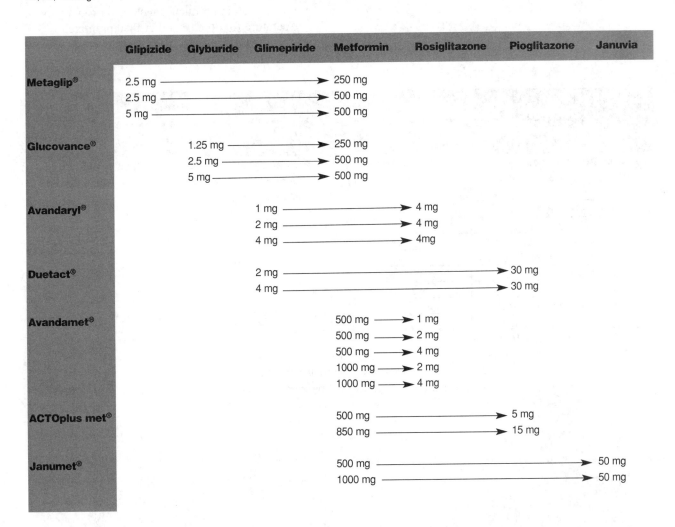

Injectable Medications for the Treatment of Diabetes Mellitus

INSULIN PRODUCTS

Mechanism of Action: At low levels, insulin causes suppression of endogenous hepatic glucose production. At higher levels, insulin promotes glucose uptake by muscle tissue.

Clinical Considerations:
- + Risk of hypoglycemia
- ↑ weight
- Should be considered as initial agent if glucose is >250mg/dL or A_{1c} is >10%
- No dosage limit
- Dosing is often started with a basal insulin (0.1-0.2 u/kg/day) and added to an existing PO regimen of 2 or more agents
- Insulin regimen should be individualized to the patient accounting for:
  - ➢ glucose readings
  - ➢ patient preferences
  - ➢ patient schedule
  - ➢ patient education / intelligence level
  - ➢ level of intensity needed
  - ➢ cost to patient

- Consider for prandial insulin coverage when:
  - ➢ Patient with fasting blood glucose target (<100), but A_{1c} ≥7%
  - ➢ A_{1c} ≥7% with evidence of frequent 2-hour post-prandial glucose values >160 mg/dL
  - ➢ Nighttime or daytime hypoglycemia with skipped/delayed meals

A_{1c} Reduction: 2.5% or more

Monthly Cost: variable depending insulin product prescribed and device (ie, pen) vs. vial/syringe used

Cautions/Contraindications:
- Dose cautiously in patients with renal and hepatic insufficiency
- Dose cautiously in elderly patients
- Do not mix the following insulins with any others: Lantus®, Levemir®, Lente®, and Ultralente®
- Patients should be counseled on signs and symptoms of hypoglycemia and how to appropriately treat
- Most insulin products are stable at room temperature for 30 days, other than premixed-insulin products (14 days) and Levemir (45 days).

Sample Titration Schedules for Basal & Prandial Insulin

Basal Insulin Titration		Prandial Insulin Titration	
Fasting Blood Glucose Levels for 3 Consecutive Days	**Adjust Basal Insulin Dose (units)**	**Preprandial or Bedtime Glucose Levels for 3 Consecutive Days**	**Adjust Rapid-Acting Insulin Dose (units)**
≥ 180 mg/dL	+8	≥ 180 mg/dL	+3
160-180 mg/dL	+6	140-180 mg/dL	+2
140-160 mg/dL	+4	140-180 mg/dL	+2
120-140 mg/dL	+2	120-140 mg/dL	+1
100-120 mg/dL	+1	100-120 mg/dL	NO CHANGE
80-100 mg/dL	NO CHANGE	80-100 mg/dL	-1
60-80 mg/dL	-2	60-80 mg/dL	-2
< 60 mg/dL	-4	< 60 mg/dL	-4

- For ↑ fasting glucose, adjust basal dose ONLY
- For ↑ preprandial / HS glucose levels: 1) if ↑ at lunchtime, adjust breakfast prandial insulin
      2) if ↑ at dinnertime, adjust lunchtime prandial insulin
      3) if ↑ at bedtime, adjust dinnertime prandial insulin

INSULIN TYPE	ONSET OF ACTION	TIME OF PEAK	DURATION OF ACTION
Rapid Acting Analogs			
glulisine (*Apidra* ®)*	15-30 min	30-90 min	1-3 hours
aspart (*Novolog* ®)**	10-15 min	30-90 min	3-5 hours
lispro (*Humalog* ®)***,+	10-15 min	30-90 min	
Intermediate Acting			
human NPH (*Novolin N* ®**,#, *Humulin N* ®***)	1-3 hours	4-12 hours	10-18 hours
human *Lente*	2-5 hours	7-15 hours	24 hours
Long Acting			
human *Ultralente*	4-8 hours	10-30 hours	18-30 hours
Basal			
glargine (*Lantus* ®)*, ^	1-2 hours	peakless	24 hours
detemir (*Levemir* ®)**	1-2 hours	6-8 hours	18-24 hours
Pre-Mixed Insulins			

NPH + Regular

*Novolin 70/30**, #*

*Humulin 70/30***

*Humulin 50/50***

Insulin Protamine + Analogs

*Novolog 70/30***

*Humalog 75/25***

*Humalog 50/50***

DEVICE AVAILABILITY: * = OptiClick pen; ** = NovoPen®; *** = Lilly pen; # = InnoLet®; ^ = SoloSTAR®
                                 += HumaPen MEMOIR™ & Luxura™ HD pens

INSULIN AVAILABILITY: U-100 = 100 units per mL [most common available concentration]
                               U-500 = 500 units per mL [used in severe insulin resistance]

INCRETIN MIMETICS

Mechanism of Action: A receptor agonist of endogenous glucagon-like peptide-1 (GLP-1) which causes: 1) increased insulin production in a glucose-dependent fashion, 2) decreased production of glucagon, 3) slowing of gastric emptying, 4) increased satiety and weight loss, and 5) improved beta-cell functioning.

Clinical Considerations:

- Minimal risk of hypoglycemia unless combined with secretagogues (consider initial reduction in secretagogue), minor increase in hypoglycemia risk if combined with TZDs
- Moderate weight loss of ~10 pounds seen after sustained use
- Dose limiting side effect is nausea – ~ 50% of patients report some degree of nausea, though ~3%-5% stop the drug secondary to the problem – this problem seems to lessen with time
- Patients should decrease meal size and carbohydrate content of meals prior to use of exenatide to lessen problem of nausea
- Dose should be given ~10-15 minutes prior to the 2 largest meals of the day that are at least 6 hours apart
- Can be stored at room temperature for 30 days after first dose is given
- Can be combined with sulfonylurea, metformin, sulfonylurea + metformin, TZDs, or metformin + TZD. Currently not indicated in combination with insulin.
- Begin with 5 mcg injected BID for 1 month, then increase to 10 mcg BID as tolerated secondary to GI toxicity
- Supplied as a pen device which contains 60 doses (1 month supply)
- Most effective to lower post-prandial glucose elevations

A_{1c} **Reduction:** 0.5%-1%

Monthly Cost: ~ $150-$200

Cautions / Contraindications:

- Should NOT be given to patients with GFR ≤30 mL/min
- Should NOT be given to patients with severe gastrointestinal disease including gastroparesis
- Should not be used in patients with DKA or type 1 DM

NAME (generic/brand/strength)	DAILY DOSE	DURATION OF ACTION	COMMENTS
Exenitide (*Byetta* ®) 5, 10 mcg pen	5-10 mcg BID	~ 8-10 hours	

AMYLIN MIMETICS

Mechanism of Action: Is an analog of endogenous amylin which when dosed at therapeutic levels causes: 1) decreased production of glucagon, 2) slowing of gastric emptying, and 3) increased satiety and weight loss

Clinical Considerations:

- Can be used in combination with insulin therapy in both type 1 and type 2 DM patients who have failed to achieve desired glucose control
- Due to significant risk of severe hypoglycemia, prandial insulin dose should be decreased by 50% when starting pramlintide
- Dose limiting side effect is nausea which seems to lessen over time
- Type 2 DM—start with 60 mcg (10 units) before meals, increase to 120 mcg before meals when no significant nausea has occurred for 3-7 days
- Type 1 DM—start with 15 mcg (2.5 units) before meals, increase to 30 to 60 mcg before meals when no significant nausea has occurred for 3-7 days
- Opened vials may be stored at room temperature for 28 days

A_{1c} **Reduction:** 0.5%-1%

Monthly Cost: ~ $100-$300/month

Cautions / Contraindications:

- Should NOT be used in the following patients:
  - ➤ severe gastrointestinal disease including gastroparesis
  - ➤ poor adherence with current insulin regimen or self-monitoring of blood glucose
  - ➤ recurrent severe hypoglycemia requiring assistance in the past 6 months
  - ➤ having an A_{1c} ≥9%
  - ➤ presence of hypoglycemia unawareness

NAME (generic/brand/strength)	DAILY DOSE	DURATION OF ACTION	COMMENTS
Pramlintide (*Symlin®*) 0.6 mg/mL – 5 mL vial	TYPE 1 DM: 15-60 mcg TID with meals TYPE 2 DM: 60-120 mcg TID with meals	4-6 hours	Dosed using an insulin syringe: 30 mcg = 5 units 60 mcg = 10 units 120 mcg = 20 units

Inhaled Medications for the Treatment of Diabetes Mellitus

Mechanism of Action: see discussion on insulin above

Clinical Considerations:
- Provides prandial insulin coverage without use of injection
- Patients should have baseline spirometry (FEV_1) prior to initiation, 6 months after beginning therapy, and yearly thereafter
- Dosing issues: 1 mg packet = 3 units
                   3 mg packet = 8 units
                   (3 X 1 mg packets DOES NOT = 1 X 3 mg packet)
- Significant education of the patient required before initially starting the medication
- Can be used in type 1 and type 2 DM patients, though long-term safety and effectiveness has not yet been established in pediatric patients
- If used in type 1 DM patients, should be used with a basal insulin product

A_{1c} Reduction: dose dependent (insulin product)
Monthly Cost: ~ $150/month

Cautions / Contraindications:
- Should NOT be used in patients with chronic lung diseases (asthma or COPD)
- Should NOT be used in patients who are active smokers or those who have stopped smoking <6 months prior to beginning Exubera® (insulin exposure rates may ↑ 2 to 5 fold compared to non-smokers)
- Patients should be counseled on signs and symptoms of hypoglycemia and how to appropriately treat
- Dose cautiously in patients with renal and hepatic insufficiency

NAME (generic/brand/strength)	DAILY DOSE	DURATION OF ACTION	COMMENTS
Insulin inhaled (*Exubera®*) 1, 3 mg	Dosed for mealtime carbohydrate coverage (see chart on next page)	6-8 hours	Onset of action is similar to analog insulins; duration of action is similar to regular insulin

Guidelines for Initial, Pre-Meal Exubera® Dose

Pt wt (in kg)	Pt wt (in lb)	Initial dose per meal	Number of 1 mg blisters per dose	Number of 3 mg blisters per dose
30-39.9	60-87	1 mg per meal	1	-
40-59.9	88-132	2 mg per meal	2	-
60-79.9	133-176	3 mg per meal	-	1
80-99.9	177-220	4 mg per meal	1	1
100-119.9	221-264	5 mg per meal	2	1
120-139.9	265-308	6 mg per meal	-	2

Approximate Equivalent IU Dose of Regular Human Insulin for Exubera®

Dose (mg)	Regular insulin dose (units)	Number of 1 mg blisters per dose	Number of 3 mg blisters per dose
1	3	1	-
2	6	2	-
3	8	-	1
4	11	1	1
5	14	2	1
6	16	-	2

3. Nondrug Therapy

- Weight loss is recommended for all diabetics who are overweight or obese
- Modest weight loss (5%) has been shown to decrease insulin resistance in type 2 diabetes
- Lifestyle changes through diet and exercise should be emphasized
- Patient education is an essential component of successful diabetes management

Medical Nutrition Therapy (MNT)
- Individualized to achieve treatment goals with consideration of usual dietary habits, metabolic profile, and lifestyle
- Monitor carbohydrate by exchanges, carbohydrate counting or experience-based estimation
- Carbohydrate (CHO) 45%-60% of total daily caloric intake; if intensive insulin therapy used with pre-meal bolus dose of insulin, then insulin should be adjusted to cover the daily CHO intake; with basal insulin therapy (when the pre-meal bolus is not used) or oral antidiabetic medications, then CHO intake must be adjusted so it is consistent with the effects of therapy
- Protein 15%-20% of total daily caloric intake; should be modified if renal function is reduced
- Saturated fat <7% of total daily calories
- Cholesterol <200 mg/d
- Fiber intake should be encouraged, but there is no reason to recommend a greater amount than that recommended for persons without DM
- Limit daily alcohol intake (adult females: one drink or less; adult males: two drinks or less)

Physical Activity/Exercise
- Regular exercise improves blood glucose control, reduces cardiovascular risk factors, and contributes to weight loss. Regular exercise may prevent type 2 diabetes in high-risk individuals
- Individualized; pre-exercise program history and detailed medical examination are essential
- Recommended 150 min/week of moderate-intensity aerobic exercise and/or at least 90 min/week of vigorous aerobic exercise distributed over at least 3 days/week
- Program should be adjusted in the presence of macro- and microvascular complications that may be worsened

* Retinopathy: Vigorous aerobic or resistance exercise may be contraindicated in the presence of proliferative diabetic retinopathy or severe non-proliferative diabetic retinopathy because of the risk of triggering vitreous hemorrhage or retinal detachment
* Peripheral neuropathy: Non-weight bearing activities may be best because decreased pain sensation in the extremities increase the risk of skin breakdown and infection
* Autonomic neuropathy: Should undergo cardiac investigation before increasing physical activity (may lead to decreased cardiac responsiveness to exercise, postural hypotension, etc.)
- SMBG necessary before and after exercise
- Fast-acting oral carbohydrates should be available during and after exercise

Diabetes Self-Management Education (DSME)
- Provides means for persons with DM to become empowered and assist with self-care
- Education content includes the disease process; acute and long-term complications; drug and nondrug treatment; monitoring; preventive measures; decision-making skills; specific self-care measures relative to foot, skin, dental and eye care; goal setting; and psychosocial adjustment

4. Key Points

- Diabetes mellitus (DM) is a group of chronic metabolic diseases exhibiting hyperglycemia resulting from defects in insulin secretion and/or action.
- The principal treatment goals include maintaining blood glucose levels in the normal or near normal range and preventing acute and chronic complications.

- Type 1 diabetes results from immune mediated β-cell destruction, which leads to absolute insulin deficiency.
- Type 2 diabetes is characterized by relative insulin deficiency and/or insulin resistance.

Comparison of Type 1 and Type 2 Diabetes Mellitus

	Type 1	Type 2
Previous names	Insulin-dependent diabetes mellitus (IDDM); juvenile-onset	Non-insulin dependent diabetes mellitus (NIDDM); adult-onset
Percentage of DM cases	5%-10%	90%-95%
Age of occurrence	<30 years of age (usually childhood or adolescence); at any age following autoimmune stimulus (eg, virus)	>30 years of age; increasing in childhood/adolescence in association with obesity and inactivity
Onset	Rapid	Gradual
Primary etiology	Autoimmune mediated mechanism with genetic predisposition	Genetic and environmental (eg, family history, ethnicity, obesity, inactivity)
Pathogenesis	Destruction of β-cells resulting in absolute insulin deficiency and abnormal glucose control	Increasing resistance of tissue (liver and skeletal muscle) to insulin; impaired insulin secretion resulting in relative deficiency of insulin; increased hepatic glucose production
Signs and symptoms	Polyuria, polydipsia, polyphagia, unexplained weight loss, fatigue, blurred vision; possibly ketoacidosis	Polyuria, polydipsia, polyphagia, obesity, fatigue, blurred vision; possibly asymptomatic
Diagnostic criteria	See Table 1	See Table 1
Ketoacidosis	Ketosis prone (diabetic ketoacidosis; DKA)	Not ketosis prone due to residual insulin (hyperglycemic hyperosmolar nonketotic syndrome [HHNS])
Treatment:		
Nondrug therapy	• Medical nutrition therapy (MNT) • Physical activity/exercise therapy approved by physician; type based on presence of factors such as retinopathy, neuropathy, and cardiovascular status	Essential adjunct to oral antidiabetic therapy; may be sufficient as monotherapy to control blood glucose
Drug therapy	Insulin monotherapy **OR** rarely oral antidiabetic drugs as adjunct to insulin therapy (if accompanied by insulin resistance)	• MNT monotherapy **OR** • Oral antidiabetic drugs **OR** • Oral antidiabetic drugs in combination therapy **OR** • Insulin monotherapy **OR** • Insulin and oral antidiabetic drugs

- Goals of diabetes therapy include achieving and maintaining glycemic control, and reaching recommended blood pressure and lipid goals.
- Outcomes of uncontrolled BG include cardiovascular, kidney, eye, and nerve disease.
- Pharmacotherapy treatment of DM should be individualized to each patient considering such factors as glucose control goals, length of time with DM, concomitant diseases, psychosocial issues including available support for the patient, patient motivation, medication and DM supply costs, as well as level of risk for complications secondary to DM control.
- Multiple studies have shown improved glycemic control delays the onset of, slows the progression of, or lowers the risk of long-term microvascular complications
- Combination therapy of either 2 or more PO therapies, PO therapies PLUS insulin, PO products PLUS GLP-1 analogs, will be required in most patients to maintain continued DM control
- Metformin
  * considered 1st-line therapy in newly diagnosed type 2 DM
  * contraindicated in renal dysfunction patients
  * low/minimal risk of hypoglycemia with monotherapy
  * GI side effects (flatulence, GI upset, abdominal pain, diarrhea, bloating) are the dose-limiting problems
  * no weight gain
  * may decrease the progression to DM in high-risk patients
- Secretagogues
  * are helpful in combination with other PO agents and injectable products
  * increases risk of hypoglycemia (sulfonylureas > meglitinides)
  * increases weight (sulfonylureas > meglitinides)
  * high rate of failure over time
  * use with caution in renally impaired and elderly patients
- Thiazoladinediones
  * helps to improve peripheral insulin resistance
  * increases weight and edema
  * low/minimal risk of hypoglycemia with monotherapy
  * contraindicated in patients with CHF
  * delayed time to see full impact on DM control
  * may decrease the progression to DM in high-risk patients

- Alpha-Glucosidase Inhibitors
  * blocks absorption of carbohydrates in small intestine
  * low/minimal risk of hypoglycemia with monotherapy
  * GI side effects (flatulence, GI upset, abdominal pain, diarrhea, bloating) are the dose-limiting problems
  * more effective for post-prandial hyperglycemia
  * minimal effect on weight
- GLP-1 / Amylin based medications
  * Byetta (GLP-1 analog)
- increases insulin production in a glucose-dependent fashion
- decreases production of glucagon
- improves beta-cell functioning
- slows gastric emptying
- increases satiety and possible weight loss
- dose-limiting side effect = nausea
- injectable product
- for use in type 2 DM
- high cost
  * Januvia (DPP-IV inhibitor)
- increases insulin production in a glucose-dependent fashion
- decreases production of glucagon
- improves beta-cell functioning
- no effect on weight
- well tolerated with few side effects
- for use in type 2 DM
- high cost
  *Symlin (Amylin mimetic)
- decreases production of glucagons
- slows gastric emptying
- increases satiety and possible weight loss
- significant risk of hypoglycemia in combination with insulin in type 1 DM
- dose-limiting side effect = nausea
- for use in type 1 & 2 DM
- high cost
- Insulin
  * essential for type 1 DM
  * often used in type 2 DM in combination with other therapies
  * should be considered initial agent if glucose is >250 mg/dL or A_{1c} >10%
  * often stated as basal therapy (0.1–0.2 units/kg/day) added to an existing PO regimen
  * should be individualized to the patient's goals and motivation
  * intensive insulin therapy (>3 doses/day or use of CSII) is replacing conventional insulin therapy (split-mix dosing: two-thirds of total daily dose [TDD]

> * Insulins vary principally by their source, appearance, time-activity profiles (onset, peak, and duration), dosing, and route of administration. The main adverse events are hypoglycemia, weight gain, and lipodystrophies. Mechanism of action is the same for all types.

- Patient education is essential for the management of DM, as it provides a means for persons with this chronic disease to become empowered, cope effectively, and engage in appropriate self-care.
- Recommend lifestyle modifications including weight management, increased physical activity, and smoking cessation.

Patient Profile #1—Institution or Nursing Home Care

Patient Name: Barbara Evens

Address:	413 Summit Street
Age:	68
Height:	5' 5"
Weight:	190 lb
Sex:	Female
Race:	African-American
Allergies:	Penicillin, sulfa drugs

Diagnosis:

Primary	1) Type 2 DM
Secondary	1) Hypertension
	2) Asthma

Lab/Diagnostic Tests:

	Date	Test
1)	2/1	LFTs
2)	2/1	Serum K
3)	5/1	LFTs
4)	5/1	Serum K
5)	6/1	A_{1c}
6)	6/1	Serum creatinine
7)	6/1	BUN
8)	6/1	Serum K

Additional Orders:

1) Referral to dietitian for weight reduction diet
2) Low impact exercise 30 mins 3 days per week

Dietary Consideration:

1) Dietary changes per dietitian consult
2) Enteral and parenteral

Pharmacist Notes and Other Patient Information:

	Date	Comment
1)	2/1	Advise patient to continue SMBG and to report any hypoglycemic episodes. Instruct patient to treat hypoglycemia with glucose or lactose products. Instruct patient to take acarbose with first bite of meal. Foot exam negative. Patient reports having 1-2 drinks of bourbon per day.
2)		Inform patient to report any changes in BG.

Medication Orders:

Date	RX No	Physician	Drug & strength	Qty	Sig	Refills
2/1	834924	Jones	Propranolol 20 mg	30	1 PO bid	3
2/1	834925	Jones	Albuterol inhaler	1	1-2 inhalations q4-6h	3
2/1	834926	Jones	Acarbose 25 mg	90	1 tab PO w/meals	2
5/1	834927	Jones	Acarbose 50 mg	90	1 tab PO w/meals	2
6/1	834928	Jones	Prednisone 10 mg	30	1 tab PO daily	0
6/1	834929	Jones	Propranolol 20 mg	30	1 tab PO bid	3
6/1	834930	Jones	Albuterol inhaler	1	1-2 inhalations q4-6h	3
6/1	834931	Jones	ASA 81 mg	30	1 tab PO daily	3

5. Questions and Answers

Use Patient Profile #1 to answer Questions 1-5.

1. Chlorpropamide would be problematic in this case for which of the following reasons?

    I.   Alcohol intake
    II.   Sulfa allergy
    III. Asthma
    IV.   Hypertension
    V.   Drug-drug interaction

    A. I only
    B. III only
    C. I and II only
    D. II, III, and IV
    E. I, II, and V

2. Due to a renal protection mechanism, the drug class of choice for B.E.'s hypertension is:

    A. β-blocker
    B. Loop diuretic
    C. Thiazide diuretic
    D. α-adrenergic blocker
    E. Angiotensin-converting enzyme inhibitor

3. One of the most common adverse drug events caused by B.E.'s oral antidiabetic agent is:

    A. Flatulence
    B. Hypoglycemia
    C. Renal failure
    D. Hyperglycemia
    E. Weight gain

4. Which of the following medications on the medication list in this case can mask the symptoms of hypoglycemia?

    A. Propranolol
    B. Albuterol
    C. Acarbose
    D. Prednisone
    E. Aspirin

5. What change in the following laboratory tests might be observed with the addition of prednisone to B.E.'s drug regimen?

    A. Increase in liver function tests (LFTs)
    B. Decrease in BUN
    C. Decrease in serum creatinine
    D. Increase in serum creatinine
    E. Increase in blood glucose

Use Patient Profile #2 to answer Questions 6-10.

6. What is the principal drug-related problem in this patient's medication record?

    A. Insulin therapy is not indicated for persons with type 2 DM
    B. Therapeutic duplication of sulfonylurea therapy
    C. Potential decrease of BG due to drug-drug interaction between phenytoin and tolazamide
    D. Potential increase of BG due to drug-drug interaction between glimepiride and itraconazole
    E. Use of an ACE inhibitor for hypertension in type 2 DM

7. All of the following monitoring parameters are necessary for T.R. except:

    A. Periodic glycosylated hemoglobin A_{1c}
    B. SMBG levels
    C. Phenytoin levels
    D. Blood pressure readings
    E. Quarterly serum C-peptide level

8. Which of the following is inappropriate treatment for a mild hypoglycemic episode?

    A. $^1/_2$ cup of diet soda
    B. 6-7 hard candies containing sugar
    C. 3 glucose tablets
    D. $^1/_2$ cup of regular soda
    E. 5 small sugar cubes

9. Persons on insulin therapy should be advised to rotate their injection sites for the following reason:

    A. Reduces the risk of infection
    B. Reduces the risk of lipoatrophy
    C. Reduces the risk of lipohypertrophy
    D. Reduces the risk of generalized myalgia
    E. This advice is outdated due to the use of human insulin

Patient Profile #2—Community

Patient Name: Tom Right
Address: 20 Blue Ridge Drive
Age: 48
Height: 5' 6"
Weight: 135 lb
Sex: Male
Race: Caucasian
Allergies: NKDA

Diagnosis:

Primary 1) Type 2 DM
2) Epilepsy
Secondary 1) Hypertension
2) Fungal infection under toenails

Pharmacist Notes and Other Patient Information:

	Date	Comment
1)	4/8	Patient should be monitored closely for hypoglycemia. Teach patient signs and symptoms of hypoglycemia and treatment measures.

Medication Orders:

Date	RX No	Physician	Drug & strength	Qty	Sig	Refills
1/6	765321	Smith	Tolazamide 250 mg	90	1 tab PO daily	0
4/8	765323	Smith	Glimepiride 2 mg	90	1 tab PO daily	0
8/6	765324	Smith	Lisinopril 5 mg	90	1 tab PO daily	0
8/6	765325	Thomas	Phenytoin extended	60	300 mg PO daily	0
8/6	765366	Smith	Itraconazole	14	50 mg PO daily	0
8/6	765367	Smith	Regular insulin	Trial	5 units SC before meals	0

10. Which of the following is the most appropriate treatment for a severe hypoglycemic episode?

A. $^1/_2$ cup of diet soda
B. 3 hard candies containing sugar
C. 1 glucose tablet
D. Glucagon injection
E. 2-3 small sugar cubes

11. Commercially available insulin (as of May 2005) may be administered by which of the following routes?

I. Intravenously
II. Subcutaneously
III. Via inhalation
IV. Transdermally
V. Sublingually

A. I only
B. II only
C. I and II only
D. II, III, and IV
E. I, II, and V

12. Insulin therapy is indicated in all of the following except:

A. Newly diagnosed type 1 DM
B. Gestational diabetes mellitus (GDM) not controlled by diet
C. Hyperglycemic hyperosmolar nonketotic syndrome (HHNS)
D. Newly diagnosed type 2 DM
E. Diabetic ketoacidosis (DKA)

13. Insulin dosing is adjusted based on the following parameters:

I. Liver function test results
II. Dietary intake
III. Physical activity/exercise
IV. Blood glucose levels
V. Ophthalmic examinations

A. I only
B. II only
C. I and II only
D. II, III, and IV
E. I, II, and V

14. Which of the following oral antidiabetic agents is a micronized formulation?

    A. Micronase®
    B. Glynase®
    C. Glucotrol XL®
    D. Amaryl®
    E. Orinase®

15. Insulin that has been stored in a refrigerator should be allowed to reach room temperature prior to administration in order to:

    A. Allow for proper mixing
    B. Minimize painful injections
    C. Prevent frosting or clumping
    D. Delay systemic absorption
    E. Prevent change in clarity

16. When mixing rapid- or short-acting insulin with intermediate- or long-acting insulin, which insulin in the list below should be drawn up first?

    A. Regular
    B. NPH
    C. Lente
    D. Ultralente
    E. Glargine

17. Uniform dispersion of insulin suspensions can be obtained by:

    A. Vigorously shaking the vial
    B. Rolling the vial gently between the hands
    C. Warming the vial in a microwave
    D. Packing the vial in dry ice
    E. Keeping the vial at room temperature (68-75°F)

18. Of the following types of insulin, which can be administered intravenously?

    A. Glargine
    B. Lente
    C. Regular
    D. Ultralente
    E. NPH

19. Diabetes mellitus is the leading cause of which of the following complications?

    A. Pancreatitis
    B. Fatty liver
    C. Blindness
    D. Stroke
    E. Deafness

20. Which of the following is an indication that a patient is developing a long-term complication from diabetes mellitus?

    A. Tachycardia
    B. Glucosuria
    C. Leukocytosis
    D. Proteinuria
    E. Tinnitus

21. What sulfonylurea has been associated with the greatest incidence of prolonged hypoglycemia in the elderly?

    A. Tolazamide
    B. Tolbutamide
    C. Chlorpropamide
    D. Glimepiride
    E. Glipizide

22. Which of the following drugs taken with alcohol is most likely to cause a disulfiram-like reaction?

    A. Chlorpropamide
    B. Acarbose
    C. NPH insulin
    D. Glucagon
    E. Pioglitazone

23. Metformin should be withheld for 48 hours prior to any procedure requiring the use of parenteral iodinated contrast media due to the potential for this adverse drug event:

    A. Optic neuritis
    B. Metabolic alkalosis
    C. Lactic acidosis
    D. Purple toe syndrome
    E. Tinnitus

24. The use of insulin in a woman with GDM helps reduce the incidence of which complication in the fetus?

    A. Macrosomia
    B. Cystic fibrosis
    C. Deafness
    D. "Soft bones"
    E. Eczema

25. Metformin would not be an option for a patient with the following diagnosis:

    A. Iron deficiency anemia
    B. Impaired renal function
    C. Hypertension
    D. Type 2 diabetes
    E. Frequent hypoglycemic episodes

26. Nocturnal hypoglycemia resulting in rebound hyperglycemia in type 1 DM is termed:

    A. Honeymoon period
    B. Somogyi effect
    C. Dawn phenomenon
    D. Hyperglycemic phase
    E. Insulin resistance syndrome

27. Which of the following is a potentially fatal adverse drug event of Glucophage®?

    A. Weight gain
    B. Frequent urination
    C. Diarrhea
    D. Lactic acidosis
    E. Angioedema

28. All of the following are true of acarbose therapy except:

    A. Contraindicated in inflammatory bowel disease
    B. Should be taken with the first bite of each meal
    C. Does not cause hypoglycemia or weight gain
    D. Hypoglycemia due to combination therapy should be treated with sucrose
    E. LFTs are monitored every 3 months during the first year and periodically thereafter (if the dose is >50 mg tid)

29. Prandin® is a nonsulfonylurea secretagogue. Adverse drug events include all of the following except:

    A. Upper respiratory infection (URI)
    B. Arthropathy
    C. Hypoglycemia
    D. Back pain
    E. Hyperglycemia

30. Patient counseling relative to meglitinides should include the following points:

    I.   Must be taken 30 minutes before main meals
    II. If a meal is omitted, do not take
    III. Enhances preprandial glucose utilization
    IV. Hyperglycemia is a potential adverse drug event
    V.   Disulfiram-like reaction possible when ingested with ETOH

    A. I only
    B. III only
    C. I and II only
    D. II, III, and IV
    E. I, II, and V

31. Which one of the following antidiabetic agents does not require liver function tests for monitoring?

    A. Glargine
    B. Miglitol
    C. Rosiglitazone
    D. Acarbose
    E. Metformin

32. Adverse drug events reported for pioglitazone (Actos), a thiazolidinedione, include all of the following except:

    A. Exacerbation of CHF
    B. Resumption of ovulation
    C. Edema
    D. Upper respiratory infection (URI)
    E. Megaloblastic anemia

33. All of the following drugs have a direct glucogenic effect except:

    A. Thiazide diuretics
    B. Corticosteroids
    C. Nicotinic acid
    D. Sympathomimetics
    E. Acetohexamide

34. Which of the following is the mechanism of action (MOA) for the sulfonylureas?

    A. Stimulate pancreatic β-cells to secrete insulin
    B. Delay carbohydrate metabolism and absorption (due to inhibition of intestinal and pancreatic enzymes)
    C. Increases hepatic insulin sensitivity and decreases hepatic glucose production
    D. Increases skeletal muscle and adipose tissue insulin sensitivity and decreases hepatic glucose production
    E. Decrease blood glucose and assists with blood glucose control by increasing glucose uptake and utilization by peripheral tissues

35. All of the following are signs or symptoms of hypoglycemia except:

    A. Tachycardia
    B. Diaphoresis
    C. Shakiness
    D. Polyuria
    E. Pallor

36. Pramlintide (Symlin®):

    A. Is a basal insulin
    B. Is an insulin analogue
    C. Is an oral insulin
    D. Is an inhaled insulin
    E. Is an injectable synthetic version of the human hormone amylin

37. Which of the following statements correctly states the current thinking on insulin storage, according to a study in *Diabetes Care*, 2003;26:2655-9?

    A. Glargine insulin (Lantus®) can safely be prefilled in a syringe and stored for up to 28 days
    B. Lispro insulin (Humalog®) should not be refrigerated since refrigeration causes crystallization
    C. Unopened insulin vials kept under refrigeration are stable until their labeled expiration dates
    D. Opened vials of any insulin product should be stored in the refrigerator and destroyed if left at room temperature for more than 3 days

Answers

1. **E.** Chlorpropamide is contraindicated in persons with a sulfa allergy. Alcohol (ETOH) ingestion with chlorpropamide could lead to a disulfiram-like reaction. Also, acute ingestion of ETOH (especially in the fasting state) includes the risk of severe hypoglycemia. Chlorpropamide and prednisone may produce a drug-drug interaction resulting in hyperglycemia. Items 3 and 4 are non-problematic in this case in relation to chlorpropamide.

2. **E.** Angiotensin-converting enzyme inhibitors (ACEIs) exhibit a renal protective mechanism in persons with DM. None of the remaining drugs exhibit such an effect.

3. **A.** The most common adverse drug events for acarbose are flatulence, abdominal pain, and diarrhea. These adverse effects may be decreased by titrating the dose gradually and taking the drug with the first bite of each meal. There may also be an increase in LFTs.

4. **A.** Propranolol (a nonselective β-blocker) can mask the symptoms of hypoglycemia (ie, tachycardia [palpitations], pallor, shakiness [tremor], paresthesia, hunger, diaphoresis [sweating], dizziness, and blurred vision). None of the remaining drugs listed have this effect.

5. **E.** The increase in LFTs may be due to acarbose, and the increase in serum creatinine may represent the development or progression of nephropathy, a long-term complication of DM. The decrease in the serum creatinine and BUN are incorrect answers. Prednisone, a corticosteroid, has a dose-dependent, direct glucogenic and glycosuric effect, and therefore an increase in BG might be observed.

6. **B.** Though tolazamide and glimepiride are first- and second-generation sulfonylureas, duplication of drug class is inappropriate. These agents are both intermediate-acting and therefore might potentiate the adverse drug event of hypoglycemia. Insulin may be indicated in the person with type 2 DM as the disease progresses. The potential drug-drug interaction between phenytoin and tolazamide could result in an increased BG level, and the potential drug-drug interaction between glimepiride and itraconazole could result in a decreased BG level. An ACEI for hypertension in type 2 DM is appropriate as this drug is renal protective.

7. **E.** The A_{1c} and SMBG tests are essential for monitoring the success of glucose control therapy. The SMBG gives an immediate determination of BG level and the A_{1c} gives an average reading over the previous 2-3 months (or 120 days, the lifespan of an RBC). Phenytoin levels are necessary for monitoring therapeutically appropriate levels, and BP readings are for monitoring the success of anti-hypertensive therapy. A serum C-peptide might be diagnostic for the determination of functioning β-cells; however, if performed, it is done very infrequently to reduce cost.

8. **A.** One-half cup of diet soda would be inappropriate, because a mild hypoglycemic episode requires a fast-acting oral carbohydrate for resolution and diet soda has none. The other options would all be appropriate for resolution of the event.

9. **C.** Lipohypertrophy (a bulging of the injection site) is due to nonrotation of injection sites. The risk of infection may be reduced by using aseptic injecting technique. Lipoatrophy (a pitting of the injection site) may be due to an antigenic response to insulin. The advice regarding rotation of injection site is not outdated.

10. **D.** Glucagon, a pancreatic hormone which is given parenterally, is the most appropriate treatment for a severe hypoglycemic episode (life-threatening), as the patient may be unconscious and not able to take a fast-acting carbohydrate by mouth. The other items represent inappropriate treatment for mild to moderate hypoglycemia (the amounts of items B, C, and E are inadequate, and the soda in item A should be regular soda).

11. **C.** Pharmaceutical research has developed an inhaled insulin product which is still being tested. Presently, the commercially available insulins may only be administered intravenously or subcutaneously.

12. **D.** Newly diagnosed type 2 DM should first have a trial with MNT and exercise, and if this nondrug therapy fails, then oral antidiabetic monotherapy should be added. Combination oral therapy would be indicated next with failure of monotherapy, and then following its failure, insulin monotherapy or in combination with oral agents is indicated. Insulin is indicated in all the other situations.

13. **D.** Dietary intake, physical activity/exercise, and blood glucose levels are the parameters used in adjusting insulin dosing (eg, if the parameters of dietary intake and blood glucose levels are decreased and physical activity/exercise is increased, then the insulin dosing would require reduction to avoid hypoglycemia). Monitoring of these parameters is critical to adjusting the insulin regimen. Items 1 and 5 are incorrect.

14. **B.** Glynase® is a micronized formulation of glyburide that is significantly absorbed (eg, a 3-mg tablet provides blood levels similar to a 5-mg conventional tablet). Micronase® is a trade name for non-micronized glyburide. Glucotrol XL® is the name of an extended formulation of glipizide. Orinase® is the trade name for tolbutamide (the only first-generation sulfonylurea listed here), and Amaryl® is the trade name for glimepiride.

15. **B.** Refrigerated insulin is allowed to reach room temperature prior to administration to minimize painful injections. Proper mixing, prevention of frosting or clumping, or maintenance of clarity have nothing to do with reaching room temperature. Systemic absorption would actually be enhanced by increasing to room temperature, not delayed.

16. **A.** Regular or clear insulin is always drawn up first (to assure that all persons mixing insulins will use the same procedure and no intermediate- or long-acting insulin will be placed in the regular insulin vial, potentially causing contamination and dose variance). Glargine is also a clear insulin; however, it is never to be mixed with other insulins due to the low pH (4.0) of its diluents.

17. **B.** Uniform dispersion of insulin suspensions can be obtained by gently rolling the vial between the hands. Insulin is a fragile molecule and all the other means listed could cause molecular degradation.

18. **C.** Of these insulins, regular is the only one that can be administered intravenously. Though glargine is clear like regular insulin, its pH is 4.0 and it should never be given intravenously. The remaining insulins are suspensions and also should never be given intravenously.

19. **C.** DM is the leading cause of new cases of blindness among adults 20-74 years of age in the U.S. There is also an increased incidence of stroke with DM, but DM is not the leading cause of this problem. The other items are incorrect.

20. **D.** Proteinuria is an indication that a patient is developing the long-term complication of nephropathy. Items A, B, and C could be related to acute complications such as DKA (glucosuria and leukocytosis) and hypoglycemia (tachycardia). Item E is incorrect.

21. **C.** Chlorpropamide has a $t_{1/2}$ of 35 hours and a duration of action of 60 hours, therefore it has been associated with prolonged hypoglycemia in the elderly (perhaps due to their declining renal function). The other sulfonylureas have reported less hypoglycemia.

22. **A.** Chlorpropamide has had the greatest reporting of this drug interaction relative to the first-generation sulfonylureas. The remaining drugs listed have not had reports of this adverse drug event.

23. **C.** Lactic acidosis can result if metformin (Glucophage) is given in this situation and it can be potentially fatal. Renal function must be evaluated following such a procedure, and it must be normal before metformin may be resumed. The other items are incorrect.

24. **A.** Macrosomia (abnormally large fetal body size) is one of the fetal complications of concern in GDM. The primary benefit of insulin therapy is reduction in the incidence of macrosomia. The other items are incorrect.

25. **B.** Contraindications for metformin are renal dysfunction for those predisposed to lactic acidosis. Metformin does not cause hypoglycemia and it is indicated in type 2 DM. Hypertension and iron deficiency anemia are incorrect answers. Metformin may cause megaloblastic anemia.

26. **B.** The Somogyi effect is rebound hyperglycemia or early morning hyperglycemia secondary to nocturnal hypoglycemia. The person with type 1 DM may experience a honeymoon period—a phase of erratic insulin secretion during destruction of β-cells by islet cell antibodies. This apparent short-lived remission lasts months to a year. The dawn phenomenon is fasting hyperglycemia (pre-breakfast) due to decreased plasma insulin during the night or the anti-insulin effect of nocturnal growth hormone. Items D and E are incorrect.

27. **D.** Lactic acidosis is a potentially fatal adverse drug event of Glucophage (metformin). It does not cause weight gain. Modest weight loss is possible and no hypoglycemia is reported when metformin is used as monotherapy. Diarrhea is an adverse drug event, but with gradual dose titration and administration with food, it decreases over time. Items B and E are incorrect.

28. **D.** Oral glucose instead of carbohydrate sources with sucrose (cane sugar) or fructose is used because absorption of these is inhibited. The remaining items are true of acarbose therapy.

29. **E.** Prandin may cause hypoglycemia like the sulfonylureas. Hyperglycemia is not one of the adverse drug events (ADEs) reported. All the other ADEs may be caused by Prandin.

30. **C.** Meglitinides should be taken 30 minutes before main meals and if a meal is omitted, the drug should not be taken. It enhances postprandial glucose utilization, hypoglycemia and not hyperglycemia may occur, and disulfiram-like reactions are not reported.

31. **A.** The α-glucosidase inhibitors (eg, acarbose), biguanides (eg, metformin), and thiazolidine-diones (eg, rosiglitazone) all require LFTs for monitoring. Glargine, a long-acting insulin, does not require LFTs for monitoring; rather it requires blood glucose monitoring.

32. **E.** Megaloblastic anemia is a reported adverse drug effect for metformin but not for Actos . All the other items listed are reported ADEs. Since troglitazone (Rezulin®), a thiazolidine-dione, was withdrawn from the market in 2000 due to severe liver toxicity, this ADE could potentially occur with Actos®; therefore LFTs should be performed periodically.

33. **E.** Acetohexamide has a hypoglycemic effect. All the other drugs listed have a direct glucogenic effect.

34. **A.** The sulfonylureas stimulate pancreatic β-cells to secrete insulin. Item B is the MOA for α-glucosidase inhibitors, item C is the MOA for the biguanide metformin, item D is the MOA for the glitizones, and item E is the MOA for insulin.

35. **D.** Polyuria (excessive urination) is one of the classic signs and symptoms of DM. All of the other answers listed are some of the signs and symptoms of hypoglycemia, which can be life threatening.

36. **E.** Pramlintide (Symlin®) was approved in March 2005 as the first new type 1 diabetes treatment in more than 80 years. It is an injectable synthetic version of the human hormone amylin.

37. **C.** Unopened insulin vials kept under refrigeration are stable until their labeled expiration dates. Glargine insulin (Lantus®) is stable in a prefilled syringe for only 2 to 3 days. Lispro insulin (Humalog®) should be refrigerated when not in use. Opened vials of any insulin product should be stored in the refrigerator and are stable for up to 28 days.

6. References

American Diabetes Association (ADA). Clinical practice recommendations 2007. *Diabetes Care.* 2007;30(suppl. 1):S1-S103.

Expert Committee on the Diagnosis and Classification of Diabetes Mellitus: Report of the Expert Committee on the Diagnosis and Classification of Diabetes Mellitus. *Diabetes Care.* 1997; 20:1183-1197.

Expert Committee on the Diagnosis and Classification of Diabetes Mellitus: Follow-up report on the diagnosis of diabetes mellitus. *Diabetes Care.* 2003; 26:3160-3167.

Bode BW (ed.): *Medical Management of Type 1 Diabetes.* Alexandria, VA. American Diabetes Association; 2004.

Burant CF (Ed.): *Medical Management of Type 2 Diabetes.* Alexandria, VA. American Diabetes Association; 2004.

Funnell MM, Brown TL, Childs BP, et al. National Standards for Diabetes Self-Management Education. *Diabetes Care.* 2007; 30(6):1630-1637.

Diabetes Control and Complications Trial Research Group. The effect of intensive treatment on the development and the progress of long-term complications in insulin-dependent diabetes mellitus. *N Engl J Med.* 1993;329:977-986.

http://www.diabetes.org/diabetes-statistics.jsp

Koda-Kimble, MA, Carlisle, BA. Diabetes mellitus. In: Koda-Kimble MA, Young LY, eds. *Applied Therapeutics: The Clinical Use of Drugs*, 8th ed. Philadelphia: Lippincott Williams & Wilkins; 2005:50-1 to 50-86.

Setter SM, White Jr JR, Campbell RK. Diabetes. In: Helms RA, Quan DJ, Herfindal ET, Gourley DR, eds. *Textbook of Therapeutics*, 8th ed. Philadelphia: Lippincott Williams & Wilkins; 2006: 1042-1105.

Stoneking K, Farr G. Early Use of Insulin in Type 2 Diabetes. Drug Topics Diabetes Supplement, October 2002.

The University Group Diabetes Program. A study of the effects of hypoglycemic agents on vascular complications in patients with adult onset diabetes. *Diabetes.* 1970;19 (suppl. 2):1-26.

UK Prospective Diabetes Study (UKPDS) Group. Intensive blood-glucose control with sulphonylureas or insulin compared with conventional treatment and risks of complications in patients with type 2 diabetes (UKPDS 33). *Lancet.* 1998;352:837-853.

UK Prospective Diabetes Study (UKPDS) Group. Effect of intensive blood-glucose control with metformin on complications in overweight patients with type 2 diabetes (UKPDS 34). *Lancet.* 1998;352:854-865.

White JR, Campbell RK. Drug/drug and drug/disease interactions and diabetes. *Diabetes Educator.* 1995;21:283-289.

14. Thyroid, Adrenal, and Miscellaneous Endocrine Drugs

Bob L. Lobo, PharmD, BCPS
Associate Professor, Department of Clinical Pharmacy
University of Tennessee College of Pharmacy

Contents

1. Thyroid

Hypothyroidism

Disease overview
Definition and epidemiology
- Hypothyroidism is a syndrome resulting from deficient thyroid hormone production that results in a slowing down of all bodily functions.
- Retardation of growth occurs in infants and children.
- Its prevalence is greater in women and increases with age; it affects 1.5%-2% of women and 0.2% of men.

Types
- Most cases are caused by thyroid gland failure (primary hypothyroidism).
- Hashimoto's disease (chronic lymphocytic thyroiditis) is the cause of 90% of primary hypothyroidism.
- Pituitary failure causes secondary hypothyroidism.
- Hypothalamic failure causes tertiary hypothyroidism.
- Iatrogenic hypothyroidism follows exposure to radiation with radioiodine or external radiation.
- Other causes may include thyroidectomy, iodine deficiency, enzymatic defects, iodine, lithium, and interferon-alfa.

Clinical presentation
- Symptoms include cold intolerance, fatigue, somnolence, constipation, menorrhagia, myalgias, and hoarseness.
- Signs include thyroid gland enlargement or atrophy, bradycardia, edema, dry skin, and weight gain.
- Myxedema coma is an end stage of hypothyroidism characterized by weakness, confusion, hypothermia, hypoventilation, hypoglycemia, hyponatremia, coma, and shock.

Pathophysiology
- Thyroxine (T_4) is the major hormone secreted by the thyroid, which is converted to the more potent triiodothyronine (T_3) in tissues.
- Thyroxine secretion is stimulated by thyroid-stimulating hormone (TSH).
- TSH secretion is inhibited by T_4, forming a negative feedback loop.
- Hashimoto's disease is an autoimmune-mediated disease resulting from cell- and antibody-mediated thyroid injury.
- Antimicrosomal antibodies are directed against thyroidal antigens.

Diagnosis
- Plasma TSH assay is the initial test of choice if hypothyroidism is suspected clinically.
- TSH levels are elevated in primary hypothyroidism.
- Low plasma-free T_4 (or T_4 index) confirms the diagnosis of hypothyroidism.

Treatment principles
- Synthetic thyroxine (levothyroxine) is the drug of choice for hypothyroidism because it is chemically stable, inexpensive, free of antigenicity, and has uniform potency.
- The typical dose is 100-125 mcg PO once daily; reduce dose to 50 mcg in the elderly and 25 mcg in patients with coronary artery disease to reduce the risk of precipitating angina.
- The goal of therapy is to maintain plasma TSH in the normal range.
- Dose changes are made at 6- to 8-week intervals until the TSH is normal.
- Overtreatment is detected by subnormal TSH and is associated with osteoporosis and atrial fibrillation.
- Failure to respond to appropriate doses is most often due to poor compliance.
- Do not use thyroid hormones to facilitate weight loss in euthyroid patients.
- Thyroid hormones have a narrow therapeutic index; careful monitoring of clinical condition and thyroid function is required.

Drug therapy of hypothyroidism (Table 1)
Mechanism of action
- Thyroid hormones enhance oxygen consumption by most tissues and increase basal metabolic rate and metabolism of carbohydrates, lipids, and proteins.

Patient counseling
- Take once daily, 30 minutes before breakfast since food may decrease absorption.
- Replacement therapy is usually to be taken for life; don't discontinue without advice of prescriber.
- Notify prescriber if you experience rapid or irregular heartbeat, chest pain, shortness of breath, nervousness, irritability, tremors, heat intolerance, or weight loss.
- Don't take antacids, calcium, or iron supplements within 4 hours of levothyroxine.

Adverse effects
- Cardiovascular: tachycardia, arrhythmia, angina, MI
- CNS: tremor, headache, nervousness, insomnia, irritability, hyperactivity
- GI: diarrhea, vomiting, cramps
- Miscellaneous: weight loss, fatigue, menstrual irregularities, excessive sweating, heat intolerance, fever,

Table 1

Thyroid Preparations for the Treatment of Hypothyroidism

Trade name	Generic name	Dosage forms	Usual dosage range
Synthroid® Levothroid® Levoxyl® Unithroid® Thyro-Tabs®	Levothyroxine sodium (T$_4$)	Tablets: 0.025, 0.05, 0.075, 0.088, 0.1, 0.112, 0.125, 0.137, 0.15, 0.175, 0.2, and 0.3 mg Injection: 200 and 500 mcg	0.1-0.15 mg PO qd for hypothyroidism (dosage is individualized); higher doses are used in treating thyroid cancer
Armour Thyroid® Nature-Throid® Westhroid®	Desiccated thyroid USP	Tablets: 15, 30, 32.4, 60, 64.8, 65, 90, 120, 129.6, 130, 180, 194.4, 195, 240, and 300 mg	60-120 mg PO qd for hypothyroidism; (dosage is individualized); higher doses used in treating thyroid cancer
Cytomel® Triostat®	Liothyronine (T$_3$)	Tablets: 5, 25, 50 mcg Injection: 10 mcg	25 mcg PO qd for hypothyroidism
Thyrolar®	Liotrix (T$_4$ and T$_3$ in a 4:1 ratio)	Tablets: 3.1/12.5 mcg, 6.25/25 mcg, 12.5/50 mcg, 25/100 mcg, 37.5/150 mcg	60-120 mg PO qd for hypothyroidism

muscle weakness, hair loss, decreased bone mineral density, hypersensitivity

Drug interactions

- Amiodarone may cause hypothyroidism or hyperthyroidism.
- Antacids decrease absorption of levothyroxine; separate administration by at least 4 hours.
- Antidiabetic agents may be less effective with levothyroxine; increase in insulin or oral hypoglycemic dose may be needed.
- Bile acid sequestrants reduce absorption of levothyroxine; separate by at least 4 hours.
- Enzyme-inducing antiepileptic agents increase hepatic degradation of levothyroxine; may need to increase thyroxine dosage.
- Estrogens may decrease response to levothyroxine; may need to increase levothyroxine dosage.
- Lithium commonly causes hypothyroidism.
- Warfarin's effect may be enhanced by levothyroxine; may need to decrease warfarin dosage.
- Digoxin levels may be reduced by levothyroxine supplementation.
- Sucralfate may decrease levothyroxine absorption; separate by at least 4 hours.
- Soybean formula decreases levothyroxine absorption.
- Sympathomimetic drugs may potentiate the effects of levothyroxine.
- Theophylline clearance may be enhanced by levothyroxine

Monitoring parameters

- Plasma TSH every 6-8 weeks until normalization
- Signs and symptoms of hypothyroidism should improve within a few weeks.
- Once the optimum replacement dose is attained, physical examination and TSH level every 6-12 months
- Patients at risk for coronary artery disease should be monitored for angina.

Pharmacokinetics

- The FDA states that all levothyroxine products should be considered therapeutically inequivalent unless equivalence (AB rating) has been established and noted in the "Orange Book."
- Levoxyl, Levothroid, Synthroid, Unithroid, and some generics are bioequivalent.
- Due to the narrow therapeutic index of levothyroxine, many experts recommend rechecking TSH concentrations 6-8 weeks after any change in formulation, even when bioequivalent.
- Oral absorption is improved by fasting but decreased by dietary fiber, drugs, and foods
- A half-life of 7 days allows once-daily dosing.
- Average bioavailability of levothyroxine products ranges from 40%-80%; when switching from oral to intravenous levothyroxine, the dosage should be reduced by 25%-50%.

Other

- Use of natural thyroid hormones such as desiccated thyroid USP is discouraged due to less predictable potency and stability compared to synthetic levothyroxine.
- Synthetic T_3 (liothyronine) has a shorter half-life than levothyroxine, a higher incidence of cardiac side effects, and is more difficult to monitor.

Hyperthyroidism

Disease overview
Definition and epidemiology

- Hyperthyroidism (thyrotoxicosis) is the clinical syndrome that results when tissues are exposed to high levels of thyroid hormone.
- Thyrotoxicosis is more common in women than men, occurring in 3 per 1000 women.

Types

- Graves' disease is the most common cause of hyperthyroidism.
- Toxic multinodular goiter (MNG), toxic adenoma, and exogenous thyroid hormone ingestion may also cause hyperthyroidism.
- Thyroid storm is a life-threatening, sudden exacerbation of all of the symptoms of thyrotoxicosis characterized by fever, tachycardia, delirium, and coma.
- Hyperthyroidism may be caused by drugs such as amiodarone and iodine.

Clinical presentation

- Symptoms include heat intolerance, weight loss, weakness, palpitations, and anxiety.
- Signs include tremor, tachycardia, weakness and eyelid lag, and warm, moist skin.
- Other manifestations include atrial fibrillation and congestive heart failure.

Pathophysiology

- Graves' disease is an autoimmune disease in which thyroid-stimulating antibodies are produced; these antibodies mimic the action of TSH on thyroid tissue.
- Toxic adenomas and MNGs are masses of thyroid tissue that secrete thyroid hormones independent of pituitary control.

Diagnosis

- Elevated T_4 or T_3 in the presence of a decreased TSH confirms the diagnosis of hyperthyroidism.

Treatment principles

- There are three primary methods for controlling hyperthyroidism: surgery, radioactive iodine (RAI), and antithyroid (thionamide) drugs.

- The goal is to minimize symptoms and eliminate excess thyroid hormone.
- RAI is often considered the treatment of choice in Graves' disease, toxic adenomas, and MNGs.
- Propylthiouracil is preferred in pregnancy; RAI is contraindicated.
- Thionamide drugs (propylthiouracil and methimazole) have no permanent effect on thyroid function.
- Adjunctive treatments for hyperthyroidism include β-adrenergic receptor blockers or calcium channel blockers in order to control tachycardia associated with hyperthyroidism.

Drug therapy of hyperthyroidism (Table 2)
Thionamides
Mechanism of action

- Propylthiouracil (PTU) and methimazole inhibit the synthesis of thyroid hormones by preventing the incorporation of iodine into iodotyrosines and by inhibiting the coupling of monoiodotyrosine and diiodotyrosine to form T_4 and T_3.
- Propylthiouracil inhibits the peripheral conversion of T_4 to T_3.

Patient counseling

- This medication prevents excessive thyroid hormone production.
- It must be taken regularly in order to be effective.
- Do not discontinue use without first consulting your physician.
- Notify physician if fever, sore throat, unusual bleeding, rash, abdominal pain, or yellowing of the skin occurs.

Adverse effects

- CNS: fever, headache, paresthesias
- General: rash, arthralgia, urticaria
- GI: jaundice, hepatitis
- Hematologic: agranulocytosis, leukopenia, bleeding

Drug interactions

- Potentiation of warfarin effect

Monitoring parameters

- Monitor for improvement in signs and symptoms of hyperthyroidism.
- Thyroid function tests, signs and symptoms of agranulocytosis (fever, malaise, sore throat)

Pharmacokinetics

- Propylthiouracil has a short half-life requiring more frequent dosing than methimazole.

Table 2

Antithyroid Medications

Drug name	Drug contains	Dosage forms	Usual dosage range
PTU	Propylthiouracil	Tablets: 50 mg	150-300 mg PO daily at 8-hour intervals
Tapazole®	Methimazole	Tablets: 5, 10 mg	5-40 mg PO in single daily dose or divided
Lugol's solution	Strong iodine solution	Solution: 5% iodine and 10% potassium iodide; delivers 6.3 mg iodine per drop	0.1-0.3 mL (3-5 drops) PO tid
SSKI	Saturated solution of potassium iodide	Solution: 1 g/mL; delivers 38 mg iodine per drop of saturated solution	1-5 drops PO tid in water or juice

Iodides

Mechanism of action
- Block hormone release, inhibit thyroid hormone synthesis
- May be used when rapid reduction in thyroid hormone secretion is desired such as in thyroid storm or to decrease glandular vascularity prior to thyroidectomy

Patient instructions
- Dilute with water or fruit juice to improve taste.
- Notify physician if fever, skin rash, metallic taste, swelling of the throat, or burning of the mouth occurs.

Adverse effects
- Rash, swelling of salivary glands, metallic taste, burning of the mouth, GI distress, hypersensitivity, goiter

Drug interactions
- Lithium potentiates antithyroid effect of iodides

Monitoring parameters
- Monitor for improvement in signs and symptoms of hyperthyroidism and for adverse effects.

2. Adrenals

Cushing's Syndrome

Disease overview

Definition and epidemiology
- Syndrome resulting from chronic glucocorticoid excess
- Incidence of 2-4 per million population cases each year

Types
- Usually iatrogenic due to therapy with glucocorticoid drugs
- Endogenous Cushing's syndrome is usually caused by overproduction of adrenocorticotropic hormone (ACTH) by pituitary gland adenomas (Cushing's disease).

Clinical presentation
- Obesity involving the face, neck, trunk, and abdomen, hypertension, hirsutism, acne, amenorrhea, depression, thin skin, easy bruising, diabetes, osteopenia, and depression

Pathophysiology
- The hypothalamus produces corticotropin-releasing hormone (CRH) which stimulates the anterior pituitary gland to release ACTH. Circulating ACTH stimulates the adrenal cortex to produce cortisol.

Diagnosis

- Based on signs and symptoms of hypercortisolism
- Dexamethasone suppression test or 24-hour urine cortisol measurement may be used.

Treatment principles

- If the syndrome is iatrogenic, minimization of corticosteroid exposure is essential.
- Pharmacotherapy of Cushing's disease is aimed at reducing cortisol production or activity with drugs, radiation, or surgery.

Drug therapy of Cushing's disease (Table 3)

Mechanism of action

- Drugs that are used to treat Cushing's disease suppress synthesis of cortisol.
- Ketoconazole inhibits cytochrome P-450–dependent enzymes and cortisol synthesis.
- Aminoglutethimide inhibits conversion of cholesterol to pregnenolone.
- Mitotane is a cytotoxic drug that suppresses ACTH secretion and reduces synthesis of cortisol.
- Metyrapone decreases cortisol synthesis by inhibition of 11-hydroxylase activity.

Patient counseling

- Ketoconazole should be taken with food; separate from antacids by at least 2 hours; notify physician if abdominal pain, yellow skin, or pale stool occurs.
- Aminoglutethimide may cause drowsiness, rash, weakness, nausea, and loss of appetite.
- Metyrapone may cause nausea, vomiting, dizziness, and sedation.
- Mitotane may cause nausea, vomiting, diarrhea, and tiredness.

Adverse effects

- Ketoconazole causes nausea, vomiting, headache, impotence, and hepatotoxicity.

- Aminoglutethimide causes drowsiness, rash, weakness, hypotension, nausea, loss of appetite, hypothyroidism, and blood dyscrasias.
- Metyrapone causes nausea, vomiting, dizziness, and sedation.
- Mitotane may cause nausea, vomiting, diarrhea, and tiredness.

Drug interactions

- Ketoconazole is a CYP450 3A4 enzyme inhibitor and may increase serum concentrations of cyclosporine, warfarin, cisapride, and triazolam; drugs that lower gastric acidity will decrease ketoconazole absorption; rifampin decreases ketoconazole levels.
- Aminoglutethimide may induce metabolism of warfarin.

Monitoring parameters

- Cortisol monitoring is required with mitotane.

Adrenal Insufficiency

Disease overview

Definition and epidemiology

- Primary adrenocortical deficiency (Addison's disease) is caused by autoimmune-mediated destruction of the adrenal cortex, and results in glucocorticoid and mineralocorticoid deficiency.
- Addison's disease occurs in 5-6 per million population per year

Types

- Primary adrenal insufficiency (Addison's disease) involves autoimmune destruction of the adrenal cortex.
- Secondary insufficiency occurs after cessation of chronic exogenous corticosteroid use.

Table 3

Drugs for Cushing's Syndrome

Trade name	Generic name	Dosage forms	Usual dosage range
Nizoral®	Ketoconazole	Tablets: 250 mg	800-1200 mg PO qd
Cytadren®	Aminoglutethimide	Tablets: 250 mg	250 mg PO q6h
Lysodren®	Mitotane	Tablets: 500 mg	9-10 g/d PO in divided doses
Metopirone®	Metyrapone	Capsules: 250 mg	1-6 g/d PO in 4-6 divided doses

- Acute adrenal insufficiency, or Addisonian crisis, is an endocrine emergency precipitated by severe stress.

Clinical presentation
- Glucocorticoid deficiency (weight loss, malaise, abdominal pain, and depression)
- Mineralocorticoid deficiency (dehydration, hypotension, hyperkalemia, and salt craving)

Pathophysiology
- Cortisol is synthesized in the adrenal cortex when cholesterol is converted to pregnenolone by ACTH.
- The adrenal cortex secretes aldosterone, cortisol, and androgenic hormones.
- Mineralocorticoids (eg, aldosterone) enhance reabsorption of sodium and water from the distal tubule of the kidney and increase urinary potassium excretion.
- Glucocorticoids affect glucose, carbohydrate, and fat metabolism; produce anti-inflammatory and immunosuppressive effects; and affect other physiologic processes.
- Chronic administration of corticosteroids produces inhibition of pituitary ACTH secretion and reduced cortisol production (hypothalamic-pituitary-adrenocortical [HPA] axis suppression).
- Abrupt cessation of steroids may precipitate adrenal insufficiency.

Diagnosis
- A cosyntropin (ACTH) stimulation test may be used to assess hypocortisolism.

Treatment principles
- Addison's disease requires lifelong glucocorticoid and mineralocorticoid replacement.
- Hydrocortisone 100 mg IV q8h is the drug of choice for acute adrenal crisis.
- "Stress doses" of corticosteroids are given for minor illness, injury, or surgery; if stress is severe, hydrocortisone 100 mg IV q8h is used.
- Gradual tapering of corticosteroids reduces the risk of adrenal insufficiency in patients with HPA axis suppression.
- Non-adrenal uses for corticosteroids are numerous, including allergic reactions; inflammatory conditions; hematologic disorders; rheumatic disorders; neurologic diseases; cancer; immunosuppression; pulmonary, renal, skin and thyroid diseases; hypercalcemia; and others.
- Fludrocortisone has minimal anti-inflammatory activity and is used only when mineralocorticoid activity is needed, such as when increased blood pressure is desired.

Drug therapy of adrenal insufficiency (Table 4)
Mechanism of action
- Glucocorticoids increase blood glucose by stimulating gluconeogenesis and glycogenolysis; fat deposition is increased.
- Catabolic effects in lymphoid, connective tissue, bone, muscle, fat, and skin
- Inhibition of inflammation and immunosuppression, vasoconstriction, reduction in prostaglandin and leukotriene synthesis, decreased neutrophils at sites of inflammation, and inhibition of macrophage function

Patient counseling
- May cause stomach upset, so take with food
- It is preferable to take the dose prior to 9 AM.
- Wear or carry identification if on chronic steroid therapy.
- May mask signs of infection
- May increase insulin or oral hypoglycemic requirements if diabetic
- Notify the physician if weight gain, muscle weakness, sore throat, or infection occurs.
- Report tiredness, stomach pain, weakness, and high or low blood sugar to your physician.
- Do not discontinue abruptly if taking long-term.

Adverse effects
- Cardiac: hypertension, sodium and fluid retention, atherosclerosis
- CNS: insomnia, anxiety, depression, psychosis
- Metabolic: obesity, hyperglycemia, hypokalemia, amenorrhea, impotence
- Ophthalmic: cataracts, glaucoma
- Immune: infections, impaired wound healing, leukocytosis
- Musculoskeletal: myopathy, osteoporosis

Drug interactions
- Rifampin and other enzyme-inducing drugs increase metabolism of corticosteroids and decrease their effectiveness.
- Concomitant use of NSAIDs and corticosteroids increases risk of peptic ulcer disease.
- Immunologic response to vaccines may be impaired by corticosteroids.
- Estrogens may increase corticosteroid clearance.
- Ketoconazole, macrolides, and other CYP450 3A4 enzyme-inhibiting drugs may decrease clearance of corticosteroids.
- Corticosteroids increase insulin and oral hypoglycemic drug requirements.

Monitoring parameters
- Weight gain, edema, increased blood pressure, electrolytes, blood glucose, infection

Table 4

Corticosteroids and Dose Equivalents

Trade name	Generic name	Anti-inflammatory potency	Sodium retaining potency	Equivalent dose (mg)	Half-life
Cortone®	Cortisone	0.8	2	25	Short
Cortef®, Hydrocortone®, Solu-Cortef®	Hydrocortisone	1	2	20	Short
Deltasone®, Liquid Pred®	Prednisone	4	1	5	Medium
Prelone®, Pediapred®, Delta-Cortef®	Prednisolone	4	1	5	Medium
Medrol®, Solu-Medrol®, Depo-Medrol®, A-Methapred®	Methylprednisolone	5	0	4	Medium
Aristocort®, Kenacort®, Kenalog®	Triamcinolone	5	0	4	Medium
Decadron®, Dexameth®, Dexone®, Hexadrol®	Dexamethasone	30	0	0.75	Long
Celestone®	Betamethasone	25	0	0.75	Long
Florinef®	Fludrocortisone	15	150	2	Medium

Pharmacokinetics

- Many dosage forms, doses, and schedules are used, including tablets, topicals, enemas, oral liquids, injections, and depot injection forms for intra-articular or intramuscular use.

3. Miscellaneous Endocrine Drugs

ACTH and Cosyntropin (Table 5)

Therapeutic uses
- For diagnosis of adrenal insufficiency and occasionally as an alternative to corticosteroids

Mechanism of action
- ACTH stimulates the adrenal cortex to secrete adrenal hormones.
- If ACTH fails to elicit an appropriate cortisol response, adrenal insufficiency is present.
- Cosyntropin is a synthetic peptide which is similar to human ACTH, but less allergenic.

Patient counseling
- Same as for corticosteroids

Adverse effects
- Same as for corticosteroids

Drug interactions
- Enzyme-inducing drugs will decrease effects.

Table 5

ACTH and Cosyntropin

Trade name	Generic name	Dosage forms	Usual dosage range
Cortrosyn®	Cosyntropin	Injection: 0.25 mg	0.25-0.75 mg for testing
Acthar® (ACTH)	Corticotropin	Injection: 25, 40 units	10-25 units for testing
H.P. Acthar Gel®		Repository injection: 40, 80 units/mL	40-80 units of repository injection every 1-3 days

Monitoring parameters
• Same as for corticosteroids

Vasopressin and Desmopressin (Table 6)

Therapeutic uses
• Vasopressin: diabetes insipidus, variceal hemorrhage, shock, ventricular fibrillation
• Desmopressin: nocturnal enuresis, diabetes insipidus, hemophilia A, von Willebrand's disease

Mechanism of action
• Vasopressin is also known as antidiuretic hormone (ADH); it increases water resorption.
• Vasopressin causes vasoconstriction in portal and splanchnic vessels (GI tract).
• Desmopressin is a synthetic derivative of vasopressin with ADH activity and only minimal vasoconstrictive properties; increases clotting factor VII levels.

Patient counseling
• Intranasal desmopressin: the bottle should be discarded after 25 or 50 doses; don't transfer solution to another bottle; may cause nasal irritation; notify physician if bleeding is not controlled or if headache, shortness of breath, or severe abdominal cramps occur; instruct on proper intranasal use.

Adverse effects
• Vasopressin: angina, MI, vasoconstriction, hyponatremia, gangrene, abdominal cramps, tissue necrosis if extravasation occurs, hypersensitivity
• Desmopressin: abdominal pain, headache, flushing, nausea, nasal irritation, vulvar pain, nosebleed, rhinitis, hypersensitivity

Drug interactions
• May enhance effects of other pressors
• Carbamazepine and chlorpropamide potentiate the effect of desmopressin on ADH.

Monitoring parameters
• Diabetes insipidus: urine volume, plasma osmolality
• von Willebrand's disease: factor VIII levels, bleeding time
• When intravenous vasopressin is used, monitor blood pressure and pulses.

Table 6

Vasopressin and Desmopressin

Trade Name	Generic name	Dosage forms	Usual dosage range
Pitressin®	Vasopressin	Injection: 20 units/mL	10-20 units IM, SC, or IV daily at 3- to 4-hour intervals or as a continuous infusion
Stimate® (DDAVP)	Desmopressin	Tablets: 0.1, 0.2 mg Nasal solution: 0.1 mg/mL, 1.5 mg/mL Injection: 4 mcg/mL	Nocturnal enuresis: 20-40 mcg intranasally qhs Diabetes insipidus: 0.1-0.2 mg PO bid, 0.1-0.4 mL intranasally in single or divided doses

Androgens and Anabolic Steroids (Table 7)

Therapeutic uses

- Hypogonadism, delayed puberty, metastatic breast cancer, anemia, AIDS wasting in HIV-infected men, corticosteroid-induced hypogonadism and osteoporosis, and moderate to severe vasomotor symptoms associated with menopause (when combined with estrogen)
- They are schedule C-III controlled substances since they are intentionally misused for performance enhancing effects and enhanced muscular development and endurance.

Mechanism of action

- Androgens promote growth and development of male sex organs and maintenance of secondary sex characteristics.
- Androgens also cause retention of nitrogen, sodium, potassium, and phosphorus; increase protein anabolism; and decrease protein catabolism.
- Androgens are responsible for the growth spurt of adolescence and termination of linear growth by fusion of epiphyseal growth centers.
- Exogenous androgens stimulate production of red blood cells and suppress endogenous testosterone release through feedback inhibition of luteinizing hormone and spermatogenesis through feedback inhibition of FSH.

Patient counseling

- May cause stomach upset; notify a physician if swelling of the ankles or persistent erections occur.
- Controlled substance; do not misuse or abuse this product.
- For females, notify physician if deepening of the voice, increased facial hair, or menstrual irregularities occur.
- Patients receiving transdermal testosterone should be provided with the manufacturer's patient instructions and carefully counseled on use and disposal of the system.

Adverse effects

- General: jaundice; hepatitis; edema; high abuse potential in an effort to enhance athletic performance; hypercholesterolemia and atherosclerosis; increased aggression and libido
- Women: hirsutism, voice deepening, acne, decreased menses, clitoral enlargement
- Men: acne, sleep apnea, gynecomastia, azoospermia, prostate enlargement, decreased testicular size

Table 7

Androgens and Anabolic Steroids

Trade name	Generic name	Dosage forms	Usual dosage range
Testoderm® Androderm®	Testosterone transdermal system	Patch: 2.5, 4, 5, 6 mg/24 h	Patch: 2.5-6 mg for 24 h
AndroGel® 1% Testim®	Testosterone	1% Gel	5 grams applied once daily
Depo-Testosterone®	Testosterone cypionate (in oil)	Injection in oil: 100 mg/mL & 200 mg/mL	50-400 mg every 2-4 weeks
Android® Testred®	Methyltestosterone	Tablets: 10, 25 mg Capsules: 10 mg	10-50 mg once daily
Halotestin®	Fluoxymesterone	Tablets: 2, 5, 10 mg	5-10 mg once daily
Anadrol-50®	Oxymetholone	Tablets: 50 mg	50-100 mg once daily
Winstrol®	Stanozolol	Tablets: 2 mg	2 mg qd-tid
Oxandrin®	Oxandrolone	Tablets: 2.5, 10 mg	2.5-10 mg qd
Deca-Durabolin®	Nandrolone decanoate	Injection: 100, 200 mg/mL (in oil)	100-200 mg once weekly

4. Key Points

- Levothyroxine is the drug of choice for hypothyroidism.
- Lower doses of levothyroxine are used in the elderly and cardiac patients.
- Overtreatment with thyroid hormones causes osteoporosis and atrial fibrillation.
- Antacids, bile acid sequestrants, sucralfate, calcium, and iron supplements decrease absorption of levothyroxine and must be separated by at least 4 hours.
- Propylthiouracil (PTU) and methimazole are thionamide derivatives that are used to treat hyperthyroidism.
- Thionamides may cause life-threatening agranulocytosis or hepatitis, so patients must report to their physician if they experience fever, sore throat, abdominal pain, or jaundice.
- Drugs used to treat Cushing's disease inhibit synthesis of cortisol.
- Corticosteroid should be used at the lowest dose for the shortest time in order to reduce the risk of HPA axis suppression and adrenal insufficiency.
- Patients with adrenal insufficiency must receive supplemental corticosteroids in times of physiologic stress.
- Vasopressin and desmopressin are antidiuretic hormones.
- Androgens and anabolic steroids are abused by athletes seeking to enhance performance.

5. Questions and Answers

Use Patient Profile #1 to answer Questions 1 and 2.

1. The Synthroid prescription dispensed to Mrs. Ricardo on 3/21 requires advising her to

   A. take 4 hours before or 4 hours after Questran®
   B. take with food
   C. watch for signs of infection
   D. take as needed to keep your desired level of energy
   E. discontinue if you experience nausea

2. Which of the following of Mrs. Ricardo's conditions could the Synthroid exacerbate?

   A. Hypercholesterolemia
   B. Anemia
   C. Coronary artery disease
   D. Hypertension
   E. Constipation

3. Excessive doses of levothyroxine may cause

   A. weight gain
   B. osteoporosis
   C. cold intolerance
   D. bradycardia
   E. sedation

4. Which of the following drugs may produce hypothyroidism?

   I. Amitriptyline
   II. Lithium
   III. Amiodarone

   A. I only
   B. III only
   C. I and II only
   D. II and III only
   E. I, II, and III

5. All of the following may decrease the effect of thyroid hormone supplementation EXCEPT

   A. antacids
   B. bile acid sequestrants
   C. estrogens
   D. sucralfate
   E. theophylline

Patient Profile #1—Corn State Community Pharmacy

Patient Name	Jasmine Ricardo				
Address	189 Jonesbourough Road				
Age	78		Height	48 in	
Sex	Female	Race Hispanic	Weight	103 lbs	
Allergies	Cats				

DIAGNOSIS	Primary	1.	Hypercholesterolemia
		2.	Anemia
		3.	Coronary artery disease
	Secondary	1.	Hypertension
		2.	

MEDICATION RECORD

Date	Rx #	Physician	Drug/Strength	Quantity	Sig	Refills
3/21	89995	Stubie	Synthroid 0.025 mg	30	1 PO qd	0
2/23	88768	Hooper	Zocor 40 mg	30	1 PO qhs	5
2/23	88769	Hooper	Questran 4 g	60	1 packet bid mix with juice	5
2/23	88770	Hooper	Tenormin 50 mg	30	1 PO qd	5
2/23	88771	Hooper	Enalapril 5 mg	60	1 PO bid	5

PHARMACIST NOTES

Date	Note
2/23	Patient reminded to continue taking aspirin 325 mg for CAD
2/23	Patient to take OTC ferrous sulfate 325 mg daily for 3 months for anemia, advised patient to begin docusate 100 mg qd if constipation occurs

6. A patient who is suffering from heat intolerance, weight loss, tachycardia, tremor, and anxiety may be treated with

   A. acetaminophen
   B. mitotane
   C. cyproheptadine
   D. propylthiouracil
   E. diazepam

7. The patient with atrial fibrillation may require a decreased warfarin dosage when which of the following drugs is initiated?

   A. Liothyronine
   B. Rifampin
   C. Methimazole
   D. Phenytoin
   E. Diphenhydramine

8. Which of the following drugs is used to treat Cushing's disease?

   I. Ketoconazole
   II. Aminoglutethimide
   III. Mitotane

   A. I only
   B. III only
   C. I and II only
   D. II and III only
   E. I, II, and III

9. Which of the following drugs works by decreasing cortisol synthesis?

   A. Cortrosyn
   B. ACTH
   C. Oxandrolone
   D. Prednisone
   E. Metyrapone

10. Decreased ketoconazole absorption may occur if it is administered concomitantly with

    A. antacids
    B. food
    C. warfarin
    D. cyclosporine
    E. CYP450 3A4 inhibitors

11. Close monitoring of adrenal hormone secretion may be required when administering

   A. methyltestosterone
   B. mitotane
   C. desmopressin
   D. iodides
   E. propylthiouracil

12. Which of the following is used to treat adrenal crisis?

   A. Cosyntropin
   B. Aminoglutethimide
   C. Fluoxymesterone
   D. Vasopressin
   E. Hydrocortisone

13. Which of the following is NOT an effect of glucocorticoids?

   A. Immunosuppression
   B. Decreased prostaglandin synthesis
   C. Inhibit glycogenolysis
   D. Decreased neutrophils at sites of infection
   E. Inhibition of macrophages

Use Patient Profile #2 to answer Questions 14 and 15.

14. Which of the following is LEAST likely to contribute to the increased blood glucose seen in this patient?

   A. Dextrose 5%/NaCl 0.9% solution
   B. Captopril
   C. Epinephrine
   D. Methylprednisolone
   E. Anaphylaxis

15. The patient in Patient Profile #2 is discharged on a new prescription for Deltasone 40 mg qd for 7 days. He should be instructed to

   A. check feet closely for wounds
   B. take ibuprofen for musculoskeletal pain
   C. take on an empty stomach
   D. take at bedtime
   E. wear identification for steroid therapy

16. Chronic administration of glucocorticoids predisposes patients to

   A. arthritis
   B. obesity
   C. Alzheimer's disease
   D. osteoporosis
   E. hepatitis

Patient Profile #2—Big Sky Hospital

Patient Name	Stuart Big	Date of Admission 4/21 @ 1526
Address	440 Mountain Lane	
Age	28	Height 5' 8"
Sex	Male	Race White
Allergies	Aspirin	Weight 178 lbs

DIAGNOSIS

Admit Diagnosis
1. Anaphylactic reaction to aspirin

Secondary
1. Type 2 diabetes mellitus
2. Hypertension

LABORATORY

Date	Time	Lab	Result	(Normal Range)
4/23	1232	Glucose	443	(60-110 mg/dL)
4/23	0620	Glucose	391	(60-110 mg/dL)
4/22	1915	Glucose	352	(60-110 mg/dL)
4/22	1221	Glucose	289	(60-110 mg/dL)
4/22	0600	Glucose	240	(60-110 mg/dL)
4/21	1920	Glucose	181	(60-110 mg/dL)
4/21	1529	Glucose	144	(60-110 mg/dL)

ACTIVE MEDICATION ORDERS

Date	Time	Name & Strength	Route	Frequency/Schedule
4/21	1530	Solu-Medrol 125 mg	IV	q6h
4/21	1530	Dextrose 5%/NaCl 0.9%	IV	200 mL/h
4/21	1530	Diphenhydramine 50 mg	IV	q6h
4/21	1703	Glipizide 5 mg	PO	bid
4/21	1703	Glucophage 850 mg	PO	bid
4/21	1703	Captopril 50 mg	PO	tid

DISCONTINUED MEDICATION ORDERS

Date	Time	Name & Strength	Route	Frequency/Schedule
4/21	1530	Epinephrine 0.1 mg	SQ	Stat
4/21	1530	Diphenhydramine 50 mg	IV	Stat

DIETARY

Date	
4/21	1800 kcal American Diabetes Association Diet

17. A patient is taking prednisone 40 mg daily for 6 months. Upon abrupt cessation, which of the following may occur?

    A. Myopathy
    B. Diabetes
    C. Infection
    D. Adrenal crisis
    E. Psychosis

18. An increased risk of peptic ulcer disease occurs when NSAIDs are combined with

    A. ranitidine
    B. ferrous sulfate
    C. dexamethasone
    D. carbamazepine
    E. acetaminophen

19. Which of the following drugs may be used to diagnose adrenal insufficiency?

    A. Desmopressin
    B. Clemestine
    C. Captopril
    D. Cosyntropin
    E. Aminoglutethimide

20. Decreased urine production is an effect of

    A. carmustine
    B. propylthiouracil
    C. ACTH
    D. desmopressin
    E. SSKI

21. Which of the following hormones is secreted by the pituitary gland?

    A. Adrenocorticotropic hormone
    B. Testosterone
    C. Cortisol
    D. Thyroxine
    E. Corticotropin-releasing hormone

22. Chronic administration of Winstrol may produce all of the following complications EXCEPT

    A. prostate enlargement
    B. increased testicular size
    C. gynecomastia in men
    D. accelerated atherosclerosis
    E. decreased menses in women

23. Androderm is administered

    A. once daily
    B. three times per week
    C. once weekly
    D. every 2 weeks
    E. monthly

24. Which of the following is NOT an acceptable indication for testosterone?

    A. Anemia
    B. Hypogonadism
    C. Delayed puberty
    D. Body building
    E. Metastatic breast cancer

Answers

1. **A.** Bile acid sequestrants reduce levothyroxine absorption and must be separated from levothyroxine administration by at least 4 hours. Levothyroxine should be administered before a meal on an empty stomach in order to maximize absorption.

2. **C.** Thyroid hormones enhance oxygen consumption and increase the oxygen demand. Mrs. Ricardo has a past medical history of coronary artery disease (CAD), and is elderly. Thyroid supplementation would actually lower her cholesterol in the long run, but may precipitate angina acutely.

3. **B.** Levothyroxine decreases bone mineral density and when given in supratherapeutic doses may cause osteoporosis. For this reason the lowest possible replacement dose should be administered.

4. **D.** Lithium and amiodarone have both been associated with hypothyroidism. Amiodarone contains iodine, and may cause hypo- or hyperthyroidism.

5. **E.** Numerous drugs are known to decrease thyroid hormone absorption, including antacids that contain divalent and trivalent cations, calcium salts, magnesium, sucralfate, and bile-acid sequestrants. Estrogens and enzyme-inducing drugs may decrease circulating thyroid hormone levels and necessitate a dose increase of thyroxine.

6. **D.** Heat intolerance, weight loss, tachycardia, tremor and anxiety are cardinal features of hyperthyroidism. Propylthiouracil is effective at reducing the excessive thyroxine level.

7. **A.** Liothyronine (Cytomel) is T$_3$, a potent thyroid hormone. In states of hypothyroidism, metabolism is decreased. However, if thyroid hormone is supplemented, blood clotting factors will be metabolized more quickly, leading to decreased warfarin requirements.

8. **E.** Ketoconazole, aminoglutethimide, and mitotane are all used to treat Cushing's disease. Ketoconazole is most commonly known as an antifungal agent, but it inhibits cortisol synthesis at high doses (800-1200 mg daily).

9. **E.** Metyrapone (Metopirone) inhibits 11-hydroxylase activity, and thus decreases cortisol synthesis.

10. **A.** Ketoconazole requires the presence of stomach acid in order to be absorbed. Any drug that decreases gastric acidity will decrease the extent of ketoconazole absorption. Food increases ketoconazole absorption since food stimulates release of gastric acid.

11. **B.** Mitotane is cytotoxic to adrenal cells and thus reduces cortisol synthesis and release. ACTH increases cortisol release. Close monitoring of cortisol levels is important when this drug is used.

12. **E.** Hydrocortisone is the drug of choice for adrenal crisis since it possesses both mineralocorticoid and glucocorticoid properties. Although cosyntropin increases cortisol release, patients with adrenal crisis may not have enough adrenal reserve to meet their increased demand.

13. **C.** Glucocorticoids have potent effects on glucose and carbohydrate metabolism. They promote glycogen breakdown, rather than inhibit it.

14. **B.** Captopril increases insulin sensitivity and would not be expected to contribute to increased blood glucose. This patient's blood glucose began rising shortly after admission. Her IV fluids contain glucose, epinephrine increases blood glucose by increasing glycogen breakdown, methylprednisolone (Solu-Medrol) promotes glycogenolysis, and anaphylaxis would be expected to increase stress response, leading to increased epinephrine release and increased blood glucose.

15. **A.** The patient has a history of diabetes and will be given prednisone, which would be expected to increase blood glucose. When diabetes is poorly controlled, infections are more likely to occur. For this reason, he should monitor more closely for wounds that may become infected. He will not be taking prednisone long enough to develop adrenal insufficiency, so there is no need for him to wear identification for steroid therapy.

16. **D.** Glucocorticoids have catabolic effects on a number of tissues, including muscle, fat, skin, and bone. Chronic administration leads to osteopenia and osteoporosis.

17. **D.** Chronic administration of glucocorticoids such as prednisone (Deltasone) will lead to feedback inhibition of pituitary ACTH release, and atrophy of the adrenal cortex. When prednisone is abruptly stopped, the adrenals will not be able to meet the body's demand for cortisol during severe stress and adrenal crisis may occur.

18. **C.** Corticosteroids such as dexamethasone (Decadron) are known to increase the risk of peptic ulcers when used in combination with NSAIDs.

19. **D.** Cosyntropin (Cortrosyn) is a synthetic analog of ACTH that is used to diagnose adrenal insufficiency. It works by stimulating the adrenal cortex to secrete cortisol. If cosyntropin administration does not result in an appropriate increase in cortisol release, adrenal insufficiency is present.

20. **D.** Desmopressin (DDAVP) is a synthetic analog of vasopressin, or antidiuretic hormone. Thus it decreases urine production by increasing water resorption.

21. **A.** Adrenocorticotropic hormone, or ACTH, is released by the pituitary and acts on the adrenal glands to increase cortisol release. Corticotropin-releasing hormone is released by the hypothalamus and acts on the pituitary to stimulate ACTH release.

22. **B.** Stanozolol (Winstrol) is an androgen that would be expected to promote growth and development of male sex organs. However, chronic administration leads to feedback inhibition of testosterone secretion which leads to testicular atrophy.

23. **A.** Testosterone transdermal systems (Andro-derm, Testoderm) are both applied once daily for 24 hours. Longer-acting androgens are available, such as nandrolone decanoate (Deca-Durabolin), for once-weekly administration.

24. **D.** Anabolic steroids may be abused by those who are seeking enhanced muscular development and endurance, such as athletes. For this reason, all of these agents are subject to the Controlled Substances Act (C-III).

6. References

American Association of Clinical Endocrinologists Medical Guidelines for Clinical Practice for the evaluation and treatment of hyperthyroidism and hypothyroidism (AACE Thyroid Task Force). *Endocr Pract.* 2002;8:457-469.

Chrousos GP, Margioris AN. Adrenocorticosteroids and adrenocortical antagonists. In: Katzung BG, ed. *Basic & Clinical Pharmacology,* 8th ed. Stamford, CT: Appleton & Lange; 2000:660-678.

Chrousos GP, Zoumakis EN, Gravanis A. The gonadal hormones and inhibitors. In: Katzung BG, ed. *Basic and Clinical Pharmacology,* 8th ed. Stamford, CT: Appleton & Lange; 2000:679-710.

Dayan CM, Daniels GH. Chronic autoimmune thyroiditis. *N Engl J Med.* 1996;335:99-106.

Dong, BJ, Hauck WW, Gambertoglio JG, et al. Bioequivalence of generic and brand name levothyroxine products in the treatment of hypothyroidism. *JAMA.* 1997;277:1205-1213.

Dong BJ. Thyroid disorders. In: Herfindal ET, Gourley DR, eds. *Textbook of Therapeutics: Drug and Disease Management.* Baltimore, MD: Lippincott Williams & Wilkins; 2000:325-358.

Fitzgerald PA. Hypothalamic and pituitary hormones. In: Katzung BG, ed. *Basic and Clinical Pharmacology,* 8th ed. Stamford, CT: Appleton & Lange; 2000:625-643.

Greenspan FG, Dong BJ. Thyroid and antithyroid drugs. In: Katzung BG, ed. *Basic and Clinical Pharmacology,* 8th ed. Stamford, CT: Appleton & Lange; 2000:644-659.

Hoffmeister AM, Tietze KJ. Adrenocortical dysfunction and clinical use of steroids. In: Herfindal ET, Gourley DR, eds. *Textbook of Therapeutics: Drug and Disease Management.* Baltimore: Lippincott Williams & Wilkins; 2000:305-324.

McEvoy GK, ed. AHFS Drug Information 2003. American Society of Health-System Pharmacists, Inc. Bethesda, MD: 2003.

15. Women's Health

Candace S. Brown, RN, CS, PharmD, BCPP, ARNP
Professor, Department of Clinical Pharmacy
University of Tennessee College of Pharmacy

Contents

1. Postmenopausal Hormone Replacement Therapy

- Menopause is permanent cessation of menses resulting from diminishing ovarian follicular function.
    * Defined as 12 consecutive months of amenorrhea
    * Median age of onset in the U.S. is 51 years of age.
    * Physiologic changes and symptoms of menopause may present up to 4 years prior to the menopause.
- Perimenopause, also called the climacteric, is the time just before the menopause and the first year following menopause. Ovarian function and production of estrogen decline during this time.

Clinical Presentation

- Cessation of menses for at least 12 consecutive months
- Symptoms of perimenopause related to declining estrogen:
    * Anovulation
    * Dysfunctional uterine bleeding
    * Extended menstrual cycle intervals
    * Oligomenorrhea
- Symptoms of menopause directly related to lack of estrogen:
    * Vaginal dryness, vulvar or vaginal atrophy
    * Hot flashes
    * Night sweats
- Symptoms associated with menopause, but without a proven link to estrogen deficiency:
    * Arthralgia
    * Depression
    * Insomnia
    * Migraines
    * Mood swings
    * Myalgia
    * Urinary frequency

Pathophysiology

- Loss of ovarian follicular activity results in endocrine, biologic, and clinical changes.
- Ovarian production of estradiol and progesterone diminishes.
- Follicle-stimulating hormone (FSH) and luteinizing hormone (LH) concentrations increase.
- Primary estrogen available is now estrone (which is converted peripherally from androstenedione and is less potent), not estradiol.

Treatment Principles

- Women with an intact uterus must be treated with estrogen plus progestin to reduce the risk of endometrial hyperplasia and endometrial cancer.
- Women who have had a hysterectomy are treated with unopposed estrogen.
- Hormone replacement therapy should be initiated on an individual basis with careful consideration of the risks and benefits.
- Contraindications to use:
    * Abnormal, undiagnosed genital bleeding
    * Breast cancer
    * Deep vein thrombosis or pulmonary embolism
    * Estrogen-dependent neoplasia
    * Pregnancy
    * Stroke or myocardial infarction in the last year
    * Thromboembolic disorder
    * Thrombophlebitis

Drug Therapy (Table 1)

Estrogen and progestin
Mechanism of action
Estrogen
- ERT = estrogen replacement therapy
- Acts as a replacement for diminished estrogen levels and restores estrogenic activity

Progestin
- HRT = hormone replacement therapy (estrogen plus progestin therapy)
- Acts as a replacement for diminished progesterone
- Protects the uterus by:
    * Decreasing nuclear estradiol receptor concentrations
    * Suppressing DNA synthesis
    * Decreasing estrogen bioavailability

Patient instructions and counseling
- Side effects due to estrogen may be diminished by starting with a low dose and may be alleviated by changing products. Fewer side effects are associated with the transdermal preparation.
- Side effects due to progestin may be alleviated or diminished by changing products or changing from a continuous to a cyclic regimen.
- Immediately report any unusual vaginal bleeding.
- Contact your physician promptly if any of the following events occur:
    * Abdominal tenderness, pain, or swelling
    * Coughing up blood
    * Disturbances of vision or speech
    * Dizziness or fainting
    * Lumps in the breast
    * Numbness or weakness in an arm or leg

Table 1

Hormone Replacement Therapy Products

Medication	Available strengths and dosing
Oral formulations	
Conjugated equine estrogens (CEE) (Premarin)	0.3, 0.45, 0.625, 0.9, 1.25, 2.5 mg qd
Micronized estradiol (Estradiol, Estrace, Gynodiol)	0.5, 1, 1.5, 2 mg qd
Estrone sulfate (Estropipate, Ortho-Est, Ogen)	0.625, 1.25, 2.5, 5 mg qd
Esterified estrogens (Estratab, Menest)	0.3, 0.625, 1.25, 2.5 mg qd
17-β-Estradiol	2 mg qd
Synthetic conjugated estrogen	0.3, 0.625, 0.9, 1.25 mg qd
Estradiol transdermal formulations	
Estradiol transdermal system (Estraderm)	0.05, 0.1 mg/24 h
Alora, Climara	0.025, 0.5, 0.075, 0.1 mg/24 h
Esclim, Vivelle, Vivelle-Dot	0.025, 0.0375, 0.5, 0.075, 0.1 mg/24 h
	Apply to skin once weekly (Climara) or twice weekly
Injectable formulations	
Estradiol valerate in oil (Delestrogen)	10, 20, 40 mg/mL in 5-mL multidose vials; dose: 10-20 mg q 4 weeks
Estradiol cypionate in oil	5 mg/mL in 5-mL vials; dose: 1-5 mg q 3-4 weeks
Vaginal estrogen formulations	
Estrace vaginal cream	0.1 mg estradiol/g; dose: 2-4 g qd for 1-2 weeks; maintenance dose: 1 g 1-3 times/week
Ogen vaginal cream	1.5 mg estropipate/g; dose: 2-4 g qd
Premarin vaginal cream	0.625 mg conjugated estrogen/g; dose: 0.5-2 g qd for 3 weeks, then 1 week off
Estring vaginal ring	2-mg estradiol ring releases 7.5 mcg/24 h; ring remains in vagina for 3 months
Vagifem vaginal tablet	25 mcg estradiol/tablet; dose: 1 tablet once daily for 2 weeks; maintenance dose: 1 tablet twice/week
Combination estrogen-progestin products	
Activella	1 mg estradiol, 0.5 mg norethindrone acetate
femhrt	2.5 or 5 mcg ethinyl estradiol, 0.5 or 1 mg norethindrone acetate
Prempro	0.3 or 0.625 mg conjugated estrogen, 1.5, 2.5, or 5 mg medroxyprogesterone
Premphase	0.625 mg conjugated estrogen, 5 mg medroxyprogesterone (2 weeks of estrogen alone, 2 weeks of combination)
Climara Pro (transdermal patch)	0.045 mg estradiol; 0.15 mg levonorgestrel
Combipatch (transdermal patch)	0.05 mg estradiol, 0.14 or 0.25 mg norethindrone acetate
Combination estrogen-androgen products	
Estratest H.S., Syntest H.S.	0.625 mg esterified estrogens, 1.25 mg methyltestosterone
Estratest, Syntest D.S.	0.625 mg esterified estrogens, 2.5 mg methyltestosterone

Adapted from Burnham et al, 2003 and Kalantaridou et al, 2002.

* Severe vomiting or headache
* Sharp chest pain or shortness of breath
* Sharp pain in the calves

Adverse drug events
• Increased risks for venous thromboembolism, stroke, coronary heart disease, and breast cancer were identified in the Women's Health Initiative (WHI) trial with postmenopausal women receiving estrogen and estrogen plus progestin products. The beneficial effects included reductions in fractures and colorectal cancer. Both ERT and HRT should be used at the lowest doses and for the shortest possible time period.

Estrogen
• Most common:
  * Breast tenderness
  * Heavy bleeding
  * Headache
  * Nausea

Progestin
- Most common:
  * Depression
  * Headache
  * Irritability

Drug-drug and drug-disease interactions
- Estrogen may exacerbate illness in the following disease states:
  * Depression
  * Diabetes (glucose intolerance has been observed with estrogen)
  * Hypertriglyceridemia
  * Hepatic adenoma
  * Thyroid disorder (patients may require an increased dose of thyroid supplement)
  * Impaired hepatic function (poor metabolism of estrogens)
  * Cardiovascular disorders (coronary heart disease and venous thromboembolism risk may be increased with estrogens)
- Interaction may result in decreased pharmacologic effect of estrogens:
  * Cytochrome P450 (CYP450) 3A4 inducers: barbiturates, carbamazepine, rifampin, St. John's wort
  * Hydantoins
  * Topiramate
- Interaction with estrogen may result in decreased pharmacologic effect of interacting drug:
  * Hydantoins
  * Thyroid hormones
  * Oral anticoagulants
- Interaction with estrogen may result in increased pharmacologic effect of interacting drug:
  * Corticosteroids
  * Tricyclic antidepressants (interaction may alter the effects and may increase toxicity of antidepressant).
- Interaction may result in increased pharmacologic effect of estrogens:
  * CYP450 3A4 inhibitors: itraconazole, ketoconazole, macrolide antibiotics, ritonavir
  * Food interaction: grapefruit juice
- Drug-drug interactions with progestins:
  * Concomitant administration with aminoglutethimide may increase the metabolism of medroxyprogesterone.
  * Concomitant administration with rifampin may increase the metabolism of norethindrone.

Parameters to monitor
- Laboratory monitoring not recommended

Androgens (testosterone)
Mechanism of action
- Androgens are the precursor hormones to estrogen production by the ovaries and peripheral sites. Ovarian testosterone production declines with menopause.
- Act at androgen receptor sites or exhibit action following conversion to estrogen
- Replaces androgen to improve deficiency-related symptoms (ie, decreased sexual desire, decreased energy, diminished well-being)

Patient instructions and counseling
- Testosterone therapy should only be administered to postmenopausal women who are receiving concurrent estrogen therapy.
- Relative contraindications to testosterone therapy
  * Androgenic alopecia
  * Clinical hirsutism
  * Moderate to severe acne

Adverse drug events
- Fluid retention
- Possible undesirable changes in lipid profile
- Virilization (lower HDL)

Parameters to monitor
- Laboratory monitoring not recommended

Nondrug Therapy

Phytoestrogens
- Plant compounds (isoflavones, lignans, coumestans)
- Food sources of phytoestrogens: soybeans, flaxseed, alfalfa sprouts
- Some studies have shown improvement in vaginal symptoms.
- No evidence supporting improvement in other symptoms of menopause (ie, hot flashes, depression, anxiety, headache, myalgia)
- May have beneficial effects on lipids

2. Birth Control: Contraceptive Options

- Contraception is the prevention of pregnancy by one of two methods:
  - * Preventing implantation of the fertilized ovum in the endometrium
  - * Inhibiting contact of sperm with mature ovum

Prescription Contraceptive Options

Oral contraceptives
- Estrogen plus progestin (combined oral contraceptives [COC])
- Progestin-only (minipill)
  - * Appropriate for use in breastfeeding women
  - * Efficacy is less than that of COCs
  - * Free of cardiovascular risks associated with estrogen-containing products
- Long-term injectables or implantation products
  - * Progestin only
- Estrogens and progestins used in prescription contraceptives (Table 2)
  - * Estrogens
    - • Ethinyl estradiol
    - • Mestranol
  - * Progestins
    - • Desogestrel
    - • Norgestrel; levonorgestrel
    - • Ethynodiol diacetate
    - • Norethindrone, norethindrone acetate, norethynodrel
- Drospirenone

Drug Therapy

Mechanism of action
Estrogens
- Prevent development of a dominant follicle by suppression of FSH; do not block ovulation

Progestin
- Blocks ovulation. Contributes to production of thick and impermeable cervical mucus. Contributes to involution and atrophy of the endometrium

Patient instructions and counseling
- Efficacy is high but dependent on proper scheduled use.
- Oral contraceptives do not prevent the transmission of sexually transmitted diseases.
- Warning signs of important complications:
  - * Severe abdominal pain
  - * Severe chest pain, shortness of breath, coughing up blood
  - * Severe headache
  - * Eye problems (ie, blurred vision, flashing lights, or blindness)
  - * Severe leg pain in the calf or thigh
- Expect changes in characteristics of the menstrual cycle.
- Use of a back-up contraceptive method is advised if more than one dose is missed per cycle.

Adverse drug events
- The World Health Organization suggests refraining from prescribing combined oral contraceptives to women with certain diagnoses (Table 3).
- For the medical conditions listed in Table 3, use of progestin-only oral contraceptives, depot medroxyprogesterone acetate, or an intrauterine device may be an appropriate contraceptive choice.
- Most common:
  - * Nausea and vomiting (usually resolves within 3 months)
  - * Breakthrough bleeding, spotting, amenorrhea, altered menstrual flow
  - * Melasma
  - * Headache, migraine
  - * Weight change, edema
- Serious and less common:
  - * Venous thrombosis, pulmonary embolism, MI, coronary thrombosis, arterial thromboembolism, cerebral thrombosis
- Potential hormonal effects associated with an imbalance in estrogen and progestin (Table 4)

Drug-drug and drug-disease interactions
- Interaction may result in decreased pharmacologic effect of oral contraceptives:
  - * Ampicillin, griseofulvin, sulfonamides, tetracycline
  - * Anticonvulsants (barbiturates, carbamazepine, felbamate, phenytoin, topiramate)
  - * Non-nucleoside reverse transcriptase inhibitors, protease inhibitors
  - * Pioglitazone
  - * Phenytoin
  - * Protease inhibitors
  - * Rifampin
  - * Theophylline
- Interaction may result in increased plasma levels of oral contraceptives:
  - * Atorvastatin
  - * Vitamin C
  - * CYP450 3A4 inhibitors
- Interaction may result in decreased pharmacologic effect of interacting drug:
  - * Anticoagulants
  - * Some benzodiazepine tranquilizers (e.g., lorazepam, oxazepam, and temazepam)

Table 2

Prescription Contraceptive Products

Product	Estrogen (mcg)	Progestin (mg)
Progestin-only oral contraceptives	—	Norethindrone (0.35)
Ortho Micronor, Errin, Nor-QD, Nora-BE, Camila		
Ovrette		
Monophasic low-dose estrogen oral contraceptives	—	Norgestrel (0.075)
Alesse, Aviane, Lessina, Levlite		
Loestrin 21 1/20, Loestrin Fe 1/20, Microgestin Fe 1/20	Ethinyl estradiol (20)	Levonorgestrel (0.1)
	Ethinyl estradiol (20)	Norethindrone acetate (1)
Yasmin		
Levlen, Levora, Nordette, Portia, Seasonale	Ethinyl estradiol (30)	Drospirenone (3)
Cryselle, Lo/Ovral, Low-Ogestrel	Ethinyl estradiol (30)	Levonorgestrel (0.15)
Apri, Desogen, Ortho-Cept	Ethinyl estradiol (30)	Norgestrel (0.3)
Ovcon-35	Ethinyl estradiol (30)	Desogestrel (0.15)
Brevicon, Modicon, Necon 0.5/35, Nortrel 0.5/35	Ethinyl estradiol (35)	Norethindrone (0.4)
Necon 1/35, Norinyl 1+35, Nortrel 1/35, Ortho-Novum 1/35	Ethinyl estradiol (35)	Norethindrone (0.5)
Kariva	Ethinyl estradiol (35)	Norethindrone (1)
Mircette	Ethinyl estradiol (20)/ ethinyl estradiol (10)	Desogestrel (0.15)
Monophasic high-dose estrogen oral contraceptives	Ethinyl estradiol (20)/ ethinyl estradiol (10)	Desogestrel (0.15)
Ovral, Ogestrel 0.5/50		
Demulen 1/50, Zovia 1/50E		
Ovcon-50	Ethinyl estradiol (50)	Norgestrel (0.5)
Necon 1/50, Norinyl 1+50, Ortho-Novum 1/50	Ethinyl estradiol (50)	Ethynodiol diacetate (1)
Biphasic oral contraceptives	Ethinyl estradiol (50)	Norethindrone (1)
Ortho-Novum 10/11, Necon 10/11	Mestranol (50)	Norethindrone (1)
Triphasic oral contraceptives		
Enpresse, Tri-Levlen, Triphasil, Trivora	Ethinyl estradiol (35)	Norethindrone (0.5 x 10 d); (1 x 11 d)
Tri-Norinyl	Ethinyl estradiol (30) x 6 d; (40) x 5 d; (30) x 10 d	Levonorgestrel (0.05) x 6 d; (0.075) x 5 d; (0.125) x 10 d
Necon 7/7/7, Ortho-Novum 7/7/7	Ethinyl estradiol (35) x 21 days	Norethindrone (0.5) x 7 d; (1) x 9 d; (0.5) x 5 d
Cyclessa	Ethinyl estradiol (35) x 21 days	Norethindrone (0.5) x 7 d; (0.75) x 9 d;(1) x 5 d
Ortho Tri-Cyclen Lo	Ethinyl estradiol (25) x 21 days	Desogestrel (0.1) x 7 d; (0.125) x 7 d; (0.15) x 7 d
Ortho Tri-Cyclen	Ethinyl estradiol (25) x 21 days	Norgestimate (0.18) x 7 d; (0.215) x 7 d; (0.25) x 7 d
Estrostep 21, Estrostep Fe	Ethinyl estradiol (35) x 21 days	Norgestimate (0.18) x 7 d; (0.215) x 7 d; (0.25) x 7 d
Transdermal contraceptive system	Ethinyl estradiol (20) x 5 d; (30) x 7 d; (35) x 9 d	Norethindrone (1) x 21 days
Ortho Evra		
Vaginal ring contraceptive system	Ethinyl estradiol (20 released per 24 hours)	Norelgestromin (0.15 released per 24 h)
NuvaRing		
Contraceptive implants		
Norplant system	Ethinyl estradiol (0.015 mg released per 24 hours)	Etonogestrel (0.12 released per 24 h)
Contraceptive injection		
Depo-Provera	—	Levonorgestrel (set of 6 capsules, each containing 36 mg)
Lunelle		
Intrauterine contraceptive systems	—	Medroxyprogesterone (150 mg/mL injection)
Progestasert	Estradiol cypionate 5 mg/mL	Medroxyprogesterone acetate 25 mg/mL
Mirena		
	—	Progesterone (unit reservoir contains 38 mg)
	—	Levonorgestrel (unit reservoir contains 52 mg)

Adapted from Burnham et al, 2003 and Dickerson et al, 2002.

Table 3

World Health Organization Contraindications for Combined Oral Contraceptive Use

- Breast cancer
- Current history of deep vein thrombosis or pulmonary embolism
- Current history of cerebrovascular accident or coronary artery or ischemic heart disease
- Diabetes with nephropathy, neuropathy, retinopathy, or other vascular disease
- Headaches
- Hypertension ($\geq$160/100 mm Hg) or hypertension with vascular disease
- Lactation (<6 weeks postpartum)
- Liver disease
- Pregnancy
- Surgery with prolonged immobilization or any surgery on the legs
- Smoker (20 or more cigarettes a day) $\geq$35 years of age
- Structural heart disease complicated by pulmonary hypertension, atrial fibrillation, or history of acute bacterial endocarditis

Adapted from Dickerson et al, 2002 and Ruggiero, 2001.

     * Hypoglycemics (tolbutamide, Diabinese, Orinase, Tolinase)
     * Methyldopa
     * Phenytoin
- Interaction may result in increased pharmacologic effect of interacting drug:
     * Tricyclic antidepressants
     * Benzodiazepine tranquilizers (other than the above benzodiazepines)
     * β-Blockers
     * Theophylline
- Interaction may result in increased toxicity of interacting drug:
     * Cortisone

Parameters to monitor
- Patients must monitor themselves for warning signs of serious complications as listed above.
- Laboratory monitoring is not recommended with use of oral contraceptives.

Nondrug Therapy

- Condoms
- Diaphragms
- Intrauterine devices
- Spermicides

Table 4

Potential Hormonal Effects Associated with an Imbalance in Estrogen or Progestin

Estrogen excess	• Breast tenderness, fullness
	• Cervical mucorrhea
	• Edema
	• Hypertension
	• Melasma
	• Migraine
	• Nausea, bloating
Progestin excess	• Acne or oily scalp
	• Breast regression
	• Depression
	• Hypomenorrhea
	• Increased appetite
	• Monilial vaginitis
	• Tiredness, fatigue
	• Weight gain
Estrogen deficiency	• Breakthrough bleeding (early or mid-cycle)
	• Hypomenorrhea
	• Spotting
Progestin deficiency	• Amenorrhea
	• Breakthrough bleeding (late)
	• Hypermenorrhea

Adapted from Burnham et al, 2003.

3. Osteoporosis

- Osteoporosis is characterized by low bone mineral density and deterioration of bone tissue, increasing fragility of bone and subsequent risk of fracture.

Types of Osteoporosis

- Postmenopausal (most common and the focus of this chapter)
- Age related
- Osteoporosis in men
- Drug-induced

Diagnostic Criteria

- T scores are used in the diagnosis and decision to treat osteoporosis.
     * The National Osteoporosis Foundation (NOF) and the American Association of Clinical

Endocrinologists (AACE) recommend initiation of therapy in the following situations:
  - T score < –2 and no risk factors
  - T score < –1.5 with risk factors
  * The National Institutes of Health (NIH) recommends choice of when to initiate therapy on an individual basis.
- The World Health Organization (WHO) classification of bone mass based on T scores:
  * Osteopenia: T score –1 to –2.5 SD below the young adult mean
  * Osteoporosis: T score ≤ –2.5 SD below the young adult mean
- Risk factors for osteoporosis:
  * Advanced age
  * Amenorrhea
  * Anorexia
  * Cigarette smoking
  * Current low bone mass
  * Estrogen deficiency as a result of menopause
  * Ethnicity (Caucasian or Asian)
  * Excessive alcohol use
  * Family history of osteoporosis or history of fracture in a primary relative
  * Female gender
  * History of fracture over the age of 50
  * Inactive lifestyle
  * Long-term use of corticosteroids or anticonvulsants
  * Low lifetime calcium intake
  * Low testosterone levels in men
  * Thin or small frame
- Medical conditions associated with increased risk of osteoporosis:
  * Acquired immunodeficiency syndrome (AIDS)
  * Cushing's disease
  * Eating disorders
  * Hyperparathyroidism
  * Inflammatory bowel disease
  * Insulin-dependent diabetes mellitus
  * Lymphoma and leukemia
  * Malabsorption syndromes
  * Rheumatoid arthritis
- Drugs associated with an increased risk of osteoporosis:
  * Anticonvulsants (phenobarbital, phenytoin)
  * Cytotoxic drugs
  * Glucocorticoids
  * Immunosuppressants
  * Lithium
  * Long-term heparin use
  * Progesterone, parenteral, long-acting
  * Supraphysiologic thyroxine doses
  * Tamoxifen (premenopausal)

- Recommendations for the initial evaluation of patients for osteoporosis are as follows:
  * AACE and NOF: screen all women 65 years of age and older; postmenopausal women less than 65 years of age with family history or clinical risk factors; and women with a fracture history unrelated to trauma
  * NIH: decision to screen is individualized

Clinical Presentation

- Shortened stature
- Vertebra, hip, or forearm fracture
- Kyphosis
- Lordosis
- Bone pain

Pathophysiology

- Two types of bone: trabecular (ie, vertebrae, wrist and ankle, and ends of long bones, which are the most susceptible to fracture) and cortical
- Osteoblasts (formation) and osteoclasts (destruction) create a constant state of bone remodeling.
- Bone formation exceeds destruction during childhood.
- Peak bone mass is reached around age 25-35, then bone density begins to decline.
  * 3-4% decline per decade in men
  * 8-12% decline per decade in women 10 years after menopause
- Following menopause (postmenopausal osteoporosis), estrogen production declines and osteoclastic activity increases.

Treatment Principles

- Adequate calcium and vitamin D intake through diet or supplementation is recommended for everyone (calcium 1000-1500 mg daily plus 400-800 IU vitamin D daily) (Table 5).
- Lifestyle modifications are recommended: weight-bearing exercise, smoking cessation, limited alcohol intake.
- Prescription drug therapy should be initiated on an individual basis, considering risk factors, bone mineral density, fracture history, and concomitant diseases and medications.

Initiation of Treatment
- Postmenopausal women who have experienced a fragility or low-impact fracture
- Postmenopausal women with bone mineral density scores less than –2 by central dual energy x-ray absorptiometry (DXA) in the absence of risk factors

Table 5

Select Calcium Supplement Products

Product	Calcium (mg)
Calcium citrate	
(24% calcium content)	
Citracal	Tablet: 200; liquitab: 500
Citracal + vitamin D	316 plus 200 IU
Calcium carbonate	
(40% calcium content)	
Caltrate 600	600
Titralac	Chewable: 168, 300;
	liquid: 400/5 mL
Tums	Chewable: 200, 300, 500
Viactiv Chews	500
Mylanta lozenges	240
Calcium carbonate + vitamin D	
Caltrate 600 + D	600 plus 200 IU
Calcilyte + vitamin D	500 plus 200 IU
Oscal + vitamin D	500 plus 125 IU
Calcium phosphate tribasic	
(39% calcium content)	
Posture	600
Posture-D	600 plus 125 IU

Adapted from Dickerson et al, 2002 and Burnham et al, 2003.

- Women with T scores less than –1.5 in the presence of one or more risk factors

Drug Therapy

Calcium and vitamin D
Mechanism of action
Calcium
- Necessary to improve bone mass; calcium is absorbed through the GI tract, stored in the skeleton, and made available when calcium levels become low.

Vitamin D
- Facilitates absorption and regulation of calcium levels

Patient instructions and counseling
- Approximately 500 mg of calcium can be absorbed from the GI tract at a time; separate doses appropriately to achieve a dose of 1000-1500 mg per day.
- Calcium carbonate contains the highest level of elemental calcium; take with food to facilitate absorption.

- Calcium citrate products may be administered without regard to meals.

Adverse drug events
- Most common:
    * GI upset (nausea, vomiting, cramping, flatulence)
    * Headache
    * Hypophosphatemia, hypercalcemia

Drug-drug and drug-disease interactions
- Concomitant administration may decrease the bioavailability of fluoroquinolones or tetracyclines.

Parameters to monitor
- Laboratory monitoring is not recommended.

Bisphosphonates: alendronate (Fosamax), risedronate (Actonel) (Table 6)
Mechanism of action
- Binds to bone (hydroxyapatite) and incorporates into bone to increase and stabilize bone mass

Patient instructions and counseling
- Bisphosphonates must be taken with a full glass of water (8 ounces) 30 minutes prior to the first meal of the day.
- Remain in an upright position for at least 30 minutes following ingestion.
- Take medication on a regularly scheduled basis.
- Compliance may be increased by once-weekly dosing.

Adverse drug events
- Most common:
    * GI: abdominal pain, dyspepsia, constipation, diarrhea, flatulence, nausea, acid regurgitation, gastritis
    * CNS: headache

Drug-drug and drug-disease interactions
- Interaction may result in decreased pharmacologic effect of bisphosphonates:
    * Calcium supplements, antacids (separate administration by 1 hour)
- Interaction may result in increased pharmacologic effect of bisphosphonates:
    * Ranitidine (IV ranitidine may double bioavailability of alendronate)
- Interaction may result in increased toxicity of interacting drug:
    * Aspirin (alendronate >10 mg/d may increase risk of upper GI side effects of aspirin)

Parameters to monitor
- Laboratory monitoring is not recommended.

Table 6

Antiresorptive Agents

Medication	Dosing	FDA indication
Bisphosphonates		
Alendronate (Fosamax®)	Prevention: 5 mg qd or 35 mg weekly; treatment: 10 mg qd or 70 mg weekly	Prevention and treatment of postmenopausal osteoporosis
Risedronate (Actonel®)	Prevention: 5 mg qd; treatment: 5 mg qd or 30 mg weekly	Prevention and treatment of osteoporosis in men
Ibandronate (Boniva®)	Prevention: 150 mg monthly Treatment: 150 mg monthly	Prevention and treatment of postmenopausal osteoporosis
Estrogen replacement therapy		
Conjugated equine estrogens (CEE) (Premarin®)	0.625 mg qd	Prevention of osteoporosis
Ethinyl estradiol (Estinyl®)	0.02 mg qd	
Estropipate (Ortho-Est®, Ogen®)	0.625 mg qd	
Esterified estrogens (Estratab®, Menest®)	0.625 mg qd	
Micronized estradiol (Estrace®)	1 mg qd	
17-β-Estradiol	2 mg qd	
Estrone sulfate	1.5 mg qd	
Transdermal estradiol (Estraderm®, Alora®, Climara®, Esclim®, Vivelle/Vivelle-Dot®)	0.05 mg qd	
Combination estrogen/progestin products:		
Prempro® (conjugated estrogens/ medroxyprogesterone acetate)	0.45/1.5 mg, 0.625/1.5 mg qd	
Premphase® (conjugated estrogens/ medroxyprogesterone acetate)	0.625 mg/5 mg qd	
femhrt 1/5 (norethindrone acetate/ ethinyl estradiol)	1 mg/ 5 mcg qd	
Activella® (estradiol/norethindrone acetate)	1/0.5 mg qd	
Selective estrogen receptor modulator		
Raloxifene (Evista®)	60 mg qd	Prevention and treatment of postmenopausal osteoporosis
Other agents		
Calcitonin (Miacalcin®)	Intranasal: 200 IU qd; IM or SC: 100 IU qd	Treatment of postmenopausal osteoporosis
Teriparatide (Forteo®)	Injection: 20 mcg qd	Treatment of postmenopausal women with osteoporosis who are at high risk for fractures or who have failed or are intolerant to other therapies; treatment of men with primary or hypogonadal osteoporosis who are at high risk for fractures

Adapted from Dickerson et al, 2002 and Burnham et al, 2003.

Estrogen replacement therapy
Mechanism of action
- Replaces the natural estrogen in postmenopausal women to restore protective skeletal benefits provided by the hormone (Table 6).

Patient instructions and counseling
- The patient must discuss and weigh benefits and risks of estrogen or combined hormone replacement therapy with her physician.

Contraindications to use of these medications
- History of thromboembolism
- History of breast or endometrial cancer
- Undiagnosed abnormal genital bleeding
- Pregnancy

Adverse drug events
- Most common:
    * Genitourinary: vaginal bleeding or spotting
    * Other: breast enlargement and tenderness, increased weight
    * Cardiovascular: increased triglycerides

Drug-drug and drug-disease Interactions
- Interaction may result in decreased serum concentrations of estrogen:
    * Rifampin
- Interaction may result in increased toxicity of interacting drug:
    * Hydrocortisone
    * Anticoagulants: increased potential for thromboembolic events

Parameters to monitor
- Laboratory monitoring is not recommended.

Selective estrogen receptor modulator: raloxifene (Evista)
Mechanism of action
- Estrogen receptor agonist at the skeleton; decreases resorption of bone and overall bone turnover

Patient instructions and counseling
- This medication may be taken without regard to food.
- Concomitant use with estrogen therapy is not recommended.
- This medication will not treat symptoms of menopause such as hot flashes.
- In the event of prolonged immobilization, discontinue raloxifene 3 days prior to and during the immobile period when possible.

Adverse drug events
- Most common:
    * Cardiovascular: hot flashes, chest pain, syncope
    * GI: nausea, diarrhea, vomiting
    * Musculoskeletal: arthralgia, myalgia
    * CNS: insomnia, neuralgia
    * Skin: rash, sweating

Drug-drug and drug-disease interactions
- Interaction may result in decreased pharmacologic effect of raloxifene:
    * Ampicillin (peak levels reduced by 28%; overall absorption reduced by 14%); coadministration is not contraindicated due to maintained systemic exposure and elimination.
    * Cholestyramine (absorption and enterohepatic cycling reduced); do not administer together.
- Interaction may result in decreased pharmacologic effect of interacting drug:
    * Warfarin (prothrombin time may decrease up to 10%)

Parameters to monitor
- Laboratory monitoring is not recommended.

Calcitonin (Miacalcin)
Mechanism of action
- Participates in the regulation of calcium and bone metabolism; inhibits bone resorption by binding to osteoclast receptors

Patient instructions and counseling
- If this medication is administered as an injection, it should be given in the upper arm, thigh, or buttocks.
- Proper education regarding administration of the injection and the nasal spray preparation is necessary.
- If you miss a shot, administer it as soon as possible. Do not administer the shot if it is almost time for your next dose.
- Store the nasal spray in the refrigerator until time for use. Warm the spray to room temperature prior to first use and then store at room temperature.

Adverse drug events
- Most common:
    * Skin: facial flushing and hand flushing (most common overall)
    * GI: nausea, diarrhea, vomiting, abdominal pain
    * Taste disorder: salty taste
    * Genitourinary: nocturia, urinary frequency
    * Nasal (with nasal spray): rhinitis, nasal dryness, irritation, itching, congestion
    * Ophthalmic: blurred vision, abnormal lacrimation

Drug-drug and drug-disease interactions
- Interaction may result in decreased pharmacologic effect of interacting drug:
    * Lithium: concomitant administration may decrease lithium levels

Parameters to monitor
• Laboratory monitoring is not recommended.

Teriparatide (parathyroid hormone, PTH) (Forteo)
Mechanism of action
• Increases the rate of bone formation by increasing the birth rate of osteoblasts and preventing apoptosis, resulting in improved bone mineral density.

Patient instructions and counseling
• Patients must read the user guide and pen manual prior to use.

Adverse drug events
• Most common:
     * Musculoskeletal: pain, arthralgia
     * CNS: paresthesias
     * GI: nausea, diarrhea, abdominal cramps
     * Taste disorder: metallic taste
     * Skin: injection pain, urticaria

Drug-drug and drug-disease interactions
• None known

Parameters to monitor
• Laboratory monitoring is not recommended.

Nondrug Therapy

• Weight-bearing exercise
• Smoking cessation
• Limited alcohol consumption
• Calcium-rich diet

4. Key Points

Postmenopausal hormone replacement therapy
• Therapy must be selected on an individual basis while considering risks and benefits, concomitant diseases, and medications. Important patient parameters to consider include menopause symptoms, risk of coronary artery disease, risk of osteoporosis, risk of breast cancer, and risk of thromboembolism.
• The primary indication for initiating hormone replacement therapy is to relieve vasomotor and other menopause symptoms to improve quality of life.
• Another indication is to continue estrogen's protective benefits, ie, the preservation of bone mass and prevention of osteoporosis.
• Hormone replacement therapy is not recommended for use in the primary prevention of any other disease states at this time.
• Estrogen plus progestin therapy is indicated in patients with a uterus.
• Estrogen alone is indicated in women who no longer have a uterus.

Contraceptives
• Oral contraceptives are highly effective and safe when used properly according to the manufacturer's recommended dose and administration.
• Selection of prescription contraceptives requires careful consideration of patient medical history, lifestyle, compliance, and preference.
• In addition to the contraceptive benefit of these products, other menstrual-related health problems may be resolved or lessened (eg, menstrual pain, irregular menses, headache, and spotting).
• Changes in dose or product are often necessary to achieve an appropriate balance of estrogen and progestin that minimizes undesirable adverse effects associated with deficiencies or excess amounts of the hormones.
• Patients must be educated to immediately report the onset of severe abdominal pain, severe chest pain, shortness of breath, severe headache, visual disturbances, or severe pain in the leg or calf.

Osteoporosis
• Women should be counseled about the following preventive measures:
     * Adequate calcium consumption, using dietary supplements if dietary sources are not adequate
     * Adequate vitamin D consumption (400-800 IU daily) and the natural sources of this nutrient
     * Regular weight-bearing and muscle-strengthening exercises to reduce falls and prevent fractures

* Smoking cessation
* Moderation of alcohol intake
* Fall prevention strategies
- Bone mineral density testing should be recommended to all postmenopausal women aged 65 years of age or older, and for postmenopausal women younger than 65 years who have one or more risk factors for osteoporosis.
- Therapy must be selected on an individual basis considering risks and benefits, concomitant diseases, and medications.
- Appropriate calcium and vitamin D intake is an important component of prevention and treatment. If this is not obtained in the diet, supplementation is recommended for all individuals, even in patients receiving prescription therapy for osteoporosis.
- First-line pharmacologic options for osteoporosis prevention are biphosphonates (alendronate and risendronate), raloxifene, and estrogen.
- First-line pharmacologic options for osteoporosis treatment are biphosphonates (alendronate and risendronate), raloxifene, calcitonin, and PTH).
- Bisphosphonates must be taken with a full glass of water 30 minutes prior to the first meal of the day. The patient must remain upright for at least 30 minutes after taking a dose.
- Estrogen replacement therapy is not approved for the treatment of osteoporosis and should not be initiated for this reason. It is approved for prevention of osteoporosis.

5. Questions and Answers

1. A.J. is a 35-year-old premenopausal woman who is concerned about her family history of osteoporosis. She states that she does not eat dairy products due to lactose intolerance. Her recent bone mineral density screening revealed a T score of 1.0. Select the appropriate therapy recommendation from the choices below.

    A. Daily estrogen replacement therapy
    B. Daily calcium and vitamin D supplementation
    C. Daily combined estrogen/progestin replacement therapy
    D. Daily teriparatide injections
    E. Daily calcitonin nasal spray

2. The pharmacist receives a prescription for Fosamax 70 mg qd for prevention of osteoporosis with instructions to take with food and remain upright for at least 30 minutes following ingestion. From the choices below, identify the errors in this prescription.

    A. The dose of Fosamax should be 35 mg weekly for prevention
    B. Fosamax should be taken at least 30 minutes prior to a meal; it should not be taken with food
    C. Patients should lie down for 1 hour following administration of Fosamax
    D. Choices B and C are correct
    E. Choices A and B are correct

3. What is the recommended dosage range of daily calcium intake for an adult?

    A. 200-400 mg
    B. 250-500 mg
    C. 300-600 mg
    D. 500-1000 mg
    E. 1000-1500 mg

4. Which dose and schedule is correct for prevention of osteoporosis?

    A. Alendronate 35 mg weekly
    B. Risedronate 5 mg weekly
    C. Alendronate 70 mg weekly
    D. Risedronate 30 mg weekly
    E. Alendronate 10 mg daily

5. Which of the following products is available in an injectable and nasal spray dosage form?

   A. Raloxifene
   B. Alendronate
   C. Teriparatide
   D. Calcitonin
   E. Prempro

6. Which of the following drugs do not increase the risk of osteoporosis?

   A. Anticonvulsants
   B. Tamoxifen
   C. Glucocorticoids
   D. Estrogen

7. What is the recommended dose of raloxifene in the prevention and treatment of postmenopausal osteoporosis?

   A. 10 mg daily
   B. 15 mg daily
   C. 40 mg daily
   D. 60 mg daily
   E. 120 mg daily

8. S.T. is a 32-year-old woman who wants to begin use of a prescription contraceptive product. S.T. is a new mother and would like to know if any products are safe for use during breastfeeding. S.T. states that she is not interested in using a device intravaginally, and experiences irritation and inflammation with condom use. Which of the following product(s) would be an appropriate choice for S.T.?

   A. Ortho Tri-Cyclen
   B. Micronor
   C. Depo-Provera
   D. A or B
   E. B or C
   F. A, B, or C

9. T.H. is a 27-year-old woman currently taking Nordette oral contraceptive pills. She presents to your pharmacy with a prescription of ampicillin 500 mg qid for 1 week. Which of the following choices describes appropriate action taken by the pharmacist?

   A. Call the physician and request a change to amoxicillin to avoid a drug interaction between Nordette and ampicillin.

   B. Dispense the ampicillin and counsel T.H. on the appropriate administration and duration of therapy for the antibiotic.
   C. Dispense the ampicillin and counsel T.H. regarding the potential for ampicillin to interfere with the efficacy of Nordette, and instruct T.H. to use a back-up method of contraception until her next menstrual period begins.
   D. Refuse to fill the ampicillin prescription, and counsel T.H. that she should never take antibiotics while she is on birth control.

10. Which of the following oral contraceptives is a biphasic product?

    A. Ortho Tri-Cyclen
    B. Ortho-Novum 10/11
    C. Ortho-Novum 1/35
    D. Mircette
    E. Alesse

11. Which of the following products is a progestin-only oral contraceptive?

    A. Nordette
    B. Ortho Tri-Cyclen
    C. Ovrette
    D. Demulen 1/50
    E. Necon 1/35

12. Which of the following triphasic oral contraceptives varies the dose of both the estrogen and progestin component?

    A. Triphasil
    B. Ortho-Novum 7/7/7
    C. Ortho Tri-Cyclen
    D. Cyclessa
    E. Tri-Norinyl

13. What is highest dose of estrogen (ethinyl estradiol) offered in an oral contraceptive?

    A. 25 mcg
    B. 30 mcg
    C. 35 mcg
    D. 40 mcg
    E. 50 mcg

14. A progestin-only oral contraceptive would be preferable over a combination oral contraceptive in all of the following cases except

    A. a smoker over 35 years old
    B. a patient with fibrocystic breast changes
    C. a lactating woman
    D. a patient with a history of thromboembolic disease

15. A.J. is a 55-year-old woman who presents to your pharmacy with a prescription for Premarin 0.625 mg daily. She has an intact uterus and has been recently diagnosed with menopause. Which of the following statements describes the appropriate action to be taken by the pharmacist?

    A. Refuse to fill the prescription and recommend a phytoestrogen supplement
    B. Call the physician and confirm that the patient has an intact uterus and recommend a product containing estrogen plus progestin
    C. Fill the prescription and counsel the patient regarding administration instructions and potential adverse effects
    D. None of the above

16. Which of the following factors is a contraindication to the use of hormone replacement therapy in postmenopausal women?

    A. Diabetes
    B. Basal cell skin cancer
    C. Thromboembolic disease
    D. Depression
    E. Obesity

17. From the choices below, please select the most common side effects associated with estrogen replacement.

    A. Breast tenderness
    B. Depression
    C. Nausea
    D. Brittle fingernails
    E. A and C

18. The Women's Health Initiative (WHI) study was terminated because both ERT and HRT increased the risk of all of the following conditions except:

    A. Breast cancer
    B. Stroke
    C. Cardiovascular disease
    D. Uterine cancer

19. Which of the following product dosing regimens is correct?

    A. Climara Transdermal: apply to skin once daily
    B. Vagifem: one tablet vaginally once daily for 2 weeks, then one tablet vaginally twice weekly
    C. Delestrogen: 10- to 20-mg injections once weekly
    D. Premarin caplets: 0.625-2.5 mg tid
    E. Ogen vaginal cream: 20-40 g vaginally once daily

20. Which of the following drug interactions may result in increased pharmacologic effect of estrogen?

    A. Macrolide antibiotics
    B. Itraconazole
    C. Ketoconazole
    D. A and C
    E. A, B, and C

Answers

1. **B.** A.J. has neither osteopenia nor osteoporosis with a T score of 1.0. At this point, preventive therapy is appropriate with adequate calcium and vitamin D intake. Prescription therapy is not indicated at this time.

2. **E.** The appropriate use of Fosamax for prevention of osteoporosis includes a 35-mg weekly or 5-mg daily dose. The 70-mg weekly dose is for treatment of osteoporosis. The medication should be taken with a full glass of water at least 30 minutes prior to ingesting food or beverage. Patients should remain in the upright position for at least 30 minutes following ingestion of Fosamax.

3. **E.** The recommended dosage range of daily calcium intake for an adult is 1000-1500 mg.

4. **A.** Choices C, D, and E are treatment doses. Choice B is not an accurate dose or frequency for treatment or prevention.

5. **D.** Injectable and nasal spray dosage forms of calcitonin are available. Teriparatide is available as an injection only. Prempro, raloxifene, and alendronate are only available in oral dosage forms.

6. **D.** Estrogen decreases rather than increases the risk of osteoporosis.

7. **D.** The approved and recommended dose of raloxifene is 60 mg once daily.

8. **E.** Micronor is a progestin only (minipill) oral contraceptive and is considered compatible with breastfeeding. Depo-Provera is an injectable progestin-only contraceptive option that is considered safe and appropriate for women who desire to breastfeed. Ortho Tri-Cyclen is a combined oral contraceptive known to decrease the quantity of breast milk available and may adversely affect the infant.

9. **C.** Ampicillin is known to interact with combined oral contraceptives. Although clinical studies have not consistently demonstrated an interaction, more than 25 case reports of unintended pregnancies have been attributed to concomitant use of ampicillin and oral contraceptives. Concomitant administration of ampicillin, as well as other antibiotics, may decrease the effectiveness of combined oral contraceptives, resulting in pregnancy. Patients must be counseled to use a back-up method of contraception until menses occurs.

10. **B.** Ortho-Novum 10/11 and Necon 10/11 are the two biphasic oral contraceptives available.

11. **C.** Ovrette is a progestin-only oral contraceptive.

12. **A.** Triphasil is a triphasic oral contraceptive that varies the dose of both the estrogen and progestin component.

13. **E.** The highest dose of estrogen (ethinyl estradiol) offered in an oral contraceptive is 50 mcg.

14. **B.** Fibrocystic breast changes are not a contraindication to using combined oral contraceptives.

15. **B.** Unopposed estrogen is not recommended in women with an intact uterus due to an increased risk of endometrial hyperplasia and endometrial cancer. Women with an intact uterus should receive a product containing estrogen plus progestin.

16. **C.** Thromboembolic disease is a definite contraindication to the use of hormone replacement therapy in postmenopausal women.

17. **E.** Breast tenderness and nausea are the most common side effects associated with estrogen replacement.

18. **D.** The Women's Health Initiative (WHI) study was not terminated because of an increased risk of uterine cancer.

19. **B.** Vagifem dosage is one tablet vaginally once daily for 2 weeks, then one tablet vaginally twice weekly.

20. **E.** Macrolide antibiotics, itraconazole, and ketoconazole may result in increased pharmacologic effect of estrogen.

6. References

Postmenopausal hormone replacement therapy
Burnham TH, Wichersham RN, Novak KK, eds. *Drug Facts and Comparisons Updated Monthly.* St Louis: Facts and Comparisons; 2003.

Hutchison TA, Shahan DR, eds. DRUGDEX® System. MICROMEDEX, Greenwood Village, CO (edition expired 6-2003).

Kalantaridou SN, Davis SR, Calis KA. Hormone replacement therapy. In: Dipiro JT, Talbert RL, Yee GC, eds. *Pharmacotherapy: A Pathophysiologic Approach,* 5th ed. New York: McGraw-Hill; 2002:1491-1504.

Loose-Mitchell DS, Stancel GM. Estrogens and pro-gestins. In: Hardman JG, Limbird LE, Goodman Gilman A, eds. *Goodman and Gilman's The Pharmacological Basis of Therapeutics,* 10th ed. New York: McGraw-Hill; 2001:1597-1622.

Sagraves R, Parent-Stevens L, Hardman J. Gynecologic disorders. In: Koda-Kimble MA, Young LY, eds. *Applied Therapeutics: The Clinical Use of Drugs,* 7th ed. Philadelphia: Lippincott Williams & Wilkins; 2001:46-32.

Warren MP. A comparative review of the risks and benefits of hormone replacement therapy regimens. *Am J Obstet Gynecol.* 2004;190:1141-1167.

Contraceptives
American College of Obstetricians and Gynecologists. The use of hormonal contraception in women with coexisting medical conditions. ACOG Practice Bulletin: Clinical Management Guidelines for Obstetrician-Gynecologists 2000; July (18):1-14.

Burnham TH, Wichersham RN, Novak KK, eds. *Drug Facts and Comparisons Updated Monthly.* St Louis: Facts and Comparisons; 2003.

Dickerson LM, Bucci KK. Contraception. In: Dipiro JT, Talbert RL, Yee GC, eds. *Pharmacotherapy: A Pathophysiologic Approach,* 5th ed. New York: McGraw-Hill; 2002:1445-1462.

Hutchison TA, Shahan DR, eds. DRUGDEX® System. MICROMEDEX, Greenwood Village, CO (edition expired 6-2003).

Loose-Mitchell DS, Stancel GM. Estrogens and pro-gestins. In: Goodman LS, Hardman JG, Limbird LE, et al, eds. *Goodman and Gilman's The Pharmacological Basis of Therapeutics,* 10th ed. New York: McGraw-Hill; 2001:1597-1629.

Ruggiero R. Contraception. In: Koda-Kimble MA, Young LY, eds. *Applied Therapeutics: The Clinical Use of Drugs,* 7th ed. Philadelphia: Lippincott Williams & Wilkins; 2001:41-43.

Osteoporosis
American Association of Clinical Endocrinologists 2001 Medical Guidelines for Clinical Practice for the Prevention and Management of Postmenopausal Osteoporosis. *Endocr Pract.* 2001;7:294-312.

American College of Obstetricians and Gynecologists. Osteoporosis. ACOG Practice Bulletin: Clinical Management Guidelines for Obstetrician-Gynecologists 2004; Jan (50):1-14.

American College of Obstetricians and Gynecologists. Selective estrogen receptor modulators. ACOG Practice Bulletin: Clinical Management Guidelines for Obstetrician-Gynecologists 2002; October (39):1-10.

Burnham TH, Wickersham RN, Novak KK, eds. *Drug Facts and Comparisons Updated Monthly.* St Louis: Facts and Comparisons; 2003.

Consensus Development Panel. Osteoporosis preven-tion, diagnosis, and therapy consensus conference. National Institutes of Health. *JAMA.* 2001;285:785-795.

Dickerson LM, Bucci KK. Contraception. In: Dipiro JT, Talbert RL, Yee GC, eds. *Pharmacotherapy: A Pathophysiologic Approach,* 5th ed. New York: McGraw-Hill; 2002:1445-1462.

Hutchison TA, Shahan DR, eds. DRUGDEX® System. MICROMEDEX, Greenwood Village, CO (edition expired 6-2003).

Marcus R. Agents affecting calcification and bone turnover. In: Hardman JG, Limbird LE, Goodman Gilman A, eds. *Goodman and Gilman's The Pharmacological Basis of Therapeutics,* 10th ed. New York: McGraw-Hill; 2001:1715-1743.

National Osteoporosis Foundation. Physician's Guide to Prevention and Treatment of Osteoporosis, 2000. Available at: http://www.nof.org/physguide. Accessed April 1, 2003.

Sagraves R, Parent-Stevens L, Hardman J. Gynecologic disorders. In: Koda-Kimble MA, Young LY, eds. *Applied Therapeutics: The Clinical Use of Drugs,* 7th ed. Philadelphia: Lippincott Williams & Wilkins; 2001:46-49.

16. Kidney Disease

Joanna Q. Hudson, PharmD, BCPS
Associate Professor, Department of Clinical Pharmacy
University of Tennessee College of Pharmacy

Contents

1. Acute Kidney Disease

- Acute kidney disease (AKD) is defined as rapid (hours to days) deterioration of kidney function resulting in azotemia (retention of nitrogenous waste products such as urea) and failure of the kidney to maintain fluid, electrolyte, and acid-base homeostasis.
- A reduced urine output is frequently seen: oliguria (urine output <400 mL/d), anuria (urine output <50 mL/d); nonoliguria indicates urine output >400 mL/d.
- Objective definition: increase in serum creatinine of 0.5 mg/dL over a 24-hour period when baseline creatinine is less than 3.0 mg/dL, or an increase of 1.0 mg/dL when baseline creatinine is greater than 3.0 mg/dL
- Characterized by 3 phases: oliguric phase (period of days to weeks when reduction in urine output may be observed), diuretic phase (period of days during which repair of renal insult occurs and urine production increases), and recovery phase (period of weeks to months when kidney function returns).

Epidemiology

Incidence and prevalence
- Community-acquired AKD accounts for 1% of hospital admissions.
- Hospital-acquired AKD occurs in 2-5% of hospitalized patients.

Mortality
- The best prognosis is when renal replacement therapy is not required.
- 10-25% mortality rate in patients who require renal replacement therapy
- >50% mortality rate in patients with multiple organ failure

Types and Classifications

- AKD is classified according to precipitating factors.

Prerenal
- Characterized by a decrease in renal perfusion with or without systemic arterial hypotension; most common type; usually reversible; *functional AKD* describes conditions that decrease glomerular ultrafiltrate production without damage to the kidney (similar to prerenal).

Intrinsic (intrarenal)
- Results from structural damage to the parenchymal tissue of the kidney; divided into vascular, glomerular, interstitial, and tubular disorders (most common)

Postrenal
- Obstruction of urine flow occurring at any level of the urinary outflow tracts

Clinical Presentation

- Changes in urine output (increased or decreased, depending on the phase of AKD)
- Signs of hypovolemia (prerenal causes): tachycardia, decreased venous and arterial pressure, orthostasis
- Unique color and composition of urine: cola-colored urine suggests bleeding; foaming is indicative of proteinuria.
- Symptoms of *uremia* (the clinical syndrome resulting from azotemia):
  * Weakness, shortness of breath, fatigue, mental confusion, nausea and vomiting, bleeding, loss of appetite, edema
- Flank pain (suggestive of swelling of the kidneys)
- Increased weight (suggesting fluid accumulation)
- Increased blood pressure (suggesting fluid accumulation)
- Signs and symptoms of electrolyte abnormalities (hyperkalemia, hypocalcemia), metabolic acidosis (see section on fluids and electrolytes)
- Bladder distention or prostate enlargement (postrenal causes)
- Other findings specific to the cause of AKD (see section on pathophysiology)

Pathophysiology

Prerenal/functional AKD
- Caused by conditions that decrease glomerular hydrostatic pressure leading to a decrease in glomerular filtration rate (GFR) (see section on etiologies)
- Hypoperfusion leads to increased sodium and water reabsorption by the kidney and stimulates compensatory mechanisms.
- Compensatory mechanisms to increase hydrostatic pressure and GFR:
  * Vasodilation of the afferent arteriole (mediated by prostaglandins)
  * Vasoconstriction of the efferent arteriole (mediated by angiotensin II)
- Alterations in afferent and efferent arteriolar tone can affect compensatory mechanisms.
- Nonsteroidal anti-inflammatory drugs (NSAIDs) and cyclooxygenase II (COX II) inhibitors can prevent compensatory vasodilation of the afferent arteriole.
- Angiotensin-converting enzyme inhibitors (ACEIs) and angiotensin receptor blockers (ARBs) can prevent compensatory vasoconstriction of the efferent arteriole.

Etiologies

Prerenal

- Intravascular volume depletion: excessive diuresis, vomiting, excessive GI fluid loss, bleeding
- Severe hypotension
- Decreased effective blood volume (volume sensed by arterial baroreceptors): congestive heart failure, cirrhosis, nephrotic syndrome, hepatorenal syndrome
- Systemic vasodilatation: sepsis, liver failure, anaphylaxis
- Large-vessel renal vascular disease: renal artery thrombosis or embolism, renal artery stenosis
- Medications: see Table 1

Intrinsic acute renal failure

- The primary anatomic sites of the kidney are prone to structural damage from prolonged ischemia and/or direct toxicity due to the high metabolic activity and concentrating ability of the kidney.

Etiologies by anatomic site
- Vascular: inflammation, emboli

- Glomerular (glomerulonephritis): systemic lupus erythematosus, medications (see Table 1)
- Interstitial: ischemia, allergic interstitial nephritis, infections, medications (see Table 1)
- Tubular: accounts for 90% of intrinsic cases
    * Intrarenal vasoconstriction, direct tubular toxicity, intratubular obstruction
    * Prolonged ischemia from prerenal causes
    * Toxins
        • Endogenous: myoglobin, hemoglobin, uric acid
        • Exogenous:
            * Medications (see Table 1): aminoglycosides are common nephrotoxins leading to nonoliguric AKD after 5-7 days of therapy.
            * Radiocontrast-induced AKD: Pretreatment of high-risk patients with oral acetylcysteine (Mucomyst®) 600 mg twice daily for 2 days (beginning the day before exposure to radiocontrast dye) may lower the risk of AKD
            * Other: ethylene glycol, pesticides

Postrenal acute kidney disease

- Obstruction of urinary flow at any level from the urinary collecting system to the urethra
- Must involve both kidneys, or one kidney in a patient with a single functioning kidney

Etiologies by anatomic site
- Renal pelves or tubules: crystal deposition
- Ureteral: tumor, stricture, stones
- Bladder neck obstruction: prostatic hypertrophy, bladder carcinoma
- Medications: Table 1

Diagnostic Criteria (Table 2)

- Physical findings: assess for signs and symptoms listed in clinical presentation
- Medication history: identify potentially nephrotoxic agents (Table 1)
- Estimate GFR: normal 100-125 mL/min/1.73 m^2
    * Consider limitations in using serum creatinine as a marker of kidney function (eg, conditions of poor muscle mass), and in using equations to estimate GFR in patients with unstable kidney function. Other assessments (eg, Jelliffe equation) are available to estimate GFR in patients with unstable kidney function.

Table 1

Drug-Induced Causes of Kidney Disease

Clinical syndrome	Causative drugs[1]
Prerenal	ACEIs, ARBs, COX-2 inhibitors, cyclosporine, diuretics, NSAIDs, radiocontrast dye, tacrolimus
Intrinsic	
Vascular	Amphetamines, cisplatin, cyclosporine, mitomycin C
Glomerular	Gold, heroin, lithium, NSAIDs, phenytoin
Interstitial nephritis	Analgesic combinations, aristolochic acid (Chinese herbs), cyclosporine, lithium, NSAIDs, penicillins, sulfonamides, tacrolimus
Acute tubular necrosis	Aminoglycosides, amphotericin B, chemotherapeutic agents, cidofovir, cocaine, foscarnet, ifosfamide, radiocontrast dye, tacrolimus
Postrenal	
Obstructive	Acyclovir, methotrexate, oxalate, sulfonamides, uric acid
Nephrolithiasis	Allopurinol, indinavir, sulfadiazine, triamterene

[1]Not inclusive of all potential nephrotoxins.

Table 2

Laboratory Findings to Differentiate Prerenal and Intrinsic Kidney Disease

Diagnostic test	Prerenal	Intrinsic
BUN:Cr ratio	>20:1	<15:1
Urinalysis	Normal with few cells or casts (hyaline casts normal)	Granular casts present with tubular epithelial cells
Urine osmolality	>500 mOsm/kg	≤300-350 mOsm/kg
Urinary Cr:Plasma Cr	>40:1	<20:1
Specific gravity	>1.020	<1.015
Urine sodium	<20 mEq/L	>40 mEq/L
FE_{Na}	<1%	>2%

Creatinine clearance (CrCl)

• Measured using urine collection methods:

$$CrCl = \frac{U_{Cr} \times V}{S_{Cr} \times t}$$

where U_{Cr} = urinary creatinine concentration (mg/dL)
V = volume of urine (mL)
S_{Cr} = serum creatinine concentration (mg/dL)
t = time period of urine collection (min)

• Estimated using the Cockcroft-Gault equation (assumes stable kidney function):

$$CrCl = \frac{(140 - age)(BW\ in\ kg)}{72 \times S_{Cr}\ (mg/dL)}$$

(multiply the result by 0.85 for females)
where BW = body weight in kg, ideal body weight (IBW) recommended if patient's BW is >30% above IBW

Blood tests

• Elevated: blood urea nitrogen, serum creatinine, electrolytes (potassium, phosphorus)
• Decreased: calcium (consider albumin concentration), bicarbonate

Urinalysis (consider whether fluids and/or diuretics were previously administered)

• Specific gravity, osmolality: high values indicate prerenal causes and stimulation of sodium and water retention.
• Proteinuria: microalbuminuria (>30 mg/d), overt proteinuria (>300 mg/d)
• Hematuria: red blood cells
• Glucose, ketones
• Urine sediment: hyaline casts normal, granular casts and cellular debris suggest structural damage.
• White blood cells: suggest inflammation
• Eosinophils: associated with acute allergic interstitial nephritis

Urine chemistries: sodium, potassium, chloride, creatinine, urinary anion gap

• Fractional excretion of sodium [FE_{Na}]: useful to differentiate prerenal from acute intrinsic renal failure; a low value (<1%) suggests retention of sodium and water (prerenal etiology) versus intrinsic cause.

$$FE_{Na} = \frac{U_{Na} \times P_{Cr} \times 100}{U_{Cr} \times P_{Na}}$$

where U_{Na} = urine sodium
U_{Cr} = urine creatinine
P_{Cr} = plasma creatinine
P_{Na} = plasma sodium

Other tests

• Radiographic procedures: ultrasound, plain film radiograph, radioisotope scan, computed tomography
• Renal biopsy: indicated for patients without cause of ARF identified by other diagnostic tests

Treatment Principles and Goals

Prevention

• Identify high-risk patients.
  * Volume depleted
  * Those undergoing surgical procedures: consider current renal function, age, cardiovascular status, volume status
  * Those receiving potentially nephrotoxic medications
  * Those with preexisting renal or hepatic disease
  * Diabetes mellitus patients
  * Those undergoing diagnostic tests (eg, radiocontrast media exposure)
• Strategies for prevention: hydration, sodium loading

Treatment

- Correct underlying causes of AKD (eg, discontinue nephrotoxic agents, correct fluid status, treat underlying infection, remove urinary tract obstructions).
- Return to baseline kidney function or highest kidney function possible.
- Prevent development of chronic kidney disease and the need for chronic renal replacement therapies (dialysis or transplantation).
- Avoid nephrotoxic agents or take measures to reduce exposure if possible (eg, acetylcysteine [Mucomyst®] to prevent radiocontrast-induced renal failure; select liposomal amphotericin B over conventional amphotericin in high-risk patients).
- Adjust doses of medications based on kidney function.
- Avoid agents contraindicated in patients with kidney disease (eg, metformin [Glucophage®])
- Address complications of AKD: eg, electrolyte abnormalities (hyperkalemia), fluid overload, metabolic acidosis (see sections on fluids and electrolytes and acid-base disorders), hyperphosphatemia (see section on chronic kidney disease).

Strategies for treatment

- Diuretic therapy (loop diuretics) and replacement fluids provide replacement fluids and supportive care by improving fluid status and maintaining urine output.

Drug Therapy (Table 3)

Diuretics

Mechanism of action

- **Loop diuretics:** delivered to the tubular lumen of the kidney by proximal tubular cells; they cause inhibition of sodium and chloride reabsorption in the thick ascending limb of the loop of Henle to promote water excretion.
- **Osmotic diuretics:** freely filtered into the tubular lumen in the proximal tubule; they increase the osmolarity of the glomerular filtrate, which inhibits tubular reabsorption of water and electrolytes and increases urinary output.

Table 3

Drug Therapy for Acute Kidney Disease by Drug Classification

Classification	Generic name (trade name)	Daily dosage range	Dosage forms	Frequency of administration
Diuretics[1]				
Loop	Furosemide (Lasix)	20-400 mg	PO	q 6-12 h
		20-200 mg (up to 1-3 g/day in AKD)	IV	
	Bumetanide (Bumex)	0.5-10 mg	PO, IV	q 12-24 h
	Torsemide (Demadex)	10-200 mg	PO, IV	q 24 h
	Ethacrynic acid (Edecrin)	50-400 mg	PO	q 8-12 h
		50-100 mg	IV	
Osmotic	Mannitol (Osmitrol, Resectisol)	Initial "test" dose: 12.5-25 g over 3-5 min; maintenance dose: 0.25-0.5 g/kg (20-200 g/day)	IV	q 4-6 h
Thiazide	Hydrochlorothiazide (Microzide™)	25-200 mg/d	PO	qd, bid
	Chlorothiazide (Diuril)	500 mg-2 g/d	PO	qd, bid
		250-1000 mg/d	IV	
Thiazide-like	Metolazone (Zaroxolyn)	5-20 mg	PO	qd
Sympathomimetic	Dopamine (Intropin)	0.5-3.0 mcg/kg per min	IV	Continuous

[1]Loop diuretics also administered as a continuous infusion. Higher dose ranges for intermittent dosing are reserved for patients unresponsive to initial smaller doses.

- **Thiazide and thiazide-like diuretics:** inhibit the Na^+-Cl^- cotransport in the early distal convoluted tubules; they are generally used in combination with loop diuretics for resistant edema and fluid overload, particularly metolazone, which is effective at GFRs <30 mL/min. Other thiazide diuretics are generally not effective when GFR is <30 mL/min.

Patient instructions and counseling
(these do not all apply in conditions of AKD)
- Take the last dose of the day early in the evening if possible to minimize nocturia (excessive urination at night).
- Follow all dietary instructions (generally a low-sodium, fluid-restricted diet).
- Move slowly from a sitting to a standing position (potential for orthostatic hypotension).
- Make note of any changes in urine output.
- Contact your health care provider if you experience hearing loss or ringing in the ears.
- This medicine may make your skin more sensitive to sunlight. Use a sunscreen when you are outdoors.
- Tell your health care provider if you have any known drug allergies, particularly to sulfa drugs.

Adverse drug events
Loop diuretics
- Hypokalemia, hypomagnesemia, hyponatremia, hypovolemia, hyperuricemia, hyperglycemia
- Hypercalciuria
- Orthostatic hypotension, dehydration
- Metabolic alkalosis (partly due to extracellular fluid volume contraction)
- Ototoxicity
- Diarrhea, nausea
- Furosemide, bumetanide, and torsemide have a sulfonamide substituent (potential for hypersensitivity reactions). Ethacrynic acid is generally reserved for patients allergic to sulfa compounds.

Osmotic diuretics
- Acute expansion of extracellular fluid volume and increased risk of pulmonary edema, acute rise in serum K^+, nausea and vomiting, headache, blurred vision, rash

Thiazide and thiazide-like diuretics (used in combination with loop diuretics)
- Hypokalemia, hyponatremia, hypercalcemia
- Hypovolemia, orthostatic hypotension
- Hyperglycemia, hypochloremic alkalosis, hyperlipidemia
- Hypersensitivity reactions from sulfonamide substituents

- Chest pain (metolazone, more common with the brand Mykrox®, which is more rapidly and extensively absorbed than Zaroxolyn)

Drug-drug and drug-disease interactions
- Loop diuretics and aminoglycosides: increased potential for ototoxicity
- Diuretics and other nephrotoxins: increased risk of nephrotoxicity if hypovolemia occurs
- Diuretics and lithium: decreased renal clearance of lithium; monitor lithium concentrations more closely.
- Diuretics and digoxin: hypokalemia from diuretic use may increase risk of toxicity with digoxin (monitor potassium and digoxin).
- Loop and thiazide diuretics and gout: potential for increased gouty attacks from hyperuricemia
- Thiazide diuretics and diabetes: hyperglycemia from thiazides; increase monitoring.
- Conditions that decrease secretion of diuretic to its site of action in the renal tubule:
    * Proteinuria (diuretic binds to protein and is not available at its site of action)
    * Decreased renal blood flow
    * Competitive inhibition of transport system (NSAIDs, probenecid, cephalosporins)

Parameters to monitor
- Blood pressure (sitting and standing), pulse, urine output, fluid intake, serum creatinine, serum electrolytes, blood urea nitrogen, bicarbonate, calcium, glucose, uric acid
- Osmotic diuretics: serum osmolality (310-320 mOsm/kg); assess urine output after initial test dose (goal urine flow at least 30-50 mL/h)

Pharmacokinetics
Loop diuretics
- Oral bioavailability: furosemide (60%), bumetanide (85%), torsemide (85%)
- PO:IV dose ratios: furosemide (1.5), bumetanide (1), torsemide (1)
- Equivalent doses: 1 mg bumetanide = 20 mg torsemide = 40 mg furosemide
- Elimination route: furosemide (primarily renal), bumetanide (hepatic and renal), torsemide (primarily hepatic), ethacrynic acid (hepatic and renal)

Thiazide and thiazide-like diuretics
- Metolazone absorption differs between brands. Mykrox (available outside the U.S.) is more rapidly and extensively absorbed than Zaroxolyn.

Other (eg, unusual storage requirements, administration, etc)

- Patients with kidney disease generally require larger doses of diuretics to achieve adequate concentrations of the drug at the site of action in the kidney.
- The brands of metolazone (Zaroxolyn and Mykrox) are not bioequivalent and should not be interchanged.

Dopamine

- *Note:* Use of dopamine in AKD is controversial, as benefits have not consistently been demonstrated.

Mechanism of action

- At low doses (1-3 mcg/kg per min) causes selective vasodilation of the renal vasculature and may cause an increase in renal blood flow and GFR. Dose is titrated to desired response.

Patient instructions and counseling

- Administered to hospitalized patients (see parameters to monitor)

Adverse drug events

- Hypotension, tachycardia, arrhythmias, dyspnea
- Headache, nausea, vomiting
- At higher doses (>10 mcg/kg per min) stimulates α- and β_1-adrenergic receptors, causing peripheral vasoconstriction and hypertension.

Drug-drug and drug-disease interactions

- Prolonged and intensified effect when given with MAO inhibitors, α- and β-adrenergic blockers, general anesthetics, and phenytoin
- Use dopamine with caution in patients with cardiovascular disease or cardiac arrhythmias and patients with occlusive vascular disease.

Parameters to monitor

- Blood pressure, pulse, urine output, ECG, heart rate
- Monitor for extravasation

Pharmacokinetics

- Onset of action: 5 minutes
- Duration: <10 minutes (continuous infusion necessary)
- Half-life: 2 minutes
- Metabolized to inactive metabolites (75%) and the active metabolite norepinephrine (25%). Metabolites are excreted in urine.

Other (eg, unusual storage requirements, administration, etc)

- Administer in large vein to prevent extravasation and tissue necrosis; phentolamine (Regitine®) used as antidote

Nondrug Therapy

Fluid management

- Fluid intake and output should be evaluated and adjustments made to maintain hemodynamic stability (consider sensible and insensible losses).
- Fluid selection and rate of correction are dependent on the clinical condition of the patient (eg, crystalloids, colloids, or normal saline).

Nutritional

- High-calorie diet generally required (patient-specific)
- Consider restriction of sodium, potassium, phosphorus

Renal replacement therapies

- These are procedures by which the blood is artificially cleared of waste and some essential metabolic products to augment the function of a failed or failing kidney. Includes **hemodialysis** and **hemofiltration,** in which the semipermeable membrane is a dialyzer, and **peritoneal dialysis,** in which the peritoneal cavity serves as this membrane. Procedures may be intermittent or continuous. Hemodialysis and hemofiltration are the most common modalities for patients with AKD. Kidney transplantation is also considered a form of renal replacement therapy.
- Consider the potential for drug removal by dialysis.

Indications for renal replacement therapy

- Any of the following refractory to more conservative measures:
  - * Acidosis
  - * Electrolyte abnormalities (hyperkalemia)
  - * Intoxication (drug-induced kidney failure), if drug can be removed by dialysis
  - * Volume overload
  - * Uremia (BUN >100 mg/dL) or uremic symptoms (pericarditis, encephalopathy, bleeding, dyscrasia, nausea, vomiting, pruritus)

2. Chronic Kidney Disease

- ***Chronic kidney disease*** (CKD) is kidney damage with or without a decrease in GFR or a GFR <60 mL/min per 1.73 m^2 for ≥3 months. ***Kidney damage*** is defined as pathologic abnormalities or markers of damage, including abnormalities in blood or urine tests or imaging studies.
- CKD is classified into five stages based on kidney damage and GFR (Table 4). End-stage kidney disease (ESKD) occurs when patients require renal replacement therapy (either dialysis or transplantation) to sustain life and is classified as stage 5 CKD.

Epidemiology of Chronic Kidney Disease

Incidence
- The number of patients with CKD is increasing, with a doubling in the number of patients with stage 5 CKD expected by the year 2010.
- Its incidence is approximately four times higher in the black population.
- The largest portion of incident patients are age 45-64.

Prevalence
- Estimated prevalence of CKD based on stage:
    * Stage 1 (5.9 million), stage 2 (5.3 million), stage 3 (7.6 million), stage 4 (400,000), stage 5 (300,000)
- Approximately 370,000 patients are being treated for ESKD (including hemodialysis, peritoneal dialysis, and transplant patients).

Mortality
- Life expectancy is four to five times shorter in dialysis patients than in the general population.
- The primary causes of death in the ESKD population are cardiac diseases and infection.
- Comorbidities, estimated GFR, and albumin at initiation of dialysis are strong predictors of mortality in the dialysis population.

Clinical Presentation

- Changes in urine output (may not occur in earlier stages of CKD)
- "Foaming" of urine: indicates proteinuria (Table 5)
    * ***Microalbuminuria:*** the presence of albumin in the urine in amounts of 30-300 mg/d
    * ***Albuminuria:*** the presence of albumin in the urine in amounts >300 mg/d
    * ***Clinical proteinuria:*** total protein in the urine in amounts greater than 300 mg/d
- Increased blood pressure (hypertension is a common etiology and result of CKD).
- Signs and symptoms of hyperglycemia and glucosuria (diabetes is a common etiology).
- Signs and symptoms associated with fluid and electrolyte abnormalities (eg, hyperkalemia, fluid overload; see section on fluids and electrolytes) and secondary complications (see secondary complications of CKD).
- Development of secondary complications of CKD
    * Anemia: decreased hemoglobin and hematocrit; may also present with iron deficiency
    * Secondary hyperparathyroidism and associated metabolic abnormalities: increased serum phosphorus, decreased serum calcium (at risk for hypercalcemia as kidney disease pro-

Table 4

Stages of Chronic Kidney Disease

Stage	Description	GFR (mL/min per 1.73 m^2)	Action
——	Increased risk	≥90 (with CKD risk factors)	Screening, CKD risk reduction
1	Kidney damage with normal or increased GFR	≥90	Diagnosis and treatment, treatment of comorbid conditions, slowing progression, CVD risk reduction
2	Kidney damage with mildly decreased GFR	60-89	Estimating progression
3	Moderately decreased GFR	30-59	Evaluating and treating complications
4	Severely decreased GFR	15-29	Preparation for kidney replacement therapy
5	Kidney failure (defined as ESKD if renal replacement therapy needed)	<15 (or need for renal replacement therapy)	Renal replacement therapy (if uremia present)

Table 5

Definitions of Proteinuria and Albuminuria

	Total protein			Albumin		
	24-hour collection (mg/d)	Spot urine dipstick (mg/dL)	Spot urine protein:SCr ratio (mg/g)	24-hour collection (mg/d)	Spot urine dipstick (mg/dL)	Spot urine albumin:SCr ratio (mg/g)
Normal	<300	<30	<200	<30	<3	<17 (men); <25 (women)
Microalbuminuria	NA	NA	NA	30-300	>3	17-250 (men); 25-355 (women)
Albuminuria or clinical proteinuria	>300	>30	>200	>300	NA	>250 (men); >355 (women)

gresses), increased intact parathyroid hormone (iPTH), vitamin D deficiency
* Metabolic acidosis: decreased serum bicarbonate, increased anion gap
* Malnutrition: decreased albumin and prealbumin (see section on nutrition)
• Signs of uremia (see section on acute renal failure) in later stages of CKD (stage 4 and 5 CKD)

Pathophysiology of Progressive Kidney Disease and Selected Secondary Complications

Progressive kidney disease
• Progressive loss of nephron function results in adaptive changes in remaining nephrons to increase single nephron glomerular filtration pressure.
• Over time the compensatory increase in single nephron GFR leads to hypertrophy from sustained increases in pressure and loss of individual nephron function.
• Proteinuria, one of the initial diagnostic signs, may also contribute to the progressive decline in kidney function.
• Loss of kidney function is usually irreversible.

Etiology of progressive kidney disease
• Each of the following may result in damage to the kidney that over time leads to a decrease in functioning nephrons and decreased total GFR:
   * Diabetes (accounts for primary cause in 45% of patients with ESKD)
   * Hypertension (accounts for primary cause in 24% of patients with ESKD)
   * Glomerulonephritis
   * Cystic kidney disease

* HIV nephropathy
* Other contributing factors (smoking, genetic factors, gender differences)

Anemia of Chronic Kidney Disease
• The primary etiology is a decrease in production of the hormone erythropoietin by the kidney as kidney disease progresses (>90% of erythropoietin production occurs in the kidney, approximately 10% by the liver)
• Results in a normochromic, normocytic anemia
• Red blood cell lifespan is also decreased from 120 days to approximately 64 days in patients with kidney failure.
• Other contributors include iron deficiency and blood loss (eg, from uremic bleeding, dialysis, etc).

Secondary hyperparathyroidism and associated metabolic abnormalities
• As kidney function declines phosphorus elimination decreases.
• Hyperphosphatemia causes a reciprocal decrease in serum calcium concentrations (hypocalcemia).
• Hypocalcemia stimulates the release of intact parathyroid hormone (iPTH) by the parathyroid glands.
• Conversion of the vitamin D precursor to the active form (1,25-dihydroxyvitamin D_3) occurs in the kidney. As kidney disease progresses there is a decline in the 1α-hydroxylase enzyme that promotes the final hydroxylation step in the kidney, resulting in a deficiency in active vitamin D. Deficiencies in the precursor form of vitamin D have also been observed in stage 3 and 4 CKD. Active vitamin D (1,25-dihydroxyvitamin D_3) promotes increased intestinal absorption of calcium and suppresses pro-

duction of PTH by the parathyroid gland; therefore, vitamin D deficiency leads to worsening secondary hyperparathyroidism.

- Increased iPTH promotes:
  * Decreased phosphorus reabsorption within the kidney
  * Increased calcium reabsorption by the kidney
  * Increased calcium mobilization from bone
- As kidney disease progresses:
  * Hyperphosphatemia and subsequent hypocalcemia progressively worsen and secondary hyperparathyroidism becomes more severe.
  * The renal effects of PTH on phosphorus and calcium are no longer maintained and PTH predominantly stimulates calcium resorption from bone.
  * Decreased production of active vitamin D worsens hypocalcemia and secondary hyperparathyroidism.
  * In more severe CKD (stage 4 and 5) patients are prone to develop hypercalcemia due in part to the use of calcium-containing phosphate binders; patients are at risk for calcifications.
- Uncontrolled secondary hyperparathyroidism leads to hyperplasia of the parathyroid gland and renal osteodystrophy (from sustained effects of iPTH on bone).

Metabolic acidosis
- Decreased excretion of acid by the kidney
- Accumulation of endogenous acids due to impaired kidney function (eg, phosphates and sulfates)

Diagnostic Criteria

Progressive kidney disease
- Progressive increase in serum creatinine: >1.1-1.2 mg/dL for females, >1.2-1.3 mg/dL for males (consider factors that may alter serum creatinine such as decreased muscle mass and nutritional status).
- Decreased GFR (see Table 4 for CKD classifications)

Measured creatinine clearance (see section on diagnostic criteria for acute renal failure)

Cockcroft-Gault equation (see section on diagnostic criteria for acute renal failure)

Modification of diet in renal disease (MDRD) abbreviated equation

$$\text{GFR} = 186 \times (\text{serum creatinine})^{-1.154} \times$$
$$(\text{age in years})^{-0.203} \times 1.210 \text{ (if patient is black)} \times 0.742$$
$$\text{(if patient is female)}$$

Schwartz equation (children)

$$\text{Creatinine clearance (mL/min)} = k \times \text{length}$$
$$\text{(in cm)/serum creatinine}$$

where k = 0.55 for children aged 1-13 years

- Microalbuminuria, albuminuria, or clinical proteinuria (Table 5)
- Abnormal serum chemistries
  * Increase in serum creatinine, BUN
  * Increased potassium, decreased serum bicarbonate, increased phosphorus, decreased calcium (indicative of secondary complications)
- Development of secondary complications (eg, anemia, secondary hyperparathyroidism)

Anemia of chronic kidney disease
- Testing for anemia is recommended in all patients with CKD
- Guidelines for anemia management in patients with CKD recommend further evaluation for anemia when hemoglobin is <12 g/dL in females and <13.5 g/dL in males.
- Iron deficiency: evaluate red blood cell indices and iron indices to identify deficiency as a contributing factor; iron deficiency manifests as a microcytic anemia.
  * Red blood cell count $<4.2 \times 10^6$ cells/mm^2
  * Mean corpuscular volume (MCV): <80 fl
  * Serum iron: <50 mg/dL
  * Total iron binding capacity (TIBC): <250 mg/dL
  * Transferrin saturation (TSat): <16%
  * Serum ferritin: <12 ng/mL
- Transferrin saturation and serum ferritin should be maintained at higher values for CKD patients receiving erythropoietin therapy (TSat >20%, serum ferritin >100 ng/mL for CKD patients not on dialysis and peritoneal dialysis patients; TSat >20%, serum ferritin >200 ng/mL in hemodialysis patients).
- Evaluate for folate and vitamin B$_{12}$ deficiencies (manifests as a macrocytic anemia), sources of blood loss (eg, GI bleeding), and confounding disease states (eg, cancer, HIV).

Secondary hyperparathyroidism and associated metabolic abnormalities
- Serum phosphorus >4.6 mg/dL (>5.5 mg/dL in stage 5 CKD)
- Calcium abnormalities:
  Hypocalcemia: corrected serum calcium <8.5 mg/dL
  Hypercalcemia becomes a concern in stage 4 and 5 CKD
  * Corrected calcium = measured serum calcium + 0.8 x (normal serum albumin – measured serum albumin); normal serum albumin = 4.0 g/dL

- Elevated calcium x phosphorus product: >55 mg^2/dL^2 (elevated product increases risk for metastatic calcifications)
- Intact parathyroid hormone (iPTH) >70 pg/mL (stage 3 CKD), >110 pg/mL (stage 4 CKD), >300 pg/mL (stage 5 CKD)
- Radiographic evidence of bone abnormalities (eg, osteitis fibrosa cystica)

Metabolic acidosis
- Serum bicarbonate (HCO$_3^-$) <20-22 mEq/L
- Typically have an increased anion gap: anion gap = [Na$^+$] − ([Cl$^-$] + [HCO$_3^-$])
- Signs and symptoms of chronic metabolic acidosis that develop as CKD progresses are generally not of the same magnitude as with acute metabolic acidosis (eg, hyperventilation and cardiovascular and CNS manifestations).

Treatment Principles and Goals

Progressive kidney disease
- Control underlying cause of progressive CKD (eg, diabetes, hypertension; see corresponding chapters on hypertension and diabetes)
    * Blood glucose: 80-120 mg/dL fasting, 100-140 mg/dL nonfasting
    * Target hemoglobin A$_{1c}$ ≤7.0%
    * BP goals:
        - BP <130/80 mm Hg for patients with evidence of kidney disease and/or diabetes
- Prevent or minimize microalbuminuria/proteinuria.
- Slow the rate of progression of CKD (by achieving diabetes and hypertension goals and minimizing proteinuria).
- Prevent drug-induced causes of kidney disease.
    * Avoid chronic use of combinations of analgesics.
    * Minimize use of agents known to cause ARF (can develop an acute-on-chronic kidney disease)
- Manage secondary complications of CKD (anemia, secondary hyperparathyroidism, electrolyte abnormalities).
- Control hyperlipidemia.
- Address cardiovascular risk factors (cardiovascular disease is the leading cause of death in the CKD population).
- Adjust drug doses based on kidney function.
- Avoid medications contraindicated in patients with reduced kidney function.
    * Example: metformin (Glucophage®) is contraindicated in patients with elevated serum creatinine (>1.5 mg/dL for men, >1.4 mg/dL for women); increased risk of lactic acidosis.

- Preparation for kidney failure and kidney replacement therapy (ie, dialysis, transplantation) as needed
- Replacement of kidney function by dialysis and transplantation, if signs and symptoms of uremia are present
- Smoking cessation

Treatment strategies
- Diuretics for fluid balance and management of hypertension (diuretic selection based on kidney function)
- Antihypertensives with diet and lifestyle modifications for control of blood pressure (see chapter on hypertension)
- Antidiabetic agents with diet and lifestyle modifications for control of blood glucose (see chapter on diabetes)
- Angiotensin-converting enzyme inhibitors (ACEIs) and angiotensin receptor blockers (ARB) to delay progression of kidney disease. Recommended for patients with diabetes and patients with hypertension and total protein creatinine ratio.
- Protein restriction to 0.6-0.8 g/kg per day
    * May consider for patients with >1 g/d proteinuria despite optimal blood pressure control with a regimen that includes an ACEI or ARB
    * Must be cautious to maintain adequate caloric intake and avoid malnutrition
    * Not to be implemented for patients <80% of their ideal body weight or with >10 g/d proteinuria
- Renal replacement therapy
    * Plans for dialysis therapy (hemodialysis or peritoneal dialysis) should be considered during stage 4 CKD (when GFR <30 mL/min) (see section on acute renal failure for general description of dialysis). Also evaluate candidacy for kidney transplantation.

Anemia of chronic kidney disease
- Target hemoglobin 11-13 g/dL
- Iron indices: Transferrin saturation >20%, serum ferritin >100 for CKD patients not on dialysis and peritoneal dialysis patients (goal serum ferritin in hemodialysis patients is >200). Note: Potential for iron overload must be considered when transferrin saturation is >50% and serum ferritin is >500 ng/mL.
- Other goals: improve symptoms of anemia (eg, fatigue, shortness of breath), improve quality of life, improve other conditions affected by decreased oxygenation (eg, heart failure)

Treatment strategies

- Erythropoietic growth factors to stimulate red blood cell production
    * Epoetin alfa (Epogen®, Procrit®): subcutaneous (SC) or intravenous (IV) administration; SC preferred for patients not on hemodialysis (ie, peritoneal dialysis and early stage CKD patients)
    * Initial doses: 50-100 U/kg IV or SC 3 times per week
    * Darbepoetin alfa (Aranesp®): initial dose 0.45 mcg/kg IV or SC administered once weekly
    * Dose conversion required from epoetin alfa (Units/week) to darbepoetin alfa (mcg/week) (Table 6)
    * Darbepoetin package insert: for patients receiving epoetin alfa 2-3 times per week, darbepoetin alfa should be administered weekly. For patients receiving epoetin alfa once per week, darbepoetin alfa should be administered every other week. In this situation, the weekly epoetin dose should be multiplied by 2 and this dose used in Table 6 to determine the appropriate darbepoetin dose.
    * Dose titration: allow at least 2-4 weeks before change in dose of epoetin alfa or darbepoetin alfa is made based on change in hemoglobin or hematocrit.
    * If change in hemoglobin <1 g/dL (hematocrit <2-3%), increase dose by 50% (epoetin alfa) or 25% (darbepoetin alfa).
    * If change in hemoglobin >2-3 g/dL (hematocrit >6-9%), reduce dose by 25% (epoetin alfa and darbepoetin alfa).
- Give iron supplementation to prevent iron deficiency as a cause of resistance to therapy with erythropoietic growth factors.

Table 6

Estimated Starting Doses of Darbepoetin Alfa Based on Previous Epoetin Alfa Dose

Weekly epoetin alfa dose (units/wk)	Weekly darbepoetin alfa dose (mcg/wk)	
	Adult	Pediatric
<1500	6.25	*
1500-2499	6.25	6.25
2500-4999	12.5	10
5000-10,999	25	20
11,000-17,999	40	40
18,000-33,999	60	60
34,000-89,999	100	100
≥90,000	200	200

* Insufficient data

- Oral iron supplementation is limited by poor absorption and is often inadequate to achieve goal iron indices. It may be reasonable for stage 3 and 4 CKD patients and the peritoneal dialysis population (patients without IV access). The recommended dose is 200 mg elemental iron per day.
- Intravenous iron supplementation is preferred to treat true iron deficiency and in hemodialysis patients with regular intravenous access. One may administer a full course of iron, typically a 1-gram total dose divided over 8-10 hemodialysis sessions (100 mg per dose for iron sucrose [Venofer®] and iron dextran [InFeD®, Dexferrum®] or 125 mg per dose for sodium ferric gluconate [Ferrlecit®]). Weekly doses of 25-125 mg may be administered as maintenance doses of iron in HD patients.
    * Iron sucrose: The 100-mg dose may be diluted in 100 mL of 0.9% NaCl administered IV over at least 15 minutes or administered undiluted over 2-5 minutes.
    * Iron dextran: The 100-mg dose may be administered over 2 minutes IV push.
    * Sodium ferric gluconate: The 125-mg dose may be diluted in 100 mL of 0.9% sodium chloride and administered IV over 1 hour or administered undiluted as an IV injection at a rate of up to 12.5 mg/min. Dosing in pediatric patients is 1.5 mg/kg in 25 mL of 0.9% NaCl over 60 min (max dose 125 mg)
- IV iron regimens differ in peritoneal dialysis patients and patients with CKD not requiring dialysis (one-gram total dose recommended for iron deficient patients; administered in divided doses. Iron sucrose has an approved regimen in these populations).
    * Iron sucrose – Nondialysis CKD patients: 200 mg over 2-5 minutes on 5 different occasions within a 14-day period. Peritoneal dialysis patients: 300 mg in 0.9% NaCl administered IV over 1.5 hours followed by a second infusion of 300 mg 14 days later, followed by a 400 mg dose administered over 2.5 hours 14 days later.
- Blood transfusions may be required for more severe anemia or when blood loss is a major contributing factor.

Secondary hyperparathyroidism and associated metabolic abnormalities

- Goal serum phosphorus 2.7-4.6 mg/dL (stages 3 and 4 CKD), 3.5-5.5 mg/dL (stage 5 CKD)
- Goal serum calcium approximately 8.5-10 mg/dL (normal range) for stage 3 and 4 CKD; 8.4-9.5 mg/dL for stage 5 CKD (recommend upper range of approximately 9.5 mg/dL in stage 5 CKD due to risk of hypercalcemia and calcifications).

- Calcium x phosphorus product <55 mg^2/dL^2
- Intact PTH (iPTH)
    * Stage 3 CKD: iPTH 35-70 pg/mL
    * Stage 4 CKD: iPTH 70-110 pg/mL
    * Stage 5 CKD: iPTH 150-300 pg/mL

Treatment strategies
- Dietary phosphorus restriction: 800-1000 mg/d phosphorus (consult with dietitian)
- Phosphate binding agents: elemental (calcium, lanthanum, aluminum, magnesium) and nonelemental (sevelamer)
    * Titrate doses based on phosphorus and calcium x phosphorus product.
    * Limit use of calcium-containing phosphate binders if hypercalcemia occurs.
    * Aluminum is not a first-line agent and should be prescribed only for short-term use (<30 days) to minimize the risk of accumulation.
- Removal of phosphorus by dialysis for stage 5 CKD patients (continue phosphorus restriction and use of phosphate binding agents with dialysis).
- Maintain goal calcium and phosphorus concentrations.
- Provide vitamin D supplementation based on stage of CKD; supplementation with the active form (calcitriol) or a vitamin D analog may be necessary in more severe stages of CKD (stages 4 and 5); supplementation with a vitamin D precursor (eg, ergocalciferol) may be sufficient in earlier stages.
- Use a calcimimetic agent [cinacalcet (Sensipar®)] to help control iPTH in stage 5 CKD. Initial dose is 30 mg PO daily. The dose of cinacalcet should be titrated no more frequently than every 2 to 4 weeks through sequential doses of 60, 90, 120, and 180 mg once daily to target iPTH (150-300 pg/mL).
- Control metabolic acidosis (causes bone demineralization if not controlled).

Metabolic acidosis
- Serum bicarbonate: 22-26 mEq/L
- pH: 7.35-7.45

Treatment strategies
- Administration of sodium bicarbonate or other alkali preparation
    * Gradual correction (over days to weeks) is usually appropriate for asymptomatic patients with mild to moderate acidosis (serum bicarbonate 12-20 mEq/L, pH 7.2-7.4).
- Dialysis: bicarbonate or lactate contained within the dialysate solution diffuses from dialysate to plasma and effectively treats metabolic acidosis.

Monitoring

Progressive kidney disease
- Patients at high risk for CKD (eg, patients with diabetes and/or hypertension) or diagnosed with CKD should have the following monitored regularly:
    * Serum creatinine (consider limitations).
    * Estimated GFR: assess rate of progression (mL/min per year)
    * Proteinuria: monitor annually in patients with type 1 diabetes with diabetes duration of ≥5 years and at diagnosis for patients with type 2 diabetes.
    * Serum electrolytes
    * Assess control of hypertension and diabetes.
    * Evaluate drug regimens and adjust based on kidney function.

Anemia of chronic kidney disease
- Hemoglobin, hematocrit: every 1-2 weeks after initiation of erythropoietic therapy or following a dose change, and every 2-4 weeks once stable target hemoglobin and hematocrit are achieved
- Iron indices (transferrin saturation, serum ferritin)
- Signs and symptoms of anemia

Secondary hyperparathyroidism and associated metabolic abnormalities
- Phosphorus
- Calcium
- Parathyroid hormone
- Consider measuring vitamin D precursor levels in patients with stage 3 and 4 CKD.

Metabolic acidosis
- Serum bicarbonate
- Potassium

Drug Therapy

Progressive kidney disease
- ACEIs, ARBs (see chapters on hypertension and diabetes)
- Antihypertensive agents (see chapter on hypertension)
- Antidiabetic agents (see chapter on diabetes)

Anemia
- Erythropoietic agents (Table 7)

Mechanism of action
- Stimulates the division and differentiation of erythroid progenitor cells and induces the release of reticulocytes from the bone marrow into the bloodstream where they mature into erythrocytes

Patient instructions and counseling

- For self-administration (subcutaneous injections):
  * Patients may experience pain at the site of injection with subcutaneous administration.
  * Always wipe the top of the vial with an alcohol pad before each use.
  * Do not shake the bottle and do not inject if you see solid material in the solution.
  * Use a new syringe with each injection.
  * Stick the needle into the rubber stopper at the top of the bottle then turn the bottle upside down and hold at eye level.
  * Pull the plunger until it lines up with the appropriate number for your dose.
  * Gently tap the syringe with your finger to make any air bubbles float to the top of the syringe.
  * Inject the medication into a different place on you body each time.
  * Store vials in the refrigerator; do not freeze.

Adverse drug events

- Hypertension
- Red blood cell aplasia
- Seizures (rare)
- Polycythemia
- Thrombocytosis

Drug-drug and drug-disease interactions

- Causes of resistance to erythropoietic therapy:
  * Iron deficiency
  * Secondary hyperparathyroidism
  * Inflammatory conditions
  * Aluminum accumulation
  * Other disease states causing anemia (eg, cancer, HIV)

Parameters to monitor

- Hemoglobin and hematocrit
- Iron indices
- Blood pressure

Pharmacokinetics

- Half-life:
  * Epoetin alfa: approximately 8.5 h IV, 24 h SC
  * Darbepoetin alfa: approximately 25 h IV, 48 h SC
- Effect on hematologic parameters observed over approximately 7 days to 6 weeks
- Steady-state dependent on lifespan of red blood cells and rate of red blood cell production stimulated by erythropoietin.

Strengths and dosage forms

- Epoetin alfa is supplied as single-dose, preservative-free solution (2000-, 3000-, 4000-, 10,000-, and 40,000-U/mL vials) and as a multidose, preserved solution (10,000- and 20,000-U/mL vials)
- Darbepoetin alfa is available in two solutions: a polysorbate solution and an albumin solution, supplied as single-dose vials (25-, 40-, 60-, 100-, 200-, 300-, and 500-mg/mL and a 150-mg/0.75-mL vial) and as single-dose prefilled syringes (25-, 40-, 60-, 100-, 150-, 200-, 300-, and 500-mg); contains no preservative.

Iron supplementation (Table 8)

Mechanism of action

- Repletes iron stores and iron available for red blood cell production in the bone marrow. It is incorporated into hemoglobin within the red cells and facilitates transport of oxygen.

Patient instructions and counseling

- Oral iron
  * May cause stools to be dark in color
  * Take between meals to increase absorption
  * May take with food if GI upset occurs
  * Do not take with dairy products or antacids

Adverse drug events

- Oral iron: stomach cramping, constipation, nausea, vomiting, dark stools
- Intravenous iron:

Table 7

Erythropoietic Growth Factors

Generic name (trade name)	Starting dose	Route of administration	Frequency of administration
Epoetin alfa (Epogen, Procrit)	50-100 units/kg	IV, SC	1-3 doses per week
Darbepoetin alfa (Aranesp)	0.45 mcg/kg	IV, SC	Once weekly or once every other week (may prolong interval to every 3-4 weeks)

* Anaphylactic reactions have occurred with iron dextran (InFed, Dexferrum); administer a 25-mg test dose prior to administration of the full dose. Reduced incidence of hypersensitivity reactions with sodium ferric gluconate (Ferrlecit) and iron sucrose (Venofer).
* All preparations: observe patients for diaphoresis, nausea, vomiting, lower back pain, dyspnea, and hypotension.
* Iron overload: may be treated with deferoxamine (Desferal®)

Drug-drug and drug-disease interactions

* Oral iron: decreased GI absorption when given with antacids, quinolones, and tetracycline; increased absorption when administered with vitamin C
* Intravenous iron: potential for increased risk of infection (administration to patients with severe systemic infections controversial)

Parameters to monitor

* Iron indices: ferritin, transferrin saturation
* Hemoglobin and hematocrit
* Monitor for anaphylactic or hypersensitivity reactions after IV administration.

Strengths and dosage forms

* Sodium ferric gluconate (Ferrlecit): supplied as colorless glass ampules containing 62.5 mg elemental iron in 5 mL (12.5 mg/mL)
* Iron sucrose (Venofer): supplied in 5-mL single-dose vials containing 100 mg elemental iron (20 mg/mL)
* Iron dextran (InFeD, Dexferrum): supplied in 2-mL single-dose vials containing 50 mg of elemental iron per milliliter

Secondary hyperparathyroidism and associated metabolic abnormalities

* Phosphate binding agents (Table 9)

Mechanism of action

* Combines with dietary phosphate in the GI tract to form an insoluble complex that is excreted in the feces

Patient instructions and counseling

* Take with meals and snacks
* Do not take with oral iron salts or certain antibiotics (quinolones, tetracyclines).
* Aluminum and magnesium products are generally for short-term use (concern of accumulation in patients with kidney disease).
* Use in conjunction with dietary phosphorus restriction

Adverse drug events

* Calcium products: hypercalcemia, nausea, vomiting, abdominal pain, constipation
* Sevelamer (Renagel): decreased LDL cholesterol, increased HDL cholesterol (may be a beneficial effect), nausea, vomiting
* Lanthanum carbonate (Fosrenol): nausea, vomiting, diarrhea, abdominal pain, constipation
* Aluminum: constipation, aluminum toxicity, chalky taste, cramps, nausea, vomiting
* Magnesium products: diarrhea, hypermagnesemia, cramps, muscle weakness
* All products: hypophosphatemia

Table 8

Iron Supplements

Generic name (trade name)	Dose	Dosage forms	Frequency of administration[1]
Ferrous sulfate (Fer-In-Sol, Feosol, Slow FE)	200 mg elemental iron per day	PO	bid-tid
Ferrous fumarate (Femiron, Vitron-C)	200 mg elemental iron per day	PO	bid-tid
Ferrous gluconate (Fergon)	200 mg elemental iron per day	PO	bid-tid
Polysaccharide iron (Hytinic, Niferec)	200 mg elemental iron per day	PO	qd-bid
Heme iron polypeptide (Proferrin)	200 mg elemental iron per day	PO	tid-qid
Sodium ferric gluconate (Ferrlecit)	62.5-125 mg	IV	Weekly, three times per week or monthly*
Iron sucrose (Venofer)	20-200 mg	IV	Weekly, three times per week or monthly*
Iron dextran (InFeD, Dexferrum)	25-1000 mg	IV	Weekly, three times per week or monthly*

[1]For oral formulations, frequency of administration dependent on amount of elemental iron per unit; must give 200 mg elemental iron per day.

*Three times per week common in iron deficient hemodialysis patients

Drug-drug and drug-disease interactions

- Calcium, lanthanum, aluminum, and magnesium are elemental compounds that may bind with antibiotics (quinolones, tetracyclines) in the GI tract, thus decreasing their absorption.
- Sevelamer (Renagel): may contribute to metabolic acidosis and decreased LDL cholesterol

Parameters to monitor

- Phosphorus, calcium, iPTH
- Aluminum, magnesium (if receiving aluminum- or magnesium-containing products)
- Sevelamer (Renagel): serum bicarbonate, LDL cholesterol

Vitamin D therapy (Table 10)
Mechanism of action (active vitamin D)

- Increases intestinal absorption of calcium, tubular reabsorption of calcium by the kidney (in patients with sufficient kidney function) and suppresses synthesis of parathyroid hormone; also increases intestinal phosphorus absorption

Patient instructions and counseling

- Use in conjunction with dietary phosphorus restriction and phosphate binding agents; therapy may need to be temporarily discontinued if calcium and phosphorus are elevated.
- Notify health care provider of any of the following signs of hypercalcemia: weakness, headache, decreased appetite, lethargy

Adverse drug events

- Hypercalcemia: decreased incidence with vitamin D analogs

- Hyperphosphatemia: decreased incidence with vitamin D analogs
- Adynamic bone disease: caused by oversuppression of PTH

Drug-drug and drug-disease interactions

- Cholestyramine may decrease intestinal absorption of oral products.
- Magnesium absorption may be increased with concomitant administration.

Parameters to monitor

- iPTH
- Calcium
- Phosphorus
- Calcium x phosphorus product: vitamin D therapy may need to be temporarily discontinued or the dose decreased if product is elevated.
- Alkaline phosphatase
- Signs of vitamin D intoxication and hypercalcemia (eg, weakness, headache, somnolence, nausea, vomiting, bone pain, polyuria)

Pharmacokinetics

- Ergocalciferol: requires hydroxylation within the liver to calcifediol and a second hydroxylation within the kidney to form active vitamin D; do not give to patients with severe kidney and/or liver disease.
- Doxercalciferol: requires conversion to its active form $1\alpha,25$-dihydroxyvitamin D_2 in the liver

Strengths and dosage forms

- Calcitriol (Calcijex®): 1- and 2-mcg/mL ampules
- Calcitriol (Rocaltrol®): 0.25- and 0.5-mcg capsules

Table 9

Phosphate Binding Agents

Generic name	Trade names	Starting dosage range[1]
Calcium carbonate (40% elemental calcium)	Tums, Os-Cal-500, Nephro-Calci, Caltrate 600, CalCarb HD, CaCO$_3$ (multiple preparations)	0.8-2 g elemental calcium
Calcium acetate (25% elemental calcium)	Phos-Lo	1334-2001 mg
Sevelamer	Renagel	800-1600 mg
Lanthanum carbonate	Fosrenol	250-500 mg
Aluminum hydroxide	AlternaGel, Amphojel, Alu-Cap, Alu-tab, Basaljel	300-600 mg
Magnesium carbonate	Mag-Carb	70 mg
Magnesium hydroxide (milk of magnesia)	Various	300-400 mg

[1]Dose per meal.

All agents are taken orally and should be taken with meals.

- Paricalcitol (Zemplar): IV: 2- and 5-mcg/mL vials; PO: 1-, 2-, and 4-mcg capsules
- Doxercalciferol: IV: 2-mcg/mL ampules; PO: 0.5- and 2.5-mg capsules

Calcimimetics: Cinacalcet (Sensipar)
- Approved for patients with stage 5 CKD on dialysis
- Used in conjunction with phosphate binder therapy and vitamin D
- Dose range 30-180 mg per day; initial dose is 30 mg titrated every 2-4 weeks based on iPTH levels.
- Do not start therapy if corrected serum calcium <8.4 mg/dL.

Mechanism of action
- Cinacalcet binds with the calcium-sensing receptor on the parathyroid gland and increases sensitivity of the receptor to extracellular calcium, thereby decreasing the stimulus for PTH secretion.

Patient instructions and counseling
- Cinacalcet should be taken with food or shortly after a meal.
- Tablets should be taken whole and should not be divided.

Adverse drug events
- Hypocalcemia (use with caution in patients with seizure disorder).
- Nausea and vomiting
- Diarrhea
- Myalgias

Drug-drug and drug-disease interactions
- Cinacalcet is metabolized by multiple cytochrome P450 enzymes, primarily CYP450-3A4, CYP450-2D6, and CYP450-1A2. Adjustments in dose may be required for patients taking agents that inhibit metabolism of cinacalcet (eg, ketoconazole). Dose

reductions of drugs with narrow therapeutic range with metabolism dependent on these enzymes may also be required (eg, tricyclic antidepressants, flecainide, and thioridazine).

Parameters to monitor
- Serum calcium and serum phosphorus should be measured within 1 week and iPTH should be measured 1-4 weeks after initiation or dose adjustment of cinacalcet. The dose of cinacalcet should be titrated no more frequently than every 2-4 weeks through sequential doses of 60, 90, 120, and 180 mg once daily to target iPTH (150-300 pg/mL).

Pharmacokinetics
- The maximum concentration (C_{max}) is achieved in approximately 2-6 hours following administration (increased with food).
- Half-life 30-40 hours
- Volume of distribution approximately 1000 L
- Cinacalcet is approximately 93-97% bound to plasma proteins
- Metabolized by primarily by CYP450-3A4, CYP450-2D6, and CYP450-1A2.

Strengths and dosage forms
- 30-, 60-, and 90-mg tablets

Metabolic acidosis
- Drug therapy: see chapter on critical care.

Vitamin supplementation (specific to the dialysis population)
- Water-soluble vitamins (Table 11)

Mechanism of action
- Replace water-soluble vitamins lost during dialysis without providing supratherapeutic amounts of fat-soluble vitamins.

Table 10

Vitamin D Therapy

Classification	Generic name (trade name)	Dosage range	Dosage forms	Frequency of administration
Vitamin D precursor	Ergocalciferol (Drisdol)	400-50,000 IU	PO	Daily, weekly, monthly
	Ergocalciferol (Calciferol)	400-50,000 IU	PO, IV	Daily, weekly, monthly
Active vitamin D	Calcitriol (Calcijex)	0.5-5 mcg	IV	Three times per week
	Calcitriol (Rocaltrol)	0.25-5 mcg	PO	Daily; every other day, three times per week
Vitamin D analogs	Paricalcitol (Zemplar)	1-4 mcg	PO	Daily, three times per week
		2.5-15 mcg	IV	Three times per week
	Doxercalciferol (Hectorol)	5-20 mcg	PO	Daily, three times per week
		2-8 mcg	IV	Three times per week

Patient instructions and counseling
- Take daily to replace water-soluble vitamins.
- Hemodialysis patients should take after dialysis.

Adverse drug events
- General: nausea, headache, pruritus, flushing (dependent on specific vitamin)
- Vitamin B_6 (pyridoxine): neuropathy, increased aspartate transaminase
- Vitamin C (ascorbic acid): hyperoxaluria, dizziness, diarrhea, fatigue, nausea
- Folic acid: headache, rash, pruritus

Drug-drug and drug-disease interactions
- Folic acid may decrease phenytoin concentrations by increasing metabolism.

Parameters to monitor
- Periodic folate levels

Nondrug Therapy

- Preparation for renal replacement therapy when patients reach stage 4 CKD:
    * Includes choice of chronic dialysis (hemodialysis or peritoneal dialysis) if patient is a candidate for both modalities and discussion of transplantation
    * Placement of dialysis access (fistula or graft or for hemodialysis, catheter for peritoneal dialysis)
- Patient education regarding choice of renal replacement therapy and complications of CKD

Diet
- Consider risks and benefits of protein restriction (0.6-0.8 g/kg per day) in patients with stage 3 and 4 CKD.

Table 11

Water-Soluble Vitamin Supplements for Dialysis Patients

Generic name (trade names)

Vitamin B complex, vitamin C, folic acid (Nephrocaps, Nephrovite, Nephrovite Rx, Renavite, Biotin Forte)

Vitamin B complex, vitamin C, folic acid, and iron (Nephrovite Rx + Iron, NephrPlex Rx)

Vitamin B complex (Allbee with C)

All these are taken orally, one capsule or tablet once a day.

- Increased protein requirements for patients on dialysis (approximately 1.2 g/kg per day), greater for peritoneal dialysis patients due to increased protein loss with the dialysis procedure
- Nutritional supplementation as needed
- Counseling by a renal dietitian may be beneficial to tailor diet based on the stage of CKD.

Renal replacement therapies
Hemodialysis
- Generally performed three times per week for 3-5 hours for patients with stage 5 kidney disease (end-stage renal disease)
- Requires a viable permanent access site (graft or fistula) or a temporary site for patients requiring immediate dialysis or with failed permanent access sites
- Complications (infection, hypotension during dialysis, clotting, dialyzer reactions)
- Drug removal: drug removal by hemodialysis most likely to occur for drugs with small molecular weight, low protein binding, and small volume of distribution.

Peritoneal dialysis
- Requires insertion of a catheter into the peritoneum
- CAPD: continuous ambulatory peritoneal dialysis
- CCPD: continuous cyclic peritoneal dialysis
- IPD: intermittent peritoneal dialysis
- Complications
    * Peritonitis
        - Most common gram-positive organisms are *Staphylococcus epidermidis* and *Staphylococcus aureus.*
        - Most common gram-negative organisms are *Enterobacteriacae* and *Pseudomonas aeruginosa*
        - Empiric therapy should include gram-positive coverage (first-generation cephalosporin) and gram-negative coverage (eg, ceftazidime, aminoglycoside).
        - Intraperitoneal administration of antibiotics is recommended.
    * Hyperglycemia from glucose content of dialysate solution
    * Malnutrition from increased protein loss

Transplantation
- See chapter on transplantation.

3. Key Points

Acute kidney disease

- Prevention of kidney dysfunction in high-risk patients is the most effective strategy to address AKD.
- Conditions that put patients at increased risk of AKD include decreased perfusion of the kidney (due to dehydration or poor effective circulating volume such as with CHF) and administration of potentially nephrotoxic agents, particularly under conditions of decreased perfusion.
- Nephrotoxic agents should be avoided when possible in patients at risk for AKD.
- Immediate recognition and treatment of AKD may prevent irreversible kidney damage.
- Goals of treatment for patients with AKD are achievement of baseline kidney function and prevention of chronic kidney disease and the need for chronic renal replacement therapy.
- Diuretics are first-line therapy in patients with AKD to maintain fluid balance and hemodynamic stability.
- A review of medications is frequently necessary to ensure appropriate dose adjustments based on kidney function (see appendix: drugs in renal failure).

Chronic kidney disease

- Chronic kidney disease is classified into stages 1 through 5 based on estimated glomerular filtration rate and evidence of pathological abnormalities or markers of kidney damage, including abnormalities in blood or urine tests or imaging studies.
- Screening for microalbuminuria and proteinuria is important for identifying patients with kidney disease and monitoring progression of the disease.
- Therapy to delay progression of kidney disease includes control of diabetes and hypertension, initiation of therapy with angiotensin-converting enzyme inhibitors or angiotensin receptor blockers, and protein restriction if indicated.
- Common secondary complications of CKD include anemia, fluid and electrolyte abnormalities, hyperphosphatemia, secondary hyperparathyroidism, and malnutrition.
- Management of anemia includes administration of erythropoietic agents (epoetin alfa [Epogen, Procrit] and darbepoetin alfa [Aranesp]) and iron supplementation with oral (multiple preparations) or intravenous iron (sodium ferric gluconate [Ferrlecit], iron sucrose [Venofer], or iron dextran [InFeD, Dexferrum]) to achieve target hemoglobin (11-13 g/dL), while preventing iron deficiency.
- Hyperphosphatemia is managed by dietary phosphorus restriction, use of phosphate binding agents (calcium-containing products, lanthanum carbonate [Fosrenol], or sevelemer [Renagel]), and dialysis.
- Management of secondary hyperparathyroidism includes control of serum calcium and phosphorus and administration of vitamin D therapy including vitamin D precursors in early CKD based on kidney function (ergocalciferol [Drisdol; Calciferol]) and active vitamin D therapy for more severe kidney disease (calcitriol [Calcijex, Rocaltrol], paricalcitol [Zemplar], or doxercalciferol [Hectorol]). The calcimimetic agent cinacalcet (Sensipar) is indicated for management of secondary hyperparathyroidism in patients with stage 5 CKD on dialysis and is used in conjunction with phosphate binders and vitamin D.
- Nutritional requirements must be re-evaluated based on severity of kidney disease (eg, protein restriction to delay progression of CKD versus increased protein requirements for patients on dialysis).

4. Questions and Answers

1. R.T. is a 45-year-old female admitted to the hospital after fainting while at work. Her past medical history includes type 2 diabetes and rheumatoid arthritis. Her only complaint is that she has had difficulty over the last 5 days keeping down anything she eats or drinks. She has also noticed a decrease in urination over the last 24 hours. Regular medications include aspirin 325 mg qd, celecoxib 200 mg qd for arthritis, metformin 500 mg qd, Triphasil® 1 qd, and Tylenol® prn headache. Laboratory values in the emergency department showed a serum creatinine of 2.0 mg/dL and BUN of 56 mg/dL, consistent with acute kidney disease. Her labs from 1 month ago at a regular check-up had been normal. The most likely etiology of R.T.'s acute kidney disease is:

   A. dehydration from poor oral intake
   B. trauma from fainting
   C. age-related decreases in kidney function
   D. kidney failure caused by diabetes
   E. obstruction of urine outflow

2. Which of the following medications may have contributed to R.T.'s acute renal failure?

   A. Aspirin
   B. Celecoxib
   C. Metformin
   D. Triphasil
   E. Tylenol

3. Which of the following diuretics may retain its effectiveness at glomerular filtration rates less than 30 mL/min?

   A. Hydrochlorothiazide
   B. Chlorothiazide
   C. Metolazone
   D. Spironolactone
   E. Aldactone

4. Which of the following fluid and electrolyte abnormalities typically occur in patients with severe kidney dysfunction (ie, creatinine clearance <15 mL/min)?

   I. Metabolic alkalosis
   II. Hyperkalemia
   III. Hyperphosphatemia

   A. I only
   B. III only
   C. I and II only
   D. II and III only
   E. I, II, and III

5. Which set of laboratory values is most consistent with a patient in acute intrinsic kidney disease?

   A. Urinary granular casts absent, FE_{Na} <1, urinary osmolality 600 mOsm/kg
   B. Urinary granular casts absent, FE_{Na} >1, urinary osmolality 600 mOsm/kg
   C. Urinary granular casts present, FE_{Na} <1, urinary osmolality 300 mOsm/kg
   D. Urinary granular casts present, FE_{Na} >1, urinary osmolality 300 mOsm/kg
   E. Acute intrinsic kidney failure can only be diagnosed by biopsy

6. Which of the following diuretics would be most appropriate for the initial treatment of a patient with acute kidney disease?

   I. Metolazone
   II. Spironolactone
   III. Furosemide

   A. I only
   B. III only
   C. I and II only
   D. II and III only
   E. I, II, and III

7. A patient with nephrotoxicity caused by gentamicin would likely present with an increase in serum creatinine

   A. immediately after starting therapy and nonoliguria
   B. immediately after starting therapy and oliguria
   C. 5-7 days after starting therapy and oliguria
   D. 5-7 days after starting therapy and nonoliguria
   E. within 24 hours with excessive diuresis

8. Lisinopril may cause hemodynamically-mediated kidney disease by preventing which of the following compensatory mechanisms by the kidney?

   A. Vasodilation of the afferent arteriole
   B. Vasoconstriction of the afferent arteriole
   C. Vasodilation of the efferent arteriole

D. Vasoconstriction of the efferent arteriole

E. Vasodilation of both the afferent and efferent arterioles

9. The estimated creatinine clearance for a 47-year-old male patient with an ideal body weight of 176 lb (less than actual body weight) and a serum creatinine of 2.2 mg/dL is

    A. 32 mL/min
    B. 40 mL/min
    C. 47 mL/min
    D. 93 mL/min
    E. 120 mL/min

10. D.K. is a 53-year-old black female (body weight = 65 kg) with hypertension and hypercholesterolemia who is seen in the outpatient nephrology clinic for evaluation of kidney disease progression. Her current BP is 156/82 mm Hg, SCr is 2.6 mg/dL, BUN is 44 mg/dL, and urinary protein is 800 mg/d. Her medications are enalapril 20 mg/d x 1 year and simvastatin 20 mg qd x 2 years. Based on D.K.'s estimated creatinine clearance, she would be classified in which of the following stages of chronic kidney disease (CKD)?

    A. Stage 1
    B. Stage 2
    C. Stage 3
    D. Stage 4
    E. Stage 5

11. The recommended target blood pressure for D.K. is

    A. <110/70 mm Hg
    B. <130/85 mm Hg
    C. <130/80 mm Hg
    D. <140/95 mm Hg
    E. <140/90 mm Hg

12. Which of the following would be most beneficial in a patient with type 1 diabetes and microalbuminuria to delay progression of CKD?

   I. Angiotensin-converting enzyme inhibitor
  II. Angiotensin receptor blocker
 III. Loop diuretic

    A. I only
    B. III only
    C. I and II only
    D. II and III only
    E. I, II, and III

13. Epoetin alfa and darbepoetin alfa stimulate erythropoiesis by which of the following?

    A. Preventing excessive red blood cell destruction
    B. Preventing degradation of bone marrow stem cells
    C. Differentiation of peritubular interstitial cells of the kidney
    D. Increasing the size of red blood cells produced in the bone marrow
    E. Differentiation of erythroid progenitor stem cells in the bone marrow

14. When administered intravenously, darbepoetin alfa has a terminal half-life approximately ___ that of epoetin alfa.

    A. equal to
    B. twofold longer than
    C. twofold shorter than
    D. threefold longer than
    E. threefold shorter than

15. One of the most commonly reported adverse reactions with epoetin alfa and darbepoetin alfa is

    A. Nausea
    B. Hypertension
    C. Constipation
    D. Anemia
    E. Anaphylaxis

16. At least _____ should be allowed to lapse before a change in dose of epoetin alfa or darbepoetin alfa is made based on change in hemoglobin and hematocrit.

    A. 1 week
    B. 2-4 weeks
    C. 6-8 weeks
    D. 2 months
    E. 4 months

17. R.A. is a 42-year-old 70-kg male on hemodialysis three times per week (tiw) who receives epoetin alfa for treatment of anemia. He has been stable on an epoetin dose of 4000 units intravenously tiw with an average hemoglobin of 11 g/dL (hematocrit of 33%). Over the last 3 months, his hematocrit has dropped to 28%. Iron indices reveal the following: ferritin 78 ng/mL and transferrin saturation 12%. The best initial treatment for RA is to

A. increase the dose of epoetin alfa to maintain a hemoglobin of 11-12 g/dL (hematocrit of 33-36%)

B. withhold epoetin alfa therapy until hemoglobin increases to 12 g/dL

C. administer intravenous iron (sodium ferric gluconate) at a maintenance dose of 125 mg per week

D. administer a 1-gram total dose of intravenous iron (sodium ferric gluconate or iron sucrose) divided over eight hemodialysis sessions

E. begin oral ferrous sulfate 325 mg three times per day

18. In the gastrointestinal tract, calcitriol promotes

A. absorption of calcium and inhibits absorption of phosphorus

B. absorption of phosphorus and inhibits absorption of calcium

C. absorption of both calcium and phosphorus

D. decreased binding of calcium and phosphorus

E. increased elimination of calcium and phosphorus

19. J.T. is a 63-year-old female with stage 5 CKD (end-stage kidney disease) receiving peritoneal dialysis. Her most recent laboratory analysis reveals the following: BUN 58 mg/dL, SCr 5.2 mg/dL, phosphorus 7.4 mg/dL, calcium 9.0 mg/dL, albumin 2.5 g/dL, and iPTH 542 pg/mL (normal 10-65 pg/mL). In addition to dietary restriction, which one of the following agents is best for initial management of J.T.'s hyperphosphatemia?

I. Sevelamer
II. Lanthanum carbonate
III. Calcium carbonate

A. I only
B. III only
C. I and II only
D. II and III only
E. I, II, and III

20. J.T. should be instructed to take her phosphate binder

A. with meals to enhance phosphorus absorption

B. with meals to minimize phosphorus absorption

C. between meals to avoid food-drug interactions

D. between meals to minimize GI side effects

E. There are no specific instructions to follow with regard to meals

21. Which of the following agents is appropriate for a patient with stage 5 CKD and secondary hyperparathyroidism requiring treatment to reduce iPTH?

I. Calcitriol
II. Paricalcitol
III. Ergocalciferol

A. I only
B. III only
C. I and II only
D. II and III only
E. I, II, and III

22. Cinacalcet is a calcimimetic that works by which of the following mechanisms?

A. It decreases the sensitivity of the calcium-sensing receptors on the parathyroid gland to calcium, which prevents secretion of PTH

B. It increases the sensitivity of the calcium-sensing receptors on the parathyroid gland to calcium, which prevents secretion of PTH

C. It stimulates the breakdown of intact PTH and prevents the effects of PTH on bone turnover

D. It inhibits the breakdown of intact PTH to provide a negative feedback system and suppress PTH synthesis

E. It increases calcium concentrations, which suppresses secretion of PTH from the parathyroid gland

23. A drug with which of the following characteristics is most likely to be removed by hemodialysis (f_u = fraction unbound, Vd = volume of distribution, MW = molecular weight)?

A. f_u 0.05, Vd 0.2 L/kg
B. f_u 0.05, Vd 0.6 L/kg
C. f_u 0.30, Vd 0.6 L/kg
D. f_u 0.95, Vd 0.2 L/kg
E. f_u 0.95, Vd 6 L/kg

24. The best antibiotic selection for empiric treatment of peritonitis in a peritoneal dialysis patient is:

A. cefazolin + vancomycin
B. cefazolin + ceftazidime
C. vancomycin alone

D. cefazolin alone

E. gentamicin alone

25. Which of the following supplements should be recommended daily in a patient with stage 5 CKD requiring chronic hemodialysis?

    A. Multivitamin
    B. Nephrocaps
    C. Vitamin A
    D. Nephrocaps + Vitamin A
    E. Folic acid only

Answers

1. **A.** Dehydration is the most likely cause of AKD in R.T. since she has had a decrease in oral intake over the last 5 days. This would be classified as a prerenal cause of AKD. Fainting was likely a result of dehydration and not the cause of her decline in kidney function. A serum creatinine of 2.0 mg/dL would not be considered normal in a 45 year old, eliminating age as a rationale for kidney disease. Diabetes would be more likely to cause a chronic decrease in her kidney function as opposed to an acute change (labs from 1 month ago were normal, ruling out evidence of chronic kidney disease). She has had some urine output in the last 24 hours, which rules out obstruction.

2. **B.** COX-II inhibitors are associated with hemodynamic changes (in particular they prevent the compensatory vasodilation of the afferent arteriole that occurs in conditions of prerenal acute kidney disease). Metformin is not a cause of AKD in this case, but would need to be discontinued at this time because of the risk of lactic acidosis in a patient with decreased kidney function (serum creatinine >1.4 mg/dL in females, >1.5 mg/dL in males).

3. **C.** There is some evidence that metolazone is beneficial in patients with kidney disease and a GFR <30 mL/min. This is not the case with other thiazide or thiazide-like diuretics or with potassium-sparing diuretics. Metolazone is frequently used in combination with loop diuretics for this reason.

4. **D.** Hyperkalemia and hyperphosphatemia are common electrolyte abnormalities observed as kidney function decreases. Metabolic acidosis is also common, not metabolic alkalosis.

5. **D.** Acute intrinsic kidney disease is generally characterized by the presence of granular casts (indicating structural damage), a fractional excretion of sodium greater than 1, and a urine osmolality similar to that of plasma osmolality (indicating changes in concentrating ability of the kidney).

6. **B.** A patient with acute kidney disease generally requires aggressive diuresis (while avoiding dehydration). Furosemide is a loop diuretic that is more potent than a thiazide-like diuretic (metolazone) or a potassium-sparing diuretic (spironolactone) and would be a rational choice for initial therapy of AKD.

7. **D.** Aminoglycoside-induced nephrotoxicity is characterized by a delay in changes in serum creatinine (approximately 5-7 days) and relatively normal urine output (nonoliguria).

8. **D.** Angiotensin-converting enzyme inhibitors may contribute to development of acute kidney disease in patients with conditions resulting in prerenal kidney disease (eg, conditions resulting in decreased perfusion of the kidney such as hypovolemia, heart failure, liver disease, etc). ACEIs (and angiotensin receptor blockers) prevent the compensatory vasoconstriction of the efferent arteriole mediated by angiotensin II that occurs in an attempt to increase GFR.

9. **C.** Using the Cockcroft-Gault equation to estimate creatinine clearance, this patient has an estimated creatinine clearance of 47 mL/min.

$$CrCl = \frac{(140 - age)\,(BW\ in\ kg)}{72 \times SCr\ (mg/dL)}$$

BW (kg) = 176 lbs/2.2 = 80 kg
SCr = 2.2 mg/dL

10. **D.** D.K.'s estimated creatinine clearance determined using the Cockcroft-Gault equation is 26 mL/min, classified as stage 4 CKD (GFR 15-29 mL/min).

$$CrCl = \frac{(140 - age)\,(BW\ in\ kg)}{72 \times SCr\ (mg/dL)}$$

with the result multiplied by .85 for a female. Note: The estimated GFR determined using the MDRD equation is 25 mL/min/1.73m^2.

11. **C.** The recommended BP for D.K. is <130/80 mm Hg since she has stage 4 chronic kidney disease.

12. **C.** ACEIs and angiotensin receptor blockers (ARBs) are advocated for patients with diabetes and microalbuminuria. The decreases in glomerular pressure caused by these agents that are detrimental in patients with acute kidney disease are beneficial in a chronic condition such as diabetes, in which sustained elevations in glomerular pressure result in worsening kidney disease over time.

13. **E.** Erythropoietic agents including epoetin alfa and darbepoetin alfa work in the bone marrow to stimulate differentiation of erythroid progenitor stem cells and result in an increase in red blood cell production (increase erythrocytes).

14. **D.** The half-life of darbepoetin alfa is three times longer than that of epoetin alfa, giving this agent the added benefit of reduced frequency of administration.

15. **B.** Hypertension is the most common adverse effect in patients receiving erythropoietic agents.

16. **B.** Stimulation of erythropoiesis by epoetin alfa and darbepoetin alfa occurs immediately; however, it will take at least 2-4 weeks before substantial changes in hemoglobin and hematocrit are observed as a result of any change in dose of erythropoietic therapy.

17. **D.** R.A. is iron deficient as indicated by his low serum ferritin (<100 ng/mL) and transferrin saturation (<20%). No change in epoetin alfa should be made until iron deficiency is corrected (this is the leading cause of resistance to epoetin alfa/darbepoetin alfa therapy). R.A. will require a full course of iron (1 g administered intravenously in divided doses with each dialysis session) as opposed to a maintenance dose, which should be administered once R.A. is iron replete. Sodium ferric gluconate may be administered in doses of 125 mg per dialysis session for 8 dialysis sessions to give the total 1-g dose (iron sucrose would be administered in 100-mg increments over 10 hemodialysis sessions). Absorption of oral iron is poor, making intravenous iron preferred in this hemodialysis patient.

18. **C.** Active vitamin D (calcitriol) promotes absorption of both calcium and phosphorus in the GI tract. This is one reason that therapy with calcitriol or a vitamin D analog may need to be withheld if the calcium x phosphorus product is elevated.

19. **C.** Sevelamer (Renagel) or lanthanum carbonate would better options than a calcium-containing binder for initial management since J.T. has a corrected calcium of 10.2 mg/dL [corrected calcium = measured serum calcium + 0.8 x (normal serum albumin – measured serum albumin)] and a calcium times phosphorus product of 75 mg^2/dL^2. This elevated product increases the risk of metastatic calcifications. She requires a phosphorus binding agent without calcium to minimize calcium absorbed in the GI tract.

20. **A.** Phosphate binders should be taken with meals to enhance binding in the GI tract and minimize phosphorus absorption from the GI tract into the systemic circulation.

21. **C.** Calcitriol and paricalcitol are active forms of vitamin D that do not require conversion in the liver or kidney. Ergocalciferol is a vitamin D precursor that does require activation and would not be recommended for a patient with stage 5 CKD without the necessary activity of the enzyme in the kidney (1α-hydroxylase) responsible for final conversion to the active form.

22. **B.** The calcimimetic agent cinacalcet (Sensipar) works by binding with the calcium-sensing receptor on the parathyroid gland and increases the sensitivity of this receptor to calcium, thereby suppressing secretion of PTH.

23. **D.** Drug characteristics that make an agent more likely to be removed by dialysis include low protein binding, small volume of distribution, and low molecular weight. Among the choices the agent that best meets these criteria is choice D, which has a high fraction unbound in the plasma and a low volume of distribution.

24. **B.** Empiric therapy should include antibiotics with gram-positive and gram-negative coverage. Choice B is most appropriate.

25. **B.** Nephrocaps include water-soluble vitamins (vitamin B complex + vitamin C + folic acid) recommended for a patient with kidney failure. Supplementation with fat-soluble vitamins is not recommended in patients with kidney failure due to toxicities associated with accumulation.

5. References

Acute renal failure and drug-induced kidney disease

Hock R, Anderson RJ. Prevention of drug-induced nephrotoxicity in the intensive care unit. *J Crit Care.* 1995;10:33-43.

Lameire N, Van Viesen W, Vanholder R. Acute renal failure. *Lancet.* 2005;365(9457):417-430.

Nolin TD, Himmelfarb J, Matzke GR. Drug-induced renal disease. In: DiPiro J, et al. eds. *Pharmacotherapy: A Pathophysiologic Approach.* 6th ed. New York: McGraw-Hill; 2005:871-890.

Wood AJJ. Diuretic therapy. *N Engl J Med.* 1998; 339:387-395.

Chronic kidney disease and progression

Abosaif NY, et al. K/DOQI clinical practice guidelines on hypertension and antihypertensive agents in chronic kidney disease. *Am J Kidney Dis.* 2004;43 (Suppl 1):S1–290.

Chobanian AV, et al and the National High Blood Pressure Education Program Coordinating committee. The Seventh Report of the Joint National Committee on Prevention, Detection, Evaluation, and Treatment of High Blood Pressure: the JNC 7 report. *JAMA.* 2003;289:2560-2572.

National Kidney Foundation. NKF-K/DOQI Clinical Practice Guidelines for Chronic Kidney Disease: Evaluation, Classification, and Stratification. *Am J Kidney Dis.* 2002;39:S1-S266.

National Kidney Foundation Task Force on CVD Report. *Am J Kidney Disease.* 1998;32:853-906.

U.S. Renal Data System, USRDS 2004 Annual Data Report; Atlas of End-Stage Renal Disease in the United States. National Institutes of Health, National Institute of Diabetes and Digestive and Kidney Diseases, Bethesda, MD: 2004.

Anemia

American Reagent Laboratories, Inc. Venofer (iron sucrose injection) package insert. Shirley, NY: American Reagent Laboratories, Inc., 2005.

Amgen Inc. Aranesp (darbepoetin alfa) package insert. Thousand Oaks, CA: Amgen Inc, 2003.

K/DOQI Clinical Practice Guidelines and Clinical Practice Recommendations for Anemia in Chronic Kidney Disease. *Am J Kidney Dis.* 2006 May;47(5 Suppl 3):S1-145.

Macdougall IC, Gray SJ, Elston O, et al. Pharmacokinetics of novel erythropoiesis stimulating protein compared with epoetin alfa in dialysis patients. *J Am Soc Nehrol.* 1999;10:2392-2395.

National Kidney Foundation. K/DOQI Clinical Practice Guidelines for Anemia of Chronic Kidney Disease. Update 2000. *Am J Kidney Dis.* 2001; 37(Suppl 1): S182-238 [erratum in *Am J Kidney Dis.* 2001;38:442].

Watson Pharmaceuticals, Inc. Ferrlecit (sodium ferric gluconate complex in sucrose injection) package insert. Corona, CA: Watson Pharmaceuticals, Inc., 2004.

Hyperphosphatemia and secondary hyperparathyroidism

Chertow GM, Dillon M, Burke SK, et al. A randomized trial of sevelamer hydrochloride (Renagel) with and without supplemental calcium. Strategies for the control of hyperphosphatemia and hyperparathyroidism in hemodialysis patients. *Clin Nephrol.* 1999;51:18-26.

Eknoyan G, Levin A, Levin NW. Bone metabolism and disease in chronic kidney disease. *Am J Kidney Dis.* 2003;42(4 Suppl 3):1-201.

Sensipar (cinacalcet HCl) tablets package insert. Thousand Oaks, CA: Amgen Inc., 2004.

Yudd M, Llach F. Current medical management of secondary hyperparathyroidism. *Am J Med Sci.* 2000; 320:100-106.

Nutrition

National Kidney Foundation. K/DOQI Clinical Practice Guidelines for Nutrition in Chronic Renal Failure. *Am J Kidney Dis.* 2000;35(suppl 2):S1-S140.

Other

Aronoff GR, Bennett WM, Berns JS, et al. *Drug Prescribing in Renal Failure: Dosing Guidelines for Adults,* 4th ed. American College of Physicians: 1999.

Ifudu O. Care of patients undergoing hemodialysis. *N Engl J Med.* 1998;339:1054-1062.

National Kidney Foundation. Kidney Disease Outcomes Quality Initiative. Clinical practice guidelines for peritoneal dialysis adequacy: update 2000. Available at http://www.kidney.org/professionals/doqi/ guidelines/doqi_uptoc.html#pd

17. Critical Care, Fluids, and Electrolytes

G. Christopher Wood, PharmD, BCPS
Associate Professor, Department of Clinical Pharmacy
University of Tennessee College of Pharmacy

Contents

1. Sedation, Analgesia, and Neuromuscular Blockade

Overview

Definition and classifications
- Pain: critically ill patients may experience acute and/or chronic pain.
- Anxiety/agitation: psychophysiologic response to real or imagined danger ("agitation" for the rest of the chapter)
- ICU delirium ("delirium" for the rest of the chapter): see clinical presentation

Clinical presentation
- Pain/agitation in patients with impaired consciousness:
  * Pulling tubes/lines, writhing, kicking, restlessness, hypertension, tachycardia, tachypnea, diaphoresis, moaning
- Delirium: fluctuating, disorganized thinking or inattentiveness not due to an obviously reversible cause; with or without agitation

Pathophysiology
- Injuries
- Medical procedures/equipment (eg, mechanical ventilation, catheters)
- Mental status changes (eg, fear, infection, hypoxia, sleep deprivation, adverse drug effects/withdrawal)
- Preexisting medical conditions (eg, chronic pain)

Diagnostic criteria
- Pain: use a verbal or visual scale to assess severity.
  * For unconscious patients, use physical signs and symptoms.
- Agitation: use a validated scale to assess (eg, Riker sedation-agitation scale)
- Delirium: use Confusion Assessment Method for the ICU (CAM-ICU) scale

Treatment goals
- Find and remove the cause of pain, agitation, and delirium.
- Achieve a balance between patient comfort, adverse effects, and ability to provide care.
- Reserve neuromuscular blocking agents (NMBs) for patients who are not controlled with maximum doses of sedation and analgesia.

Mechanism of action (Table 1)
- Opiates, NSAIDs: see chapter on pain management.
- Benzodiazepines, haloperidol: see chapter on psychiatric disease.
- Propofol: unknown, possible GABA-related activity

- NMBs: postsynaptic cholinergic receptor antagonists; they do not provide analgesia or sedation.

Patient instructions
- Patient-controlled analgesia (PCA) pumps; make sure the patient understands how to activate the device.

Adverse drug events
- Opiates, NSAIDs: see chapter on pain management.
- Benzodiazepines, haloperidol: see chapter on psychiatric disease.
- Propofol: respiratory depression, hypotension, hypertriglyceridemia; max. dose 5 mg/kg/h
- Neuromuscular blockers: respiratory depression, prolonged weakness/paralysis after discontinuation, tachycardia with pancuronium

Drug interactions
- Opiates, NSAIDs: see chapter on pain management.
- Benzodiazepines, haloperidol: see chapter on psychiatric disease.
- Propofol: actions potentiated by other sedatives
- Neuromuscular blockers: actions potentiated by corticosteroids, aminoglycosides, clindamycin, calcium channel blockers, anesthetics; actions inhibited by anticholinesterase inhibitors (eg, neostigmine)

Parameters to monitor
- Opiates, NSAIDs: use visual or verbal scale to assess efficacy; also monitor HR, BP, RR (also see chapter on pain management).
- Benzodiazepines, haloperidol: use validated scale; also monitor HR, BP, RR (also see chapter on psychiatric disease).
- Propofol: use validated scale; also monitor BP, HR, RR, ICP, and serum triglycerides at baseline and 1-2 times a week during long-term use.
- Neuromuscular blockers: movement/spontaneous breathing; also monitor BP, HR, ICP (acute increases may indicate suboptimal sedation/analgesia).
  * Peripheral nerve stimulation monitoring ("train of four") highly recommended.
- In patients with continuous sedation, a daily wakening and assessment period results in decreased sedative use and ICU length of stay.

Kinetics
- Opiates, NSAIDs: see chapter on pain management.
- Benzodiazepines, haloperidol: see chapter on psychiatric disease.
- Propofol: highly lipophilic (may accumulate long term), rapid onset (1 min), short duration (~10 min)
- Neuromuscular blockers:
  * Onset for all <5 min

Table 1

Select Drug Therapy Based on Guidelines for Use in ICU Patients

Generic (trade) name	Dosage range	Forms[1]	Schedule[2]	Notes on usage
Morphine sulfate (generic)	0.5-10 mg	IV, IM, PO	Continuous; q6h	General opiate of choice
Hydromorphone (Dilaudid®)	0.3-1.5 mg	IV	Continuous; q6h	Use in morphine intolerance, hemodynamic instability, or renal dysfunction
Fentanyl (Sublimaze®)	50-200 mcg/h	IV	Continuous	Same as hydromorphone
Acetaminophen (Tylenol®)	Up to 4 g/d	PO, PR	q4-6h	NSAIDs may be added to opiates
Ketorolac (Toradol®)	10-30 mg	IV, IM, PO	q6h	Maximum use 5 days
Lorazepam (Ativan®)	0.5-4 mg	IV, PO	Continuous; q6h	Long-term sedation (>24-72 h)
Midazolam (Versed®)	1-5 mg	IV	Continuous; q2h	Acute and short term (<24-72 h)
Propofol (Diprivan®)	1-8 mg/kg/h	IV	Continuous	Use when rapid awakening needed
Haloperidol (Haldol®)	2-5 mg	IV, PO	q1-4h	Drug of choice for delirium
Pancuronium (Pavulon®)	0.05-0.1 mg/kg	IV	Continuous; q2h	General NMB of choice (low cost); causes tachycardia
Vecuronium (Norcuron®)	0.05-0.1 mg/kg	IV	Continuous; q1h	Use in hemodynamic instability, renal dysfunction, cardiac disease
Cisatracurium (Nimbex®)	0.05-0.1 mg/kg	IV	Continuous; q1h	Use in renal and hepatic dysfunction

[1]Long-acting drugs and dosage forms generally not used in ICU (eg, fentanyl patch, controlled-release morphine, doxacurium).

[2]Continuous analgesia and sedation with frequent titration (PCA pump, IV infusion, or scheduled) preferred to prn therapy alone. NMBs used prn are preferred.

* Duration: pancuronium, 60-90 min; vecuronium, cisatracurium, 30-60 min
* Excretion: pancuronium, mostly renal; vecuronium, ~50:50 hepatic:renal; cisatracurium, not organ dependent

Other
- Propofol is in a lipid vehicle (provides 1 kcal/mL; use with caution in egg allergy)
  * Potential growth medium for bacteria; 12-hour maximum hang time for a bottle
- *New agent:* dexmedetomidine (Precedex®)
  * Central α_2 agonist indicated for sedation <24 h (continuous IV infusion)
  * Potential advantage: less respiratory depression than other agents
  * Adverse events: hypotension, bradycardia

2. Traumatic Brain Injury

Overview

Definition
- Neurologic deficit secondary to brain trauma

Classifications
- Severe
- Mild/moderate

Clinical presentation
- Use Glasgow Coma Scale (GCS) for assessment; sum of eye, motor, and verbal scores (range 3-15).
- Wide range of presentation from mild confusion to totally nonresponsive coma

Pathophysiology
- Motor vehicle accidents (most common), falls/accidents, assaults, gunshot wounds
- Most common in 15- to 24-year age group; 375,000 cases and 75,000 deaths per year
- Consists of direct neuronal damage ± edema ± secondary ischemia-related neuronal death

Diagnostic criteria
- CT scan
- GCS
- Intracranial pressure (ICP) monitoring in severe patients (GCS score 3-8)

Treatment goals
- Improved outcomes with cerebral perfusion pressure (CPP) >60 mm Hg and ICP <20 mm Hg (CPP = mean arterial pressure – ICP)
- Seizure prevention

Strategies to decrease ICP
- Osmotic agents/diuretics
    * Mannitol 0.25-1 g/kg IV q4h
    * Loop diuretics IV (eg, furosemide)
    * Hypertonic NaCl IV (eg, 3%, 7.5%)
- Sedation: short-acting agent preferred to allow frequent patient assessment (eg, propofol, fentanyl)
    * Pentobarbital 1-3 mg/kg/h IV: long-acting agent for refractory intracranial hypertension
- NMBs: short-acting agent preferred (vecuronium); used for refractory intracranial hypertension

Nondrug interventions
- Raise the head of the bed 30°.
- Ventricular drainage of CSF via ventriculostomy
- Mild/moderate hyperventilation (pCO_2 30-35 mm Hg)
- Surgery

Strategies to increase MAP
- Maximize fluid status; overall goal is euvolemia.
- Vasopressors/inotropes may be used in shock after fluid status is optimized.

Seizure prevention (may be started based on severity and type of injury)
- Phenytoin (Dilantin®, generic) 20 mg/kg IV loading dose + 4-8 mg/kg/d for 7 days
    * Continue beyond 7 days if the patient has a seizure.
    * Alternative agent: carbamazepine
- See chapter on epilepsy for mechanism of action, adverse drug events, drug interactions, and kinetics.

Parameters to monitor
- Overall goal of CPP >60 mm Hg and ICP <20 mm Hg; drug classes are covered elsewhere.

Other
- Nimodipine (Nimotop®): calcium channel blocker given for 21 days; indicated for treating aneurysmal subarachnoid hemorrhage; may also provide some benefit in traumatic subarachnoid hemorrhage

3. Acute Spinal Cord Injury

Overview

Definition
- Traumatic spinal cord injury with neurologic impairment

Classifications
- Complete: total loss of motor and sensory function in affected areas
- Incomplete: some motor and/or sensory function retained in affected areas
- Paraplegia: neurologic deficit in the lower extremities
- Quadriplegia: neurologic deficit in the upper and lower extremities
- Central cord syndrome: atypical symptoms

Clinical presentation
- Loss of motor and/or sensory function from nerves distal to level of vertebral injury
- Symptoms are usually bilaterally symmetrical.

Pathophysiology
- See traumatic brain injury

Diagnostic criteria
- Physical examination consistent with SCI plus CT and/or radiographic evidence of injury

Treatment goals
- Preservation/restoration of motor and sensory function

Drug therapy
- Methylprednisolone: 30 mg/kg IV loading dose, then 5.4 mg/kg/h IV infusion:
    * Continued for a total of 24 hours if loading dose given within 3 hours of injury
    * Continued for a total of 48 hours if loading dose is given 3-8 hours from injury
- No methylprednisolone if >8 hours from injury or for penetrating injuries.

Mechanism of action
- Unknown; thought to protect neurons by inhibiting lipid peroxidation

Adverse drug effects
- Increased infections (48 h worse than 24 h)
- Hyperglycemia

Parameters to monitor
- Neurologic status
- Serum glucose

4. Venous Thromboembolism Prophylaxis

Overview

Definition
- Venous thromboembolism (VTE): pathogenic blood clot formation

Classifications
- Deep venous thrombosis (DVT): VTE in a large vein, generally in a lower extremity
- Pulmonary embolism (PE): DVT that has embolized to the pulmonary vasculature (much less common)

Clinical presentations
- DVT: often asymptomatic
    * Unilateral leg symptoms: swelling, pain, tenderness, erythema, warmth, ± palpable cord
    * Pain behind the knee upon dorsiflexion (Homans' sign)
- PE: often asymptomatic
    * Pulmonary symptoms: chest pain, cough, dyspnea, tachypnea, hemoptysis
    * May proceed rapidly to life-threatening shock and hypoxia

Pathophysiology
Three general risk factors
- Hypercoagulable states
    * Clotting factor deficiencies/abnormalities (eg, protein C or S deficiency)
    * Malignancy, pregnancy, estrogen use
- Direct vessel trauma
- Venous stasis: poor blood flow allows clot formation

Specific risk factors
- Age: risk increases with age (Table 2)
- Immobility, previous VTE, cancer, obesity, CHF, pregnancy, estrogen therapy, smoking
- Major surgery or trauma: worse in lower extremity, pelvis; GU, neurologic injury

Epidemiology
- ~600,000 hospitalizations in the U.S. yearly with ~60,000 deaths (10% mortality)
- Incidence of DVT ranges from 2-80% depending on risk factors.

Diagnostic criteria
- Radiocontrast dye studies (venography for DVT, pulmonary angiography for PE)
    * Invasive, expensive, requires expertise, adverse events common (eg, nephropathy)
* Ventilation/perfusion scan (for PE): less invasive, but inconclusive results are common.

Table 2

Drug and Nondrug Therapy for Prevention of Venous Thromboembolism

Patient group	Recommended therapy
Medical conditions	
General medical patient with risk factor	LDUH or LMWH; alternatives: IPC, ES
Acute MI	LDUH or full dose IV heparin
Ischemic stroke	LDUH or LMWH; alternatives: IPC, ES
General surgery: begin preoperatively, generally continue until ambulatory or discharged	
Low risk	
Minor procedure without risk factors	Early ambulation
Moderate to high risk	
Minor procedure + risk factor or >40 years old; major procedure	LDUH or LMWH; alternatives: IPC, ES
Highest risk	
Major procedure + multiple risk factors or >40 years old; minor procedure + multiple risk factors or >60 years old	LDUH or LMWH + IPC and/or ES (combine drug + mechanical)
Orthopedic surgery or trauma (recommended duration if available)	
Hip replacement (28-35 d)	LMWH or fondaparinux or warfarin (INR 2-3) ± IPC or ES
Knee replacement (minimum 10 d); hip fracture (28-35 d)	LMWH or fondaparinux or warfarin (INR 2-3); alternative: IPC
Neurosurgery	IPC ± ES; add LDUH or LMWH when bleeding is stopped
Major trauma (until discharge)	LMWH; alternative: IPC ± ES if bleeding risk; may use warfarin (INR 2-3) during rehabilitation if major impairment
Acute spinal cord injury (throughout rehabilitation)	LMWH ± IPC, ES; convert to warfarin (INR 2-3) in rehabilitation

ES, elastic compression stockings (may add to efficacy of drugs); IPC, intermittent pneumatic compression (may add to efficacy of drugs but noncompliance is high); LDUH, low-dose unfractionated heparin (generic) dosing: 5000 units SC q8-12h.
Low molecular weight heparin (LMWH) dosing:
   Dalteparin (Fragmin®): 2500-5000 units SC qd; enoxaparin (Lovenox®): 30 mg SC q12h or 30-40 mg SC qd.

Fondaparinux (Arixtra®) dosing: 2.5 mg SC qd.
Major trauma: start within 36 h of injury; routine vena cava filter placement not recommended.

- Ultrasonography (for DVT)
  * Noninvasive, inexpensive, performed at the bedside, but less sensitive
- Serum D-dimer concentrations: normal levels may rule out VTE

Treatment goals
- Decrease morbidity (VTE recurrence, progression to PE), mortality, and costs of VTE
- VTE prophylaxis is underused: only 35-50% of at-risk patients receive it.

Drug Therapy to Treat Venous Thromboembolism

- Full-dose IV heparin (80 U/kg load + 18 U/kg/h) or full-dose low molecular weight heparin (LMWH) SC (eg, enoxaparin 1 mg/kg q12h or 1.5 mg/kg qd)
  * LMWH may be used outpatient in stable DVT patients.
  * May give full-dose heparin SC bid (rarely done)
- Warfarin: begin concurrently, discontinue heparin/LMWH when the INR is therapeutic (usually 2-3) and stable.

* Duration: reversible risk factor - 3 months; idiopathic - 6-12 months (consider longer); high risk - 12 months to indefinite
* Direct thrombin inhibitors: use in place of heparin for heparin-induced thrombocytopenia
* Thrombolytic therapy: reserve for very severe cases; highly individualized
* Inferior vena cava filter: reserve for select patients with contraindication to anticoagulation

Drug Therapy to Prevent Venous Thromboembolism (Table 2)

Mechanism of action
* Heparin: binds to antithrombin and potentiates its anticoagulation (anti IIa activity > anti Xa)
* LMWHs: same as heparin but anti Xa activity > anti IIa
    * There is some controversy over the interchangeability of these drugs because of differences in Xa:IIa activity ratios.
* Fondaparinux: factor Xa inhibitor
* Warfarin: see chapter on arrhythmias
* Direct thrombin inhibitors (lepirudin [Refludan®], bivalirudin [Angiomax®], argatroban): directly inhibit thrombin

Patient instructions and counseling
* Heparin, fondaparinux, thrombin inhibitors, thrombolytics: not applicable
* LMWHs, fondaparinux: patients can be taught to self-inject after hospital discharge
    * Monitor for signs and symptoms of bleeding or VTE recurrence.
    * Avoid NSAIDs
* Warfarin: see chapter on arrhythmias.

Adverse drug events
* Bleeding: all agents
    * Low-dose unfractionated heparin (LDUH) and low-dose LMWH have similar bleeding risks
    * Protamine sulfate reverses heparin, LMWH
* Thrombocytopenia (heparin-induced thrombocytopenia [HIT]): heparin, LMWH
    * Early: occurs about in first week; transient; no therapy needed
    * Late: immune mediated; if severe must discontinue heparin/LMWH; less frequent with LMWH
        * Switch to direct thrombin inhibitor
        * May result in severe thrombosis/limb amputation
        * May happen immediately upon rechallenge with heparin or LMWH

* Spinal hematoma with epidural catheters: LMWH or full anticoagulation worse than LDUH; do not use LMWH
* Osteoporosis: heparin worse than LMWH; occurs with long-term therapy
* Hypersensitivity (reexposure): lepirudin

Drug interactions
* NSAIDs may increase bleeding risk with all agents.
* Warfarin: see chapter on arrhythmias.

Parameters to monitor
* Heparin (full-dose IV) and thrombin inhibitors:
    * Goal PTT that corresponds to an anti Xa level of 0.3-0.7 IU/mL (check with each lab for therapeutic range); monitor q6h until therapeutic; then once or twice daily
    * LDUH doesn't affect PTT
* LMWHs: anti Xa levels (goal 0.6-1 units/mL)
    * No routine monitoring; may monitor in renal impairment, obesity, prolonged use, pregnancy
* Fondaparinux: no monitoring; affects anti Xa levels
* Direct thrombin inhibitors:
    * Argatroban: goal PTT 1.5-3 times control; falsely elevates INR
    * Bivalirudin: no recommendations in HIT; elevates PTT and INR
    * Lepirudin: goal PTT 1.5-2.5 times control
* Warfarin: see chapter on arrhythmias

Kinetics
* Heparin: cleared by endothelial cell enzymes ($t_{1/2}$ ~90 min); higher doses also renally cleared
* LMWHs: renally cleared; $t_{1/2}$ 2-4 times longer than heparin
* Fondaparinux: renally cleared; longer $t_{1/2}$ (~24 h)
* Direct thrombin inhibitors: $t_{1/2}$ 30-90 min; lepirudin renally cleared; others hepatically cleared

5. Stress Ulcer Prophylaxis

Overview

Definition and classifications
- GI mucosal damage related to metabolic stress in the ICU

Clinical presentation
- Similar to peptic ulcer disease (see chapter on gastrointestinal disorders).

Pathophysiology
- Shunting of blood from the GI tract to vital organs during critical illness results in breakdown of gastric mucosal defenses (eg, bicarbonate production, epithelial cell turnover)

Risk factors
- Mechanical ventilation >48 h
- Coagulopathy
- Other disease states/organ dysfunction where GI perfusion may be compromised (eg, sepsis, burns, traumatic brain injury)

Diagnostic criteria
- Based on signs/symptoms; diagnosis can be confirmed with endoscopy.

Treatment goals
- Prevent stress ulcers

Drug Therapy

- See the chapter on gastrointestinal disorders for full drug information.
- Histamine$_2$ (H$_2$) antagonists or sucralfate are traditional standards of therapy; H$_2$ antagonists may be more effective.
    * Sucralfate administration can be difficult in ICU patients.
- Proton pump inhibitors: equivalent to H$_2$ antagonists
- Optimal duration of therapy is unknown (usually until risk factors have resolved or transfer from ICU).
- Antacids: less effective; not recommended; higher aspiration risk; require frequent dosing

6. Severe Sepsis and Septic Shock

Overview

Definition
- Severe sepsis is sepsis (see chapter on infectious diseases) plus dysfunction of one or more major organs (eg, hypotension responsive to fluids, oliguria, acute mental status change, lactic acidosis, respiratory insufficiency, coagulopathy).
- Septic shock is severe sepsis plus hypotension that is not fully responsive to fluids (ie, requires vasopressor therapy).

Classifications
- Severe sepsis
- Septic shock

Clinical presentation
- See sepsis criteria (see chapter on infectious diseases) and definitions above.

Pathophysiology
- Progression of the systemic manifestations of sepsis; imbalances in the inflammatory, immune, and coagulation systems lead to organ hypoperfusion and organ dysfunction with or without refractory hypotension.
- Causative organisms vary by institution, but broad patterns are known:
    * Common community-acquired organisms include *Streptococcus pneumoniae, Staphylococcus aureus, Haemophilus influenzae, Escherichia coli*, and "atypicals" (*Mycoplasma pneumoniae, Chlamydia pneumoniae, Legionella* spp.)
    * Common nosocomial/health care-associated organisms include *Pseudomonas aeruginosa, S aureus* (methicillin resistance more common), *Enterobacter* spp., *Klebsiella* spp., *Proteus* spp., *Citrobacter* spp., *Serratia* spp., and *Candida* spp.

Diagnostic criteria
- See sepsis criteria (see chapter on infectious diseases) and definitions above.

Treatment goals
- Rapid stabilization of hemodynamic parameters and organ dysfunction within 6 hours
- Identification of causative organism(s), starting appropriate antimicrobial therapy within 1 hour, and elimination of the source of infection if applicable (eg, vascular or urinary catheter, abscess); duration of antimicrobial therapy is typically 7-14 days.

- Modulation of inflammatory, coagulating, and hormonal derangements if applicable

Drug and Nondrug Therapy

- See chapter on infectious diseases for antimicrobial information (mechanism of action, dosing, adverse effects, etc).
- Empiric antimicrobial selection is also covered in the chapter on infectious diseases; definitive therapy should be streamlined to a narrower-spectrum agent if possible, based on the final culture and sensitivity reports.
- See section on fluid and electrolytes for details on fluid therapy; fluid therapy for severe sepsis and septic shock can be colloids and/or isotonic crystalloids; vasopressors should only be used after appropriate fluid therapy fails to adequately normalize BP (Table 3).

Mechanism of action

- Vasopressors/inotropes: adrenergic receptor agonists
- Drotrecogin alfa: recombinant human activated protein C (an endogenous anticoagulant); the exact MOA is unknown; modulates coagulation and inflammatory cascades

Adverse drug events

- Vasopressors/inotropes: tachycardia, arrhythmias, organ and extremity ischemia, hypertension
- Drotrecogin alfa: bleeding
    * Contraindicated in active internal bleeding, recent trauma, stroke, or other clinical condition at high bleeding risk, presence of epidural catheter

Drug-drug interactions

- Vasopressors/inotropes: none
- Drotrecogin alfa: increased bleeding risk with concomitant anticoagulation or antiplatelet therapy

Parameters to monitor

- Vasopressors/inotropes: BP, HR, cardiac output, urine output, extremity perfusion on physical exam
- Drotrecogin alfa:
    * Signs and symptoms of bleeding on physical exam, BP, HR
    * Improvement in signs and symptoms of infection; temperature, WBC, organ dysfunction
    * May prolong aPTT

Kinetics

- Drotrecogin alfa: dose adjustment is not required in renal or hepatic dysfunction.

Table 3

Vasopressors and Inotropes Used in Severe Sepsis and Septic Shock

Name	Dosage range	Adrenergic receptor activity	Comments
Dopamine	<5 mcg/kg/min	Increased renal perfusion (dopaminergic receptors)	Preferred agent; use of low-dose "renal tonic" dopamine is not recommended
	5-10 mcg/kg/min	Increased CO/HR (β_1) > increased BP (α_1)	
	10-20 mcg/kg/min	Increased CO/HR and BP	
Norepinephrine	0.01-3 mcg/kg/min	Increased BP (α_1) > increased CO/HR (β_1)	Preferred agent
Epinephrine	0.01-0.5 mcg/kg/min	Increased CO/HR and BP (all receptors)	Second-line agent (due to tachycardia, gut ischemia)
Phenylephrine	0.01-5 mcg/kg/min	Increased BP only (α_1)	
Dobutamine	5-20 mcg/kg/min	Increased CO/HR (β_1)	

Immunomodulator used in severe sepsis and septic shock

Drotrecogin alfa (Xigris®)	Dosing regimen: 24 mcg/kg/h x 96 h IV infusion		Add to antimicrobial therapy within 48 h of onset of severe sepsis; decreases mortality; limit use to highly severe illness (ie, APACHE II score >25); monitor for bleeding; very expensive but likely cost effective

APACHE, Acute Physiology, Age, and Chronic Health Evaluation.
Note: All vasoactive agents are given as continuous IV infusions and are titrated to effect.

Other

- Low-dose hydrocortisone (200-300 mg x 7 days ± fludrocortisone 50 mcg/d) is recommended for patients with septic shock based on mortality reduction in a recent trial; patients with a poor response to cosyntropin stimulation testing (serum cortisol increase of <9 mcg/dL) respond better to corticosteroid supplementation.
- Vasopressin infusion (0.01-0.04 U/min) may be used to increase BP in patients refractory to high doses of traditional pressors; doses >0.04 U/min are associated with severe adverse events (eg, cardiac arrest).

7. Fluid and Electrolyte Abnormalities in Critically Ill Patients

(See chapter on nutrition; chapter on renal disorders for hyperphosphatemia; and chapter on oncology for hypercalcemia.)

Overview

Definition
- Pathologic alterations in fluid and electrolyte homeostasis

Classifications
- Classified by electrolyte (see below)

Clinical presentation
- *FOR ALL:* Mild to moderate abnormalities are usually asymptomatic.

Sodium (normal range: 135-145 mEq/L)
- Hyponatremia or hypernatremia: lethargy, nausea, headache, dry mucous membranes, poor skin turgor (depends on hydration status), confusion
- Coma, seizures, or central pontine myelinolysis may occur in severe hyponatremia or if sodium increases or decreases rapidly (>12 mEq/L/d)

Chloride (normal range: 96-106 mEq/L)
- Symptoms are related to acid-base or fluid abnormalities, not chloride itself.

Water (moves osmotically with sodium)
- Dehydration: dry mucous membranes, poor skin turgor, lethargy, nausea, headache, hypotension, tachycardia, seizures/coma/death if severe, decreased urine output, metabolic acidosis, hypotension, tachycardia
- Edema/fluid overload: see chapter on heart failure.

Potassium (normal range: 3.5-5.0 mEq/L)
- Hypokalemia: confusion, muscle cramps, weakness, cardiac arrhythmias
- Hyperkalemia: muscle cramps, weakness, cardiac arrhythmias

Magnesium (normal range: 1.5-2.2 mEq/L)
- Hypomagnesemia: similar to hypocalcemia
- Hypermagnesemia: lethargy, weakness, cardiac arrhythmias, coma if severe

Phosphorus (normal range: 2.6-4.5 mg/dL)
- Hypophosphatemia: confusion, anxiety, weakness, respiratory depression, paresthesias, lethargy; seizures and coma if severe

- Hyperphosphatemia: see chapter on kidney disorders.

Calcium (normal range: 8.5-10.5 mg/dL)
- Hypocalcemia: confusion, anxiety, paresthesias, muscle cramps, tetany; coma and cardiac arrhythmias if severe
- Hypercalcemia: see chapter on oncology.

Pathophysiology
Normal distribution of fluids and electrolytes
- Electrolytes with high serum concentrations are primarily extracellular (Na, Cl); those with low serum concentrations are mostly intracellular or in bone (K, P, Mg, Ca)
- Total body water is ~60-70% of total body weight (differs by age, gender, disease states).
    * Of all water: intracellular ~$2/_3$, extracellular ~$1/_3$
    * Of extracellular: ~$3/_4$ is interstitial and ~$1/_4$ is intravascular (plasma)
- Fluid requirements: typical requirements for adults ~35 mL/kg/d, can be much higher in critical illness due to extrarenal losses (GI tract, wounds) and fluid shifts (trauma, sepsis).
- Primary hormonal controls: aldosterone (Na retention), antidiuretic hormone (water retention)

Hyponatremia (the first three below are hypotonic)
- Hypovolemic (high urine osmolality): Na and water loss
    * Extrarenal fluid losses (GI, wounds), diuretics, adrenal insufficiency
- Euvolemic: moderate water retention
    * SIADH, renal failure, carbamazepine, NSAIDs, chlorpropamide
- Hypervolemic: Na and water retention
    * CHF, cirrhosis, nephrotic syndrome, glucocorticoids
- Hypertonic: dilutional effect of abnormal osmotic agents in the vasculature (severe hyperglycemia)

Hypernatremia: water loss or excessive Na intake (eg, from IV fluids)
- Extrarenal fluid losses (GI, wounds), diabetes insipidus

Hypochloremia
- GI losses

Hypokalemia
- Diuretics, β_2 agonists, amphotericin B, glucocorticoids, cisplatin, GI losses

Hyperkalemia
- Renal dysfunction, acidosis, ACE inhibitors, K-sparing diuretics, trimethoprim, PO salt substitutes, adrenal insufficiency

Hypomagnesemia
- GI losses, diuretics, amphotericin B, alcohol, cisplatin
    * Treat prior to treating hypokalemia; Na-K-ATPase pumps require Mg to work.

Hypermagnesemia
- Renal dysfunction, Mg-containing antacids, adrenal insufficiency, hyperparathyroidism

Hypophosphatemia
- Refeeding syndrome, phosphate binders, diuretics, hypercalcemia, vitamin D deficiency, glucocorticoids

Hypocalcemia
- Hypoparathyroidism, hypomagnesemia, vitamin D deficiency, loop diuretics
    * Total Ca artificially low in hypoalbuminemia (Ca is highly albumin bound)

Diagnostic criteria
- Serum concentration, signs, and symptoms
- Sodium analysis may use urine Na, urine osmolality

Treatment goals
- Find and treat the underlying cause of abnormality.
- Treat abnormality to avoid sequelae.

Drug and Nondrug Therapy

Fluid replacement
- Crystalloids: salt solutions—$1/_2$ or $1/_4$ NS ± dextrose 5% ± KCl 20 mEq/L (approximates urine electrolytes), NS (154 mEq/L of Na), lactated Ringer's, $1/_4$ NS, or D_5W chosen based on Na and fluid needs; NS or LR typically used for fluid resuscitation (Na is the major osmotic cation in plasma).
- Colloids: osmotic agents—albumin 5-25%, hetastarch, used for fluid resuscitation or to raise oncotic pressure (eg, cirrhosis)
- Vasopressors ± isotropic activity may be used after fluids are optimized (see chapter on heart failure).

Edema
- Fluid restriction ± diuretics (see chapters on heart failure and kidney disorders).

Hyponatremia
- If severe, titrate 3% NaCl to maximum serum Na increase of 12 mEq/d.

* Hypovolemic: replace fluid losses with IV NS (0.9% NaCl, 154 mEq/L)
* Euvolemic (SIADH): fluid restriction ± demeclocycline
* Hypervolemic: fluid restriction ± diuretics
* Hypertonic: correct hyperglycemia

Hypernatremia

* Titrate low Na fluids (eg, D_5W, $^1/_4$ NS) to a normal serum Na
    * Diabetes insipidus: use DDAVP

Hyperchloremia

* Give Na acetate or LR instead of NS, especially if acidemic (acetate is converted to bicarbonate by the liver).

Hypokalemia

* IV (KCl) or PO (KCl, K phosphate, or K acetate); each 10-mEq dose increases serum K ~0.1 mEq/L
    * IV administration faster than 10 mEq/h requires ECG monitoring for arrhythmias

Hyperkalemia

* K removal (slower onset of action): Na polystyrene sulfonate (Kayexalate®) PO or PR, loop diuretics, hemodialysis (if severe)
* Intracellular K shifting (rapid onset of action): regular insulin + dextrose IV, albuterol, Na bicarbonate
* K antagonism of cardiac effects (rapid onset of action): IV calcium

Hypomagnesemia

* Large percentage of dose is renally wasted; repletion requires 3-5 days of treatment.
    * IV: 0.5-1 mEq/kg/d (8 mEq = 1 g), administration rate = 8 mEq/h
    * Can give IM but painful
    * PO: Mg-containing antacid or laxative tid-qid as tolerated or Mg oxide 300-600 mg bid-qid

Hypermagnesemia

* Diuretics, IV Ca, hemodialysis (similar to hyperkalemia)

Hypophosphatemia

* If severe, IV Na or K phosphate 0.16-0.64 mmol/kg at 7.5 mmol/h to avoid K overdose (if K phosphate is used) and/or Ca precipitation
    * PO: 1-2 g/d (5-60 mmol/d) eg, Neutra-Phos®, Neutra-Phos-K®, Fleet Phospho-soda®

Hyperphosphatemia

* See chapter on kidney disorders.

Hypocalcemia

* If symptomatic, IV Ca gluconate (2-3 g) or IV Ca chloride (1 g) over 10 min
    * ± IV infusion of 0.5-2.0 mg/kg/h of elemental Ca
    * PO: calcium salts (eg, calcium carbonate) 1-3 g elemental Ca/d ± vitamin D

Patient counseling

* PO administration: advise patient about potential adverse events (see below).

Adverse drug events

* Sodium: edema, central pontine myelinolysis if serum Na changes rapidly (>12 mEq/d)
* Crystalloids: vein irritation with hypotonic ($^1/_4$ NS, $^1/_2$ NS) or hypertonic fluids (3% NaCl)
    * D_5W is approximately isotonic; often added to low-Na fluids
* Potassium: cardiac arrhythmias (>10 mEq/h), vein irritation (IV), GI upset (PO; worse with wax matrix controlled-release tablets), bad taste (PO liquid)
    * Na polystyrene sulfonate: constipation (usually mixed with sorbitol)
* Magnesium: diarrhea (PO), flushing, sweating (IV), vein irritation (IV)
* Phosphorus: diarrhea (oral), Ca phosphate precipitation (IV)
* Calcium: IV Ca gluconate less irritating than Ca chloride, cardiac dysfunction if administered >60 mg/min (elemental Ca), Ca phosphate precipitation (IV), constipation (oral)

Drug interactions

* Hypokalemia and/or hypomagnesemia predisposes to digoxin toxicity.
* Binding of drugs in the GI tract by Ca, Mg (see nutrition chapter).

Parameters to monitor

* Serum concentrations
* Resolution of signs and symptoms
* Fluid replacement (normalization of the following): BP, HR, urine output (goal >0.5 mL/kg/h), skin turgor, mucous membrane hydration, edema, cardiac output, pulmonary artery wedge pressure (see chapter on heart failure), serum lactate/base deficit

Other/miscellaneous

* Glucose control in critically ill patients (hyperglycemia increases infection risk).
    * Tight glucose control (80-110 mg/dL) with insulin infusion has been shown to reduce mortality in one large trial; however, it is not practical in many centers to use insulin infusions

routinely (labor intensive, risk of hypoglycemia).
  * Some benefit may occur at glucose <150 mg/dL.

- Anemia of critical illness
  * Common complication due to blood loss, bone marrow dysfunction (eg, erythropoietin resistance), and hemodilution.
  * RBC transfusion is not recommended until hemoglobin is <7.0 g/dL (unless symptomatic); no benefit to transfusing sooner and transfusions are associated with increased infections and higher mortality.
  * Recombinant erythropoietin (40,000 units SC per week) has been shown to decrease the need for RBC transfusions by ~20% in a large trial.
  * Until further data are available, erythropoietin is not recommended for routine use in the ICU; may be used if patient has another indication for it (eg, renal failure).

8. Key Points

- Appropriate sedation and analgesia are essential because pain and agitation are common in critically ill patients. Drug selection should be based on clinical guidelines and patient parameters.
- Sedation and analgesia should be monitored using a validated assessment tool.
- Neuromuscular blockers should only be used after sedation and analgesia have been maximized.
- Neuromuscular blockade should be monitored using peripheral nerve stimulation in addition to clinical signs and symptoms.
- Appropriate stress ulcer prophylaxis (H_2 antagonists or sucralfate) is recommended in patients at risk.
- Appropriate VTE prophylaxis is recommended for patients at risk. Optimal therapy is determined by clinical guidelines and patient risk factors.
- High-dose methylprednisolone therapy within 8 hours of injury may improve outcomes after acute spinal cord injury.
- ICP and CPP should be optimized after severe traumatic brain injury using drug and nondrug therapies. Phenytoin is effective at preventing early posttraumatic seizures.
- Severe sepsis and septic shock are progressions of sepsis. Therapy includes hemodynamic stabilization, appropriate antimicrobial agents, and removal of infectious foci if possible.
- Drotrecogin alfa may decrease mortality as an adjunctive agent in patients with severe sepsis and a high severity of illness.
- Maintaining adequate fluid status is vital to maintaining tissue perfusion and organ function. However, many clinical factors can affect fluid and electrolyte status in critically ill patients. Finding and treating underlying causes of fluid and electrolyte abnormalities is essential.
- Fluid and electrolyte abnormalities are generally asymptomatic unless severe.
- Fluid and electrolyte therapy should be monitored closely because of patient instability and the risk of iatrogenic abnormalities (eg, cardiac arrhythmias, fluid overload).

9. Questions and Answers

1. In most critically ill patients, the opiate of choice for analgesia is

   A. morphine
   B. hydromorphone
   C. fentanyl
   D. acetaminophen
   E. ketorolac

2. In which situations should hydromorphone or fentanyl be used for analgesia in critically ill patients?

   I. Morphine allergy
   II. Renal dysfunction
   III. Hemodynamic instability

   A. I only
   B. III only
   C. I and II only
   D. II and III only
   E. I, II, and III

3. What is the maximum duration of therapy for ketorolac?

   A. 5 days
   B. 7 days
   C. 14 days
   D. 30 days
   E. There are no restrictions on length of use

4. Which agent is recommended for general long-term sedation in the ICU (>24-72 hours)?

   A. Diazepam
   B. Propofol
   C. Midazolam
   D. Pentobarbital
   E. Lorazepam

5. In most critically ill patients, the NMB agent of choice is

   A. propofol
   B. vecuronium
   C. cisatracurium
   D. pancuronium
   E. any agent may be used first-line

6. The primary advantage of cisatracurium over pancuronium and vecuronium is

   A. elimination is not organ dependent
   B. shorter duration of action
   C. longer duration of action
   D. more effective
   E. doesn't require monitoring

7. Which of the following is preferred as a first-line sedative agent for ICP control in patients with traumatic brain injury?

   A. Pentobarbital
   B. Lorazepam
   C. Propofol
   D. Vecuronium
   E. Sedation is not recommended

8. The regimen of choice for posttraumatic seizure prophylaxis is

   A. phenytoin indefinitely
   B. phenytoin x 7 days
   C. carbamazepine x 7 days
   D. benzodiazepines prn if seizures occur
   E. propofol x 7 days

9. Which of the following best describes the use of high-dose methylprednisolone in acute spinal cord injury?

   A. Duration of therapy is 24 hours if started within 12 hours of injury
   B. Duration of therapy is 48 hours if started within 8 hours of injury
   C. Duration of therapy is 24 hours if started 0-3 hours from injury and 48 hours if started 3-8 hours from injury
   D. High-dose methylprednisolone may be started at any time after injury
   E. Both blunt and penetrating spinal cord injuries should be treated with high-dose methylprednisolone

Use this case to answer Questions 10 and 11:

Patient name:	DG
Address:	N/A
Age:	24 years
Race:	Caucasian
Sex:	M
Height:	5'10"
Allergies:	NKDA
Weight:	70 kg
Diagnosis:	Motor vehicle accident
	Multiple rib fractures
	Moderate liver contusion

Lab/diagnostic tests:	CT scan of liver shows no active bleeding
Medication orders:	Cimetidine 300 mg IV q8h
	Morphine 1-4 mg IV q1h prn pain
Additional orders:	Pharmacy consult for VTE prophylaxis
Dietary:	N/A
Pharmacist notes:	N/A

10. Which of the following is the most appropriate VTE prophylaxis regimen for DG?

    A. Low-dose LMWH
    B. Heparin 5000 units SC q12h
    C. Full-dose IV heparin infusion
    D. Warfarin to INR 2-3
    E. Intermittent pneumatic compression and elastic stocking

11. The following day DG requires placement of an epidural catheter for pain control for his rib fractures. Which of the following is true regarding VTE prophylaxis in DG?

    A. LMWH should be started and monitored closely with anti Xa levels
    B. LMWH should be avoided because of the risk of perispinal hematoma
    C. Full-dose IV heparin should be used for VTE prophylaxis
    D. Warfarin should be started
    E. A full-dose direct thrombin inhibitor should be started

Use this case to answer Questions 12 and 13:

Patient name:	AC
Address:	N/A
Age:	65 years
Race:	Caucasian
Sex:	F
Height:	5'4"
Allergies:	Penicillin (rash)
Weight:	60 kg

| *Diagnosis:* | Severe community-acquired pneumonia |
| | Acute pain and swelling in left leg 7 days after admission |

| *Lab/diagnostic tests:* | Bedside ultrasound shows acute DVT in left leg |

Below is a comparison of AC's CBC on admission and day 7:

	Admission	Day 7
WBC	18.0	4.0
% neutrophils/% bands	80/10	60/0
Hematocrit (%)	42	48
Platelets	175,000	8000

Medication orders:	Ranitidine 50 mg IV q8h
	Heparin 5000 units SC q12h changed to IV heparin infusion 1100 U/h after DVT is diagnosed
	Gatifloxacin 400 mg IV qd
Additional orders:	N/A
Dietary:	N/A
Pharmacist notes:	N/A

12. Which of AC's hematologic changes over time is most likely due to heparin?

    A. Leukopenia
    B. Leukocytosis
    C. Increased hematocrit
    D. Bandemia (left shift)
    E. Thrombocytopenia

13. What should be done regarding heparin therapy in AC?

    A. Switch to a direct thrombin inhibitor
    B. Continue heparin; monitor CBC closely
    C. Switch to high-dose LMWH
    D. Switch to aspirin
    E. Discontinue heparin; do not anticoagulate

14. In most patients with an acute DVT who are hemodynamically stable, what is the initial treatment of choice?

    A. Heparin 5000 units SC q12h
    B. Full-dose IV heparin or full-dose LMWH
    C. Thrombolytic therapy (eg, recombinant tissue plasminogen actovator)
    D. Aspirin
    E. Low-dose LMWH

15. All of the following are risk factors for the development of stress ulcers EXCEPT

    A. sepsis
    B. coagulopathy
    C. mechanical ventilation
    D. age >40 years
    E. burns

16. Which of the following is correct regarding stress ulcer prophylaxis?

   A. H$_2$ antagonists or sucralfate are equally effective and considered drugs of choice
   B. Proton pump inhibitors are more effective than H$_2$ antagonists or sucralfate
   C. Antacids have the most direct effect on gastric pH and are considered drugs of choice
   D. Sucralfate is more effective and causes less pneumonia than H$_2$ antagonists
   E. All agents (H$_2$ antagonists, sucralfate, PPIs, and antacids) are equally effective

17. Which of the following is the most likely adverse event associated with drotrecogin alfa use in severe sepsis?

   A. Renal dysfunction
   B. Allergy/anaphylactic shock
   C. Tachycardia
   D. Bleeding
   E. Rash

18. Which of the following will NOT increase blood pressure via α_1 adrenergic activation?

   A. Phenylephrine
   B. Dopamine
   C. Epinephrine
   D. Norepinephrine
   E. Dobutamine

19. MW is a 25-year-old pregnant female who is admitted to the medical ICU following several days of severe nausea and vomiting. She is hypotensive, tachycardic, and confused, and her urine output is very low. Her serum sodium is 128 mEq/L. Which of the following should be given to treat her fluid and sodium abnormality?

   A. IV normal saline or lactated Ringer's
   B. IV 5% dextrose in water
   C. PO water
   D. IV furosemide
   E. Desmopressin

20. Common fluid and electrolyte abnormalities associated with loop diuretics include all of the following EXCEPT

   A. hypokalemia
   B. hyperkalemia
   C. hypomagnesemia
   D. dehydration
   E. hypocalcemia

21. RT is a 40-year-old male admitted to the medical ICU following a severe asthma exacerbation. RT's serum phosphorus is 0.9 mEq/L and his body weight is 70 kg (100% of ideal). Which of the following acute phosphorus supplementation regimens is most appropriate?

   A. 45 mmol of sodium phosphate IV over 6 hours
   B. 45 mmol of sodium phosphate IV over 10 minutes
   C. 15 mmol of PO phosphorus (eg, Neutra-phos®) over the next 24 hours
   D. 15 mmol of IV sodium phosphate over 2 hours
   E. No acute phosphorus therapy is required

22. The most common electrolyte abnormality associated with ACE inhibitors is

   A. hypomagnesemia
   B. hypokalemia
   C. hyperkalemia
   D. hyperphosphatemia
   E. hypernatremia

23. All of the following are useful in the rapid treatment of severe hyperkalemia EXCEPT

   A. potassium restriction
   B. IV calcium
   C. IV regular insulin and dextrose
   D. IV sodium bicarbonate
   E. PO Kayexalate

24. The most common electrolyte abnormalities associated with amphotericin B are

   I. hypokalemia
   II. hypomagnesemia
   III. hypocalcemia

   A. I only
   B. III only
   C. I and II only
   D. II and III only
   E. I, II, and III

25. All of the following are side effects of potassium replacement therapy EXCEPT

   A. constipation (PO)
   B. GI upset (PO)
   C. cardiac arrhythmias (IV)

D. vein irritation (IV)

E. poor taste (PO liquid)

26. Which of the following best describes GI side effects of antacids containing magnesium and calcium salts?

A. Mg causes constipation; Ca causes diarrhea

B. Mg causes diarrhea; Ca causes constipation

C. Both cause diarrhea

D. Both cause constipation

E. Neither has GI side effects

Answers

1. **A.** Morphine is recommended by the current Society of Critical Care Medicine (SCCM) guidelines on sedation and analgesia as the opiate of choice for most critically ill patients. Morphine is inexpensive, relatively short-acting, and well tolerated by many patients.

2. **E.** Based on SCCM guidelines, hydromorphone or fentanyl is recommended for critically ill patients with any of the three conditions mentioned. Morphine may cause more hemodynamic instability than hydromorphone or fentanyl because of more histamine release. In addition, morphine has a renally-excreted, partially active metabolite that may accumulate in renal dysfunction. Hydromorphone and fentanyl do not have such a metabolite. The reason for using these agents in morphine allergy is self-explanatory.

3. **A.** Per the manufacturer, ketorolac should not be used longer than 5 days due to the high risk of GI bleeding with this drug.

4. **E.** Based on SCCM guidelines, lorazepam is the sedative of choice in most critically ill patients requiring long-term sedation. Lorazepam is less expensive than propofol and has a longer duration of action than propofol or midazolam.

5. **D.** Based on SCCM guidelines, pancuronium is the NMB of choice for most critically ill patients. Pancuronium is less expensive than other agents.

6. **A.** Cisatracurium is metabolized by nonspecific plasma esterases, while pancuronium and vecuronium have varying degrees of hepatic and renal elimination. Thus, cisatracurium is recommended by SCCM guidelines for use in patients with renal and hepatic dysfunction.

7. **C.** Based on SCCM guidelines, propofol is the sedative of choice for patients that require neurologic assessment often. Traumatic brain injury patients may require multiple neurologic assessments daily. The short duration of action of propofol allows rapid wakening.

8. **B.** Based on the Brain Trauma Foundation guidelines, phenytoin for 7 days postinjury is the regimen of choice for posttraumatic seizure prophylaxis in patients requiring such therapy.

9. **C.** This regimen is based on the results of the NASCIS III trial. There is some controversy regarding the study design of this trial and the actual efficacy of the drug for this indication; however, most clinicians treat acute SCI with high-dose methylprednisolone.

10. **A.** Based on American College of Chest Physicians (ACCP) guidelines, low-dose LMWH is the drug of choice for VTE prophylaxis in a patient with multiple trauma. LMWH is acceptable in this patient because the organ injury is not actively bleeding. If the patient had active bleeding, then mechanical methods (intermittent pneumatic compression and elastic stocking) would be indicated instead of LMWH.

11. **B.** Manufacturers of LMWHs do not recommend using these agents in patients with epidural catheters because of case reports of clinically significant spinal hematomas. Full anticoagulation should also be avoided.

12. **E.** Thrombocytopenia is a common hematologic side effect of heparin. A severe drop in platelets during the first 7-14 days is a typical presentation.

13. **A.** Based on ACCP guidelines, all forms of heparin must be discontinued. However, this patient requires acute, full anticoagulation for treatment of an active DVT. A direct thrombin inhibitor should be started. These agents do not cross react with heparin and potentiate thrombocytopenia.

14. **B.** Based on ACCP guidelines, rapid, full anticoagulation with IV heparin or SC LMWH is recommended in most patients with uncomplicated DVT. Thrombolytic therapy is only recommended in selected patients with hemodynamic instability or a massive VTE.

15. **D.** Increased age is not an independent risk factor for stress ulcers.

16 **A.** Based on ASHP guidelines, H_2 antagonists and sucralfate are generally considered to be equally effective and the drugs of choice. However, there is some controversy over the effect of H_2 antagonists on pneumonia development. Because of this, some clinicians prefer sucralfate.

17. **D.** Drotrecogin alfa is a recombinant form of the endogenous anticoagulant activated protein C. The anticoagulant activity increases the risk of bleeding.

18. **E.** Dobutamine has no α_1 adrenergic (vasoconstriction) activity.

19. **A.** MW is hyponatremic and her clinical signs and symptoms indicate severe dehydration from GI losses of water and sodium. She requires rapid fluid resuscitation with a fluid that has an approximately physiologic amount of sodium (either NS 154 mEq/L or LR 130 mEq/L). This amount of sodium will increase her serum sodium into the normal range over time and the osmotic effect will hold water in the extracellular compartment (the vasculature and interstitium) to help restore organ perfusion.

20. **B.** Loop diuretics enhance renal excretion of water, K, Mg, and Ca.

21. **A.** RT is severely hypophosphatemic and requires high-dose IV therapy (0.64 mmol/kg x 70 kg = 44.8 mmol). The dose should be infused at 7.5 mmol/h (total time ~6 h) to avoid precipitation with Ca.

22. **C.** ACE inhibitors cause hyperkalemia because of aldosterone inhibition.

23. **E.** Oral Kayexalate does not act very quickly. It requires transit time through the intestines to bind potassium and create a gradient that pulls more potassium into the lumen of the GI tract.

24. **C.** Amphotericin B causes renal wasting of potassium and magnesium.

25. **A.** Oral potassium replacement therapy does not normally cause constipation. Cardiac arrhythmias are a concern if IV potassium is given faster than 10 mEq/h.

26. **B.** Magnesium salts (eg, milk of magnesia) are often used as osmotic laxatives and may cause diarrhea. Calcium salts may cause constipation.

10. References

Allen ME, Kopp BJ, Erstad BL. Stress ulcer prophylaxis in the postoperative period. *Am J Health Syst Pharm.* 2004;61:588-596.

ASHP Commission on Therapeutics. ASHP therapeutic guidelines on stress ulcer prophylaxis. *Am J Health Syst Pharm.* 1999;56:347-379.

Boucher BA, Clifton GD, Hanes SD. Critical care therapy. In: Herfindal ET, Gourley DR, eds. *Textbook of Therapeutics: Drug and Disease Management,* 7th ed. Philadelphia: Lippincott Williams & Wilkins; 2000:2077-2094.

Boucher BA, Phelps SJ. Acute management of the head injury patient. In: DiPiro JT, Talbert RL, Yee GC, et al, eds. *Pharmacotherapy: A Pathophysiologic Approach,* 5th ed. New York: McGraw-Hill; 2002:1077-1088.

Bracken ME, Shepard MJ, Holford TR, et al. Administration of methylprednisolone for 24 or 48 hours or tirilazad mesylate for 48 hours in the treatment of acute spinal cord injury. Results of the Third National Acute Spinal Cord Injury Randomized Controlled Trial. National Acute Spinal Cord Injury Study. *JAMA.* 1997;277:1597-1604.

Brain Trauma Foundation, American Association of Neurologic Surgeons. The Joint Section on Neurotrauma and Critical Care. Management and prognosis of severe traumatic brain injury. New York: Brain Trauma Foundation; 2003.

Brain Trauma Foundation, American Association of Neurologic Surgeons. Update Notice. Guidelines for the management of severe traumatic brain injury: Cerebral perfusion pressure. New York: Brain Trauma Foundation; 2003.

Brophy DF, Gehr TWB. Disorders of potassium and magnesium homeostasis. In: DiPiro JT, Talbert RL, Yee GC, et al, eds. *Pharmacotherapy: A Pathophysiologic Approach,* 5th ed. New York: McGraw-Hill; 2002:981-994.

Corwin HL, Gettinger A, Pearl RG, et al. Efficacy of recombinant human erythropoietin in critically ill patients: a randomized trial. *JAMA.* 2002;288:2827-2835.

Dellinger RP, Carlet JM, Masur H, et al. Surviving Sepsis Campaign guidelines for management of severe sepsis and septic shock. *Crit Care Med.* 2004;32:858-873.

Geerts WH, Pineo GF, Heit JA, et al. Prevention of venous thromboembolism. *Chest.* 2004;126:338S-400S.

Jacobi J, Fraser GL, Coursin DB, et al. Clinical practice guidelines for the sustained use of sedatives and analgesics in the critically ill adult. *Crit Care Med.* 2002;30:119-141.

Joy MS, Hladik GA. Disorders of sodium, water, calcium, and phosphorus homeostasis. In: DiPiro JT, Talbert RL, Yee GC, et al, eds. *Pharmacotherapy: A Pathophysiologic Approach,* 5th ed. New York: McGraw-Hill; 2002:953-980.

Kang-Birken SL, DiPiro JT. Sepsis and septic shock. In: DiPiro JT, Talbert RL, Yee GC, et al, eds. *Pharmacotherapy: A Pathophysiologic Approach,* 5th ed. New York: McGraw-Hill; 2002:2029-2041.

Lau A, Chan LN. Electrolytes, other minerals, and trace elements. In: Lee M, ed. *Basic Skills in Interpreting Laboratory Data,* 3rd ed. Bethesda, MD: American Society of Health-System Pharmacists; 2004:183-232.

Murray MJ, Cowen J, DeBlock H, et al. Clinical practice guidelines for sustained neuromuscular blockade in the critically ill patient. *Crit Care Med.* 2002;30:142-156.

18. Nutrition

Rex O. Brown, PharmD, BCNSP
Professor and Executive Vice Chair,
Department of Clinical Pharmacy
University of Tennessee College of Pharmacy

Contents

1. Overview

General Nutrition

U.S. dietary guidelines (food pyramid)
- Maintain healthy weight
- Low-fat diet (<30% of total calories)
- Plenty of fruits, vegetables, and grain products
- Salt, sugar, and alcohol in moderation

Malnutrition
- Causes of undernutrition (protein-calorie malnutrition)
  * Depressed intake of nutrients (starvation, semi-starvation)
  * Alteration in nutrient metabolism (trauma, major infection)
- Obesity and its causes
  * Excessive caloric intake (especially carbohydrate and fat)
  * Alteration in nutrient metabolism (genetic predisposition)
  * Sedentary lifestyle

Dietary reference intakes (DRIs) of selected nutrients
- Fiber: 20-35 g per day (many people find this goal unpalatable).
- Calcium: 1200-1500 mg/d in adolescents and young adults; 1000 mg/d in men until age 65 and women until age 50; 1200-1500 mg/d for life (usually requires supplements)
- Multivitamins help to meet daily requirements of pregnant and lactating women, elderly persons, and those who eat vegetarian or low-calorie diets.

Nutritional assessment components
History and physical examination
- Dietary intake (anorexia, hyperphagia, taste alterations)
- Underlying pathology affecting nutrition (cancer, burns)
- End-organ effects (diarrhea, constipation)
- General appearance (edema, cachexia)
- Skin appearance (scaling skin, decubitus ulcers)
- Musculoskeletal (depressed muscle mass, growth retardation)
- Neurologic (depressed sensorium, encephalopathy)
- Hepatic (jaundice, hepatomegaly)

Anthropometrics
- Skinfold measurements for assessment of fat (triceps, calf)
- Arm muscle circumference for assessment of skeletal muscle
- Weight for height to determine undernutrition or obesity
- Head circumference in infants to document appropriate growth
- Percentage of ideal body weight (IBW) after calculation of IBW for patient
  * IBW of males (kg) = 50 + (2.3 x height in inches over 5 feet)
  * IBW of females (kg) = 45.5 + (2.3 x height in inches over 5 feet)
- Body mass index (BMI) for assessment of undernutrition or obesity calculated from body weight (kg) and height (meters): $BMI = wt (kg)/ht (m)^2$

Biochemical assessment
Serum albumin concentration
- Good prognostic indicator and good for assessment of long-term nutritional status
- Poor for repletion marker because of long half-life (21 days) and large body pool
Serum prealbumin concentration
- Good for short-term assessment of nutrition support because of short half-life (2 days) and small body pool
- Serum transferrin concentration is also good for short-term assessment because of short half-life (7 days) and small body pool
  * Elevated in iron-deficiency anemia
Creatinine height index
- Requires 24-hour urine collection to determine levels of creatinine

Immune assessment
- Total lymphocyte count from complete blood count with differential (insensitive)
- Cell-mediated immunity
- Skin test with common antigens, eg, *Candida*, mumps (usually takes 48-72 hours for skin induration to occur to give positive response)
Other methods of nutritional assessment
- Muscle strength testing
- Bioelectrical impedance (ie, a low-grade electrical current runs through the body to identify body protein stores and fat stores)

Types of malnutrition
Marasmus
- Features depleted fat and muscle stores, normal biochemical measurements, and intact immune status

Kwashiorkor
- Features normal or elevated fat and body weight with abnormally low biochemical measurements and depressed immune function

Kwashiorkor-marasmus mix
• All measurements are depressed.

Obesity
• Demonstrated as elevated body weight to at least 120% of IBW, or BMI >27.8 (male) and >27.3 (female)
    * Class I obesity: BMI >30 and <35
    * Class II obesity: BMI >35 and <40
    * Class III obesity: BMI >40

Selected definitions
• Hypermetabolism: An increase in energy expenditure above normal (usually >10% above normal)
• Hypercatabolism: An increase in protein losses above normal (usually via urinary excretion of urea nitrogen)
• Specialized nutrition support: Parenteral nutrition (PN) or enteral nutrition (EN)
• Basal energy expenditure (BEE): A calculation of normal energy needs of healthy adult men or women using gender, age, height, and weight (Harris-Benedict equations)
    * Male (kcal/d) = 66 + 13.7 (wt in kg) + 5 (ht in cm) – 6.8 (age in years)
    * Female (kcal/d) = 655 + 9.6 (wt in kg) + 1.8 (ht in cm) – 4.7 (age in years)
• Resting energy expenditure (REE): A measured value of energy expenditure (generally ~10% above BEE in health, can be 100% above BEE in severe burns)
• Respiratory quotient (RQ): The value that results when carbon dioxide production (VCO_2) is divided by oxygen consumption (VO_2)
    * RQ for carbohydrate oxidation = 1
    * RQ for fat oxidation = 0.7
    * RQ for protein oxidation = 0.8
    * RQ for fat synthesis = 8
• Body cell mass: Lean, metabolically active tissue (skeletal muscle, body organs)
• Lean body mass: Body cell mass, extracelluar fluid, and extracellular solids (bone, serum proteins)
• RDI: Recommended daily intake

2. Nutritional Requirements

Calorie Requirements

• Most clinicians dose specialized nutrition support in total calories (ie, using carbohydrate, fat, and protein calorie contributions to obtain the desired dose).
    * 25 kcal/kg/d for adults with little stress (eg, elective surgery)
    * 30 kcal/kg/d for patients with infections, skeletal trauma
    * 35 kcal/kg/d for patients with major trauma (head injury, long-bone fractures)
    * 40 kcal/kg/d for patients with major thermal injury (>50% total body surface area burn)
• Multiply basal energy expenditure (BEE) times the stress factor to determine calorie requirements.
    * 1 x BEE for patients with little stress
    * 1.3 x BEE for patients with minor trauma, infections
    * 1.5 x BEE for patients with major trauma
    * 2 x BEE for patients with severe thermal injury
• Measurement of the resting energy expenditure (REE) via indirect calorimetry for calorie requirements

Caloric contribution of the major macronutrients
• Glucose: 3.4 kcal/g because hydrated glucose is used in PN (glucose powder would be 4 kcal/g)
• Fat: 9 kcal/g
• Protein: 4 kcal/g
    * Protein requirements are usually dosed in grams per kilogram per day.
    * 0.8 g/kg/d is the adult recommended daily allowance (RDA) for protein in the U.S.
    * 1 g/kg/d for patients with minor stress (elective operations)
    * 1.5 g/kg/d for patients with major trauma, infection
    * 2 g/kg/d for patients with severe head injury, sepsis, severe thermal injury

Measurement of Nutritional Efficacy Using Nitrogen Balance (NB)

NB = nitrogen in – nitrogen out
• Nitrogen in (grams) is determined by dividing the grams of protein taken in on the day of balance divided by 6.25.
• Nitrogen out (grams) is determined by measuring the grams of urea nitrogen excreted during a 24-hour urine collection and then adding a factor of 2 or 4 g for insensible nitrogen loss/stool loss.

- Positive nitrogen balance can be used to document adequacy of nutritional support.
    * +4 to 6 g/d is desired in undernourished patients.
    * Nitrogen equilibrium (–2 to +2 g/d) is usually adequate in critically ill patients.

Other Requirements During Nutrition Support

Water
- Up to 35 mL/kg/d for average-sized adults
- 40 mL/kg/d for smaller adults and adolescents
- >40 mL/kg/d for patients with extra-renal losses (eg, gastrointestinal drains)

Electrolytes
- Sodium requirements
    * 60-100 mEq/d in adults
    * 2-6 mEq/kg/d in children
- Chloride requirements
    * 60-100 mEq/d in adults
    * 2-6 mEq/kg/d in children
- Potassium requirements
    * 60-100 mEq/d in adults
    * 2-5 mEq/kg/d in children
- Calcium requirements
    * 5-15 mEq/d in adults
    * 2-3 mEq/kg/d in children
- Phosphorus requirements
    * 20-45 mmol/d in adults
    * 1-2 mmol/kg/d in children
- Magnesium requirements
    * 10-20 mEq/d in adults
    * 0.25-1 mEq/kg/d in children

Vitamins
- Vitamins are provided daily in both PN (added) and EN (endogenous).
    * Most enteral formulations provide the RDI for vitamins in a volume of 1000-1500 mL.
- Parenteral vitamin products
    * Adult products contain 12 (MVI-12) or 13 vitamins (Infuvite Adult, MVI-Adult®); vitamin K is added separately when the product with 12 vitamins is used.
    * Pediatric products (MVI-Pediatric®, Infuvite Pediatric®) contain all 13 vitamins.

Trace elements
- Zinc: 3-5 mg/d in adults with PN; 50-250 mcg/kg/d in children with PN
- Copper: 0.5-1.2 mg/d in adults with PN; 20 mcg/kg/d in children with PN (maximum of 300 mcg/d)
- Chromium: 10-15 mcg/d in adults with PN; 0.14-0.2 mcg/kg/d in children with PN (maximum of 5 mcg/d)
- Manganese: 50-100 mcg/d in adults with PN; 1 mcg/kg/d in children with PN (maximum of 50 mcg/d)
- Selenium: 40-80 mcg/d in adults with PN; 1.5-3 mcg/kg/d in children with PN

3. Specialized Nutrition Support

Parenteral Nutrition

Indications: PN is generally used for patients who cannot be fed via the gastrointestinal tract.

Severe acute pancreatitis
- Oral or tube feeding will usually exacerbate this condition.

Short bowel syndrome
- Requires PN from a few weeks to lifelong as needed

Ileus
- Secondary to lack of bowel function (eg, acute renal failure secondary to sepsis)

Other indications
- Crohn's disease exacerbation with fistula or obstruction
- Neonates who cannot eat in the first day of life
- Preoperatively for undernourished patients who are undergoing an elective operation and there is no direct access to the GI tract (eg, partial small bowel obstruction from cancer)
- Pregnancy with severe hyperemesis gravidarum (ie, there is an inability to tolerate oral or enteral nutrition)
- Gastrointestinal fistulae where oral or enteral nutrition should be restricted

Components of parenteral nutrition
Protein
- Protein should be included in all PN formulations.
- Standard amino acids from 10%, 15%, or 20% stock solutions can be used for most patients.
- Final concentrations in the PN formulation vary from 2-7%.
- Rarely need doses >2 g/kg/d

Fat
- Fat is provided as intravenous fat emulsion either as a separate infusion or admixed with the rest of the PN formulation, making a total nutrient admixture (TNA).
- Products are manufactured as 10%, 20%, and 30% fat emulsions (30% can be used only for TNAs, not for direct infusion in the U.S.).
- Provides essential fatty acids to the patient who is most likely not eating by mouth
- Provides nonprotein calories other than glucose
- Common doses used in adults are ~1 g/kg/d (9-10 kcal/kg/d).

- Intravenous fat emulsions contain phospholipid to emulsify the product and glycerol to make the emulsion isotonic (both of these components provide modest calories).

Dextrose
- Common doses of dextrose in critically ill patients: 3-4 mg/kg/min (~15-20 kcal/kg/d)
- In all PN formulations for obligate needs (CNS, renal medulla, WBCs, RBCs, and wound healing)
- PN formulations are usually made from 70% dextrose in water.
- Final concentrations in the PN formulation vary from $D_{10}W$ to $D_{35}W$.
- Should never exceed a dose of 5 mg/kg/min (~25 kcal/kg/d)

Sodium
- Can be provided as chloride, acetate, or phosphate salts in PN
- After phosphate addition, the remaining anions are added based on acid-base status (eg, acetate with metabolic acidosis, chloride with metabolic alkalosis).
- Requirements can be increased when the patient has extra-renal losses from nasogastric suction, abdominal drains, or ostomy losses.

Potassium
- Can be provided as chloride, acetate, or phosphate salts in PN
- Requirements can be increased with administration of potassium-wasting drugs (diuretics, steroids) or in severe undernutrition.
- Like sodium, the remaining potassium can be added as acetate or chloride after the proper dose of phosphate is determined.

Calcium
- Most practitioners add calcium as the gluconate salt.
- Higher doses of calcium (~20-25 mEq/d) are needed in patients receiving long-term PN to help prevent metabolic bone disease.
- Addition of calcium is limited in PN formulations because of the potential to precipitate with phosphate salts, which ultimately results in insoluble calcium phosphate.

Phosphate
- Added as the sodium or potassium salt
- Higher doses of phosphorus (eg, 30 mmol/L) are needed to prevent refeeding syndrome in severely undernourished patients.
- Phosphorus should be decreased or removed in patients with renal failure.

- Addition of phosphorus is limited in PN formulations because of the potential to precipitate with calcium or magnesium salts to form an insoluble compound.

Magnesium
- Most practitioners add magnesium as the sulfate salt.
- Higher doses should be used in patients with alcoholism or large bowel losses, or in patients receiving drugs causing renal wasting of magnesium (cisplatin, amphotericin B, aminoglycosides, loop diuretics).
- Magnesium should be restricted or deleted in patients with renal failure.

Multivitamins
- Given daily as part of PN
- Parenteral multivitamin preparations contain 12 or 13 vitamins (vitamin K should be administered separately if the 12-vitamin preparation is used).
- Additional thiamine and folic acid are often given to alcoholic patients who are receiving PN.
- Additional folic acid (at least 600 mcg/d) should be given to pregnant patients receiving PN.

Trace elements
- Given daily as a cocktail of four or five trace metals
- Extra zinc should be given in patients with ostomy or diarrhea losses.
- Copper and manganese should be reduced or eliminated in patients with cholestasis.
- Extra selenium is usually needed in home-bound PN patients.

Total nutrient admixtures (TNAs) versus 2-in-1 admixtures
Advantages of TNAs
- Decreased nursing time for administration
- Potentially decreased touch contamination
- Decreased pharmacy preparation time (assuming a 24-hour hangtime)
- Financial savings (use of only 1 pump and 1 intravenous administration set)
Disadvantages of TNAs
- Better media for bacterial growth than 2-in-1 admixtures
- Impossible to visualize particulate matter
- Cannot filter formulation with a 0.22-micron filter
- Some additives like calcium and phosphorus are less compatible in TNAs.

Central vein PN versus peripheral vein PN
Advantages of central vein PN
- Can maximize caloric intake
- Can volume-restrict patients
- Long-term catheter can be maintained

Disadvantages of central vein PN
- Mechanical complications during catheter placement (eg, pneumothorax)
- Potential hyperosmolar complications (eg, from using hypertonic dextrose)
- Potential septic catheter complications
Advantages of peripheral vein PN
- Easier to place the catheter (ie, peripheral vein stick)
- Avoid hyperosmolar complications because dilute formulations must be used.
Disadvantages of peripheral vein PN
- High incidence of thrombophlebitis
- Requires frequent vein rotation
- Energy intake is limited
- Volume restriction is not possible (using dilute formulations)
- Higher cost because more lipid calories are generally used (lipids are isotonic)

Parenteral nutrition calculations
$D_{20}W$ (final concentration of PN formulation)
- $D_{20}W$ = 20% dextrose = 20 g/100 mL = 200 g/L x 3.4 kcal/g = 680 kcal/L
- 2 L/d of $D_{20}W$ (final concentration of PN) = 1360 kcal/d

Amino acids 5% (final concentration of PN formulation)
- 5% amino acids = 5 g/100 mL = 50 g/L x 4 kcal/g = 200 kcal/L
- 2 L/d of 5% amino acids = 100 g/d = 400 kcal/d

Lipid 2% (final concentration of TNA formulation)
- 2% lipid will deliver 200 kcal/L (includes calories from glycerol/phospholipid).
- 2 L/d of lipid 2% = 400 kcal/d

Lipid 20% infused at 20 mL/h x 24 h (separate infusion given with 2-in-1 PN)
- 20% lipid = 2 kcal/mL
- 20 mL/h x 24 h = 480 mL/d
- 480 mL/day x 2 kcal/mL = 960 kcal/d

Example: $D_{30}W$; amino acids 4%; lipid 3%, at 60 mL/h
- 60 mL/h x 24 h/d = 1440 mL/day (1.44 L/d)
- $D_{30}W$ = 30% dextrose = 300 g/L x 3.4 kcal/g = 1020 kcal/L x 1.44 L = 1469 kcal
- 4% amino acids = 40 g/L = 160 kcal/L x 1.44 L = 230 kcal
- 3% lipid = 300 kcal/L x 1.44 L = 432 kcal
- 1469 kcal + 230 kcal + 432 kcal = 2131 total kcal/d

Example: dextrose 400 g; amino acids 100 g; lipids 40 g; at 85 mL/h
- Dextrose 400 g x 3.4 kcal/g = 1360 kcal/d

- Amino acids 100 g x 4 kcal/g = 400 kcal/d
- Lipids 40 g x 10 kcal/g (includes phospholipid and glycerol) = 400 kcal/d

General principles of compounding parenteral nutrition

- Each component of the PN prescription should be reviewed to ensure a balanced PN formulation is provided.
- Each component should be assessed for dose and potential compatibility programs.
- All compounded PN formulations should be visually inspected to ensure no gross contamination or precipitation is present.
- Manufacturers of automated compounders should provide the additive sequence to ensure safety in PN preparation.

General principles of stability and compatibility of parenteral nutrition

- Parenteral multivitamins should be added shortly before dispensing and administering the PN formulation because vitamins A and C degrade fairly quickly.
- Preparation of TNAs using dual-chambered bags (lipid is kept in a separate compartment until administration) can enhance the shelf life of a PN formulation.
- Dibasic calcium phosphate ($CaHPO_4$) can precipitate in PN formulations if the amounts of calcium gluconate and sodium or potassium phosphate are excessive.
- Generally, phosphate should be added first to the PN formulation.
- Generally, calcium should be added last to the PN formulation.
- Calcium chloride should not be used in PN because it is highly reactive with phosphate.
- Iron dextran can be added to 2-in-1 PN formulation, but should not be added to TNAs.

Parenteral nutrition filtration

- Filters are used to prevent administration of particulate matter, microorganisms, and air.
- Use a new 0.22-micron filter each day with 2-in-1 PN formulations (0.22-micron filters with positive charged nylon can be used for up to 96 hours in 2-in-1 PN formulations).
- Use a new 1.2-micron filter each day with TNAs.

Complications of parenteral nutrition
Metabolic
Hyperglycemia
- Patients with stress of trauma or infection or those with diabetes often need regular human insulin added to the PN to control hyperglycemia.

Electrolyte disorders
Hypokalemia
- Patients often require extra potassium in PN (eg, 60 mEq/L).
Hypophosphatemia
- Patients often require extra phosphorus in PN (eg, 30 mmol/L).
Hypomagnesemia
- Patients often require extra magnesium in PN (eg, 16 mEq/L).
Hyponatremia
- Diagnosis of electrolyte disorders must include an assessment of extracellular fluid status (ie, volume status).
  - * Volume depleted: Add sodium and water to PN or increase intravenous fluid administration.
  - * Volume overloaded: Remove sodium from PN and concentrate the formulation.
  - * Euvolemic: Generally, water restriction is first-line therapy (PN concentration).

Acid-base disorders
- Increase acetate anions if the patient has metabolic acidosis.
- Increase chloride anions if the patient has metabolic alkalosis.

Essential fatty acid deficiency
- During PN, at least 4% of total calories need to be provided as intravenous lipid (easily attained when lipid is used daily as a calorie source).

Trace element disorders
- Patients with increased ostomy output or chronic diarrhea need extra zinc.
- Hold copper and manganese in patients with cholestasis.

Hepatic steatosis
- Fatty infiltration of the liver has been reported with long-term PN.
- Thought to be primarily caused by administration of excessive dextrose calories
- The key to prevention is via administration of an appropriate dose of dextrose (eg, <5 mg/kg/min).

Mechanical complications
- Pneumothorax (punctured lung) can occur during central vein access.
- Subclavian artery injury can occur when the artery is cannulated instead of the vein.
- Subclavian vein thrombosis can occur with long-term central vein access (heparin is used in some PN patients to prevent this).

Infectious complications
- Usually due to catheter-related breakdown in sterile technique
- Rarely solution-related

Monitoring of parenteral nutrition
- Frequency and intensity of monitoring is based on the patient's condition, as assessed by:
  * Electrolytes and glucose
  * Acid-base status via arterial blood gases
  * Intake and output for assessment of fluid balance
  * Serum prealbumin concentrations and/or nitrogen balance to document efficacy

Enteral Nutrition

Indications
- Generally used in patients who cannot or will not eat, but have a functional and accessible gastrointestinal tract
- Neonates should begin EN as early as possible, even if receiving PN.
- Elderly patients without the ability to ingest food orally

Cardiac
- May need fluid-restricted EN with fluid overload

Pulmonary failure
- Used frequently in patients receiving mechanical ventilation

Hepatic failure
- EN is used frequently in this population.
- In severe hepatic encephalopathy, use a formulation with high branched-chain amino acids and low aromatic amino acids.
- In the absence of encephalopathy or mild encephalopathy, use EN with standard protein.

Gastrointestinal failure
- In short-bowel syndrome, EN is used to enhance small bowel hypertrophy after major resection.
- Inflammatory bowel syndrome: preferred method of nutrition support in these patients

Neurologic impairment
- EN is preferred because the patient may not be able to eat, but the gastrointestinal tract is functional and accessible.

Cancer/HIV infection
- Use EN (if possible) in these patients to prevent or treat undernutrition.

Types of enteral access
Feeding enterostomy
- Usually placed for long-term EN
- Gastrostomy: G-tube or PEG (percutaneous endoscopic gastrostomy)
- Jejunostomy: Requires an exploratory laparotomy to place.

Oral route (by drinking supplements)

Nasal tube feeding
- Usually placed for short-term EN
- Nasogastric tube
- Nasoduodenal tube
- Nasojejunal tube

Products for enteral nutrition
- Polymeric, nutritionally-complete tube feeding for patients with normal digestive processes (eg, 1 kcal/mL)
- Concentrated, nutritionally-complete tube feeding for patients who need severe fluid restriction (eg, 2 kcal/mL)
- Polymeric, nutritionally-complete, oral supplements to supplement an oral diet (eg, 1 or 1.5 kcal/mL)
- Chemically-defined, nutritionally complete tube feeding for patients with impaired digestive processes like short bowel syndrome or pancreatic insufficiency (eg, 1 kcal/mL)
- Fiber-containing, nutritionally-complete tube feeding is beneficial in patients who receive long-term tube feeding (can prevent diarrhea and constipation; eg, 1 or 1.2 kcal/mL).
- Concentrated, low-protein, low-electrolyte tube feeding is generally used for patients with renal failure.
- High branched-chain amino acid, low aromatic amino acid EN formula is used for patients with liver failure and severe hepatic encephalopathy (eg, 1 or 1.5 kcal/mL).
- High-fat, low-carbohydrate, nutritionally-complete tube feeding is helpful in management of diabetic or other glucose-intolerant patients (eg, 1 kcal/mL).
- Immune-enhancing formulas that contain arginine, glutamine, and omega-3 fatty acids are marketed and used in patients with high metabolic stress (eg, severe trauma or infection; 1 or 1.3 kcal/mL).

Complications of enteral nutrition
Pulmonary (eg, aspiration pneumonia)
- The most severe complication of EN
- Caused by regurgitation of gastric contents into the lung (with or without tube feeding)
- Prevention is important.
  * Elevate the head of the bed to 30° if possible.
  * Frequently assess the patient's abdomen to ensure tolerance.

* Frequently assess the placement of the feeding tube (especially nasally placed tubes).

Gastrointestinal

- Diarrhea is often associated with the administration of EN, but it is not necessarily the cause of the diarrhea.

Increased frequency or volume of stools

- Pharmacotherapy is often the cause, due to sorbitol in liquid vehicles; lack of fiber and excessive infusion rate advancements can also be causes.
- Decreasing (or at least not advancing) the infusion rate is appropriate.
- Change to a fiber-containing formulation if the patient is not receiving one.
- Pseudomembranous enterocolitis from antibiotic therapy
- Use pharmacotherapeutic treatment if the above factors are ruled out (bismuth subsalicylate, loperamide).

Constipation (decrease in stool frequency)

- Lack of fiber can be a cause.
- Lack of water can be a cause.
- Poor mobility and drugs with anticholinergic activity can contribute.
- Keep patient well hydrated and use a fiber-containing EN formulation.

Mechanical complications of EN

- In the event of nasal necrosis, use a small-bore feeding tube and do not tape it too firmly to the nose.
- In the event of esophageal injury, use a small-bore feeding tube.
- In the event of tube clogging, frequently flush the feeding tube with warm water.
- In the event of tube displacement, discourage removing the tube; the tube may have to be anchored with a bridle.

Metabolic complications of EN

Hyperglycemia

- Use regular human insulin.
- Consider a high-fat, low-carbohydrate EN formulation.

Hypokalemia

- Provide additional potassium as an IV or per tube supplement.
- Some institutions allow the addition of potassium salts to the EN formulation.

Hypophosphatemia

- Provide additional phosphorus as an IV supplement (eg, potassium phosphate).
- Some institutions allow the addition of phosphorus salts to the EN formulation (eg, Fleet® Phospho-Soda, 5 or 10 mL/L).

Monitoring of enteral nutrition

- The intensity of monitoring will be dictated by the condition of the patient.
    - * Electrolytes and glucose
    - * Acid-base status via arterial blood gases (critical care only)
    - * Intake and output for assessment of fluid balance

Assessment of the patient's abdomen

- Positive bowel sounds usually should be present.
- The abdomen should be soft, nontender, and nondistended in most cases.
- A profoundly distended abdomen usually requires the EN to be decreased or discontinued temporarily.
- Serum prealbumin concentrations and/or nitrogen balance to document efficacy

Home Nutrition Support

Parenteral nutrition

- Can be given from weeks to a lifetime (eg, severe short bowel syndrome)
- Usually cycled at night over 10-16 hours
- Must be monitored closely for iron deficiency because iron supplementation is not routinely added to PN
- Regular assessment of hemoglobin, hematocrit, and MCV
- Serum iron, TIBC, and ferritin are commonly used in the diagnosis of iron deficiency.
- Metabolic bone disease is another long-term complication of home PN.
    - * Supplemental calcium in the PN formulation is usually required (15-25 mEq/d).
    - * Adequate vitamin K for osteocalcin is important on a long-term basis.

Enteral nutrition

- Can be given indefinitely as full nutrition support or as a supplement to an oral diet
- Permanent feeding ostomies are used almost exclusively in home EN.
- Patients in nursing homes and extended-care facilities usually receive EN as a continuous infusion over 12-24 hours.
- Patients who receive home EN via gastrostomy usually receive bolus feeding (eg, two 240-mL cans tid via PEG).
- Patients who receive home EN as a supplement to oral intake are often cycled at night (eg, 1000 mL at 85 mL/h from 7 pm to 7 am each night).

4. Major Drug-Nutrient Interactions

Phenytoin and enteral tube feeding
- It has been demonstrated that enteral feeding will bind to phenytoin, thus impairing the absorption dramatically (possibly due to the protein component of EN [caseinates]).

Management of phenytoin/enteral nutrition interaction
- Hold the EN 2 hours before and after the daily dose of phenytoin capsules.
- Hold the EN 1 hour before and after each dose of phenytoin suspension (usually given bid or tid).
- Increase the EN infusion rate to allow the desired nutritional dose of EN to be given (ie, to make up the lost time while the EN is being held for drug administration).

Warfarin and enteral tube feeding
- It has been reported that adequate anticoagulation with warfarin is very difficult to achieve with concurrent EN (low INRs).

Management of warfarin/enteral nutrition interaction
- Some practitioners hold EN 1 hour before and after the daily warfarin dose. If this is done, the EN rate should be increased to attain the desired nutritional dose.

Grapefruit juice interacts with many drugs (eg, amlodipine, carbamazepine, cyclosporine)
- Grapefruit juice from frozen concentrate has been reported to inhibit gastrointestinal cytochrome P450-3A4, resulting in enhancement of oral absorption of some drugs (toxicity).

Management of grapefruit juice/drug interaction
- When taking drugs that are known to interact with grapefruit juice, patients should be advised to avoid these products (ie, substitute another fruit juice such as apple or orange juice).

5. Key Points

- Malnutrition can present as either undernutrition or obesity.
- The components of a nutritional assessment include a history and physical exam, anthropometric measurements, biochemical tests, and immune competence assessment.
- An increase in energy expenditure (energy needs) is defined as hypermetabolism, and an increase in nitrogen excretion (protein needs) is defined as hypercatabolism.
- Most patients receiving specialized nutrition support (parenteral or enteral nutrition) require from 25-30 kcal/kg/d and 1-2 g protein/kg/d.
- Water requirements for most adult patients without substantial extra-renal losses is from 30-40 mL/kg/d.
- Parenteral nutrition (PN) should be reserved for patients whose gastrointestinal tracts are not functional or accessible (eg, severe acute pancreatitis, severe short bowel syndrome).
- Total nutrient admixtures (TNAs) contain dextrose, amino acids, lipid emulsion, electrolytes, vitamins, and trace elements in one container.
- The advantages of TNAs include decreased nursing administration time, decreased potential for touch contamination, and reduced expense (the patient needs only 1 pump and 1 intravenous administration set).
- The advantages of central vein PN over peripheral vein PN include the ability to concentrate the formulation, administer adequate calories and protein, and use the catheter for long-term administration.
- For PN calculations: 1 g hydrated dextrose = 3.4 kcal, 1 g amino acids = 4 kcal, and 1 g lipid = 9 kcal (intravenous fat emulsion actually provides 10 kcal/g because it includes calories provided as glycerol and phospholipid).
- All PN formulations should be filtered during administration (0.22-micron filter for 2-in-1 PN formulations and 1.2-micron filter for TNAs).
- Enteral nutrition support is generally used in patients who cannot or will not eat, but have a functional and accessible gastrointestinal tract.
- Enteral tube feeding can be provided by one of the following methods: nasogastric, nasoduodenal, nasojejunal, gastrostomy, or jejunostomy.
- Diarrhea associated with enteral tube feeding is often caused by pharmacotherapy (eg, sorbitol in liquid drug preparations as a vehicle).
- Patients receiving phenytoin or warfarin concurrently with enteral tube feeding should have the tube feeding held at least 1 hour before and after each dose.

6. Questions and Answers

1. What is the most appropriate calcium intake (mg/d) for adults >65 years of age?

   A. 600-800 mg
   B. 800-1000 mg
   C. 1000-1200 mg
   D. 1200-1500 mg
   E. 1500-1800 mg

Use this case for Questions 2 and 3.

A patient presents for a comprehensive nutritional assessment. She is 35 years old, 5'8", and weighs 52 kg. She has a history of Crohn's disease involving both the small bowel and colon. She has had no surgeries, but has intermittent diarrhea.

Medications:
Prednisone 5 mg qod
Mesalamine 1 g tid
Loperamide 2 mg q6h prn diarrhea

Measurements:
Triceps skinfold = 3 mm (normal, 10-14 mm)
Calf skinfold = 4 mm (normal, 10-15 mm)
Serum albumin concentration = 2.5 g/dL
Serum prealbumin concentration = 13 mg/dL
(normal, 15-45 mg/dL)

2. The triceps skinfold measurement for this patient is an anthropometric measurement for assessment of

   A. somatic protein stores
   B. fat stores
   C. visceral protein stores
   D. immune competence
   E. body cell mass

3. What type of malnutrition does this patient have?

   A. Kwashiorkor
   B. Marasmus
   C. Obesity
   D. Kwashiorkor-marasmus mix
   E. Fat overload syndrome

4. A patient with a bone fracture and gram-negative pneumonia excretes 15 g (normal, 6-8 g/d) of urea nitrogen during a 24-hour urine collection. Based on these data, the patient is

   A. hypercatabolic
   B. hypermetabolic
   C. hypocatabolic
   D. hypometabolic
   E. euvolemic

5. During nutritional assessment, the measurement of body cell mass includes

   A. bone
   B. interstitial fluid
   C. skeletal muscle
   D. intravascular fluid
   E. extracellular fluid solids

Use this case for Questions 6-9:

Following major gastrointestinal resection, a patient with severe short bowel syndrome is started on parenteral nutrition (PN). It is anticipated that this patient may need this therapy for 6 months to 1 year. The PN prescription for this patient includes:

- $D_{20}W$ amino acids 5% (final concentrations) at 105 mL/h (2500 mL/d)
- Intravenous fat emulsion 20% at 10 mL/h x 24 hours (240 mL/d)
- 0.45% sodium chloride injection at 50 mL/h x 24 hours (1200 mL/d)

6. How many calories from dextrose will this patient receive each day?

   A. 1100
   B. 1300
   C. 1500
   D. 1700
   E. 1900

7. How many grams of protein will this patient receive each day?

   A. 25
   B. 50
   C. 75
   D. 100
   E. 125

8. How many calories from intravenous lipid will this patient receive each day?

   A. 240
   B. 360
   C. 480
   D. 600
   E. 720

9. Calculate the daily nitrogen balance (grams per day) in this patient if she excretes 12 g of urea nitrogen during the urine collection and 4 g is used as insensible and stool loss each day.

    A. –4
    B. –2
    C. 0
    D. 2
    E. 4

10. What would be an appropriate water/fluid requirement for a 60-kg patient with no extra-renal fluid losses?

    A. 800 mL
    B. 1200 mL
    C. 2400 mL
    D. 3600 mL
    E. 4800 mL

11. Which of the following disease states or clinical conditions would usually require the administration of parenteral nutrition?

    A. Severe acute pancreatitis
    B. Motor vehicle crash resulting in femur fracture and head injury
    C. 20% body surface area burn from a house fire
    D. Laparoscopic cholecystectomy
    E. Acute exacerbation of hepatic encephalopathy

12. What is the maximum dose (in kilocalories per kilogram per day) of dextrose in parenteral nutrition for adult patients?

    A. 5
    B. 10
    C. 15
    D. 20
    E. 25

13. In a patient with metabolic acidosis, what anion salt would you use to add the majority of sodium and potassium to a PN formulation?

    A. Chloride
    B. Gluconate
    C. Phosphate
    D. Acetate
    E. Sulfate

14. If excessive amounts of calcium are added to a standard parenteral nutrition formulation, it will likely precipitate with

    A. phosphate
    B. gluconate
    C. magnesium
    D. chloride
    E. sodium

15. Which vitamin should be supplemented during nutrition support of a pregnant patient?

    A. Cyanocobalamin
    B. Folic acid
    C. Biotin
    D. Chromium
    E. Pantothenic acid

16. Which of the following is an advantage of central vein parenteral nutrition over peripheral vein parenteral nutrition?

    A. Easier catheter placement
    B. Does not require a pump for administration
    C. Allows for fluid restriction
    D. Does not have to be filtered
    E. Dilute formulations are used in most cases

17. Which component of a total nutrient admixture should be added last before storing it in a refrigerator?

    A. Phosphorus
    B. Magnesium
    C. Trace elements
    D. Calcium
    E. Intravenous fat emulsion

18. The advantages of using a 0.22-micron filter when administering a 2-in-1 parenteral nutrition formulation include:

    I.   Traps particulate matter
    II. Prevents precipitates from entering the patient
    III. Filters most bacteria

    A. I only
    B. III only
    C. I and II only
    D. II and III only
    E. I, II, and III

19. Which trace element should be reduced or removed in patients with cholestasis who are receiving parenteral nutrition?

    A. Zinc
    B. Chromium
    C. Selenium

D. Copper

E. Iodine

20. A 70-year-old female who has mild congestive heart failure, GERD, type II diabetes mellitus, and rheumatoid arthritis had a recent CVA. She will not regain her premorbid degree of mental status, so it is decided to give her long-term nutritional support. Which method would be most appropriate for this patient?

   A. Central parenteral nutrition
   B. Nasogastric tube feeding
   C. Peripheral parenteral nutrition
   D. Jejunostomy tube feeding
   E. Nasoduodenal tube feeding

21. A common cause of diarrhea in patients receiving enteral nutrition is from the

   A. osmotic load of the enteral nutrition formulation
   B. sorbitol in drug vehicles
   C. addition of fiber to the enteral nutrition formulation
   D. solute load from the protein component of the enteral nutrition formulation
   E. improper placement of a nasogastric feeding tube

22. What is the drug of choice for enhancing gastric emptying in a patient receiving enteral nutrition support?

   A. Bismuth subsalicylate
   B. Azithromycin
   C. Metoclopramide
   D. Loperamide
   E. Acyclovir

23. A patient is receiving phenytoin capsules 300 mg each day for seizure control. She requires tube feeding with a 1 kcal/mL formulation at 85 mL/h (2000 mL/d). What would be the most appropriate intervention to maintain a therapeutic drug concentration and maintain the required nutrition support?

   I. Increase the dose of phenytoin to 600 mg/d.
   II. Hold the enteral nutrition 2 hours before and after the dose.
   III. Increase the enteral nutrition to 100 mL/h x 20 hours.

   A. I only
   B. III only

C. I and II only
D. II and III only
E. I, II, and III

24. What is the mechanism for grapefruit juice to inhibit the metabolism of some drugs that can result in drug toxicity?

   A. Decreased renal excretion of drug
   B. Inhibition of gastrointestinal cytochrome P450-3A4
   C. Decreased systemic clearance of drug
   D. Inhibition of hepatic cytochrome P450-3A4
   E. Expanded apparent volume of distribution

Answers

1. **D.** Calcium requirements are 1000 mg/d for male adults until age 65, when they increase to 1200-1500 mg/d. Calcium requirements are 1000 mg/d for female adults until age 50, when they increase to 1200-1500 mg/d.

2. **B.** Skinfold measurements measure body fat stores, which assess the lipid component of the body. Visceral protein stores are serum proteins. Body cell mass and somatic protein stores assess skeletal muscle and visceral organs. Immune competence assessment requires a skin test with a common antigen.

3. **D.** All measurements of nutritional assessment are depressed (ie, weight for height, anthropometric measurements, and biochemical serum markers of protein status).

4. **A.** Catabolism is related to loss of body protein. Since it is increased, the patient would be considered hypermetabolic in this case.

5. **C.** Lean body mass includes bone, skeletal muscle, visceral organs, and extracellular solids. Body cell mass includes only the lean, metabolically active tissue like skeletal muscle and visceral organs (eg, liver).

6. **D.** $D_{20}W$ = 20 g/100 mL = 200 g/L x 2.5 L/d = 500 g/d x 3.4 kcal/g = 1700 kcal/d.

7. **E.** 5% amino acids = 5 g/100 mL = 50 g/L x 2.5 L/d = 125 g/d.

8. **C.** Intravenous lipid emulsion 20% = 2 kcal/mL x 240 mL/d = 480 kcal/d.

9. **E.** The nitrogen intake is calculated by dividing the protein intake (125 g) by 6.25, which results in 20 g. The nitrogen output would be the sum of the urinary urea nitrogen and insensible losses (12 g + 4 g = 16 g/d). Therefore, the nitrogen balance would be 20 g – 16 g = 4 g. A nitrogen balance of +4 would be suggestive of nutritional adequacy with this PN formulation.

10. **C.** Water requirements are 30-40 mL/kg/d for patients without extra-renal fluid losses: 60 kg x 40 mL/kg/d = 2400 mL/d.

11. **A.** It is difficult to feed patients with severe pancreatitis enterally unless there is access to the small bowel (eg, jejunostomy). The other clinical conditions like trauma and burns would occur in patients in whom the gastrointestinal tract could and should be used for nutrition support. A patient receiving laparoscopic cholecystectomy would not need nutrition support. Most patients with hepatic encephalopathy can be fed enterally if they require nutrition support.

12. **E.** The dose of dextrose in PN should never exceed 5 mg/kg/min in adult patients. This can be converted to 25 kcal/kg/d.

13. **D.** Acetate is converted to bicarbonate in the liver and would thus help or at least not exacerbate the metabolic acidosis.

14. **A.** Calcium phosphate is a relatively insoluble compound, so manufacturer guidelines for the concentrations of these two elements must be followed closely to prevent precipitation. The order of mixing these components in the PN formulation is also important.

15. **B.** Folic acid should be given at a dose of at least 600 mcg/d during pregnancy. Many practitioners administer 1 mg/d above what the patient is eating or receiving via nutrition support. This has been shown to prevent neural tube defects in the newborn.

16. **C.** Hyperosmolar nutrients (dextrose, amino acids) can be used to concentrate the PN formulation, but it would have to be administered via a central vein.

17. **D.** If calcium is added last, the PN formulation will contain the final volume including all other nutrients. The chance of calcium causing a precipitate will be decreased since all other components (eg, phosphorus) are diluted in the entire volume of the PN.

18. **E.** A 0.22-micron filter will do all three. In contrast, a 1.2-micron filter (used with TNAs) will not filter most bacteria.

19. **D.** Copper is excreted via the biliary tract. Patients with severe cholestasis should have copper removed during short-term parenteral nutrition. In long-term PN, copper may be required in reduced doses to prevent anemia. Serum copper concentrations should be monitored regularly in long-term patients who have cholestasis.

20. **D.** She is not a candidate for long-term PN because her gastrointestinal tract would be accessible and functional. Nasogastric and nasoduodenal methods are only used for short-term use of enteral nutrition. A jejunostomy would be ideal because she also has GERD and perhaps gastroparesis from her diabetes.

21. **B.** Several liquid preparations for drugs contain sorbitol as a pharmaceutical vehicle. These liquid preparations are commonly used in patients with tubes because the drugs can be given easily this way, especially if the patient cannot swallow. Most enteral nutrition formulations are close to being isotonic, ie, the osmotic load or solute load are not big factors in causing diarrhea. Fiber will prevent or improve diarrhea in most cases.

22. **C.** Metoclopramide enhances gastric emptying and is used commonly in patients with gastro-intestinal intolerance. This is true in both diabetics and nondiabetics.

23. **D.** Phenytoin absorption is markedly impaired when it is given concurrently with enteral tube feeding. The enteral tube feeding should be held 2 hours before and after the daily dose of phenytoin capsules. To maintain the current dose of enteral nutrition, the rate of feeding should be increased to 100 mL/h x 20 h (2000 mL/d).

24. **B.** Drugs such as amlodipine, carbamazepine, and cyclosporine are profoundly metabolized in the gastrointestinal tract before absorption. Grapefruit juice from frozen concentrate has been shown to inhibit gastrointestinal CYP 450-3A4 and thus allows more of the drug to be absorbed. This has caused drug toxicity for drugs with a narrow therapeutic index.

7. References

Brown RO, Dickerson RN. Drug-nutrient interactions. *Am J Managed Care.* 1999;5:345-351.

Brown RO. Parenteral and enteral nutrition in adult patients. In: Herfindal ET, Gourley DR, eds. *Textbook of Therapeutics: Drug and Disease Management,* 7th ed. Philadelphia: Lippincott, Williams & Wilkins; 2001:193-211.

Chessman KH, Teasley-Strausburg KM. Assessment of nutrition status and nutrition requirements. In: Dipiro JT, Talbert RL, eds. *Pharmacotherapy: A Pathophysiologic Approach,* 5th ed. New York: McGraw-Hill; 2002:2445-2463.

DeHart RM, Worthington MA. Nutritional considerations in major organ failure. In: Dipiro JT, Talbert RL, eds. *Pharmacotherapy: A Pathophysiologic Approach,* 5th ed. New York: McGraw-Hill; 2002:2519-2542.

Guidelines for the use of parenteral and enteral nutrition in adult and pediatric patients. *J Parenter Enteral Nutr.* 2002;26(1 Suppl):1SA-138SA.

Janson DD, Chessman KH. Enteral nutrition. In: Dipiro JT, Talbert RL, eds. *Pharmacotherapy: A Pathophysiologic Approach,* 5th ed. New York: McGraw-Hill; 2002:2495-2517.

Malone M. General nutrition. In: Herfindal ET, Gourley DR, eds. *Textbook of Therapeutics: Drug and Disease Management,* 7th ed. Philadelphia: Lippincott, Williams & Wilkins; 2001:163-174.

Mattox TW. Parenteral nutrition. In: Dipiro JT, Talbert RL, eds. *Pharmacotherapy: A Pathophysiologic Approach,* 5th ed. New York: McGraw-Hill; 2002:2475-2494.

Reiter PD, Sacks G. Prevalence and significance of malnutrition. In: Dipiro JT, Talbert RL, eds. *Pharmacotherapy: A Pathophysiologic Approach,* 5th ed. New York: McGraw-Hill; 2002:2465-2474.

Task Force for the Revision of Safe Practices for Parenteral Nutrition. Safe practices for parenteral nutrition. *J Parenter Enteral Nutr.* 2004;28:S39-S70.

Van Den Berghe G, Wouters P, Weekers F, et al. Intensive insulin therapy in critically ill patients. *N Engl J Med.* 2001;345:1359-1367.

19. Oncology

J. Aubrey Waddell, PharmD, FAPhA, BCOP
Associate Professor
University of Tennessee College of Pharmacy - Knoxville
Oncology Pharmacist
Blount Memorial Hospital
Maryville, TN

Contents

1. Overview

Definition

- Oncology can be defined as the science dealing with the etiology, pathogenesis, and treatment of cancers (synonymous with malignant neoplasms).
- It encompasses more than 100 different diseases that share characteristics of uncontrollable cell proliferation, invasion of local tissues, and metastases (eg, spread from original site).
- In the United States, men have roughly a 1 in 2 cumulative lifetime risk of developing cancer and women have a 1 in 3 risk. In 2007, approximately 1,444,920 new cases of cancer will develop and 559,650 cancer deaths will occur. The most common types of cancer are prostate, lung, and colorectal in men and breast, lung, and colorectal in women.

Classifications

- Neoplastic malignancies arise from four tissue types (epithelial, connective, lymphoid, and nerve) and are classified based on this origin. Table 1 lists the tis-

Table 1

Tissue Origin of Malignant Tumor Types

Origin	Tissue type	Malignant tumor
Epithelial	Surface epithelium	Carcinoma
	Glandular tissue	Adenocarcinoma
Connective	Fibrous	Fibrosarcoma
	Bone	Osteosarcoma
	Smooth/striated muscle	Leiomyosarcoma/ rhabdomyosarcoma
	Fat	Liposarcoma
Lymphoid	Bone marrow	Leukemia
	Lymphoid	Hodgkin, non-Hodgkin lymphoma
	Plasma	Multiple myeloma
Neural	Glial	Glioblastoma, astrocytoma
	Nerve sheath	Neurofibrosarcoma
	Melanocytes	Malignant melanoma
Mixed	Gonadal tissue	Teratocarcinoma

Adapted from Balmer et al, 2002.

Table 2

Warning Signs of Cancer in Adults

Change in bowel or bladder habits
A sore that does not heal
Unusual bleeding or discharge
Thickening of lump in breast or elsewhere
Indigestion or difficulty swallowing
Obvious change in wart or mole
Nagging cough or hoarseness

sue origin of each type of malignancy and the corresponding medical terminology.

Clinical Presentation

- The first signs and symptoms of cancer develop when the tumor has grown to approximately 10^9 cells (1 cm in diameter or 1 g mass).
- The type of cancer determines the presentation of signs and symptoms, which vary widely across tumor types.
- Positive screening tests (see section on nondrug therapy) or generalized signs of anorexia, fatigue, fever, weight loss, and anemia must also be evaluated.
- Tables 2 and 3 show the American Cancer Society's seven warning signs of cancer for adults and the warning signs for children.

Pathophysiology and Etiology

- Cancer promoting factors include:
  - * External factors: tobacco, chemicals, radiation, infectious organisms, diet

Table 3

Warning Signs of Cancer in Children

Continued, unexplained weight loss
Headaches with vomiting in the morning
Increased swelling or persistent pain in bones or joints
Lump or mass in abdomen, neck, or elsewhere
Development of a whitish appearance in the pupil of the eye
Recurrent fevers not caused by infection
Excessive bruising or bleeding
Noticeable paleness or prolonged tiredness

* Internal factors: genetics, hormones, immune conditions
* Development of cancer is genetically regulated and is a multistage process:
    * Initiation: normal cells are exposed to chemical, physical, or biological carcinogens. This results in irreversible damage, genetic mutations, and selective growth advantages.
    * Promotion: reversible environmental changes favor the growth of the mutated cells.
    * Transformation: the cells become cancerous.
    * Progression: additional genetic changes occur resulting in increased cancerous proliferation. Tumors invade local tissues and metastasis occurs.
* Genetic alterations are necessary for the development and growth of cancer. Some of the most common are:
    * Oncogenes promote growth advantages in mutated cells and cause excessive proliferation (eg, ras, c-myc).
    * Inactivation of tumor suppressor genes (TSGs) results in inappropriate cell growth, as TSGs normally regulate the cell cycle (eg, p53).
    * Activation of anti-apoptotic genes (eg, bcl-2).
    * Reduced activity of DNA repair genes.
* Malignant tumor cells do not resemble their tissue of origin (in contrast to benign tumors). They are unstable and are incapable of performing normal cell functions.

Diagnostic Criteria

* A sample of suspected malignant tissues or cells is needed for a definitive diagnosis. This can be done with a biopsy, fine-needle aspiration, or exfoliative cytology.
* Radiation or chemotherapy should not begin without pathological staging. Further pathological imaging may include:
    * Chest x-ray: evaluates spread to bones or lungs
    * Computed tomography (CT): assesses the size, shape, and position of tumor; detects masses in lymph nodes, brain, or adrenal glands via a three-dimensional view
    * Magnetic resonance imaging (MRI): evaluates spread to the brain or spinal cord
    * Positron emission tomography (PET): evaluates lymph and other metastatic involvement
    * Bone scanning: assesses for the presence of bone metastasis
* Laboratory work may include: complete blood counts (CBCs), blood chemistries, and tumor markers (see section on nondrug therapy).
* If a diagnosis of cancer is made, the malignancy will need to be staged or categorized based on severity of the disease and the results of the pathological staging tests. Staging guides the oncology practitioner in determining the prognosis and the treatment regimen for the patient.
    * The TNM staging system is the most commonly used tool for solid tumors. Tumors are scored numerically based on the size of the tumor (T), the extent of lymph node involvement (N), and presence or absence of metastases (M). This allows classification of tumors by stage, from stage 0 to stage IV, with stage IV denoting the presence of metastasis (eg, most severe disease). A stage 0 tumor is called a carcinoma *in situ*, where the malignancy has not yet invaded the basement membrane of the epithelial surface.
    * Lymphoid tumors are staged differently and are beyond the scope of this review. Refer to Balmer et al, 2002, Chaps. 129, 131, and 132, for more information.

Treatment Principles and Goals

* Treatment regimens are based on the type of cancer, stage, the age of the patient, and other prognostic factors (eg, presence of a tumor marker, poor performance status, and ethnicity, among others).
* Primary therapy is the initial and mainstay approach to treat cancer. It usually consists of removal of the tumor or debulking through surgery.
* *Neoadjuvant therapy* is therapy given prior to the primary therapy. The goal is to shrink the tumor, thereby increasing the efficacy of the primary treatment. Examples include chemotherapy or radiation.
* *Adjuvant therapy* is additional therapy given after the main treatment. The goal is to make sure that all residual disease has been eradicated.
* The four main cancer treatments include: surgery, radiation, chemotherapy, and biologic therapy. Most regimens are a combination of modalities.
    * Surgery alone is reserved for solid localized tumors, where the entire cancer can be resected. It may also be combined with other modalities in later stages of disease. This is not an option for patients with lymphoid-based disease (eg, Hodgkin disease).
    * Radiation alone is also reserved for curing localized tumors, as it treats a very focused area. It also can be combined with other treatments as neoadjuvant or adjuvant therapy to reduce disease-related symptoms or to reduce the incidence of disease recurrence.
    * Chemotherapy is a means of systemic treatment, in contrast to the two types of local treatment just described. It can be used to treat the primary tumor as well as metastases. This is

generally not administered to patients with local disease that can be fully resected.

* Biologic therapy is another systemic treatment and includes agents such as monoclonal antibodies, interferons, interleukins, and tumor vaccines. It is a new type of treatment and acts by stimulating the host immune system.

- The goals of cancer therapy are based on the type and stage of cancer, as well patient characteristics (eg, an older patient with a short life expectancy may not be offered intense treatment that may impair quality of life).
  - * *Localized or regional disease* (ie, stages 0, I, II, and early III): curative intent, inhibit recurrence of disease
    - Stage 0 diseases are often not treated, but monitored until clinically apparent.
  - * *Advanced or metastasized disease* (ie, advanced stage III and all stage IV): palliate symptoms, reduce tumor load, prolong survival, and increase quality of life

Survival and response to treatment

- In 2007, more than 1500 people a day will die of a cancer, which accounts for one in four deaths.
- Survival depends on patient characteristics, type of disease, stage of disease, and treatment regimen. Older patients with more severe disease, a poor performance status, and faster-growing tumors have a poor prognosis.
- Response to treatment modalities for solid tumors are classified as:
  - * Cure: 5 years of cancer-free survival for most tumor types
  - * Complete response (CR): absence of all neoplastic disease for a minimum of 1 month after cessation of treatment
  - * Partial response (PR): ≥50% decrease in tumor size or other disease markers for a minimum of 1 month
  - * Stable disease: no change or criteria for PR or progression are not met
  - * Progression: ≥25% increase in tumor size or new lesion
- Response to treatment for hematologic cancers are measured by the elimination of abnormal cells, a decrease in tumor markers to normal, and the improved function of affected cells.

2. Drug Therapy

Chemotherapy

- Chemotherapeutic agents have a very narrow therapeutic index and a toxic side-effect profile.
- They are generally more effective in combination due to synergism through biochemical interactions.
  - * It is important to choose drugs with different mechanisms of action, resistance, and toxicity profiles to get the full benefit of combination therapy.
- Chemotherapy has the greatest effect on rapidly-dividing cells, as most of the potent chemotherapy drugs act by damaging DNA.
  - * These agents are more active in different phases of the cell cycle. A therapeutic effect is seen on cancer cells, but adverse effects are also seen on human cells that rapidly divide (eg, hair follicles, gastrointestinal tract, blood cells).
  - * Agents can be phase-specific or phase-nonspecific. Nonspecific agents are effective in all phases.

Cell Cycle Phase

- G_0 = resting phase: no cell division occurs and cancer cells are generally not susceptible to chemotherapy. This is problematic for slow-growing tumors that exist primarily in this phase.
- G_1 = postmitotic phase: enzymes for DNA synthesis are manufactured; lasts 10-24 hours.
- S = DNA synthesis phase: DNA separation and replication occurs; lasts 10-20 hours.
- G_2 = premitotic phase: specialized proteins and RNA are made; lasts 2-10 hours.
- M = mitosis: actual cell division occurs; lasts 30-60 minutes.

Drug Classes

There are numerous chemotherapy agents. Drugs are grouped by class. Please refer to the corresponding table for each class of drugs.

Alkylating agents (Table 4)
Mechanism of action
- Covalent bond formation of drugs to nucleic acids and proteins; results in the cross-linking of one or two DNA strands and inhibition of DNA replication. These are non–phase specific agents. The most commonly used agents include: cyclophosphamide (C), ifosfamide (I), carmustine, dacarbazine, and temozolomide.

Table 4

Alkylating Agents

Generic name (trade name)	Dosage range	Dosage forms	Frequency	Diseases[1]
Nitrogen mustard				
Mechlorethamine (Mustargen®)	6-10 mg/m^2	IV	Days 1, 8	HL, NHL
Cyclophosphamide (Cytoxan , Neosar®)	500-2000 mg/m^2, 40-500 mg/m^2	IV, PO	qd 2-5 days, qd	ALL, CLL, HL, NHL, myeloma, testis, neuroblastoma, breast, ovary, lung, cervix
Ifosfamide (Ifex®)	1.2 g/m^2, 4 g/m^2	IV	qd x 5 days q 3 wk, qd x 6 d	HL, NHL, lung, bladder, sarcoma
Melphalan (Alkeran®)	16 mg/m^2, 6 mg	IV, PO	q 2 wk x 4, 2-3 wk	Myeloma, breast, ovary
Chlorambucil (Leukeran®)	0.1-0.2 mg/kg	PO	qd x 3-6 wk	CLL, HL, NHL
Ethylenimines and methylmelamines				
Altretamine (Hexalen®)	260 mg/m^2	PO	qd x 14-21 d	Ovarian
Thiotepa (Thioplex®)	10-20 mg/m^2	IV	q 3-4 wk	Bladder, breast, ovarian, HL, NHL
Alkyl sulfonates				
Busulfan (Myleran , Busulfex®)	4-8 mg/kg	IV, PO	qd	CML, BMT
Nitrosureas				
Carmustine (BICNU)	150-200 mg/m^2	IV,	q 6 wk	HL, NHL, brain, myeloma
Streptozocin (Zanosar)	500 mg/m^2	IV	qd 5 d	Islet cell carcinoma
Polifeprosan 20 with carmustine implant (Gliadel®)	7.7-mg implant	—	Implant	Glioblastoma multiforme

[1]Does not indicate FDA approval.

ALL, acute lymphocytic leukemia; BMT, bone marrow transplant; CLL, chronic lymphocytic leukemia; CML, chronic myelogenous leukemia; HL, Hodgkin lymphoma; NHL, non-Hodgkin lymphoma.

Patient instructions and counseling

- All drugs are carcinogenic, teratogenic, and mutagenic. Medications may cause sterility. Let your dentist know you are on chemotherapy, due to an increased risk of bleeding and infections. Hydration and mesna therapy are recommended for C and I. Let your doctor know if you have burning upon urination.

Adverse drug events

- Myelosuppression, primarily leukopenia; mucosal ulceration; pulmonary fibrosis (carmustine) and interstitial pneumonitis; alopecia; nausea and vomiting; amenorrhea and azoospermia; hemorrhagic cystitis with C and I; encephalopathy with I; seizures (polifeprosan/carmustine).

Drug interactions

- Drugs with specific interactions of moderate to major severity include:
  * Altretamine: tricyclic antidepressants, monoamine oxidase inhibitors
  * Busulfan: itraconazole, phenytoin, acetaminophen
  * Carmustine: cimetidine, ethyl alcohol, phenytoin, amphotericin B
  * Cyclophosphamide: allopurinol, barbiturates, digoxin, phenytoin, warfarin
  * Ifosfamide: allopurinol, phenytoin, warfarin
  * Streptozocin: nephrotoxic agents

Monitoring parameters

- Pulmonary function tests; renal and hepatic tests; chest x-ray; CBC with differential (baseline and expected nadir prior to next cycle) and electrolytes; urinalysis for RBC detection from hemorrhagic cystitis; signs of bleeding (bruising, melena); infection (sore throat, fever); nausea or vomiting

Antimetabolites: S-phase–specific (Table 5)
Mechanism of action

- Structural analogues of natural metabolites. Act by falsely inserting themselves in place of a pyrimidine or purine ring, causing an interference in nucleic acid synthesis. Phase-specific agents are most active

Table 5

Antimetabolites

Generic name (trade name)	Dosage range	Dosage forms	Frequency	Disease[1]
Folic acid antagonists	500-600 mg/m²	IV	q 21 d	Malignant mesothelioma,
Pemitrexed (Alimta®)	10-100 mg/m², 1-2,	IV, PO, IM, SC,	qd	NSCLC Breast, NHL,
Methotrexate	10-12 mg/m²	intrathecal,		sarcoma, ALL
(Rheumatrex®)		intra-arterial		
Pyrimidine analogs	75-100 mg/m²	SC	qd x 7 d	Myelodysplastic syndrome
Azacitidine (Vidaza®)	450 mg/m²	IV	qd x 5 d	Colorectal, breast, head,
Fluorouracil, 5-FU	100-300 mg/m², 50 mg	IV, intrathecal	qd x 7 d, q 14d	neck
(Adrucil®)				ALL, AML, CML
Cytarabine (Cytosar-U®,	2500 mg/m²	PO	qd x 14 d q 3 wk	
DepoCyt®)	1000-1250 mg/m²	IV	q wk	Breast, colorectal
Capecitabine (Xeloda®)	15 mg/m²	IV	q8h x 3 d, q 6W	Pancreatic, NSCLC, bladder
Gemcitabine (Gemzar®)				Myelodysplastic syndrome
Decitabine (Dacogen®)	52 mg/m²	IV	qd x 5 d	
	1.5-2.5 mg/kg	PO	qd	Acute lymphoblastic
Purine analogs				leukemia (pediatric)
Clofarabine (Clolar®)	2-3 mg/kg	PO	qd	ALL
Mercaptopurine	4 mg/m²	IV	q 2 wk	ALL, AML
(Purinethol®)	0.09-0.1 mg/kg	IV	qd x 7 d	CLL, hairy cell leukemia, ALL
Thioguanine (Tabloid®)	25 mg/m²	IV	qd x 5 d	NHL, hairy cell leukemia,
Pentostatin (Nipent®)				CLL
Cladribine (Leustatin®)				CLL, NHL
Fludarabine (Fludara®)				
Guanosine Analogs	Children: 650	IV	qd xd, q 21 d	T-cell ALL/NHL
Nelarabine (Arranon®)	mg/m²/day			
	Adults: 1500	IV	d 1, 3, 5, q 21 d	
	mg/m²/day			

[1]Does not indicate FDA approval.

ALL, acute lymphocytic leukemia; AML, acute myelogenous leukemia; CLL, chronic lymphocytic leukemia; CML, chronic myelogenous leukemia; NHL, non-Hodgkin lymphoma; NSCLC, non–small cell lung cancer.

in the S phase and in tumors with a high growth fraction. They are subdivided into three groups: folate, purine, and pyrimidine antagonists.

Patient instructions and counseling
- Avoid crowds and sick people. You may be asked to chew ice if receiving fluorouracil (5-FU). This is to reduce damage to the mucosal lining in your mouth. Contact your MD if you have uncontrollable nausea or vomiting, excessive diarrhea, or pain, swelling, or tingling in palms and soles of feet (hand-foot syndrome). Call your doctor if you feel dizzy, lightheaded, or have trouble urinating (clofarabine). You should be receiving folic acid and vitamin B_{12} injections if you are receiving pemetrexed.
- Nelarabine may cause sleepiness and dizziness.

Adverse drug events
- Hand-foot syndrome, stomatitis (5-FU, capecitabine); severe diarrhea, GI mucosal damage, nausea, vomiting, fatigue, myelosuppression, alopecia, neurotoxicity (nelarabine, cytarabine, fludarabine, methotrexate); rash and fever, flu-like symptoms (gemcitabine); renal toxicity, mucositis (5-FU, methotrexate); conjunctivitis (cytarabine); hemolytic uremic syndrome (gemcitabine); opportunistic infections (cladribine, fludarabine); tumor

lysis syndrome, systemic inflammatory response syndrome (SIRS), or capillary leak with clofarabine.

Interactions
- Specific interactions include:
  - * Capecitabine: warfarin, phenytoin
  - * Cytarabine: digoxin
  - * Fluorouracil: warfarin
  - * Mercaptopurine: warfarin, allopurinol
  - * Methotrexate: NSAIDs, amiodarone, amoxicillin, sulfasalazine, doxycycline, erythromycin, hydrochlorothiazide, mercaptopurine, omeprazole, phenytoin, folic acid
  - * Pentostatin: cyclophosphamide, fludarabine

Monitoring parameters
- Note any complaints of mucositis or mouth soreness, monitor for neurotoxicity (eg, ask the patient to write their name); CBC with differential prior to each dose of drug; hepatic and renal function; monitor for tingling or swelling of palms and soles of hands and feet; bruising or bleeding; INR (capecitabine); monitor weight and question patient

about diarrhea, jaundice, and hepatomegaly (mercaptopurine). Continuous IV fluids and allopurinol should be administered for clofarabine patients and prophylactic corticosteroids for SIRS and capillary leak. Plasma homocysteine with pemetrexed, and dexamethasone should be given to prevent cutaneous reactions.

Antitumor antibiotics: (Table 6)
Mechanism of action
- Anthracyclines block DNA and RNA transcription through the intercalation (insertion) of adjoining nucleic acid pairs in DNA, which results in DNA strand breakage. They also inhibit the topoisomerase II enzyme. Mitomycin is an alklyating-like agent that cross-links DNA. Dactinomycin blocks RNA synthesis. Bleomycin inhibits DNA synthesis in mitosis and G_2 stages of growth. Bleomycin is the only cell cycle–specific agent.

Patient instructions and counseling
- Contact doctor for fast, slow, or irregular heartbeats and/or breathing difficulties; anthracyclines may cause a change of urine color or whites of eyes to a

Table 6

Antitumor Antibiotics

Generic name (trade name)	Dosage range	Dosage forms	Frequency	Disease[1]
Anthracyclines				
Doxorubicin (Adriamycin®, Doxil® [liposomal])	60-75 mg/m², 20-50 mg/m² (lipo)	IV	q 3 wk	ALL, AML, NHL, HL, solid tumors of every major organ
Daunorubicin (Cerubidine®, Daunoxome® [liposomal])	45 mg/m², 40-100 mg/m² (lipo)	IV	qd x 3 d, q 2-3 wk	ALL, AML, NHL
Epirubicin (Ellence®, Pharmarubicin®)	60-120 mg/m²	IV	q 3 wk	Breast, bladder, lung, ovarian, gastric
Idarubicin (Idamycin®)	12 mg/m²	IV	qd x 3 d	AML, ALL, breast
Mitoxantrone (Novantrone®)	12-14 mg/m²	IV	qd x 3 d	Prostate, NHL, AML, breast
Valrubicin (Valstar®)	800 mg	Intravesically	q wk x 6 wk	Bladder
Alkylating-like				
Mitomycin (Mutamycin®)	10-20 mg/m²	IV	q 6-8 wk	Bladder, breast, NSCLC, cervix, pancreatic, colon
Chromomycin				
Dactinomycin (Cosmegen®)	12-15 mcg/kg	IV	qd x 5 d	Wilms', testis, sarcoma
Miscellaneous				
Bleomycin (Blenoxane®)	10-20 USP U/m²/wk	IV, IM, SC	q wk	HL, NHL, testis, head, neck, lung, skin

[1]Does not indicate FDA approval.

ALL, acute lymphocytic leukemia; AML, acute myelogenous leukemia; HL, Hodgkin lymphoma; NHL, non-Hodgkin lymphoma; NSCLC, non–small cell lung cancer.

bluish-green or orangish-red. Bleomycin may cause a change in skin color or nail growth.

Adverse drug events

- Severe nausea and vomiting, alopecia, and stomatitis; anthracyclines: cardiac toxicity, acute or chronic (doxorubicin = daunorubicin > idarubicin > epirubicin > mitoxantrone). All anthracyclines have limits on cumulative lifetime dosing, are vesicants, and are associated with secondary acute myelogenous leukemia (AML); avoid in patients with a cardiac history. Myelosuppression risk with all agents, although mitomycin demonstrates a delayed effect. Dactinomycin: renal toxicity, leukopenia, increased pigmentation of previously radiated skin; bleomycin: pulmonary fibrosis and interstitial pneumonitis

Interactions

- Specific interactions include:
  * Bleomycin: phenytoin, digoxin
  * Doxorubicin: cisplatin, digoxin, paclitaxel, phenytoin, phenobarbital, trastuzumab, zidovudine
  * Epirubicin: cimetidine, trastuzumab
  * Idarubicin: probenecid, trastuzumab

Monitoring parameters

- Hepatic, renal, CBC with differential monitoring; pulmonary function tests pre- and post-treatment with bleomycin; cardiac monitoring via left ventricular ejection fraction (LVEF) measurements for anthracyclines as well as monitoring the cumulative lifetime dose; extravasation and necrosis with anthracyclines. Adjust anthracycline dosing based on elevated total bilirubin.

Pharmacokinetics

- Anthracyclines are extensively bound in the tissue, have large volumes of distribution and long half-lives, and are excreted in the bile. They need dosing adjustments in hepatic impairment. Bleomycin is renally excreted and needs dosing adjustments in impaired patients.

Other

- Lifetime doses of doxorubicin should not exceed 450-550 mg/m^2, taking into account other anthracycline agents received; lifetime maximum of epirubicin is 900 mg/m^2, idarubicin <150 mg/m^2.

Hormones and antagonists (Table 7)
Mechanism of action

- A diverse group of compounds that act on hormone-dependent tumors by inhibiting or decreasing the production of the disease-causing hormone.

Patient instructions and counseling

- Avoid use in pregnant women; several agents may cause weight gain and menstrual irregularities in women. Be aware of leg swelling or tenderness (eg, signs of a deep vein thrombosis), breathing problems, and sweating. Transient muscle or bone pain, problems urinating, and spinal cord compression may occur initially in patients receiving LHRH agonists. Take exemestane after meals.

Adverse drug events

- Edema, menstrual disorders, hot flashes, transient muscle or bone pain, tumor flare, transient increase in serum testosterone (LHRH) thromboembolic events, gynecomastia, elevated liver enzymes, nausea and vomiting, diarrhea, erectile impotence, decreased libido, endometrial cancers with tamoxifen, bone loss (LHRH, aromatase inhibitors); black box warning for hypotension and syncope with abarelix; also risk of ventricular arrhythmias and QT prolongation

Interactions

- Specific interactions include:
  * Abarelix: amiodarone, procainamide, quinidine, sotalol
  * Aminoglutethimide: dexamethasone, warfarin, tamoxifen, theophylline
  * Bicalutamide: warfarin
  * Flutamide: warfarin
  * Megestrol: dofetilide contraindication
  * Medroxyprogesterone acetate: aminoglutethimide, rifampin
  * Nilutamide: alcohol
  * Tamoxifen: anticoagulants, cyclophosphamide
  * Toremifene: cyytochrome P450 (CYP450) 3A4 inducers (carbemazepine, phenytoin)
  * Fluoxymesterone: cyclosporine, anticoagulants, valerian

Monitoring parameters

- Check WBCs with differential, platelets, liver function tests, thyroid function, and serum creatinine regularly. Note any weight changes, abnormal vaginal bleeding, body or bone pain, galactorrhea, or decreased libido. Monitor for embolic disorders and uterine cancer (in females). Check PSA and testosterone levels in males; bone mineral density for LHRH agonist and aromatase inhibitors.

Pharmacokinetics

- The majority of agents are available orally with longer half-lives, allowing once-daily dosing.

Table 7

Hormones and Antagonists

Generic name (trade name)	Dosage range	Dosage forms	Frequency	Disease[1]
Adrenocorticoids				
Aminoglutethimide (Cytadren®)	250 mg	PO	qd	Adrenal, breast, prostate
Progestins				
Megestrol acetate (Megace®)	40 mg, 40-320 mg	PO	qid, qd divided	Breast, endometrial
Medroxyprogesterone acetate (Provera , Depo-Provera®)	400-1000 mg	IM	qw	Endometrial
Estrogens				
Ethinyl estradiol (Estinyl®)	150 mcg-3 mg, 100 mcg to 1 mg	PO	qd	Prostate, breast
Antiestrogen				
Tamoxifen (Nolvadex®)	20-40 mg	PO	qd	Breast
Fulvestrant (Faslodex®)	250 mg	IM	q mo	Breast
Toremifene (Fareston®)	60 mg	PO	qd	Breast
Aromatase inhibitors				
Exemestane (Aromasin®)	25 mg	PO	qd	Breast
Anastrozole (Arimidex®)	1 mg	PO	qd	Breast
Letrozole (Femara®)	2.5 mg	PO	qd	Breast
Androgens				
Testosterone propionate (Delatestryl®)	200-400 mg	IM	qd	Breast
Fluoxymesterone (Halotestin®)	10-40 mg	PO	q 2-4 wk	Breast
Antiandrogens				
Flutamide (Eulexin®)	750 mg	PO	tid	Prostate
Bicalutamide (Casodex®)	50 mg	PO	qd	Prostate
Nilutamide (Nilandron®)	300 mg	PO	qd	Prostate
LHRH agonists				
Triptorelin (Trelstar®)	3.75, 11.25 mg	IM	q 28 d, q 34 d	Prostate
Leuprolide (Lupron®, Eligard®)	7.5, 22.5, 30 mg	IM, SC	q mo, q 3 mo, q 4 mo	Prostate, breast
Goserelin (Zoladex®)	3.6, 10.8 mg	SC	q mo, q 3 mo	Prostate, breast
GNRH agonist				
Abarelix (Plenaxis®)	100 mg	IM	q 2 w	Prostate

[1]Does not indicate FDA approval.

GNRH, gonadotropin-releasing hormone; LHRH, luteinizing hormone–releasing hormone.

Other

• Agents are often contraindicated if the patient has more than one hormone-dependent tumor. With the exception of tamoxifen and LHRH agonists, the majority of agents are not indicated for first-line therapy.

Plant alkaloids (Table 8)

Mechanism of action

• Inhibit the replication of cancerous cells; taxanes and vincas interfere with microtubule assembly in the M phase; camptothecins and epipodophyllotoxins inhibit topoisomerase I and II enzymes, respectively, causing DNA strand breaks. Topoisomerase I and II affect G_2 and S phases, respectively.

Alkaloids

Generic name (trade name)	Dosage range	Dosage forms	Frequency	Disease[1]
Taxanes				
Docetaxel (Taxotere®) gastric	60-100 mg/m²	IV	q 3 wk	NSCLC, breast, ovarian, head, neck, gastric
Paclitaxel (Taxol®)	135-175 mg/m²	IV	q 3 wk	NSCLC, breast, ovarian, head
Paclitaxel (Abraxane®)	260 mg/m²	IV	q w wk	Breast
Epipodophyllotoxins				
Etoposide (VePesid®)	100 mg/m², 50 mg/m²	IV, PO	qd x 4-5 d, qd x 21 d	SCLC, testis, NSCLC
Teniposide (Vumon®)	165 mg/m²	IV	q wk x 4 doses	ALL, SCLC
Camptothecins				
Irinotecan (Camptosar®)	100-125 mg/m²	IV	q wk x 4 doses	Colorectal, NSCLC, SCLC
Topotecan (Hycamtin®)	1.5 mg/m²	IV	qd x 5 d q 21 d	Ovarian, lung, AML, cervical
Vinca alkaloids				
Vincristine (Oncovin®)	1.4 mg/m²	IV	q wk	ALL, HL, NHL, CLL
Vinblastine (Velban®)	6 mg/m²	IV	q wk	HL, NHL, testis
Vinorelbine (Navelbine®)	25-30 mg/m²	IV	q wk	NSCLC, breast, ovarian

[1]Does not indicate FDA approval.

ALL, acute lymphocytic leukemia; CLL, chronic lymphocytic leukemia; HL, Hodgkin lymphoma; NHL, non-Hodgkin lymphoma; NSCLC, non–small cell lung cancer; SCLC, small cell lung cancer.

Patient instructions and counseling
- Contact doctor for uncontrollable diarrhea (irinotecan), nausea or vomiting, or signs and symptoms of an infection; should receive prophylaxis for emesis, pretreatment for anaphylaxis or peripheral edema (taxanes); you should receive a prescription for loperamide and atropine with irinotecan therapy.

Adverse drug events
- Myelosuppression, mucositis, nausea and vomiting, alopecia, edema (docetaxel); hypotension/hypersensitivity upon administration (paclitaxel); neurotoxicity (vincristine); diarrhea, headache, secondary malignancies (topoisomerase II inhibitors); syndrome of inappropriate ADH secretion (SIADH) (vinca alkaloids)

Interactions
- Specific interactions include:
    * Docetaxel: CYP450 3A4 inducers and inhibitors
    * Etoposide: cyclosporine, St. John's wort, warfarin
    * Irinotecan: St. John's wort
    * Paclitaxel: CYP450 3A4 inducers and inhibitors
    * Teniposide: CYP450 3A4 inducers and inhibitors
    * Vincas: CYP450 3A4 inhibitors; itraconazole, voriconazole
    * Vincristine: phenytoin, l-asparaginase, carbamazepine, digoxin, filgrastim, nifedipine, zidovudine
    * Vinblastine: phenytoin, erythromycin, mitomycin, zidovudine

Monitoring parameters
- Monitor WBCs with differential for all agents; peripheral neuropathy, liver and renal function, painful mouth sores, blood pressure (taxanes and epipodophyllotoxins); acute and late-onset diarrhea or dyspnea on exertion (irinotecan); bilirubin elevations (taxanes and camptothecins); fluid retention (docetaxel); neuropathy, shortness of breath, bronchospasm, and SIADH (vincas)

Pharmacokinetics
- Taxanes and epipodophyllotoxins are extensively bound to plasma and tissues.

Other
- Drug resistance may occur via p-glycoprotein pumps for all agents; topotecan needs dose adjustments for

Table 9

Biologic Response Modifiers and Monoclonal Antibodies

Generic name (trade name)	Dosage range	Dosage forms	Frequency	Disease[2]
Immune therapies				
Aldesleukin (Proleukin®)	600,000 U/kg	IV	q8h x 14 doses	Metastatic renal cell, metastatic melanoma
Interferon-alfa 2b (Intron A®)	10-20 x 10^6 U, 2 x 10^6 U (hairy)	IV and SC	qd x 5 d per wk,[1] 3 x wk x 6 mo	Malignant melanoma, hairy cell leukemia
Thalidomide (Thalomid®)	200 mg	PO	qd	Multiple myeloma, erythema nodosum leprosum
Lenalidomide (Revlimid®)	10 mg	PO	qd	
	25 mg	PO	qd d 1-21 q 28 d	Myelodysplastic syndrome Multiple myeloma
Monoclonal antibodies				
Rituximab (Rituxan®)	375 mg/m^2	IV	q wk x 4-8 doses	NHL, CLL _CD20⊕_
Trastuzumab (Herceptin®)	2-4 mg/kg	IV and SC	q wk	Metastatic breast _HER2⊕_
Gemtuzumab (Mylotarg®)	9 mg/m^2	IV	q 2 wk	AML
Alemtuzumab (Campath®)	3-10 mg	IV	qd, then 30 mg/d 3 x wk	B-cell CLL
Bevacizumab (Avastin®)	5-10 mg/kg	IV	q 2 wk	Colorectal, NSCLC
Cetuximab (Erbitux®)	250-500 mg/m^2	IV	qw x 7 wk	Colorectal, head and neck _rash_
Denileukin diftitox (Ontak®)	9 or 18 mcg/kg	IV	qd x 5 d	T cell lymphoma
Ibritumomab tiuxetan (Zevalin®)[3]				NHL
Tositumomab (Bexxar®)[3]				NHL

[1]Induction dose.

[2]Does not indicate FDA approval.

[3]See package insert for dosing information.

AML, acute myelogenous leukemia; CLL, chronic lymphocytic leukemia; NHL, non-Hodgkin lymphoma.

patients with a CrCl <40 mL/min; vincas are vesicants and need close monitoring for extravasation; vincristine should not be administered intrathecally or in doses higher than 2 mg.

Biologic response modifiers and monoclonal antibodies (Table 9)

Mechanism of action

• Biologic response modifiers activate the body's immune-mediated host defense mechanisms to malignant cells. In contrast to immunotherapy, these agents have direct biological effects on malignancies. Monoclonal antibodies bind to specific antigens and kill malignant cells through the activation of apoptosis, an antibody-mediated toxicity, or complement-mediated lysis.

Patient instructions and counseling

• Let your doctor know if you have severe fatigue, trouble breathing, or irregular heart rhythms. Chills, fever, depression, and flu-like symptoms are common. Taste and smell alterations occur with levamisole. Monoclonal antibodies can cause infusion-related reactions such as fever and chills. If you receive bevacizumab, you should have your blood pressure checked regularly and have tests checking for protein in your urine. You should wear sunscreen and avoid excessive sunlight if receiving cetuximab. You should receive medication for your thyroid if you are going to receive tositumomab. Do not try to conceive until 12 months after finishing therapy for both men and women.

• With thalidomide and lenalidomide, do not get pregnant. Two forms of birth control must be used, including men on the drug that have sexual contact with women of childbearing age.

Adverse drug events

- Hypotension and hypersensitivity upon infusion, cardiac, pulmonary, and renal impairment; avoid in patients with autoimmune disorders. Mental status changes (eg, depression), fever, chills, nausea, and musculoskeletal pain with all agents; tumor lysis syndrome with rituximab; bleeding, hemorrhage, hypertension, proteinuria, skin rash with bevacizumab; cutaneous and severe infusion reactions, interstitial lung disease with cetuximab; hypothyroidism with tositumomab
- Neurotoxicity with thalidomide, neutropenia with thalidomide and lenalidomide, deep vein thrombosis and pulmonary embolism with thalidomide and lenalidomide

Interactions

- Specific drug interactions include:
  * Aldesleukin: glucocorticoids, NSAIDs, antihypertensives
  * Interferon-alfa 2b: zidovudine, theophylline, phenytoin, phenobarbital
  * Ibritumomab: antiplatelets, anticoagulants
  * Levamisole: warfarin, alcohol
  * Tositumomab: antiplatelets, anticoagulants
  * Trastuzumab: anthracyclines, cyclophosphamide, warfarin

Monitoring parameters

- Baseline and follow-up pulmonary, cardiac, and renal function tests; check CBCs with differential, LFTs, TSH, electrolytes, and glucose regularly. Premedicate with acetaminophen and diphenhydramine for monoclonal antibodies. Observe blood pressure during infusion (hypotension concerns) for all agents. Perform blood pressure monitoring (hypertensive concerns) and urine dipstick analysis for bevacizumab. Monitor for vital signs, itching, and swelling. Trouble breathing with cetuximab and ibritumomab.

Other

- Make sure correct form of interferon alfa is being used (four forms). Do not administer gemtuzumab and alemtuzumab as an IV push or bolus.

Miscellaneous (Table 10)

Platinum compounds

- Alklyating-like agents causing the inhibition of DNA synthesis. These include: cisplatin, carboplatin, and oxaliplatin. Adverse effects include: nephrotoxicity, peripheral neurotoxicity, myelosuppression, ototoxicity, nausea, and vomiting.
  * Cisplatin: hydration therapy and premedications are needed. Interactions: doxorubicin,

Table 10

Miscellaneous Agents

Generic name (trade name)	Dosage range	Dosage forms	Frequency	Disease[1]
Platinum compounds				
Cisplatin (Platinol-AQ®)	50-100 mg/m^2	IV	q 3-4 wk	NSCLC, ovarian, testis, bladder, head, neck, lung
Carboplatin (Paraplatin®)	300-400 mg/m^2	IV	q 3-4 wk	Ovarian, testis, NSCLC, head, neck, lung
Oxaliplatin (Eloxatin®)	85-200 mg/m^2	IV	qd x 2 d q 2 wk	Colorectal
Enzymes				
Asparaginase (Elspar®)	6000-10,000 IU/kg	IV	q 3 d x 9 doses	ALL
Cell-specific				
Hydroxyurea (Hydrea®)	20-30 mg/kg	PO	qd	CML, AML, head, neck
Tyrosine kinase inhibitor				
Imatinib mesylate (Gleevec®)	400-600 mg	PO	qd	CML, gastrointestinal stromal tumors
Erlotinib (Tarceva®)	150 mg	PO	qd	NSCLC
Gefitinib (Iressa®)	250-500 mg	PO	qd	NSCLC
Sutinib (Sutent®)	50 mg	PO	qd x 28 d, 14 d off	Kidney, gastrointestinal stromal tumors
Dasatinib (Sprycel®)	70 mg	PO	bid	CML or AML resistant to or intolerant to imatinib
Sorafenib (Nexavar®)	400 mg	PO	bid	renal cell
26S Proteasome inhibitor	1.3 mg/m^2	IV	Days 1, 4, 8, 11	Multiple myeloma
Bortezomib (Velcade®)				

[1]Does not indicate FDA approval.

AML, acute myelogenous leukemia; CML, chronic myelogenous leukemia; NSLC, non-small cell lung cancer.

rituximab, tacrolimus, topotecan, amino-
glycosides
* Carboplatin: monitor for thrombocytopenia.
  Interactions: aminoglycosides
* Oxaliplatin: unique neurotoxicities (eg,
  bronchial spasms)

Sorafenib

• Inhibits multiple tyrosine kinases. Used for treatment of advanced renal cell cancer. Take tablets on
  an empty stomach. Causes diarrhea, fatigue, rash,
  hand-foot syndrome, hypertension, nausea/vomiting,
  neurtropenia, alopecia. Can decrease doxorubicin
  and irinotecan levels.

Sunitinib

Inhibits multiple tyrosine kinases. Used for treatment
of advanced renal cell cancer and gastrointestinal stro-
mal tumors. Take with or without food. Causes neutropenia, rash changes in skin color, fatigue, myalgia,
headaches, hypertension, nausea/vomiting, diarrhea,
increased liver enzymes. Extensively metabolized by
CYP3A4; CYP3A4 inhibitors may increase levels,
CYP3A4 inducers may decrease levels. Ketoconazole
increases levels, rifampin reduces levels.

Table 11

Common Toxicities of Chemotherapeutic Agents

Toxicity	Causative drugs[1]	Recommended therapy
Alopecia	Cyclophosphamide, doxorubicin, paclitaxel, mechlorethamine	N/A
Cardiac toxicity	Anthracyclines	Limit cumulative doses
Diarrhea	Irinotecan, fluorouracil	Premedicate with atropine (irinotecan); treat with loperamide
Extravasation	Anthracyclines, mitomycin, vinca alkaloids, paclitaxel, mechlorethamine	Treat with heat packs for vincas, cold compresses for all other causes or instill normal saline to dilute drug
Hemorrhagic cystitis	Cyclophosphamide, ifosfamide	Premedicate with hydration therapy, mesna
Hepatotoxicity	Asparaginase, cytarabine, mercaptopurine, methotrexate	N/A
Hypersensitivity	Paclitaxel, asparaginase, cisplatin, carboplatin, etoposide, teniposide	Premedicate with ranitidine or cimetidine, diphenhydramine, dexamethasone or test dose; treat with emergency resuscitation
Infertility	Cyclophosphamide, chlorambucil, melphalan, mechlorethamine	N/A
Myelosuppression	Alklyating agents, fluorouracil, methotrexate, lomustine, cyclophosphamide, methotrexate	Treat with G-CSF, platelet transfusions, erythropoietin-stimulating agents
Nausea and vomiting	Cisplatin, cyclophosphamide, cytarabine, dacarbazine, ifosfamide, melphalan, mitomycin, mechlorethamine	Premedicate with dexamethasone, phenothiazines (eg, compazine), 5-HT$_3$-receptor antagonists (eg, granisetron), neurokinin-1 antagonists
Neurotoxicity	Paclitaxel, cisplatin, cytarabine, methotrexate, vincristine, asparaginase	N/A
Pulmonary toxicity	Bleomycin, busulfan, carmustine, mitomycin	Treat with corticosteroids
Renal toxicity	Cisplatin, ifosfamide, methotrexate, streptozocin	Premedicate with hydration therapy, mannitol
Stomatitis	Fluorouracil, methotrexate	Hold ice chips in mouth; palifermin[2]
Edema	Docetaxel	Prophylactic dexamethasone

[1]Adverse effects are not limited to the listed drugs.
[2]For hematologic malignancies requiring myelotoxic therapy requiring hematopoietic agents only.

Table 12

Pharmacologic Management for the Prevention of Acute Chemotherapy-Induced Nausea and Vomiting

Generic name (trade name)	Dosage range	Dosage forms	Frequency	Side effects
5-HT₃ receptor antagonists				
Dolasetron (Anzemet®)	100-200 mg	PO	30 min before treatment	Headache, dizziness, constipation, blurred vision,
Granisetron (Kytril®)	5-20 mg	PO	30 min before treatment	elevated liver enzymes
Ondansetron (Zofran®)	10-25 mg	PO	30 min before treatment	
Palonosetron (Aloxi®)	0.25 mg	IV	Day 1 (not to be repeated within 7 d)	Diarrhea, headache, fatigue, insomnia, arrhythmias
Phenothiazines				
Prochlorperazine (Compazine®)	10-25 mg	PO	q4h prn	Sedation, hypotension, extrapyramidal effects,
Chlorpromazine (Thorazine®)	1.25-5 mg	PO	q4-6h prn	lethargy
Promethazine (Phenergan®)	1-4 mg	PO	q4-6h prn	
Butyrophenones				
Droperidol (Inapsine®)	10-20 mg	IV	q4h prn	Sedation, tachycardia, hypotension
Haloperidol (Haldol®)	5-15 mg/m²	IV, IM, PO	q4-6h prn	
Corticosteroids				
Dexamethasone (Decadron®)	0.5-2 mg	PO	Varies	Anxiety, insomnia, GI upset, psychosis
Cannabinoids				
Dronabinol (Marinol®)	10-20 mg	PO	q3-6h	Drowsiness, euphoria, dry mouth
Nabilone (Cesamet®)	1-2 mg	PO	bid	Drowsiness, euphoria, dry mouth
Benzodiazepines				
Lorazepam (Ativan®)	2 mg	PO	q6h	Sedation, amnesia
Benzamides				
Metoclopramide (Reglan®)	24 mg	PO	tid-qid	Diarrhea, sedation, agitation
Neurokinin-1 antagonist				
Aprepitant (Emend®)	80-125 mg	PO	Day 1 (125 mg) Days 2-3 (80 mg daily)	Somnolence, fatigue, diarrhea

[1]*Note:* Most agents are available in more than one dosage form. Due to space limitations, oral dosing has been given preference.

Dasatinib

Specifically targets BCR-ABL mutations, including those resistant to imatinib, inhibiting leukemic cell growth. Used for treatment of CML and pH+ ALL. Causes rash neutropenia, thrombocytopenia, edema, diarrhea, nausea/vomiting, weight changes, arthralgia, myalgia, cough, shortness of breath, infection, electrolyte changes, arrythmias. Significant drug interactions with CYP3A4 inhibitors, avoid concurrent use or reduce dose. Avoid acid reduction therapies as they will reduce absorption, avoid medications which prolong QT interval.

Asparaginase

• Removes exogenous asparagines from leukemic cells, which are required for their survival. Intradermal skin testing is needed due to severe anaphylactic reactions. Myelosuppression, hyperuricemia, hyperglycemia, and renal problems; interactions: methotrexate, prednisolone, prednisone, vincristine

Hydroxyurea

• Inhibits DNA synthesis without interfering with RNA and protein synthesis. Myelosuppression (leukopenia), development of secondary leukemias, nausea, vomiting, diarrhea, constipation, mucositis, and rare fatal hepatotoxicity and pancreatitis; interactions: didanosine, stavudine.

Imatinib mesylate

• Selective inhibitor of the Philadelphia chromosome (biomarker in CML); causes hepatotoxicity, fluid retention (pleural effusions, weight gain), neutropenia, GI effects, muscle cramps, nausea, and vomiting; interactions: CYP450 3A4 substrates (cyclosporine, simvastatin, erythromycin, itraconazole), CYP450 2C9 substrates (warfarin)

Erlotinib

- Human epidermal growth factor receptor type 1 (HER-1), epidermal growth factor receptor (EGFR) tyrosine kinase inhibitor; oral therapy; take pills 1 hour before or 2 hours after meals. Causes rash, diarrhea, anorexia, stomatitis, intersitital lung disease; interactions: CYP450 3A4 inducers, inhibitors; monitor hepatic function.

Gefitinib

- EGFR tyrosine kinase inhibitor; third-line agent for NSCLC; causes diarrhea, rash, acne, dry skin; interactions: CYP450 3A4 inducers and inhibitors, warfarin

Bortezomib

- Inhibits the 26S proteasome; stabilizes regulatory proteins causing apoptosis and disrupting cell proliferation; causes nausea, vomiting, thrombocytopenia, neuropathy, hypotension, diarrhea

Common Toxicities and Treatments

- Common toxicities of chemotherapeutic agents are outlined in Table 11. These can be classified as acute or subacute, chronic and/or cumulative. Rapidly dividing cells, including mucous membranes, hair, skin, GI tract, and bone marrow are the most common acute toxicities. Examples of delayed or cumulative toxicities include: nephrotoxicity, neurotoxicity, cardiomyopathy, pulmonary fibrosis, and secondary malignancies.
- The prevention and treatment of chemotherapy-induced nausea and vomiting (CINV) is an important area in which pharmacists may play a role in drug selection in oncology patients. The selection of antiemetic agents should be based primarily on the emetogenic potential of the drug regimen. Other factors that increase the risk of CINV include: female gender, young age, prior chemotherapy exposure, lack of chronic alcohol use, combination chemotherapy, high dosage and numerous cycles, and short infusion times. It is important that patients also receive prescriptions to prevent delayed CINV.
- Table 12 summarizes the pertinent antiemetic drugs used in the prophylactic setting.
- For highly to moderately emetogenic drug regimens, dexamethasone and 5-HT$_3$ receptor antagonists are recommended at a minimum for the prevention of acute CINV. Aprepitant should also be considered.
- For low-risk to unlikely emetogenic drug regimens, dexamethasone and a phenothiazine are recommended.

Table 13

American Cancer Society Screening Recommendations

Disease[1]	Sex	Age (y)	Procedure	Frequency
Colorectal	M and F	50+	Fecal occult blood test (FOBT)	Every year
	M and F	50+	Flexible sigmoidoscopy OR colonoscopy OR double contrast barium enema	Every 5 years OR every 10 years OR every 5 years
Breast	F	20+	Breast self-exam	Every month
	F	20-39 OR 40+	Clinical breast exam	Every 3 years OR every year
	F	40+	Mammography	Every year
Cervical	F	21+[2]	Pap smear and pelvic exam	Every 3 years
Prostate	M	50+	Digital rectal exam (DRE)	Every year
	M	50+	Prostate-specific antigen (PSA) test	Every year

[1]No specific screening recommendations have been made for lung, skin, and testicular cancer in patients with average risk. However, after the age of 40, it is recommended that all men and women receive health counseling and a physical exam every year.

[2]Earlier if sexually active.

Adapted from the American Cancer Society.

Table 14

Common Tumor Markers and Associated Cancers

Tumor marker	Abnormal level	Cancer
Alpha-fetoprotein (AFP)	>20 ng/mL	Hepatocellular, ovarian
β-2 Microglobulin (β2M)	>3 ng/mL	Multiple myeloma, lymphoma
CA 15-3	>25 U/mL	Breast
CA 125	>30 U/mL	Ovarian
CA 19-9	>37 U/mL	Pancreatic, colorectal
Calcitonin[1]	>70 pg/mL	Thyroid
Carcinoembryonic antigen (CEA)	>5 U/mL	Colorectal, breast, non–small cell lung
Chromogranin A	>76 ng/mL (men); >51 (women)	Neuroendocrine, lung, prostate
Gamma globulin	>2-3 g/100 mL	Multiple myeloma
Her-2/neu	>450 fmol/mL	Breast
Human chorionic gonadotropin (HCG)	>5 mIU/mL	Testicular
Prostate-specific antigen (PSA)[1]	>4-10 ng/mL	Prostate
Thyroglobulin	>10 ng/mL	Thyroid

[1]Can be used to diagnose early disease.

- For delayed CINV (>24 hours after administration of chemotherapy), metoclopramide and dexamethasone are recommended, at a minimum.
- All patients receiving agents with emetogenic potential should receive prophylactic therapy for CINV with rescue medication readily available.

Miscellaneous Commonalities Across Chemotherapy Agents

- All patients should not receive live and rotavirus vaccines during chemotherapy due to their suppressed immune systems.
- The majority of agents are teratogenic and mutagenic.
- Patients should avoid becoming pregnant or breast-feeding during and immediately after chemotherapy.
- Patients should receive lab work on a regular basis to check for common toxicities, such as myelosuppression, renal and hepatic impairment, and electrolyte disturbances.

3. Nondrug Therapy

- As mentioned above, cancer treatment is generally a combination of modalities. Chemotherapy is an important component, as most patients present with advanced disease upon diagnosis.
- Surgery plays a role in resecting primary tumors or metastases. It can also be used diagnostically to biopsy tumors or for other exploratory purposes.
- Radiation is used to shrink primary tumors in local disease or metastases. It can be used in both neoadjuvant therapy to downsize tumors and in adjuvant therapy to eradicate residual disease.
- Screening is also an important part of cancer therapy, as it can allow the detection of disease in very early stages, when the survival rates are much more acceptable. Table 13 refers to American Cancer Society (ACS) screening recommendations for patients at average risk of developing cancer.
- Tumor markers are additional screening and monitoring tests. They are found in the plasma, serum, or other body fluids, and may be used to identify neoplastic growth.
  * These markers are often not sensitive to diagnose cancer and may produce false-positive results (ie, falsely identify people with a disease that do not have the disease).
  * They are helpful in identifying the recurrence of advanced disease in patients that had elevated levels upon diagnosis. Table 14 lists some commonly used tumor markers.

4. Key Points

- Oncology includes over 100 diverse diseases that share properties of abnormal and detrimental cell growth.
- Diseases are classified based on the tissue they originate in (eg, breast cancer metastasized to the brain is classified as breast cancer).
- Signs and symptoms of cancer do not follow a specific pattern. A health care provider should evaluate any unusual or persistent change in body appearance or function.
- Before a diagnosis of cancer can be made and systemic treatment can begin, a positive biopsy or blood examination must confirm the presence of the disease.
- Further imaging and lab work-up should be done to evaluate the extent of the disease (ie, determine the stage of disease).
- Cancer therapy must be individualized to each patient based on the type and severity of disease, patient characteristics, and patient and family preferences.
- Surgery, radiation, chemotherapy, and biologic therapy are all cancer treatment modalities that are often used in combination.
- Pharmacists can impact patients' chemotherapy and biologic therapy by counseling the patients and educating health care providers on details of the individual drug regimens.
- Chemotherapy is often employed in combinations to take advantage of different mechanisms of action, avoid resistance, and minimize toxicities.
- Most chemotherapy is aimed at rapidly proliferating cancerous cells. However, many chemotherapy-related side effects occur in normal highly proliferative cells of the body, such as hair follicles, the GI tract lining, and blood cells.
- Patients should be aware of expected toxicities of chemotherapy, which are not limited to alopecia, diarrhea, nausea and vomiting, infertility, myelosuppression, neurotoxicity, nephrotoxicity, hepatotoxicity, stomatitis, and pulmonary toxicity.
- Lab work and the importance of follow-up appointments to treatment should be stressed to the patient.
- All prophylactic and post-treatment medications for chemotherapy-related complications should be made available to the patient. Counsel the patient to keep a diary of events that occur prior to and after treatments. Use this record to make interventions and monitor the patient's quality of life.

- All pharmacists should be aware of the accepted cancer screening recommendations and discuss these with all pertinent patients. Many diseases can be cured if they are caught early enough.
- It is the pharmacist's responsibility to make sure that the patient and family are educated enough to participate in making decisions about their care.

5. Questions and Answers

Use Patient Profile #1 to answer Questions 1-5

1. Which of the following agents that Ms. Tiny is taking can be used to treat breast and prostate cancer?

   I. Zoladex®
   II. Tamoxifen
   III. Celebrex®

   A. I only
   B. III only
   C. I and II only
   D. II and III only
   E. I, II, and III

2. When the patient presents with the tamoxifen prescription, you notice that the directions are missing. You call the doctor to clarify what the instructions are. Which of the following is a CORRECT choice?

   A. 10 mL PO qd
   B. 20 mL PO qd
   C. 40 mg PO bid
   D. 20 mg PO qd
   E. 5 mg PO bid

3. Ms. Tiny presents to your pharmacy with complaints of lower leg calf pain that is tender to the touch and red. You suspect a deep vein thrombosis. Which of the following agents is MOST likely to be associated with this?

   I. Megace®
   II. Goserelin
   III. Tamoxifen

   A. I only
   B. III only
   C. I and II only
   D. II and III only
   E. I, II, and III

Patient Profile #1—Medication Profile: Community

Patient Name	Tina Tiny		
Address	234 Small St.		
Age	33	Height	5'8"
Sex	Female	Weight	150 lb
Allergies	Sulfa, penicillin		

DIAGNOSIS
1. Diagnosed on 12/03 with metastatic breast cancer
2. Mastectomy to right breast on 12/15/03
3. Weight loss of 20 lb
4. Allergies

MEDICATION RECORD

Date	Rx #	Physician	Drug/Strength	Quantity	Sig	Refills
12/03	12345	Buford	Percocet 325/5	30	1-2 q4h prn	0
03/04	12347	Buford	Tamoxifen 20 mg	30	1 PO qd	2
03/04	12349	Buford	Megace 40 mg/mL	80 mg/d	—	2
03/04	12350	Charles	Celebrex 10 mg	30	1 PO qd	2

PHARMACIST NOTES

Date	Note
01/04	Patient complained of soreness after mastectomy and swelling of right arm
03/04	Patient did not pick up birth control last month (2/01)
03/04	Patient is receiving Zoladex 3/6 mg SC q28d at oncology clinic. Received dose today.

4. Ms. Tiny calls you 2 days after her 03/04 visit to your pharmacy. She has been feeling a lot of bone pain and describes an "achy, creaky feeling all over." She is worried that her cancer has spread to her bones. What advice can you give her?

I. She should call her oncology caretaker and be formally evaluated
II. This could be a side effect of her Zoladex therapy and the pain should subside
III. This could be a side effect of her Celebrex therapy and the pain should subside

A. I only
B. III only
C. I and II only
D. II and III only
E. I, II, and III

5. Ms. Tiny's mother (age 59) is worried that she will develop breast cancer like her daughter. Which of the following is NOT an appropriate initial screening test for breast cancer?

A. Monthly breast self-examination
B. Clinical breast examination
C. Mammography
D. Biopsy
E. Mammography and clinical breast examination

6. Which of the following classes of agents is best known for causing infusion-related reactions, such as fever and chills?

I. Monoclonal antibodies
II. Alkylating agents
III. Vinca alkaloids

A. I only
B. III only
C. I and II only
D. II and III only
E. I, II, and III

7. Your patient has just received 5-FU and irinotecan for the treatment of colorectal cancer. Before he leaves the clinic, you make sure that he has a prescription to prevent and/or treat which of the following side effects from irinotecan?

A. Nausea with Aloxi®
B. Diarrhea with loperamide
C. Headache with aspirin
D. Delayed allergic reaction with epinephrine
E. Change in urine color: no treatment available

8. Which of the following drugs is an oral prodrug of 5-FU?

A. Fluorouracil
B. Xeloda®
C. Fludara®
D. Cytoxan
E. Alkeran®

9. An elderly male patient comes to your pharmacy and is worried that he might have prostate cancer. He just had some lab work done and his doctor told him that some level was abnormal, indicating potential prostate cancer. Which lab test might he be talking about?

I. PSA
II. Cortisol
III. ESR

A. I only
B. III only
C. I and II only
D. II and III only
E. I, II, and III

10. Stomatitis is the clinical term for which of the following chemotherapy-related adverse effects?

I. Nausea and projectile vomiting
II. Obstruction of the lower esophageal sphincter
III. Inflammation of the mucosal lining of the mouth

A. I only
B. III only
C. I and II only
D. II and III only
E. I, II, and III

11. Which of the following does not describe characteristics of most chemotherapy agents?

A. A wide therapeutic index
B. Interfere with DNA synthesis and replication
C. More effective in combination
D. Acute adverse effects occur primarily in rapidly dividing normal cells
E. Phase-specific and non–phase specific actions

Use Patient Profile #2 to answer Questions 12-17.

12. A nurse would like to know if she can administer the diphenhydramine and the cimetidine in the same IV line simultaneously. Which of the following resources will provide you with this information?

    I. Facts and Comparisons™
    II. Trissel's
    III. Micromedex®

    A. I only
    B. III only
    C. I and II only
    D. II and III only
    E. I, II, and III

13. Which of the following agents that Mr. Migash is taking requires the premedication regimen of dexamethasone, diphenhydramine, and ranitidine or cimetidine to prevent an anaphylactic reaction?

    I. Taxotere
    II. Paraplatin
    III. Taxol

    A. I only
    B. III only
    C. I and II only
    D. II and III only
    E. I, II, and III

Patient Profile #2—Medication Profile: Institution

| Patient Name | Cassimer Migash |
| Address | 579 Hunter's Ridge |

Age	60		Height	180 cm
Sex	Male		Weight	200 lb
Allergies	NKDA			

DIAGNOSIS	1. Diagnosed on 02/04 with metastatic non–small cell lung cancer
	2. Chronic obstructive pulmonary disease
	3. Asthma

LABS AND DIAGNOSTIC TESTS

Date	Test
05/04	WBC: 2500/microliter
05/04	RBC: $2.8 \times 10^6/mm^3$
05/04	PLT: 100×10^3/microliter
05/04	Theophylline: 10 mcg/mL
05/04	Hgb: 9 g/dL
05/04	Hct: 30%

MEDICATION RECORD

Date	Route	Drug	Sig
04/04	IV	Paclitaxel 135 mg/m^2	135 mg/m^3 over 3 h q 3 wk
04/04	IV	Carboplatin AUC 6	AUC 6 over 2 h q 3 wk
04/04	PO	Theophylline SR 400 mg	1 tab PO bid
04/04	INH	Albuterol inhaler	2 puffs prn
04/04	INH	Cromolyn inhaler	1 puff qid
04/04	INH	Beclomethasone inhaler	2 puffs qid
04/04	PO	Dexamethasone 20 mg	1 tab 12 h and 6 h prior to chemo
4/03	IV	Diphenhydramine 50 mg	Infuse 30 min and 60 min prior to chemo
4/03	IV	Cimetidine 300 mg	Infuse 30 min and 60 min prior to chemo

14. Based on the patient's weight and height, you calculate Mr. Migash's body surface area to be 2.1 m². Paclitaxel is supplied as 6 mg/mL in 5-mL, 16.7-mL, and 50-mL vials. Your pharmacy has all quantities available. What is the best way to correctly dose this patient?

    A. One 50-mL vial
    B. One 50-mL vial and one 5-mL vial
    C. Two 16.7-mL vials
    D. Two 16.7-mL vials and one 5-mL vial
    E. Three 16.7-mL vials

15. You are concerned that Mr. Migash will develop nausea and vomiting from his chemotherapy regimen. Which of the following regimens would be suitable to prevent acute CINV?

    A. Dexamethasone, granisetron, and aprepitant
    B. Granisetron and prochlorperazine
    C. Metoclopramide, dexamethasone, and aprepitant
    D. Palonsetron and granisetron
    E. Lorazepam and droperidol

16. Based on the patient's lab values, which of the following adverse reactions appear to have occurred as a likely result of the chemotherapy?

    I.   Thrombocytopenia
    II. Leukopenia
    III. Anemia

    A. I only
    B. III only
    C. I and II only
    D. II and III only
    E. I, II, and III

17. The goal of Mr. Migash's treatment regimen is:

    I.   to cure his disease
    II. to palliate his disease-related symptoms
    III. to increase his quality of life

    A. I only
    B. III only
    C. I and II only
    D. II and III only
    E. I, II, and III

18. Doxorubicin is an antineoplastic agent that:

    A. is not related to epirubicin and daunorubicin
    B. interacts with the microtubules of cells during mitosis
    C. has an oral dosage form commercially available
    D. causes cumulative cardiac toxicity
    E. can also be used to treat tuberculosis

19. Which of the following agents is used in cancer regimens, but is not considered an antineoplastic agent?

    A. Methotrexate
    B. Levamisole
    C. Doxorubicin
    D. Cyclophosphamide
    E. Gemcitabine

20. Methotrexate (Rheumatrex®) is not available as which of the following dosage forms?

    A. An intravenous injection
    B. An oral tablet or capsule
    C. An intrathecal injection
    D. An ointment
    E. An intramuscular injection

Answers

1. **A.** Zoladex (goserelin) is an LHRH agonist that can be used to treat both breast and prostate cancer. LHRH agonists are FDA approved for premenopausal women, as they inhibit estrogen production from the ovaries.

2. **D.** 20 mg PO qd is the FDA approved dose for breast cancer therapy. The drug is not available in a liquid form.

3. **E.** All three agents are hormonal products and are associated with thromboembolic side effects. It is important that patients on these products are aware of the signs and symptoms of DVTs.

4. **C.** While the bone pain is most likely a side effect of her Zoladex therapy, she should notify her oncology practitioner so they can document this side effect. If other factors point to metastatic disease, this patient may need additional evaluation.

5. **D.** Biopsies should never be performed as initial screening tests. However, if results from the mammography and other tests point to disease, a biopsy is needed to make a diagnosis. There is some debate about the usefulness of clinical breast examinations (CBEs) for women that are reluctant to perform breast self-examinations; CBEs should be offered.

6. **A.** Monoclonal antibodies are commonly associated with infusion-related reactions. Patients should receive premedication, such as acetaminophen, to prevent this.

7. **B.** Diarrhea is a dose-limiting toxicity of irinotecan. Late diarrhea can be life threatening. All patients should receive a prescription for loperamide to treat delayed-onset diarrhea. Patients should be instructed to take 2 mg PO q2h while awake and 4 mg PO q4h during the night until the diarrhea has stopped for at least 12 hours. Acute-onset diarrhea can be treated with atropine.

8. **B.** Xeloda, generic name capecitabine, is an oral prodrug of 5-FU. Fluorouracil is another name for 5-FU. Fludara is the brand name for fludarabine and is used to treat CLL and NHL intravenously. Cytoxan is the brand name for cyclophosphamide and is available in IV and PO dosage forms. Alkeran is the brand name for melphalan and is also available in IV and PO dosage forms.

9. **A.** PSA is a lab test that is commonly done in men over the age of 40. It should be tested annually in men over the age of 50 to check for prostate cancer. PSA stands for prostate-specific antigen.

10. **B.** Stomatitis is used to describe an irritation or ulceration of the mucosal lining. This side effect is common with fluorouracil and methotrexate. Having the patient hold ice chips in their mouth during treatment can prevent it. The cold is thought to cause vasoconstriction of the lining and prevent damage.

11. **A.** Chemotherapy agents have a very narrow therapeutic index. This is one of the main reasons why there are so many toxic effects with these drugs. They can be phase–specific or non–phase specific drugs and cause many adverse reactions to normal cells that undergo rapid proliferation.

12. **D.** Both Trissel's *Handbook of Injectable Drugs* and the Micromedex IV compatibility tool can be used to assess whether the diphenhydramine and cimetidine are compatible.

13. **B.** Taxol is the brand name of paclitaxel. This agent has been shown to cause hypersensitivity reactions in patients. It is unclear if these reactions are due to the drug itself or the drug's vehicle (Cremophor®). All patients receiving paclitaxel should receive a premedication regimen of dexamethasone, diphenhydramine, and ranitidine or cimetidine. Taxotere is the brand name of docetaxel. This agent also requires premedications with a minimum of a corticosteroid. However, this is to prevent peripheral edema, not an anaphylactic reaction.

14. **A.** The patient requires 283.5 mg of drug, which can be rounded up to 300 mg. Both choices A and E will provide 300 mg of drug; however, using one large vial is more economical than using three smaller vials.

15. **A.** This patient's regimen contains carboplatin and paclitaxel. Together these agents have a high likelihood of causing acute (and delayed) CINV. The patient should receive a corticosteroid, a 5-HT$_3$ antagonist, and a neurokinin-1 inhibitor. Aprepitant is approved in combination with a corticosteroid and a 5-HT$_3$ antagonist, making choices B and C incorrect. Choice D contains two 5-HT$_3$ antagonists. Therapy should include more than one class of agent. Choice E agents are not efficacious in moderate to severe CINV.

16. **E.** Myelosuppression is a common adverse reaction to most chemotherapy agents. Both paclitaxel and carboplatin can cause anemia, thrombocytopenia, and leukopenia. It is very important to monitor blood levels in these patients. If myelosuppression is too severe, the length of time between chemotherapy cycles may be increased so all or some of the blood cells can return to normal levels.

17. **D.** Mr. Migash has metastatic disease. Anytime a solid tumor is diagnosed as stage IV, this is representative of the fact that their disease is incurable. The treatment goals for these patients include relieving any disease-related symptoms, minimizing toxicity from treatments, and increasing the patient's quality of life through treatment or supportive care measures.

18. **D.** Doxorubicin is an antitumor antibiotic related to epirubicin and daunorubicin. These agents act by binding tightly to DNA via intercalation and by inhibiting the topoisomerase II enzyme. Doxorubicin does have a liposomal IV product, but it is not available orally. All anthracyclines are associated with cardiac toxicity and have cumulative dosing limits to prevent this.

19. **B.** Levamisole is an anthelmintic agent that is approved for combination therapy with 5-FU in the treatment of colorectal cancer.

20. **D.** Methotrexate is not commercially available for topical use. It is available in all of the other dosage forms.

6. References

American Cancer Society. Cancer Facts and Figures 2007. Available at *www.cancer.org.* Accessed 9 August 2007.

ASHP Therapeutic Guidelines on the Pharmacologic Management of Nausea and Vomiting in Adult and Pediatric Patients Receiving Chemotherapy or Radiation Therapy or Undergoing Surgery. *Am J Health Syst Pharm.* 1999;56:729-764.

Balmer CM, Valley AW. Cancer treatment and chemotherapy. In: Dipiro JT, Talbert RL, Yee GC, et al, eds. *Pharmacotherapy: A Pathophysiologic Approach,* 5th ed. New York: McGraw-Hill; 2002:2175-2222.

Calabresi P, Chabner BA. Chemotherapy of neoplastic diseases. In: Hardman JG, Limbird LE, eds. *Goodman & Gilman's: The Pharmacological Basis of Therapeutics,* 10th ed. New York: McGraw-Hill; 2001:1381-1388.

Chabner BA, Ryan DP, Paz-Ares L, Garcia-Carbonero R, Calabresi P. Antineoplastic agents. In: Hardman JG, Limbird LE, eds. *Goodman & Gilman's: The Pharmacological Basis of Therapeutics,* 10th ed. New York: McGraw-Hill; 2001:1389-1459.

DeVita VT, Hellman S, Rosenberg SA, eds. *Cancer: Principles & Practices of Oncology,* 6th ed. Philadelphia: Lippincott Williams & Wilkins; 2001.

Dorr RT, Fritz WL. *Cancer Chemotherapy Handbook.* New York: Elsevier North Holland; 1980.

Mueller BA, Schumock GT, Bertch KE, et al, eds. *Pharmacotherapy Self-Assessment Program,* 4th ed. Book 10, Hematology Oncology. Kansas City: American College of Clinical Pharmacy; 2002.

National Comprehensive Cancer Network (NCCN). NCCN Clinical Practice Guidelines in Oncology— Antiemesis. Available at *www.nccn.org.* Accessed 19 August 2007.

20. Solid Organ Transplantation

Benjamin Duhart, Jr, MS, PharmD
Assistant Professor, College of Pharmacy
Director, Transplant Pharmacy Services
University of Tennessee Health Science Center

Contents

1. **Organ Transplantation**

2. **Immunosuppressants**

3. **Key Points**

4. **Questions and Answers**

5. **References**

1. Organ Transplantation

Principles of Transplantation

Types of allografts
- Heart: first successfully transplanted in 1968; in 2002, 3196 heart transplants were performed in the U.S.
- Intestinal: first successfully transplanted in 1987; in 2002, 108 intestinal transplants were performed in the U.S.
- Kidney: first successful cadaveric transplant in 1954; in 2002, 15,641 kidney transplants were performed in the U.S.
- Liver: first successful cadaveric transplant in 1967; in 2002, 5329 liver transplants were performed in the U.S.
- Lung: first successful cadaveric single-lung transplant in 1983; in 2002, 2084 lung transplants were performed in the U.S.
- Pancreas: first successful solitary pancreas transplant in 1968; in 2002, 1457 pancreas transplants were performed in the U.S.

Goal
- Improve patients' quality of life and survival by stabilizing and/or improving end-organ failure–related complications

Outcome
- See Table 1.

Definitions
- *acute rejection:* a systemic immunologic response to donor antigens primarily mediated by T lymphocytes
- *adaptive immunity:* involves stimulation of cells and soluble mediators in response to specific antigens with a markedly enhanced response on repeat exposure
- *complement:* an enzyme system that is a crucial part of the basic immune response on primary exposure to an antigen, and also provides augmented signaling during memory immunity
- *human leukocyte antigen (HLA):* antigen binding proteins that rescue protein fragments from intracellular catabolism (class I or II) or select antigens from the extracellular milieu that are then presented to lymphocytes (class II)
- *innate immunity:* involves stimulation of cells and soluble mediators that nonspecifically recognize antigens and have no ability to alter response with repeat exposure
- *major histocompatibility complex (MHC):* a group of genes that encode for human leukocyte antigens class I and II
- *opsonization:* occurs when antigens or immune complexes become coated with a molecule that facilitates binding with a phagocyte
- *panel reactive antibody (PRA):* a test that quantitates a patient's immunologic reactivity to a given pool of antigens
- *phagocytosis:* process by which recognized antigens are engulfed and subsequently undergo intracellular catabolism

Table 1

Kaplan-Meier Patient and Graft Survival Rates for Transplants Performed: 1996-2001

Organ	Patient survival (%)	Graft survival (%)
Heart		
1 year	85.3	84.9
3 years	78.1	77.4
Intestinal		
1 year	71.3	66.7
3 years	53.8	46.9
Kidney: cadaveric		
1 year	94.4	88.3
3 years	89.3	77.8
Kidney: living		
1 year	97.7	94.4
3 years	94.9	87.7
Liver: cadaveric		
1 year	85.3	80.0
3 years	77.7	70.6
Liver: living		
1 year	87.9	77.7
3 years	80.1	71.6
Lung: cadaveric		
1 year	76.6	76.1
3 years	57.7	56.6
Lung: living		
1 year	73.4	72.2
3 years	50.7	49.2
Pancreas		
1 year	95.0	78.5
3 years	86.9	60.5

Based on the Organ Procurement and Transplantation Network data as of February 7, 2003.

Basic Immunology and Acute Rejection

Fundamental types of immunity
Innate immunity
Cellular components
- Macrophages: phagocytic cells found throughout the body, which may function as antigen-presenting cells
- Neutrophils: highly motile cells whose major physiologic role is the destruction of invading microorganisms via phagocytosis/opsonization
- Natural killer cells: a subset of non-B, non-T lymphocytes that survey for the normal biosynthesis and expression of HLA class I, making them important in immunity against viral infection and malignancy

Humoral component
- Complement: activation leads to formation of lipophilic complexes, called membrane-attack complexes, in the cell membrane of the target cell and results in osmotic leakage
    * Physiologic function: defense against pyogenic bacterial infections
    * Bridges innate and adaptive immunity
    * Mediates disposal of immune complexes
    * Acute phase proteins

Adaptive immunity
Cellular components
- Thymus-derived lymphocytes (T cells): mature T cells become activated when they encounter an antigen-presenting cell presenting an antigen; T cells do not recognize antigens directly:
    * CD4$^+$ T cells ("T helper cells") recognize antigen presented via HLA class II
    * CD8$^+$ T cells ("cytotoxic T cells") recognize antigen presented via HLA class I
- Bone marrow–derived lymphocytes (B cells): B cells encounter the antigen to which their surface immunoglobulin has specificity, through either its APC function or via interaction with an activated CD4$^+$ T cell. B-cell/CD4$^+$ T-cell interaction is required for translocation into a follicle within secondary lymphoid tissue, where a germinal center forms and where high-affinity memory B cells and plasma cells are produced/selected (somatic hypermutation).

Humoral components
- Complement: as above
- Immunoglobulins (Ig): complex proteins of various isotypes formed as a consequence of B-cell activation for the purpose of binding and elimination of the activating antigen

Acute rejection
Pathophysiology
- During transplantation, the recipient is exposed to donor antigens to which he or she has no previous exposure. While undesirable, acute rejection is the normal physiologic response of the immune system to these donor antigens. This response can be divided into 5 basic phases:
1. Recognition: recognition of foreign antigen via self/nonself recognition mediated via MHC
2. Presentation: upon recognition, antigen-presenting cells present antigens in association with native HLA class II to inactive CD4$^+$ T cells.
3. Activation/proliferation: activation is dependent on antigen/HLA binding to the T-cell receptor (TCR) complex and the subsequent binding of a second signal or "co-stimulatory pathway." Subsequently, the active CD4$^+$ T cell produces and releases various lymphokines, particularly interleukin-2 (IL-2), important for activation and proliferation of numerous lymphocyte lineages.
4. Recruitment: recruitment is mediated via several lymphokines produced as a consequence of lymphocyte activation.
5. Antigen/tissue destruction: tissue injury is mediated via induction of polyclonal immune response.

Incidence
- The incidence is organ specific and dependent on many pre- and post-transplant factors. There are several known factors that increase risk:
    * Increasing HLA mismatch
    * Factors affecting previous sensitization: history of pregnancy, previous transplantation, previous rejection, or panel reactive antibody >20%
    * Ethnicity: African-American recipients
    * Age: pediatric recipients
    * Donor source: cadaveric donor
    * Prolonged preservation time
    * Noncompliance

Immunosuppressive Strategies

Balance of immunosuppression
- Selection of an immunosuppression regimen for the prevention of acute rejection should be individualized based on known risk and potential for toxicity. Subsequent adjustment must focus on the balance of the triad: rejection, infection, and toxicity.

Phases of preventive immunosuppression
Induction
- The early phase is intended to provide highly potent, multi-focal suppression of the immune system for

several days to a few weeks. Commonly used agents include:
  * Corticosteroids
  * Monoclonal antibody: muromonab, basiliximab, daclizumab
  * Polyclonal antibody: antithymocyte globulin (equine or rabbit)

Maintenance

- The immunosuppression regimen is designed to provide chronic, balanced immunodeficiency. Some commonly used regimens include:
  * Double therapy:
    • Calcineurin inhibitor + steroids
    • Calcineurin inhibitor + antimetabolite
    • Calcineurin inhibitor + mTOR inhibitor
    • mTOR inhibitor + steroids
    • mTOR inhibitor + antimetabolite
    • Antimetabolite + steroids
  * Triple therapy:
    • Calcineurin inhibitor + antimetabolite + steroids
    • mTOR inhibitor + calcineurin inhibitor + steroids
    • mTOR inhibitor + antimetabolite + steroids

Phases of immunosuppression during treatment
Treatment

- Selection of the agents is organ specific and dependent on the severity of acute rejection. Commonly used agents include:
  * Corticosteroids
  * Calcineurin inhibitor: tacrolimus may be used as the primary treatment of acute rejection in liver recipients; may also have a role as adjuvant therapy in refractory acute rejection in various other solid organ recipients
  * Monoclonal antibody: muromonab
  * Polyclonal antibody: antithymocyte globulin (horse or rabbit)

Maintenance re-evaluation

- The decision to heighten maintenance immunosuppression is dependent on the cause for rejection (ie, failure of regimen versus noncompliance).

Immunosuppressive Complications

Infectious

- Infectious complications are an important cause of early morbidity and mortality. The incidence is organ specific and closely linked to the net degree of immunodeficiency. Prevention is a key management strategy post-transplant.

Bacterial
- Tuberculosis: *Mycobacterium tuberculosis*
- Nocardiasis: various species of *Nocardia*

Fungal
- Aspergillosis: various species of *Aspergillus*
- Blastomycosis: *Blastomyces dermatitidis*
- Candidiasis: various species of *Candida*
- Coccidioidomycosis: *Coccidioides immitis*
- Cryptococcosis: *Cryptococcus neoformans*
- Histoplasmosis: *Histoplasma capsulatum*
- Mucormycosis: various species of *Mucor*
- *Pneumocystis carinii*

Parasitic
- Toxoplasmosis: *Toxoplasma gondii*

Viral
- Cytomegalovirus
- Epstein-Barr virus: including post-transplant lymphoproliferative disease (PTLD)
- Herpes simplex virus
- Varicella-zoster virus
- Human herpes viruses (ie, HHV-6, HHV-8)
- Parvovirus
- Polyomavirus

Noninfectious
- The noninfectious complications are specific to the agents included in the immunosuppressive regimen.

2. Immunosuppressants

- See Table 2.

Calcineurin Inhibitors

Cyclosporine
Mechanism of action
- Inhibits calcineurin-dependent translocation of the cytosolic subunit of NFAT, the promoter gene for IL-2, into the nucleus, thereby inhibiting transcription and synthesis of IL-2; thus it inhibits IL-2–mediated monoclonal T-cell proliferation and polyclonal T-cell activation.

Administration
- Intravenous
    * 5-6 mg/kg per day divided every 12 h or as a continuous infusion; each milliliter of IV concentrate should be diluted in 20-100 mL of NS or D_5W in a glass container. For bolus dosing, the dose should be infused over 2-6 h.
- Oral
    * Capsules: administer the daily dose as two equally divided doses every 12 h with meals.
    * Oral solution: administer the daily dose as two equally divided doses every 12 h with meals. The solution may be diluted with chocolate milk or orange juice in a glass container. Additional diluent should be used to rinse the container to assure administration of the total dose.

Drug-drug interactions
- Metabolized primarily via cytochrome P450 3A isoenzymes; substances known to alter functionality of these enzymes will alter bioavailability and elimination of this drug (Table 3).
- Drug interactions leading to altered exposure of other drugs by cyclosporine (Table 4)

Drug-disease interactions
- Altered biliary flow: diversion of biliary flow can significantly reduce adsorption. This more profoundly affects cyclosporine USP compared to cyclosporine USP (modified).
- Diabetes mellitus: administration worsens glycemic control in patients with pre-existing diabetes.
- Vaccination: in general, immunosuppressants may affect efficacy of vaccinations. The use of live vaccines should be avoided.

Adverse drug reactions
- CNS: seizure, hallucinations, insomnia, tremor, paresthesias
- HEENT: gingival hyperplasia
- CV: hypertension
- GI: hepatotoxicity
- Renal: nephrotoxicity
- Endocrine and metabolic: diabetes mellitus, hyperlipidemia, hyperuricemia, hyperkalemia, hypomagnesemia
- Dermatologic: hirsutism, hypertrichosis, acne

Patient instructions
- Keep cyclosporine stored in its original container. Take the prescribed dose twice daily with meals. Keep timing of dosing consistent. Make sure you take or do not take your medication at the appropriate time prior to therapeutic drug monitoring. Many medications interact with this medication. Do not take anything prescribed by another physician until you verify that there are no drug interactions.

Monitoring
- C_0 (trough): goals dependent on multifactorial risk assessment and assay type
- C_2: concentration 2 hours after dose; goals dependent on multifactorial risk assessment and assay type

Pharmacokinetics
- Cyclosporine USP: highly lipoprotein bound
    * Bioavailability: significant intra- and interpatient variability
    * Mean F = 30%, range 5-92%
    * Elimination: $t_{1/2}$ = 19 h, range 10-28 h (increased with hepatic dysfunction)
- Cyclosporine USP, (modified): highly lipoprotein bound
    * Bioavailability: improved and more consistent absorption (60-70% increased C_{max})
    * Elimination: $t_{1/2}$ = 8 h, range 5-18 h (increased with hepatic dysfunction)

Tacrolimus
Mechanism of action
- Inhibits translocation of the cytosolic subunit of NFAT, the promoter gene for IL-2, into the nucleus via its binding with FKBP-12 and a calcium-calmodulin-calcineurin complex, thereby inhibiting transcription and synthesis of IL-2; thus it inhibits IL-2–mediated monoclonal T-cell proliferation and polyclonal T-cell activation.

Administration
- Intravenous
    * Dilute in NS or D_5W to a concentration between 0.004 and 0.02 mg/mL and administer as a continuous infusion via PVC-free container and tubing

Table 2

Immunosuppressant Drugs

Trade name	Generic name	Dosage forms	Dose	Generic products
Calcineurin inhibitors				
Sandimmune®	Cyclosporine USP	Injection: 50 mg/mL; oral solution: 100 mg/mL; capsules: 25, 50, 100 mg	**Intravenous:** 5-6 mg/kg/d; **oral:** 8-14 mg/kg/d divided q12h; **adjusted to desired trough concentration**	Injection 50 mg/mL; capsules 25 and 100 mg
Neoral®	Cyclosporine USP (modified)	Oral solution 100 mg/mL; capsules 25 and 100 mg	**Oral:** 5-10 mg/kg/d divided q12h; **adjusted to desired trough concentration**	Oral solution: 100 mg/mL; capsules: 25 and 100 mg
Prograf®	Tacrolimus	Injection: 5-mg ampules; capsules: 0.5, 1, and 5 mg	**Intravenous:** 0.03-0.05 mg/kg/d as continuous infusion; **oral:** 0.1-0.2 mg/kg/d divided q12h; **adjusted to desired trough concentration**	Not available
mTOR inhibitors				
Rapamune®	Sirolimus	Oral solution: 1 mg/mL; tablets: 1, 2 mg	**Initial:** 6-15 mg PO; **maintenance:** 2-5 mg PO qd; **adjusted to desired trough concentration**	Not available
Antiproliferative agents				
Imuran®	Azathioprine	Injection: 100 mg vial; tablets: 50 mg	**Initial:** 3-5 mg/kg IV or PO; **maintenance:** 1-2 mg/kg IV or PO qd	Injection: 100 mg vial; tablets: 50 mg
CellCept®	Mycophenolate mofetil	Injection: 500 mg vial; oral suspension: 200 mg/mL; capsules: 250 mg; tablets: 500 mg	**Maintenance:** Adults: 2-3 g/d divided q8-12h IV or PO; pediatrics: 1200 mg/m^2 divided q8-12h IV or PO	Not available
Myfortic®	Mycophenolate sodium	Tablets: 180, 360 mg	**Maintenance:** Adults: 720 mg PO q12h; pediatrics: 400 mg/m^2 PO q12h (maximum dose of 720 mg PO q12h)	Not available
Arava®	Leflunomide	Tablets: 10, 20, and 100 mg	**Initial:** 100 mg PO qd x 3; **maintenance:** 10-20 mg PO qd	Not available
Monoclonal antibodies				
Orthoclone OKT 3®	Muromonab-CD3	Injection: 5-mg ampules	**Induction:** 2-5 mg IV qd x 7-10 d; **acute rejection:** 5-10 mg IV qd x 10-14 d	Not available
Simulect®	Basiliximab	Injection: 10- and 20-mg vials	**Induction:** adults and pediatrics >35 kg: 20 mg IV on day 0 and day 4; pediatrics <35 kg: 10 mg IV on day 0 and day 4	Not available
Zenapax®	Daclizumab	Injection: 25-mg vials	**Induction:** 1 mg/kg IV q 2 wk x 5	Not available
Polyclonal antibodies				
Atgam®	Anti-thymocyte globulin (equine)	Injection: 50-mg vials	**Induction:** 15 mg/kg IV qd x 7-10 d; **acute rejection:** 10-15 mg/kg IV qd x 14 d	Not available
Thymoglobulin®	Anti-thymocyte globulin (rabbit)	Injection: 25-mg vials	**Induction:** 1.5 mg/kg IV qd x 3-7 d; **acute rejection:** 1.5 mg/kg IV qd x 7-10 d	Not available

Table 3

Drug Interactions Leading to Altered Exposure of Cytochrome P450 3A Isoenzyme Substrates[1]

Cytochrome P450 3A4 enzyme inducers: *Inducers result in increased metabolism and decreased bioavailability of substrates of the same system*	Cytochrome P450 3A4 enzyme inhibitors: *Inhibitors result in decreased metabolism and increased bioavailability of substrates of the same system*
Anticonvulsants: phenytoin, phenobarbital, carbamazepine	Antidepressants: nefazodone
Antimicrobial agents: rifampin, rifabutin	Antiviral agents: delavirdine, indinavir, nelfinavir, ritonavir, saquinavir
Antiviral agents: nevirapine, efavirenz	Azole antifungal agents: ketoconazole, fluconazole, itraconazole, clotrimazole
Herbal products: St. John's wort	Calcium channel blockers: diltiazem, nicardipine, verapamil
	Macrolide antimicrobial agents: erythromycin, clarithromycin, troleandomycin
	Food-drug interaction: grapefruit juice

[1]These are examples only. Numerous other interactions are associated with CYP450 3A4 substrates. See current journals or drug interaction texts for a more detailed list.

- Oral
  - * Two equally divided doses PO every 12 h consistently with or without food

Drug-drug interactions
- Metabolized primarily via cytochrome P450 3A isoenzymes; substances known to alter functionality of these enzymes will alter bioavailability and elimination of this drug (Table 3).

Drug-disease interactions
- Diabetes mellitus: administration worsens glycemic control in patients with pre-existing diabetes.
- Vaccinations: in general, immunosuppressants may affect efficacy of vaccinations. The use of live vaccines should be avoided.

Adverse drug reactions
- CNS: seizure, hallucinations, insomnia, tremor, depression, psychosis, anorexia
- HEENT: alopecia
- CV: hypertension
- GI: hepatotoxicity
- Renal: nephrotoxicity
- Endocrine and metabolic: diabetes mellitus, hyperlipidemia, hyperkalemia, hypercalcemia, hypomagnesemia, hypophosphatemia
- Hematologic: anemia

Patient instructions
- Take the prescribed dose at a consistent time twice daily. It may be taken with or without food, but should be taken the same way to maintain consistency. Make sure you do not take your medication

Table 4

Drug Interactions Leading to Altered Exposure of Other Drugs by Cyclosporine[1]

Mechanism	Drug	Comment
Cytochrome P450 3A4 enzyme substrates	HMG-CoA reductase inhibitors: lovastatin, simvastatin, atorvastatin	Co-administration of these agents with CsA results in significant increases in HMG-CoA reductase inhibitor exposure and may place patients at increased risk of rhabdomyolysis
Cytochrome P450 3A4 enzyme substrates	Sirolimus	Simultaneous administration increased C_{max} and AUC of sirolimus by 120-500% and 140-230%, respectively; administration 4 hours apart increased C_{max} and AUC of sirolimus by 30-40% and 35-80%, respectively
Alteration in enterohepatic recycling	Mycophenolate mofetil	CsA co-administration inhibits MPAG excretion via hepatocytes, thus interfering with MPA enterohepatic recycling, leading to reduced exposure of the active metabolite, MPA

CsA, cyclosporine A; HMG-CoA, 3-hydroxy-3-methyglutaryl coenzyme A; MPA, mycophenolic acid; MPAG, phenolic glucuronide of MPA.
[1]These are examples only. See current journals or drug interaction texts for detailed lists.

prior to therapeutic drug monitoring. Many medications interact with this medication. Do not take anything prescribed by another physician until you verify that there are no drug interactions.

Monitoring
- C_0 (trough): goals dependent on multifactorial risk assessment; in general, 5-20 ng/mL

Pharmacokinetics
- Highly protein bound
- Bioavailability: F = 14-32%
- Elimination: $t_{1/2}$ = 8 h, range 6-11 h (increased with hepatic dysfunction)

mTOR Inhibitor

Sirolimus
Mechanism of action
- Binds to FKBP-12 to form a complex that binds and inhibits activation of its target protein, mTOR (mammalian target of rapamycin), a kinase that is critical in IL-2–mediated cell cycle progression

Administration
- To limit variability, administer consistently with or without food.
- Tablets: administer daily dose PO once a day.
- Oral solution: dilute the dose in 2 ounces of water or orange juice, stir vigorously, and drink at once. Then refill container with 4 ounces of the chosen fluid, stir vigorously, and drink.

Drug-drug interactions
- Metabolized primarily via cytochrome P450 3A isoenzymes; substances known to alter functionality of these enzymes will alter bioavailability and elimination of this drug (Table 3).
- Additionally, the pharmacokinetic profile of sirolimus is significantly altered by concomitant cyclosporine (Table 4).

Drug-disease interactions
- Liver transplantation: associated with increased incidence of mortality, graft loss, and hepatic artery thrombosis in de novo liver transplant recipients.
- Lung transplantation: there have been cases of fatal bronchial anastomotic dehiscence in de novo lung transplant recipients.
- Vaccinations: in general, immunosuppressants may affect efficacy of vaccinations. The use of live vaccines should be avoided.

Adverse drug reactions
- CNS: anorexia
- HEENT: oral ulcers

- GI: diarrhea, esophagitis, gastritis, gastroenteritis, hepatotoxicity, hepatic artery thrombosis in de novo liver transplant recipients
- Renal: synergistic nephrotoxicity with calcineurin inhibitors
- Endocrine and metabolic: hyperlipidemia, hypertension, hyperkalemia
- Dermatologic: rash, acne
- Hematologic: leukopenia, thrombocytopenia, pancytopenia, thrombosis
- Other: lymphocele, pneumonitis, bronchial anastomotic dehiscence in de novo lung transplant recipients

Patient instructions
- Take the prescribed dose at a consistent time once daily. It may be taken with or without food, but should be taken the same way to maintain consistency. Make sure you do not take your medication prior to therapeutic drug monitoring. Many medications interact with this medication. Do not take anything prescribed by another physician until you verify that there are no drug interactions.

Monitoring
- C_0 (trough): goal dependent on multifactorial risk assessment and assay type; in general, 5-20 ng/mL

Pharmacokinetics
- Bioavailability: tablet: F = 27%; oral solution: F = 15%
- Elimination: $t_{1/2}$ = 57-63 h (increased with hepatic dysfunction)

Antiproliferative Agents

Azathioprine
Mechanism of action
- Azathioprine is a purine analogue prodrug, which is cleaved to 6-mercaptopurine. 6-Mercaptopurine is activated intracellularly to several active metabolites, which can be incorporated directly into DNA as thiopurine, as well as interfere with the RNA and DNA biosynthesis directly and via feedback inhibition.

Administration
- Intravenous: dilute dose in NS or D_5W and administer IV infusion over 5-60 minutes.
- Oral: administer daily dose PO once a day

Drug-drug interactions
- Allopurinol: xanthine oxidase is responsible for the elimination of the active metabolites of azathioprine. Concomitant use of allopurinol with azathioprine results in significantly increased azathioprine-

induced toxicity. Reduce dose of azathioprine by 65-75%.

Drug-disease interactions
- Renal insufficiency: bioavailability is significantly reduced in uremic patients.
- Vaccinations: in general, immunosuppressants may affect efficacy of vaccinations. The use of live vaccines should be avoided.

Adverse drug reactions
- HEENT: retinopathy
- GI: nausea, vomiting, diarrhea, anorexia, pancreatitis, hepatotoxicity
- Dermatologic: rash, skin cancer
- Hematologic: leukopenia, thrombocytopenia, pancytopenia

Patient instructions
- Take the prescribed dose at a consistent time once daily. It may be taken with or without food, but should be taken the same way to maintain consistency. Do not take anything prescribed by another physician until you verify that there are no drug interactions.

Monitoring
- No clinically important pharmacokinetic or pharmacodynamic monitoring is needed.

Pharmacokinetics
- Bioavailability: F = 41-47%; in uremic patients, F = 17%

Mycophenolate mofetil
Mechanism of action
- Metabolized to mycophenolic acid (MPA), which causes noncompetitive, reversible inhibition of inosine monophosphate dehydrogenase (IMPDH), a critical enzyme in the de novo pathway of purine synthesis, which is crucial during lymphocyte activation and proliferation.

Administration
- Intravenous: dilute in D_5W to a concentration of 6 mg/mL and infuse over at least 2 h
- Oral: administer as equally divided doses PO every 8-12 h consistently with or without food

Drug-drug interactions
- Cyclosporine: see Table 4
- Cholestyramine: due to the interruption of enterohepatic recirculation, administration can decrease MPA exposure.
- Colestipol and colesevelam: simultaneous administration can decrease MPA exposure
- Antacids: simultaneous administration with magnesium- or aluminum-containing antacids reduces absorption and decreases MPA exposure
- Efficacy of oral contraceptives may decrease with therapy. Additional birth control methods are recommended.

Drug-disease interactions
- Severe renal impairment: reduces protein binding of MPA
- Vaccinations: in general, immunosuppressants may affect efficacy of vaccinations. The use of live vaccines should be avoided.

Adverse drug reactions
- GI: nausea, vomiting, diarrhea, abdominal pain
- Hematologic: leukopenia, thrombocytopenia, anemia, pancytopenia

Patient instructions
- Take the prescribed dose at consistent times during the day. It may be taken with or without food, but should be taken the same way to maintain consistency. Make sure you do not take your medication prior to therapeutic drug monitoring.

Monitoring
- No clinically important pharmacokinetic or pharmacodynamic monitoring is needed.

Pharmacokinetics
- MPA is highly protein bound.
- Bioavailability: F = 94%
- Elimination: $t_{1/2}$ = 16-18 h

Mycophenolate sodium
Mechanism of action
- Delayed-release tablets that deliver mycophenolic acid (MPA), which causes noncompetitive, reversible inhibition of inosine monophosphate dehydrogenase (IMPDII), a critical enzyme in the de novo pathway of purine synthesis, which is crucial during lymphocyte activation and proliferation

Administration
- Oral: administer as equally divided doses PO every 12 h consistently without food

Drug-drug interactions
- Cholestyramine: administration interrupts enterohepatic recirculation, and decreases MPA exposure
- Antacids: simultaneous administration with magnesium- or aluminum-containing antacids reduces absorption and decreases MPA exposure.

- Efficacy of oral contraceptives may decrease with therapy. Additional birth control methods are recommended.

Drug-disease interactions
- Severe renal impairment: reduces protein binding of MPA
- Vaccinations: in general, immunosuppressants may affect efficacy of vaccinations. The use of live vaccines should be avoided.

Adverse drug reactions
- GI: nausea, vomiting, diarrhea, abdominal pain
- Hematologic: leukopenia, thrombocytopenia, anemia, pancytopenia

Patient instructions
- Take the prescribed dose at consistent times during the day. It may be taken either 30 minutes before or 2 hours after meals, but it should be taken the same way each day to maintain consistency. Make sure you do not take your medication prior to therapeutic drug monitoring.

Monitoring
- No clinically important pharmacokinetic or pharmacodynamic monitoring is needed.

Pharmacokinetics
- MPA is highly protein bound.
- Bioavailability: F = 72-92%
- Elimination: $t_{1/2}$ = 8-16 h

Leflunomide
Mechanism of action
- Metabolized to an active metabolite, A77 1726, which inhibits de novo pyrimidine synthesis by selective inhibition of dihydro-orotate dehydrogenase (DHODH); inhibits proliferation of stimulated lymphocytes.

Administration
- Administer the daily dose PO once a day.

Drug-drug interactions
- Cholestyramine: reduces biliary recycling, which significantly shortens $t_{1/2}$; should not be used during leflunomide therapy.

Drug-disease interactions
- Renal insufficiency: bioavailability is significantly reduced in uremic patients.
- Vaccinations: in general, immunosuppressants may affect efficacy of vaccination. The use of live vaccines should be avoided.

Adverse drug reactions
- CNS: headache, dizziness, neuralgia, neuritis
- HEENT: alopecia
- GI: nausea, vomiting, diarrhea, anorexia, gastroenteritis, esophagitis, colitis
- Endocrine and metabolic: diabetes mellitus, hyperlipidemia, hyperthyroidism
- Patient instructions: take the prescribed dose at a consistent time once daily. It may be taken with or without food.

Monitoring
- No clinically important pharmacokinetic or pharmacodynamic monitoring is needed.

Pharmacokinetics
- A77 1726 is highly protein bound.
- Bioavailability: F = 80%
- Elimination: $t_{1/2}$ = 11-14 d

Corticosteroids

Selection of agent
- Selection of the corticosteroid used is based on the ratio of glucocorticoid to mineralocorticoid potency.

Intravenous
- Methylprednisolone, dexamethasone

Oral
- Prednisone, prednisolone, dexamethasone

Mechanism of action
- Corticosteroids bind to cytosolic glucocorticoid receptors, which translocate to the nucleus where the complexes bind to regulatory DNA sequences, glucocorticoid-responsive elements (GREs), within the promoter section of various genes. Activation of these GREs modifies activities of promoter genes such as NFAT, AP-1, and NF-κB. This results in downregulation of expression of HLA and numerous cell adhesion molecules, as well as decreased synthesis of numerous lymphokines responsible for activation, proliferation, and migration (ie, IL-1, IL-2, IL-6, IL-8, IFN-γ, TNF-α).

Administration
- Dependent on the individual agent

Drug-drug interactions
- Metabolized primarily via cytochrome P450 3A isoenzymes. Substances known to alter functionality of these enzymes will alter bioavailability and elimination of these drugs (Table 3).

Drug-disease interactions
- Diabetes mellitus: administration worsens glycemic control in patients with pre-existing diabetes.
- Osteopenia/osteoporosis: administration alters calcium and phosphate absorption and excretion, as well as osteoblast activity, resulting in progression of bone loss that is common in metabolic diseases such as end-stage renal disease and liver failure.
- Vaccinations: in general, immunosuppressants may affect efficacy of vaccinations. The use of live vaccines should be avoided.

Adverse drug reactions
- The incidence and extent of most adverse drug reactions with corticosteroids depend on the ratio of glucocorticoid to mineralocorticoid potency.
- CNS: seizure, psychosis, delirium, hallucinations, mood swings, insomnia, pseudotumor cerebri
- HEENT: cataracts, glaucoma
- CV: hypertension, cardiomyopathy
- GI: increased appetite, GERD, PUD, pancreatitis
- Renal: edema, alkalosis, hyperkalemia
- Endocrine and metabolic: diabetes mellitus, hyperlipidemia, hypothalamic-pituitary-adrenal axis suppression, growth suppression
- Dermatologic: hirsutism, acne, skin atrophy, impaired wound healing
- Hematologic: transient leukocytosis
- Musculoskeletal: arthralgia, myopathy, osteoporosis, avascular necrosis

Patient instructions
- When taking orally, take daily dose in the morning with food. Many drugs interact with these agents. Do not take anything prescribed by another physician until you verify that there are no drug interactions.

Monitoring
- No clinically important pharmacokinetic or pharmacodynamic monitoring is needed.

Pharmacokinetics
- Dependent on the individual agent

Monoclonal Antibodies

Orthoclone OKT3
Mechanism of action
- Murine monoclonal IgG that binds to and facilitates removal of cell lines expressing CD3. CD3, part of the TCR complex, is an important molecule that distinguishes T cells. CD3 is important in antigen recognition and antigen-specific signal transduction.

Administration
- Premedication:
  * Dose 1: intravenous steroids, acetaminophen, and antihistamines taken 1 h prior are strongly recommended to modify first-dose reactions.
  * Subsequent doses: acetaminophen and antihistamines taken 1 h prior with steroids as needed for infusion-related reactions
- Dosing: prior to administration, volume status must be carefully assessed. Patients with evidence of volume overload or uncompensated CHF on chest x-ray should not receive this drug. The dose should be administered via IV bolus over less than a minute.

Drug-drug interactions
- No clinically significant interactions occur.

Drug-disease interactions
- Uncompensated CHF/volume overload: risk of fatal pulmonary edema
- Vaccinations: in general, immunosuppressants may affect efficacy of vaccinations. The use of live vaccines should be avoided.

Adverse drug reactions
- CNS: dizziness, headache
- HEENT: photophobia
- CV: tachycardia
- Hematologic: transient lymphopenia, pancytopenia
- Musculoskeletal: rigor, tremor
- Other: fever, chills, dyspnea, pulmonary edema

Patient instructions
- Report any shortness of breath, palpitations, lightheadedness, tremor, fever, or itching to your nurse immediately.

Monitoring
- CD3: suppression of CD3 lineage <25 cells/mm^3

Pharmacokinetics
- Elimination: $t_{1/2}$ = 18 h

Basiliximab
Mechanism of action
- Chimeric (murine/human), monoclonal IgG that specifically binds to the subunit, CD25, of the human high-affinity IL-2 receptor, which is only expressed on activated lymphocytes; in this way basiliximab competitively inhibits IL-2 and facilitates preferential elimination of activated lymphocytes.

Administration

- Dilute to a concentration of 0.4 mg/mL in NS or D_5W; administer peripherally or centrally as a bolus or continuous infusion over 20-30 minutes

Drug-drug interactions

- No clinically significant drug interactions occur.

Drug-disease interactions

- Vaccinations: in general, immunosuppressants may affect efficacy of vaccinations. The use of live vaccines should be avoided.

Adverse drug reactions

- Severe acute hypersensitivity reactions including anaphylaxis may occur within the 24 hours following administration of the initial dose or on repeat exposure.

Patient instructions

- Report any shortness of breath, palpitations, light-headedness, or itching to your nurse immediately.

Monitoring

- No clinically important pharmacokinetic or pharmacodynamic monitoring is needed.

Pharmacokinetics

- Adults: following a 20-mg IV infusion over 20 minutes:
    * Mean C_{max} = 7.1 ± 5.1 mg/L
    * Mean $t_{1/2}$ = 7.2 ± 3.2 days
    * Pediatrics: mean $t_{1/2}$ = 11.5 ± 6.3 days

Pharmacodynamics

- Adults: CD25 saturation at or above serum concentration of 0.2 mcg/mL
    * Mean duration of saturation is dependent on concomitant immunosuppressive regimen.
- Pediatrics: CD25 saturation similar to that seen in adults

Daclizumab
Mechanism of action

- Humanized monoclonal IgG that specifically binds to the subunit, CD25, of the human high-affinity IL-2 receptor, which is only expressed on activated lymphocytes; in this way daclizumab competitively inhibits IL-2 and facilitates preferential elimination of activated lymphocytes.

Administration

- Dilute in 50 mL of NS and administer peripherally or centrally as a continuous infusion over 15 minutes

Drug-drug interactions

- No clinically significant drug interactions occur.

Drug-disease interactions

- Vaccinations: in general, immunosuppressants may affect efficacy of vaccination. The use of live vaccines should be avoided.

Adverse drug reactions

- Severe acute hypersensitivity reactions including anaphylaxis have rarely occurred within the 24 hours following administration of the initial dose or on repeat exposure.

Patient instructions

- Report any shortness of breath, palpitations, light-headedness, or itching to your nurse immediately.

Monitoring

- No clinically important pharmacokinetic or pharmacodynamic monitoring is needed.

Pharmacokinetics

- Adults: at recommended dosing:
    * Mean C_{max}: dose 1 = 21 ± 14 mg/mL; dose 5 = 32 ± 22 mg/mL
    * Mean C_{min}: dose 5 = 7.6 ± 4.0 mg/mL
    * $t_{1/2}$ = 20 days
- Pediatrics: at recommended dosing:
    * Mean C_{max}: dose 1 = 16 ± 12 mg/mL; dose 5 = 21 ± 14 mg/mL
    * Mean C_{min}: dose 5 = 5.0 ± 2.7 mg/mL
    * $t_{1/2}$ = 13 days

Pharmacodynamics

- Adults: CD25 saturation at serum concentrations of 5-10 mg/mL
    * At recommended dosing, saturation occurs for approximately 120 days.
- Pediatrics: CD25 saturation at serum concentrations of 5-10 mg/mL
    * At recommended dosing, saturation occurs for approximately 90 days.

Polyclonal Antibodies

Antithymocyte globulin (equine)
Mechanism of action

- Purified, sterile, polyclonal IgG harvested from horses immunized with human thymocytes. This preparation includes IgG directed against cell surface markers such as CD2, CD3, CD4, CD8, CD11a, and CD18. In this way horse antithymocyte globulin targets multiple phases of immunity, including T-cell activation, homing, and cytotoxic activities.

Administration
- Premedication
  - * Dose 1: Giving intravenous steroids, acetaminophen, and antihistamines 1 hour prior to the dose is strongly recommended to modify first-dose reactions.
  - * Subsequent doses: acetaminophen and antihistamines 1 h prior with steroids as needed for infusion reactions.
- Dose: Dilute the dose to a concentration not to exceed 4 mg/mL in $^{1}/_{2}$NS or D_5W and administer centrally over 4-6 h.

Drug-drug interactions
- No clinically significant drug interactions occur.

Drug-disease interactions
- Vaccinations: in general, immunosuppressants may affect efficacy of vaccinations. The use of live vaccines should be avoided.

Adverse drug reactions
- Most adverse drug reactions with antithymocyte globulin (equine) are infusion-related reactions (ie, fever, chills, dyspnea), leukopenia, thrombocytopenia, and/or rash.

Patient instructions
- Report any shortness of breath, palpitations, lightheadedness, tremor, fever, or itching to your nurse immediately.

Monitoring
- CD2: the goal for treatment of acute rejection is suppression of CD2 lineage to <50 cells/mm^3.

Pharmacokinetics
- Elimination: $t_{1/2}$ = 36 h-12 d

Antithymocyte globulin (rabbit)
Mechanism of action
- Purified, pasteurized, polyclonal IgG harvested from pathogen-free rabbits immunized with human thymocytes; this preparation includes IgG directed against cell surface markers such as TCRab, CD2, CD3, CD4, CD5, CD6, CD7, CD8, CD11a, CD18, CD28, CD45, CD49, CD54, CD58, CD80, CD86, HLA class I, and β_2 microglobulin. In this way, rabbit antithymocyte globulin targets multiple phases of immunity, including T-cell activation, homing, and cytotoxic activities.

Administration
- Premedication
  - * Dose 1: giving intravenous steroids, acetaminophen, and antihistamines 1 hour prior to the dose is strongly recommended to modify first-dose reactions.
  - * Subsequent doses: acetaminophen and antihistamines 1 h prior with steroids as needed for infusion reactions
- Dose: dilute dose to a concentration of 0.5 mg/mL in NS or D_5W and administer centrally over 4-6 h.

Drug-drug interactions
- Immunoglobulin: administration may decrease the degree of lymphocyte depletion achieved.

Drug-disease interactions
- Vaccinations: in general, immunosuppressants may affect efficacy of vaccinations. The use of live vaccines should be avoided.

Adverse drug reactions
- Most adverse drug reactions with antithymocyte globulin (rabbit) are infusion-related reactions (ie, fever, chills, dyspnea), leukopenia, thrombocytopenia, and/or rash.

Patient instructions
- Report any shortness of breath, palpitations, lightheadedness, tremor, fever, or itching to your nurse immediately.

Monitoring
- CD2: the goal for treatment of acute rejection is suppression of CD2 lineage to <50 cells/mm^3.

Pharmacokinetics
- Two-compartment model; terminal elimination: $t_{1/2}$ = 2-3 days for first dose; range 14-45 days with multiple doses

3. Key Points

- The goal of solid organ transplantation is to improve patients' quality of life and survival by stabilizing and/or improving end-organ failure–related complications.
- The immune system is a highly intricate system with mechanisms for antigen recognition in a highly specific manner, as well as a nonspecific manner.
- Acute rejection is a normal physiologic immune response to transplantation of donor antigens.
- The incidence of acute rejection is organ specific and dependent on multiple pre- and post-transplant factors.
- Selection of the post-transplant immunosuppression regimen for prevention of acute rejection should be individualized based on known risk and potential toxicity.
- Adjustment in the post-transplant immunosuppression regimen should focus on the balance between acute rejection, infection, and toxicity.
- Selection of the agent to be used to treat acute rejection is organ dependent and dependent on the severity of acute rejection.
- Immunosuppressive complications, both infectious and noninfectious, are an important cause of early morbidity and mortality and require close management post-transplant.
- Many agents commonly included in immunosuppression regimens require a clinician with expertise in immunosuppressive therapeutic drug monitoring to optimize efficacy and/or reduce toxicity.
- Many agents commonly included in immunosuppression regimens have the potential for numerous pharmacokinetic and pharmacodynamic drug interactions.

4. Questions and Answers

Use the patient profile provided below to answer Questions 1-4.

Patient name: Doe, John   Age: 52
Address: 101 South First Street
Gender: Male   Ethnicity: African-American
Height: 5'11"   Weight: 240 lb
Allergies: Sulfa
Diagnoses: h/o ESRD s/p cadaveric renal transplant 3 mo ago
DM x 20 yrs
HTN x 30 yrs
Drug-induced hyperkalemia 1/2003
Laboratory: 3/20/03 SCr = 1.2, K = 4.8, WBC 3.8, Plt 120
Medications:

1/20/03	Prograf 4 mg PO bid
	Amaryl 4 mg PO bid
	Cellcept 750 mg PO bid
	Metoprolol 100 mg PO bid
	Diflucan 200 mg PO qd
	Dapsone 100 mg PO qd
	Valcyte 450 mg PO qd
	EC ASA 81 mg PO qd
	Prednisone 5 mg PO qd
2/1/03	Lasix 40 mg PO bid
	Imuran 100 mg PO qd

1. Which medication(s) should be given with caution due to the patient's sulfonamide allergy?

I. Lasix
II. Dapsone
III. Amaryl

   A. I only
   B. II only
   C. I and III only
   D. II and III only
   E. I, II, and III

2. Which of the following combinations of drugs represent therapeutic duplication?
   A. Prograf and Imuran
   B. Azathioprine and CellCept
   C. Dapsone and Valcyte
   D. Amaryl and Tacrolimus
   E. Prednisone and CellCept

3. Which of the following combinations of drugs interact?

I. Diflucan and tacrolimus
II. Diflucan and Valcyte
III. Dapsone and Lasix

A. I only
B. II only
C. I and II only
D. II and III only
E. I, II, and III

4. In the above case, the patient was diagnosed with drug-induced hyperkalemia in 1/2003. Which medication on his profile could be responsible for this?

   A. CellCept
   B. Lasix
   C. Prednisone
   D. Prograf
   E. EC ASA

5. Which medication(s) is/are classified as a calcineurin inhibitor?

   A. Rapamune
   B. Cyclosporine
   C. Tacrolimus
   D. B and C
   E. A and C

6. Which medication(s) cause myelosuppression?

   A. Sirolimus
   B. Mycophenolate mofetil
   C. Valcyte
   D. All of the above
   E. B and C

7. Which medication(s) require bile for emulsification and absorption?

   A. Imuran
   B. Cyclosporine
   C. Prograf
   D. Prednisone
   E. All of the above

8. All of the following are known adverse effects of cyclosporine EXCEPT

   A. hirsutism
   B. nephrotoxicity
   C. oral ulceration
   D. gingival hyperplasia
   E. hyperlipidemia

9. All of the following are contraindications or precautions associated with Rapamune EXCEPT

   A. de novo lung transplant recipient
   B. hyperlipidemia
   C. diabetes mellitus
   D. de novo liver transplant recipient
   E. allergy to sirolimus

10. What is the generic name for Arava?

    A. Leflunomide
    B. Azathioprine
    C. Daclizumab
    D. Tacrolimus
    E. Alemtuzumab

11. Which of the immunosuppressive medication(s) listed may cause diabetes mellitus?

    A. Prednisone
    B. Azathioprine
    C. Tacrolimus
    D. A and C
    E. All of the above

12. Which medication(s) requires therapeutic drug monitoring via trough concentrations?

    A. Mycophenolate mofetil
    B. Prograf
    C. Daclizumab
    D. Leflunomide
    E. A and B

13. Which medication(s) selects for destruction of activated lymphocytes by binding to the CD25 subunit of the high affinity IL-2 receptor?

    A. Anti-thymocyte globulin (rabbit)
    B. Anti-thymocyte globulin (equine)
    C. Zenapax®
    D. A and B
    E. All of the above

14. All of the following increase the risk of acute rejection EXCEPT

    A. pediatric recipient
    B. HLA mismatch
    C. living donor
    D. noncompliance
    E. history of previous transplantation

15. Which of the following produces a significant pharmacokinetic interaction when administered with azathioprine?

   A. Allopurinol
   B. Diflucan
   C. Sirolimus
   D. Probenecid
   E. A and D

16. Which of these conditions alter the pharmacokinetic profile of cyclosporine?

   A. Biliary obstruction
   B. Malnutrition
   C. Hyperglycemia
   D. A and B
   E. All of the above

17. Which of the following medication(s) interacts with leflunomide?

   A. Erythromycin
   B. Prevalite®
   C. Diltiazem
   D. A and C
   E. B and C

18. Which of the following immunosuppressants should not be administered at the same time secondary to an interaction related to timing of doses?

   A. Prograf® and mycophenolate mofetil
   B. Rapamune® and cyclosporine
   C. Neoral® and leflunomide
   D. None of these interact
   E. B and C

19. Which type of immunity involves stimulation of cells and soluble mediators that nonspecifically recognize alloantigens with no altered response on repeat exposure?

   A. Autoimmunity
   B. Innate immunity
   C. Adaptive immunity
   D. Acute rejection
   E. Hyperacute rejection

20. Which group of genes encodes for antigens that are responsible for self/nonself recognition?

   A. Class I human leukocyte antigen (HLA)
   B. Class II human leukocyte antigen (HLA)
   C. Major histocompatibility complex (MHC)
   D. A and B
   E. All of the above

21. Upon binding of antigen displayed by the APC to the T-cell receptor complex, what additional step is required for T-helper cell activation?

   A. Binding of the co-stimulatory pathway (ie, CD58/CD2)
   B. Activation of the promoter gene NFAT
   C. Transcription of the IL-2 gene
   D. No additional step is required
   E. Both B and C

22. Which cytokine released by activated CD4$^+$ lymphocytes plays a major role in the subsequent activation of numerous lymphocyte lineages?

   A. Interleukin-1 (IL-1)
   B. Tumor necrosis factor-α (TNF-α)
   C. Interleukin-2 (IL-2)
   D. Interferon-γ (IFN-γ)
   E. Complement

23. Which solid organ was the first to be successfully transplanted?

   A. Heart
   B. Liver
   C. Kidney
   D. Lung
   E. Pancreas

24. What is the 1-year patient survival rate for renal transplant recipients?

   A. >90%
   B. 60-70%
   C. 25-50%
   D. <25%
   E. Limited data available; currently an experimental procedure

Answers

1. **C.** Lasix and Amaryl are structurally similar to sulfonamides and would be expected to elicit a similar allergic response. Dapsone is a sulfone and would not be expected to elicit an allergic response.

2. **B.** Both azathioprine and CellCept are classified as antiproliferative agents. Both agents inhibit purine biosynthesis and would not act synergistically.

3. **A.** Diflucan is an inhibitor of cytochrome P450 3A isoenzymes, which is the enzyme system that is responsible for metabolism of tacrolimus.

4. **D.** Hyperkalemia (incidence 20-40%) is a well-documented adverse drug reaction with Prograf.

5. **D.** Both cyclosporine and tacrolimus are calcineurin inhibitors.

6. **D.** All of the above-listed agents have myelosuppressive properties when administered individually. When administered concurrently the myelosuppression is synergistic.

7. **B.** Cyclosporine is highly lipophilic and requires bile for emulsification and absorption.

8. **C.** Hirsutism, nephrotoxicity, gingival hyperplasia, and hyperlipidemia are known adverse effects of cyclosporine. Oral ulceration is not an adverse effect of cyclosporine.

9. **C.** The use of Rapamune in de novo lung and liver transplant recipients is contraindicated due to an increased incidence of fatal adverse drug reactions. Additionally, use of Rapamune in patients with uncontrolled hyperlipidemia is strongly discouraged due to its profound effects on lipid biosynthesis and catabolism.

10. **A.** Leflunomide is the generic name for Arava.

11. **D.** Prednisone and tacrolimus may cause diabetes mellitus. Azathioprine does not produce a diabetogenic effect.

12. **B.** Prograf requires therapeutic drug monitoring via trough concentrations in order to obtain desired therapeutic effects.

13. **C.** Zenapax® selects for destruction of activated lymphocytes by binding to the CD25 subunit of the high-affinity IL-2 receptor.

14. **C.** Of the listed parameters, all are considered to increase the risk of acute rejection except living donor as donor source.

15. **A.** Xanthine oxidase is responsible for the elimination of the active metabolites of azathioprine. Concomitant use of allopurinol with azathioprine results in significantly increased azathioprine-induced toxicity. Reduce the dose of azathioprine by 65%-75%.

16. **D.** Both biliary obstruction and severe malnutrition would change the pharmacokinetic profile of cyclosporine. Cyclosporine requires bile for emulsification and absorption. If bile flow is obstructed, then the bioavailability is significantly decreased. Additionally, cyclosporine is a highly lipoprotein bound drug. In severe malnutrition, total protein stores are depleted, thereby increasing the total free drug.

17. **B.** Cholestyramine reduces biliary recycling which significantly shortens $t_{1/2}$.

18. **B.** Simultaneous administration increases C_{max} and AUC of sirolimus by 120%-500% and 140%-230%, respectively. Administration 4 hours apart increases C_{max} and AUC of sirolimus by 30%-40% and 35%-80%, respectively.

19. **B.** Innate immunity is the fundamental type of immunity in which antigens are recognized in a nonspecific manner. This type of immunity is not augmented on repeat exposure.

20. **C.** Class I and II HLA are the actual antigens important for self/nonself recognition. The group of genes that encode for these antigens is the major histocompatibility complex (MHC).

21. **A.** Activation is dependent on antigen/HLA binding to the T-cell receptor complex and the subsequent binding of a second signal or "co-stimulatory pathway."

22. **C.** Active CD4+ T cells produce and release various lymphokines, particularly IL-2, important for activation and proliferation of numerous lymphocyte lineages.

23. **C.** The kidney was the first organ to be successfully transplanted, in 1954.

24. **A.** Currently, the 1-year patient survival rate after renal transplantation is 94.4%, based on Organ Procurement and Transplantation Network data.

5. References

Budde K, Curtis J, Knoll G, et al. Enteric-coated mycophenolate sodium can be safely administered in maintenance renal transplant patients: results of a 1-year study. *Am J Transplant.* 2003;4:237-243.

Christians U, Jacobsen W, Benet LZ, Lampen A. Mechanisms of clinically relevant drug interactions associated with tacrolimus. *Clin Pharmacokinet.* 2002;41:813-851.

Cotts WG, Johnson MR. The challenge of rejection and cardiac allograft vasculopathy. *Heart Fail Rev.* 2001;6:227-240.

Delves PJ, Roitt IM. The immune system—first of two parts. *N Engl J Med.* 2000;343:37-49.

Delves PJ, Roitt IM. The immune system—second of two parts. *N Engl J Med.* 2000;343:108-117.

Dunn CJ, Wagstaff AJ, Perry CM, Plosker GL, Goa KL. Cyclosporin: an updated review of the pharmacokinetic properties, clinical efficacy and tolerability of a microemulsion-based formulation (Neoral)1 in organ transplantation. *Drugs.* 2001;61:1957-2016.

Galley BJ, Perez RV, Ramsamooj R. Acute renal transplant injury and interaction between antithymocyte globulin and pooled human immunoglobulin. *Clin Transplant.* 2004;18:327-331.

Kelly P, Kahan BD. Review: metabolism of immunosuppressant drugs. *Curr Drug Metab.* 2002;3:275-287.

Klupp J, Holt DW, van Gelder T. How pharmacokinetic and pharmacodynamic drug monitoring can improve outcome in solid organ transplant recipients. *Transpl Immunol.* 2002;9:211-214.

Neuberger J. Incidence, timing, and risk factors for acute and chronic rejection. *Liver Transpl Surg.* 1999;5(Suppl 1):S30-S36.

Salvadori M, Holzer H, de Mattos A, et al. Enteric-coated mycophenolate sodium is therapeutically equivalent to mycophenolate mofetil in de novo renal transplant patients. *Am J Transplant.* 2003;4:231-236.

Tejani A, Emmett L. Acute and chronic rejection. *Semin Nephrol.* 2001;21:498-507.

Williams JW, Mital D, Chong A, et al. Experience with leflunomide in solid organ transplantation. *Transplantation.* 2002;15:358-366.

21. Gastrointestinal Diseases

Christa M. George, PharmD, BCPS
Assistant Professor, Department of Clinical Pharmacy
University of Tennessee College of Pharmacy

Contents

1. Peptic Ulcer Disease

Definition and Incidence

- Peptic ulcer disease (PUD) is a group of disorders of the upper gastrointestinal tract characterized by ulcerative lesions dependent on acid and pepsin for their formation.
- Approximately 1.5-2 million Americans have an active ulcer at any given time.
- 500,000 new cases are diagnosed in the U.S. annually.
- The U.S. lifetime prevalence of PUD ranges from 11-20% for men and 8-11% for women.
- The cost of PUD in the U.S. is $20 billion per year.

Classification

- Ulcers are either duodenal or gastric in nature (duodenal ulcers are more common).
- Duodenal and gastric ulcers are classified as *Helicobacter pylori*–related, nonsteroidal anti-inflammatory drug (NSAID)–related, non–*H pylori*-related, non–NSAID related, or stress related.

Clinical Presentation

- Epigastric pain occurring 1-3 hours after meals that is relieved by ingestion of food or antacids is the classic presentation of PUD.
- Pain typically occurs in episodes lasting weeks to months, and may be followed by variable periods of spontaneous remission and recurrence.
- Ten percent of patients with PUD present with complications and have no prior history of pain.

Pathophysiology

- Duodenal ulcers result from the imbalance between duodenal acid load and the acid-buffering capacity of the duodenum.
- Duodenal ulcers are more frequently associated with an antrum-predominant gastritis.
- *H pylori* is a gram-negative microaerophilic bacterium that inhabits the area between the mucosal layer and epithelial cells in the stomach. It can be found anywhere gastric epithelium is present.
  - * Over 50% of the world's population is colonized by *H pylori,* but only 15% of colonized individuals develop clinical symptoms of PUD. The prevalence of *H pylori* is decreasing in developed countries.
  - * *H pylori* causes duodenal inflammation, increases duodenal acid load, and impairs duo-

denal bicarbonate secretion, which leads to duodenal ulcers.
  - * *H pylori* causes inflammation of gastric epithelium, particularly in the antrum-corpus area. This disrupts mucosal defense, which also leads to gastric ulcers.
- NSAIDs are the leading cause of PUD in patients negative for *H pylori* infection.
  - * NSAIDs are directly toxic to gastric epithelium and inhibit the synthesis of prostaglandins.
  - * Inhibition of prostaglandin synthesis leads to decreased bicarbonate secretion, the presence of epithelial mucus, mucosal perfusion, epithelial proliferation, and mucosal resistance to injury.
  - * NSAIDs may cause gastric or duodenal ulcers (more frequently gastric).
- Gastric ulcers are associated with a corpus-predominant (ie, diffuse-predominant) gastritis.
- This pattern of gastritis is associated with low acid output, gastric atrophy, and adenocarcinoma.

Diagnostic Criteria

- Upper gastrointestinal endoscopy is used to diagnose PUD. The procedure is usually reserved for patients with clinical features that suggest PUD complications (eg, gastric cancer, bleeding).

- Patients who initially present with clinical symptoms of PUD may be treated for *H pylori* if a test is positive for *H pylori* infection.
  - * *H pylori* may be detected noninvasively by serology, urea breath test (UBT), a fecal antigen test, and/or a urine antibody test. The UBT is the test of choice and is commercially available for use in medical offices.
  - * Gastric mucosal biopsies may be obtained during endoscopy for culture, rapid urease tests, and histology.

Treatment Principles and Goals

- The goals of PUD therapy include healing the ulcer and eliminating the cause of the ulcer.
- Additional considerations include preventing complications and relieving symptoms.
- Use of proton pump inhibitors (PPIs) is associated with faster healing rates and symptom relief than treatment with histamine$_2$-receptor antagonists (H$_2$RAs). (Note: H$_2$RAs are less expensive.)
- Choice of PUD therapy is based on the etiology of the case. For *H pylori*–related PUD, antibacterial therapy is used with antisecretory therapy.

* Eradication of *H pylori* reduces the recurrence of PUD, and is of prime importance.
* The ideal treatment regimen for *H pylori* has not been identified.
* Treatment regimens consist of triple or quadruple drug therapy (eg, with a PPI or an H$_2$RA, bismuth, and one or two antibiotics for 10-14 days). Average cure rates range from 86-94%, depending on the regimen used.
* The eradication of *H pylori* should be confirmed with UBT or fecal antigen testing 2-4 weeks after completing therapy.
* If resistance to clarithromycin is suspected, replace it with metronidazole, and vice versa. Often metronidazole resistance can be overcome by increasing the dose.
* If both clarithromycin and metronidazole resistance is suspected, furazolidone may be substituted (as part of a quadruple drug regimen).
• For NSAID-related PUD, discontinuation of the offending agent is imperative.
* Antisecretory therapy should be instituted to promote healing and to relieve symptoms.
* If *H pylori* is also present, antibacterial therapy should be initiated. Eradication of *H pylori* does not prevent NSAID-related complications or recurrence.

* PPIs, H$_2$RAs, or misoprostol should be used to prevent PUD in patients who require chronic NSAIDs and who are at risk of developing PUD (eg, patients who are elderly and/or have concomitant cardiovascular disease, patients with a history of PUD, patients using high-dose NSAID therapy, and/or patients who concomitantly use corticosteroids or anticoagulants).
* If chronic anti-inflammatory therapy is required, replacing the NSAID with a COX-2 inhibitor should be considered since it may reduce the risk of PUD.
• Sucralfate may also be used to aid in ulcer healing, but it requires multiple daily dosing and is associated with many significant drug interactions.
• Non–*H pylori,* non-NSAID–related PUD should be treated with antisecretory therapy.

Drug Therapy

Mechanism of action
• PPIs suppress gastric acid secretion specifically by inhibiting the H$^+$-K$^+$-ATPase enzyme system of the secretory surface of the gastric parietal cell (Table 1).
• H$_2$RAs suppress gastric acid secretion by reversibly blocking histamine$_2$ receptors on the surface of the gastric parietal cell.

Table 1

Selected Medications Used in Peptic Ulcer Disease

Generic name (trade name)	Classification	Dosage range and frequency	Dosage forms
Omeprazole (Prilosec®)	Proton pump inhibitor	20-40 mg qd	C
Esomeprazole (Nexium®)	Proton pump inhibitor	20-40 mg qd	C, IV
Lansoprazole (Prevacid SoluTab®)	Proton pump inhibitor	15 mg qd-30 mg bid	C, DT, L, ST
Rabeprazole (Aciphex®)	Proton pump inhibitor	10-20 mg qd	T
Pantoprazole (Protonix®)	Proton pump inhibitor	40-80 mg qd	T, IV
Cimetidine (Tagamet®)	H$_2$-receptor blocker	300 mg qid-800 mg hs	T, L, IV
Ranitidine (Zantac®)	H$_2$-receptor blocker	150 mg bid-300 mg hs	T, L, IV, C, EfT
Nizatidine (Axid®)	H$_2$-receptor blocker	150 mg bid-300 mg hs	C, L
Famotidine (Pepcid®)	H$_2$-receptor blocker	20 mg bid-40 mg hs	T, L, DT, IV
Ranitidine bismuth citrate (Tritec®)	H$_2$-receptor blocker + bismuth	400 mg bid x 10-14 d	T
Clarithromycin (Biaxin®)	Antibacterial	500 mg bid x 10-14 d	T, L
Amoxicillin (Amoxil®)	Antibacterial	1 g bid x 10-14 d	C, L
Metronidazole (Flagyl®)	Antibacterial	250-500 mg tid x 10-14 d	T, IV
Tetracycline (various)	Antibacterial	500 mg qid x 10-14 d	C
Furazolidone (Furoxone®)	Antibacterial	100 mg tid x 10-14 d	T
Sucralfate (Carafate®)	Cytoprotective	1 g qid	T, L

T, tablet; C, capsule; L, liquid; EfT, effervescent tablet; DT, delayed-release tablet; IV, intravenous; ST, SoluTab

- Clarithromycin, amoxicillin, metronidazole, tetracycline, bismuth subsalicylate, and furazolidone exhibit antibacterial effects against *H pylori*.
- When exposed to gastric acid, sucralfate forms a viscous adhesive that binds positively-charged protein molecules in the ulcer crater. This forms a protective barrier, which protects against back-diffusion of hydrogen ions.

Patient counseling

- Educate patients about the importance of completing the entire course of therapy to ensure the eradication of *H pylori* and to avoid bacterial resistance.
- PPIs are best taken before eating. Lansoprazole granules may be sprinkled onto applesauce for patients who have trouble swallowing pills. Omeprazole capsules should be swallowed whole.
- If antacids are being used to control breakthrough symptoms, the dose should be taken no less than 1-2 hours before or after taking an H$_2$RA. H$_2$RAs may be taken without regard to meals.
- Amoxicillin, clarithromycin, and metronidazole may be taken without regard to meals; however, taking clarithromycin and metronidazole with meals often reduces the incidence of stomach upset.
- Tetracycline is best taken on an empty stomach. Antacids, dairy products, or iron-containing products should be taken 2 hours before or after taking tetracycline.
- Sucralfate should be taken 1 hour before meals and at bedtime.

Adverse drug effects

- Side effects occur in 15-20% of patients, but they are usually minor.
- PPIs and H$_2$RAs are generally well-tolerated, but headache, diarrhea, and nausea have been reported.
- Antibiotics may cause diarrhea, nausea, dysgeusia, rash, and monilial vaginitis.
- Bismuth subsalicylate may cause black, tarry stools.
- Constipation is the most common side effect of sucralfate.
- Furazolidone may cause nausea, vomiting, headache, tachycardia, and hypertension.
- PPIs may alter the bioavailability of drugs that require an acidic environment for absorption (eg, ketoconazole, digoxin, and iron).

Drug interactions

- Omeprazole inhibits the cytochrome P450 enzyme system, which decreases the elimination of warfarin, phenytoin, diazepam, and cyclosporine. Lansoprazole has been reported to increase theophylline clearance by approximately 10%.
- Cimetidine is a potent inhibitor of the cytochrome P450 enzyme system, which decreases the elimination of numerous drugs (eg, warfarin, theophylline, and phenytoin).
- Amoxicillin and tetracycline may decrease the effectiveness of oral contraceptives.
- Clarithromycin is a potent inhibitor of the cytochrome P450 enzyme system, which decreases the elimination of warfarin, digoxin, cyclosporine, carbamazepine, theophylline, and cisapride (no longer on the market).
- Tetracycline may decrease the effectiveness of oral contraceptives. Antacids, iron products, and dairy products bind to tetracycline, decreasing its effectiveness. Tetracycline can also increase the therapeutic effect of warfarin. Tetracycline can increase or decrease lithium levels.
- Metronidazole produces a disulfiram-like reaction when ingested with alcohol, and increases the therapeutic effect of warfarin and lithium.
- Sucralfate leads to the absorption of small amounts of aluminum, which may accumulate if given to patients with renal insufficiency (especially when combined with aluminum-containing antacids).
- Sucralfate alters the absorption of numerous drugs, including warfarin, digoxin, phenytoin, ketoconazole, quinidine, and quinolones.
- Furazolidone is a monoamine oxidase inhibitor (MAOI). In order to avoid hypertensive crisis, furazolidone should not be administered with selective serotonin reuptake inhibitors (SSRIs), tricyclic antidepressants (TCAs), or tyramine-containing foods.
- Disulfiram-like reactions have been reported with the concurrent ingestion of alcohol and furazolidone.

Monitoring parameters

- Patients should monitor for the return of PUD symptoms and for the side effects of medications as discussed in the earlier sections.

Pharmacokinetics

- Several medications are substrates for or have effects on the cytochrome P450 enzyme system in the liver. Please see discussion in the drug interactions section.

Nondrug Therapy and Complications

- Patients should be counseled to decrease psychological stress and to discontinue smoking, taking NSAIDs, and ingesting food or beverages that may exacerbate PUD symptoms.
- Major complications occur in approximately 25% of patients with PUD (hemorrhage, perforation, penetration, and obstruction).
  - * Patients with active bleeding should initially undergo endoscopic hemostasis, as the proce-

dure is associated with a lower mortality rate than emergency surgery.
* Due to its safety, laparoscopic repair is beginning to replace laparotomy in the treatment of perforated ulcers.
* Surgery is reserved for those patients who have refractory ulcers (or hemorrhage or perforation) that cannot be managed with endoscopy or laparoscopic repair.

2. Gastroesophageal Reflux Disease

Definition and Incidence

- Gastroesophageal reflux disease (GERD) is defined as chronic symptoms or mucosal damage produced by the abnormal reflux of gastric contents into the esophagus.
- The prevalence of GERD is highest in Western countries. It occurs equally in men and women, except during pregnancy, when its incidence is higher in women. The incidence of GERD is higher and more frequently severe in Caucasians than in African Americans. Obesity has also been strongly correlated to the incidence of GERD. GERD may also occur in children. The risk of experiencing complications from GERD increases with age.
- Approximately 20% of the population experiences heartburn or regurgitation of gastric acid weekly.
- Approximately 30-50% of pregnant women have symptomatic esophageal reflux; 50% experience heartburn daily.

Classification

- Nonerosive reflux disease (NERD), erosive esophagitis (EE), and Barrett's esophagus (BE) are types of GERD. Esophageal adenocarcinoma rarely develops (2-4 cases per 100,000 persons per year). Patients with BE have an increased risk of developing esophageal adenocarcinoma.

Clinical Presentation

- Symptoms of GERD may be classified as typical, atypical, or complicated.
- The hallmark symptom of GERD is heartburn (pyrosis), which is described as substernal burning or pain that may radiate to the neck, back, or throat.
- Symptoms usually occur shortly after meals or when reclining after meals, or upon lying down at bedtime. Patients are often awakened from sleep by symptoms.
- Symptoms are exacerbated by eating a large meal (especially a high-fat meal), bending over, and occasionally by exercising.
- Additional typical symptoms include hypersalivation, belching, and regurgitation.
    * Typical symptoms are usually relieved with antacids.
- Atypical symptoms (or extraesophageal symptoms) include chronic cough, hoarseness, nonallergic asthma, pharyngitis, and chest pain that resembles angina.

- Symptoms suggestive of complications from GERD include continuous pain, dysphagia, odynophagia, bleeding, unexplained weight loss, and choking.
    * Complications include esophageal ulcers, strictures, and adenocarcinoma.
- Symptom severity does not correlate with the degree of esophagitis present on endoscopy, but severity usually does correlate with the duration of reflux.

Pathophysiology

- The effortless movement of gastric contents into the esophagus is a physiologic process that occurs numerous times daily throughout life and does not produce symptoms. This occurs more frequently in patients with GERD.
- The pathophysiology of GERD involves the prolonged contact of esophageal epithelium with refluxed gastric contents containing acid and pepsin.
- Prolonged contact between esophageal epithelium and gastric contents can overwhelm esophageal defense mechanisms and produce symptoms.
- Higher-potency gastric refluxate may produce symptoms during times of esophageal contact of normal duration.
- The presence of refluxate in an esophagus with impaired defense mechanisms may also produce symptoms.
- Esophageal defenses consist of the antireflux barrier, luminal clearance mechanisms, and tissue resistance.
    * Components of the antireflux barrier are the lower esophageal sphincter (LES) and the diaphragm. The LES is a thickened ring of circular smooth muscle localized to the distal 2-3 centimeters of the esophagus. It is contracted at rest, thereby serving as a barrier to refluxate. The diaphragm encircles the LES and acts as a mechanical support, especially during physical exertion.
    * Luminal clearance factors include gravity, esophageal peristalsis, and salivary and esophageal gland secretions (which contain acid-neutralizing bicarbonate).
    * The three areas of tissue resistance are pre-epithelial, epithelial, and postepithelial defense. Pre-epithelial and epithelial tissues limit the rate of diffusion of H^+ between cell membranes. Postepithelial defense is provided by the blood supply, which removes HCl and supplies oxygen, nutrients, and bicarbonate.

Diagnostic Criteria

- For patients who present with typical symptoms of GERD, a trial of empiric therapy is appropriate. A diagnosis of GERD may be assumed for patients who respond to empiric treatment.
- Further diagnostic testing (usually with endoscopy) should be considered for patients who do not respond to empiric therapy, patients who present with atypical symptoms or alarm symptoms, patients with chronic symptoms at increased risk for developing BE, patients with the need for continuous chronic therapy, elderly patients, and patients taking esophagotoxic medications (ie, NSAIDs, bisphosphonates).
    * Endoscopy is the preferred method for evaluating the esophageal mucosa for esophagitis and for evaluating for the presence of complications (eg, ulcers, strictures, BE).
    * Endoscopy is a highly specific test, but it is not extremely sensitive. Patients with symptoms may have normal esophageal mucosa (NERD).
    * Ambulatory pH monitoring may be used to confirm the diagnosis of GERD in patients with persistent symptoms (and no esophagitis present on endoscopy [NERD]), patients with noncardiac chest pain (or pulmonary symptoms), and in patients with refractory symptoms.
    * Ambulatory pH monitoring is performed by passing a small electrode to measure pH intranasally to the level of 5 cm above the LES. This allows patient symptoms to be correlated with the timing of episodes of decreased pH levels in the esophagus. This test may not be available at all institutions.
    * The Bernstein test of mucosal sensitivity to acid is highly specific for GERD and is the most commonly used provocative test of the esophagus.
    * Esophageal manometry consists of passing a multilumen tube into the stomach and subsequently measuring pressures as the tube is pulled back across the LES, esophagus, and pharynx.
    * Esophageal manometry is often performed to facilitate placement of ambulatory pH probes. It is always performed to aid in determining the best procedure in antireflux surgery candidates.

Treatment Principles and Goals

- Goals of therapy are to alleviate or eliminate symptoms, decrease frequency and duration of reflux, promote healing of the injured mucosa, and prevent the development of complications.
- Therapy is directed at increasing lower esophageal pressure, improving esophageal acid clearance and gastric emptying, protecting esophageal mucosa, decreasing the acidity of refluxate, and decreasing the amount of gastric contents being refluxed.

- Acid suppression is the mainstay of therapy for GERD. Proton pump inhibitors (PPI) provide the fastest symptomatic relief and heal esophagitis in the highest number of patients.
- Therapy for patients with GERD may be divided into three phases. Phase I consists of lifestyle modifications and patient-directed therapy with OTC H_2RAs and/or antacids. Phase II consists of continuation of lifestyle modifications and therapy with standard or high-dose antisecretory agents. Phase III consists of surgical intervention.
- Phase I therapy is appropriate for patients with mild typical symptoms of GERD. If symptoms persist after 2 weeks of therapy, phase II therapy is appropriate.
- For patients who present with mild to moderate typical symptoms, phase II therapy is appropriate. If atypical symptoms or symptoms suggestive of complications develop, patients should undergo endoscopic evaluation.
- H_2RAs are effective for patients with mild GERD. Patients with more severe symptoms (or patients with documented esophagitis) should receive PPI therapy. PPIs provide faster symptomatic relief and heal esophagitis much more effectively than H_2RAs.
- The addition of prokinetic agents to antisecretory drugs may offer modest improvements in symptoms compared to standard doses of H_2RAs. This addition is not routinely recommended, however, due to the increased incidence of side effects, higher cost, and only modest improvement of symptoms. Prokinetic agents are not appropriate for monotherapy of GERD.
- The decision to progress to phase III (surgery) should be individualized. There is no medical evidence to support medical or surgical therapy as the best treatment for GERD. Surgery should be considered in patients who are intolerant of medical therapy due to side effects, in patients who respond poorly to medical therapy, and in patients who desire a permanent solution to free them from chronic medication regimens.
* Three endoscopic procedures were recently approved by the Food and Drug Administration for the treatment of GERD. They include thermal ablation (Stretta® procedure), endoscopic suturing (plication), and endoscopic injection of inert materials. Data are currently limited on the overall efficacy of these procedures. Current guidelines recommend using these procedures only in select patient populations until more data are available from larger studies.
- GERD is considered a chronic condition, and most patients will require chronic therapy with antisecretory agents. For patients with more severe symptoms (with or without esophagitis) or for patients with complications, maintenance therapy with PPIs is preferred.
- GERD in patients with BE should be managed no differently than GERD in patients without BE. Aggressive GERD therapy for patients with BE is controversial. Patients with BE, no GERD symptoms, and no esophagitis do not require antisecretory therapy.

Drug Therapy

Mechanism of action

- For information on H_2RAs and PPIs, see Table 1 in the section on PUD.
- Antacids neutralize gastric acid (which increases LES tone) and inhibit the conversion of pepsinogen to pepsin, thus raising the pH of gastric contents.
- Alginic acid reacts with sodium bicarbonate in saliva to form sodium alginate viscous solution, which floats on the surface of gastric contents. The solution acts as a barrier to protect the esophagus from the corrosive effects of gastric reflux (Table 2).

Patient counseling

- Antacids and alginic acid are appropriate for the management of mild symptoms of GERD (phase I therapy). Symptoms persisting longer than 2 weeks require further evaluation and treatment with prescription medications.
- Refrigeration of liquid antacids may aid in palatability. Chewable tablets may be more effective than liquids due to increased adherence of antacid and saliva to the distal esophagus. Antacids must be taken at least 2 hours apart from tetracyclines, iron, and digoxin. Antacids and quinolones should be taken 4-6 hours apart.
- Alginic acid is effective for the relief of GERD symptoms, but there are no data to indicate esophageal healing on endoscopy. Alginic acid is ineffective if the patient is in the supine position, and must not be taken at bedtime.

Adverse drug effects

- Magnesium-containing antacids frequently cause diarrhea. Aluminum-containing antacids frequently cause constipation and bind to phosphate in the gut. This can lead to bone demineralization. Antacids may also cause acid-base disturbances.
- Magnesium and aluminum toxicity may occur when used chronically in patients with renal insufficiency. Sodium bicarbonate may cause sodium overload, particularly in patients with hypertension, congestive heart failure, and chronic renal failure. It may also lead to systemic alkalosis. It should be used on a short-term basis, if at all.

Table 2

Selected Antacids and Absorbents

Generic name (trade name)	Classification	Dosage range and frequency	Dosage forms
Magnesium hydroxide (milk of magnesia)	Antacid	15-30 mL prn	T, L
Aluminum hydroxide (Amphojel®, ALternaGEL®)	Antacid	15-30 mL prn	T, L
Aluminum carbonate (Basaljel®)	Antacid	15-30 mL prn	T, L
Magnesium hydroxide + aluminum hydroxide (Maalox®)	Antacid	15-30 mL prn	T, L
Magaldrate (Riopan®)	Antacid	15-30 mL prn	T, L
Calcium carbonate (Tums®, Titralac®)	Antacid	15-30 mL prn	T, L
Sodium bicarbonate (various)	Antacid	15-30 mL prn	T, L
Alginic acid + aluminum hydroxide + magnesium hydroxide (Gaviscon®)	Absorbent + antacid	15-30 mL prn; 2 after meals	T, L

T, tablet; L, liquid.

Drug interactions

- When taken with antacids, the absorption and effectiveness of tetracycline, ferrous sulfate, and quinolones is reduced, as the antacids form chelates with them. Antacids decrease the absorption of azoles and sucralfate by increasing gastric pH. Antacids increase urine pH, which decreases the renal clearance of quinidine. Antacids decrease the systemic absorption of digoxin and H_2RAs when taken concomitantly with them. Large doses of antacid may decrease the absorption of phenytoin.
- Digoxin and phenytoin levels should be monitored frequently when antacids are used concomitantly. Suspected adverse effects of antacids should be reported to a health care provider.

Monitoring parameters

- Patients should monitor for the return of GERD symptoms and for the side effects of medications as discussed in the earlier section.

Pharmacokinetics

- Several medications are substrates for or have effects on the cytochrome P450 enzyme system in the liver. Please see discussion under drug interactions in the PUD section.

Nondrug Therapy

- While lifestyle modifications alone are unlikely to control GERD symptoms, they should be initiated and maintained throughout the course of GERD therapy.
- Lifestyle modifications include elevating the head of the bed, decreasing fat intake, quitting smoking, avoiding lying down within 3 hours of eating, losing weight, avoiding foods or medications that can exacerbate GERD, avoiding alcohol, and eating smaller meals.
- Fats, chocolate, alcohol, peppermint, and spearmint reduce LES pressure and may exacerbate GERD symptoms. Spicy foods, orange juice, tomato juice, and coffee have direct irritant effects on the esophageal mucosa.

- Calcium channel blockers, β-blockers, nitrates, barbiturates, anticholinergics, and theophylline decrease LES pressure. Tetracyclines, NSAIDs, aspirin, bisphosphonates, iron, quinidine, and potassium chloride have direct irritant effects on the esophageal mucosa.

3. Inflammatory Bowel Disease

Definition and Incidence

- Idiopathic inflammatory bowel disease (IBD) is divided into two major types: (1) ulcerative colitis (UC) and (2) Crohn's disease (CD).
- UC is defined as a mucosal inflammatory condition confined to the rectum and colon.
- CD is defined as a transmural inflammation of the gastrointestinal (GI) tract that can affect any part of the GI tract from mouth to anus.
- The prevalence of UC is approximately 37.5-229 cases per 100,000 persons; the prevalence of CD is approximately 26-198.5 cases per 100,000 persons.
- There are approximately 1.3 million people with UC in North America, and each year 7000-43,000 new cases of UC are diagnosed in this region.
- Approximately 9000-44,000 new cases of CD are diagnosed each year; UC is slightly more predominant in men; CD is more predominant in women.
- North America, Scandinavia, and Great Britain have the highest incidence rates for IBD.
- UC typically occurs between age 30 and 40. CD typically occurs between age 20 and 30. Both may be diagnosed at any stage in life, but of all cases of IBD, 10-15% are diagnosed before adulthood.
- The incidence of IBD is low for Hispanic and Asian-Americans. Its incidence in African-Americans has increased and is equal to that of Caucasians. In addition, its incidence rate is high among the Jewish population in North America, Europe, and Israel.

Classification

- There are two major types of idiopathic inflammatory bowel disease (IBD): ulcerative colitis (UC) and Crohn's disease (CD).
- Clinical presentation and diagnostic tests help to distinguish one form from the other.

Clinical Presentation

- IBD is characterized by acute exacerbations of symptoms followed by periods of remission that are spontaneous or secondary to changes in medical therapy.
- The hallmark clinical symptom of UC is bloody diarrhea that is often accompanied by rectal urgency and tenesmus.
- The extent and severity of UC is characterized by clinical and endoscopic findings. Clinical symptoms are categorized as mild, moderate, severe, and fulminant. Endoscopic findings are categorized as distal

(limited to below the splenic flexure) or extensive (extending proximal to the splenic flexure).

Mild
- Mild UC is characterized by less than four stools per day with or without blood, without systemic disturbance, and with a normal erythrocyte sedimentation rate (ESR).

Moderate
- Moderate UC is characterized by more than four stools per day with minimal signs of toxicity.

Severe
- Severe UC is characterized by more than six stools per day with blood, systemic disturbance (eg, fever, tachycardia, anemia), and ESR greater than 30.

Fulminant
- Fulminant UC is characterized by more than 10 bowel movements per day, continuous bleeding, toxicity, abdominal tenderness and distension, blood transfusion requirement, and colonic dilation on abdominal plain films.
- The presentation of CD is variable and its onset is often insidious. Typical symptoms include chronic or nocturnal diarrhea and abdominal pain. Additional typical symptoms include weight loss, fever, and rectal bleeding.
- Symptoms differ depending on the site and severity of inflammation.
    * Mild to moderate: patients tolerate oral alimentation without dehydration, toxicity (fever, rigors, or prostration), abdominal tenderness, painful mass, and/or obstruction, or weight loss >10%.
    * Moderate to severe: patients fail to respond to treatment for mild to moderate disease or have fever, weight loss, abdominal pain, nausea, vomiting (without obstruction), or anemia.
    * Severe to fulminant: patients have persistent symptoms despite the use of steroids (as outpatients); or individuals presenting with high fever, persistent vomiting, evidence of obstruction, rebound tenderness, cachexia, or abscess.
    * The ileum and colon are the most commonly affected sites. Ileitis may mimic appendicitis. Intestinal obstruction and inflammatory masses or abscesses may also develop. Patients with colonic CD commonly have rectal bleeding, perianal lesions, and extraintestinal manifestations (eg, spondylarthritis, peripheral arthritis, erythema nodosum, pyoderma gangrenosum, uveitis, fatty liver, chronic active hepatitis, cirrhosis, primary sclerosing cholangitis, gall-

stones, cholangiocarcinoma, and hypercoagulability).

* Oral CD is characterized by lesions ranging from a few aphthous ulcers to deep linear ulcers with edema and induration. Gastroduodenal involvement may mimic PUD.

Pathophysiology

- The etiology of UC and CD is unclear, but similar factors may contribute to both diseases. These include infectious agents, genetics, environmental factors, immune deficits, and psychologic factors. Major etiologic theories involve a combination of infectious and immunologic factors.
- UC is confined to the rectum and colon and only affects the mucosa and submucosa. The primary lesion of UC is a crypt abscess, which forms in the crypts of the mucosa. CD most commonly affects the terminal ileum and involves extensive damage to the bowel wall.
- UC and CD complications can be local or systemic. Local complications of UC include hemorrhoids, anal fissures, and perirectal abscesses. Toxic megacolon can lead to perforation and is a major complication that affects 1-3% of patients with UC or CD. Colonic strictures and hemorrhage may also occur. Small bowel strictures, obstruction, and fistulae are common in CD. Systemic complications (extraintestinal) can occur with UC and CD.

Diagnostic Criteria

- UC is diagnosed based on clinical symptoms, proctosigmoidoscopy or colonoscopy, tissue biopsy, and bacteria-negative stool studies. CD is diagnosed based on clinical symptoms, contrast radiography or endoscopy, tissue biopsy, and bacteria-negative stool studies. Abdominal ultrasonography, computed tomography, and magnetic resonance imaging aid in the identification of masses, abscesses, and perianal complications in UC and CD.

Treatment Principles and Goals

- Treatment of IBD involves medications that target inflammatory mediators and alter immuno-inflammatory processes. These medications include anti-inflammatory agents and immunosuppressive agents.
- Nutritional considerations are also important since many patients with IBD may be malnourished.
- Goals of therapy for UC and CD include the induction and maintenance of remission of symptoms; improved quality of life; resolution of complications and systemic symptoms; and prevention of future complications. For patients with CD, remission

means that patients are asymptomatic or without inflammatory sequelae. This includes patients who have responded to medical intervention. Patients who require steroids to maintain their condition are considered "steroid dependent," not in remission.

- In UC patients, remission is likely to last at least 1 year with medical therapy. Without medical therapy, up to two-thirds of patients will relapse within 9 months. For mild CD, up to 40% of patients improve in 3-4 months with observation alone. Most will remain in remission for prolonged periods without medical therapy.
- The treatment of choice for distal UC that only involves the rectum (proctitis) is topical therapy with aminosalicylates.
  * Treatment is initiated with a nightly suppository or enema. Improvement usually occurs within 2-3 weeks. Most patients will require maintenance therapy with topical aminosalicylates in order to remain in remission.
  * Rectally administered steroids may be used in combination with aminosalicylates when patients do not respond to aminosalicylates alone.
  * For patients who do not respond to or cannot tolerate topical therapy, oral therapy with steroids and/or aminosalicylates is necessary.
  * Mild to moderate distal colitis may be treated with oral aminosalicylates, topical mesalamine, or topical steroids; however, topical aminosalicylates are more effective than topical steroids or oral aminosalicylates.
  * Combining oral and topical aminosalicylates is more effective than using them individually.
  * Patients who are refractory to maximum doses of these agents may require oral steroid treatment.
  * For the maintenance of remission, mesalamine enemas may be used every third night. Oral aminosalicylates are also effective for maintaining remission. Combining oral and topical aminosalicylates is more effective at maintaining remission than using them individually. Topical steroids are not effective at maintaining remission.
- For moderate to severe distal colitis, twice-daily enemas are required. Combining oral and topical aminosalicylates may also be required.
- For severe distal colitis, combining oral and topical aminosalicylates is required.
  * Oral corticosteroids are reserved for patients who fail initial aminosalicylate therapy.
  * Corticosteroids are tapered once remission is achieved, and topical and oral aminosalicylates are continued as maintenance therapy.

- Extensive UC (pancolitis) requires oral therapy; however, topical therapy is still a useful adjunct in controlling rectal disease.
    * For mild to moderate extensive UC, oral aminosalicylates are first-line therapy.
    * Patients who fail to respond require the addition of high-dose oral corticosteroid therapy.
    * Azathioprine and 6-mercaptopurine may be used in patients who do not respond to, or cannot be weaned from, corticosteroids. They may also be used to maintain remission.
    * Corticosteroid tapering should begin only when complete remission is achieved.
    * Corticosteroids do not have a role in maintenance therapy, as aminosalicylates are usually effective at maintaining remission.
    * For patients who fail oral therapy, hospitalization and intravenous steroid therapy is necessary.
- For moderate-to-severe UC refractory to conventional therapy, infliximab may be used to avoid or reduce corticosteroid use and to induce remission.
- For severe or fulminant colitis, hospitalization and complete bowel rest are required.
    * Intravenous steroids are the mainstays of therapy.
    * Topical therapy may be added for patients with significant rectal symptoms.
    * In patients who do not respond to 7 days of IV steroids, surgery or intravenous cyclosporine should be considered. Patients who respond to IV cyclosporine are converted to oral cyclosporine and a steroid taper.
    * Azathioprine may be added to maintain remission.
- Abdominal x-ray should be performed to exclude toxic megacolon. Surgery is often required for patients with toxic megacolon, and preoperative antibiotics are recommended to reduce the chance of septic complications.
- For mild to moderate CD, oral aminosalicylates are appropriate initial therapy.
    * Rectal aminosalicylates are often used to treat distal colonic CD; however, controlled studies showing efficacy are lacking.
    * Alternatively, metronidazole or ciprofloxacin may be used as first-line therapy.
    * Both aminosalicylates and antibiotics are more effective for colonic CD than ileal CD.
    * In studies, controlled-release budesonide produces a higher remission rate than mesalamine in treating mild to moderate ileal CD. Results of studies comparing budesonide with oral steroids are conflicting.
    * No controlled data exist regarding the treatment of mild to moderate oral CD. Lidocaine lozenges may provide symptomatic relief. Lesions will respond to systemic steroids or azathioprine in 50% of patients.

    * For mild to moderate cases of gastroduodenal CD, acid suppression therapy with H_2RAs or PPIs is recommended.
    * Once remission is achieved, maintenance therapy should be initiated. For patients who do not respond, progression to therapy for moderate-to-severe disease should be considered.
- For patients with moderate to severe disease, oral corticosteroids are the mainstay of therapy.
    * Prednisone or budesonide may be used as first-line agents. Steroids are not appropriate maintenance therapy.
    * For steroid-refractory patients, azathioprine or 6-mercaptopurine should be added.
    * Alternatively, methotrexate may be added for maintenance therapy. Infliximab is also effective therapy, but requires IV infusion at least every 8 weeks.
    * Total parenteral nutrition and enteral nutrition with elemental nutrient formulas are also effective in inducing remission.
- For severe to fulminant CD, hospitalization for intravenous steroids and hydration is required.
    * Anemic patients may require blood transfusions.
    * Intestinal obstructions related to adhesions should be managed with bowel rest and nasogastric tube suctioning. Obstructions related to inflammatory strictures require antibiotic therapy and IV steroids. Surgery should be considered if obstructive symptoms do not respond to therapy.
    * Abscesses should be drained and appropriate antibiotic therapy instituted.
    * High-dose metronidazole or ciprofloxacin may be used in the management of fistulas.
    * Azathioprine, 6-mercaptopurine, infliximab, and PPIs in combination with octreotide may also be used in the management of fistulas.
    * If patients do not respond to IV steroids after 5-7 days of therapy, cyclosporine or tacrolimus therapy may be instituted.
    * Maintenance therapy with azathioprine is usually required.
    * Patients who do not respond to therapy require surgical intervention.
- 6-Mercaptopurine is the best agent for preventing relapse of CD after surgical intervention.

Drug Therapy (Table 3)

Mechanism of action
- Sulfasalazine is cleaved to sulfapyridine (excreted in the urine) by bacteria in the gut and mesalamine (the active component). The sulfapyridine molecule is

Table 3

Selected Medications Used in Inflammatory Bowel Disease

Generic name (trade name)	Classification	Dosage range and frequency	Dosage forms
Sulfasalazine (Azulfidine®)	Aminosalicylate	4-6 g/d	T
Mesalamine (Asacol®,	Aminosalicylate	2.4-4.8 g/d	DT
Pentasa®, Rowasa®		2-4 g/d	DC
Salofalk®, Claversal®)		1-4 g/d	EN, SU
Balsalazide (Colazal®)	Aminosalicylate	6.75 g/d	DC
Metronidazole (Flagyl®)	Antibacterial	10-20 g/d (Crohn's)	T, IV
Ciprofloxacin (Cipro®)	Antibacterial	500 mg bid (Crohn's)	T, IV
Prednisone (various)	Corticosteroid	40-60 mg/d	T
Methylprednisolone (Solu-Medrol®)	Corticosteroid	16 mg q8h	IV
Budesonide (Entocort EC®)	Corticosteroid	9 mg qd	C
Azathioprine (Imuran®)	Immunosuppressive	1-2.5 mg/kg/d	T, IV
6-Mercaptopurine (Purinethol®)	Immunosuppressive	1.5 mg/kg/d	T
Methotrexate (Abitrexate®)	Antimetabolite	25 mg/wk	IM, SQ
Infliximab (Remicade®)	Immunomodulator	5 mg/kg q 8 weeks	IV
Cyclosporine (Neoral®, Sandimmune®)	Immunosuppressive	4 mg/kg/d	IV, C, L

T, tablet; C, capsule; L, liquid; DT, delayed-release tablet; DC, delayed-release capsule; IV, intravenous; IM, intramuscular; SQ, subcutaneous; EN, enema; SU, suppository.

responsible for the many side effects associated with sulfasalazine.

- Mesalamine's mechanism of action is poorly understood. Mesalamine inhibits cyclooxygenase and may also inhibit production of cyclooxygenase, thromboxane synthetase, platelet-activating factor synthetase, and interleukin-1 in macrophages. It may also act as a superoxide free-radical scavenger.
- Corticosteroids have immunomodulatory effects and inhibit the production of cytokines and other inflammatory mediators.
- Corticosteroids, azathioprine, 6-mercaptopurine, cyclosporine, and tacrolimus are immunosuppressive agents. For full discussion of mechanism of action, patient counseling, side effects, drug interactions, and pharmacokinetics, the reader is referred to the chapter on transplantation.
- The exact mechanism of action of metronidazole and ciprofloxacin in IBD is not known. One theory suggests that antibacterials interrupt the role of bacteria in the inflammatory process.
- Methotrexate inhibits dihydrofolate reductase and purine synthesis, reduces the production of leukotriene B_4 and interleukins 1 and 2, and may induce T-cell apoptosis.
- Infliximab is a chimeric monoclonal antibody that inhibits tumor necrosis factor.

Patient counseling

- Sulfasalazine should be taken after meals. Patients should avoid sun exposure while taking sulfasalazine. Folic acid supplementation should be given during sulfasalazine treatment to avoid anemia. Sulfasalazine may cause orange discoloration of urine and skin. Mesalamine tablets should be swallowed whole. Suppositories should not be handled excessively and foil wrappers should be removed before insertion. Suspension enemas should be shaken well before use.
- Antacids and ciprofloxacin should be taken 4-6 hours apart. Iron- or zinc-containing products should be taken 4 hours before or 2 hours after taking ciprofloxacin. Patients should avoid excessive exposure to sunlight.
- Patients taking methotrexate should avoid alcohol, salicylates, and prolonged exposure to sunlight. Female patients of childbearing age should be counseled on appropriate contraceptive measures during methotrexate therapy.
- Patients receiving therapy with infliximab should be counseled on the possibility of infusion reactions. Live vaccines should not be administered to patients taking infliximab.

Adverse drug effects

- Sulfasalazine may cause nausea, vomiting, anorexia, and headaches. The sulfapyridine moiety leads to hypersensitivity reactions (eg, rash, fever, agranulocytosis, pancreatitis, nephritis, and hepatitis) and altered spermatogenesis in males.
- Mesalamine is better tolerated than sulfasalazine. Olsalazine may cause self-limited watery diarrhea. Balsalazide may cause abdominal pain in 10% of patients.
- Ciprofloxacin may cause nausea, diarrhea, headache, and vaginal candidiasis.
- Methotrexate frequently causes nausea and leukopenia. Asymptomatic elevations in liver function tests may occur.
- Infliximab may cause acute and delayed infusion reactions, autoantibody development, and lupus.

Drug interactions

- Sulfasalazine may decrease the bioavailability of digoxin.
- Allopurinol enhances the effect of azathioprine. The azathioprine dose should be lowered by 50% when the agents are used concurrently.
- Ciprofloxacin binds with antacids, zinc, and iron products. It also increases the therapeutic effects of warfarin, cyclosporine, and theophylline.
- The use of methotrexate and concurrent NSAIDs has caused fatal interactions. Methotrexate may increase levels of 6-mercaptopurine.

Monitoring parameters

- Serum creatinine, complete blood counts, liver function tests, blood glucose concentrations, ESR, response to therapy, and the presence of adverse effects should be monitored.

Pharmacokinetics

- Several medications are substrates for or have effects on the cytochrome P450 enzyme system in the liver. Please see discussion in drug interactions section.

Nondrug Therapy

- Patients with UC and CD are often malnourished due to malabsorption or maldigestion caused by chronic bowel inflammation, "short gut" syndrome from multiple bowel surgeries, or bile salt deficiency in the gut. The catabolic effects of the disease process can also lead to malnutrition.
- Individuals should eliminate foods that exacerbate symptoms. Patients with lactase deficiency should avoid dairy products or take lactase supplements to avoid symptoms.
- Fish oil supplementation may improve weight gain and reduce the rate of relapse in CD.

- Enteral or parenteral supplementation may also be used in patients with severe UC or CD.
- Surgery may be necessary for patients with severe UC or CD. Surgery (proctocolectomy) is curative for UC, but not for CD.
    * Surgery involves removing diseased segments of bowel, repairing fistulas, and draining abscesses.
    * In UC, surgery is indicated for patients who fail maximum medical therapy to correct complications (perforation, strictures, obstruction, hemorrhage, toxic megacolon). It is also used and as prophylaxis against the development of cancer (in patients with long-standing UC) and in patients with premalignant changes found on bowel biopsies.
    * In CD, surgery is reserved for patients with complications from the disease. There is a high recurrence rate after surgery for CD. Other indications for surgery are colon cancer, inflammatory mass, or perforations.

4. Irritable Bowel Syndrome

Definition and Incidence

- Irritable bowel syndrome (IBS) is defined as abdominal discomfort associated with altered bowel habits. It is characterized by symptoms of abdominal pain or discomfort.
- IBS is classified according to the Rome II diagnostic criteria.
- IBS is the most prevalent digestive disease; it constitutes 12% of visits to primary care physicians and 28% of referrals to gastroenterologists.
- The medical expenses of patients with IBS are 1.6-fold higher than the expenses of an asymptomatic individual. They miss three times as many days of work per annum as persons without IBS. IBS significantly decreases the quality of life of most patients who seek medical care.
- Most cases of IBS are diagnosed before age 45. Women develop IBS 2-3 times more often than men. IBS is less common in Asians and Hispanics than in other ethnic groups.

Classifications

- IBS may be classified according to the Rome II diagnostic criteria (see pathophysiology section).
- IBS is usually classified as either diarrhea-predominant, constipation-predominant, or alternating between diarrhea and constipation, depending upon the patient's clinical presentation.
  - * Patients are also categorized as having mild, moderate, or severe disease.

Clinical Presentation

- IBS is a heterogeneous disorder with various clinical presentations.
  - * Abdominal pain is generally described as crampy or achy, and the intensity and location is highly variable. It may be exacerbated by meals and may last from 1-3 hours. Stress and emotional turmoil can also exacerbate pain.
  - * Patients typically present with diarrhea, constipation, or alternating periods of both.
  - * Upper gastrointestinal symptoms occur more frequently in patients with constipation (heartburn, dyspepsia, early satiety, and nausea). Women experience abdominal distention, bloating, and nausea more often than men.
  - * Extraintestinal symptoms are common.
    - • They include genitourinary symptoms (eg, pelvic pain, dysmenorrhea, dyspareunia, urinary frequency, nocturia, and sensation of incomplete bladder evacuation), impaired sexual function (eg, decreased libido), and musculoskeletal complaints (eg, lower back pain, headaches, and chronic fatigue).

Pathophysiology

- The pathogenesis is multifactorial and includes abnormal gut sensorimotor activity, central nervous system (CNS) dysfunction, psychologic disturbances, genetic predisposition, enteric infection, and other luminal factors.
  - * Colonic motor abnormalities commonly occur in IBS. Patients with IBS may exhibit an exaggerated gastrocolonic response lasting up to 3 hours.
  - * Small intestinal motor patterns are frequently disturbed in patients with IBS. Small intestinal transit is delayed in constipation-predominant IBS and is accelerated in diarrhea-predominant IBS.
  - * Bloating may be the result of abnormal retrograde reflux of intestinal gas, enhanced perception of the presence of intestinal gas, or obstructive intestinal motor patterns.
  - * Motor dysfunction of other smooth muscles may occur in IBS. The following abnormalities may also be found: lowered LES sphincter pressures, abnormal esophageal body peristalsis, gastric slow-wave dysrhythmias, delayed gastric and gallbladder emptying, and dysfunction of the sphincter of Oddi.
  - * It is theorized that IBS results from sensitization of visceral afferent fibers, which causes normal physiologic events to be perceived as painful. It is unknown if sensorineural dysfunction is generalized or localized to the gut afferent fibers.
  - * It is unknown whether IBS is primarily a CNS disorder with centrally directed changes in gut sensorimotor function, or primarily a gut disorder with inappropriate CNS input. Further investigation is needed in this area.
  - * Eighty percent of patients with IBS exhibit psychiatric disturbances. The onset of psychiatric disturbances usually predates or occurs concurrently with the onset of IBS. Psychological stress triggers symptoms in many patients. IBS is also associated with a history of sexual abuse.
  - * Other factors that may contribute to IBS are alterations in gut flora (controversial), antecedent gastrointestinal infection, carbohydrate malabsorption, food allergies, neurohumoral disturbances, genetic factors, and abnor-

mal stool characteristics (low concentrations of bile or short-chain fatty acids).

- IBS may be categorized using the Rome II diagnostic criteria.
    * Abdominal discomfort or pain present for at least 12 weeks (not necessarily consecutive weeks) in the preceding 12 months, that has two of these three features:
        - It is relieved with defecation; and/or
        - Its onset is associated with a change in frequency of stool; and/or
        - Its onset is associated with a change in the form (appearance) of the stool
    * Symptoms that cumulatively support the diagnosis of IBS include the following:
        - Abnormal stool frequency (ie, more than three bowel movements per day and fewer than three bowel movements per week)
        - Abnormal stool form (lumpy/hard or loose/watery stool)
        - Abnormal stool passage (straining, urgency, or feeling of incomplete evacuation)
        - Passage of mucus
        - Bloating or feeling of abdominal distention
- Weight loss, bleeding, fever, or palpable masses are warning signs of organic disease and are not common in IBS.
- Relief of pain with defecation, looser stool with pain onset, more frequent stools with pain onset, and abdominal distention are significantly more common in IBS than in organic disease.

Diagnostic Criteria

- Physical examination is usually normal.
    * Although the incidence of organic disease is low in patients with IBS, the following diagnostic tests may be used to exclude the presence of organic disease in patients presenting with IBS symptoms: complete blood count; serum electrolytes; erythrocyte sedimentation rate (ESR) and thyroid hormone levels; fecal occult blood testing; stool tests for ova and parasites; colonoscopy; and testing for celiac sprue.
    * The American College of Gastroenterology states that the aforementioned tests may be not be necessary unless the patient presents with alarm symptoms. Alarm symptoms are: onset of symptoms in patients aged >50; unexplained weight loss; GI bleeding; progressive or unrelenting pain; nocturnal or large-volume diarrhea; and family history of colon cancer, IBD, or iliac sprue.

- In patients with diarrhea, hydrogen breath testing may be used to exclude lactase deficiency (an empiric trial of lactose restriction may also be used).
- Sigmoidoscopy or colonoscopy may be performed for patients under age 50 with constipation to exclude obstruction and in patients with diarrhea to exclude IBD.
- In patients over age 50, colonoscopy should be performed to exclude colonic neoplasm.

Treatment Principles and Goals

- Treatment should be offered to patients seeking medical care if the patient and physician believe that the IBS symptoms decrease the quality of life of the patient.
    * Goals of therapy include improving IBS symptoms and improving patient quality of life.
    * There is inconsistent evidence from small clinical trials regarding the effectiveness of anticholingergic/antimuscarinic agents (dicyclomine and hyoscyamine) in the management of IBS; however, they are often used as first-line therapy in patients with mild symptoms. They may be effective in some patients, and should be used with caution in patients with constipation.
    * Bulking agents (calcium polycarbophil and psyllium) have little effect on IBS symptoms; however, they may be useful in some patients with constipation-predominant IBS.
    * Loperamide significantly improves stool consistency and decreases stool frequency in patients with diarrhea-predominant IBS. It has no effect on abdominal pain or global IBS symptoms.
    * Tegaserod improves global IBS symptoms, bloating, abdominal pain, and altered bowel habits in patients with constipation-predominant IBS.
    * There are no randomized controlled trials evaluating the effectiveness of osmotic laxatives in patients with IBS; however, they are often used as adjunctive agents in patients with constipation-predominant IBS.
    * Tricyclic antidepressants improve abdominal pain in patients with IBS. They also improve global IBS symptoms in patients with diarrhea-predominant IBS, but not constipation-predominant IBS.
    * Selective serotonin reuptake inhibitors (SSRIs) improve abdominal pain in patients with IBS and are also effective in the treatment of comorbid psychiatric disorders in patients with IBS. SSRIs are recommended for patients with moderate to severe abdominal pain, or those

with psychiatric comorbidities. Several types of psychological counseling/therapy are also effective in some patients with IBS.
  * Alosetron improves global IBS symptoms, abdominal discomfort, stool consistency, and stool frequency in women with diarrhea-predominant IBS.

Drug Therapy (Table 4)

Mechanism of action
* The antispasmodic agent dicyclomine decreases GI motility by relaxing smooth muscle in the gut.
* Hyoscyamine is an anticholinergic agent that decreases GI motility by decreasing smooth muscle tone through antimuscarinic activity in the gut.
* TCAs (eg, amitriptyline) delay intestinal transit and may blunt perception of visceral distention. The effect of TCAs on the cerebral processing of visceral pain is unknown.
* Tegaserod maleate, a partial 5-HT$_4$ agonist that stimulates the peristaltic reflex and intestinal secretion, inhibits visceral sensitivity by binding to 5-HT$_4$ receptors in the gut.
* Lactulose, milk of magnesia, and polyethylene glycol solutions are osmotic laxatives that aid in the treatment of IBS patients with constipation.
* Fiber supplements (bulk laxatives) increase stool bulk and water content.
* Loperamide inhibits peristalsis by directly affecting the circular and longitudinal muscles of the intestinal wall. Diphenoxylate is a meperidine congener

that has a direct effect on the circular smooth muscle in the gut, which slows GI transit time.
* Alosetron is a selective 5-HT$_3$–receptor antagonist that inhibits activation of nonselective cation channels in the gut, thereby modulating the enteric nervous system.
* Selective serotonin reuptake inhibitors (SSRIs) inhibit the neuronal uptake of serotonin in the CNS. Citalopram has peripheral effects on colonic tone and sensitivity. Paroxetine has potent anticholinergic effects.

Patient counseling
* Antispasmodics and anticholinergic agents are best used on an as-needed basis up to three times per day during acute attacks or before meals when postprandial symptoms are present.
* Patients taking a TCA should avoid prolonged exposure to sunlight and avoid concurrent use of CNS depressants.
* Tegaserod should be taken before meals and should not be initiated during an acute exacerbation of IBS.
* Osmotic laxatives should be used on an as-needed basis. Lactulose may be mixed with water or juice to increase palatability. Patients should drink plenty of water.
* Patients must be enrolled in the manufacturer prescribing program in order to receive alosetron. Patients should not initiate therapy with alosetron if they are currently constipated. Alosetron should be discontinued if no improvement in symptoms is seen after 4 weeks of therapy.

Table 4

Selected Medications Used in Irritable Bowel Syndrome

Generic name (trade name)	Classification	Dosage range and frequency	Dosage forms
Dicyclomine (Bentyl®)	Antispasmodic, anticholinergic	10-20 mg qid prn	T, C, L
Hyoscyamine (various)	Anticholinergic	0.25-0.5 mg bid-qid	T, L
Amitriptyline (Elavil®)	Tricyclic antidepressant	10-50 mg qhs	T
Paroxetine (Paxil®)	Selective serotonin-reuptake inhibitor	10-60 mg/d	T, L, DT
Tegaserod (Zelnorm®)	Serotonin (5-HT$_4$) receptor antagonist	6 mg bid	T
Lactulose (various)	Osmotic laxative	30-45 mL bid-qid prn	L
Polycarbophil (Fibercon®)	Bulking agent	1 g qd-qid prn	T
Polyethylene glycol (various)	Osmotic laxative	250 mL q 10 min up to 4 L	L
Alosetron (Lotronex®)	Serotonin (5-HT$_3$) receptor antagonist	1 mg qd-bid	T
Loperamide (Imodium®)	Antidiarrheal	2 mg after each loose stool; max 16 mg/d	T, C, L
Diphenoxylate/atropine (Lomotil®)	Antidiarrheal	15-20 mg/d of diphenoxylate in 3-4 divided doses	T, L

T, tablet; C, capsule; L, liquid; DT, delayed release tablet.

- See the chapter on psychiatric disease for a full discussion of SSRIs.

Adverse drug effects
- Dicyclomine, hyoscyamine, and TCAs may cause anticholinergic side effects (CNS depression, dry mouth, urinary retention, constipation, and decreased sweating).
- Tegaserod may cause diarrhea, nausea, headache, and abdominal pain.
- Osmotic laxatives may cause abdominal pain and cramping.
- Alosetron may cause constipation, abdominal pain, and nausea. Intestinal obstruction, perforation, toxic megacolon, ischemic colitis, and death have occurred.

Drug interactions
- Anticholinergics and antispasmodics may decrease the effectiveness of antipsychotic medications. Anticholinergic side effects are increased when given concurrently with a TCA.
- TCA concentrations may be increased or decreased by medications that induce or inhibit the activity of the cytochrome P450 enzyme system in the liver. TCAs should not be given concurrently with monoamine oxidase inhibitors or sympathomimetic agents.
- No significant drug interactions with tegaserod have been reported.
- Other medications should not be taken within 1 hour of the start of therapy with osmotic laxatives.
- Drugs that induce or inhibit the cytochrome P450 enzyme system may affect serum concentrations of alosetron. The clinical significance of this is unknown.

Monitoring parameters
- Patients should monitor for the presence of IBS symptoms and for the side effects of medications as discussed in the earlier section.

Pharmacokinetics
- Several medications are substrates for or have effects on the cytochrome P450 enzyme system in the liver.

Nondrug Therapy

- An effective physician-patient relationship is necessary for successful treatment.
- Education regarding disease pathophysiology and treatment and reassurance that the symptoms are real should be provided.
- Patients should be counseled to avoid foods that exacerbate symptoms. Foods commonly implicated are fatty foods, beans, gas-producing foods, alcohol, caffeine, and lactose (in lactase-deficient individuals), and occasionally excess fiber.
  * Several types of psychological counseling/therapy are effective in some patients with IBS.

5. Key Points

Peptic ulcer disease

- Peptic ulcer disease (PUD) is a group of disorders of the upper gastrointestinal tract characterized by ulcerative lesions that require acid and pepsin for their formation.
- Duodenal and gastric ulcers are classified as *Helicobacter pylori*–related, NSAID-related, non-*H pylori*–related, non-NSAID–related, or stress-related.
- Epigastric pain occurring 1-3 hours after meals that is relieved by ingestion of food or antacids is the classic symptom of PUD.
- *H pylori* is a gram-negative microaerophilic bacterium inhabiting the area between the mucous layer and epithelial cells in the stomach. It can be found anywhere gastric epithelium is present.
- NSAIDs are the leading cause of PUD in patients who are negative for *H pylori* infection. NSAIDs are directly toxic to gastric epithelium and inhibit the synthesis of prostaglandins.
- PUD is diagnosed with upper gastrointestinal endoscopy. This is usually reserved for patients with clinical features suggestive of complications from PUD (eg, gastric cancer or bleeding).
- *H pylori* may be detected noninvasively by serology, urea breath test (UBT), fecal antigen testing, and urine antibody testing. UBT is the test of choice and is commercially available for use in medical offices.
- The goals of PUD therapy are ulcer healing and eliminating the cause. Additional considerations are prevention of complications and relief of symptoms.
- For patients with *H pylori*-related PUD, a triple or quadruple drug regimen consisting of a PPI or an H_2RA, bismuth, and antibiotics should be used for 7-14 days. *H pylori* eradication reduces the risk of recurrence of PUD. The ideal treatment regimen for *H pylori* has not been identified.
- For NSAID-related PUD, treatment consists of discontinuing the offending agent and issuing antisecretory therapy for symptom relief. If *H pylori* is present, eradication therapy should be used. A PPI, an H_2RA, or misoprostol should be used for prevention of PUD in patients requiring chronic NSAIDs who are at risk for developing PUD.
- Patients with active bleeding should initially undergo endoscopic hemostasis. Laparoscopic repair or surgery may be used to repair perforations. Open surgery is reserved for those patients with refractory ulcers or for hemorrhage/perforations that cannot be managed endoscopically or with laparoscopy.
- Patients should be counseled on the importance of adherence to treatment regimens, proper dosing, and the side effects of medications.
- Patients should be counseled to decrease psychological stress, to discontinue smoking and use of NSAIDs, and to avoid food or beverages that exacerbate PUD symptoms.

Gastroesophageal reflux disease

- Gastroesophageal reflux disease (GERD) is defined as chronic symptoms or mucosal damage produced by the abnormal reflux of gastric contents into the esophagus.
- Approximately 20% of the population experience heartburn or regurgitation of gastric acid weekly.
- Patients with GERD may be classified as having nonerosive reflux disease (NERD), erosive esophagitis (EE), or Barrett's esophagus (BE). Adenocarcinoma is rare.
- Symptoms of GERD may be classified as typical, atypical, or complicated. The hallmark symptom of GERD is heartburn (pyrosis), which is described as substernal burning or pain that may radiate to the neck, back, or throat.
- Atypical symptoms (or extraesophageal symptoms) include chronic cough, hoarseness, nonallergic asthma, pharyngitis, and chest pain that resembles angina. Symptoms that are suggestive of complications of GERD include continuous pain, dysphagia, odynophagia, bleeding, unexplained weight loss, and choking. Complications include ulcers, strictures, and adenocarcinoma.
- The pathophysiology of GERD involves the prolonged contact of esophageal epithelium with refluxed gastric contents that contain acid and pepsin.
- Esophageal defenses consist of the antireflux barrier, luminal clearance mechanisms, and tissue resistance. Increased contact time of refluxate and esophageal mucosa or impaired defense mechanisms can lead to the symptoms of GERD.
- For patients who present with typical symptoms of GERD, a trial of empiric therapy is appropriate. A diagnosis of GERD may be assumed for patients who respond to empiric treatment.
- Further diagnostic testing should be considered for patients who do not respond to empiric therapy, patients who present with atypical symptoms or alarm symptoms, patients with chronic symptoms at increased risk for developing BE, patients with the need for continuous chronic therapy, elderly patients, and patients taking esophagotoxic medications.
- Goals of therapy are to alleviate or eliminate symptoms, decrease frequency and duration of reflux, promote healing of the injured mucosa, and prevent the development of complications.
- Acid suppression is the mainstay of therapy for GERD. Proton pump inhibitors (PPIs) provide the

fastest symptomatic relief and heal esophagitis in the highest number of patients.

* Therapy for patients with GERD may be divided into three phases. Phase I consists of lifestyle modifications and patient-directed therapy with OTC H$_2$RAs and/or antacids. Phase II consists of continuation of lifestyle modifications and therapy with standard or high-dose antisecretory agents. Phase III consists of surgical intervention.

- Patients should be counseled on medication dosing and administration, side effects, drug interactions, monitoring of GERD symptoms, and lifestyle modifications.
- Lifestyle modifications should be initiated and maintained throughout the course of GERD therapy. These include elevating the head of the bed, decreasing fat intake, smoking cessation, avoiding lying down within 3 hours of eating, losing weight, avoiding foods or medications that can exacerbate GERD, avoiding alcohol, and eating smaller meals.
- GERD is considered a chronic condition, and most patients will require chronic therapy with antisecretory agents.

Inflammatory bowel disease

- Idiopathic inflammatory bowel disease (IBD) is divided into two major types: (1) ulcerative colitis (UC) and (2) Crohn's disease (CD).
- UC is defined as a mucosal inflammatory condition confined to the rectum and colon.
- CD is defined as a transmural inflammation of the gastrointestinal (GI) tract that can affect any part (mouth to anus).
- The hallmark clinical symptom of UC is bloody diarrhea, often with rectal urgency and tenesmus.
- Clinical symptoms are categorized as mild, moderate, or severe. Endoscopic findings are categorized as distal (limited to below the splenic flexure) or extensive (extending proximal to the splenic flexure).
- Typical symptoms of CD include chronic or nocturnal diarrhea and abdominal pain. Additional typical symptoms include weight loss, fever, and rectal bleeding.
- Symptoms differ depending on the site of inflammation, and are categorized as mild, moderate, or severe.
- The etiology of IBD is unclear, but similar factors may contribute to both UC and CD. The diagnosis of IBD is made based on negative stool evaluation for infectious causes.
- Treatment of IBD involves medications that target inflammatory mediators and alter immuno-inflammatory processes. These medications include anti-inflammatory agents and immunosuppressive agents.

- Goals of therapy for UC and CD include the induction and maintenance of remission of symptoms, improving quality of life, resolution of complications and systemic symptoms, and prevention of future complications.
- Patients should be counseled on medication dosing and administration, side effects, drug interactions, monitoring of IBD symptoms, and proper nutrition.
- Patients with IBD are often malnourished due to malabsorption or maldigestion caused by chronic bowel inflammation, "short gut" syndrome from multiple bowel surgeries, or bile salt deficiency in the gut.
- Surgery may be necessary for patients with severe UC or CD. Surgery (proctocolectomy) is curative for UC, but not for CD.

Irritable bowel syndrome

- Irritable bowel syndrome (IBS) is a functional bowel disorder characterized by symptoms of abdominal pain or discomfort associated with disturbed defecation.
- IBS is the most prevalent digestive disease, representing 12% of visits to primary care physicians and 28% of referrals to gastroenterologists.
- IBS is a heterogeneous disorder with various clinical presentations.
- The pathogenesis is multifactorial, including abnormal gut sensorimotor activity, central nervous system (CNS) dysfunction, psychologic disturbances, genetic predisposition, enteric infection, and other luminal factors.
- IBS may be categorized using the Rome II diagnostic criteria. IBS is typically categorized as being diarrhea-predominant, constipation-predominant, or alternating between diarrhea and constipation. It is also categorized as mild, moderate, or severe. Weight loss, bleeding, fever, or palpable masses are warning signs of organic disease, and are not common in IBS.
- Treatment should be offered to patients seeking medical care if the patient and physician believe that the IBS symptoms decrease the quality of life of the patient.

* Goals of therapy include improving IBS symptoms and patient quality of life.
* Anticholinergic/antimuscarinic agents may be effective in patients with mild symptoms. Bulking agents and osmotic laxatives may be useful in some patients with constipation-predominant IBS. Loperamide decreases stool frequency in patients with diarrhea-predominant IBS. TCAs improve abdominal pain in IBS patients. SSRIs are recommended for patients with moderate to severe abdominal pain and/or psychiatric comorbidities. Tegaserod improves

global IBS symptoms, bloating, abdominal pain, and altered bowel habits in patients with constipation-predominant IBS. Alosetron improves global IBS symptoms, abdominal discomfort, stool consistency, and stool frequency in women with diarrhea-predominant IBS.

- Patients should be counseled on medication dosing and administration, side effects, drug interactions, and monitoring of IBS symptoms.
- An effective physician-patient relationship is necessary for successful treatment.
- Education regarding disease pathophysiology and treatment, and reassurance that the symptoms are real should be provided.
- Patients should be counseled to avoid foods that exacerbate symptoms.

6. Questions and Answers

1. H.B. is a 59-year-old black male recently diagnosed with PUD on endoscopy. Tissue biopsy is positive for *H pylori*. Which of the following is the ideal therapeutic regimen for *H pylori*-related PUD in H.B.?

   A. Omeprazole, bismuth, tetracycline, furazolidone
   B. Omeprazole, amoxicillin, clarithromycin
   C. Omeprazole, amoxicillin
   D. Omeprazole, bismuth, clarithromycin, furazolidone
   E. Omeprazole, sucralfate, clarithromycin, furazolidone

2. H.B. does not respond to the initial treatment regimen. Which of the following modifications to H.B.'s treatment regimen should be made?

   A. Clarithromycin should be replaced by tetracycline
   B. Clarithromycin should be replaced by metronidazole
   C. Clarithromycin dosage should be increased
   D. Clarithromycin should be replaced by furazolidone
   E. Clarithromycin should be replaced by amoxicillin

3. Which one of the following is the leading cause of PUD in *H pylori*–negative patients?

   A. Mineralocorticoids
   B. NSAIDs
   C. DMARDs
   D. Antibiotics
   E. Corticosteroids

4. Which of the following is true of NSAIDs?

   I. They inhibit production of prostaglandins
   II. They are directly toxic to gastroduodenal epithelium
   III. They require dose adjustments in renal insufficiency
   IV. They only cause gastric ulcers
   V. They allow healing of PUD during continued therapy

   A. I, II, and III only
   B. I and III only
   C. II and IV only
   D. V only
   E. All are correct

5. Which of the following are goals of therapy for PUD?

I. Reduce episodes of diarrhea
II. Eliminate symptoms
III. Reduce risk of gastric cancer
IV. Heal ulcerations
V. Avoid spreading *H pylori*

   A. I, II, and III only
   B. I and III only
   C. II and IV only
   D. V only
   E. All are correct

6. The test of choice for identifying *H pylori* infection is:

   A. Serology
   B. Urine antigen test
   C. Urea breath test
   D. Endoscopic biopsy
   E. Blood culture

7. A.B. is a 45-year-old white female with a past medical history significant only for seizure disorder. She has experienced heartburn soon after meals for 2 weeks. It becomes worse upon reclining at bedtime. Her medications include phenytoin 300 mg hs. A.B. wishes to self-treat with an OTC H_2RA. Which one of the following should NOT be recommended to A.B.?

   A. Alginic acid
   B. Cimetidine
   C. Famotidine
   D. Ranitidine
   E. Magnesium hydroxide

8. A.B.'s symptoms are not relieved after 2 weeks of OTC treatment with famotidine and lifestyle modifications. Which one of the following is the best choice?

   A. Add the prokinetic agent metoclopramide to famotidine
   B. Endoscopy should be performed since A.B. is at high risk for complications
   C. Add alginic acid 2 tablets qhs to famotidine
   D. Switch to high-dose omeprazole 60 mg qd
   E. Continue lifestyle modifications and switch to famotidine 20 mg bid

9. Which of the following is an atypical symptom of GERD?

I. Heartburn
II. Regurgitation
III. Belching
IV. Hypersalivation
V. Hoarseness

   A. I, II, and III only
   B. I and III only
   C. II and IV only
   D. V only
   E. All are correct

10. Which of the following diagnoses carries an increased risk for developing esophageal adenocarcinoma?

I. Moderate erosive esophagitis
II. Mild nonerosive reflux disease
III. Mild erosive esophagitis
IV. Moderate nonerosive reflux disease
V. Barrett's esophagus

   A. I, II, and III only
   B. I and III only
   C. II and IV only
   D. V only
   E. All are correct

11. Which one of the following may exacerbate GERD symptoms by lowering the LES pressure?

   A. Quinidine
   B. Iron
   C. Potassium chloride
   D. Diltiazem
   E. Tetracycline

12. Which of the following is the best choice for the initial (phase I) treatment of a patient with mild GERD?

   A. Nizatidine 75 mg bid
   B. Pantoprazole 40 mg bid
   C. Metoclopramide 10 mg qid
   D. 3-month trial of lifestyle modifications
   E. Lansoprazole 30 mg bid

13. A.Y. is a 32-year-old white male who presents with bloody diarrhea (less than four stools per day) for 2 days. Complete blood counts and ESR are normal. Physical exam is normal. Colonoscopy reveals distal colitis. Which of the following is the best choice for initial therapy for A.Y.?

    A. Prednisone 40 mg PO qd
    B. Sulfasalazine 4-6 g PO qd
    C. Mesalamine 1-4 g PR qhs
    D. Mesalamine 4-6 g PO qd
    E. Methylprednisolone 16 mg IV q8h

14. A.Y. continues to have bloody diarrhea (without systemic disturbances). Which one of the following is the best choice?

    A. Add prednisone 40 mg PO qd and discontinue enema
    B. Add mesalamine 2-4 g PO qd and continue enema
    C. Add methylprednisolone 16 mg IV q8h until remission is achieved
    D. Add mesalamine 2-4 g PO qd and discontinue enema
    E. Add azathioprine 1-2.5 mg/kg per day and discontinue enema

15. Which of the following is true for UC?

    I. Aminosalicylates are the drugs of choice for maintenance therapy
    II. Oral corticosteroids are the drugs of choice for maintenance therapy
    III. Azathioprine often allows reduction in corticosteroid dose
    IV. Topical aminosalicylates are the drugs of choice for severe or fulminant disease
    V. Ciprofloxacin is alternative first-line therapy for mild to moderate disease

    A. I, II, and III only
    B. I and III only
    C. II and IV only
    D. V only
    E. All are correct

16. Which of the following is true for CD?

    I. Infliximab is the drug of choice for mild to moderate disease
    II. Oral corticosteroids are the drugs of choice for maintenance therapy
    III. Topical aminosalicylates are the drugs of choice for mild to moderate disease

IV. Oral cyclosporine is the drug of choice for maintenance therapy
V. Ciprofloxacin is an alternative drug of choice for mild to moderate disease

    A. I, II, and III only
    B. I and III only
    C. II and IV only
    D. V only
    E. All are correct

17. Which of the following is true for moderate to severe CD?

    A. Azathioprine is the drug of choice for initial therapy
    B. Budesonide is appropriate maintenance therapy
    C. Oral corticosteroids are the drugs of choice for initial therapy
    D. Methotrexate has no role in CD therapy
    E. Topical aminosalicylates are appropriate maintenance therapy

18. Which one of the following may be used in the management of fistulas?

    A. Prednisone
    B. Sulfasalazine
    C. Mesalamine
    D. Methotrexate
    E. Infliximab

19. J.J. is a 39-year-old female who presents with intermittent abdominal pain for 14 weeks and four episodes of diarrhea per day (worsened after meals). J.J. has no significant past medical history and occasionally misses days from her full-time job. Which one of the following is the best choice for initial therapy?

    I. Paroxetine 10 mg qd
    II. Amitriptyline 10 mg hs
    III. Tegaserod 6 mg bid
    IV. Alosetron 1 mg qd
    V. Dicyclomine 10 mg qid after meals

    A. I, II, and III only
    B. I and III only
    C. II and IV only
    D. V only
    E. All are correct

20. J.J.'s symptoms are controlled for several months until she loses her job. Her abdominal pain has returned, she has five episodes of diarrhea per day, and complains of fatigue and insomnia. Which of the following is the most appropriate for J.J.?

I. Psychological counseling should be initiated
II. Amitriptyline 10-50 mg hs
III. Add loperamide 2 mg after each loose stool (16 mg/d max)
IV. Add alosetron 1 mg qd
V. Start paroxetine 10-40 mg qd

   A. I, II, and III only
   B. I and II only
   C. II and IV only
   D. V only
   E. All are correct

21. Which of the following is indicated for constipation-predominant IBS?

   A. Tegaserod 6 mg bid
   B. Alosetron 1 mg bid
   C. Loperamide 2-16 mg/d
   D. Paroxetine 10-40 mg qd
   E. Diphenoxylate + atropine 2 tabs qid

22. Which of the following is affected by medications that induce or inhibit the cytochrome P450 enzyme system?

   A. Tegaserod
   B. Alosetron
   C. Fibercon
   D. Hyoscyamine
   E. Amitriptyline

23. Which life-threatening complication caused the restriction of alosetron?

   A. Stevens-Johnson syndrome
   B. Toxic epidermal necrolysis
   C. Aplastic anemia
   D. Ischemic colitis
   E. Chronic diarrhea

24. Alosetron is indicated for which group of IBS patients?

   A. Women with diarrhea-predominant IBS
   B. Men with diarrhea-predominant IBS
   C. Women with constipation-predominant IBS
   D. Men with constipation-predominant IBS
   E. Children with diarrhea-predominant IBS

Answers

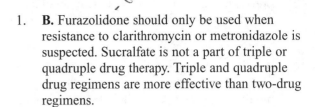

1. **B.** Furazolidone should only be used when resistance to clarithromycin or metronidazole is suspected. Sucralfate is not a part of triple or quadruple drug therapy. Triple and quadruple drug regimens are more effective than two-drug regimens.

2. **B.** Furazolidone should only be used when resistance to clarithromycin or metronidazole is suspected. Increasing dose does not overcome resistance to clarithromycin.

3. **B.** NSAIDs are the leading cause of PUD in patients who are negative for *H pylori* infection.

4. **A.** NSAIDs inhibit production of prostaglandins and are directly toxic to gastroduodenal epithelium. NSAIDs require dose adjustments in renal insufficiency. NSAIDs may cause gastric or duodenal ulcers, and must be discontinued to allow for ulcer healing.

5. **C.** Elimination of symptoms and healing of ulcerations are goals of therapy for PUD.

6. **C.** The urea breath test is commercially available for in-office use and is the test of choice for identifying *H pylori.*

7. **B.** Cimetidine is a potent inhibitor of the cytochrome P450 enzyme system and will increase serum concentrations of phenytoin in A.B.

8. **E.** Prokinetic agents are useful mainly in patients with concurrent gastric motility disorders and are not routinely recommended. Alginic acid is ineffective when the patient is lying in the supine position. High-dose omeprazole is used to confirm the diagnosis of GERD in patients not responding to initial therapy with prescription medications.

9. **D.** Hoarseness, chronic cough, nonallergic asthma, pharyngitis, and chest pain that resembles angina are atypical symptoms of GERD.

10. **D.** Patients with Barrett's esophagus have an increased risk of developing esophageal adenocarcinoma.

11. **D.** Calcium channel blockers decrease LES pressure. Quinidine, iron, potassium chloride, and tetracycline have direct irritant effects on the esophageal mucosa.

12. **A.** GERD therapy may be divided into three phases. Phase I therapy consists of lifestyle modifications and patient-directed therapy with OTC histamine-receptor antagonists and/or antacids. Nizatidine 75 mg bid is appropriate for patients with mild typical GERD symptoms. If symptoms persist after 2 weeks, phase II therapy is appropriate. Phase II therapy is for patients with mild to moderate typical GERD symptoms and consists of continuous lifestyle modifications and standard or high-dose antisecretory (prescription strength) medications. Phase III therapy consists of surgical intervention and is reserved for patients with severe symptoms.

13. **C.** Topical aminosalicylates (answer C) are more effective than oral aminosalicylates (answer B) and topical steroids for mild distal UC (although oral aminosalicylates or topical steroids may be used first-line if the patient prefers). Oral and IV steroids (answers A and E) are reserved for more severe cases of UC, or cases that do not respond to oral and topical aminosalicylates. The oral dose of mesalamine in answer D is incorrect.

14. **B.** Oral aminosalicylates should be added if no response is achieved with topical aminosalicylates. Oral and IV steroids are reserved for moderate to severe UC or for patients with systemic disturbances. Azathioprine may be added if UC is refractory to aminosalicylates, and to allow corticosteroid dose reduction.

15. **B.** Aminosalicylates are the drugs of choice for maintenance therapy of UC, not corticosteroids. Azathioprine often allows a reduction in dose of corticosteroids in the management of active UC. Severe or fulminant UC requires oral, not topical, therapy. Ciprofloxacin may be used as an alternative first-line therapy in the treatment of mild to moderate CD, not UC.

16. **D.** Ciprofloxacin or metronidazole is an alternative first-line agent for mild to moderate disease. Infliximab is reserved for moderate to severe disease, or patients who do not respond to initial therapy. Oral cyclosporine is not effective maintenance therapy. Topical aminosalicylates may be used as an adjunct to oral therapy.

17. **C.** Moderate to severe disease initially requires oral corticosteroid therapy. Corticosteroids have no role in maintenance therapy. Topical aminosalicylates may be used as adjuncts in colonic CD. Methotrexate is used as maintenance therapy for moderate to severe CD.

18. **E.** Infliximab, high-dose metronidazole, ciprofloxacin, or azathioprine may be used in the management of fistulas.

19. **D.** J.J. has mild, diarrhea-predominant IBS. Symptomatic treatment with dicyclomine is appropriate initial therapy. A TCA may be added to dicyclomine if needed. Tegaserod is indicated for constipation-predominant IBS. Alosetron is reserved for severe, diarrhea-predominant disease. Paroxetine may be added if initial therapies are ineffective, or if J.J. develops psychiatric comorbidities.

20. **A.** Alosetron is reserved for patients with severe, diarrhea-predominant IBS (FDA-restricted use). SSRIs are recommended for patients with severe abdominal pain and/or psychiatric comorbidities. Several types of cognitive therapy have been shown to be effective in IBS. TCAs improve abdominal pain in IBS. Loperamide may be used on an as-needed basis for diarrhea.

21. **A.** Alosetron is approved for restricted use in diarrhea-predominant IBS. Loperamide and diphenoxylate + atropine are antidiarrheal medications that will exacerbate constipation. Paroxetine is an SSRI with potent anticholinergic effects, which could worsen constipation. Another should be chosen if an SSRI is needed for depression.

22. **E.** TCA serum concentrations are affected by drugs that alter cytochrome P450 activity.

23. **D.** Severe constipation, ischemic colitis, and death have been reported with alosetron.

24. **A.** Alosetron is approved for women with diarrhea-predominant IBS. It was not found to be effective in men, and is not approved for use in children.

7. References

Peptic ulcer disease
Berardi R. Peptic ulcer disease. In: Dipiro JT, Talbert RL, Yee GC, et al, eds. *Pharmacotherapy: A Pathophysiologic Approach,* 5th ed. Stamford, CT: McGraw-Hill/Appleton & Lange; 2002:603-624.

Chan FKL, Leung WK. Peptic ulcer disease. *Lancet.* 2002;360:933-941.

Current European concepts in the management of *Helicobacter pylori* infection. The Maastricht Consensus Report. European Helicobacter Pylori Study Group. *Gut.* 1997;41:8-13.

Del Valle J. Peptic ulcer disease and related disorders. In: Braunwald E, Fauci AS, Casper DL, et al, eds. *Harrison's Principles of Internal Medicine,* 15th ed. New York: McGraw-Hill; 2001:1649-1661.

Henderson RP. Acid-peptic disorders and intestinal gas. In: Berardi RR, DiSimone EM, Newton GD, eds. *Handbook of Nonprescription Drugs,* 13th ed. Washington: American Pharmaceutical Association; 2002:243-272.

Henderson RP, Lander RD. Peptic ulcer disease. In: Herfindal ET, Gourley DR, eds. *Textbook of Therapeutics: Drug and Disease Management,* 7th ed. Philadelphia: Lippincott Williams & Wilkins; 2000:515-531.

NIH Consensus Conference. *Helicobacter pylori* in peptic ulcer diseases. NIH Consensus Development Panel on Helicobacter Pylori in Peptic Ulcer Disease. *JAMA.* 1994;272:65-69.

Shiotani A, Graham DY. Pathogenesis and therapy of gastric and duodenal ulcer disease. *Med Clin North Am.* 2002;86:1447-1466.

Singh G, Triadafilopoulos G. Epidemiology of NSAID-induced GI complications. *J Rheumatol.* 1999;26(Suppl 26):18-24.

Wolfe MM, Lichtenstein DR, Singh G. Gastrointestinal toxicity of nonsteroidal anti-inflammatory drugs. *N Engl J Med.* 1999;340:1888-1889.

Gastroesophageal reflux disease
Cappell MS. Clinical presentation, diagnosis, and management of gastroesophageal reflux disease. *Med Clin North Am.* 2005;89:243-291.

DeVault KR, Castell DO, et al. Updated guidelines for the diagnosis and treatment of gastroesophageal reflux disease. *Am J Gastroenterology.* 2005;100:190-200.

Fass R. Gastroesophageal reflux disease revisited. *Gastroenterol Clin North Am.* 2002;31(Suppl 4):S1-S10.

Goyal RK. Diseases of the esophagus. In: Fauci AS, Braunwald KJ, Wilson JD, et al, eds. *Harrison's Principles of Internal Medicine,* 15th ed. New York: McGraw-Hill; 2001:1642-1649.

Henderson RP. Acid-peptic disorders and intestinal gas. In: Berardi RR, DeSimone EM, Newton GD, et al. *Handbook of Nonprescription Drugs: An Interactive Approach to Self-Care,* 13th ed. Washington: American Pharmaceutical Association; 2002:243-272.

Henderson RP, Lander RD. Peptic ulcer disease. In: Herfindal ET, Gourley DR, eds. *Textbook of Therapeutics: Drug and Disease Management,* 7th ed. Baltimore: Lippincott Williams & Wilkins; 2000:515-531.

Locke GR. Natural history of nonerosive reflux disease: Is all gastroesophageal reflux the same? What is the evidence? *Gastroenterol Clin North Am.* 2002;31(Suppl 4):S59-S66.

Locke GR, Talley NH, Fett SL, et al. Prevalence and clinical spectrum of gastroesophageal reflux: a population-based study in Olmstead county. *Gastroenterology.* 1997;112:1448-1456.

Orlando RC. Pathogenesis of gastroesophageal reflux disease. *Gastroenterol Clin North Am.* 2002;31(Suppl 4):S35-S44.

Spechler SJ. Barrett's esophagus and esophageal adenocarcinoma: pathogenesis, diagnosis, and therapy. *Med Clin North Am.* 2002;86:1423-1445.

Waring JP. Surgical and endoscopic treatment of gastroesophageal reflux disease. *Gastroenterol Clin North Am.* 2002;31(Suppl 4):S89-S109.

Williams DB. Gastroesophageal reflux disease. In: Dipiro JT, Talbert RL, Yee GC, et al, eds. *Pharmacotherapy: A Pathophysiologic Approach,* 5th ed. Stamford, CT: McGraw-Hill/Appleton & Lange; 2002:585-601.

Inflammatory bowel disease

Ardizzone S, Porro GB. Inflammatory bowel disease: new insights into pathogenesis and treatment. *J Intern Med.* 2002;252:475-496.

Banerjee S, Peppercorn MA. Inflammatory bowel disease: Medical therapy for specific clinical presentations. *Gastroenterol Clin North Am.* 2002;31:185-202.

Berardi RR. Inflammatory bowel disease. In: Herfindal ET, Gourley DR, eds. *Textbook of Therapeutics: Drug and Disease Management,* 7th ed. Philadelphia: Lippincott Williams & Wilkins; 2000:533-551.

DiPiro JT, Schade RR. Inflammatory bowel disease. In: Dipiro JT, Talbert RL, Yee GC, et al, eds. *Pharmacotherapy: A Pathophysiologic Approach,* 5th ed. Stamford, CT: McGraw-Hill/Appleton & Lange; 2002:625-639.

Friedman S, Blumberg RS. Inflammatory bowel disease. In: Braunwald E, et al, eds. *Harrison's Principles of Internal Medicine,* 15th ed. New York: McGraw-Hill; 2001:1679-1692.

Hanauer SB, Sandborn W, et al. Management of Crohn's disease in adults. Practice guidelines. *Am J Gastroenterol.* 2001;96:635-643.

Hanauer SB, Sandborn W, et al. Practice guidelines: Management of Crohn's disease in adults. *Am J Gastroenterol.* 2001;96:635-643.

Harrison J, Hanauer SB. Medical treatment of Crohn's disease. *Gastroenterol Clin North Am.* 2002;31:167-184.

Jani N, Regueiro MD. Medical therapy for ulcerative colitis. *Gastroenterol Clin North Am.* 2002;31:147-166.

Kornbluth A, Sachar DB. Ulcerative colitis practice guidelines in adults (update): American College of Gastroenterology, Practice Parameters Committee. *Am J Gastroenterol.* 2004;99:1371-1385.

Lichtenstein GR, Hanauer MD, Kane SV, et al. Crohn's is not a 6-week disease: Lifelong management of mild to moderate Crohn's disease. *Inflamm Bowel Dis.* 2004;10:S2-S10.

Irritable bowel syndrome

American College of Gastroenterology Functional Gastrointestinal Disorders Task Force. Evidence-based position statement on the management of irritable bowel syndrome in North America. *Am J Gastroenterol.* 2002;97:S1-S5.

Brandt LJ, Bjorkman D, Fennerty MB, et al. Systematic review on the management of irritable bowel syndrome in North America. *Am J Gastroenterol.* 2002;97(Suppl 11):S7-S26.

Cash BD, Chey WD. Diagnosis of irritable bowel syndrome. *Gastroenterol Clin North Am.* 2005;34:205-220.

Drossman DA, Camilleri M, Mayer EA, Whitehead WE. AGA technical review on irritable bowel syndrome. *Gastroenterology.* 2002;123:2108-2131.

Hasler WL. The irritable bowel syndrome. *Med Clin North Am.* 2002;86:1525-1551.

Owyang C. Irritable bowel syndrome. In: Braunwald E, et al, eds. *Harrison's Principles of Internal Medicine,* 15th ed. New York: McGraw-Hill; 2001:1692-1695.

Palsson OS, Drossman DA. Psychiatric and psychological dysfunction in irritable bowel syndrome and the role of psychological treatments. *Gastroenterol Clin North Am.* 2005;34:281-303.

Schoenfeld P. Efficacy of current drug therapies in irritable bowel syndrome: what works and does not work. *Gastroenterol Clin North Am.* 2005;34:319-335.

Spruill WJ, Wade WE. Diarrhea, constipation, and irritable bowel syndrome. In: Dipiro JT, et al, eds. *Pharmacotherapy: A Pathophysiologic Approach,* 5th ed. New York: McGraw-Hill; 2002:655-669.

Talley NJ, Spiller R. Irritable bowel syndrome: a little understood organic bowel disease? *Lancet.* 2002;360:555-564.

Viera AJ, Hoag S, Shaughnessy J. Management of irritable bowel syndrome. *Am Fam Physician.* 2002;66:1867-1874.

22. Rheumatoid Arthritis, Osteoarthritis, Gout, and Lupus

Kevin L. Freeman, PharmD, BCNSP
Assistant Professor, Department of Clinical Pharmacy
University of Tennessee College of Pharmacy

Contents

1. Rheumatoid Arthritis

- Rheumatoid arthritis (RA) is a highly variable, chronic autoimmune disorder of unknown etiology characterized by symmetric, erosive synovitis. Manifestations may extend to extra-articular sites.

Incidence

- RA affects 1% of the population and is two to three times more common in women than in men. RA has a peak incidence in women between 30 and 60 years of age. There is a greater incidence of RA in certain families, monozygotic twins, and people with specific HLA genetic markers, which suggests a genetic predisposition.

Clinical Presentation

- The onset of RA is unpredictable and varies from rapid to insidious progression.
- The course of the disease is likewise variable. Ten to twenty percent of patients have a short course with remission, 70-80% have mild to moderate disease with cyclic exacerbations, and 10-20% develop progressively destructive disease.
- RA usually affects diarthrodial joints such as the proximal interphalangeal (PIP) joints, metacarpophalangeal (MCP) joints, metatarsophalangeal (MTP) joints, wrists, and ankles. Also commonly involved are the elbows, shoulders, sternoclavicular joints, temporomandibular joints, hips, and knees.
- The initial complaints may include generalized fatigue and multiple joint pain.
- Morning stiffness is a hallmark of RA. Patients describe it as a gel-like sensation in the joints that occurs after attempting to move upon awakening.
- Ulnar deviation, swan-neck deformities, boutonnière deformities, hammer toe formation, and ankylosis are common irreversible joint abnormalities that occur in RA.
- The extra-articular features that occur in RA include rheumatoid nodules, vasculitis, anemia, thrombocytopenia, Felty's syndrome, and Sjögren's syndrome.

Etiology

- The cause of RA remains a mystery. Factors that may be responsible are of environmental, genetic, endocrinologic, gastrointestinal, atmospheric, and infectious origin.
- It is widely held that RA has a strong genetic component. This assertion is supported by the fact that a greater prevalence of RA is found in patients with the major histocompatibility complex (MHC) antigen HLA-DR4. This is a class II antigen expressed on the surface of helper T lymphocytes and macrophages. In combination with environmental factors, an inappropriate immune response may occur, resulting in chronic inflammation.
- It has been demonstrated that patients with RA have increased antibody titers to *Mycobacterium tuberculosis, Proteus mirabilis, Escherichia coli, Klebsiella pneumoniae,* normal human gut flora antigen, Epstein-Barr virus, and the superantigen staphylococcal enterotoxin B.
- There is a greater risk of RA in female patients after breastfeeding, which supports that there are endocrinologic risk factors.
- Gastrointestinal factors may be responsible for hyperactivity of the immune system, ie, antibodies to enteric organisms and gluten develop in the GI tract.
- Atmospheric changes are associated with symptomatic changes in the disease course.

Pathophysiology

- Due to causes still unknown, the body's immune system (starting with macrophages) attacks the cells within the joint capsule, thereby causing synovitis (as indicated by the warmth, swelling, redness, and pain associated with RA). Specifically, helper T lymphocytes stimulate B cells to attack antigen (in this case, the body's own collagen). In addition, helper T lymphocytes release cytokines (interleukins and tumor necrosis factor) which cause further inflammation and injury in the joints. During the inflammatory process, the cells of the synovium grow and divide abnormally, causing a normally thin synovium to become thick (pannus).
- These abnormal synovial cells begin to invade and destroy the cartilage and bone within the joint.
- The above effects are responsible for the pain and deformities seen in patients with RA.

Diagnostic Criteria

- Patients meeting four of the following criteria are classified as having rheumatoid arthritis:
    - * Morning stiffness of or near joints lasting 1 hour before maximum improvement. This must be present for 6 weeks.
    - * Three or more joint areas, including the right or left proximal interphalangeal (PIP) joint, metacarpophalangeal (MCP) joint, wrist, elbow, metatarsophalangeal (MTP) joint, ankle, or knee joint must have arthritis as demonstrated by soft tissue swelling or fluid. This must be present for at least 6 weeks and observed by a physician.

* Arthritis as demonstrated by soft tissue swelling or fluid in the hand joints (MCP, PIP, or wrist) must be present for at least 6 weeks and observed by a physician.
* Symmetric arthritis must occur in the areas noted in the second criterion. This must be present for at least 6 weeks and observed by a physician.
* Subcutaneous nodules (rheumatoid nodules) over bony prominences, extensor surfaces, or in juxta-articular regions
* Positive rheumatoid factor (antibodies that collect in the synovium of the joint) as demonstrated by a positive test in less than 5% of normal subjects
* Radiologic changes of the hands or wrists, eg, erosions or bone decalcification in or next to involved joints

Treatment Goals

* According to the American College of Rheumatology, the goals in managing RA are to prevent or control joint damage, prevent loss of function, and decrease pain (Figure 1).

Monitoring

* At each visit, the patient should be evaluated for subjective evidence of active disease based on the following criteria:
  * Degree of joint pain
  * Duration of morning stiffness
  * Duration of fatigue
  * Presence of actively inflamed joints on examination
  * Limitation of function
* Periodically, the patient should be evaluated for disease activity or progression:
  * Evidence of disease progression on physical examination (loss of motion, instability, malalignment, and/or deformity)
  * Erythrocyte sedimentation rate or C-reactive protein elevation
  * Progression of radiographic damage of involved joints
* Other parameters for assessing response to treatment (outcomes):
  * Physician's global assessment of disease activity
  * Patient's global assessment of disease activity
  * Functional status or quality-of-life assessment using standardized questionnaires
* The majority of clinical studies use a benchmark of 20% improvement in the criteria above, also known as ACR 20.

Drug Therapy

* Currently the most popular approach to the pharmacological treatment of RA is the "inverted pyramid," which refers to utilizing aggressive therapy with disease-modifying antirheumatic drugs (DMARDs) (Table 1). Some patients start out immediately with DMARDs with or without nonsteroidal anti-inflammatory drugs (NSAIDs). Others start DMARDs after 3 months if NSAIDs have not relieved symptoms (Table 2).

Nonsteroidal anti-inflammatory drugs (NSAIDs)

* Salicylates, NSAIDs, and selective cyclooxygenase-2 (COX-2) inhibitors are agents with analgesic and anti-inflammatory properties useful in the management of RA. These agents reduce joint pain and swelling; however, they do not inhibit joint destruction or otherwise alter the course of the disease. For this reason, they should not be considered as a sole treatment option. These agents act by inhibiting prostaglandin synthesis and release. Cyclooxygenase is present in many cells, including platelets, endothelial cells, and cells of the gastric and intestinal mucosa. The initial choice of agent is based on the efficacy, safety, cost, and convenience for any given patient. There is a wide range of interpatient variability with regard to clinical effect; several NSAIDs may need to be tried before achieving patient satisfaction.

Aspirin
Mechanism of action
* Aspirin prevents prostaglandin formation by inhibiting the action of the enzyme cyclooxygenase. The antithrombotic effect of aspirin occurs by an irreversible inhibition of platelet cyclooxygenase. This irreversible inhibition is unique to aspirin, because the remaining NSAIDs do so in a reversible manner.

Dosage
* The usual daily dosage needed to achieve anti-inflammatory effects is 3-5 g per day.

Patient instructions
* Aspirin should be taken with food or milk to decrease gastrointestinal intolerance. Patients should report any dark or black stools, abdominal pain, or swelling to his or her physician immediately.

Adverse drug events
* Aspirin irreversibly inhibits platelet activity and serious bleeding may result. Dyspepsia, gastrointestinal bleeding, tinnitus, hepatitis, and renal damage have been reported.

Figure 1.

Outline of the management of rheumatoid arthritis.

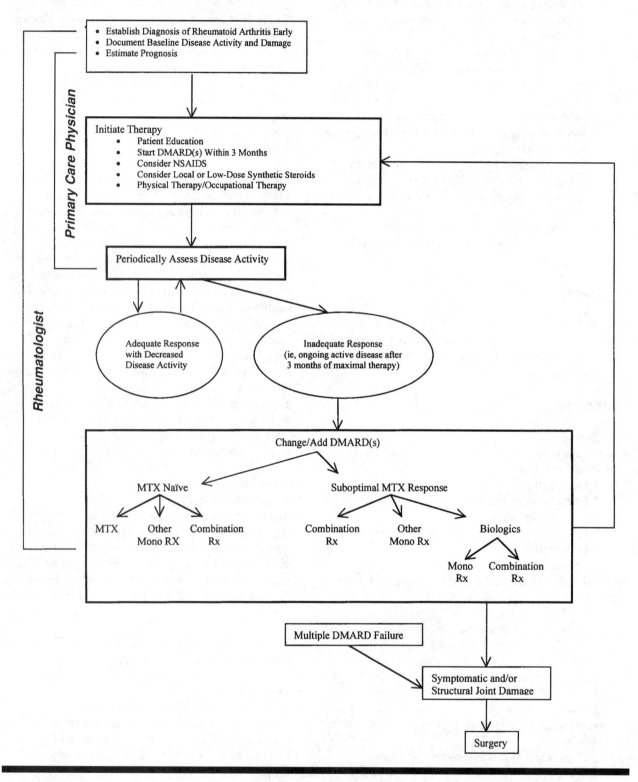

Boxes with heavy borders represent major decision points in management. A suboptimum response to methotrexate is defined as intolerance, lack of satisfactory efficacy with a dosage of up to 25 mg/week, or a contraindication to the drug.

DMARD, disease-modifying antirheumatic drug; NSAID, nonsteroidal anti-inflammatory drug; mono Rx, monotherapy; combination Rx, combination therapy.

Reprinted with permission from American College of Rheumatology Subcommittee on Rheumatoid Arthritis Guidelines. Guidelines for the Management of Rheumatoid Arthritis. *Arthritis Rheum.* 2002;46:328-346.

Table 1

Disease-Modifying Antirheumatic Drugs (DMARDs)

Generic name (trade name)	Dosage range	Administration schedule	Dosage forms
Hydroxychloroquine (Plaquenil®)	200-400 mg	1-2 doses per day	PO
Sulfasalazine (Azulfidine®)	2000-4000 mg	2-3 doses per day	PO
Methotrexate (Rheumatrex®)	7.5-25 mg	Once weekly	PO, IM, SC, IV
Gold sodium thiomalate (Myochrysine®)	25-50 mg	Every 2-4 weeks	IM
Auranofin (Ridaura®)	3-6 mg	1-2 doses per day	PO
Azathioprine (Imuran®)	50-150 mg	1-2 doses per day	PO, IV
Penicillamine (Cuprimine®)	250-750 mg	2-3 doses per day	PO
Minocycline (Minocin®)	100-200 mg	2 doses per day	PO
Leflunomide (Arava®)	10-20 mg	1-2 doses per day	PO
Etanercept (Enbrel®)	25 mg	Twice weekly or 50 mg once weekly	SC
Infliximab (Remicade®)	3 mg/kg	Weeks 0, 2, and 6, then every 8 weeks	IV
Anakinra (Kineret®)	100 mg	1 dose per day	SC
Adalimumab (Humira®)	40 mg	Every other week	SC

Table 2

Drug Therapy with Nonsteroidal Anti-Inflammatory Drugs (NSAIDs)

Generic name (trade name)	Dosage range (mg/d)	Administration schedule (doses/d)	Available dosage forms
Acetic acids			
Diclofenac (Voltaren®)	150-200	3-4	PO, ophth
Diclofenac (Votaren XR®)	100-200	1-2	PO
Etodolac (Lodine®)	800-1200	3-4	PO
Etodolac (Lodine XL®)	400-1200	1-2	PO
Indomethacin (Indocin®)	100-200	2-3	PO, IV, supp
Indomethacin (Indocin SR®)	75-150	1-2	PO
Nabumetone (Relafen®)	1000-2000	1-2	PO
Tolmetin (Tolectin®)	1600-2000	3-4	PO
Sulindac (Clinoril®)	300-400	2	PO
Propionic acids			
Fenoprofen (Nalfon®)	1600-3200	3-4	PO
Flurbiprofen (Ansaid®)	200-300	2-4	PO
Ibuprofen (Motrin®)	1600-3200	3-4	PO
Ketoprofen (Orudis®)	150-300	3-4	PO
Ketoprofen SR (Oruvail®)	100-200	1	PO
Naproxen (Naprosyn®)	500-1500	2-3	PO
Oxaprozin (Daypro®)	1200-1800	1	PO
Fenamates			
Meclofenamate (Meclomen®)	300-400	3-4	PO
Oxicams			
Piroxicam (Feldene®)	10-20	1	PO
COX-2 selective			
Celecoxib (Celebrex®)	200-400	1-2	PO

Drug-drug and drug-disease interactions
- Warfarin: aspirin may enhance the hypoprothrombinemic effects of warfarin.
- Uricosuric agents: the uricosuric effects of agents such as probenecid are antagonized by aspirin.
- Methotrexate: aspirin may displace methotrexate from its protein binding sites thereby increasing serum methotrexate concentrations.

Parameters to monitor
- Complete blood count as well as creatinine should be monitored at least yearly.

Other nonsteroidal anti-inflammatory drugs (NSAIDs)
Mechanism of action
- See aspirin, above.

Patient instructions
- See aspirin, above. Studies indicate that the optimal times for taking an NSAID might be after the evening meal and immediately upon awakening. Patients with a hypersensitivity to aspirin should not take NSAIDs.

Adverse drug events
- Compared to patients with osteoarthritis, patients with RA on NSAID therapy are at increased risk for a serious complication.
    * As with aspirin, NSAIDs cause platelet dysfunction. Unlike aspirin, however, this effect is readily reversible with discontinuation of the medication.
    * All NSAIDs are capable of causing gastrointestinal intolerance and peptic ulceration. Risk factors for the development of peptic ulcer disease include advanced age, history of previous ulcer, concomitant use of corticosteroids or anticoagulants, higher dosage of NSAID, use of multiple NSAIDs, or serious underlying disease. Options to decrease the risk of developing GI ulceration include adding a high-dose histamine blocker such as ranitidine or a proton pump inhibitor such as lansoprazole to the patient's regimen. Lansoprazole is the only proton pump inhibitor with FDA approval for reducing the risk of NSAID-induced gastric ulcers in those patients with a previous risk of ulceration and who continue to require NSAID treatment. Also misoprostol, an oral prostaglandin analogue, may be added at a dose of 100-200 mcg four times daily to prevent ulceration. Misoprostol is available in combination with diclofenac and sold under the trade name Arthrotec®. There is also some evidence that compared to other NSAIDs, ibuprofen, nabumetone, and naproxen carry lower risks of ulceration and GI symptoms. Piroxicam, on the other hand, appears to carry a higher risk of serious GI consequences.
    * Hepatic failure has been reported with NSAID use.
    * Renal blood flow can be decreased by NSAIDs, which may lead to permanent renal damage. Prostaglandins are responsible for maintaining the patency of the afferent renal tubule. Inhibition by NSAIDs decreases glomerular filtration pressure, resulting in decreased blood flow. Due to this mechanism, patients with hypertension, severe vascular disease, kidney or liver problems, and those taking diuretics must be monitored closely.
    * Central nervous system side effects such as dizziness, drowsiness, and confusion may occur with all NSAIDs.
    * Within the class, there are some drug-specific adverse reactions. Meclofenamate, for example, has a high incidence (>10%) of abdominal cramping and diarrhea. Paradoxically, indomethacin tends to have more severe CNS adverse effects such as headache.
    * There is concern about NSAIDs and their risk of cardiovascular events. The FDA now requires that manufacturers include a box warning regarding the potentially serious cardiovascular and GI adverse events associated with these drugs.

Drug-drug interactions
- See aspirin, above. It appears that ibuprofen may diminish the antiplatelet mechanism of aspirin if it is taken before aspirin or taken daily on a scheduled basis. It is recommended to take aspirin 2 hours before taking ibuprofen.

Cyclooxygenase-2 (COX-2) inhibitors
- COX-1 is the isoenzyme constitutively found in most tissues that produce the prostaglandins PGI_2 and PGE_2, which protect the gastric barrier, and thromboxane A_2, which is responsible for platelet function. COX-2 is the inducible isoenzyme present at sites of inflammation. COX-2 is also found in the brain, kidneys, and reproductive organs. Celebrex® has been shown to lower the incidence of endoscopically demonstrated gastroduodenal lesions compared to ibuprofen, naproxen, and diclofenac. It appears that the lower risk for GI complications is eliminated when patients take low-dose aspirin concomitantly.

Celebrex (celecoxib)
Mechanism of action

- Selectively inhibits prostaglandin synthesis by specifically targeting the COX-2 isoenzyme

Patient instructions

- Patients with a history of allergic reaction to sulfonamides should avoid the use of celecoxib.

Adverse drug events

- Although the rates of GI ulceration have been demonstrated to be lower with COX-2 inhibitors compared to traditional NSAIDs, the risk is not completely eliminated. In addition, the risk of dyspepsia, abdominal pain, and nausea is not significantly less with COX-2 inhibitors compared to traditional NSAIDs. Celecoxib now contains a black box warning regarding CV and GI risk associated with its use (see below for more information).

Drug-drug interactions

- See above interactions associated with aspirin.

Parameters to monitor

- Complete blood count as well as creatinine should be monitored at least yearly.

Other

- Recently the FDA recommended the voluntary removal of valdecoxib (Bextra®) from the market due to the lack of adequate data on the cardiovascular safety of its long-term use and the recent data demonstrating increased cardiovascular risk in short-term coronary artery bypass graft (CABG) patients. This is in addition to its risk of potentially life-threatening skin reactions. Merck recently removed rofecoxib (Vioxx®) from the market because its use was shown to be associated with an increased cardiovascular risk in the VIGOR, APPROVE, and VICTOR trials. The FDA has concluded that the benefits of celecoxib outweigh the risks in properly selected and informed patients. It will contain a black box warning about CV and GI risk. Patients with a high risk of cardiovascular events should not use celecoxib, including CABG patients. Low doses of celecoxib (200 mg per day) do not seem to be associated with increased risk.

Disease-modifying antirheumatic drugs (DMARDs)

- Unlike the NSAIDs, DMARDs have the ability to reduce or prevent joint damage and preserve joint integrity and function. The American College of Rheumatology recommends that the initiation of DMARD therapy not exceed 3 months from the diagnosis of RA in patients who have ongoing joint pain despite adequate treatment with NSAIDs, significant morning stiffness, active synovitis, persistent elevation of ESR or CRP level, or radiographic evidence of joint damage. Methotrexate is typically selected for initial therapy due to its track record to induce long-term response. This is in addition to its record of acceptable toxicity and low cost. Unfortunately, all DMARDs tend to lose effectiveness over time. It is rare for a patient to use one medication for longer than 2 years.

Plaquenil (hydroxychloroquine)
Mechanism of action

- May inhibit interleukin-1 release by monocytes, thereby decreasing macrophage chemotaxis and phagocytosis

Patient instructions

- Beneficial effect may not be seen until 1-6 months of use; patients should report any changes in vision to their physician immediately.

Adverse drug events

- The most serious potential adverse effect associated with hydroxychloroquine is retinal damage that can lead to vision loss. This is caused by the deposition of the drug in the melanin layer of the cones. A cumulative dose of 800 g and age >70 years increases the risk. Hydroxychloroquine may also cause rash, abdominal cramping, diarrhea, myopathy, skin pigment changes, and peripheral neuropathy.

Parameters to monitor

- Ophthalmic evaluations should be performed every 6-12 months. It is unnecessary to perform a baseline evaluation if the patient is under 40 years of age. Those patients receiving the drug for over 7 years should have monthly visual field and color vision testing.

Dose

- 6-7.5 mg/kg of lean body weight daily or 200 mg bid (maximum dose)

Azulfidine (sulfasalazine)
Mechanism of action

- The intestinal flora breaks sulfasalazine down to 5-aminosalicylic acid and sulfapyridine, the active moiety in RA. Sulfapyridine likely inhibits endothelial cell proliferation, reactive oxygen species, and cytokines. In addition, it has been shown to slow radiographic progression of RA.

Patient instructions

- Sulfasalazine may produce effects more quickly (within 1 month) than hydroxychloroquine. A coated tablet form may help reduce GI adverse effects.

Adverse drug events

- The most common adverse reactions associated with sulfasalazine include headache, GI intolerance, dysgeusia, rash, leukopenia, and thrombocytopenia.

Drug-drug interactions

- Sulfasalazine may inhibit the absorption of folic acid.

Parameters to monitor

- Patient tests should include baseline CBC, liver function tests, and G6PD levels. Patients should then have a CBC drawn every 2-4 weeks for the first 3 months, then every 3 months thereafter.

Dose

- Begin with 500 mg daily titrated up to 1-3 g per day divided tid or qid.

Rheumatrex (methotrexate)

Mechanism of action

- Methotrexate inhibits dihydrofolate reductase. It reduces dihydrofolate to tetrahydrofolate, which can be utilized as a carrier of single carbon units for the synthesis of nucleotides and thymidylate. Therefore, methotrexate interferes with DNA synthesis, repair, and cellular replication.

Patient instructions

- Never change the amount of methotrexate you take without first consulting your physician.

Adverse drug events

- Liver: methotrexate may cause liver damage. People with diabetes, liver problems, obesity, psoriasis, and those who are elderly or alcoholic are at higher risk; if LFTs (liver function tests) are more than three times the upper limit of normal, methotrexate should be discontinued.
- Bone marrow: leukopenia, thrombocytopenia, and pancytopenia are rare but serious adverse events associated with methotrexate therapy.
- Pulmonary toxicity occurs in up to 5% of people who take methotrexate. Risk factors for the development of pulmonary toxicity include age, diabetes, rheumatoid involvement of the lungs, protein in the urine, and previous use of sulfasalazine, oral gold, or penicillamine.
- GI: nausea, vomiting, and stomatitis occur with an incidence of 5-30%.

Drug-drug interactions

- Aspirin and other NSAIDs may increase methotrexate concentrations by as much as 30-35%. Trimethoprim-sulfamethoxazole may cause additive

hematologic abnormalities due to its similar affinity for dihydrofolate reductase.

Parameters to monitor

- CBC, AST, albumin, and creatinine should be monitored every 4-8 weeks.

Other

- Taking folate supplements may help to minimize adverse effects like liver toxicity. Folic acid in doses up to 3 mg per day has proven effective and does not diminish methotrexate activity.

Dose

- 7.5-25 mg once weekly

Arava (leflunomide)

Mechanism of action

- Leflunomide inhibits dihydro-orotate dehydrogenase (an enzyme involved in de novo pyrimidine synthesis) and has antiproliferative activity. Several in vivo and in vitro experimental models have demonstrated its anti-inflammatory effect.

Patient instructions

- Leflunomide is under pregnancy category X. Women taking leflunomide who wish to become pregnant should follow the drug elimination procedure outlined below.

Adverse drug events

- Diarrhea, elevated LFTs, alopecia, hypertension, and rash have been reported with leflunomide therapy.

Drug-drug interactions

- There is an increased risk of liver toxicity when leflunomide is used in conjunction with methotrexate. Rifampin causes a 40% increase in levels of leflunomide's active metabolite, M1.

Parameters to monitor

- It is recommended that liver function tests be monitored at baseline, monthly (initially), and periodically thereafter. If ALT exceeds two times the upper limit of normal, reduce the dose of leflunomide to 10 mg per day.

Kinetics

- After absorption, 80% of the parent compound is converted to the active metabolite, M1, which is responsible for all of leflunomide's activity. Since the half-life is 2 weeks, a loading dose is necessary. In addition, M1 undergoes extensive enterohepatic recirculation.

Other

- Begin a drug elimination procedure if a patient decides to become pregnant. It is as follows: 8 g of cholestyramine three times daily for 11 days; plasma levels of M1 <0.02 mg/L must be verified on two separate occasions at least 14 days apart. Many randomized controlled trials have established leflunomide as an alternative to methotrexate as monotherapy.

Dose

- 100 mg daily for 3 days (loading dose), then 20 mg daily

Cuprimine (D-penicillamine)

Mechanism of action

- It is currently unknown how penicillamine induces therapeutic effects in RA. It is known, however, that it significantly reduces IgM rheumatoid factor and appears to suppress disease activity.

Patient instructions

- Penicillamine should be taken on an empty stomach and at least 2 hours from any dose of antacids or iron supplements.

Adverse drug events

- Bone marrow: penicillamine may cause thrombocytopenia and leukopenia approximately 6 months into therapy. Rarely, aplastic anemia develops and is associated with its use.
- Renal: proteinuria may occur in up to 32% of patients on penicillamine therapy.
- Dermatologic: skin rash may occur 6-9 months after starting therapy.
- Other: penicillamine causes stomatitis, dysgeusia, and polymyositis.

Drug-drug interactions

- Absorption decreases approximately 70% with concomitant administration of antacids, iron, and zinc. Penicillamine may increase digoxin levels. In addition, penicillamine's chelating effects in combination with oral gold compounds may cause gold from deep tissue compartments to mobilize, which can increase toxicity.

Parameters to monitor

- Patients should have CBC, platelet count, creatinine, and urine dipstick for protein lab testing done before initiating therapy. Afterwards, the patient should have a CBC and urine dipstick for protein every 2 weeks until the dosage is stable, then every 1-3 months.

Other

- It may take up to 1 year for penicillamine to be effective. Note that more than half of the patients who take it withdraw due to side effects.

Dose

- Begin with 125-250 mg daily and increase by 125-250 mg/day every 8-10 weeks, not to exceed a maximum dose of 750 mg per day.

Gold compounds (gold sodium thiomalate [Myochrysine®; given IM] and aurothioglucose [Solganal®; given IM], and auranofin [Ridaura®; given PO])

Mechanism of action

- The MOA of gold compounds is currently unknown; they appear to suppress the synovitis seen in RA. Current research indicates that they may stimulate specific protective factors such as interleukins 6 and 10.

Patient instructions

- Patients receiving gold therapy should avoid prolonged sun exposure, which may increase the risk of serious rash.

Adverse drug events

IM gold

- Patients may experience an immediate "nitroid reaction," ie, flushing, weakness, dizziness, sweating, syncope, and hypotension. Rash is the single largest adverse effect associated with gold therapy. The rash may range from simple erythema to exfoliative dermatitis. Gold therapy may also cause proteinuria or microscopic hematuria. Rarely, immunologic glomerulonephritis may occur, in which case gold therapy should be permanently discontinued. Leukopenia and thrombocytopenia may occur with a 1-3% incidence.

PO gold

- Adverse reactions are similar to those associated with the IM formulation. However, GI complaints of nausea, diarrhea, emesis, and dysgeusia are higher.

Drug-drug interactions

- Patients receiving concomitant penicillamine therapy may be subject to an increased risk of toxicity associated with gold therapy. The risk of rash is higher when gold therapy is used with hydroxychloroquine.

Parameters to monitor

- At baseline, all patients should have a CBC, platelet count, creatinine, and urine dipstick for protein checked. For patients receiving IM therapy, a CBC, platelet count, and urine dipstick are recommended every 1-2 weeks for the first 20 weeks, and then again at the time of each (or every other) injection. Those on oral therapy should have a CBC, platelet count, and urine dipstick for protein every 4-12 weeks.

Other
- Aurothioglucose may have a lower rate of injection reactions; its sesame seed formulation slows absorption.

Dosing
IM gold
- A 10-mg test dose IM followed by a 25-mg test dose on week two, then weekly 50-mg doses until a cumulative dose of 1 g is achieved; maintenance regimen: 50 mg every 2 weeks for 3 months or until 1.5 g is given, then every 3 weeks, then monthly

PO gold
- 3 mg bid up to 3 mg tid

Anti–tumor necrosis factor therapy (Remicade® [infliximab], Enbrel® [etanercept], and Humira® [adalimumab])
Mechanism of action
- Composed of human constant and murine variable regions, infliximab binds specifically to human tumor necrosis factor (TNF).
- Similarly, by binding specifically to TNF, etanercept binds and blocks its interaction with the cell surface's TNF receptors. It is produced via recombinant technology in Chinese hamster ovaries.
- Adalimumab is a recombinant human IgG$_1$ monoclonal antibody that binds to TNF with high affinity.

Patient instructions
- Patients should not receive live vaccines during treatment. Therapy should be temporarily discontinued in the event of an acute infection.

Adverse drug events
- Therapy has been associated with serious mycobacterial, fungal, and opportunistic infectious complications, eg, sepsis and tuberculosis. Other adverse reactions include rash, headache, nausea, and cough. Although rare, both etanercept and infliximab have been associated with nerve damage that resembles the disease process in multiple sclerosis. Lymphoma has been reported with all three TNF antagonists.

Drug-drug interactions
- Live vaccines

Parameters to monitor
- Be clinically alert for tuberculosis, histoplasmosis, and other opportunistic infections.

Other
- Patients should be tested for tuberculosis before initiating therapy. Currently, infliximab is only approved for therapy in combination with methotrexate. Increased mortality in heart failure patients taking infliximab has been shown.

Dose
Infliximab
- 3 mg/kg IV initially, at weeks 2 and 6, then every 8 weeks in combination with methotrexate

Etanercept
- 25 mg SC twice weekly or 50 mg SC once weekly

Adalimumab
- 40 mg SC every second week

Kineret (anakinra)
Mechanism of action
- Anakinra blocks the biologic activity of IL-1 by competitively inhibiting IL-1 binding to the interleukin-1 type I receptor (IL-1RI).

Patient instructions
- Kineret is supplied as a single-use, prefilled syringe that should be stored in the refrigerator. Any syringe left unrefrigerated for over 24 hours should be discarded.

Adverse drug events
- Similarly to the anti-TNF agents, anakinra increases the risk of serious infections. Injection site reactions are extremely common. Headache, nausea, diarrhea, sinusitis, flu-like symptoms, and abdominal pain have also been reported.

Drug-drug interactions
- Live vaccines

Parameters to monitor
- Patients should have a CBC checked at baseline, then monthly for 3 months, followed by every 3 months for the first year of therapy.

Dose
- 100 mg daily SC

Other agents
Imuran (azathioprine)
- This agent is a purine analogue immunosuppressive agent generally reserved for refractory RA. It is

associated with dose-related bone marrow suppression, stomatitis, diarrhea, rash, and liver failure. Patients must have a baseline CBC, creatinine, and liver profile. Patients should then have a CBC and platelet count drawn every 1-2 weeks after any change in dosage and every 1-3 months thereafter. Azathioprine should not be administered with allopurinol since xanthine oxidase metabolizes 6-mercaptopurine.

Sandimmune® (cyclosporine A)

- By blocking T-cell activation, this agent produces powerful immunosuppressive effects and is beneficial as monotherapy in the treatment of RA. Serious adverse effects such as hypertension, nephrotoxicity, glucose intolerance, and hepatotoxicity have limited its use.

Corticosteroids

- Low-dose oral corticosteroids (<10 mg per day of prednisone or the equivalent) and local injections of glucocorticoids are highly effective. Studies indicate that corticosteroids decrease the progression of RA. They may be useful for acute flare-ups and in patients with significant systemic manifestations of RA. RA is associated with an increased risk of osteoporosis (independent of steroid therapy), and the addition of said agents increases the risk. Patients on glucocorticoids should receive 1500 mg of elemental calcium per day and 400-800 IU of vitamin D per day.

Nondrug Therapy

Surgery/Prosorba®
Prosorba column
- A device called the Prosorba column removes inflammatory antibodies from the patient's blood.

Joint surgery

- Patients may have arthroscopy performed to clean out the bone and cartilage fragments that cause pain within the joint capsule. Patients may eventually require complete joint replacement surgery.

Lifestyle modifications
- Mild exercise
- Diet: there is some evidence to suggest a moderate increase in daily protein intake may be beneficial in RA.
- Psychological: patients with RA benefit from a formal support group.

2. Osteoarthritis

- Osteoarthritis (OA), a disease that affects the weight-bearing joints of the peripheral and axial skeleton, is the most common form of arthritis in the U.S. OA is also known as degenerative joint disease (DJD).

Incidence
- Based on radiologic evidence, approximately 60-80% of people over the age of 65 have OA. Before the age of 50, men have a higher incidence; however, after the age of 50, women have a higher incidence.

Clinical Presentation

- Pain is a common initial finding in patients with OA. This pain typically worsens with weight-bearing activity and improves with rest of the affected joint.
- Changes in weather and barometric pressure tend to influence the severity of pain.
- Joint stiffness, including morning stiffness, is another common complaint. This stiffness differs from that of RA; it is relatively short in duration, is related to periods of inactivity, and resolves with movement.
- Crepitus is common, especially when the knee joint is involved.
- Joint deformities also occur in OA. Heberden's nodes, Bouchard's nodes, and osteophytes on the DIP and PIP joints are commonly seen.

Pathophysiology

- Although the causes of OA are not completely understood, biomechanical stresses affecting the articular cartilage and subchondral bone are thought to be the primary factors in the development of OA. In addition, inflammatory, biochemical, and immunologic components play a role. The function of the normal cartilage, ie, to dissipate the force and stress caused by normal weight-bearing activity, is impaired in OA.
1. Collagen fibers are destroyed and subsequently release proteoglycans. The hydration of the cartilage increases, and the cartilage becomes thick.
2. Metalloproteinases, which degrade the proteoglycans, are released to initiate the reparation process. This degradation causes an increase in chondrocyte activity.
3. The resulting cartilage is thin because the chondrocyte activity cannot match the rate at which proteoglycan degradation occurs.
4. With this ever-thinning layer of cartilage now exposing bone, the grinding motion stimulates

osteoclast/osteoblast activity, thereby causing bone resorption and vascular changes. Ultimately, this leads to the formation of osteophytes.

Diagnostic Criteria

Osteoarthritis of the hip (American College of Rheumatology Classification Criteria)
• See Table 3.

Osteoarthritis of the knee (American College of Rheumatology Classification Criteria)
• See Table 4.

Treatment Principles

• Treatment of patients with OA focuses on symptom control; there are currently no therapeutic options known to change the course of the disease (Tables 5 and 6).

Drug Therapy

• Pain relief is the primary treatment goal for patients with OA. The recommended initial drug of choice is acetaminophen. For those patients that do not respond fully, the addition of an NSAID (see discussion of this class in the RA section) is made.

Acetaminophen
Mechanism of action
• Acetaminophen centrally inhibits prostaglandin synthesis.

Table 3

Traditional Means of Diagnosing Osteoarthritis of the Hip

Hip pain and at least two of the following three:
• Erythrocyte sedimentation rate <20 mm/h
• Radiographic femoral or acetabular osteophytes
• Radiographic joint space narrowing

Other criteria:
• Hip pain and radiographic femoral or acetabular osteophytes
or
• Hip pain and radiographic joint space narrowing and erythrocyte sedimentation rate <20 mm/h

Table 4

Traditional Means of Diagnosing Osteoarthritis of the Knee

Knee pain, radiographic osteophytes, and at least one of the following three:
• Age >50 years
• Morning stiffness ≤30 minutes in duration
• Crepitus on motion

Other criteria:
• Knee pain and radiographic osteophytes
or
• Knee pain and age ≥40 years, morning stiffness ≤30 minutes in duration, and crepitus on motion

Patient instructions
• Patients with hepatic disease or viral hepatitis are at risk of toxicity from chronic acetaminophen use.

Adverse drug events
• Hepatotoxicity is the most severe side effect associated with acetaminophen therapy. For this reason,

Table 5

Medical Management of Patients with Osteoarthritis of the Hip

Nonpharmacologic therapy
  Patient education
    Self-management programs (eg, arthritis self-help course)
  Health professional social support via telephone contact
  Weight loss (if overweight)
  Physical therapy
    Range-of-motion exercises
    Strengthening exercises
    Assistive devices for ambulation
  Occupational therapy
    Joint protection and energy conservation
    Assistive devices for ADLs and IADLs
  Aerobic aquatic exercise programs

Pharmacologic therapy
  Nonopioid analgesics (eg, acetaminophen)
  Nonsteroidal anti-inflammatory drugs
  Opioid analgesics (eg, propoxyphene, codeine, oxycodone)

ADLs, activities of daily living; IADLs, instrumental ADLs.

Table 6

Medical Management of Patients with Osteoarthritis of the Knee

---

Nonpharmacologic therapy

    Patient education

        Self-management programs (eg, arthritis self-help course)

    Health professional social support via telephone contact

    Weight loss (if overweight)

    Physical therapy

        Range-of-motion exercises

        Quadriceps strengthening exercises

        Assistive devices for ambulation

    Occupational therapy

        Joint protection and energy conservation

        Assistive devices for ADLs and IADLs

    Aerobic exercise programs

Pharmacologic therapy

    Intra-articular steroid injections

    Nonopioid analgesics (eg, acetaminophen)

    Topical analgesics (eg, capsaicin and methylsalicylate creams)

    Nonsteroidal anti-inflammatory drugs

    Opioid analgesics (eg, propoxyphene, codeine, oxycodone)

ADLs, activities of daily living; IADLs, instrumental ADLs.

patients should not ingest more than 4 g of acetaminophen per day. Long-term therapy has also been linked to renal failure.

Other

- Acetaminophen is generally considered the initial drug of choice; however, there have been no clinical trials comparing its side effects, potential toxicity, or pain-relieving properties with those of NSAIDs.

Topical agents (capsaicin)

Mechanism of action

- Derived from the pepper plant, capsaicin works by exciting the nociceptive C-afferent neurons, which in turn causes the release of substance P, which is responsible for transmitting pain from the peripheral to the central nervous system.

Patient instructions

- Patients should avoid contact with eyes. It is important to wash hands thoroughly after use.

Adverse drug events

- Patients will experience mild burning and stinging at the site of application.

Other

- Patients usually derive benefit after several weeks of application. Capsaicin is often used in conjunction with oral agents.

Glucosamine sulfate and chondroitin

Mechanism of action

- Glucosamine is found naturally in articular cartilage and acts as a substrate in the synthesis of proteoglycans. Chondroitin, another constituent in the cartilage, attracts and retains water, which provides shock absorption. In addition, chondroitin prevents the breakdown of cartilage and stimulates RNA synthesis of chondrocytes.

Patient instructions

- Patients taking anticoagulants concomitantly may be at increased risk of bleeding.

Adverse drug events

- Adverse events tend to be mild but include dyspepsia and euphoria.

Other

- This combination is available over the counter and has some clinical literature to support its use. The Arthritis Foundation, however, does not currently recognize it as a treatment for OA.

Other agents

- Hyaluronic acid derivatives have been approved by the FDA for the treatment of pain associated with OA of the knee. These agents may be an option after all conventional therapies for OA have been exhausted. The injection of this product into the synovium appears to replenish the viscosity to the space, thus enabling normal tissue to regenerate.

Nondrug Therapy

- See Table 7.

Table 7

Nondrug Therapy for Osteoarthritis

Patient education
Self-management programs (eg, Arthritis Foundation
  Self-Management Program)
Personalized social support through telephone contact
Weight loss (if overweight)
Aerobic exercise programs
Physical therapy (ie, range-of-motion exercises)
Muscle-strengthening exercises
Assistive devices for ambulation
Patellar taping
Appropriate footwear
Lateral-wedged insoles (for genu varum); bracing
Occupational therapy
Joint protection and energy conservation
Assistive devices for ADLs

ADLs, activities of daily living.

3. Gout

- Gout, a systemic disease caused by the build-up of uric acid in the joints, causes inflammation, swelling, and pain. Hyperuricemia is defined as a urate level >8 mg/dL in men and 7 mg/dL in women.

Incidence

- Gout has been known as "the disease of kings and the king of diseases," and can be traced to the time of Hippocrates. Gout occurs in approximately 1% of the population; the vast majority of these are men.

Clinical Presentation

- Pain in one joint of the lower extremity is the most common first symptom of gout. The initial period of pain, usually monarticular and self-limiting, is followed by a period in which the patient is completely asymptomatic.
- Termed intercritical periods, the time between acute gouty arthritis attacks may be 3 months to 2 years; the length of time shortens as the disease progresses.
- The first attack is typically at night or in the early morning.
- Gout commonly affects the ankle, heel, knee, wrist, finger, elbow, and instep. The most common site of

the initial attack is the first MTP joint, and is known as podagra.
- The patient may experience fever, chills, and malaise during an acute gouty arthritis attack. Left untreated, the attack may last 1-2 weeks.
- The skin over the affected joint becomes red, hot, swollen, and tender. As the patient recovers from the attack, local desquamation may occur.

Pathophysiology

- Uric acid is the end product of purine metabolism (Figure 2).
- Xanthine oxidase is the rate-limiting step in the formation of uric acid.
- Uric acid, which serves no known biological function, has a body content of 1-1.2 g.
- Approximately 70% of uric acid is excreted via the kidneys.
- At physiologic pH, uric acid primarily exists as monosodium urate salt.
- Approximately 95% of serum uric acid is filtered across the glomerulus. Of this filtered amount, almost 100% is reabsorbed in the early part of the

Figure 2.

Ribose-uric acid pathway.

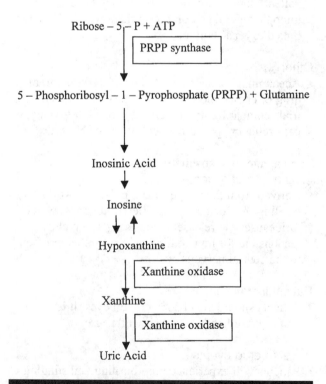

proximal tubule, only to be secreted back into the lumen in the more distal part of the tubule.
- Primary gout is a result of an innate defect in purine metabolism or uric acid excretion.
  * In this case, hyperuricemia may result from uric acid overproduction (in "overproducers"), impaired renal clearance of uric acid (in "underexcreters"), or a combination of both.
  * In rare instances, enzyme defects of either hypoxanthine guanine phosphoribosyltransferase (HGPRT) or 5-phosphoribosyl-1-pyrophosphate (PRPP) may cause primary gout (Figure 2).
- Secondary gout is associated with increased nucleic acid turnover, decreased renal function, increased purine production, or drug-induced decreased elimination of uric acid.
  * Hematologic disorders that are lymphoproliferative and myeloproliferative in nature are known causes of secondary hyperuricemia.
  * Salicylates such as aspirin may inhibit tubular secretion of uric acid at low doses.
  * All diuretics, with the exception of spironolactone, may cause hyperuricemia.
  * Ethambutol, pyrazinamide, nicotinic acid, ethanol, niacin, and cyclosporine are known to cause an increase in serum uric acid.
- Acute gout attacks are caused by the deposition of monosodium urate crystals (MSU) in the synovium of the joint.
- This deposition results in the stimulation of the body's inflammatory cascade. The MSU crystals undergo phagocytosis by polymorphonuclear leukocytes. These leukocytes, damaged by the sharp crystals, burst and release their contents (interleukin-1, lysosomes, and prostaglandins) into the synovium. This results in the inflammatory reaction, ie, pain, swelling, and erythema.
- If left untreated, deposits of MSU crystals, also known as tophi, lead to joint deformity and disability. Ultimately, patients may develop one of two types of renal disease—urate nephropathy or uric acid nephropathy. Urate nephropathy results from the deposition of MSU crystals in the renal interstitium; uric acid nephropathy results from the deposition of uric acid in the collecting tubules.

Diagnostic Criteria

- The American Rheumatism Association lists the following criteria for the diagnosis of gout:
  * Definite: Sodium urate crystals in affected joint appear negatively birefringent when viewed through a polarized light source.
  * Suggestive: A minimum of six of the following criteria should be met.

- More than one attack of arthritis
- Development of maximum inflammation within 1 day
- Oligoarthritis attack
- Redness over joint
- Painful or swollen first metatarsophalangeal joint
- Unilateral attack on first metatarsophalangeal joint
- Unilateral attack on tarsal joint
- Tophus
- Hyperuricemia
- Asymptomatic swelling within a joint

  * It is also important to rule out pseudogout. In pseudogout, crystals deposited into the joint synovium cause intense pain and inflammation, but the culprit is calcium pyrophosphate dihydrate, not monosodium urate.

Treatment Goals

- Relieve pain and inflammation
- Reduce serum uric acid concentration
- Prevent recurrent gout attacks

Drug Therapy

- See Table 8.

Acute gouty arthritis attack

- There are three treatments available: colchicine, NSAIDs (indomethacin in particular), and corticosteroids. It is best to avoid treatments that affect serum uric acid concentrations during an acute attack.

Colchicine
Mechanism of action

- Colchicine inhibits the phagocytosis of urate crystals by leukocytes. Colchicine also inhibits the release of chemotactic factor, thus reducing the adhesion of polymorphonuclear leukocytes. The net result makes colchicine an anti-inflammatory agent without analgesic activity.

Patient instructions

- Patients should immediately stop taking colchicine once abdominal cramping and/or diarrhea occurs. Patients should never exceed a total of 8 mg during an acute gouty arthritis attack.

Adverse drug events

- Nausea, bloating, emesis, and diarrhea occur in up to 80% of patients taking colchicine. Rarely, it may cause bone marrow suppression. This effect occurs with a higher incidence in those patients with under-

Table 8

Drugs for the Treatment of Gout

Generic name (trade name)	Classification	Normal dose	Comments	Dosage forms
Colchicine	Anti-inflammatory	0.6-1.2 mg PO every 1-2 hours until resolution of symptoms, severe GI symptoms occur, or a max of 8 mg reached	May be used for chronic suppressive therapy; must adjust dose for renal insufficiency	PO, IV
Probenecid (Benemid®)	Uricosuric agent	250-500 mg bid	Avoid salicylates; take with plenty of water	PO
Sulfinpyrazone (Anturane®)	Uricosuric agent	50-200 mg bid	Avoid salicylates; take with plenty of water	PO
Allopurinol (Zyloprim®)	Xanthine oxidase inhibitor	100-300 mg qd	May cause rash; reduce dosage in renal failure	PO
Indomethacin (Indocin)	NSAID	50 mg tid-qid	May cause fluid retention, GI bleeding	PO, IV, supp

lying renal or hepatic dysfunction. When colchicine is given intravenously, possible extravasation may cause local skin necrosis.

Drug-drug and drug-disease interactions
- Patients with active peptic ulcer disease should not take colchicine.

Parameters to monitor
- With long-term therapy, patients should have a serum creatinine test, liver function test, and complete white blood cell count check periodically.

Dose
- For the treatment of an acute gouty arthritis attack, patients should take 0.6-1.2 mg orally every 2 hours until pain relief is achieved, diarrhea occurs, or a maximum dose of 8 mg is reached. When given intravenously, an initial dose of 2 mg is given followed by two additional doses of 1 mg at 6-hour intervals. The dose should never exceed 4 mg.

Other
- Colchicine is most effective when initiated within 12-36 hours of the attack.

Indomethacin
- (Please see review of NSAIDs in RA section.) Indomethacin is the most extensively studied NSAID in the treatment of an acute gouty arthritis attack. Unlike colchicine, indomethacin is effective at any point during the acute attack.

Corticosteroids
- For the treatment of acute gout pain, corticosteroids are effective when given intra-articularly, intravenously, or orally. Their use is limited to treatment failures of colchicine and NSAIDs. Intramuscular corticotropin (ACTH) is also effective when given (40 U) to treat an acute gouty arthritis attack.

Gout prophylaxis (intercritical period)
- Patients with asymptomatic hyperuricemia should not be routinely treated with pharmacologic agents. These patients should undergo a work-up to determine the cause of hyperuricemia. The use of low-dose (0.6-1.2 mg/d) colchicine can prevent subsequent attacks of gout. Patients in the intercritical period (after an acute gouty arthritis attack) are candidates for long-term prophylactic therapy directed at affecting serum uric acid levels. Choice of therapy is based on the patient's pathophysiologic cause of hyperuricemia. Patients are generally classified as "overproducers" or "underexcreters." Placing the patient on a purine-restricted diet and performing a 24-hour urine collection to measure uric acid concentration may identify overproducers of uric acid. Those patients who excrete more than 600 mg of uric acid are considered overproducers. Once this diagnosis is made, patients are treated with one of two classes of agents: xanthine oxidase inhibitors or uricosurics.

Benemid (probenecid)

Mechanism of action

- Probenecid is a uricosuric agent that promotes the excretion of uric acid by blocking its reuptake at the proximal convoluted tubule.

Patient instructions

- Patients should drink at least 2 liters of water per day in order to decrease the risk of uric acid stone formation. Patients should take probenecid with food if GI intolerance occurs.

Adverse drug events

- Probenecid is generally well-tolerated and is associated with very few adverse side effects. Up to 10% of patients receiving probenecid therapy develop uric acid stones. Probenecid may cause abdominal discomfort, but this is often avoided by taking it with food.

Drug-drug interactions

- Since probenecid prevents the tubular secretion of many weak organic acids, it has potential drug interactions, eg, with the penicillins, cephalosporins, nitrofurantoin, and rifampin. Although the interaction between probenecid, penicillins, and cephalosporins has been utilized therapeutically, its interaction with nitrofurantoin reduces nitrofurantoin's effectiveness. Aspirin interferes with uric acid secretion and therefore should never be used in conjunction with probenecid. Additionally, the diuretic effects of furosemide and hydrochlorothiazide are magnified when probenecid is taken concomitantly. Finally, patients receiving sulfonylureas should be monitored closely for hypoglycemia when started on probenecid.

Other

- Patients should never begin uricosuric therapy during an acute gouty arthritis attack due to the risk of exacerbating the attack. Probenecid should not be used in patients with a creatinine clearance less than 50 mL/min.

Anturane (sulfinpyrazone)

Mechanism of action

- Sulfinpyrazone is a uricosuric agent that promotes the excretion of uric acid by blocking its reuptake at the proximal convoluted tubule.

Patient instructions

- Patients should drink at least 2 liters of water per day in order to decrease the risk of uric acid stone formation. Patients should take sulfinpyrazone with food if GI intolerance occurs. Patients who are sensitive to aspirin should not take this agent due to the risk of bronchoconstriction.

Adverse drug events

- Like probenecid, sulfinpyrazone is generally well-tolerated. The most common reported adverse effects are GI discomfort and uric acid stone formation. In addition, rarely it has been associated with bone marrow suppression and immunoallergic interstitial nephritis.

Drug-drug interactions

- Sulfinpyrazone decreases the effectiveness of nitrofurantoin. When sulfinpyrazone is taken with aspirin, the effect of sulfinpyrazone is lessened.

Parameters to monitor

- Patients should have complete blood work periodically due to the rare risk of bone marrow suppression associated with sulfinpyrazone therapy.

Other

- Patients should never start uricosuric therapy during an acute gouty arthritis attack; it may exacerbate the attack. When increasing the dose of sulfinpyrazone, titrate upward slowly to minimize the risk of uric acid stone formation. Since uricosuric therapy may precipitate an acute gouty arthritis attack, patients should take an NSAID or colchicine for the first 6-12 months of therapy. Patients with a creatinine clearance of less than 50 mL/min should not use sulfinpyrazone.

Zyloprim (allopurinol)

Mechanism of action

- Allopurinol and its metabolite, oxypurinol, inhibit xanthine oxidase formation (XO), which is the rate-limiting step in uric acid synthesis. This facilitates the clearance of the more water soluble precursors of uric acid, oxypurines.

Patient instructions

- Patients should immediately report any signs of rash to their health care providers. Allopurinol should be taken with food to minimize GI discomfort.

Adverse drug events

- Allopurinol is generally well tolerated; the overall occurrence of adverse effects is less than 1%. Patients should be advised that rash, the most common adverse effect, might occur at any time during therapy. The rash may be as simple as a maculopapular eruption or as serious as the life-threatening Stevens-Johnson syndrome (which is exfoliative and erythematous). Rarely, allopurinol may cause alopecia, neutropenia, and hepatitis.

Drug-drug interactions

- The chemotherapeutic agents azathioprine and 6-mercaptopurine are metabolized via the xanthine oxidase pathway; therefore, allopurinol and its metabolite oxypurinol may increase serum levels of these agents. The concomitant administration of ampicillin or amoxicillin with allopurinol increases the risk of rash to approximately 20%.

Parameters to monitor

- Patients should be encouraged to report the first signs of rash to their physicians immediately. Patients should have serum creatinine as well as liver function tests drawn periodically.

Kinetics

- With a half-life of 30 hours, allopurinol is rapidly converted to its active metabolite (oxypurinol). This allows for once-daily dosing.

Other

- To reduce the risk of precipitating an acute gouty arthritis attack, allopurinol should be initiated at a dose of 100 mg per day and increased at 100-mg intervals weekly to an average dose of 300 mg per day. Patients with renal insufficiency require a dose adjustment. Assuming the target dose is 300 mg per day, patients with a creatinine clearance of 10-20 mL/min should receive 200 mg per day. Those with a clearance of less than 10 mL/min should receive 100 mg per day.

Secondary hyperuricemia

- As discussed earlier, hyperuricemia may be caused by lymphoproliferative and myeloproliferative disorders, as well as their chemotherapeutic treatments (eg, tumor lysis syndrome). It is common to add allopurinol to the prescribed chemotherapeutic regimen to prevent complications of hyperuricemia, eg, an acute gouty arthritis attack. Elitek® (rasburicase) is a newly approved therapeutic agent used to prevent hyperuricemia in children with leukemia, lymphoma, and solid tumor malignancies. Rasburicase is a recombinant urate oxidase enzyme that converts uric acid to allantoin, thereby allowing it to be eliminated. Patients with G6PD deficiency should not use rasburicase.

4. Systemic Lupus Erythematosus

- SLE is a chronic autoimmune inflammatory disorder that can affect any system in the body, including the skin, joints, and internal organs.

Classification

- SLE is broken down into three types: (1) discoid lupus, which affects the skin; (2) drug-induced lupus, which generally resolves after discontinuing the offending medication; and (3) overlap syndrome, in which the patient has features that overlap with another rheumatic disease process.

Clinical Presentation

- Signs and symptoms consistent with SLE include:
    * Malar rash (a butterfly-shaped rash over the cheeks and across the bridge of the nose)
    * Discoid rash (scaly, disk-shaped sores on the face, neck, and/or chest)
    * Photosensitivity
    * Oral ulcers
    * Arthritis
    * Serositis (inflammation of the lining around the heart, lungs, and/or abdomen that causes pain and shortness of breath)
    * Proteinuria
    * Central nervous system problems
    * Antinuclear antibodies (autoantibodies that react against the body's own cells)
    * Anemia
    * Fatigue
    * Fever
    * Skin rash
    * Muscle aches
    * Nausea
    * Vomiting and diarrhea
    * Anorexia
    * Raynaud's phenomenon
    * Weight loss

- Patients typically present with chronic fatigue and depression. Dermatitis and arthritis (in multiple joints) are the most common clinical manifestations. The arthritic pain patients describe is generally out of proportion to the amount of synovitis present. Although it is rare, serious renal abnormalities can occur in patients with SLE. Central nervous system involvement, also rare, can be serious. Lupus-related encephalopathy may occur due to scarring of arterioles in the subcortical white matter. In addition, patients with SLE are at risk of stroke due to the thromboembolic nature of the antiphospholipid antibody.

Pathophysiology

- The exact pathophysiology of SLE remains unknown. It is an autoimmune disease (type III hypersensitivity) in which patients have an overactivity of B cells. The result is hypergammaglobulinemia that ultimately precipitates immune complexes on the vascular membranes, thereby causing activation of complement. Drugs, procainamide being the most predominant, may also cause SLE. Other such medications include phenytoin, chlorpromazine, hydralazine, quinidine, methyldopa, and isoniazid.

Diagnostic Criteria

- See Table 9.

Therapy

- Therapy for each case of SLE is based on the particular symptoms of any given patient. Arthritis is commonly treated with NSAIDs or glucocorticoids. Dermatologic complications can be treated with hydroxychloroquine (see RA section). Thrombocytopenia generally responds to glucocorticoid therapy. Refractory cases may respond to cyclophosphamide therapy and/or splenectomy. Finally, plasmapheresis has been used with some degree of success.

Table 9

Criteria for Diagnosing Systemic Lupus Erythematosus

1. Characteristic rash across the cheek(s)
2. Discoid lesion rash
3. Photosensitivity
4. Oral ulcers
5. Arthritis
6. Inflammation of membranes in lungs, heart, or abdomen
7. Evidence of kidney disease
8. Evidence of severe neurologic disease
9. Blood disorders, including low red blood cell, white blood cell, and platelet counts
10. Immunologic abnormalities
11. Positive antinuclear antibody

Note: A patient must experience four of the criteria before a classification of SLE can be made. These criteria, proposed by the American College of Rheumatology, should not be the sole characteristics for diagnosis, however.

5. Key Points

- Rheumatoid arthritis (RA), a highly variable autoimmune disease characterized by symmetric, erosive synovitis, often affects extra-articular sites.
- RA usually affects diarthrodial joints, eg, the proximal interphalangeal (PIP) joints, metacarpophalangeal (MCP) joints, metatarsophalangeal (MTP) joints, wrists, and ankles. Also commonly involved are the elbows, shoulders, sternoclavicular joints, temporomandibular joints, hips, and knees.
- Morning stiffness is the hallmark of RA.
- According to the American College of Rheumatology, the goals in managing RA are to prevent or control joint damage, prevent loss of function, and decrease pain.
- The American College of Rheumatology recommends the use of DMARDs within 3 months of diagnosis of RA.
- Unlike the NSAIDs, DMARDs have the ability to reduce or prevent joint damage and preserve joint integrity and function. DMARDs carry the risk of various toxicities and they must be monitored on a regular basis.
- Osteoarthritis is the most common form of arthritis in the United States.
- Joint stiffness, a common complaint in osteoarthritis, differs from RA in that it is relatively short in duration and resolves with movement.
- Unlike RA, pain relief is the primary treatment goal in osteoarthritis. The initial drug of choice is acetaminophen.
- Gout, a systemic disease caused by the build-up of uric acid in the joints, causes inflammation, swelling, and pain.
- Primary gout is a result of an innate defect in purine metabolism or uric acid excretion.
- Patients with gout are classified as overproducers or underexcreters based on measuring 24-hour uric acid concentration levels.
- Treatment of an acute gouty arthritis attack involves the use of colchicine, NSAIDs, or glucocorticoids.
- Uricosuric agents and/or xanthine oxidase inhibitors are used to prevent further gout attacks. These agents should not be used during an acute gouty arthritis attack.
- Systemic lupus erythematosus is a chronic autoimmune inflammatory disorder that can affect any system in the body.
- Therapy for SLE is primarily driven by the clinical manifestations of the disease.

6. Questions and Answers

A 45-year-old man presents to his local physician with a complaint of extreme stiffness in the morning that lasts until noon on most days. He also states that he feels "drained" all the time and both of his knees are swollen and painful. Upon examination, the physician documents the presence of rheumatoid nodules. The patient's laboratory work-up is significant for thrombocytopenia and a positive rheumatoid factor. He states that he has been taking over-the-counter ibuprofen at a dose of 200 mg 2-3 times daily without relief.

1. Which of the following represents the best drug therapy option for this patient?

   A. Increase the dose of ibuprofen to 800 mg three times daily
   B. Increase the dose of ibuprofen and add methotrexate 25 mg twice daily
   C. Increase the dose of ibuprofen and add celecoxib 100 mg twice daily
   D. Increase the dose of ibuprofen and add leflunomide at a dose of 100 mg daily for 3 days followed by 20 mg daily

2. Which of the following represents the best way to decrease potential liver toxicity with methotrexate while achieving optimal therapeutic benefit?

   A. Add 1-3 mg of folic acid per day to the patient's regimen
   B. Decrease the dose of methotrexate to 25 mg once monthly
   C. Add monthly injections of leucovorin to the patient's regimen
   D. Add leflunomide to the patient's regimen

3. As combination DMARD therapy may be more efficacious in the refractory RA population, which of the following represents the BEST choice for combination therapy?

   A. Arava 20 mg once daily + Rheumatrex 25 mg once weekly
   B. Remicade 3 mg/kg IM + Rheumatrex 25 mg once weekly
   C. Myochrysine IM + Plaquenil 200 mg twice daily
   D. Remicade 3 mg/kg IV + Rheumatrex 25 mg once weekly

4. A physician inquires about the recommended monitoring parameters for patients started on Ridaura. Which of the following represents the most appropriate response?

   A. Baseline ophthalmologic exam, CBC, and serum creatinine, followed by a yearly CBC, serum creatinine, and ophthalmologic exam
   B. Baseline liver function tests, CBC, and albumin, followed by monthly liver function tests
   C. Baseline CBC, serum creatinine, and urine dipstick for protein, followed by a CBC and urine dipstick for protein every 1-2 months
   D. There are no recommended monitoring parameters at this time

5. All of the following represent methods used to decrease the GI toxicity associated with NSAIDs except

   A. changing patients from a nonselective cyclooxygenase inhibitor to a type II–specific inhibitor such as Celebrex
   B. adding a proton pump inhibitor such as Prevacid to the patient's NSAID
   C. adding Cytotec to the patient's NSAID
   D. instructing the patient to take his or her NSAID at night, when acid secretion is limited

6. Which of the following is (are) true concerning diclofenac?

   I. It is available as an extended-release product, Voltaren XR
   II. It is available as an injectable product, Voltaren IM
   III. It is available in combination with misoprostol, Arthrotec

   A. I only
   B. I and II only
   C. I, II, and III
   D. I and III only

7. Which of the following would be a contraindication for the use of Enbrel?

   A. Renal insufficiency
   B. Active infection
   C. Persons over the age of 65
   D. Patients with congestive heart failure

8. Regarding therapies designed to target tumor necrosis factor and interleukin-1 in the treatment of RA, the following statements are correct EXCEPT

   A. Kineret is packaged as a single-use prefilled syringe that should be kept in the refrigerator
   B. patients should have a tuberculin skin test completed before initiating Enbrel or Remicade
   C. kineret is a soluble receptor that binds tumor necrosis factor
   D. Enbrel is approved for use as a single agent

9. The use of glucocorticoids is associated with numerous adverse effects and long-term consequences. All of the following are initiatives to treat and/or prevent/minimize these adverse effects EXCEPT

   A. instruct patients to take the glucocorticoid once daily versus dividing the total daily dose into two to four doses
   B. instruct patients on long-term therapy to add 1500 mg of elemental calcium and 400-800 IU of ergocalciferol to their regimen
   C. suggest adding a bisphosphonate to their therapy
   D. inform patients that stopping glucocorticoid abruptly is contraindicated

10. A young lady enters your pharmacy and informs you that she is planning on becoming pregnant and would like you to review her medication profile to see if any would be potentially harmful. Upon review of her profile, you notice that she is taking Arava for RA. Which is the most appropriate response?

    A. Arava is a category C drug, and could potentially harm the fetus. She should discuss the risks and benefits of becoming pregnant with her physician first
    B. Arava is a category X drug, and she should undergo the drug-elimination procedure with cholestyramine before trying to become pregnant
    C. Arava is a category X drug with no active metabolites and a short half-life; therefore she should discontinue the drug and wait 1-2 weeks before trying to become pregnant
    D. Arava is a category B drug and the risk of toxicity to the fetus is extremely low

11. R.Y. is a 67-year-old man with chief complaints of a swollen big left toe and extreme pain. The area is erythematous and tender. Laboratory analysis reveals a uric acid level of 10 mg/dL. Review of R.Y.'s past medical history reveals hypertension and congestive heart failure. A diagnosis of gout is made. Which is the best choice for the treatment of R.Y.'s acute gouty arthritis attack?

    A. Probenecid 500 mg now followed by 500 mg twice daily
    B. Indomethacin 50 mg now followed by 50 mg three to four times daily
    C. Allopurinol 100 mg once daily
    D. Colchicine 0.6 mg every hour until resolution of symptoms, development of diarrhea, or a cumulative dose of 8 mg is reached

12. The following comments are consistent with the diagnosis of gout EXCEPT

    A. The presence of negatively birefringent crystals in the affected synovial joint fluid
    B. The presence of calcium pyrophosphate in the affected synovial joint fluid
    C. Presence of tophi
    D. Presence of hyperuricemia

13. Which of the following best describes Benemid?

    A. Like allopurinol, it decreases the body's production of uric acid
    B. Like Anturane, it is a uricosuric agent that aids in the tubular reabsorption of uric acid
    C. It blocks the excretion of uric acid in the urine
    D. Like Anturane, it is a uricosuric agent that blocks reuptake of uric acid at the proximal convoluted tubule

14. Which of the following represents a therapeutically ineffective combination that should be avoided?

    A. Benemid + penicillin G
    B. Benemid + aspirin (>2 g per day)
    C. Anturane + Macrobid
    D. Benemid + colchicine

15. All of the following statements are true regarding Zyloprim EXCEPT

    A. it works to decrease the formation of uric acid by inhibiting xanthine oxidase
    B. it does not require dosage adjustment in patients with renal insufficiency
    C. skin reactions, including Stevens-Johnson syndrome, have been reported with its use
    D. it should not be used for the treatment of an acute gouty arthritis attack

16. Which of the following represent potentially dangerous drug interactions with Zyloprim?

    I. Amoxicillin
    II. Imuran
    III. Essidrex

    A. I only
    B. I and II only
    C. I, II, and III
    D. III only

17. All of the following are consistent with the diagnosis of osteoarthritis EXCEPT

    A. the presence of morning stiffness that is not associated with immobility and may last for several hours
    B. pain is a common initial finding that typically worsens with weight-bearing activity and subsides with rest
    C. it commonly occurs in the knees or the hips
    D. crepitus is common

18. Which of the following medications is(are) suggested for the treatment of osteoarthritis by the American College of Rheumatology?

    I. Tylenol
    II. Capsaicin
    III. Glucosamine sulfate and chondroitin

    A. All of the above
    B. II only
    C. III only
    D. I and II only

19. Concerning treatment of osteoarthritis, which of the following statements is incorrect?

    A. Tylenol is generally considered the initial drug of choice
    B. Tylenol is considered safe and effective, and has minimal adverse effects, especially in doses greater than 4 g per day
    C. Muscle-strengthening exercises may be helpful
    D. Hyaluronic acid derivatives have been approved by the FDA for the treatment of pain associated with osteoarthritis

20. The following medications are considered to be DMARDs EXCEPT

    A. Plaquenil
    B. Cuprimine
    C. Myochrysine
    D. Nalfon

Answers

1. **D.** Although the patient currently has room to increase his dose of NSAID, he is demonstrating signs and symptoms of systemic RA. This indicates that the addition of DMARD therapy is necessary. Methotrexate represents a viable option; however, the dose of 25 mg twice daily is excessive (it should be dosed once weekly). The addition of leflunomide is the best choice.

2. **A.** The addition of folic acid to the methotrexate regimen has been demonstrated to reduce the risk of liver toxicity. Lowering the dose of methotrexate is likely to decrease risk, but is also likely to decrease its effectiveness. Leucovorin, an injectable formulation of folate, is used only to reverse methotrexate toxicity.

3. **D.** Arava plus methotrexate may be a very efficacious combination, but it increases the risk of liver toxicity significantly. Gold therapy in combination with Plaquenil increases the risk of rash. Remicade, only approved for use in combination with Rheumatrex, is given IV and not IM; this combination represents the best choice.

4. **C.** Gold therapy is associated with glomerulonephritis, thrombocytopenia, and leukopenia; therefore, a baseline renal evaluation and periodic testing should occur during the entire course of therapy.

5.   **D.** Adding a proton pump inhibitor, Cytotec, or changing to a selective COX-II inhibitor has been demonstrated to lower the risk of significant GI adverse effects. Timing of the dose of an NSAID has never been demonstrated to affect the risk of GI toxicity.

6.   **D.** Diclofenac is available as an immediate-release product, an extended-release product, and in combination with misoprostol. It is not available in an injectable formulation.

7.   **B.** Due to its effects on tumor necrosis factor, Enbrel may decrease a patient's ability to fight infection. Enbrel is contraindicated in patients with an active infection. Its use should be temporarily discontinued until the acute process has resolved.

8.   **C.** Kineret targets interleukin-1, not tumor necrosis factor. Kineret is available as a single-use prefilled syringe. Unlike Remicade, Enbrel is approved as monotherapy.

9.   **A.** Patients taking glucocorticoids are at risk of developing osteoporosis. Efforts to minimize this adverse effect include the addition of calcium and vitamin D to the patient's regimen as well as adding a bisphosphonate, eg, Fosamax, to suppress bone resorption. Due to adrenal suppression that occurs with long-term glucocorticoid therapy, patients should taper off the agent.

10.   **B.** Since Arava is a teratogenic agent with an active metabolite with a long half-life, a drug-elimination procedure should be performed before becoming pregnant.

11.   **D.** Both Probenecid and allopurinol may exacerbate an acute gouty arthritis attack and should only be reserved for the prevention of further attacks. Indomethacin is an option for the treatment of an acute gouty arthritis attack; however, due to NSAIDs' tendency to cause fluid retention in the renal tubules, it would not be the ideal agent in a patient with congestive heart failure. Colchicine represents the best option from this list.

12.   **B.** The presence of calcium pyrophosphate is consistent with the diagnosis of pseudogout, not gout.

13.   **D.** Benemid is a uricosuric agent that blocks reuptake of uric acid at the proximal convoluted tubule. It does not affect the body's ability to produce uric acid. Response B is incorrect because Benemid does not promote the reabsorption of uric acid.

14.   **C.** Benemid does prevent the tubular secretion of penicillin. However, this interaction is therapeutically utilized to increase the duration of action of a single dose of penicillin. Although low doses of aspirin may inhibit the tubular secretion of uric acid, larger doses (>2 g per day) do not have the same effect. The combination of Benemid and colchicine (marketed under the trade name Colbenemid®) has been therapeutically utilized to prevent the manifestation of an acute gouty arthritis attack. Finally, a combination of Anturane and Macrobid will inhibit Macrobid from reaching its site of action, thus diminishing its therapeutic efficacy.

15.   **B.** Zyloprim must be adjusted in patients with renal insufficiency. Its use has been associated with serious skin reactions that may occur at any point during therapy. Zyloprim should never be used in the treatment of an acute gouty arthritis attack.

16.   **B.** The co-administration of amoxicillin and allopurinol increases the risk of rash up to 20%. Imuran is metabolized via xanthine oxidase, whose activity is inhibited by allopurinol. This increases the risk of toxicity associated with Imuran. Although Essidrex may increase uric acid levels, there is no direct drug-drug interaction associated with allopurinol.

17.   **A.** The morning stiffness associated with osteoarthritis is usually of short duration, is associated with periods of inactivity, and resolves with movement.

18.   **D.** Both Tylenol and capsaicin are effective and recommended by the American College of Rheumatology as treatment options for osteoarthritis. Although there is some clinical data to support its use, glucosamine sulfate and chondroitin are not currently recommended by the American College of Rheumatology.

19.   **B.** Tylenol is generally considered to be safe and effective; however, its use is associated with hepatic failure and the rare incidence of renal failure. Patients should be advised to take LESS than 4 g per day to limit the risk of hepatic failure.

20.   **D.** Nalfon, also known as fenoprofen, is an NSAID, not a DMARD.

7. References

Rheumatoid arthritis

Olsen NJ, Stein CM. New drugs for rheumatoid arthritis. *N Engl J Med.* 2004;21:2167-2179.

Boyce EG. Rheumatoid arthritis. In: Herfindal ET, Gourley DR, et al, eds. *Textbook of Therapeutic Drugs and Disease Management,* 7th ed. Baltimore: Lippincott Williams & Wilkins; 2000:641-666.

Goekoop YP, Allaart CF, Breedveld FC, et al. Combination therapy in rheumatoid arthritis. *Curr Opin Rheumatol.* 2001;30:249-254.

Kremer JM. Rational use of new and existing disease-modifying agents in rheumatoid arthritis. *Ann Intern Med.* 2001;134:695-706.

Kwoh CK, Anderson LG, Greene JM, et al. Guidelines for the management of rheumatoid arthritis. *Arthritis Rheum.* 2002;46:328-346.

Sims RW, Kwoh CK, Anderson LG, et al. Guidelines for monitoring drug therapy in rheumatoid arthritis. *Arthritis Rheum.* 1996;39:723-731.

Schuna AA, Schmidt MJ, Pigarelli DW. Rheumatoid arthritis. In: Dipiro JT, Talbert RL, et al, eds. *Pharmacotherapy: A Pathophysiologic Approach,* 4th ed. New York: McGraw-Hill; 1997:1427-1440.

Wolfe F, Rehman W, Lane NE, et al. Starting a disease-modifying antirheumatic drug or a biologic agent in rheumatoid arthritis: Standards of practice for RA treatment. *J Rheumatol.* 2001;28:1704-1711.

Osteoarthritis

Altman RD, Hochberg MC, Moskowitz RW, et al. Recommendations for the medical management of osteoarthritis of the hip and knee. *Arthritis Rheum.* 2000;43:1905-1915.

Boh LE. Osteoarthritis. In: Dipiro JT, Talbert RL, et al, eds. *Pharmacotherapy: A Pathophysiologic Approach,* 4th ed. New York: McGraw-Hill; 1997:1441-1459.

Roberts LJ, Morrow JD. Analgesic-antipyretic and antiinflammatory agents and drugs employed in the treatment of gout. In: Hardman JG, Limbird LE, et al, eds. *Goodman and Gilman's The Pharmacological Basis of Therapeutics,* 10th ed. New York: McGraw-Hill; 2001:687-732.

Whitaker AL, Small RE. Osteoarthritis. In: Herfindal ET, Gourley DR, et al, eds. *Textbook of Therapeutic Drug and Disease Management,* 7th ed. Baltimore: Lippincott Williams & Wilkins; 2000:667-678.

Gout

American College of Rheumatology Fact Sheet 2000. Gout. http://www.rheumatology.org/patients/factsheet/gout.html.

Emmerson BT. The management of gout. *N Engl J Med.* 1996;334:445-451.

Hawkins DW, Rahn DW. Gout and hyperuricemia. In: Dipiro JT, Talbert RL, et al, eds. *Pharmacotherapy: A Pathophysiologic Approach,* 4th ed. New York: McGraw-Hill; 1997:1460-1465.

Kelley WN, Schumaker HR, Jr. Gout. In: *Textbook of Rheumatology,* 6th ed. Philadelphia: WB Saunders; 2001.

Maloley PA, Westfall GR. Gout and hyperuricemia. In: Herfindal ET, Gourley DR, et al, eds. *Textbook of Therapeutic Drug and Disease Management,* 7th ed. Baltimore: Lippincott Williams & Wilkins; 2000:679-690.

Terkeltaub RA, Edwards NL, Pratt PW, et al. Gout. In: Klippel JH, ed. *Primer on the Rheumatic Diseases,* 11th ed. Atlanta: Arthritis Foundation; 1998:230-243.

Systemic lupus erythematosus

Burlingame MB, Delafuente JC. Systemic lupus erythematosus. In: Dipiro JT, Talbert RL, et al, eds. *Pharmacotherapy: A Pathophysiologic Approach,* 4th ed. New York: McGraw-Hill; 1997:1378-1392.

Fuller SH, Camara C. Systemic lupus erythematosus. In: Herfindal ET, Gourley DR, et al, eds. *Textbook of Therapeutic Drug and Disease Management,* 7th ed. Baltimore: Lippincott Williams & Wilkins; 2000:691-708.

The Lupus Foundation of America. Lupus. http://www.lupus.org/

23. Pain Management and Migraines

Elizabeth S. Miller, PharmD
Assistant Professor, Department of Clinical Pharmacy
University of Tennessee College of Pharmacy

Contents

1. Pain

Definitions

- *Pain:* any unpleasant sensory and emotional experience associated with actual or potential tissue damage, or defined in terms of such damage or both
- Chronic pain is a largely unrecognized problem in American society.
    * Currently, about 75 million individuals suffer from some form of chronic benign pain.
    * Between one-third and one-half of chronic pain sufferers have pain severe enough to require daily medication.

Types and Clinical Presentation

- Pain can be classified as acute, chronic benign, or malignant.
- Acute pain is caused by an injury, illness, or surgery.
    * Acute pain responds to medications and usually resolves when the underlying cause has been treated or healed.
    * It is often associated with physiologic symptoms such as tachycardia, hypertension, diaphoresis, and mydriasis.
- Chronic benign pain exists beyond an expected time for healing, typically 3-6 months or more.
    * It is often associated with psychological effects including social isolation, depression, and anxiety.
    * Chronic pain syndromes are often not responsive to traditional analgesics and require the use of adjuvant medications.
- Malignant pain may be acute, chronic, or intermittent, and is often related to cancer progression or chemotherapy.
- Pain is also defined by source. Such a classification divides pain into somatic, visceral, and neuropathic pain.
- Somatic pain originates from the skin, muscles, tendons, ligaments, and bones.
    * Somatic pain is localized and described as sharp, stabbing, throbbing, or aching in nature.
    * While somatic pain can be severe, it tends to respond well to treatment with opioids.
- The body's internal organs such as the liver, intestines, or stomach generate visceral pain.
    * Visceral pain tends to be poorly localized and more likely to generate referred pain felt some distance away from the actual problem.
    * Opioids are not as effective for visceral pain as they are for somatic pain.

- Neuropathic pain results when the nerves themselves are damaged.
    * Neuropathic pain is typically burning in nature, although it may also be numb, aching, or cause a sensation like an electric shock.
    * Opioid medications are often ineffective for treating neuropathic pain and adjuvant analgesics play a significant role in treatment.

Pathophysiology

- Nociception, the pain sensation, begins when a sensory nerve ending is stimulated and sends repetitive signals to the spinal cord along ascending nerve fibers. An individual nerve does not transmit directly to the brain, but instead connects to secondary nerves in the dorsal horn of the spinal cord. The secondary nerves eventually connect to nerve cells in the brain stem.
- A descending antinociceptive pathway also exists. Neurotransmitters from the descending fibers inhibit the transmission of the pain signal. Opioids chemically resemble these neurotransmitters.
- Chronic pain is not a prolonged version of acute pain. As pain signals are repeatedly generated, neural pathways undergo changes that make them hypersensitive to pain signals and resistant to antinociceptive input.

Diagnostic Criteria

- The individual's self-report of pain is the primary source of information in acute pain.
- Chronic pain assessment should include a detailed history of the pain's intensity and characteristics, a physical examination emphasizing the neurological exam, and a psychosocial assessment (Figure 1).
- The purpose of diagnostic tests, such as x-rays, CT or MRI scans, or laboratory tests differs between chronic benign pain and acute pain or malignant pain.
    * In cancer patients, the major purpose of diagnostic testing is to visualize the disease progression.
    * In chronic benign pain, the major purpose of diagnostic testing is to rule out the presence of any diseases for which there is a curative treatment.

Goals of Pain Management

Acute pain
- The goal in acute pain management is to provide patients with pain relief that allows them to rest comfortably and to rehabilitate them postsurgery or postinjury. This can be accomplished with short-acting prn medications.

Figure 1.

Algorithm for comprehensive evaluation and management of chronic pain.

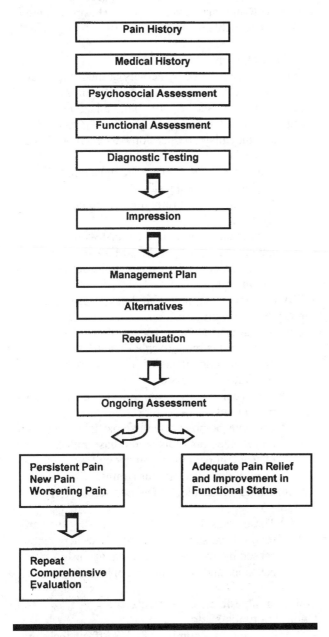

From the Pain Management Center of Paducah, Paducah, KY. Used with permission.

Malignant pain
- A major goal of cancer pain management is to relieve the patient's pain without inducing disabling side effects.
- The World Health Organization has developed a three-step hierarchy for analgesic pain management

in cancer pain patients (Figure 2). In general, this includes using nonopioid analgesics as a baseline, supplementing with opioid analgesics as needed, and adding adjunctive medications when appropriate.
- Cancer patients may suffer from constant pain that continues for months or years. For this reason, treatment with long-acting agents is more appropriate than treatment with short-acting medications. However, short-acting agents, referred to as "breakthrough" or "rescue" doses, are often available in addition to the long-acting medications.

Chronic benign pain
- The goal of chronic benign pain treatment is to restore the patient to the highest degree of function possible.
- Multimodal therapy, the use of several different types of treatment, is usually required. Multimodal therapies include nerve blocks, rehabilitation, physical therapy, pharmacotherapy, acupuncture, and psychotherapy.
- Basic pharmacotherapy follows the World Health Organization guidelines for treating cancer pain (Figure 2). Analgesics are categorized into nonopioid analgesics, opioid analgesics, and adjuvant analgesics.

Figure 2.

The WHO's three-step hierarchy for analgesic pain management in cancer patients.

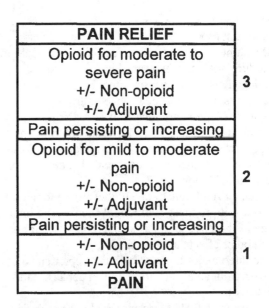

Reproduced with permission from WHO, 1996.

- Nonopioid analgesics such as acetaminophen and nonsteroidal anti-inflammatory drugs (NSAIDs) relieve all types of mild to moderate pain.
  - Unless contraindicated, all pain patients should first be given a trial of nonopioid analgesics.
  - Nonopioids and opioids relieve pain via different mechanisms. Thus, combination therapy offers the potential for improved relief with fewer side effects.
  - Nonopioids do not produce tolerance, physical dependence, or addiction.
- Adjuvant analgesics are drugs with a primary indication other than pain. Commonly used analgesic adjuvants include antiepileptic drugs, tricyclic antidepressants, and local anesthetics.

Principles of opioid use
- Opioids have no ceiling effect of analgesia.
- Oral medications should be used whenever possible. Intramuscular injections are painful and should be avoided.
- When patients have constant or near-constant pain, analgesics should be given around the clock. This is often accomplished with the use of long-acting opioid analgesics.
- The use of short-acting opioids as rescue medication is controversial in chronic benign pain. If allowed, doses of rescue medications should range from 10-15% of the total daily long-acting opioid dose.
- Mixed agonist-antagonist opioids are not used in chronic pain. They may induce a withdrawal syndrome in patients tolerant to opioids.

Drug Therapy

Mechanism of action
Opioid receptors
- Morphine and other opioid agonists are thought to produce analgesia by mimicking the action of endogenous opioid peptides that bind at opioid receptors in the antinociceptive pathway.
- Opioid receptors are located in the CNS, pituitary gland, and GI tract. They are abundant in the periaqueductal gray matter of the brain and the dorsal horn of the spinal cord, two areas that are very active in pain reduction.
- When a drug binds to one of these receptors as an agonist, it produces analgesia. When a drug binds to one of these receptors as an antagonist, analgesia and other effects are blocked.
- The three major types of opioid receptor sites involved in analgesia are mu (μ), kappa (κ), and delta (δ).
  - Binding to the μ receptor produces analgesia, sedation, euphoria, respiratory depression, physical dependence, constipation, and other effects.

- Activation of the κ receptor produces analgesia and respiratory depression. In addition, psychotomimetic effects such as anxiety, strange thoughts, nightmares, and hallucinations are more common.
- Activation of δ receptors produces analgesia without many adverse events. However, there is no available δ-receptor agonist.

Opioid analgesics
- Opioids are classified by activity at the receptor site, ie, they are classified as pure opioid agonists, agonist-antagonists, or pure opioid antagonists.
- Pure opioid agonists primarily activate μ receptors, although they may produce some κ-receptor activation (Table 1).
  - Pure opioid agonists are the most clinically useful opioid analgesics.
  - Morphine is the prototypical pure opioid agonist.
  - Methadone is an opioid agonist with additional antagonist activity at the NMDA receptor. The NMDA receptor is believed to be active primarily in chronic pain.
- Mixed agonist-antagonists bind as agonists at the κ receptor, producing weak analgesia. They bind as weak antagonists at the μ receptor (Table 2).
  - The result is more dysphoria and psychotomimetic effects with a lower risk of respiratory depression.
  - Pentazocine is the prototypical agonist-antagonist opioid.
  - Buprenorphine is actually a partial agonist at μ and κ receptors. This opioid has limited efficacy in pain management and is primarily used in detoxification programs.
- Opioid antagonists block the μ and κ receptors (Table 3).
  - These drugs do not produce analgesia. They are used to reverse respiratory and CNS depression caused by overdose with opioid agonists.
  - Naloxone and naltrexone are opioid antagonists.

Opioid analgesic adverse effects
Central nervous system
- Opioids produce a number of CNS effects including sedation, euphoria, dysphoria, changes in mood, and mental clouding. Confusion, disorientation, and cognitive impairment are also possible.
- Chronic sedation can be treated with CNS stimulants such as methylphenidate or dextroamphetamine. Modafinil also promotes daytime wakefulness.
- Mild to moderate muscle jerks are common in patients on high doses of opioids. Myoclonus can be treated by changing the opioid dose, changing the opioid, or giving low doses of a benzodiazepine.

Table 1

Starting Doses for Strong Opioids for Severe Pain in Adults

Generic name	Common product name and strength	Dosing interval (h)	IV starting dose (mg)		Oral starting dose
			IV	Oral	
Pure mu agonists					
Fentanyl (synthetic)	Injection (INJ): Sublimaze® 50 mcg/mL	INJ: 0.5-2	0.1	Not available	Transmucosal: Start with 100 to 200 mcg and titrate to effect
	Transdermal (TD): Duragesic® 12, 25, 50, 75, 100 mcg/h	TD: q 2-3 days			
	Transmucosal lozenge (LOZ): Actiq® 200, 400, 600, 800, 1200, 1600 mcg; Oralet® 100, 200, 300, 400 mcg	LOZ: prn			
Hydromorphone (semisynthetic)	Dilaudid®: Tablet: 2, 4, 8 mg	PO/PR 3-6;	1.5	7.5	4-8
	Liquid: 1 mg/mL	IV 6-8			
	Injection: 1, 2, 4 mg/mL and high potency (HP) 10 mg/mL				
	Suppository: 3 mg				
Levorphanol (semisynthetic)	Levo-Dromoran®: Tablet: 2 mg	PO 6-8	2	4	2-4
	Injection: 2 mg/mL	IV 3-4			
		IM/SC 6-8			
Meperidine (synthetic)	Demerol®: Tablet: 50 mg	3-4	75	300	50-150
	Liquid: 10 mg/mL				
	Injection: 25, 50, 75, 100 mg/mL				
Methadone (synthetic)	Tablet: Dolophine®/Methadose® 5, 10 mg; Methadose 40 mg dispersible	3-8	5	10	5-10
	Liquid: Methadone 2, 5, 10 mg/mL; Methadose 10 mg/mL				
	Injection: Methadone 10 mg/mL		10 acute; 2-4 chronic		
Morphine (natural)	Tablet: MSIR® 15, 30 mg				
	Liquid: Roxanol®/MSIR 2, 4 mg, 20, 100 mg/mL	2-4			
	Injection: 0.5, 1, 2, 4, 8, 10, 15, 25, 50 mg/mL		10	30	15-30
	Controlled-release: Oramorph SR® 15, 30, 60, 100 mg; MS Contin® 15, 30, 60, 100, 200 mg; Kadian® 20, 30, 50, 60, 100 mg; Avinza® 30, 60, 90, 120 mg	Oramorph SR 8-12 MS Contin 8-12 Kadian 12-24 Avinza 24			
Oxycodone (semisynthetic)	Capsule: OxyIR® 5 mg	3-4			
	Tablet: Roxicodone® 5, 15, 30 mg				
	Liquid: Roxicodone 1, 20 mg/mL; OxyFAST® 20 mg/mL		Not available	20	15-30
	Oxycodone/acetaminophen tablet: (mg): Percocet® 2.5/325, 5/325, 7.5/325, 10/325; Roxicet® 5/325, 5/500, Tylox® 5/500				
	Controlled-release tablet: OxyContin® 10, 20, 40, 80 mg	OxyContin 12			
Oxymorphone (semisynthetic)	Injection: 1, 1.5 mg/mL	3-6	1	10 rectal	Not available
	Suppository: Numorphan® 5 mg				

Table 2

Opioid Dosing for Mild to Moderate Pain in Adults

Generic name	Common product name and strength	Dosing interval (h)	IV starting dose (mg)	Oral starting dose (mg)
Moderate-mild opioids				
Codeine (natural)	Tablet: 15, 30, 60 mg (CII)			
	Acetaminophen/codeine tablet: Tylenol with Codeine® #1 = 300/7.5, #2 = 300/15, #3 = 300/30, #4 = 300/60 mg	4-6	15-30	30-60
	Liquid: 5 mg/mL			
	Injection: 30, 60 mg/mL			
Hydrocodone (semisynthetic)	Hydrocodone/APAP tablet (mg): Vicodin® 5/500; Vicodin ES® 7.5/750; Lorcet® or Vicodin HP® 10/650; Lortab® 2.5/500, 5/500, 7.5/500, 10/500; Norco® 5/325, 7.5/325, 10/325	4-8	Not available	5-10
	Hydrocodone/ibuprofen tablet (mg): Vicoprofen® 7.5/200			
Propoxyphene (synthetic)	Propoxyphene/acetaminophen tablet (mg): Darvocet-N® 50 (50/325), Darvocet-N® 100 (100/650)	4-6	Not available	65-130; max 600 mg/day
	Capsule: Darvon® 32, 65 mg			
Agonists-antagonists				
Pentazocine	Pentazocine 50 mg tablet: Talwin®	3-4		50
	Pentazocine 50/naloxone 0.5 mg tablet: Talwin NX®		30-60 mg; max 360 mg/day	50-100; max
	Pentazocine 12.5/aspirin 325 tablet: Talwin Compound®	3-4		600 mg/day
Butorphanol	Injection: 30 mg/mL			
	Injection: Stadol® 1, 2 mg/mL	3-4	IV 0.5-2 mg	Not available
	Nasal spray: Stadol NS® 10 mg/mL		NS 1 mg followed by 2nd dose in	
Nalbuphine	Injection: Nubain® 10, 20 mg/mL	3-6	60-90 min prn	
Buprenorphine	Injection: Buprenex® 0.3 mg/mL	6-8	10	Not available
Dezocine	Injection: Dalgan® 5, 10, 15 mg/mL	IM 3-6; IV 2-4	0.3-0.6	Not available
			5-20 mg IV; 2.5-10 mg IV	Not available
Miscellaneous				
Tramadol	Tablet: Ultram® 50 mg	4-6	Not available	50-100; max 400 mg/day
	Tramadol/acetaminophen tablet: Ultracet® 37.5/325 mg	4-6	Not available	1-2 tabs; max 8 tabs/day
	Extended release tablet: Ultram® ER 100, 200, 300 mg	24	Not available	100; max 300 mg/day

Neuroendocrine
- Morphine acts in the hypothalamus to inhibit the release of gonadotropin-releasing hormone (GnRH) and corticotropin-releasing factor (CRF), thus decreasing levels of luteinizing hormone (LH), follicle-stimulating hormone (FSH), ACTH, and β-endorphins.
- Changes in hormone levels may cause decreased levels of testosterone and cortisol, disturbances in menstruation, and sexual dysfunction.
- High doses of morphine and related opioids produce convulsions. Most convulsions occur at doses far in excess of those required to produce analgesia.

Respiratory
- Respiratory depression is the most serious opioid-induced adverse effect.
- Opioids depress respiration by a direct effect on the brain stem respiratory centers, making the brain stem less responsive to carbon dioxide.

Table 3

Opioid Antagonists

Generic name	Common product name and strength	Dosing interval (h)	IV starting dose (mg)	Oral starting dose (mg)
Naloxone	Injection: Narcan® 0.02, 0.4, 1 mg/mL	Every 2-3 min	Opioid overdose 0.4-2 mg; postoperative narcotic depression 0.1-0.2 mg qd, qod, or q3d	Not available
Naltrexone	Tablet: Trexan®/ReVia® 50 mg (approved for alcohol dependence and narcotic addiction)			Alcoholism 50 mg qd; narcotic addiction 50 mg qd, 100 mg qod, or 150 mg q3d
Nalmefene	Injection: Revex® 0.1, 1 mg/mL	Every 2-5 min	Opioid overdose 0.5-1 mg; postoperative respiratory depression 0.25 mcg/kg	Not available

- The μ receptor is the primary receptor involved in respiratory depression, although activation of the κ receptor also contributes.
- At equianalgesic doses, all of the pure opioid agonists depress respiration to the same degree. The agonist-antagonists have a ceiling effect (ie, a dose beyond which no further respiratory depression or analgesia is produced), but this is usually above recommended doses.
- Opioids depress cough by inducing a direct effect on the cough reflex in the medulla.

Cardiovascular
- Therapeutic doses of many opioids produce peripheral vasodilation, reduced peripheral resistance, and inhibition of the baroreceptor reflexes.
- Peripheral vasodilation results primarily from opioid-induced release of histamine. Orthostatic hypotension and fainting can result.
- The naturally occurring and semisynthetic products are potent histamine releasers. Fentanyl has little propensity to release histamine.
- Recently, methadone has been associated with torsades de pointes, an atypical rapid ventricular tachycardia, at an average daily dose of 400 mg.

Gastrointestinal
- All clinically significant μ agonists produce some degree of nausea and vomiting by direct stimulation of the chemoreceptor trigger zone in the medulla, sensitization of the vestibular system, and slowing of GI motility.
- Nausea and vomiting commonly occur in ambulatory patients (15-40% of patients with nausea and vomiting are ambulatory). Both can be pretreated with an antiemetic such as promethazine or prochlorperazine.
- Opioids promote constipation by delaying gastric emptying, slowing bowel motility, and decreasing peristalsis. Opioids may also reduce secretions from the colonic mucosa. At its worst, gastrointestinal dysfunction results in ileus, fecal impaction, and obstruction.
- Because transdermal delivery bypasses absorption from the GI tract, constipation has been reported to be less frequent than with other opioids.
- Patients on opiates do not develop tolerance to constipation. All patients taking around-the-clock opioid analgesics should be placed on prophylactic bowel regimens. Bowel regimens include increased fluid and fiber intake, daily stool softeners, and mild laxatives.
- Manage severe constipation with osmotic laxatives such as magnesium citrate and milk of magnesia.

Genitourinary tract
- Opioids increase smooth muscle tone in the bladder and ureters and may cause bladder spasm and urgency.
- An opioid-induced increase in sphincter tone can make urination difficult. Urinary retention is most common in elderly men.

Biliary
- Opioids increase smooth muscle tone in the biliary tract, especially in the sphincter of Oddi, which regulates the flow of bile and pancreatic fluids.
- This can result in a decrease in biliary and pancre-

atic secretions and a rise in the bile duct pressure. Patients may experience epigastric distress and occasionally biliary spasm.

- All opioids are capable of causing constriction of the sphincter of Oddi and the biliary tract. Although morphine may cause more biliary constriction in animals than other opioids, this has never been shown to be clinically useful in humans.

Skin and eyes

- Therapeutic doses of morphine dilate cutaneous blood vessels, which causes flushing on the face, neck, and upper thorax. Sweating and pruritus may also occur.
  - * These changes may be due in part to release of histamine.
  - * Histamine release may induce or worsen asthmatic attacks in predisposed patients and can lead to wheezing, bronchoconstriction, and status asthmaticus.
- Skin rash around the transdermal fentanyl patch is a common side effect caused by the patch adhesive.
- Following a toxic dose of μ agonists, miosis is marked and pinpoint pupils are pathognomonic; however, mydriasis occurs when asphyxia intervenes.

Overdose

- Acute overdose with opioids is manifested by respiratory depression, somnolence progressing to stupor or coma, skeletal muscle flaccidity, cold and clammy skin, constricted pupils, and sometimes pulmonary edema, bradycardia, hypotension, and death.
- An opioid antagonist may be given to block opioid receptors and reverse the effects of overdose.
- Antagonist administration may cause a complete reversal of opioid effects and precipitate an acute withdrawal syndrome in persons physically dependent on opioids.
- Antagonists are dosed to patient response every few minutes. If no response is observed after 10 mg, the diagnosis of opioid-induced toxicity should be questioned.
- Infusion may be useful in cases of overdose with long-acting drugs such as methadone. The infusion rate for adults is approximately 100 mL/h (0.4 mg/h).

Tolerance and physical dependence

- Opioids often have their use limited by concerns regarding tolerance, physical dependence, and addiction.
- Tolerance can be defined as a state in which a larger dose is required to produce the same response that could formerly be elicited by a smaller dose.

- Tolerance to analgesia is demonstrated by the need for an increased dosage of a drug to produce the same level of analgesia. Tolerance to analgesia develops more slowly than tolerance to other opioid effects.
- Tolerance to adverse effects of opioids occurs after 2-3 weeks of continuous administration. Tolerance to the constipating and neuroendocrine effects of opioids does not occur.
- Physical dependence is the occurrence of a withdrawal syndrome after an opioid is stopped or quickly decreased without titration. Warn patients to avoid abrupt discontinuation of such drugs.
- Addiction is the psychological dependence on the use of substances for psychic effects and is characterized by compulsive use. Consider addiction if patients no longer have control over drug use and continue to use drugs despite the harm they promote.

Pharmacokinetics of Selected Opioids

Morphine

- Compared with other opioids, morphine is relatively insoluble in lipids (ie, in adults, only small amounts of the drug cross the blood-brain barrier).
- Morphine does not accumulate in tissues when given in normal doses, and therefore does not cause increasing toxicity with frequent dosing.
- Morphine is primarily metabolized by glucuronidation during the first pass through the liver. Approximately 50% of morphine is converted by the liver to morphine-3-glucuronide (M3G) and 15% to morphine-6-glucuronide (M6G). The pharmacologic effects of morphine (both analgesia and side effects) are due in part to M6G.
- Much of an oral dose is inactivated during this first pass through the liver; consequently, oral doses need to be much larger than parenteral doses to produce the same analgesic effects.

Fentanyl

- Fentanyl is highly soluble in lipids. It accumulates in skeletal muscle and fat and is slowly released into the blood. Plasma half-life is 3-4 hours after parenteral administration.
- Fentanyl is rapidly metabolized, primarily by dealkylation, to inactive metabolites in the liver. This process is mediated through the cytochrome P450 (CYP450) 3A4 hepatic enzyme system. The presence of inactive metabolites makes it a preferred drug in patients with liver dysfunction.
- It is not used orally because of low oral bioavailability.

Transdermal fentanyl

- The uptake of fentanyl through the skin is relatively slow and constant. The skin does not metabolize the drug and 92% of the dose is delivered into the bloodstream as intact fentanyl.
- An increase in body temperature to 40°C (104°F) theoretically may increase serum fentanyl concentrations by approximately one-third. This is due to temperature-dependent increases in fentanyl release from the patch system as well as increased skin permeability.
- Fentanyl is absorbed into the upper layers of the skin forming a depot. Fentanyl then becomes available to systemic circulation. Serum fentanyl concentrations are measurable within 2 hours after application of the first patch, and analgesic effects can be observed 8-16 hours after application. Steady state is reached after several sequential patch applications.

Transmucosal fentanyl citrate

- The absorption pharmacokinetics of fentanyl from the oral transmucosal dosage form is a combination of initial rapid absorption from buccal mucosa and a delayed absorption of fentanyl from the GI tract. Normally 25% of the total dose is available by buccal absorption, and 25% is available from the GI tract, making the total bioavailability 50%.
- Analgesia begins in 10-15 minutes, peaks in 20 minutes, and persists for 1-2 hours.

Methadone

- After therapeutic doses, about 90% of methadone is bound to plasma protein and is widely distributed in tissues. Methadone is found in low concentrations in the blood and the brain, with higher concentrations in the kidney, spleen, liver, and lung. Terminal half-life is extremely variable (15-55 hours); therefore, accumulation is possible and dosing intervals need to be carefully monitored.
- Methadone is extensively metabolized in the liver, mainly by N-demethylation. This appears to be mediated by several CYP450 enzymes. The major metabolites are excreted in the bile and urine.
- Analgesic efficacy does not correspond to the half-life of the drug. Methadone may be dosed every 3 hours for pain control.

Oxycodone

- Oxycodone is metabolized to noroxycodone, oxymorphone, and their glucuronides via the CYP450 2D6 enzyme system. The major circulating metabolite is noroxycodone. Noroxycodone is reported to be a weaker analgesic than oxycodone. Oxymorphone, although possessing analgesic activity, is present in the plasma only in low concentrations.

Hydromorphone

- Hydromorphone is metabolized to 3 major metabolites: hydromorphone 3-glucuronide, hydromorphone 3-glucoside, and dihydroisomorphine 6-glucoside. It is not known whether hydromorphone is metabolized by the cytochrome CYP450 system. Hydromorphone is a poor inhibitor of CYP450 isoenzymes and is not expected to inhibit the metabolism of other drugs.

Meperidine

- Normeperidine, a metabolite of meperidine, produces anxiety, tremors, myoclonus, and generalized seizures when it accumulates with repetitive dosing. Patients with compromised renal function are particularly at risk. Naloxone does not reverse this hyperexcitability. For these reasons, meperidine should not be used in patients with renal or CNS disease, for more than 48 hours, or at doses greater than 600 mg/24 hours.

Propoxyphene

- Propoxyphene is appropriate for short-term mild to intermittent pain. It produces a toxic metabolite, norpropoxyphene, with effects similar to normeperidine.

Drug Interactions and Drug-Disease Interactions

Drug interactions

- All drugs with CNS depressant actions (barbiturates, benzodiazepines, alcohol) can intensify sedation and respiratory depression caused by morphine and other opioids.
- Antihistamines, tricyclic antidepressants, and atropine-like drugs can exacerbate morphine-induced constipation and urinary retention.
- Antihypertensive drugs and others that lower blood pressure can exacerbate opioid-induced hypotension.
- The combination of meperidine and a monoamine oxidase inhibitor has produced a syndrome characterized by excitation, delirium, hyperpyrexia, convulsions, and severe respiratory depression. Death has also occurred. Although this syndrome has not been reported with other opioids, combinations containing opioids and monoamine oxidase inhibitors should be avoided.
- Agonists-antagonists can precipitate a withdrawal syndrome if administered to an individual who is physically dependent on a pure opioid agonist.

Cytochrome P450 substrates, inhibitors, and inducers

- CYP450 enzymes metabolize codeine, hydrocodone, fentanyl, methadone, and oxycodone. Although not well documented, drug interactions through this system may exist.

- Codeine, hydrocodone, and oxycodone require metabolism through CYP450 2D6 to active drug (Table 4). Approximately 7% of Caucasians, 3% of African-Americans, and 1% of Asians are poor metabolizers of CYP450 2D6; they produce no CYP450 2D6 or produce undetectable levels of it. Poor metabolizers may experience little to no analgesia from drugs requiring 2D6 for conversion to active metabolites.
- About 5% have multiple copies of the CYP450 2D6 gene, making them ultrafast metabolizers. The clearance of some opioids may be increased, making it necessary to dose the medications more often.

Drug-disease interactions
- In view of their extensive hepatic metabolism, the effects of opioids may be increased in patients with liver disease, particularly those with severe liver failure. Most opioids require dose reduction in severe liver disease.
- Fentanyl, morphine, and methadone require dosing adjustment in renal impairment. Doses of fentanyl and morphine should be reduced 25% when CrCl is 10-50 mL/min and by 50% when CrCl is <10 mL/min. The dosing interval of methadone should be increased to at least every 6 hours when CrCl is 10-50 mL/min and to every 8 hours when CrCl is <10 mL/min.
- Renal impairment slows the clearance of morphine conjugates, resulting in accumulation of the active metabolite M6G (morphine-6-glucuronide). For this reason, dosage reduction may be advisable in the presence of clinically significant renal impairment.
- Methadone appears to be firmly bound to protein in various tissues, including the brain. After repeated

administrations, there is gradual accumulation in tissues. The risk of accumulation is greater in patients with impaired renal or hepatic function, since both organs are involved with the metabolism of methadone.

Patient Counseling

- Respiratory depression is increased by concurrent use of other drugs with CNS depressant activity (eg, alcohol, barbiturates, and benzodiazepines). Outpatients should be warned against the use of alcohol with all other CNS depressants.
- Inform patients about symptoms of hypotension (lightheadedness, dizziness). Minimize hypotension by moving slowly when changing from a supine to an upright position.

Transdermal patch
- The fentanyl transdermal patch must be applied to a clean, nonhairy site on the upper torso. Use only water to clean the area. Do not use soap or alcohol because this can increase the effects of the medication. Do not apply the patch to oily, broken, burned, cut, or irritated skin.
- It must be held in place for a minimum of 30 seconds to ensure adhesion.
- Apply each new patch to a different area of skin to avoid irritation. If a patch comes off or causes irritation, remove it and apply a new patch to a different site.
- To dispose of the patch, fold in half and flush down the toilet.
- Do not cut or damage the patch.
- Temperature dependent increases in fentanyl release from the patch could result in an overdose. Advise patients to avoid exposing the patch to direct external heat sources such as heating pads, electric blankets, heat lamps, saunas, hot tubs and heated water beds. In addition, patients who develop a high fever while wearing the patch should contact their physician immediately.

Long-acting opioid formulations
- The long-acting formulations should be swallowed whole (ie, not broken, chewed, or crushed).
- Avinza, a long-acting morphine capsule formulation, contains fumaric acid. Doses above 1600 mg per day contain a quantity of fumaric acid that has not been demonstrated to be safe, and which may result in serious renal toxicity.
- Kadian and Avinza (long-acting morphine sulfate) may be opened and the beads ingested with a small amount of applesauce (sprinkle administration). In addition, Kadian is approved for sprinkle administration through a gastrostomy tube.

Table 4

Cytochrome P450 2D6 Enzyme Activity

Substrates	Inhibitors	Inducers
Oxycodone	Celecoxib	Carbamazepine
Tramadol	Cimetidine	Ethanol
Hydrocodone	Citalopram	Phenobarbital
Codeine	Sertraline	Phenytoin
Meperidine	Paroxetine	Rifampin
Propoxyphene	Fluoxetine	
Methadone	Propoxyphene	
	Methadone	

Oral transmucosal fentanyl citrate lozenge

- The lozenge is used by placing it in the mouth between the cheek and gum. Consumption of the lozenge should take 15 minutes. Another lozenge may be used 30 minutes after the start of the first one. Tell the patient not to bite or chew transmucosal fentanyl citrate.
- To dispose of a finished lozenge, discard the handle in a place that is out of the reach of children and pets. If medicine remains on the handle, place the handle under hot running tap water until the medicine is dissolved. Never leave unused or partly used lozenges where children or pets can get to them.

Parameters to monitor

- Evaluate for pain control 1 hour after opioid administration. If analgesia is insufficient, consider a dosage increase. Patients taking opioids chronically should be evaluated regularly for adequate doses.
- Monitor the patient for respiratory depression. Higher risk for respiratory depression exists in patients who are not tolerant to opioid analgesics. Consider treatment when the respiratory rate is less than 8-12 respirations per minute for 30 minutes or longer despite stimulation and/or if oxygen saturation is less than 90%.
- If a patient is easily arousable, he or she is unlikely to have respiratory depression.

Tramadol

- Tramadol is an analog of codeine whose mechanism of action is not completely understood. It appears that analgesia is likely mediated by binding of the parent molecule and the O–desmethyl tramadol (M1) active metabolite to μ opioid receptors, as well as by weak inhibition of neuronal uptake of norepinephrine and serotonin.
- The liver extensively metabolizes tramadol. The formation of the M1 active metabolite is dependent on CYP450 2D6. M1 appears to be up to 6 times more potent than tramadol in producing analgesia and 200 times more potent in binding to μ opioid receptors.
- Tramadol is not a federally controlled substance.
- The most common adverse effects are sedation, dizziness, headache, dry mouth, and constipation. Respiratory depression is minimal. Seizures have been reported; avoid its use in patients with seizure disorders or recognized risk for seizure (such as head trauma, metabolic disorders, alcohol and drug withdrawal, CNS infections).

2. Nonpharmacologic Treatment of Pain

General Principles of Nonpharmacologic Treatment

- Nonpharmacologic strategies used in combination with appropriate drug regimens may improve pain relief by enhancing the therapeutic effects of medications and permitting lower doses to be used.
- Nonpharmacologic interventions should not be a substitute for analgesic use.

Physical Interventions

Physical therapy

- Physical therapy is most commonly used to help restore physical strength and functioning after injury or surgery.
- Physical therapy can also provide pain relief for patients with musculoskeletal pain, some types of neuropathic pain, and sympathetically mediated pain.
- The National Institutes of Health recognize the benefit of acupuncture as an adjunct treatment of painful conditions.

Transcutaneous electrical nerve stimulation (TENS)

- In TENS, a controlled, low-voltage electrical current is applied through electrodes placed on the skin. Theoretically, the current will interfere with the ability of nerves to transmit pain signals to the spinal cord and brain.
- Even after several decades of research, it still is not clear if TENS provides any better pain relief than placebo.

Neurostimulation

- Neurostimulation involves implanting a computerized generator and electrodes near the spinal cord, peripheral nerves, or within the brain.
- Stimulators are most effective for patients with neuropathic pain, and are not very beneficial in other types of pain.

Behavioral Techniques

Biofeedback

- In biofeedback, electrodes connected to amplifiers are placed on the body or scalp. During biofeedback sessions, a therapist helps the patient learn to mentally control and change the signals from the electrodes, which helps the patient gain conscious control over normally unconscious functions.
- Biofeedback is most commonly used to relax muscles and reduce stress.

- Its advantages are that it is noninvasive, inexpensive, and safe; however, usually between 5 and 15 sessions are required before effective control is achieved.

Distraction and relaxation
- Distraction and relaxation assist the patient in refocusing attention on nonpainful stimuli.
- Both are believed to improve mental health, which translates into improved pain control.

3. Migraines

Definition

- Migraine is a chronic neurovascular disorder characterized by recurrent attacks of severe headache and autonomic nervous system dysfunction. Some patients also experience aura with neurologic symptoms.
- An estimated 18% of women and 6% of men experience migraine.

Clinical Presentation and Diagnostic Criteria

- Migraine classification is based on whether an aura of visual or sensory symptoms is present. Migraine with aura is less common than migraine without aura.
- Migraine headache manifests as moderate or severe throbbing pain that is localized in the temple or around the eye. It is accompanied by nausea in 90% of patients and vomiting in about half of patients.
- Photophobia (increased sensitivity to light) and phonophobia (increased sensitivity to sound) also are frequent complaints. A prodrome of mood changes, stiff neck, fatigue, or other symptoms may occur hours or days before the onset of the headache.

Criteria for diagnosing migraine without aura
- At least five headaches lasting 4-72 hours each
- The headaches have at least two of the following four characteristics:
    * Unilateral location
    * Pulsating quality
    * Moderate or severe intensity (inhibits or prohibits daily activities)
    * Aggravation with walking stairs or similar routine physical activity
- During the headache, at least one of the following symptoms occurs: nausea or vomiting, photophobia, or phonophobia.
- Symptoms cannot be consistent with other headache types.

Criteria for diagnosis of migraine with aura
- At least two attacks with three of the following four criteria:
    * One or more completely reversible aura symptoms indicating focal cerebral cortical or brain stem dysfunction (or both)
    * At least one aura symptom develops gradually (>4 minutes) or two or more symptoms occur in succession.

* No aura symptom lasts >60 minutes.
* Headache follows aura in <1 hour.
• There is no evidence of related organic disease.

Pathophysiology

Migraine and the brain
• The pathogenesis of migraine is unclear and is thought to be multifactorial. The current thinking is that a primary neuronal dysfunction originates in the Central Nervous System (CNS), leading to a sequence of changes that account for the different stages of migraine.
• The Cortical Spreading Depression (CSD) theory explains that a wave of depolarization spreads across the cerebral cortex from occipital to frontal regions, resulting in brain ion dysfunction and secondary vasoconstrictor vascular events. These changes account for the progression and variety of symptoms that occur in patients with prodromal or aura phase.
• The headache phase is probably related to trigemino-vascular activation with the release of inflammatory neuropeptides such as substance P, neurokinin A and calcitonin gene-related peptide in the trigeminal vascular system. This, in turn, causes vasodilation.
• It is suggested that the pain of headache is due to vasodilation as well as direct stimulation via the thalamus of the cortical pain areas situated in higher centers of the CNS. Not all migraneurs experience aura, so both direct effects and the secondary vasoactive responses account for the headache in patients who have migraine attacks without the aura.
• The pathophysiology of the postdrome is unknown, but may be due to a gradual recovery from the extreme neurologic disruption that occurs during migraine.
• Individuals prone to migraine may have a genetic migraine threshold that renders them susceptible to a migraine attack upon exposure to some or any of a range of patient-specific triggers. Hormonal influences, environmental and physiologic stressors, low blood sugar, and fatigue are all thought to affect this threshold. Once the threshold is exceeded, trigeminovascular activation is thought to be responsible for inducing a migraine.

Treatment Principles

Abortive therapy
• The U.S. Headache Consortium identifies the following goals for successful treatment of acute attacks of migraine:
    * Treat attacks rapidly and consistently and prevent recurrence.
    * Restore the patient's ability to function.
    * Minimize the use of rescue medication.
    * Optimize self-care and reduce subsequent use of resources.
    * Promote cost-effective therapies with minimal adverse effects.
• Successful treatment of migraine depends on early intervention in relation to onset of headache and adequate dosing.

Preventive therapy
• Preventive therapy should be considered in the following situations:
    * Attacks unresponsive to abortive medication
    * Attacks causing substantial disability
    * Attacks occurring twice or more monthly
    * Patient is at risk for rebound headache
    * Trend in increasing frequency of attacks
• Two-thirds of patients taking preventive medication will have a 50% decrease in the frequency of attacks. Note: Use of abortive therapies should be limited to 2-3 days per week.
• The goals of migraine preventive therapy are as follows:
    * Reduction of attack frequency, severity, and duration
    * Improve responsiveness to treatment of acute attacks.
    * Improve function and reduce disability.

Rebound headaches
• Persons who take abortive medications daily can develop drug rebound headaches, or headaches that begin upon discontinuation of a medication.
• Essentially all of the medications, with the possible exception of the triptans, cause rebound headache.

Drug Therapy

Abortive therapy: Nonprescription medications
• Aspirin, acetaminophen, ibuprofen, and other aspirin-like analgesics provide adequate relief of mild to moderate migraines.

Combinations with caffeine
• Combination products containing aspirin, acetaminophen, or both with caffeine are available without a prescription.
• Caffeine has analgesic and possibly anti-inflammatory properties. It may also increase gastric acidity and perfusion, enhancing the absorption of aspirin.
• Excedrin Migraine® (acetaminophen 250 mg, aspirin 250 mg, and caffeine 65 mg) is the only nonprescription preparation that carries a specific indication for migraine relief.

Abortive therapy:
Nonspecific prescription medications
- Combination products containing an analgesic, caffeine, and butalbital or codeine are available.
  - * The butalbital may be useful for its sedative properties.
  - * Excessive use of these products can cause physical dependence and rebound headaches.
- A combination of the vasoconstrictor isometheptene, the sedative dichloralphenazone, and acetaminophen (Midrin®) may be useful for mild to moderate migraines and is generally well tolerated.
- It is well recognized that opioids are good analgesics, but there is good evidence only for the efficacy of butorphanol nasal spray for migraine. Although opioids are commonly used, surprisingly few studies of opioid use in headache pain document whether overuse and the development of dependence are as frequent as clinically perceived.
- Given intravenously, the antiemetic metoclopramide may be appropriate as monotherapy for acute attacks, particularly in patients with significant nausea. Chlorpromazine and prochlorperazine may also be considered. Serotonin receptor antagonists (5-HT$_3$) have not been shown to be useful migraine treatments.

Abortive therapy: Ergotamine
Mechanism of action
- In cranial arteries, ergotamine acts directly to promote constriction and reduce the amplitude of pulsations. In addition, the drug can affect blood flow by depressing the vasomotor center. Antimigraine effects are possibly due to agonist activity at serotonin receptor subtypes 5-HT$_{1B}$ and 5-HT$_{1D}$.
- Because of the risk of dependence, ergotamine should not be taken daily on a long-term basis.
- Multiple ingredients are added to ergotamine to enhance efficacy (Table 5). Caffeine enhances vasoconstriction and ergotamine absorption. Pentobarbital provides sedation. The belladonna alkaloids suppress emesis.

Pharmacokinetics
- Oral ergotamine has poor bioavailability due to extensive first-pass metabolism. Sublingual administration may not provide therapeutic blood levels.
- Although the half-life of ergotamine is only 2 hours, pharmacologic effects can be seen for 24 hours after administration.
- The drug is eliminated primarily by hepatic metabolism. Metabolites are excreted in the bile.

Adverse effects
- Ergotamine is well tolerated at usual therapeutic doses.

- The drug can stimulate the chemoreceptor trigger zone to cause nausea and vomiting in about 10% of patients. Concurrent treatment with metoclopramide or a phenothiazine antiemetic can help suppress this response.
- Other common side effects include weakness in the legs, myalgia, numbness and tingling in the periphery, angina-like pain, tachycardia, and bradycardia.

Overdose
- Acute or chronic overdose can cause serious toxicity (ergotism).
- Symptoms include ischemia, myalgias, and paresthesias. Ischemia can progress to gangrene.
- The risk of ergotism is highest in patients with sepsis, peripheral vascular disease, and renal or hepatic impairment.

Drug-drug and drug-disease interactions
- Ergotamine should not be combined with selective serotonin receptor agonists due to the risk of a prolonged vasospastic reaction.
- Separate doses of ergotamine and serotonin agonists by at least 24 hours.
- Ergotamine is contraindicated for patients with hepatic or renal impairment, sepsis, coronary artery disease, and peripheral vascular disease.

Patient counseling
- Monitor patients to avoid overuse of the medication.
- Ergotamine and its derivatives are FDA pregnancy category X. They should not be taken during pregnancy due to their ability to promote uterine contractions and cause fetal harm or abortion.
- Teach patients to recognize signs of ergotism. Muscle pain, paresthesias, and cold or pale extremities should be reported immediately.

Dihydroergotamine (DHE)
Mechanism of action
- The action of dihydroergotamine is similar to that of ergotamine. Like ergotamine, dihydroergotamine alters transmission at serotonergic, dopaminergic, and α-adrenergic junctions.
- In contrast to ergotamine, dihydroergotamine causes minimal peripheral vasoconstriction, little nausea and vomiting, and no physical dependence. However, diarrhea is prominent.
- Contraindications are the same as for ergotamine: coronary artery disease, peripheral vascular disease, sepsis, pregnancy, and hepatic or renal impairment.
- As with ergotamine, do not administer dihydroergotamine within 24 hours of a serotonin agonist.

Table 5

Agents Used in Migraine Treatment

Drug	Available strengths	Maximum daily dose (weekly maximum)	Dosing instructions
Ergot alkaloids			
Ergotamine	SL tablet: Ergomar® 2 mg		
	Tablet: Ergostat® 2 mg, Wigrettes® 2 mg	PO: 6 mg (10 mg)	1 tablet at onset; then 1 every 30 min prn
	Injection: Gynergen® 0.5 mg/mL	INJ: 1 mg per week	IM 125-500 mcg, repeated if needed to weekly maximum
	Inhalation: Medihaler-Ergotamine® 9 mg/mL	INH: 820 mcg (5.4 mg)	1 inhalation (360 mcg) followed by one inhalation after 30-60 min
Ergotamine 1 mg/caffeine 100 mg tablet	Cafergot®, Wigraine®	Ergotamine 6 mg (10 mg)	2 tablets at onset; then 1 every 30 min prn
Ergotamine 0.3 mg/pentobarbital 20 mg/bellafoline 0.1 mg tablet	Bellergal®	Ergotamine 6 mg (10 mg)	2 tablets at onset; then 1 every 30 min prn
Ergotamine 0.6 mg/pentobarbital 40 mg/belladonna 0.2 mg tablet	Bellamine®, Bellamine S®, Bellaspas®, Bellaphen S®, Bellergal-S®, Duragal-S®	Ergotamine 6 mg (10 mg)	2 tablets at onset; then 1 every 30 min prn
Ergotamine 1 mg/pentobarbital 30 mg/belladonna 0.125 mg/caffeine 100 mg tablet	Cafergot PB®	Ergotamine 6 mg (10 mg)	2 tablets at onset; then 1 every 30 min prn
Ergotamine 1 mg/belladonna 0.1 mg/caffeine 100 mg/phenacetin 130 mg suppository	Wigraine®	Ergotamine 4 mg (10 mg)	Insert 1 at onset; repeat in 1 hour prn
Ergotamine 2 mg/phenobarbital 60 mg/belladonna 0.25 mg/caffeine 100 mg suppository	Cafergot PB®, Wigraine-PB®	Ergotamine 4 mg (10 mg)	Insert 1 at onset; repeat in 1 hour prn
Ergotamine 2 mg/caffeine 100 mg suppository	Cafergot®	Ergotamine 4 mg (10 mg)	Insert 1 at onset; repeat in 1 hour prn
Dihydroergotamine (DHE)	Injection: 1 mg/mL D.H.E. 45®	DHE 2 mg (6 mg IV or 3 mg IM)	0.5-1 mg IV/IM every hour as needed
	Nasal spray: Migranal® 4 mg/mL	DHE 2 mg (6 mg)	Administer one spray (0.5 mg) in each nostril, followed in 15 min by an additional spray in each nostril
Miscellaneous agents			
Isometheptene 65 mg/dichloralphenazone 100 mg/acetaminophen 325 mg capsule	Midrin®	5 capsules within a 12-hour period	2 capsules at once, followed by 1 capsule every hour until headache is relieved

Table 6

Selective Serotonin Receptor Agonists (Triptans)

Drug	Available strengths	Dosage (maximum daily dose)	Half-life (h)	Onset (min)	Metabolism
Almotriptan (Axert®)	Tablet: 6.25, 12.5 mg	12.5 mg; repeat in 2 hours (25 mg)	3.5	60	CYP450; MAO
Sumatriptan (Imitrex®)	Tablet: 25, 50, 100 mg	50 to 100 mg; repeat in 2 hours (200 mg)	2.5	60-120	MAO
	Nasal: 5, 20 mg	5 or 20 mg; repeat in 2 hours (40 mg)		15-20	
	Injection: 6 mg/mL	6 mg; repeat in 1 hour (12 mg)		10-15	
Eletriptan (Relpax®)	Tablet: 20, 40 mg	20 mg; repeat in 2 hours (80 mg)	5	60	CYP450 3A4
Frovatriptan (Frova®)	Tablet: 2.5 mg	2.5 mg: repeat in 2 hours (7.5 mg)	25	60-120	Renal 50%
Rizatriptan (Maxalt®)	Tablet/wafer: 5, 10 mg	5 or 10 mg; repeat in 2 hours (30 mg)	2-3	30	MAO
Zolmitriptan (Zomig®)	Tablet/wafer: 2.5, 5 mg	2.5 or 5 mg; repeat in 2 hours (10 mg)	2.5-4	45	CYP450; MAO
	Nasal: 5 mg	5 mg; repeat in 2 hours (10 mg)	3	10-15	CYP450; MAO
Naratriptan (Amerge®)	Tablet: 1, 2.5 mg	1 or 2.5 mg; repeat in 4 hours (5 mg)	6	60	Renal 70%; CYP450

CYP450, cytochrome p450 hepatic enzyme system; MAO, monoamine oxidase.

Pharmacokinetics
- Dihydroergotamine is not active orally due to extensive first-pass metabolism.
- An active metabolite, 8'-hydroxydihydroergotamine, contributes to its therapeutic effects. The half-life of dihydroergotamine plus its active metabolite is about 21 hours.

Abortive therapy: Selective serotonin receptor agonists (triptans)
- The selective serotonin receptor agonists, also known as triptans, are first-line drugs for terminating a migraine attack (Table 6).
- The triptans all activate $5\text{-HT}_{1B}/5\text{-HT}_{1D}$ and to a lesser extent 5-HT_{1A} or 5-HT_{1F} receptors. Triptans have no known affinity for 5-HT_2 or 5-HT_3 and other 5-HT receptor subclasses, nor do they bind to adrenergic, dopaminergic, muscarinergic, or histaminergic receptors.

Pharmacokinetics
- The pharmacokinetics of the different triptans vary somewhat. However, all are generally well tolerated and efficacious at appropriate doses.
- Subcutaneous sumatriptan injection has the fastest onset of action when compared with other triptans. Sumatriptan nasal spray has a slightly slower onset than the injection.
- The onset of the majority of oral triptans, including the dissolving wafers, is similar among the available agents. Rizatriptan may have a slightly faster onset of action at 1-1.5 hours.
- Migraine recurrence rates may be lower with long half-life triptans such as naratriptan and frovatriptan. However, triptans with longer half-lives tend to have a slower onset of action.

Adverse effects
- Triptans are generally well tolerated. Most side effects are mild and transient.
- The triptans differ slightly from one another in terms of tolerability but not in terms of safety.
- The most frequent side effects are tingling and paresthesias, and sensations of warmth in the head, neck, chest, and limbs.
- Less frequent effects are dizziness, flushing, and neck pain or stiffness.

Chest symptoms
- About 50% of patients on sumatriptan experience unpleasant chest symptoms usually described as "heavy arms" or "chest pressure" rather than pain.
- These symptoms are transient and not related to ischemic heart disease.
- Possible causes are pulmonary vasoconstriction, esophageal spasm, intercostal muscle spasm, and bronchoconstriction.

Coronary vasospasm
- Rarely, sumatriptan causes angina secondary to coronary vasospasm.
- Electrocardiographic changes have been observed in patients with CAD or Prinzmetal's (vasospastic) angina.
- To reduce the risk of angina, do not give sumatriptan to patients who have risk factors for CAD. These

patients include postmenopausal women, men over 40, smokers, and patients with hypertension, hyper-cholesterolemia, obesity, diabetes, or a family history of CAD.

Other adverse effects
- Mild reactions include vertigo, malaise, fatigue, and tingling sensations.
- Transient pain and redness may occur at sites of SC injection.
- Intranasal administration may cause irritation in the nose and throat as well as an offensive or unusual taste.

Drug-drug and drug-disease interactions
Ergot alkaloids and other triptans
- All triptans and ergot alkaloids cause vasoconstriction. Accordingly, if one triptan is combined with another or with an ergot alkaloid, excessive and prolonged vasospasm could result.
- Do not use triptans within 24 hours of an ergot derivative or another triptan.
- Monoamine oxidase inhibitors (MAOIs) can suppress degradation of triptans, which causes plasma levels to rise and toxicity to result. Furthermore, triptans should not be administered within 2 weeks of stopping an MAOI.
- Triptans are contraindicated for patients with a history of ischemic heart disease, myocardial infarction, uncontrolled hypertension, or other heart disease.
- Do not use triptans during pregnancy.

Patient counseling
- Patients should be counseled to contact a physician if pain or tightness in the chest occurs.
- Patients should not exceed daily maximum doses. If migraines occur more than three times a month, prophylactic treatment should be considered.
- Pain at the sumatriptan injection site should last less than 1 hour.

Migraine Prophylactic Therapy (Table 7)

β-Adrenergic blocking agents
- Propranolol is one of the drugs of choice for migraine prophylaxis. This agent can reduce the

Table 7

Selected Migraine Preventive Treatments

Drug	Dose	Selected side effects
β-Adrenergic receptor antagonists		
Propranolol	40-120 mg twice daily	Reduced energy, tiredness, postural
Metoprolol	100-200 mg daily	symptoms
Antidepressants		
Amitriptyline	25-75 mg at bedtime	Drowsiness
Fluoxetine	10-20 mg daily	Headache, nausea, nervousness, insomnia, drowsiness
Serotonin antagonists		
Methysergide	1-6 mg daily (treatment must be discontinued for 1 month every 6 months)	Drowsiness, leg cramps, hair loss, retroperitoneal fibrosis
Calcium channel blockers		
Diltiazem	90-180 mg daily	Headache
Verapamil	160-320 mg daily	Constipation, peripheral edema, cardiac conduction disturbances
Anticonvulsants		
Divalproex	400-600 mg twice daily	Drowsiness, weight gain, tremor, hair loss, hematologic and liver abnormalities, teratogenicity
Gabapentin	900-2400 mg daily	Somnolence, dizziness
Topiramate	100 mg day in 2 divided doses	Confusion, paresthesias, weight loss

Adapted from Goadsby et al, 2002.

number and intensity of attacks in about 70% of patients.

- Not all β-blockers are active against migraines. Recommended first-line agents include propranolol and timolol. Additional agents with demonstrated efficacy include atenolol, metoprolol, and nadolol.
- Since not all β-blockers are effective, it would appear that a mechanism other than β-blockade is responsible for the beneficial effects.

Anticonvulsants

- There is good evidence for the efficacy of divalproex sodium and sodium valproate. Adverse events with these therapies include weight gain, hair loss, tremor, and teratogenic potential, such as neural tube defects. Both are considered first line for prevention.
- Topiramate has traditionally been considered efficacious based on clinical experience, but had lacked evidence of efficacy. Recently completed clinical trial data provided the scientific evidence needed for topiramate to gain FDA approval for migraine prevention. Side effects associated with use include paresthesia, fatigue, nausea, dizziness, and difficulty concentrating. Anorexia and weight loss may also occur.
- There is limited evidence for moderate efficacy of gabapentin.
- Clonazepam and carbamazepine have not been shown to be an effective migraine prevention treatment.

Antidepressants

- Amitriptyline has been more frequently studied than the other antidepressants and is the only one with consistent support for efficacy in migraine prevention. It is considered a first line treatment. There is no evidence for the use of other TCAs such as nortriptyline, protriptyline, doxepin, clomipramine, or imipramine.
- Drowsiness, weight gain, and anticholinergic symptoms are frequently reported with the TCAs.
- Limited evidence exists that supports using fluoxetine at dosages ranging from 20 mg every other day to 40 mg per day. Although benefit may be seen in clinical practice, controlled trials offer no evidence for the use of fluvoxamine, paroxetine, sertraline, bupropion, mirtazapine, trazodone, or venlafaxine in this manner.

Calcium channel blockers

- Several calcium channel blockers are moderately effective at reducing migraine attacks. These include verapamil, nifedipine, and nimodipine.
- Beneficial effects develop slowly, reaching a maximum in 1-2 months.
- Calcium channel blockers cause side effects in 20-60% of patients. Constipation and orthostatic hypotension are most common. Vascular headache develops in about 25% of patients taking nifedipine.

Methysergide

- Methysergide is an ergot alkaloid used in migraine prophylaxis. It is not effective for aborting an ongoing attack.
- It is more efficacious than propranolol but has significantly more side effects.
- The drug seems to activate serotonin receptors in the CNS. Suppression of pain pathways by this mechanism may explain its usefulness.
- Methysergide causes a number of adverse effects.
    * With long-term therapy, methysergide can cause retroperitoneal, pleuropulmonary, and cardiac fibrosis. Fibrotic changes, although rare, are most serious.
    * Other adverse effects include vascular insufficiency, insomnia, altered mood, depersonalization, hallucinations, nightmares, and GI disturbances such as nausea, vomiting, and diarrhea.
    * Ergot alkaloids, serotonin receptor agonists, β-adrenergic blockers, dopamine, and drugs that inhibit the CYP450 3A4 subclass of hepatic metabolizing enzymes increase the risk of arterial spasm.

4. Nonpharmacologic Treatment of Migraines

General Principles of Nonpharmacologic Therapies

- Nonpharmacologic approaches may be well suited to patients who have exhibited a poor tolerance or poor response to drug therapy, who have a contraindication to drug therapy, and/or who have a history of long-term, frequent, or excessive use of analgesics or other acute medications.
- Nonpharmacologic interventions may also be useful in patients who are pregnant, are planning to become pregnant, or are nursing.

Treatment Recommendations

- Patients with migraine pain may experience relief by resting or sleeping in a cool, quiet, dark environment. Half of migraine patients experience considerable relief by applying a cold compress to the head.
- Relaxation training, thermal biofeedback combined with relaxation training, electromyographic (EMG) biofeedback, and cognitive-behavioral therapies are somewhat effective in preventing migraine.
- Evidence pertaining to the treatment of migraine with acupuncture is limited and the results are mixed. Similarly, limited evaluation has been conducted with hypnosis, TENS, cervical manipulation, and hyperbaric oxygen.

Trigger Management

- Trigger management is important in preventing migraine attacks. Triggering factors can cause migraine, and if recognized and/or avoided, may impede an impending attack.
- Triggers vary from person to person. Examples of triggers include changes in weather or air pressure, bright sunlight, glare, fluorescent lights, chemical fumes, menstrual cycles, and certain foods such as processed meats, red wine, beer, dried fish, broad beans, fermented cheeses, aspartame, and MSG.

5. Key Points

Pain management

- Opioids relieve pain by mimicking the actions of endogenous opioid peptides at μ, κ, and δ receptors.
- Opioids fall into three categories: pure μ agonists, agonist-antagonists, and pure antagonists. Pure μ agonists are the most pharmacologically useful.
- Addiction is a behavior pattern involving the continued use of a substance for nonmedical reasons despite harm. Physical dependence refers to the occurrence of an abstinence syndrome if the opioid is abruptly discontinued.
- With prolonged use, tolerance develops to analgesia, euphoria, sedation, respiratory depression, and other adverse effects, but not to constipation.
- Opioid overdose induces coma, respiratory depression, and pinpoint pupils. Naloxone and other pure opioid antagonists are used in cases of overdose to reverse most effects of opioids.
- Alcohol and other CNS depressants can intensify opioid-induced sedation and respiratory depression. Tricyclic antidepressants and antihistamines may worsen opioid-induced constipation and urinary retention.
- Hydrocodone, codeine, fentanyl, methadone, and oxycodone are metabolized by the cytochrome P450 system. Thus, drug interactions through the CYP450 enzymes may exist.
- The liver extensively metabolizes opioids; dose adjustments may be required in liver dysfunction. Fentanyl, morphine, and methadone require dosing adjustments in renal dysfunction.

Migraine

- The pathogenesis of migraine is unclear and is thought to be multifactorial. The current thinking is that a primary neuronal dysfunction originates in the Central Nervous System (CNS), leading to a sequence of changes that account for the different stages of migraine.
- The goal of abortive therapy is to eliminate headache pain and associated nausea and vomiting. The goal of preventive therapy is to reduce the incidence of migraine attacks.
- Nonopioid analgesics are effective for abortive therapy of mild to moderate pain.
- Opioid analgesics are reserved for severe migraine that has not responded to other drugs.
- Ergotamine is used for abortive therapy but should not be used daily. Overdose with ergotamine can cause ergotism, a serious condition in which generalized constriction of peripheral arteries and arterioles causes severe tissue ischemia.

- Triptans are drugs of choice for abortive therapy of migraines. They activate $5\text{-HT}_{1B}/5\text{-HT}_{1D}$ receptors, thereby causing constriction of cranial blood vessels and suppression of inflammatory neuropeptides.
- Triptans can cause coronary vasospasm and are contraindicated in patients with ischemic heart disease, prior myocardial infarction, and uncontrolled hypertension. If a triptan is combined with another triptan or with an ergot alkaloid, excessive prolonged vasospasms could result. Due to increased triptan toxicity, monoamine oxidase inhibitors (MAOIs) should not be administered concurrently with a triptan or for 2 weeks after MAOI discontinuation.
- The most recently published clinical practice guidelines consider propranolol, amitriptyline, divalproex sodium, and timolol first line for prevention of migraines. Since the publication of the guidelines, topiramate has gained an FDA indication for migraine prevention.

6. Questions and Answers

1. Approximately how many people in the United States experience severe chronic pain?

   A. 10 million
   B. 23 million
   C. 40 million
   D. 50 million
   E. 75 million

2. Addiction is currently understood to be

   I. characterized by compulsive use of drugs
   II. synonymous with physical dependence on a medication
   III. the use of a substance for psychic effects

   A. I only
   B. III only
   C. I and III only
   D. II and III only
   E. I, II, and III

3. The World Health Organization analgesic hierarchy emphasizes

   A. concurrent use of nonopioids, opioids, and adjuvant medications
   B. avoiding opioid use
   C. reserving opioid use only for severe pain
   D. using single agents rather than a combination of medications
   E. using nonopioids only for treatment of mild pain

4. All of the following adverse effects are manifestations of μ opioid agonists except

   A. constipation
   B. respiratory depression
   C. atrial flutter
   D. nausea
   E. miosis

5. The preferred route of opioid administration is

   A. oral
   B. intravenous
   C. subcutaneous
   D. rectal
   E. intramuscular

6. Which of the following opioids has the longest duration of analgesic effect?

A. Methadone
B. Controlled-release morphine
C. Hydromorphone
D. Transdermal fentanyl
E. Controlled-release oxycodone

7. All of the following opioids are metabolized through the cytochrome P450 hepatic enzyme system except

    A. hydrocodone
    B. oxycodone
    C. morphine
    D. methadone
    E. fentanyl

8. The clearance of which opioid may be increased in patients with multiple copies of the CYP450 2D6 gene?

    A. Methadone
    B. Oxycodone
    C. Fentanyl
    D. Morphine
    E. Hydromorphone

9. Which of the following statements regarding methadone pharmacokinetics is true?

    A. The half-life corresponds to analgesic efficacy
    B. It is highly plasma protein bound and widely distributed in tissue
    C. The clearance of methadone is rapid, resulting in frequent dosing
    D. Methadone has low bioavailability from the GI tract and therefore is not useful when given orally
    E. Methadone is metabolized by hepatic glucuronidation

10. Which agent can be used to reverse respiratory effects caused by opioid overdose?

    A. Naloxone
    B. Pentazocine
    C. Buprenorphine
    D. Naltrexone
    E. Tramadol

11. Which of the following opioids is not appropriate for use as an around-the-clock medication in chronic pain?

    A. Morphine
    B. Oxycodone
    C. Fentanyl

D. Hydromorphone
E. Methadone

12. Which of the following opioids has a toxic metabolite that can accumulate in renal dysfunction?

    A. Oxycodone
    B. Fentanyl
    C. Meperidine
    D. Hydromorphone
    E. Methadone

Use Case Study 1 to answer Questions 13 and 14.

13. Which of her medications is most likely to worsen opioid-induced constipation?

    A. Paxil
    B. Zocor
    C. Lotensin
    D. Premarin
    E. Elavil

14. The physician recommends changing her opioid to one that is less constipating. Which of the following medications is least likely to cause constipation?

    A. Morphine extended-release
    B. Methadone
    C. Oxycodone extended-release

Case Study 1

Patient Name:	Mary Martin
Address:	815 Elm Street
Age:	65
Sex:	Female
Allergies:	NKDA

Diagnosis: Chronic low back pain, hypertension, hypercholesterolemia, and chronic constipation.

Medications:

3/3	Paxil® 20 mg qd
3/3	Zocor® 40 mg qd
3/3	Lotensin® 20 mg qd
3/3	Premarin® 0.625 mg
3/3	Morphine sulfate extended-release 60 mg bid
3/3	Senokot S®
3/28	Elavil® 50 mg qhs
4/1	Milk of magnesia

    D. Transdermal fentanyl patch
    E. Hydromorphone

15. The rationale of adding caffeine to a simple analgesic for migraine treatment is to

  I. decrease the required dose of acetaminophen and aspirin
  II. cause cerebral arterial vasoconstriction
  III. increase gastric acidity and perfusion, enhancing aspirin absorption

    A. I only
    B. III only
    C. I and III only
    D. II and III only
    E. I, II, and III

16. Which of the following agents is a selective serotonin agonist?

    A. Sumatriptan
    B. Ketorolac
    C. Dihydroergotamine
    D. Metoclopramide
    E. Caffeine

17. Which is true regarding the adverse effects of ergotamine?

    A. Ergotamine inhibits the chemoreceptor trigger zone to minimize nausea and vomiting
    B. Ergotamine has minimal risk of dependence
    C. Muscle weakness is an uncommon side effect of ergotamine
    D. Angina-like pain reported with the triptans is not seen with ergotamine use
    E. Overuse of ergotamine can result in ischemia

18. Which statement about triptans is correct?

    A. There are few contraindications to the use of triptans
    B. Triptans are contraindicated in ischemic cardiovascular disease
    C. Triptans are preferred for migraine treatment during pregnancy
    D. Patients taking ergot alkaloids can use triptans concomitantly
    E. Triptans are strictly contraindicated in patients with hypertension

19. Which of the following statements is true regarding the use of opioids for migraines?

    A. Opioid use is not associated with rebound headaches
    B. Butorphanol nasal spray is efficacious in migraine abortive therapy
    C. Opioids in combination with butalbital and caffeine do not produce physical dependence
    D. Opioids scheduled around the clock are useful for migraine prophylaxis
    E. Opioids are not commonly prescribed for migraine treatment

20. Which of the following agents is most likely to cause pulmonary fibrosis?

    A. Methysergide
    B. Amitriptyline
    C. Carbamazepine
    D. Propranolol
    E. Valproic acid

21. Which statement about Midrin is correct?

  I. Midrin can be used concomitantly with over-the-counter products containing acetaminophen
  II. Midrin dose is limited to 5 capsules per 12 hours
  III. Midrin may cause sedation

    A. I only
    B. III only
    C. I and III only
    D. II and III only
    E. I, II, and III

22. Dihydroergotamine differs from ergotamine in which of the following ways?

    A. Lower incidence of nausea and vomiting
    B. Higher incidence of physical dependence
    C. No contraindications for ischemic cardiovascular disease
    D. Higher incidence of diarrhea
    E. It can be administered concomitantly with a triptan

Use Case Study 2 to answer Questions 23 and 24.

23. Which of the following statements is true regarding initiation of prophylactic migraine therapy in Mr. Hunt?

    A. Mr. Hunt is at high risk for rebound headaches due to excessive sumatriptan use
    B. Mr. Hunt is limiting his sumatriptan use to 3 days per week and is not a candidate for prophylactic treatment

Case Study 2

Patient Name:	James Hunt	
Address:	817 Elm Street	
Age:	45	
Sex:	Male	
Allergies:	NKDA	

Diagnosis: Migraine with aura, controlled hypertension

Medications:

1/1	sumatriptan 100 mg tablet	oral	use as directed	#9 tabs
1/1	lisinopril 10 mg tablet	oral	qd	#30 tabs
2/1	sumatriptan 100 mg tablet	oral	use as directed	#9 tabs
2/1	lisinopril 10 mg tablet	oral	qd	#30 tabs
3/1	sumatriptan 100 mg tablet	oral	use as directed	#9 tabs
3/1	lisinopril 10 mg tablet	oral	qd	#30 tabs
3/9	sumatriptan 100 mg tablet	oral	use as directed	#9 tabs
3/14	sumatriptan 100 mg tablet	oral	use as directed	#9 tabs

    C. Mr. Hunt is a candidate for prophylactic therapy due to the increasing frequency of attacks

    D. Mr. Hunt requires prophylactic therapy because his hypertension is a contraindication to using abortive therapies

    E. Prophylactic treatment is contraindicated in migraines with aura

24. Which medication is appropriate to give Mr. Hunt for migraine prophylaxis?

    A. Butorphanol
    B. Propranolol
    C. Dihydroergotamine
    D. Acetaminophen
    E. Hydrocodone

Answers

1. **E.** Currently, about 75 million individuals suffer from some form of chronic benign pain.

2. **C.** Physical dependence is the occurrence of a withdrawal syndrome after an opioid is stopped or quickly decreased without titration. Addiction is the psychological dependence on the use of substances for psychic effects and is characterized by compulsive use.

3. **A.** The WHO analgesic hierarchy involves choosing among three stepped levels of treatment. Mild pain may respond to nonopioid drugs alone. Combining a low-dose opioid with a nonopioid can relieve pain of moderate severity. More severe pain requires the addition of a higher-dose opioid preparation to the nonopioid. At any step, analgesic adjuvants may be useful.

4. **C.** Atrial flutter is not a documented adverse effect of opioids. However, therapeutic doses of many opioids produce peripheral vasodilation, reduced peripheral resistance, and inhibition of the baroreceptor reflexes. Recently, methadone has been associated with torsades de pointes, an atypical rapid ventricular tachycardia.

5. **A.** Oral medications should be used whenever possible because of convenience, flexibility, and steady serum levels.

6. **D.** Transdermal fentanyl provides analgesia for up to 72 hours. The analgesic effects of methadone do not correlate with its long half-life.

7. **C.** Morphine is metabolized by hepatic glucuronidation.

8. **B.** Oxycodone is metabolized through CYP450 2D6 to active metabolites. Fast metabolizers, those with multiple copies of the CYP450 2D6 gene, would clear oxycodone and its metabolites quickly.

9. **B.** About 90% of methadone is bound to plasma protein and is widely distributed in tissues. Methadone has a long terminal half-life resulting in slow clearance. This half-life does not correspond to analgesic dosing. It is metabolized via the CYP450 enzyme system.

10. **A.** Naloxone is a μ antagonist useful in opioid overdose. Naltrexone is also a μ antagonist, but it is reserved for use in alcoholism and opioid addiction.

11. **D.** Hydromorphone is an opioid with a short half-life with no available long-acting formulation. Thus it is not useful as an around-the-clock medication.

12. **C.** Normeperidine, a metabolite of meperidine, can accumulate with chronic use, renal impairment, and when the dose exceeds 600 mg/24 hours.

13. **E.** The anticholinergic effects of tricyclic antidepressants such as Elavil can exacerbate opioid-induced constipation and urinary retention.

14. **D.** Because transdermal delivery bypasses absorption from the GI tract, constipation has been reported to be less frequent than with other opioids.

15. **C.** Caffeine has analgesic and possibly anti-inflammatory properties. Therefore, reduced doses of acetaminophen and aspirin may be required. Caffeine may also increase gastric acidity and perfusion, enhancing the absorption of aspirin.

16. **A.** Sumatriptan is a selective serotonin agonist.

17. **E.** Adverse effects of ergotamine include nausea and vomiting, physical dependence, muscle weakness, and angina-like pain. Overuse of ergotamine can result in ischemia that may progress to gangrene.

18. **B.** Triptans are contraindicated in pregnancy and ischemic cardiovascular disease. They cannot be used within 24 hours of another triptan or ergot alkaloid.

19. **B.** There is good evidence for the efficacy of butorphanol nasal spray in migraine abortive therapy. Although opioids are commonly used for abortive therapy, they may be associated with rebound headaches and physical dependence.

20. **A.** With long-term therapy, methysergide can cause retroperitoneal, pleuropulmonary, and cardiac fibrosis. Fibrotic changes, although rare, are serious.

21. **D.** Midrin may be useful for mild to moderate migraines. It is generally well tolerated but may cause sedation. Due to its acetaminophen content, use of other acetaminophen products should be limited.

22. **D.** In contrast to ergotamine, dihydroergotamine causes minimal peripheral vasoconstriction, little nausea and vomiting, and no physical dependence. However, diarrhea is prominent.

23. **C.** Prophylactic therapy should be considered since his migraines occur more than twice monthly and there is a trend toward increasing frequency of attacks.

24. **B.** Propranolol has shown to be effective for migraine prophylaxis. This agent can reduce the number and intensity of attacks in about 70% of patients. Butorphanol, acetaminophen, dihydroergotamine, and hydrocodone are not approved for migraine prophylaxis.

7. References

Pain

American Pain Society. *Principles of Analgesic Use in the Treatment of Acute Pain and Cancer Pain,* 5th ed. Glenview, IL: American Pain Society; 2003.

Baumann TJ. Pain management. In: DiPiro JT, Talbert PE, Hayes PE, et al, eds. *Pharmacotherapy: A Pathophysiologic Approach,* 4th ed. New York: Elsevier; 1999:1014-1025.

Bonica JJ, ed. *The Management of Pain,* 2nd ed. Philadelphia: Lea & Febiger; 1990.

Brookoff D. Chronic pain: 1. a new disease. *Hosp Pract (Off Ed).* 2000;35:45-52, 59.

Duragesic package insert. Titusville, NJ: Janssen Pharmaceutical Products, L.P.; February 2005.

Holdsworth M, Forman W, Killilea T, et al. Transdermal fentanyl disposition in elderly subjects. *Gerontology.* 1994;40:32-37.

Hutchison TA, Shahan DR, eds. DRUGDEX® System. MICROMEDEX, Greenwood Village, CO (volume expired 3/2003).

IASP Task Force on Taxonomy. Merskey H, Bogduk N, eds. *Classification of Chronic Pain,* 2nd ed. Seattle: IASP Press; 1994:209-214.

Jacox A, Carr DB. Management of Cancer Pain. Clinical Practice Guideline No. 9. Rockville, MD: Agency for Health Care Policy and Research, U.S. Department of Health and Human Services, Public Health Service, 1994:34. AHCPR Publication No. 94-0492.

JCAHO. *Pain Assessment and Management. An Organizational Approach.* Oakbrook Terrace, IL: Joint Commission on Accreditation of Healthcare Organizations; 2000.

National Institute of Health. NIH Consensus Statement on Acupuncture, Vol. 15, No. 5, November 3-5, 1997; available online at http://odp.od.nih.gov/consensus/cons/107/107_statement.htm

NIH American Pain Society. Acupuncture. *Principles of Analgesic Use in the Treatment of Acute Pain and Cancer Pain,* 4th ed. Glenview, IL: American Pain Society; 1999.

Portenoy RK. Opioid therapy for chronic nonmalignant pain: A review of the critical issues. *J Pain Symptom Manage.* 1996;11:203-217.

Practice guidelines for chronic pain management: A report by the American Society of Anesthesiologists Task Force on Pain Management, Chronic Pain Section. *Anesthesiology.* 1997;86:995-1004.

Public policy statement on definitions related to the use of opioids in pain treatment. American Society of Addiction Medicine. *J Addict Dis.* 1998;17:129-133.

The Use of Opioids for the Treatment of Chronic Pain. A consensus statement from the American Academy of Pain Medicine and the American Pain Society. *Clin J Pain.* 1997;13:6.

Turk DC, Melzack R, eds. *Handbook of Pain Assessment,* 2nd ed. New York: Guilford Press; 2001.

Ultram ER package insert. Raritan, NJ: PriCara, a unit of Ortho-McNeil, Inc.; January 2006.

World Health Organization. *Cancer Pain Relief: With a Guide to Opioid Availability,* 2nd ed. Geneva: World Health Organization; 1996.

Migraines

Anthony M, Rasmussen BK. Migraine without aura. In: Olesen J, Tfelt-Hansen P, Welch KMA, eds. *The Headaches.* New York: Raven Press; 1993:255-261.

Barbanti P, Fabbrini G, Pesare M, Cerbo R. Unilateral cranial autonomic symptoms in migraine. *Cephalalgia.* 2002;22:256-259.

Brandes JL, Saper JR, Diamond M, et al. Topiramate for migraine prevention: a randomized controlled trial. *JAMA.* 2004 Feb 25;291(8):965-73.

Cady RK, Schreiber CP. Sinus headache or migraine? Considerations in making a differential diagnosis. *Neurology.* 2002;58(suppl 6):S10-S14.

Campbell JK, Penzien DB, Wall EM. Evidence-based guidelines for migraine headache: behavioural and physical treatments, 2000. Accessed at http://www.aan.com/professionals/practice/guidelines.cfm.

Couch JR. Sinus headache: a neurologist's viewpoint. *Semin Neurol.* 1988;8:298-302.

Diamond M. The role of concomitant headache types and non-headache comorbidities in the underdiagnosis of migraine. *Neurology.* 2002;58(suppl 6):S3-S9.

Drug Treatments for the Prevention of Migraine Headache. Technical Review 2.3. February 1999. Prepared for the Agency for Healthcare Policy and Research (contract no. 290-94-2025). Available from the National Technical Information Service (NTIS Accession No. 127953).

Goadsby P, Lipton R, Ferrari M. Migraine—current understanding and treatment. *N Engl J Med.* 2002;346:257-270.

Hargreaves RJ, Shepheard SL. Pathophysiology of migraine—new insights. *Can J Neurol Sci.* 1999;26(suppl 3):S12-S19.

Headache Classification Committee of the International Headache Society. Classification and diagnostic criteria for headache disorders, cranial neuralgias and facial pain. *Cephalalgia.* 1988;8(suppl 7):1-96.

Hutchison TA, Shahan DR, eds. DRUGDEX® System. MICROMEDEX, Greenwood Village, CO (edition expired 3/2003).

International Headache Society Web site. Revised classification proposal. Accessed at: http://216.25.100.131/members/Sections/members/login/Temp_Frame/frameset_26_06_02.htm.

Kaniecki RG, Totten J. Cervicalgia in migraine: prevalence, clinical characteristics, and response to treatment. Poster presented at 10th Congress of the International Headache Society, New York; 2002.

Lipton RB, Diamond S, Reed M, Diamond ML, Stewart WF. Migraine diagnosis and treatment: results from the American Migraine Study II. *Headache.* 2001;41:638-645.

Lipton RB, Stewart WF, Diamond S, et al. Prevalence and burden of migraine in the United States: data from the American Migraine Study II. *Headache.* 2001;41:646-657.

Matchar DB, Young WB, Rosenberg JH, et al. Evidence-based guidelines for migraine headache in the primary care setting: pharmacological management of acute attacks, 2000. Accessed at http://www.aan.com/professionals/practice/guidelines.cfm.

Pietrobon D, Striessnig J. Neurobiology of migraine. *Nat Rev Neurosci.* 2003;4(5):386-98.

Ramadan NM, Silberstein SD, Freitag FG, Gilbert TT, Frishberg BM. Evidence-based guidelines for migraine headache in the primary care setting: pharmacological management for prevention of migraine, 2000. Accessed at http://www.aan.com/professionals/ practice/guidelines.cfm.

Rasmussen BK, Jensen R, Schroll M, Olesen J. Interrelations between migraine and tension-type headache in the general population. *Arch Neurol.* 1992;49:914-918.

Silberstein SD. Practice parameter: evidence-based guidelines for migraine headache (an evidence-based review): report of the Quality Standards Subcommittee of the American Academy of Neurology. *Neurology.* 2000;55(6):754-62.

Silberstein SD. Topiramate in migraine prevention: evidence-based medicine from clinical trials. *Arch Neurol.* 2004;61:490-495.

Smith TR. Pitfalls in migraine diagnosis and management. *Clin Cornerstone.* 4(3), 2001. Accessed at http://www.medscape.com/viewarticle/418183.

Snow V, Weiss K, Wall EM, Mottur-Pilson C. Pharmacological management of acute attacks of migraine and prevention of migraine headache. *Ann Intern Med.* 2002;137:840-849.

Spierings ELH, Ranke AH, Honkoop PC. Precipitating and aggravating factors of migraine versus tension-type headache. *Headache.* 2001;41:554-558.

Tepper S, Newman L, Dowson A, et al. The prevalence and diagnosis of migraine in a primary care setting in the United States—insights from the Landmark Study. Poster presented at the Annual Scientific Meeting of the American Headache Society, June 21-23, 2002, Seattle, Washington.

Topamax package insert. Ortho-McNeil Neurologics, Inc.; Titusville, NJ: June 2005.

24. Seizure Disorders

Stephanie J. Phelps, PharmD, BCPS
Professor, Departments of Clinical Pharmacy and Pediatrics
University of Tennessee College of Pharmacy

Contents

1. Epilepsy

- Neurons become depolarized and repetitively fire action potentials.
- Involuntary and episodic
- The term is applied after two unprovoked seizures.
- A seizure does not mean a person has epilepsy; however, epilepsy means a person has seizures.
- Anticonvulsants do not cure epilepsy.

Terminology

- *aura:* a subjective sensation or motor phenomenon that marks a seizure onset and is generally associated with sensations that are localized in a particular region of the brain
- *automatisms:* purposeless movement seen with partial seizures
- *postictal:* symptoms and signs seen after a seizure

Types of Epilepsy

- There are two main types of epilepsy: partial seizures and generalized seizures.

Partial seizures

- Begins in one hemisphere of the brain; unilateral, asymmetric movements; generally associated with an aura. Complex partial seizures are accompanied by altered consciousness

Drugs for new-onset seizures

- Monotherapy: carbamazepine (DOC), phenytoin, valproic acid, gabapentin, lamotrigine, topiramate, oxcarbazepine, phenobarbital
- Adjunctive therapy: carbamazepine, gabapentin, lamotrigine, topiramate, oxcarbazepine, zonisamide, levetiracetam

Drugs for refractory seizures

- Monotherapy: carbamazepine, phenytoin, valproic acid, phenobarbital, lamotrigine, topiramate
- Adjunctive therapy: carbamazepine, gabapentin, lamotrigine, topiramate, oxcarbazepine, levetiracetam

Generalized seizures

- Begins simultaneously in both brain hemispheres; bilateral movements; no aura

Absence seizures

- Type of generalized seizure that has a sudden onset; brief (seconds); blank stare, upward rotation of the eyes, lip smacking (confused with daydreaming); 3-per-second spike and wave on EEG; can be precipitated by hyperventilation

Drugs of choice

- Ethosuximide; if patient has both absence and generalized tonic-clonic seizures, then valproic acid if >2 years old; lamotrigine

Primary generalized tonic-clonic seizure

- There are two phases to this seizure type.

Tonic phase

- Rigid, violent, sudden muscular contractions (stiff or rigid); cry or moan; deviation of the eyes and head to one side; rotation of the whole body and distortion of features; suppression of respiration; fall to the ground, loss of consciousness; tongue biting; involuntary urination

Clonic phase

- Repetitive jerks; cyanosis continues; foaming at the mouth; small grunting respirations between seizures, but deep respirations as all muscles relax at the end of the seizure

Drugs of choice for tonic-clonic seizures

- Phenytoin, carbamazepine, topiramate, valproic acid

Second-line agents

- Lamotrigine, phenobarbital, primidone

Juvenile myoclonic epilepsy (JME)

- Myoclonic seizures precede generalized tonic-clonic seizure; generally occur upon awakening; sleep deprivation and alcohol commonly precipitate; lifelong treatment required (valproic acid, lamotrigine)

Other less common seizure types

Catamenial epilepsy

- Associated with hormonal changes during menstruation; may be treated with acetazolamide

Infantile spasms

- Begin in the first 6 months of life; occur in clusters, several times a day; parents describe symptoms that sound like colic; high mortality and morbidity; treated with ACTH or oral steroids

Post-traumatic epilepsy

- Seizures that occur after head trauma; patients may be started on phenytoin for a period of 7 days; if no seizures occur, it should be discontinued.

Etiologies for Epilepsy

- Mechanical: birth injuries; head trauma; tumors; vascular abnormalities (stroke)
- Metabolic: electrolyte disturbances; glucose abnormalities; inborn errors of metabolism
- Genetic: benign familial neonatal seizures (chromosome 20); juvenile myoclonic epilepsy (chromosome 6); Baltic myoclonic (chromosome 21)
- Other: fever; infection

Medications
- Recreational (alcohol; cocaine/crack; ephedra; narcotics; methylphenidate)
- Carbapenems (imipenem); lindane; local anesthetics (lidocaine); metoclopramide; theophylline; tricyclic antidepressants
- Meperidine: the metabolite normeperidine can cause seizures in patients with renal failure who receive normal doses.
- Anticonvulsants that are used for treatment of a non-indicated seizure type (Table 1)

Criteria for Treating Epilepsy

- Almost no child should be treated after one seizure.
- Treat adults who have structural brain damage, a first seizure that was severe, or those with an occupation that places them at risk of injury should a second seizure occur.

Principles in the Treatment of Epilepsy

- Monotherapy (1 agent): always preferred
- Polytherapy (2 agents): add an anticonvulsant with a different mechanism of action, provided serum concentrations and doses of the first anticonvulsant have

been maximized. Begin to slowly reduce the dose of the first drug. This is important if the patient has developed side effects or if the patient has not responded to the first anticonvulsant.

- Polytherapy (≥3 agents): although rarely needed, add a third anticonvulsant if: (1) a combination of anticonvulsants is tolerated and significantly reduces seizure frequency or severity, but greater control might be achieved; or (2) the two anticonvulsants have been maximized. Reassess response and discontinue unnecessary anticonvulsants as soon as possible.

Reasons for Treatment Failure

- Incorrect diagnosis
- Wrong anticonvulsant selected
- Inappropriate dose, route, or formulation
- Altered pharmacokinetics that require a dosage alteration
- Poor patient adherence
- Seizures are refractory to therapy

Patient Counseling Information Applicable to All of the Anticonvulsants

- It is important that you keep a diary of your seizure(s) and keep regular appointments with your doctor, so it can be determined if your medication is working properly and if you are experiencing unwanted side effects.
- The full effects of this medication may not be seen for several weeks. Continue to take the medication unless directed otherwise by your physician.
- Take with food or milk if upset stomach occurs.
- Do not drink alcohol or take CNS depressants or illegal drugs with this medication.
- If this medication causes blurred vision or drowsiness, do not drive or operate heavy machinery while taking this medication until you have become accustomed to its effects (exception: gabapentin).
- Consult with your physician if you anticipate pregnancy, become pregnant, or plan to breast-feed while taking this medication.
- Some medications decrease the effectiveness of birth control pills. You should discuss this with your physician or pharmacist, who may recommend that you use a back-up birth control method to prevent pregnancy.
- *It is extremely important if you are a woman capable of having children that you take 1 mg of folic acid a day.*
- Do not stop taking this medication unless your doctor advises you to do so; some medicines have to be stopped slowly. Let your doctor or pharmacist know

Table 1

Seizures Caused by Anticonvulsants

Anticonvulsant	Seizure type		
	Absence	Generalized tonic-clonic	Myoclonic
Carbamazepine (Tegretol®)	Causes		Causes
Ethosuximide (Zarontin®)		Causes	
Phenytoin (Dilantin®)	Causes		
Phenobarbital	Causes		Causes

if you stop taking this medication.

- Check with your pharmacist or doctor before taking or starting any new medication (prescription, over-the-counter, or herbal product).
- Missed doses: if you miss a dose, take it as soon as you remember unless it is almost time for the next dose. If it is almost time for the next dose, then skip the missed dose and resume your regular schedule. Do not take extra or double doses. If you miss two or more doses contact your physician for further instructions.
- Contact your physician immediately if skin rash occurs.

Mechanisms of Action of the Anticonvulsants

- Anticonvulsants work through a variety of mechanisms including:
    * Enhancement of sodium channel inactivation
    * Reducing current through T-type calcium channels
    * Enhancement of GABA activity
    * Antiglutamate activity

2. Medications Used to Treat Epilepsy

Phenobarbital

- Indications: neonatal seizures, generalized seizures (except absence); other anticonvulsants are more effective in complex partial seizures (Table 2)

Pharmacokinetics
- Bioavailability: excellent
- Protein binding: not clinically important
- Metabolism: hepatic
- Renal elimination: low; can increase with alkalinization of the urine
- Half-life: long (20-150 hours)
- Reference range: 15-40 mg/L
- Other: primidone is an active anticonvulsant that is metabolized to phenobarbital.

Side effects
- *On initiation:* drowsiness, dizziness, light headedness, incoordination, headaches, or nervousness
- *With chronic therapy:*
    * Hyperactivity, primarily in children; however, rarely necessitates discontinuation of therapy
    * Cognition: lower memory and concentration abilities, slightly lowers IQ
    * Folate deficiency may cause megaloblastic anemia
    * Vitamin K–deficient hemorrhagic disease: administer vitamin K to the mother before delivery and to the newborn
- *Severe life-threatening:*
    * Hepatic failure: discontinue phenobarbital if liver function tests increase to >3 times above normal
    * Stevens-Johnson syndrome: refer patient to a physician if signs or symptoms of a rash develop. The physician may suggest holding a single dose until the rash is evaluated.
- Teratogenic (phenobarbital syndrome): developmental delay, short noses, low nasal bridges, low-set ears, wide mouths, protruding lips, distal digital hypoplasia; pregnancy category D

Drug-drug interactions: (inducer)
- Drugs that increase the serum concentration or effect of phenobarbital: chloramphenicol, felbamate, ketoconazole, methylphenidate, valproic acid
- Drugs that decrease the anticonvulsant effect of phenobarbital: phenytoin
- Phenobarbital may increase the serum concentration or effect of: alcohol, caffeine, and MAO inhibitors.
- Phenobarbital may decrease the serum concentration or effect of rifampin, birth control pills, cortico-

Table 2

Dosage Forms, Normal Maintenance Doses, and Dosing Interval for Older Anticonvulsants

Generic name	Trade name	Dosage form	Adult oral maintenance dose[1]	Interval[2]
Carbamazepine	Tegretol®	Suspension (100 mg/5 mL) Chewable tablet (100 mg) Tablet (200 mg) Extended-release tablet (Tegretol XR®: 100, 200, 400 mg)	800-1200 mg/d	Suspension: qid Chewable tablet: tid-qid Tablet (200 mg): bid Extended-release tablet: bid
	Carbatrol®	Extended-release capsule (200, 300 mg) (not available in liquid)		Extended-release capsule: bid
Ethosuximide	Zarontin®	Capsule (250 mg)	25-1500 mg/d	bid
Fosphenytoin	Cerebyx®	Injection (150 mg/2 mL; 750 mg/10 mL) 150 mg of fosphenytoin = 100 mg phenytoin	Not applicable	
Phenobarbital	Barbital®	Elixir (15 mg/5 mL, 20 mg/5 mL)	3-120 mg/d	bid-tid
	Luminal®	Tablet (8, 15, 16, 30, 32, 60, 65, 100 mg)		
	Solfoton®	Capsule (16 mg); powder for injection (120 mg); injection (30, 60, 65, 130 mg/mL)		
Phenytoin	Dilantin®	Suspension (125 mg/5 mL); chewable tablet (50 mg); prompt-release capsule (30, 100 mg); extended-release capsule (30, 100 mg); injection (50 mg/mL)	100-600 mg/d	qd-tid
Primidone	Mysoline®	Suspension (250 mg/5 mL); tablet (50, 125, 250 mg); chewable tablet (125 mg)	250-750 mg/d	tid-qid
Valproic acid	Depacon®	Injection (100 mg/mL)	250-4000 mg/d	bid-tid
Sodium valproate	Depakene®	Syrup (250 mg/5 mL)		
Divalproex sodium	Depakene	Gel capsule (125, 250 mg)		
	Depakote Sprinkles®	Capsule (125 mg)		
	Depakote®	Delayed-release tablet (125, 250, 500 mg)		
	Depakote ER®	Extended-release tablet (250, 500 mg)		qd

[1]With the exception of the intravenous dosage forms, these anticonvulsants are begun at low doses and slowly titrated to a dose that will control the patient's seizures.

[2]Interval may either decrease or increase in the presence of medications that induce or inhibit metabolism, respectively.

steroids, cyclophosphamide, cyclosporine, delavirdine, griseofulvin, haloperidol, lamotrigine, metronidazole, propranolol, quinidine, ritonavir, saquinavir, theophylline, and warfarin.

Patient counseling (see general counseling information)
Counseling specific to this medication
- This medication decreases the effectiveness of birth control pills. Use a supplemental birth control method to prevent pregnancy while taking phenobarbital or contact your physician about a "high" estrogen oral contraceptive.

Phenytoin

- Indications: all seizure types except absence and febrile seizures

Pharmacokinetics

- Bioavailability: slow, variable, decreased in children, and formulation-dependent
- Protein binding: very high (90-95%)
- Metabolism: hepatic
- Renal elimination: low (<5%)
- Half-life: phenytoin exhibits capacity-limited or saturable (ie, Michaelis-Menten) pharmacokinetics.
- Reference range: 10–20 mg/L

Side effects

- *Upon initiation:* nausea, vomiting, drowsiness, and dizziness
- *With chronic therapy:*
  - * Peripheral neuropathy
  - * Hydantoin facies (thickening of subcutaneous tissues, enlargement of nose and lips)
  - * Acne, hirsutism, and gingival hyperplasia (suggest good oral hygiene)
  - * Osteomalacia (treat with vitamin D if alkaline phosphatase increase and 25-hydroxycholecalciferol decreases)
  - * Vitamin K–deficient hemorrhagic disease: administer vitamin K to the mother before delivery and to the newborn
  - * Folate deficiency causing megaloblastic anemia
- **Severe life-threatening:**
  - * Hepatic failure: discontinue if liver function tests increase >3 times above normal
  - * Stevens-Johnson syndrome: refer patient to a physician if signs or symptoms of a rash develop. The physician may suggest holding a single dose until the rash is evaluated.
- Teratogenic (fetal hydantoin syndrome): craniofacial anomalies, broad nasal bridges, short upturned noses, low-set and prominent ears, distal digital hypoplasia, intrauterine growth restriction, pregnancy category D

Drug-drug interactions

- Drugs that increase the serum concentration or effect of phenytoin: acute alcohol use, amiodarone, chloramphenicol, chlordiazepoxide, diazepam, disulfiram, estrogens, felbamate, histamine antagonists (eg, cimetidine), halothane, isoniazid, methylphenidate, phenothiazines, phenylbutazone, salicylates, succinimides, sulfonamides (sulfadiazine, sulfamethoxazole, and sulfisoxazole), tolbutamide, trazodone, warfarin, zidovudine
- Drugs that decrease the effect of phenytoin: antacids, bleomycin, cisplatin, nevirapine, rifampin, ritonavir, vinblastine, zidovudine, and the herbals shankhapushpi, kava kava and valerian
- Phenytoin may increase the serum concentration or effect of valproic acid.

- Phenytoin may decrease the serum concentration or effect of phenobarbital.

Drug-nutrient interactions

- Patients receiving tube feedings and oral phenytoin at the same time may have a significant decrease in absorption of phenytoin. If possible, discontinue feeding 2 hours before and after a dose of phenytoin.

Patient counseling (see general counseling information)

Specific to phenytoin

- Do not break, crush, or chew capsule before swallowing; swallow whole. Shake suspension well.
- This medication may alter your gums. Brush and floss daily, and have regular visits with your dentist.

Carbamazepine

- Indications: most widely used anticonvulsant in adults and children; drug of choice for complex partial seizures; effective in most generalized seizures; ineffective in absence seizures and febrile seizures

Pharmacokinetics

- Bioavailability: good; dispense in moisture-proof containers because studies show decreased bioavailability with high humidity (ie, medicine cabinets)
- Protein binding: low
- Metabolism: hepatic
- Renal elimination: low
- Half-life: about a day if used as monotherapy; about 12 hours if given with >1 anticonvulsant
- Reference range: 4-12 mg/L (monotherapy = 8-12 mg/L; polytherapy = 4-8 mg/L)

Other

- Carbamazepine is metabolized to a 10,11 carbamazepine epoxide, which is both effective as an anticonvulsant and capable of causing toxicity.
- Carbamazepine is one of a few drugs that can induce its own metabolism (ie, autoinduction). Mean time to onset is 21 days (range: 17-31 days)

Side effects

- *Upon initiation:* dose-related, transient, and reversible rash that rarely cause the drug to be discontinued; nausea, vomiting, drowsiness, dizziness, and neutropenia
- *With chronic therapy:*
  - * SIADH (hyponatremia and water retention)
  - * Osteomalacia (treat with vitamin D if alkaline phosphatase increase and 25-hydroxycholecalciferol decreases)
  - * Folate deficiency causing megaloblastic anemia

- *Severe or life-threatening:*
  * Direct hepatotoxicity (*FDA Black Box Warning*): generally presents within 1 month; fever; rash; fatalities may occur even if drug is discontinued; stop carbamazepine if liver function tests increase >3 times above normal.
  * Aplastic anemia (*FDA Black Box Warning*): recommended to discontinue carbamazepine if WBC <2000-3000 or neutrophils <1000-1500
- Teratogenic (fetal carbamazepine syndrome): epicanthal folds; short nose, long philtrum, hypoplastic nails, microcephaly, developmental delay, pregnancy category D

Drug-drug interactions
- Drugs that increase the serum concentration or effect of carbamazepine: erythromycin, cimetidine, lithium, propoxyphene
- Drugs that decrease the anticonvulsant effect of carbamazepine: phenobarbital, primidone, phenytoin
- Carbamazepine may increase the serum concentration or effect of felbamate; felbamate will increase concentration of the 10,11 epoxide metabolite and cause toxicity.
- Carbamazepine may decrease the serum concentration or effect of: cyclosporine, doxycycline, haloperidol, oral contraceptives, theophylline

Patient counseling (see general counseling information)
- Shake suspension well.
- Do not use with monoamine oxidase inhibitors.

Valproic Acid

- Indications: all types of generalized and partial seizures; along with ethosuximide this is the drug of choice for absence seizures. Rarely used in children <2 years of age.

Pharmacokinetics
- Bioavailability: excellent
- Protein binding: high
- Metabolism: hepatic
- Renal: low
- Reference range: 50-150 mg/L (curvilinear relationship between serum concentration and protein binding)

Side effects
- *Upon initiation:* nausea and vomiting
- *With chronic therapy:*
  * Weight gain: at times significant enough to warrant discontinuing the medication

  * Alopecia: partial or total (to prevent/treat supplement with zinc and selenium)
  * Tremor: dose-dependent (treat by decreasing the dose, discontinuing the drug, or adding propranolol)
  * Thrombocytopenia: dose-dependent decrease in platelets
  * Elevation in liver enzymes: may be transient and responds to discontinuation of valproic acid
- *Severe or life-threatening:*
  * Fatal hepatotoxicity (*FDA Black Box Warning*): most common in children <2 years of age who have severe epilepsy and are receiving multiple anticonvulsants
  * Fatal hemorrhagic pancreatitis (*FDA Black Box Warning*)
- Teratogenic (*FDA Black Box Warning*): (fetal valproate syndrome): craniofacial anomalies, small inverted noses, shallow philtrum, flat nasal bridge, long upper lip, congenital liver disease, and spina bifida, pregnancy category D.
- There is an association between folic acid deficiency and spina bifida, so all women with epilepsy who are of childbearing age should be on daily folic acid (1 mg).

Drug-drug interactions
- Drugs that increase the serum concentration or effect of valproic acid: felbamate, phenytoin, salicylates
- Drugs that decrease the anticonvulsant effect of valproic acid: carbamazepine, felbamate, lamotrigine, phenytoin, phenobarbital, primidone
- Valproic acid may increase the serum concentration or effect of: amitriptyline, carbamazepine, ethosuximide, felbamate, lamotrigine, phenobarbital, primidone, zidovudine
- Valproic acid may decrease the serum concentration or effect of: phenytoin

Patient counseling (see general counseling information)
- You may take this medication with food or milk to reduce stomach irritation. Do not take with carbonated drinks.
- Valproic acid capsules: swallow whole with water only; do not break, chew, or crush.
- Divalproex sodium delayed-released capsules: swallow whole or sprinkle the contents on a small amount of cool, soft food (eg, applesauce or pudding) and swallow without chewing immediately after preparation.
- Divalproex sodium delayed-release tablets: swallow the tablets whole; do not break, chew, or crush.
- Valproic acid syrup: you may mix the syrup with any liquid or add it to a small amount of food.

- Report any sore throat, fever, fatigue, bleeding, or bruising that is severe or persists to the patient's physician.
- Your doctor may monitor your liver function with blood tests every 1-2 weeks initially, and periodically thereafter.

Felbamate (Rarely Used)

- Indications: Lennox-Gastaut syndrome; tonic-clonic, tonic-myoclonic, and refractory partial seizures with or without secondary generalization (Table 3)

Pharmacokinetics
- 50% renally eliminated

Side effects
- *With chronic therapy:* weight loss significant enough to warrant discontinuing the medication
- *Severe or life-threatening:*
     * Hepatotoxicity: (*FDA Black Box Warning*)
     * Aplastic anemia: (*FDA Black Box Warning*)

Drug-drug interactions
- Inhibitor and inducer: if a patient on carbamazepine has symptoms of toxicity and their carbamazepine serum concentration is low, they likely have an increased concentration of the active metabolite (10,11 epoxide). Reduce the dose of carbamazepine.

Patient counseling (see general counseling information)
- The patient or legal guardian should sign a consent form before taking this medication.
- Your doctor may monitor your liver function with blood tests every 1-2 weeks initially, and periodically thereafter and may also do urine testing.

Gabapentin

- Indications: partial seizures; this drug is used most often for peripheral neuropathies and not epilepsy.

Pharmacokinetics
- Bioavailability: poor
- Renal elimination: 100%

Side effects
- *Severe life-threatening:* None

Drug-drug interactions
- No interactions that affect metabolism; aluminum- and/or magnesium-containing antacids may decrease the absorption; not a true drug interaction, but combination with carbamazepine may cause dizziness (reduce the dose of carbamazepine).

Patient counseling (see general counseling information)
- Food may decrease the extent of absorption.

Table 3

Dosage Forms, Normal Maintenance Doses, and Dosing Intervals for the Newer Anticonvulsants

Generic name	Trade name	Dosage form	Oral maintenance dose[1]	Interval[2]
Felbamate	Felbatol®	Suspension (500 mg/5 mL), tablet (400, 600 mg)	1200-3600 mg/d	tid-qid
Gabapentin	Neurontin®	Capsules (100, 300, 400 mg), suspension (50 mg/mL)	900-3600 mg/d[3]	tid
Lamotrigine	Lamictal®	Chewable tablet (5, 25 mg), tablet (25, 100, 150, 200 mg)	50-400 mg/d	qd-bid
Levetiracetam	Keppra®	Tablet (250, 500, 750 mg), solution (100 mg/mL)	1000-3000 mg/d	bid
Oxcarbazepine	Trileptal®	Tablet (150, 300, 600 mg)	600-2400 mg/d	bid
Tiagabine	Gabitril®	Tablet (4, 12, 16, 20 mg)	4-56 mg/d	bid-qid
Topiramate	Topamax®	Sprinkle capsule (15, 25 mg), tablet (25, 50, 100, 200 mg)	200-400 mg/d[4]	bid
Zonisamide	Zonegran®	Capsule (100 mg)	100-600 mg/d	qd

[1]With the exception of gabapentin, these anticonvulsants are begun at low doses and slowly titrated over weeks to a dose that will control the patient's seizures.

[2]Interval may either decrease or increase in the presence of medications that induce or inhibit metabolism, respectively.

[3]Much larger doses have been given.

[4]The recommended maintenance doses for initial monotherapy and adjunctive therapy are 400 mg/d and 200-400 mg/d, respectively. Doses >400 mg are no more effective than doses ≤400 mg.

- If you take antacids, wait at least 2 hours before taking gabapentin.
- Missed dose: take as soon as possible; if <2 hours until the next dose, take the missed dose and then take the next dose 1-2 hours later, resuming your normal regimen. If you miss more than one dose, call your pharmacist or doctor for instructions.

Lamotrigine

- Indications: partial seizures; primary and secondary generalized tonic-clonic seizures; absence, atypical absence, atonic, and myoclonic seizures; and seizures associated with Lennox-Gastaut syndrome

Pharmacokinetics
- None unique

Side effects
- *Severe life-threatening:*
  * Skin rash (*FDA Black Box Warning*): refer patient to a physician if signs or symptoms of a rash develop. The physician may suggest holding a single dose until the rash is evaluated. Must titrate a patient to a maintenance dose very slowly. This is especially true if they are also receiving valproic acid.

Drug-drug interactions
- Drugs that increase the serum concentration or effect of lamotrigine: valproic acid
- Drugs that decrease the anticonvulsant effect of lamotrigine: carbamazepine, phenytoin, phenobarbital, primidone
- Lamotrigine may increase the serum concentration or effect of: none
- Lamotrigine may decrease the serum concentration or effect of: valproic acid
- Not a true drug-drug interaction, but the combination with carbamazepine may cause dizziness (reduce the dose of carbamazepine).

Patient counseling (see general counseling information)
- Notify your physician *immediately* if a skin rash occurs.

Topiramate

- Indications: As initial monotherapy (>10 years of age) for the treatment of partial onset seizures or primary generalized tonic-clonic seizures; as adjunctive therapy for adults and pediatric patients ages 2-16 years with partial onset seizures or primary generalized tonic-clonic seizures; and in patients 2 years of age and older with seizures associated with Lennox-Gastaut syndrome

Pharmacokinetics
- Elimination: primarily renal

Side effects
- *Upon initiation:* drowsiness, dizziness, difficulty with concentration, loss of appetite, mood changes, paresthesias; monitor use in children in hot climates.
- *With chronic therapy:*
  * Metabolic acidosis
  * Acute myopia and secondary angle closure glaucoma
  * Kidney stones (caution patient that adequate hydration may reduce stone formation)
  * Paresthesia
  * Word finding difficulties/CNS effects
  * Significant weight loss
- *Severe or life-threatening:*
  * Oligohidrosis (may not sweat): children taking topiramate may not sweat as needed and could develop hyperthermia. Caution the patient about getting overheated and to drink plenty of water.

Drug-drug interactions
- Drugs that increase the serum concentration or effect of topiramate: CNS depressants (alcohol, morphine, codeine), carbonic anhydrase inhibitors (acetazolamide)
- Drugs that decrease the anticonvulsant effect of topiramate: phenobarbital, phenytoin, valproic acid
- Topiramate may increase the serum concentration or effect of: metformin
- Topiramate may decrease the serum concentration or effect of: oral contraceptives, valproic acid

Patient counseling (see general counseling information)
- If using the Topamax sprinkle capsules, sprinkle the contents on a small amount of cool, soft food (eg, applesauce or yogurt) and swallow immediately without chewing.
- Drink plenty of fluids.

Tiagabine

- Indications: partial seizures

Pharmacokinetics
- Protein binding: high
- Metabolism: hepatic

Side effects
- *Severe life-threatening:* none

Drug-drug interactions
- Drugs that increase the serum concentration or effect of tiagabine: valproic acid

- Drugs that decrease the anticonvulsant effect of tiagabine: carbamazepine, phenobarbital, primidone, phenytoin
- Tiagabine may increase the serum concentration or effect of: none
- Tiagabine may decrease the serum concentration or effect of: valproic acid

Patient counseling
- None unique

Zonisamide

- Indications: partial seizures

Side effects
- *Chronic therapy:* (very similar to topiramate)
  * Kidney stones (contraindicated in patients with a history of kidney stones; should be adequately hydrated)
  * Weight loss
  * Reversible or irreversible psychosis (rare)

- *Severe or life-threatening:*
  * Oligohidrosis (may not sweat) (*FDA Bold Warning*): children taking zonisamide may not sweat as needed and could develop hyperthermia. Warn patients of the need to be aware of getting overheated and to drink plenty of water.

Drug-drug interactions
- Drugs that decrease the effect of zonisamide: carbamazepine, phenobarbital, phenytoin, valproic acid

Patient counseling (see general counseling information)
- Notify your pharmacist or physician if you are allergic to sulfa medications.
- Drink plenty of fluids to help prevent kidney stones.
- Contact your doctor if your child is not sweating as usual.

Levetiracetam

- Indications: partial seizures

Side effects
- *Upon initiation:* dizziness, fatigue, sedation
- *With chronic therapy:* none
- *Severe life-threatening:* none

Drug-drug interactions
- No significant interactions noted to date.

Patient counseling (see general counseling information)
- None

3. Other Issues

Nondrug Treatment of Epilepsy

- Ketogenic diet
- Vagal nerve stimulator
- Surgical correction

Withdrawal of Anticonvulsants
- Over half of patients who remain seizure-free for 2 years can have their anticonvulsant successfully withdrawn. Most who are seizure-free for 4 years can be successfully withdrawn.
- Unless the patient is experiencing a severe or life-threatening adverse effect, **never** abruptly discontinue an anticonvulsant; taper slowly over 2-6 months.

Status Epilepticus

- Defined as a seizure that lasts longer than 5 minutes or ≥2 discrete seizures between which there is incomplete recovery of consciousness.
- Status epilepticus is a medical emergency.
- See Table 4 for suggested order of therapies.

Benzodiazepines
- First-line agents; diazepam or lorazepam; lorazepam is preferred)

Phenytoin (intravenous)
- Can only be mixed with normal saline
- Loading dose: if an individual is not already receiving phenytoin, give 15-20 mg/kg. Because phenytoin contains propylene glycol and is in itself cardiotoxic, do not infuse faster than 50 mg/min.
- Maintenance dose: if the maintenance dose is to be given every 12 hours, give the first dose 12 hours after the end of the loading dose. If the maintenance dose is to be given every 24 hours, give the first dose 24 hours after the end of the loading dose.
- Not only is the bioavailability of phenytoin reduced, but its alkaline pH precludes its administration by the IM route.

Fosphenytoin
- Phenytoin prodrug which is converted to phenytoin within minutes after infusion
- Can be admixed with any IV solution
- Must be dosed in PE (phenytoin equivalents): 1 mg of phenytoin = 1.5 mg of fosphenytoin
- Can be given at a rate of 150 mg/min (three times faster than phenytoin)

Table 4

Treatment of Status Epilepticus

As soon as possible	• Assess cardiorespiratory status; insert oral airway and administer oxygen as needed • Place secure IV and start infusion of normal saline • Obtain medical history; perform neurological examination • Obtain the following test: If the patient has been on anticonvulsants as an outpatient, obtain blood for serum drug concentrations; chemistry panel including electrolytes, glucose, BUN, and urine drug screen • Administer 25 g of glucose and 100 mg of thiamine IV
If still seizing:	• Administer either diazepam or lorazepam up to maximum dosage until seizure stops
If still seizing:	• Load with IV phenytoin (provided patient was not on phenytoin at home or has low serum concentrations) and begin maintenance doses • Monitor blood pressure and EEG
If still seizing:	• Load with IV phenobarbital or begin a continuous infusion of midazolam
If still seizing:	• Begin medically-induced coma • Adjust EEG to burst-suppression • Avoid hypotension during infusion of the barbiturate

Phenobarbital

• May cause respiratory depression/arrest (likelihood may be increased if benzodiazepines have been given)
• Sedation may eliminate the ability to perform an accurate neurologic assessment.

Midazolam

• Continuous infusion due to short half-life

Medically-induced coma

• Usually achieved with pentobarbital
• Use for severe refractory status epilepticus
• Give loading dose (20-40 mg/kg) over 1-2 hours, followed by continuous infusion (1-4 mg/kg per hour).
• If hypotension occurs, begin dopamine or slow the rate of infusion.
• Titrate to burst suppression (isoelectric) on EEG.

Other therapies used for refractory status epilepticus

• Propofol
• Topiramate
• Magnesium
• Lidocaine
• IV immune globulin

Febrile Seizures

• A benign seizure occurring in the absence of CNS infection in a child with fever
• Most common seizure disorder in childhood
• Age of onset: 4 months to 5 years (peak at 14-18 months)
• Risk factors (≥2 of the following):
  * A first- or second-degree relative with a history of a febrile seizure
  * Developmental delay
  * Delayed discharge (>28 days) from a newborn center
  * Day care attendance
• Risk for developing epilepsy:
  * Overall, the development of epilepsy is rare (1-2%).
  * About 15% of children who have a complex febrile seizure will go on to develop epilepsy.
• There are two types of febrile seizures:
  * Simple febrile seizure:
    • Benign
    • A primary generalized seizure
    • <15 minutes in duration
    • Does not recur within 24 hours
  * Complex febrile seizure:
    • Focal (involves an arm, leg, or face on one side only or eye deviation towards one side)

• Prolonged (>15 min) and/or recurring within 24 hours of the initial seizure

Acute treatment of a simple or complex partial seizure

• Seizure control: drugs of choice for prolonged febrile seizure are rectally administered benzodiazepines (rectal diazepam [Valium®] or lorazepam [Ativan®])
• Diastat®: commercially available as a gel of diazepam to be given rectally

Prophylaxis for a simple or complex partial seizure

• If temperature is >38C° give a non-aspirin antipyretic.
• Daily anticonvulsants are not indicated for the prevention of recurrent febrile seizures.

Maintenance therapy

• *Not* generally used
• An anticonvulsant (ie, phenobarbital) may be considered after a complex febrile seizure if epilepsy is suspected.
• Carbamazepine and phenytoin are *not* effective in the prevention of recurrent febrile seizures.

4. Key Points

• Phenytoin can only be mixed with normal saline and should not be given faster than 50 mg/min.
• Gabapentin and levetiracetam are not associated with any significant drug interactions.
• As of January 2003, the following anticonvulsants carry a "black box" warning: carbamazepine (aplastic anemia, hepatic failure), valproic acid (liver failure, teratogenicity, pancreatitis), felbamate (aplastic anemia, hepatic failure), and lamotrigine (serious rash). Zonisamide and topiramate have been reported to cause oligohidrosis and hyperthermia.
• Although absence seizures are frequently treated with ethosuximide or valproic acid if ≥2 years of age), lamotrigine is also acceptable.
• Carbapenems (eg, imipenem) and normeperidine (a metabolite of meperidine that accumulates in renal failure) may cause seizures.
• Carbamazepine undergoes autoinduction (ie, it induces its own metabolism) and phenytoin has capacity-limited or saturable (ie, Michaelis-Menten) pharmacokinetics.
• Because of the potential for severe life-threatening liver toxicity, valproic acid is generally not used in a patient ≤2 years of age.
• There is an association between folic acid deficiency and spina bifida; hence, all women and especially those with epilepsy who are of childbearing age should be on daily folic acid (1 mg).
• Unless a patient is experiencing a life-threatening adverse effect, an anticonvulsant should not be abruptly discontinued.
• Topiramate may cause significant weight loss and valproic acid may cause significant weight gain.
• Topiramate and zonisamide may cause kidney stones.
• Patients with an allergy to sulfa medications should not be given zonisamide

5. Questions and Answers

1. Which of the following is true regarding phenytoin?

   A. The maximum rate of intravenous administration is 50 mg/min
   B. If intravenous access can't be established, phenytoin can be given IM
   C. Because phenytoin contains propylene glycol it is soluble is any IV fluid
   D. It is an inhibitor of the cytochrome P450 system
   E. A major limitation to the use of the product in pediatric patients is the lack of a commercially available liquid formulation

2. A 50-kg patient with no history of epilepsy presents in status epilepticus. The patient is given an adequate dose of lorazepam and is about to be given a loading dose of intravenous phenytoin. Assuming a phenytoin Vd of 0.6 L/kg, what dose of phenytoin should be given to achieve a serum phenytoin concentration of ~16-18 mg/L?

   A. 18 mg/kg
   B. 500 mg
   C. 30 mg/kg
   D. 50 mg
   E. 5 g

3. Which of the following is true regarding a patient with refractory status epilepticus who is placed in a medically-induced coma with a barbiturate?

   A. If the patient is mechanically ventilated, the barbiturates will induce respiratory arrest
   B. The goal of a coma that is medically-induced with a barbiturate is to induce burst suppression (isoelectric) on EEG
   C. If hypotension develops, the patient should be given nitroprusside
   D. The barbiturates are not associated with drug interactions
   E. A major problem with this type of therapy is kidney failure

4. Which of the following is associated with autoinduction?

   A. Phenobarbital
   B. Phenytoin
   C. Carbamazepine
   D. Gabapentin
   E. Levetiracetam

5. Which of these agents reduces the likelihood of congenital malformations in epileptic women receiving valproate?

   A. Folic acid
   B. Vitamin B_{12}
   C. Gingko biloba
   D. Iron
   E. Selenium

6. A 33-year-old woman is being started on an anticonvulsant. The woman is already slightly overweight and is very concerned about the effects of the various medications on her weight. Which of the following is true regarding anticonvulsants and their effect on weight?

   I. Valproic acid increases weight
   II. Topiramate decreases weight
   III. Phenytoin increases weight

   A. I
   B. I and II
   C. II
   D. III
   E. I, II, and III

7. A 24-year-old with complex partial seizures is currently controlled with valproic acid, gabapentin, and topiramate. She calls your pharmacy to ask if any of her medications can cause nosebleeds since she has had 1-2 in the past week. You refer her to her local medical doctor, where her platelet count is reported to be 95,132/mm^3. Which of the following is true?

   A. None of her anticonvulsants cause thrombocytopenia
   B. Valproate can cause a dose-related thrombocytopenia
   C. Gabapentin has inhibited the metabolism of topiramate, and the elevated concentration of topiramate is responsible for the thrombocytopenia
   D. Gabapentin can cause idiosyncratic thrombocytopenia
   E. Topiramate can cause thrombocytopenia

8. A patient has hypertension, diabetes mellitus, and chronic renal failure (serum Cr 6.8), and has developed seizures. Which of the following anticonvulsants would require dosage adjustment in this patient?

   A. Gabapentin, topiramate
   B. Lamotrigine, felbamate
   C. Phenobarbital, gabapentin
   D. Phenytoin, valproic acid
   E. Phenobarbital, levetiracetam

9. Which of the following anticonvulsants is metabolized to phenobarbital?

   A. Ethosuximide
   B. Primidone
   C. Zonisamide
   D. Levetiracetam
   E. Carbamazepine

10. A 7-year-old on valproic acid for partial complex seizures with secondary generalization that are refractory to phenobarbital, phenytoin, carbamazepine, and gabapentin, continued to have seizures and was started on lamotrigine 2 weeks ago. Today he presents with a diffuse maculopapular erythematous rash with lesions on the lips. Which of the following is correct?

   A. A rash associated with lamotrigine generally occurs within the first few days; hence the rash is not associated with an anticonvulsant
   B. The patient should be given diphenhydramine and the lamotrigine should be continued
   C. Lamotrigine should be discontinued
   D. The rash is secondary to a drug interaction between gabapentin and carbamazepine
   E. All of the anticonvulsants are associated with life-threatening rash. In order to prevent status epilepticus associated with abrupt discontinuation of the anticonvulsants, the medications should be slowly discontinued

11. A new anticonvulsant has just been approved by the FDA. Its bioavailability is >95% and it is highly protein bound to α_1-acid glycoprotein. It undergoes extensive hepatic metabolism by CYP450 2C9. Less than 5% is excreted unchanged in the urine. It is known to inhibit CYP450 3A4. A patient on this anticonvulsant has developed significant depression and is being started on an antidepressant that is 93% bound to albumin and is a potent inhibitor of CYP450 2C19. The antidepressant is metabolized by CYP450 3A4 to an active metabolite that is hepatically cleared by CYP450 2C9. The neurologist wants to know if any drug interactions may occur that would necessitate a reduction in drug dosage.

   A. No drug interactions should occur in this patient
   B. The dose of the anticonvulsant should be reduced because of a potential protein binding interaction that would increase the serum concentration of the anticonvulsant
   C. The dose of the anticonvulsant should be increased
   D. The dose of the antidepressant should be reduced
   E. Because of an interaction in the gut that decreased bioavailability, the dose should be increased

12. Which of the following are not associated with any drug-drug interactions?

   I. Gabapentin
   II. Carbamazepine
   III. Levetiracetam

   A. I
   B. II
   C. I and III
   D. II and III
   E. I and II
   F. III

13. A 42-year-old woman has been successfully treated with valproic acid for years, but she has experienced some undesirable side effects. She is slowly titrated onto a new anticonvulsant and the valproic acid is slowly discontinued. She presents to the ED with severe flank pain and is diagnosed with a kidney stone. Which of the following may have precipitated her current situation?

   A. Gabapentin
   B. Lamotrigine
   C. Levetiracetam
   D. Topiramate
   E. Phenytoin

14. Which of the following drugs carries a black box warning?

I. Carbamazepine
II. Felbamate
III. Levetiracetam

A. II
B. III
C. I
D. I and II
E. II and III

15. Which of the following carries a black box warning for pancreatitis?

A. Carbamazepine
B. Felbamate
C. Zonisamide
D. Valproic acid
E. Phenytoin

16. What is the drug of choice for absence seizures in a child <2 years of age?

A. Phenytoin
B. Phenobarbital
C. Ethosuximide
D. Valproic acid
E. Primidone

17. Diastat is given by which of the following routes?

A. Rectally
B. Intramuscularly
C. Intravenously
D. Intranasally
E. Subcutaneously

18. Which of the following is true?

A. Febrile seizures must be accompanied by a CNS infection
B. Complex febrile seizures last >15 minutes
C. Most children who have a febrile seizure go on to develop epilepsy
D. The drug of choice for a simple febrile seizure is carbamazepine
E. Simple febrile seizures should never be treated

19. Which of the following anticonvulsants are available in a liquid, chewable tablet, and intravenous formulation?

I. Carbamazepine
II. Phenytoin
III. Valproic acid

A. II
B. III
C. I
D. I and II
E. I, II, and III

20. Patients should be told to drink plenty of fluid when taking which of the following?

A. Carbamazepine
B. Topiramate
C. Levetiracetam
D. Gabapentin
E. Phenytoin

21. Which of the following medications may cause seizures in an adult patient with renal failure?

A. Meperidine
B. Phenobarbital
C. Carbamazepine
D. Lamotrigine
E. Theophylline

22. Which of the following is associated with Michaelis-Menten pharmacokinetics?

A. Carbamazepine
B. Valproic acid
C. Topiramate
D. Phenytoin
E. Phenobarbital

23. A patient on this medication should be made aware of the importance of good oral hygiene.

A. Felbamate
B. Phenytoin
C. Zonisamide
D. Phenobarbital
E. Levetiracetam

Answers

1. **A.** Because phenytoin contains propylene glycol and is itself cardiotoxic, the IV formulation should not be infused faster than 50 mg/min. Phenytoin is extremely alkaline (pH ~13). Not only is IM administration associated with tissue damage, it is erratically absorbed. Phenytoin can only be admixed with normal saline, is an inducer, and is also available as a suspension and a chewable tablet.

2. **B.** The equation for calculation of a loading dose is as follows: dose = Cp desired x Vd. So Cp desired is ~17 x (0.6 L/kg x 50 kg) ≈510 mg.

3. **B.** The goal is to produce a "flat" EEG. If the patient is mechanically ventilated, the effect of a medication on respiration is not a factor in its administration. Although pentobarbital may cause hypotension if given too rapidly, nitroprusside is a vasodilator used to treat hypertension. The barbiturates are known inducers. Coma that is medically induced with a barbiturate does not cause kidney failure.

4. **C.** Carbamazepine induces its own metabolism, with peak effects seen about 21 days after beginning the medication or following an increase in dosage. Phenobarbital and phenytoin are inducers. Gabapentin and levetiracetam are not cleared hepatically.

5. **A.** Many of the anticonvulsants can cause folic acid deficiency. There is an association between folic acid deficiency and spina bifida; hence all women with epilepsy who are of childbearing age should receive supplemental folic acid every day (1 mg).

6. **B.** Topiramate can cause significant weight loss and valproate can cause significant weight gain. Phenytoin does not significantly affect weight.

7. **B.** Valproic acid can cause clinically significant thrombocytopenia. Gabapentin is not associated with any drug interaction that affects metabolism, and it does not cause a decrease in platelets. Topiramate does not cause thrombocytopenia.

8. **A.** Gabapentin and topiramate would require dosage adjustment since they are renally eliminated.

9. **B.** Primidone (Mysoline) is an active anticonvulsant, but it is also metabolized to phenobarbital.

10. **C.** Lamotrigine has a black box warning for severe rash. Since this patient has a diffuse rash and lesions on the lips, the lamotrigine should be discontinued. Because the incidence of severe rash may be higher in children than adults, current practice would be to discontinue lamotrigine and not "treat through" the rash with diphenhydramine. Gabapentin does not interact with lamotrigine. However, the combination of valproic acid and lamotrigine is associated with a higher incidence of rash. While abrupt discontinuation of an anticonvulsant may induce status epilepticus, an anticonvulsant may be abruptly discontinued in the face of a life-threatening event.

11. **D** is correct because the new anticonvulsant inhibits CYP450 3A4 and the antidepressant is metabolized by this enzyme.

12. **C.** At this time, neither gabapentin nor levetiracetam are associated with significant drug-drug interactions. The absorption of gabapentin may be reduced by concurrent administration of aluminum- and/or magnesium-containing antacids; hence antacids should be given 2 hours before or after a dose of gabapentin. Carbamazepine is an inducer that is associated with numerous drug-drug interactions.

13. **D.** Both topiramate and zonisamide may cause kidney stones. Although neither agent is contraindicated in an individual with a history of kidney stones, these drugs should be used cautiously in such patients. Patients should be counseled to remain adequately hydrated since this may decrease the risk of stone formation.

14. **D.** Both carbamazepine and felbamate are associated with aplastic anemia and hepatic failure. Levetiracetam has no black box warning.

15. **D.** Valproic acid may cause fatal hemorrhagic pancreatitis.

16. **C.** Although valproic acid is extremely effective and is frequently used as monotherapy for absence seizures, it should not be given to a patient ≤2 years of age.

17. **A.** Diastat is a commercially available gel form of diazepam that is given rectally.

18. **B.** Unlike simple febrile seizures that last a brief period, complex febrile seizures are prolonged (>15 minutes) and/or recur within 24 hours of the initial seizure. Febrile seizures must occur in the absence of CNS infection in a child with fever. Most febrile seizures are benign and children do not go on to develop epilepsy. Carbamazepine is ineffective in febrile seizures.

19. **A.** Only phenytoin is available as a liquid (125 mg/5 mL), chewable tablet (50 mg), and in an intravenous dosage form. Carbamazepine is not available in an IV dosage form and valproic acid is not available as a chewable tablet.

20. **B.** Because topiramate may cause kidney stones, patients should be encouraged to drink plenty of fluids. This would also be true for zonisamide.

21. **A.** Normeperidine, a metabolite of meperidine, can accumulate in patients with renal failure who receive normal doses and cause seizures. The other agents listed are not eliminated renally in adults.

22. **D.** Phenytoin has capacity-limited or saturable (ie, Michaelis-Menten) pharmacokinetics.

23. **B.** Phenytoin may cause gingival hyperplasia (ie, overgrowth of the gums). Hence patients should be instructed to brush and floss daily, and have regular visits with the dentist.

6. References

American Academy of Neurology. Quality Standards Subcommittee. Practice Parameter: A guideline for discontinuing antiepileptic drugs in seizure-free patients—summary statement. *Neurology.* 1996;47:660-702.

Anderson GD. A mechanistic approach to antiepileptic drug interactions. *Ann Pharmacother.* 1998;32:554-563.

Baumann RJ, Duffner PK. Treatment of children with simple febrile seizures: the AAP practice parameter. American Academy of Pediatrics. *Pediatr Neurol.* 2000;23:11-17.

Brunbech L, Sabers A. Effect of antiepileptic drugs on cognitive function in individuals with epilepsy: a comparative review of newer versus older agents. *Drugs.* 2002;62:593-604.

Carroll MC, Yueng-Yue KA, Esterly NB, et al. Drug-induced hypersensitivity syndrome in pediatric patients. *Pediatrics.* 2001;108:485-492.

Commission on antiepileptic drugs, International League Against Epilepsy. Guidelines for therapeutic monitoring on antiepileptic drugs. *Epilepsia.* 1993;34:585-587.

Deckers CL, Knoester PD, de Haan GJ, et al. Selection criteria for the clinical use of the newer antiepileptic drugs. *CNS Drugs.* 2003;17:405-421.

Johannessen SI, Battino D, Berry DJ, et al. Therapeutic drug monitoring of the newer antiepileptic drugs. *Ther Drug Monit.* 2003;25:347-463.

Perucca E. The clinical pharmacokinetics of the new antiepileptic drugs. *Epilepsia.* 1999;40(suppl 9):S7-S13.

Working Group on Status Epilepticus. Treatment of convulsive status epilepticus: Recommendations of the Epilepsy Foundation of America's Working Group on Status Epilepticus. *JAMA.* 1993;270:854-859.

25. Psychiatric Disease

Jason Carter, PharmD
Associate Professor of Psychopharmacology
University of Tennessee College of Pharmacy

Contents

1. Schizophrenia

Schizophrenia is a psychiatric disorder characterized by a profound disruption in perception, cognition, and emotion.

Epidemiology

- Approximately 1% of the U.S. adult population has schizophrenia.
- 200,000 new cases are reported yearly.
- No gender or racial differences
- Earlier onset in males (average age, 18-24) than females (average age, late 20s to early 40s)

Types and Classifications

Paranoid
- Prominent preoccupation with hallucinations (usually auditory) and one or more delusions

Disorganized
- Disorganized speech and behavior
- Blunted, flat, or inappropriate affect

Catatonic
- Psychomotor disturbances that may involve catalepsy or stupor, excessive motor activity, rigid posture, mutism, peculiar or repetitive movements, and/or echolalia or echopraxia

Undifferentiated
- Hallucinations/delusions are present but without prominent paranoid, disorganized, or catatonic symptoms.

Residual
- Hallucinations/delusions are not prominent, but there is continued evidence of an ongoing disturbance (flat affect, poverty of speech, or avolition).

Clinical Presentation

- The onset of schizophrenia is typically characterized by deterioration in occupational and social situations over a period of 6 months or more.

Symptoms
- Hallucinations (auditory, visual, tactile, olfactory, and/or gustatory)
- Delusions (usually persecutory and/or grandiose)
- Disorganized thoughts and/or speech
- Impaired cognition, attention, concentration, judgment, and motivation

- Symptoms are commonly referred to as positive (hallucinations or delusions), negative (flat affect, avolition, anhedonia, and poverty of thought), or disorganized (disorganized speech and/or behavior).
- Most patients fluctuate between acute episodes and remission, but complete remission without any symptoms is uncommon.

Associated Features
Morbidity
- There are many comorbid disease states (mental and medical), eg, substance abuse is found in 60%-70% of persons with schizophrenia.

Mortality
- Shortened life expectancy
- Increased risk of suicide (10% commit suicide).
- Risk factors for suicide:
  * Male gender, social isolation, comorbid psychiatric disorders, unemployed, <30 years of age

Etiology (Most Likely Multifactorial)

Genetic

Neurobiologic

Developmental
- Season of birth, viral, traumatic

DSM-IV Diagnostic Criteria

- Two or more of the following symptoms prevail for at least 1 month:
  * Hallucinations
  * Delusions
  * Disorganized speech
  * Grossly disorganized or catatonic behavior
  * Negative symptoms
  * Anhedonia
  * Flat affect
  * Avolition
- Significant social dysfunction
  * Signs of the disturbance are continuous and persist for 6 months.
  * Schizoaffective disorders and mood disorders, mental retardation, substance abuse, and other causative medical disorders have been ruled out.

Treatment Principles and Goals

- All antipsychotics are equally effective if used properly.
- Clozapine is the only agent proven effective in treating refractory schizophrenia.

- Basis for choosing an antipsychotic medication:
    * Past history of response (patient's response or a family member's response to a medication)
    * Side-effect profile of the antipsychotic
- Therapy with a trial of antipsychotics (at least 4-6 weeks at recommended doses)
- Do everything possible to simplify the drug regimen.
- Consider long-acting injectable preparations in situations of poor compliance.

Drug Therapy (Tables 1 and 2)

Mechanism of action
- These drugs block postsynaptic dopamine-2 receptors. They share anticholinergic, antihistaminic, and α-blocking properties.

Other conventional agents (not commonly used)
- Perphenazine (Trilafon®), thiothixene (Navane®), trifluoperazine (Stelazine®), and loxapine (Loxitane®)

Management of adverse effects
Sedation
- The level of sedation depends on the drug used; low-potency drugs in this class are more sedating than high-potency drugs.

- Sedation effects are worse initially, but become more tolerable over time.

Orthostasis
- Severity depends on the drug used; low-potency formulations promote more orthostasis than high-potency formulations.
- Especially problematic in elderly patients

Weight gain
- Very prominent in this population
- Use low doses; appropriate diet and exercise is encouraged to offset weight gain.

Anticholinergic
- Severity depends on the drug used; low-potency drugs of this type are more sedating than high-potency ones.
- Dry mouth, blurred vision, constipation, and/or urinary hesitancy may occur.
- Use high-potency agents in patients bothered by anticholinergic side effects.

Extrapyramidal symptoms (EPS)
- Most likely attributed to an imbalance in dopamine and acetylcholine; antipsychotics cause a hypodopaminergic state.

Table 1

Typical (Conventional or Older) Antipsychotics

Drug and form	Potency	Dosage range	Equivalent oral dose	Clinical pearls
Chlorpromazine (Thorazine®) 10, 25, 50, 100, 200 mg tabs; 30, 75, 150, 200, 300 mg SR caps; 10 mg/5 mL syrup; 30 mg/mL, 100 mg/mL concentrate; 25 mg, 100 mg rectal supp.; 25 mg/mL injection	Low	50-2000 mg/d	100 mg	First antipsychotic used clinically; contributed to deinstitutionalization of many patients in the 1950s; 100 mg of chlorpromazine is equivalent to 2 mg of haloperidol
Thioridazine (Mellaril®) 10, 15, 25, 50, 100, 150, 200 mg tabs; 25 mg/5 mL, 100 mg/5 mL susp.; 30 mg/mL, 100 mg/mL concentrate	Low	50-800 mg/d	100 mg	Pigmentary retinopathy at daily doses >800 mg/d; black box warning: QT prolongation
Fluphenazine (Prolixin®) 1, 2.5, 5, 10 mg tabs; 25 mg/mL decanoate injection; 2.5 mg/mL injection; 2.5 mg/5 mL elixir; 5 mg/mL concentrate	High	1-65 mg/d (PO); 12.5-75 mg IM (decanoate) every 2 weeks	2 mg	Decanoate injection given every 2 weeks; immediate-release injection, 5-10 min onset
Haloperidol (Haldol®) 0.5, 1, 2, 5, 10, 20 mg tabs; 2 mg/mL concentrate; 50, 100 mg/mL decanoate injection; 5 mg/mL injection	High	1-100 mg/d (PO); 50-300 mg IM (decanoate) every 4 weeks	2 mg	Decanoate injection given every 4 weeks; immediate-release injection, 5-10 min onset

Table 2

Adverse Effects of Typical Antipsychotic Medications

Drug	EPS	Sedation	Orthostasis	Weight gain	Anticholinergic
Chlorpromazine	+	+++	+++	+++	+++
Thioridazine	+	+++	+++	+++	+++
Fluphenazine	++++	+	+	+	+
Haloperidol	++++	+	+	+	+

EPS, extrapyramidal symptoms.

Dystonic reactions
- Usually occur within 24-96 hours of initiating or changing dose
- Present as painful, involuntary muscle spasms in skeletal muscles (most commonly in the facial/neck muscles; may also occur in back, arm, and leg muscles)
- Treatment: benztropine (Cogentin®) 1-2 mg IM or diphenhydramine (Benadryl®) 25-50 mg IM every 30 minutes until relieved
- Prophylaxis with oral therapy is usually initiated.

Akathisia
- Usually occurs within a few weeks of initiating antipsychotic therapy
- Described as a subjective feeling of discomfort usually seen as motor restlessness of the legs (inability to stand still or sit still)
- Treatment: lipophilic β-blockers (eg, propranolol), benzodiazepines, clonidine, and anticholinergics

Pseudoparkinsonism
- Usually occurs within months to years of therapy
- Resembles Parkinson's symptoms (eg, cogwheel rigidity, bradykinesia, tremor, shuffling gait)
- Treatment: amantadine (Symmetrel®) 100 mg bid or anticholinergics

Other adverse effects
Tardive dyskinesia (TD)
- Irreversible drug-induced movement disorder that occurs after years of antipsychotic therapy
- Due to long-term suppression of dopamine

Triad of symptoms
* Choreoathetosis: splayed, writhing fingers
* Oral/buccal movements: grimacing, bruxism, lip-smacking
* Protrusion of tongue

- Only treatment is prevention (ie, only use lowest effective dose of antipsychotic).
- Various therapies (vitamin E, lecithin, and vitamin B_6) may help alleviate symptoms.
- Monitor for TD by administering the Abnormal Involuntary Movement Scale (AIMS) to all patients taking antipsychotics.

Neuroleptic malignant syndrome (NMS)
- Low incidence, high mortality
- Thought to be due to dopamine blockade

Clinical presentation
* Rapid progression (<24 hours)
* Body temperature >104° F
* Lead-pipe rigidity
* Hypertension
* Diaphoresis
* Increased HR
* Incontinence
* Increased LFTs, CPK, WBCs
- Treatment: emergency room STAT, discontinue antipsychotic, administer supportive therapy (cooling blankets, hydration), bromocriptine (dopamine agonist), dantrolene (smooth muscle relaxant)

Endocrine and metabolic effects
- Amenorrhea, galactorrhea, and/or gynecomastia due to hyperprolactinemia
  * Dopamine regulates prolactin release; when dopamine is blocked, prolactin is elevated.
- Weight gain
- Decreased glucose tolerance

Dermatologic effects
(especially in long-term therapy)
- Allergy to medication, photosensitivity, pigmentation problems

Hypothalamic effects
- Temperature dysregulation, ie, sensitivity to extreme temperatures

Cardiac effects
- QT prolongation possible
- More common with thioridazine (black box warning)
- Recommendation: obtain an ECG for all patients on antipsychotics.

Ophthalmologic effects
- Pigmentary retinopathy is associated with daily thioridazine doses >800 mg; melanin deposits on cornea and may lead to blindness.

Atypical (newer) antipsychotics (Table 3)
- No universally accepted definition of "atypical"
  - * Less severe side effects (little or no EPS, minimal to no prolactin increase, less risk of TD)
  - * More weight gain, lipid abnormalities, and risk of diabetes

Table 3

Atypical Antipsychotics

Drug	Usual dose	Adverse effects	Clinical pearls
Clozapine (Clozaril®) 25, 100 mg tabs FazaClo® (disintegrating clozapine tabs) 25, 100 mg tabs **Note:** Indicated for refractory schizophrenia only	12.5 mg titrated up to 300-900 mg/d	Sedation; weight gain; hypersalivation (procyclidine [Kemadrin®] 5 mg may help); seizure risk (>600 mg/d); agranulocytosis; no EPS or TD	Weekly CBC w/differential required; WBC <3500 or ANC <1500 **must** discontinue; if stable CBC w/differential for 6 months, may go to biweekly; if stable and additional 6 months may go to every 4 weeks.
Risperidone (Risperdal®) 0.25, 0.5, 1, 2, 3, 4 mg tabs; 1 mg/mL concentrate Risperdal-M® (disintegrating risperidone tabs) 0.5, 1, 2 mg Risperdal Consta® (long-acting injection) 25, 37.5, 50 mg	1 mg bid up to 4-6 mg/d; max dose 16 mg/d	Dose-related EPS (>8 mg/d); +/– weight gain; +/– sedation; prolactin elevation; orthostasis sedation; weight gain; possible dose-related EPS	Available in concentrate; don't mix with teas or colas; used commonly in dementia (0.25-1 mg); must overlap Consta with oral risperidone for at least 3 weeks
Olanzapine (Zyprexa®) 2.5, 5, 7.5, 10, 15, 20 mg tabs Zyprexa Zydis® (disintegrating olanzapine tabs) 5, 10, 15, 20 mg 10 mg/mL injection	10-20 mg/d; higher doses have been reported 10 mg IM x 1 repeat in 2 and 4h, max IM daily dose 30 mg	Sedation; orthostasis Sedation; weight gain; or thostasis	Olanzapine is also indicated for acute manic episodes of bipolar disorder; Zydis useful for patients who are unable to swallow or are "cheeking" meds
Quetiapine (Seroquel®) 25, 100, 200, 300 mg tabs	300-800 mg/d; higher doses have been reported		Low EPS and prolactin elevation risk
Ziprasidone (Geodon®) 20, 40, 60, 80 mg caps; 20 mg/mL injection	40-160 mg/d (PO); 20 mg IM x 1 dose (may repeat in 4 h; max IM daily dose 40 mg)	+/– Sedation; +/– weight gain; QT prolongation warning in package insert	Use caution with other meds that prolong QT interval
Aripiprazole (Abilify®) 2, 5, 10, 15, 20, 30 mg tabs 1 mg/mL concentrate	10-30 mg/d	Possible insomnia; +/– weight gain	Once daily dosing benefit; partial dopamine agonist
Paliperidone (Invega®) 3, 6, 9 mm extended release tabs	6 mg/d; max dose 12 mg/d	Headache; tachycardia; somnolence; anxiety	Sustained release tablet: do not crush or chew; tablet shell may be seen in stool

* Decreased affinity for the dopamine receptor
* Black box warning for increase in mortality with atypical antipsychotics in elderly patients with dementia, also atypical antipsychotics are not approved for the treatment of patients with dementia-related psychosis

Mechanism of action

* These drugs are weak dopamine and dopamine-2 receptor blockers that block serotonin and α-adrenergic, histaminic, and muscarinic receptors in the central nervous system.

Treatment Strategies

Acute schizophrenia

* Decrease danger to self and/or others
* May use haloperidol or fluphenazine (immediate-release) 5-10 mg IM and lorazepam 2 mg IM q4h prn for psychosis/agitation; an anticholinergic may also be needed (eg, benztropine or diphenhydramine for EPS)
* May use olanzapine 10 mg IM, can repeat in 2 hours and again 4 hours later, maximum of 30 mg per day for psychosis/agitation
* May use ziprasidone 10 mg IM administered every 2 hours or 20 mg IM administered every 4 hours to a maximum of 40 mg/day for psychosis/agitation

Maintenance

* Start an atypical antipsychotic at a recommended dose or continue conventional agent (if it was effective for patient before hospital admission).
* Positive symptoms will respond first.
* Monitor for side effects; emphasize compliance.
* Lifelong therapy is usually needed.
* Use lowest effective dose to decrease risk of side effects (eg, TD)

Recommended monitoring for patients on atypical antipsychotics

* Fasting glucose and lipids, blood pressure at baseline and 12 weeks
* Weight (BMI) at baseline, 4 weeks, 8 weeks, 12 weeks, then quarterly
* Waist circumference baseline then annually

Noncompliance and alternative dosing

Haloperidol decanoate (Haldol-D®)

* Conversion from PO to IM: PO daily dose x 10 = IM dose every 4 weeks
    * Example: 20 mg daily dose x 10 = 200 mg every 4 weeks
    * Reaches steady state in 8-12 weeks

Fluphenazine decanoate (Prolixin-D®)

* Conversion from PO to IM: 1 mg PO = 1.25 mg IM
    * Example: 20 mg daily dose x 1.25 mg = 25 mg IM every 2 weeks
    * Reaches steady state in approximately 6 weeks

Depot administration technique

* Both medications are suspended in sesame seed oil (they are very viscous; ensure no allergy to sesame seed oil)
* Must administer in gluteal or deltoid muscle with a 16- or 18-gauge needle

Risperidone long-acting injection (Risperdal Consta®)

* Must overlap with PO medication for 3 weeks
* Reaches steady state in approximately 8 weeks
* Must use diluent and needle supplied in the pack to reconstitute and administer injection

2. Bipolar Disorder

Bipolar disorder (manic-depressive illness) is a recurrent mood disorder with a lifetime prevalence of 0.8%-1.6%

- Associated with significant morbidity and mortality
- Incidence is equal in women and men.
- Onset is usually between the ages of 18 and 44.
- The first episode for women is usually marked by a depressive episode; for men, a manic episode.

Types and Classifications

Bipolar I
- Characterized by the occurrence of manic episodes and major depressive episodes

Bipolar II
- Characterized by the occurrence of hypomanic episodes and major depressive episodes

Cyclothymia
- Defined as numerous episodes of hypomania and depressive episodes that cannot be classified as major depressive episodes; diagnosis requires that cyclothymia occur for at least a 2-year period

Clinical Presentation
(see *DSM-IV* for complete diagnostic criteria)

Mania
- Characterized by heightened mood (euphoria), flight of ideas, rapid or pressured speech, grandiosity, increased energy, decreased need for sleep, irritability, and impulsivity
- Judgment is significantly impaired, eg, increased risk-taking behavior.
- Marked impairment in social and/or occupational functioning
- Psychotic features are usually present; hospitalization is needed.
- Changes in sleeping patterns (especially insomnia) commonly initiate manic episodes

Hypomania
- Less severe form of mania
- Usually does not cause marked impairment in social and/or occupational functioning
- Many patients find this state highly desirable because they experience a great sense of well-being and feel productive, creative, and/or confident.

Dysphoric (or mixed) mania
- Characterized by manic and depressive features, mood variability, and mood lability
- Symptoms usually include agitation, insomnia, suicidal ideation, psychosis, and appetite disturbances

Major depression
- See section on depression

Rapid cycling
- Patient experiences >4 mood episodes in a year
- Mood episodes may occur in any combination.
- Rapid cycling primarily occurs in women (70%-90%).
- Usually poor prognosis

Etiology

- Unknown
- The leading hypothesis supports genetic etiology.
- Other theories include neurotransmitter involvement, circadian rhythm, and kindling hypothesis.

Clinical Course

- Mean age of onset is 21 years
- First episode for women is usually depression, and for men, mania
- Untreated episodes may last from weeks to months.
- High mortality rate due to suicide
- Comorbid substance abuse is very common (60%-70%).

Treatment Principles and Goals

Acute
- Control the current episode (slow patient down, reduce harm to self and/or others).

Maintenance
- Prevent or minimize future episodes.
- Maintain drug therapy and reduce adverse effects.
- Prevent drug interactions.
- Educate the patient and family about the disorder.
- Provide adequate follow-up services (including substance abuse treatment).
- Maximize the patient's functional status and quality of life.

Drug Therapy (Table 4)

Lithium
Indications
- Acute treatment and prophylaxis of manic episodes associated with bipolar disorders; effective for both the manic and depressive components

Table 4

Mood Stabilizers

Drug and form	Usual dose	Adverse effects	Clinical pearls
Lithium (Lithobid®, Eskalith CR®) 150, 300, 600 mg caps; 300 mg, 450 mg (CR) tabs; 300 mg (SR) tabs; syrup, as citrate 300 mg/5 mL (Cibalith-S®)	Starting: 900-1200 mg in divided doses; titrate to desired response/level	Tremor; polydipsia/polyuria; nausea/diarrhea; weight gain; hypothyroidism; mental dulling	Many drug interactions; toxicity is a concern (pregnancy category D); monitor blood levels—acute: 0.6-1.2 mEq/L; maintenance: 0.8-1.0 mEq/L
Divalproex sodium (Depakote®) 125, 250, 500 mg tabs; 250, 500 mg (ER) tabs	Starting: 500 mg; bid-tid or 15 mg/kg; max dose 60 mg/kg per day	GI upset; sedation, tremor; weight gain; alopecia; transient elevation in LFTs	Black box warnings: hepatotoxicity; hemorrhagic pancreatitis; teratogenicity (pregnancy category D); monitor blood levels—50-125 mcg/mL
Carbamazepine (Tegretol®) (see text for contraindications) 200 mg tabs; 100 mg chew tabs; 100, 200, 400 mg ER tabs; 100 mg/5 mL susp.	Starting: 200 mg bid; increase to 800-1200 mg/d (tid-qid doses); usual range 400-1600 mg/d	Ataxia; dizziness; sedation; slurred speech; aplastic anemia	Many drug interactions (pregnancy category C); monitor blood levels—4-12 mcg/mL
Lamotrigine (Lamictal®) 25, 100, 150, 200 mg tabs; 2 , 5, 25 mg chew tabs	Starting: 25 mg/day weeks 1 & 2; 50 mg/day week 5; 200 mg/day week 6; 200 mg/day usual dose	Dizziness; headache; ataxia; nausea; diplopia; rash	Black box warning: sever rashes such as Stevens-Johnson Syndrome; start at 25 mg titrate to 200 mg over 6 weeks to help prevent rash

Mechanism of action
- Unknown
- Various theories: lithium facilitates gamma-aminobutyric acid function, alters cation transport across cell membranes in nerve and muscle cells, and/or influences reuptake of 5-HT and/or norepinephrine (NE).

Contraindications
- Renal disease, severe cardiovascular disease, history of leukemia, first trimester of pregnancy, hypersensitivity to lithium

Precautions
- Use with caution in patients with thyroid disease, sodium depletion, patients receiving diuretics, or dehydrated patients.

Monitoring (baseline/follow-up)
Thyroid panel
- Lithium may cause hypothyroidism; baseline and TSH every 6-12 months or as clinically indicated.

SCr/BUN
- Lithium is 100% renally eliminated; baseline and every 3 months for patients with renal dysfunction; every 12 months otherwise or as clinically indicated.

CBC w/differential
- Lithium may cause leukocytosis and may reactivate leukemia; baseline and every month for 3 months, then as clinically indicated.

Electrolytes
- In the event of hyponatremia, lithium toxicity may occur.

ECG
- Lithium causes flattened or inverted T waves, which is reversible; baseline and every 6-12 months or as clinically indicated

Urinalysis
- Lithium may decrease specific gravity.

Pregnancy test
- Lithium may cause cardiovascular defects (eg, Ebstein's anomaly).

Table 5

Drug Interactions with Lithium

Increase level of lithium	Decrease level of lithium
NSAIDs	Theophylline
ACE inhibitors	Caffeine
Fluoxetine	Pregnancy
Metronidazole	Osmotic diuretics (mannitol, urea)
Diuretics (eg, thiazides)	
Sodium depletion	
Low sodium diet	
Excessive	
exercise/sweating	
Vomiting/diarrhea	
Salt deficiency	

Lithium level
- Reaches steady-state levels in 4-5 days ($t_{1/2}$ = ~24 h); obtain level 2-8 hours post-dose (acute: 0.6-1.2 mEq/L; maintenance: 0.8-1.0 mEq/L); draw level weekly for 4 weeks then monthly for 3 months or as clinically indicated.

Drug Interactions (Table 5)

Toxicity concerns
Mild toxicity (serum levels 1.5-2.0 mEq/L)
- GI upset (nausea/vomiting/diarrhea), muscle weakness, fatigue, fine hand tremor, difficulty with concentration and memory

Moderate toxicity (serum levels 2.0-2.5 mEq/L)
- Ataxia, lethargy, nystagmus, worsening confusion, severe GI upset, coarse tremors, increased deep tendon reflexes

Severe toxicity (serum levels >3.0 mEq/L)
- Severely impaired consciousness, coma, seizures, respiratory complications, death

Treatment of toxicity
- Discontinue lithium and initiate gastric lavage.
- Correct electrolyte and fluid imbalances.
- Monitor neurologic changes.
- Give supportive care.
- Give dialysis if indicated.

Patient information
- Monitoring serum lithium levels routinely is important; maintain a steady salt and fluid intake; do not crush or chew extended- or slow-release dosage forms.

Divalproex sodium
Indication (as related to bipolar disorder)
   Acute manic episodes
- *Note:* Considered first-line treatment; unlabeled use for prophylaxis of manic episodes; effective for rapid cyclers and patients with dysphoric mood; helpful in the management of agitation/aggression

Mechanism of action
- Unknown, but divalproex sodium is thought to increase GABA or mimic its action at the postsynaptic receptor site.

Contraindications
- Hepatic dysfunction
- Pregnancy
  - * Valproic acid may cause neural tube defects; if benefit outweighs risk, supplement with 4-5 mg/d of folic acid to decrease risk of fetal damage
- Hypersensitivity to divalproex sodium
- Patients <2 years old

Monitoring
- Valproic acid level reaches steady state in 3-5 days ($t_{1/2}$ = 9-16 h); 50-125 mcg/mL optimal.
- Draw level weekly for 2-3 weeks, then every 3 months or as clinically indicated.

   LFTs
- Baseline and every month for 6 months, then every 6 months or as clinically indicated
- Divalproex sodium is hepatically eliminated; carries black box warning for hepatotoxicity

   CBC with differential
- Baseline and every month for 6 months, then every 6 months or as clinically indicated
- Valproic acid may cause thrombocytopenia.

Drug interactions
- Cytochrome P450 (CYP450) 2C19 enzyme substrate; CYP450-2C9 and -2D6 inhibitor, weak CYP450-3A3/4 inhibitor
- Carbamazepine, lamotrigine, and phenytoin
  - * Increased sedative effects with phenobarbital and benzodiazepines.

Patient information
- Take with food to avoid GI upset; take a multivitamin with selenium and zinc if alopecia (hair loss) occurs.
- Important to monitor VPA levels routinely

Carbamazepine (CBZ)
- Considered second-line therapy for acute and prophylactic treatment of bipolar disorder

Mechanism of action
- Unknown

Monitoring
- CBC with differential, electrolytes, LFTs, SCr/BUN, ECG (if age >40 or pre-existing heart disease)
- CBZ is an autoinducer; monitor levels routinely, especially during first few months of therapy.
- 4-12 mcg/mL = optimal

Contraindications
- History of previous bone marrow depression, hypersensitivity to CBZ

Drug interactions
- CYP450-2C8 and -3A3/4 enzyme substrate
- CYP450-1A2, -2C, and -3A3/4 inducer
- CBZ may induce the metabolism of benzodiazepines, clozapine, corticosteroids, oral contraceptives, VPA, warfarin, phenytoin, and tricyclic antidepressants (plus others).
- Cimetidine, clarithromycin, diltiazem, propoxyphene, verapamil, metronidazole, and lamotrigine (plus others) inhibit CBZ.

Lamotrigine (Lamictal®)
- Approved for maintenance treatment of Bipolar I disorder
- Titration of dose is required to monitor for signs/symptoms of severe and potentially life-threatening skin rashes (co-administration with VPA increases risk)

Atypical antipsychotics
- Approved for treatment of bipolar disorder; olanzapine/Fluoxetine (Symbyax®) is indicated for the treatment of depressive episodes associated with bipolar disorder

Drug interactions and effects
- CBZ, phenytoin, oral contraceptives, rifampin, and phenobarbital decrease lamotrigine concentrations
- Valproic acid increases lamotrigine concentrations
- Adverse effects: nausea, headache, tremor/anxiety, and sedation

Other therapies
Gabapentin (Neurontin®)
- May be useful as adjunctive therapy for bipolar disorder
- No significant drug interactions
- No required drug serum level monitoring

- Renally eliminated
- Mild sedative effects (sedation, ataxia, fatigue)

Oxcarbazepine (Trileptal®)
- Structurally similar to CBZ (keto-analogue of CBZ)
- At times utilized as a mood stabilizer in some patients with bipolar disorder, but further studies are needed.
- No autoinduction problems, no drug serum levels to monitor
- Appears to have fewer drug-drug interactions than CBZ

Topiramate (Topamax®)
- May be useful for treatment of bipolar disorder, but further studies are needed.
- Doses are usually lower than those indicated for treating seizure disorders.
- May cause weight loss

Calcium channel blockers
- Usually reserved as last-line therapy
- Data in the literature are inconsistent about using verapamil for mania (other CCBs may be effective).
- Not routinely utilized
- Possible for use in pregnancy

3. Major Depression

Major depression is a prevalent and serious illness in the U.S.

- It affects 10-14 million people of all ages.
- It is treatable but grossly undertreated.
- Most cases go unrecognized, which may be due to the social stigma surrounding depression.
- Several myths contribute to the problem of under-treatment (eg, that it is due to personal weakness or an inability to handle life's problems).

Epidemiology

- Lifetime prevalence rate is 17%.
    * 1 out of 4 females (10%-24%)
    * 1 out of 8 males (5%-12%)
- Most common between the ages of 25 and 44 years

Risk factors
- Family history
- Female gender
- Previous depressive episode
- Previous suicide attempt
- Comorbid medical or substance abuse disorder

Etiology

- Unknown
- There are many different hypotheses, including:
    * Dysregulation of neurotransmitters
    * Decreased concentration of certain neuro-transmitters
    * Genetic basis for the disorder

Clinical Presentation

Physical findings
- Fatigue
- Pain (ie, headaches, back pain, GI upset)
- Sleep disturbances (usually insomnia)
- Appetite disturbances (usually decreased appetite)
- Psychomotor retardation or agitation

Emotional symptoms
- Anhedonia
- Depressed mood for most of the day
- Hopelessness/helplessness
- Inappropriate feelings of guilt and worthlessness
- Anxiety/worry
- Suicidal ideation

Cognitive symptoms
- Decreased ability to concentrate
- Indecisiveness

Laboratory studies
- There are no diagnostic laboratory tests for depression, but the following lab work should be conducted to rule out other medical illnesses that may manifest as depressive symptoms:
    * CBC with differential
    * Thyroid function tests
    * Rapid plasma reagin (RPR) (test for syphilis)
    * Urine drug screen (UDS)
- Medical conditions that may contribute to the development or worsening of depression:
    * MI, CVA, Parkinson's, MS, SLE, HIV, RA, thyroid abnormalities, DM, cancer, vitamin deficiency
- Possible drug-induced causes of depression should also be ruled out:
    * Corticosteroids, oral contraceptives, propranolol, clonidine, methyldopa

Prognosis

- 70% of patients are responsive to antidepressant therapy.
- Following the first episode, 50%-60% of patients will have another episode; following the second episode, 70%-80% will have a third; following the third, 90% will have another.
- If untreated, an episode may resolve spontaneously within 6 to 24 months
- Approximately 15% of patients will commit suicide.
    * Risk factors for suicide: male gender, >50 years old, unemployed status, recent loss of job/spouse, social isolation, presence of a weapon, comorbid substance abuse
    * *Note:* Males are more likely to commit suicide; females are more likely to attempt suicide; males commonly use more violent means of suicide (eg, firearms, hanging) than females (eg, slashing of wrists, drug overdoses).

DSM-IV Diagnostic Criteria

- At least five symptoms (see clinical presentation section above) must be present mostly every day for a 2-week period and represent a change from previous functioning; at least one of the symptoms must be depressed mood or anhedonia.

Treatment Principles and Goals

- Improve patient's ability to function and quality of life.
- Reduce or eliminate target symptoms with an antidepressant.
- Incorporating psychotherapy is optimal.
- Prevent relapse

- All antidepressants are equally effective in a given population.
    * Response varies from person to person.
    * Each differs in side-effect and drug-interaction profiles.
    * None are "speed" or "uppers."
- *Note:* The FDA now requires all antidepressant drugs to include boxed warnings about increased risk of suicidal ideation and behavior in children and adolescents, and young adults (up to age 24), and a medication guide highlighting these risks is to be distributed with each new or refilled prescription for antidepressants in this population.

Basis for choosing an agent
- Past history of a patient's response or a family member's response to certain agent(s)
- Side-effect profile and how it relates to any given patient's situation

Monitoring parameters
First week
- Patient should demonstrate decreased anxiety.
- Trend towards normalization of appetite and sleep pattern

Second to third week
- Increase in energy
- *Note:* There is an increased risk for suicide at this time because the patient has the energy to carry out any ideations.
- Improvement in concentration and memory
- Improvement in somatic symptoms

Four to six weeks
- Improvement in mood
- Decreased suicidal ideation
- Increased libido

Duration of therapy
Acute phase
- The duration is usually 6-12 weeks or the length of time needed to stabilize depressive symptoms.

Maintenance phase
- Maintain therapeutic doses of antidepressant.
- Usually 1-year duration; may taper antidepressant for a period of time and monitor for signs of relapse
- The goal is to prevent relapse.

Prophylaxis
- Chronic antidepressant therapy may be necessary for certain patients.
- Those with a first-degree relative with bipolar disorder or recurrent depression

- Onset before age 20 or after age 60
- Recurrence within 1 year after medication discontinuation
- Severe, sudden, or life-threatening depression

Drug Therapy (Table 6)

Tricyclic antidepressants
Mechanism of action
- TCAs increase the synaptic concentration of 5-HT and/or norepinephrine in the CNS, ie, TCAs inhibit the presynaptic neuronal membrane's reuptake of 5-HT and/or NE.

Other information about TCAs
- Doses may be titrated to full dose range over 1-3 weeks.
- Many patients are dosed half-strength due to sedative effects; however, for patients with insomnia, the sedating effects may be helpful.
- Deadly in overdose (blocks sinoatrial node in the heart)
- Drug serum levels are not commonly utilized in guiding therapy, but monitoring may be useful in patients taking amitriptyline, desipramine, imipramine, or nortriptyline.

Adverse effects
- Orthostatic hypotension, tachycardia, sedation, anticholinergic effects, arrhythmias (prolonged QT interval), weight gain, sexual dysfunction
- Tertiary amines (eg, amitriptyline, imipramine, doxepin, and clomipramine) have more intense adverse effects compared to secondary amines (eg, nortriptyline, desipramine).

Contraindications
- Concomitant use of an MAOI within the last 14 days, pregnancy, lactation, and narrow-angle glaucoma

Precautions
- Use with caution in patients with cardiac conduction disturbances, seizure disorders, hyperthyroidism, and renal or hepatic impairment; avoid abrupt withdrawal in patients with prolonged use

Drug interactions
- Increase in TCA level increases the levels of SSRIs (selective serotonin reuptake inhibitors), cimetidine, diltiazem, verapamil, labetalol, propoxyphene, quinidine, haloperidol, and methylphenidate
- Decrease in TCA level affects CBZ, phenytoin, and barbiturate metabolism
- Administration with MAOIs may cause serotonin syndrome.

Table 6

Tricyclic Antidepressants (TCAs)

Drug and form	Indications	Initial dose (mg/d)	Dose range (mg)
Amitriptyline (Elavil®) 10, 25, 50, 75, 100, 150 mg tabs; 10 mg/mL injection (pregnancy category D)	Depression; chronic and neuropathic pain; migraine prophylaxis; peripheral neuropathy	50-75	75-300
Nortriptyline (Pamelor®, Aventyl®) 10, 25, 50, 75 mg caps; 10 mg/5 mL injection (pregnancy category D)	Depression; chronic pain	25-50	40-200
Imipramine (Tofranil®) 75, 100, 125, 150 mg pamoate capsule (Tofranil-PM®); 10, 25, 50 mg tabs; 12.5 mg/mL injection (pregnancy category D)	Depression; childhood enuresis; chronic and neuropathic pain	50-75	75-300
Doxepin (Sinequan®) 10, 25, 50, 75, 100, 150 mg caps; 10 mg/mL concentrate; 5% cream (pregnancy category C)	Depression; anxiety; unlabeled: chronic and neuropathic pain	75 (in divided doses)	75-300
Clomipramine (Anafranil®) 25, 50, 75 mg (pregnancy category C)	Obsessive-compulsive disorder; depression; panic attacks; chronic pain	25-100 mg qd, titrated up for 1-2 weeks	Usual effective dose 200-250 mg/d; max dose 250 mg due to dose-related increased risk of seizure
Desipramine (Norpramin®) 10, 25, 50, 75, 100, 150 mg tabs (pregnancy category C)	Depression; chronic pain; unlabeled: peripheral neuropathy	50-75	75-300

- Monitoring BP, pulse, ECG changes, and mental status changes is prudent; drug serum monitoring may be useful for amitriptyline, desipramine, imipramine, and nortriptyline.

Monoamine oxidase inhibitors (MAOIs) (Table 7)
Mechanism of action
- MAOIs increase the synaptic concentration of NE, 5-HT, and DA by inhibiting the breakdown enzyme, monoamine oxidase.
- *Note:* May be useful for patients who do not respond to other antidepressants and/or to treat atypical depression; MAOIs are rarely utilized due to the need for dietary restrictions, side-effect profile, and potentially dangerous interactions with other medications.

Adverse effects
- Orthostatic hypotension, weight gain, sexual dys-

function, anticholinergic effects, and hypertensive crisis

Contraindications
- Renal or hepatic dysfunction, CVD, concomitant sympathomimetic therapy (eg, pseudoephedrine, ephedra); MAOIs cannot be used within 5 weeks of fluoxetine or within 2 weeks of any other SSRI.

Precautions
- Drug-food interaction with tyramine-containing foods (eg, red wine, aged cheeses, and marmite)

Drug interactions
- TCAs, SSRIs, sympathomimetics, and meperidine

Table 7

Monoamine Oxidase Inhibitors (MAOIs)

Drug	Initial dose	Dose titration	Dose range
Phenelzine (Nardil®) 15 mg tabs	15 mg tid (>16 years old)	Increase by 15 mg/week	60-90 mg/d
Tranylcypromine (Parnate®) 10 mg tabs	30 mg/d in divided doses	Increase by 10 mg/d every 1-3 weeks	30-60 mg/d

Selective serotonin reuptake inhibitors (Table 8)

Mechanism of action

- These agents selectively inhibit the reuptake of 5-HT.
- *Note:* All SSRIs should be tapered upon discontinuing treatment (over 2-4 weeks), except fluoxetine; side effects with abrupt withdrawal include flu-like symptoms, dizziness, nausea, tremor, anxiety, and palpitations.

Adverse effects

- GI complaints, nervousness, insomnia, headache, fatigue, and sexual dysfunction, but safer in overdose compared to TCAs

Drug interactions

- TCAs, MAOIs, and SSRIs (variable depending on which SSRI; escitalopram and citalopram reportedly have fewer drug interactions)

Other classes of antidepressant medication

Venlafaxine (Effexor®, Effexor XR®)

Mechanism of action

- Inhibits the reuptake of 5-HT and NE (and also DA at higher doses); it is frequently referred to as a serotonin-norepinephrine reuptake inhibitor (SNRI);

Table 8

Selective Serotonin Reuptake Inhibitors (SSRIs)

Drug and form	Initial dose	Usual dose	Clinical pearls
Citalopram (Celexa®) 10, 20, 40 mg tabs; 10 mg/5 mL syrup	10 mg	20-40 mg/d; max dose 60 mg/d	Used in geriatric patients; fewer drug interactions
Escitalopram (Lexapro®) 5, 10, 20 mg tabs	10 mg	10-20 mg/d	S-isomer of citalopram; 40 mg Celexa = 10 mg Lexapro
Fluvoxamine (Luvox®) 50, 100 mg tabs	50 mg	100-300 mg/d	Available in generic; primarily used for OCD drug interactions
Paroxetine (Paxil®) 10, 20, 30, 40 mg tabs; 10 mg/5 mL susp.	10-20 mg	10-40 mg; max dose 50 mg/d	Least-activating SSRI
Paroxetine (Paxil CR®) 12.5, 25, 37.5 mg tabs	12.5-25 mg	25-37.5 mg	CR formulation associated with fewer side effects; 10 mg Paxil = 12.5 mg Paxil CR
Fluoxetine (Prozac®, Sarafem®) 10, 20, 40 mg caps; 10, 20 mg tabs; 20 mg/5 mL syrup; 90 mg caps	10-20 mg	20-80 mg/d	Longer $t_{1/2}$, so tapering unnecessary; 90 mg formulation given once weekly
Sertraline (Zoloft®) 25, 50, 100 mg tabs; 20 mg/mL concentrate	25-50 mg	50-100 mg/d; max dose 200 mg/d	Used in geriatric patients; fewer drug interactions

anticholinergic and antihistaminic effects are negligible; as dose increases, NE and DA reuptake are more pronounced.

Adverse effects

- GI upset, anxiety, insomnia, headache, elevation in BP possible (use with caution in patients with uncontrolled hypertension); XR formulation is available to minimize GI upset; other side effects are similar to those with SSRIs; withdrawal symptoms may occur if abruptly discontinued

Drug interactions

- Cimetidine inhibits venlafaxine metabolism; cyproheptadine induces venlafaxine metabolism; "serotonin syndrome" seen in combination with sibutramine, sumatriptan, tramadol, and trazodone; PT/INR elevations have been seen when adding venlafaxine to patients taking warfarin
- *Note:* Indicated for both generalized anxiety disorder (GAD) and major depression; not recommended in patients with uncontrolled hypertension or recent MI or CV disorders

Duloxetine (Cymbalta®)
Mechanism of action

- Similar to venlafaxine; potent inhibitor of 5-HT and NE; no significant affinity for dopaminergic, adrenergic, cholinergic, or histaminergic receptors

Adverse effects

- GI upset, dry mouth, dizziness, decreased appetite, elevation in blood pressure, other similar side effects to those of SSRIs; urinary hesitation; may have withdrawal symptoms with abrupt withdrawal

Drug interactions

- CYP1A2 inhibitors (eg, cimetidine, quinolone antibiotics) and CYP2D6 inhibitors (eg, fluoxetine, quinidine) increase duloxetine levels; combination of duloxetine with triptans and serotonergic drugs may cause "serotonin syndrome"
- *Note:* Indicated for both major depression (20 or 30 mg bid or 60 mg qd) and diabetic peripheral neuropathic pain (60 mg qd); metabolized by CYP450-1A2 and 2D6, and inhibitors may increase plasma levels of duloxetine, causing increased side effects; contraindicated in uncontrolled narrow-angle glaucoma

Bupropion (Wellbutrin®, Wellbutrin SR®, Wellbutrin XL®, Zyban®)
Mechanism of action

- Bupropion, an inhibitor of NE and DA reuptake (effects on 5-HT reuptake are minimal), is referred to as a norepinephrine-dopamine reuptake inhibitor (NDRI).

Adverse effects

- GI upset, insomnia, anxiety, headache, and psychosis (rare); it is associated with less sexual dysfunction than SSRIs and other classes; it decreases the seizure threshold (see Note, below).

Drug interactions

- Cimetidine and ritonavir inhibit bupropion metabolism; CBZ induces bupropion metabolism.
- *Note:* There is an increased risk of seizure with bupropion, especially in patients with a seizure disorder, eating disorder, or electrolyte imbalance; maximum daily dose is 450 mg (400 mg SR); titrate the dose slowly to minimize seizure risk; bupropion is marketed as Zyban® for smoking cessation.

Trazodone (Desyrel®)
Mechanism of action

- Inhibits 5-HT reuptake and blocks 5-HT$_{2A}$ receptors

Adverse effects

- Extremely sedating, orthostatic hypotension, and priapism; there are no anticholinergic or cardiotoxic effects

Drug interactions

- Fluoxetine and ritonavir inhibit trazodone metabolism.

- *Note:* Due to excessive sedation, trazodone is not clinically used as an antidepressant; rather, it is commonly used to treat insomnia (usually dosed 25-150 mg qhs for insomnia).

Nefazodone (Serzone®)
Mechanism of action

- Inhibits 5-HT and NE uptake and blocks 5-HT$_{2A}$ receptors

Adverse effects

- GI upset, sedation, dry mouth, constipation, lightheadedness; it is associated with minimal sexual dysfunction and/or orthostatic hypotension.

Drug interactions

- Potent inhibitor of CYP3A4 isoenzyme; use with caution with drugs metabolized via this enzyme (eg, buspirone, HMG-CoA reductase inhibitors, alprazolam, triazolam, and digoxin); ritonavir inhibits nefazodone metabolism.
- *Note:* Usually dosed bid due to short half-life; there is a black box warning for hepatotoxicity.

Mirtazapine (Remeron®, Remeron Soltab®)
(7.5, 15, 30, and 45 mg tabs)

Mechanism of action

- Antagonizes presynaptic α_2 autoreceptors and heteroreceptors that prevent the release of 5-HT and NE (resulting in increased 5-HT and NE in the synapses); it antagonizes 5-HT_{2A} and 5-HT_3 receptors, resulting in less GI upset and less anxiety.

Adverse effects

- Sedation, increased appetite, weight gain, constipation; elevation in LFTs, increase in TGs; there is a small risk of agranulocytosis or neutropenia.
- *Note:* May be useful in geriatric patients since it causes increased appetite, is sedating, and there are no significant drug interactions.

Selegiline (Emsam®)
(6, 9, and 12 mg/24hr patches)

Mechanism of action

- Not fully understood, believe to be linked to selegiline irreversibly inhibiting monoamine oxidase

Adverse effects

- Headache, insomnia, application site reaction, diarrhea, dry mouth
- *Note:* No dietary restrictions for 6 mg dose

Psychostimulants

- Methylphenidate has been used to treat depression (especially in the geriatric population) and has been shown to increase activity level as well as improve mood symptoms; it may cause GI upset, insomnia, and CV effects; use with caution in anxious or psychotic patients; it inhibits TCA metabolism.

Nonpharmacologic Treatments

- Psychotherapy is especially useful combined with drug therapy.

Electroconvulsive therapy (ECT)

- Very safe and effective for treating depression
- Believed to physically "reset" receptors in the brain
- Usually reserved for refractory or psychotic patients

Procedure

- Patient is anesthetized and paralyzed in an outpatient setting.
- Patient is monitored via EEG during the procedure, and a seizure is induced for 30-90 seconds.

Acute treatment

- Administered every other day for 6-9 treatments

- Maintenance treatment is variable for each patient, but ECT is usually administered monthly after acute treatment.

Adverse effects

- Short-term memory loss, confusion on the day of treatment

Relative contraindications

- Increases intracranial pressure, and therefore is not recommended in patients with recent MI, intracerebral hemorrhage, or cerebral lesions

4. Anxiety Disorders

Anxiety disorders are serious, debilitating mental illnesses that include a group of conditions that share extreme anxiety as the primary mood disturbance.

Epidemiology

- It affects approximately 19 million adults in the U.S.
- There are no racial or cultural differences; gender differences depend on the specific anxiety disorder.
- There is significant comorbidity with other psychiatric illnesses (eg, substance abuse).

Types and Classifications

Generalized anxiety disorder (GAD)
- Characterized by unprovoked excessive worry and tension; anxiety usually consumes the patient's day, thereby affecting social and occupational functioning; physical complaints (eg, GI upset, headache, muscle tension, tremors, insomnia, and/or fatigue) are common; incidence is higher in females than in males

Panic disorder with or without agoraphobia (PD)
- Characterized by feelings of terror that suddenly strike without warning and usually last for approximately 10-15 minutes

Physical symptoms
- Increased HR, sweating, tremors, shortness of breath, chest pain, and/or dizziness; patient feels as if death is imminent.
- Agoraphobia (fear of open or public places) usually develops later in the illness, especially if PD is not treated; agoraphobic patients associate panic attacks with certain places and occasions, so they avoid going out and remain at home; agoraphobia is more prevalent in females than in males.

Obsessive-compulsive disorder (OCD)
- Characterized by intrusive, recurrent, and repetitive thoughts that severely interfere with the patient's social and occupational functioning (eg, preoccupation with contamination, order, counting, cleanliness, and/or safety)
- Compulsions (eg, repetitive washing of hands, checking and rechecking) are acts that must be performed in an attempt to decrease the anxiety felt about the obsessions. There is equal male and female prevalence.

Social anxiety disorder (SAD)
- Characterized by feelings of anxiety in social situations (eg, speaking in front of others, social gatherings); patients feel as though everyone is staring and judging them; affected persons usually do not seek treatment and will instead self-medicate with alcohol; there is equal male and female prevalence.

Table 9

Benzodiazepines (BZDs)

Drug	Time to peak plasma concentration (h)	Half-life (h)	Usual daily dose (mg/d)	Metabolic pathway
Alprazolam (Xanax®, Niravam™)	1-2	12-15	0.5-4	Oxidation
Chlordiazepoxide (Librium®)	2-4	5-30	5-200	Oxidation
Clonazepam (Klonopin®)	1-2	18-50	1-3	Nitro reduction
Clorazepate (Tranxene®)	1-2	Not significant	15-60	Oxidation
Diazepam (Valium®)	0.5-2	20-80	2-40	Oxidation
Estazolam (ProSom®)	2	10-24	0.5-2	Oxidation
Flurazepam (Dalmane®)	0.5-2	Not significant	15-30	Oxidation
Halazepam (Paxipam®)	1-3	7-14	80-160	Oxidation
Lorazepam (Ativan®)	1-6	10-20	2-6	Conjugation
Oxazepam (Serax®)	2-4	5-20	30-120	Conjugation
Prazepam (Centrax®)	6	1.2	20-60	Oxidation
Quazepam (Doral®)	2	25-41	7.5-30	Oxidation
Temazepam (Restoril®)	2-3	10-40	15-30	Conjugation
Triazolam (Halcion®)	1	1.5-5	0.125-0.5	Oxidation

Simple (or specific) phobias
- Defined as specific fears (eg, heights, dogs, mice, spiders, and needles) that cause an extreme anxiety response; affected persons usually do not seek treatment and instead will avoid situations that involve the phobia.

Treatment
- Exposure therapy to the perceived threat is common therapy; incidence in females is greater than in males.

Posttraumatic stress disorder (PTSD)
- Characterized by severe anxiety that is caused by an event outside of normal human experience (eg, war, rape, and natural disasters); symptoms include vividly reliving the event to the extent that anxiety symptoms (ie, flashbacks, nightmares/night terrors, extreme mood changes, feelings of fright) commonly occur; PTSD is often associated with strong guilt feelings, impaired relationships, social withdrawal, and personality changes; there is a greater prevalence in females than in males.

Anxiety due to a medical disorder
- Anxiety is likely to be related to evidence of a medical condition (eg, CHF, hyperthyroidism, COPD).

Substance-induced anxiety disorder
- Anxiety symptoms are likely to be a direct result of use of an agent (eg, amphetamines, toxin, and medication); symptoms may also occur with intoxication or withdrawal.

Associated features
- High comorbidity with other psychiatric illnesses (especially depression)
- High comorbidity with alcohol/substance abuse
- Associated with chronic medical illnesses (eg, chronic pain syndromes, long-term illnesses, GI distress, headaches)

Etiology
- Presently unknown
- Most current evidence suggests the cause is primarily biologic (imbalance of GABA, 5-HT, NE) with genetic predisposition.

Drug Therapy

Benzodiazepines (BZDs) (Table 9)
- Most commonly utilized anxiolytics

Mechanism of action
- BZDs potentiate the actions of GABA by increasing the influx of chloride ions into neurons; it is hypothesized that through their effects on neurons mediated by receptor complexes, BZDs reduce neuronal firing and thus the symptoms of anxiety.
- *Notes:* The rate of absorption varies with BZDs; the more lipophilic compounds (ie, alprazolam, diazepam, chlorazepate, and flurazepam) are rapidly absorbed and result in quicker onset of action; the less lipophilic BZDs are chlordiazepoxide, clonazepam, and lorazepam.

Adverse effects
- Sedation, dizziness, confusion, blurred vision, diplopia, syncope, residual daytime sedation, reduced psychomotor and cognitive dysfunction

Metabolism
- Lorazepam, oxazepam, and temazepam (LOT) are conjugated and are preferred in patients with hepatic dysfunction and elderly patients.

Drug interactions
- BZDs metabolized by CYP3A4 (eg, alprazolam, diazepam, and triazolam) have decreased clearance if taken concomitantly with CYP3A4 inhibitors (eg, ketoconazole, erythromycin, and nefazodone); BZDs are deadly in overdose if taken concomitantly with alcohol.

Clinical pearls
- May cause a paradoxical reaction in children, cognitively impaired elderly patients, mentally retarded patients, and post–head injury patients
- Never abruptly discontinue BZDs, as this may precipitate status epilepticus; always taper the dose to avoid seizure risk and withdrawal symptoms.
- In elderly patients, the BZDs of choice are those that are conjugated (LOT); there is an increased risk of falls in this population.
- Best to avoid in pregnancy (especially first trimester) due to risk of cleft palate; BZDs are also present in breast milk and should be avoided in nursing women.
- The abuse potential is great; BZDs are not recommended for patients with substance abuse issues.
- Tolerance is common and increasing doses are needed to control anxiety levels.
- Alprazolam extended-release (Xanax XR®) is dosed once daily; do not crush, chew, or break; also available as an orally disintegrating tablet (Niravam®).

Buspirone (BuSpar®)
Mechanism of action
- Poorly understood; 5-HT$_{1A}$ is a partial agonist and buspirone reportedly stimulates presynaptic 5-HT$_{1A}$ receptors; in addition, the agent has a moderate affinity for D$_2$ receptors.
- Does not interact with the BZD-GABA receptor complex
- Onset of anxiolytic effect is longer than BZD (2-3 weeks)

Adverse effects
- GI upset, headache, nervousness
- Possible benefits over BZDs
    * Usually less sedating than BZDs
    * Little to no psychomotor or cognitive impairment
    * Has not been associated with withdrawal symptoms, abuse, or physical dependence
    * Not cross-tolerant with BZDs or alcohol

Antidepressants as treatment for anxiety disorders
- TCAs are usually used third line due to side effects and the danger of overdose; clomipramine is effective for OCD.
- MAOIs are usually used third-line due to side effects and drug/food interactions.
- SSRIs and SNRIs are used first line for many anxiety disorders (especially in patients with comorbid depression and substance abuse problems).
- Titrate doses of antidepressants slowly to decrease risk of initial anxiety symptoms; ultimately, higher doses are commonly utilized for anxiety disorders.

Other classes of drugs used to treat anxiety disorders
- β-Blockers (eg, propranolol, atenolol) ease peripheral symptoms of anxiety and may be useful for panic disorders and SAD.
- Hydroxyzine reduces anxiety and is often used in patients with substance abuse issues.

Nonpharmacologic Treatment

- Supportive psychotherapy (individual, group, family)
- Cognitive behavioral therapy (CBT)
    * Focuses on coping with the fear of the symptoms of anxiety
- Relaxation techniques
- Exercise and/or lifestyle modifications (reduce caffeine and simple sugars)

5. Eating Disorders

Anorexia Nervosa (AN)

Characteristics
- A refusal to maintain body weight at or above a minimal, normal weight for age and height (85% or less of expected body weight)
- Intense fear of gaining weight or becoming fat, although patient is underweight
- Disturbance in self-perception of body weight, size, proportion, and attractiveness
- Amenorrhea for at least three consecutive cycles

Types
- Restricting and binge eating/purging types

Bulimia Nervosa (BN)

Characteristics
- Recurrent episodes of binge eating (often followed by intense feelings of guilt); patient may consume as much as 5000-20,000 calories over 2-8 hours
- Recurrent and inappropriate compensatory behavior in order to prevent weight gain
- Average of 2 binges/week for 3 months
- Person's self evaluation is primarily influenced by body shape and weight

Types
- Purging (vomiting, abuse of laxatives/diuretics) and nonpurging (excessive exercise, fasting)

Binge Eating Disorder

Characteristics
- Recurrent episodes of binge eating (patients usually obese)
- Eating when not physically hungry; eating more rapidly than normal; feeling disgusted with oneself
- Marked distress is present regarding binge eating.
- Binge eating episodes occur, on average, at least 2 days/week for 6 months.

Etiology and Prevalence

- The etiology is essentially unknown, but there are various theories (genetic predisposition, environmental/societal issues, chemical imbalance in the brain).
- There is usually a defined event or situation that begins the disorder (eg, a significant stressor such as starting college, divorce, or death of a loved one).
- Most commonly seen in Caucasian, middle- to upper-class females

Age of onset
- Anorexia nervosa: 13-20 years old
    * Male-to-female ratio, 1:10-20
- Bulimia nervosa: 16-18 years old
    * Male-to-female ratio, 1:10

Medical Complications and Signs of Disease

- Eating disorders produce states of semistarvation and noticeable malnutrition, especially in anorexia; in bulimia, patients are more difficult to identify because they are commonly of normal body weight.
- Dehydration
- High incidence of comorbid anxiety, depression, OCD, and substance abuse
- Dental caries/enamel erosion due to stomach acid exposure
- Calluses on dorsum of hand and/or fingers due to induction of vomiting
- Mortality rate ~10% from starvation (primarily due to electrolyte imbalances), arrhythmia, or suicide
- Long-term complications: endocrine/metabolic, cardiovascular, renal, gastroenterologic, hematologic, pulmonary, musculoskeletal, immunologic, dermatologic

Treatment

- Psychotherapy is the mainstay of treatment; therapy can be individual, group, family, supportive, cognitive-behavioral, or insight-oriented.
- Primary objectives: define and examine extent of problem; patient learns to accept condition; treatment results in a reconstruction of self-identity and self-confidence.
- Dietary intake is slowly normalized with goal of restoring normal body weight; nutritional counseling is utilized.
- Distorted ideas about caloric intake and body shape are corrected.
- Relapse prevention focuses on developing and using coping mechanisms and avoiding high-risk situations.

Drug therapy

Antidepressants
- SSRIs are primarily utilized and may be more effective for patients with bulimia. Antidepressants don't appear to be beneficial in helping severely malnourished AN patients gain weight, but may help maintain weight after weight has been gained.
- Fluoxetine (Prozac®) is indicated for the treatment of bulimia nervosa; higher doses used, titrate to 60 mg/day every morning.

- Topiramate (Topamax®) and zonisamide (Zonegran®) may be beneficial in binge-eating disorder and bulimia nervosa
- Ideal treatment includes both psychotherapy and pharmacotherapy.

6. Key Points

Schizophrenia

- Patients with schizophrenia have positive (hallucinations, delusions), negative (flat affect, avolition, anhedonia, poverty of thought), and disorganized (speech, behavior) symptoms; positive symptoms usually respond to drug therapy first.
- Antipsychotics (conventional or atypical) are essential treatment for schizophrenia; atypical medications (risperidone, olanzapine, quetiapine, ziprasidone, aripiprazole and paliperidone) have been considered first-line medical treatment because they lower EPS and TD risk more than conventional medications and appear to be more beneficial for negative symptoms. Recent evidence has shown that schizophrenic patients discontinue medications frequently regardless of whether they are taking second generation or first generation antipsychotics, and question whether the atypical antipsychotics are more effective at treating negative symptoms than the typical medications.
- Atypical antipsychotics (especially olanzapine) are associated with weight gain, lipid and glucose abnormalities (ziprasidone and aripiprazole do not appear to have the weight gain and metabolic abnormalities)
- Low-potency conventional agents (chlorpromazine, thioridazine) are more often used that high-potency agents (haloperidol, fluphenazine)
- Low-potency agents have more sedation, orthostatic hypotension (OH), and anticholinergic (AC) side effects and fewer extrapyramidal symptoms (EPS) compared to high-potency agents; high-potency agents have more EPS and less sedation, OH, and AC effects.
- Extrapyramidal symptoms consist of dystonic reactions (to be remedied by diphenhydramine 25-50 mg IM or benztropine 1-2 mg IM every 30 minutes until resolution), akathisia (to be treated with lorazepam, clonidine, or propranolol), and pseudoparkinsonism (ameliorated by amantadine or benztropine).
- Clozapine is the only agent proven effective for refractory schizophrenia.
- Consider long-acting injectable preparations in situations of poor compliance.

Bipolar disorder

- The acute treatment for bipolar disorder focuses on slowing the patient down and reducing harm to self and others; maintenance treatment focuses on prevention and/or reducing the number of future episodes.
- A mood stabilizer is an essential component in the treatment of bipolar disorder; first-line mood stabilizers include lithium and divalproex sodium (or valproic acid).
- The risk of lithium side effects and toxicity can be prevented by monitoring the patient for signs and symptoms of problems and by obtaining regular blood level readings.
- Other drug therapies that may be used to treat the patient with bipolar disorder include atypical antipsychotics, gabapentin, carbamazepine, oxcarbazepine, topiramate, and lamotrigine (especially if depressed).

Major depression

- All antidepressants are equally effective in a given population.
- Response varies from person to person; antidepressants differ in side-effect and drug-interaction profiles; none are "speed" or "uppers."
- Choice of agent depends on the history of response of other family members to certain antidepressants (if available) and the particular side-effect profile (as it relates to any given patient).
- First-line agents include SSRIs, bupropion, venlafaxine, and duloxetine; second-line agents may include mirtazapine and nefazodone; third-line agents may include TCAs and MAOIs.
- Reduce or eliminate target symptoms with an antidepressant; incorporating psychotherapy is optimal.
- The goal of treatment of depression is to improve the patient's ability to function and his or her quality of life.

Anxiety disorders

- Anxiety disorders are serious, debilitating mental illnesses that have extreme anxiety as the primary mood disturbance.
- Various drug therapies include benzodiazepines, buspirone, antidepressants (especially SSRIs and venlafaxine), β-blockers, and hydroxyzine.
- Nonpharmacologic therapy of anxiety disorders is an important aspect of care (eg, supportive therapy, cognitive behavioral therapy, relaxation techniques, and exercise/lifestyle modifications).

Eating disorders

- Anorexia nervosa is characterized by a refusal to maintain body weight (at or above a minimal normal weight for age and height), an intense fear of gaining weight, a disturbance in self-perception of body weight, and amenorrhea for at least three consecutive cycles.
- Bulimia nervosa is characterized by recurrent episodes of binge eating, recurrent and inappropriate compensatory behavior in order to prevent weight gain, an average of two binges/week for 3 months, and self-evaluation that is primarily influenced by

body shape and weight.
- Eating disorders most commonly occur in young, Caucasian, middle- to upper-class females.
- Medical complications and comorbid psychiatric disorders (eg, anxiety, depression, and substance abuse) are extremely common in this population.
- Medications such as antidepressants may be helpful in treating eating disorders (especially bulimia); optimal therapy should include psychotherapy in combination with drug therapy.

7. Questions and Answers

Select the single best response for Questions 1 through 4.

1. S.J. is a 30-year-old white female with a 10-year history of schizophrenia. Her current therapy includes haloperidol 10 mg PO bid. The psychiatrist wants to convert her to haloperidol decanoate. What would be the appropriate equivalent monthly dose of haloperidol decanoate?

   A. 100 mg
   B. 10 mg
   C. 500 mg
   D. 200 mg
   E. 12.5 mg

2. B.T. reports to the nursing station with his head pulled sharply to the side and rear. He complains of severe pain in his neck and back area. The most appropriate diagnosis and treatment would be:

   A. Akathisia; propranolol 20 mg IM until resolution
   B. Dystonic reaction; diphenhydramine 50 mg IM every 30 minutes until resolution
   C. Tardive dyskinesia; physical therapy
   D. Dystonic reaction; lorazepam 2 mg IM every 30 minutes until resolution
   E. None of the above

3. Negative symptoms in schizophrenia could include all of the following except:

   A. Flat affect
   B. Anhedonia
   C. Avolition
   D. Persecutory delusions
   E. Poverty of thought

4. A 48-year-old black male arrives at the ED seeking his "nerve pill." He has a 27-year history of paranoid schizophrenia with multiple hospitalizations. In recent years, he has been effectively maintained on fluphenazine 10 mg PO bid. He now states that he feels "really bad today." His arms and jaws are stiff, his temperature is 104°F, his BP is 176/110, and his WBC is 19,000. LFTs and CPK are ordered STAT. While you await the test results, you would:

A. Discontinue oral fluphenazine and begin quetiapine
B. Discontinue oral fluphenazine
C. Continue oral fluphenazine and add bromocriptine
D. Discontinue oral fluphenazine and give fluphenazine decanoate 25 mg IM STAT
E. Do nothing; labs need to be evaluated first

For Questions 5 through 8, one or more of the answers given may be correct. Answer each question as follows:

A. I only
B. II only
C. I and III only
D. II and III only
E. I, II, and III

A 25-year-old white male has been increasingly disruptive at home. He has been claiming that he is the President of the United States and has been staying awake all night planning bills for Congress. He has been argumentative and threatening with his friends and family. Though he appears extremely tired physically, he is constantly active.

5. The psychiatrist has decided to initiate Eskalith CR 450 mg bid in this patient. Which of the following lab tests will need to be performed for this patient before starting this drug therapy regimen?

I. Pregnancy test
II. Thyroid function tests
III. SCr

6. As the pharmacist on the treatment team, you alert the patient's family to the common side effects of lithium, which include:

I. Polyuria
II. Alopecia
III. Elevated hepatic enzymes

7. Which of the following statements are correct regarding the treatment of bipolar disorder?

I. Lithium and divalproex sodium are considered first-line therapy options for mood stabilization.
II. When treating a patient with lithium, the WBC and ANC must be monitored due to lithium's propensity to cause agranulocytosis.
III. Patients diagnosed with bipolar I disorder exhibit intermittent cycles of mania and major depression.

8. Which of the following therapies have been used for the treatment of bipolar disorder?

I. Olanzapine
II. Topiramate
III. Calcium channel blockers

Select the single best response for Questions 9 through 16.

9. Insomnia, GI upset, and headache are common side effects of which of the following antidepressants?

A. Phenelzine
B. Amitriptyline
C. Fluoxetine
D. Trazodone
E. Both B and C

10. A 29-year-old depressed black female has shown little improvement with fluoxetine treatment so the psychiatrist decides to change her medication to tranylcypromine. What is your recommendation for the switch?

A. Gradually decrease fluoxetine dosage over a 4-week period and then start tranylcypromine
B. Wait 2 weeks after stopping fluoxetine and then begin tranylcypromine
C. Over 6 weeks, gradually decrease fluoxetine dosage as you gradually increase the tranylcypromine dosage
D. Wait 5 weeks after stopping fluoxetine before initiating tranylcypromine
E. Maintain fluoxetine dosage and start tranylcypromine; stop the fluoxetine when the tranylcypromine has achieved a therapeutic level

11. Which of the following has been shown to induce or worsen depression?

A. Oral contraceptives
B. Amoxicillin
C. Thiamine
D. Methylphenidate
E. Phenelzine

12. Which of the following is correct regarding electroconvulsive therapy (ECT)?

    A. For maximum effectiveness, seizures should last 5-10 minutes
    B. Contraindicated in patients with COPD
    C. Effective treatment for pregnant females with major depression
    D. Memory loss lasting 1-2 weeks is common
    E. ECT may cause amenorrhea in female patients

13. A 33-year-old waitress is experiencing symptoms of anxiety, including night terrors and mood lability. She reports no past psychiatric history but admits that these symptoms started about 2 weeks after armed and masked gunmen robbed her restaurant. She is most likely experiencing:

    A. LSD
    B. PTSD
    C. GAD
    D. OCD

14. A new patient presents to your clinic. He reports that it took him 3 hours to get ready for this appointment and that he returned home several times in order to check to see if the door was locked. During the interview, he straightens up your desk, making sure all square items are at right angles to each other. He would most likely be diagnosed with:

    A. PTSD
    B. PCP
    C. OCD
    D. GAD

15. Which of the following statements regarding the use of SSRIs in anxiety disorders is most accurate?

    A. SSRIs are not usually effective in the treatment of anxiety
    B. SSRI doses for anxiety should be started lower than initial doses for depression
    C. SSRIs should only be used after a failed treatment trial with benzodiazepines
    D. SSRIs may be used on a prn basis when anxiety symptoms emerge

16. Which of the following statements are not correct regarding benzodiazepines?

    A. Potentiate the effect of gamma-aminobutyric acid
    B. Highly lipophilic
    C. Cross tolerant with alcohol
    D. Similar pharmacologic action to buspirone
    E. Risk of seizure if abruptly discontinued

For Questions 17 through 20, one or more of the following answers given are correct. Answer each question as follows:

    A. I only
    B. II only
    C. I and III only
    D. II and III only
    E. I, II, and III

17. Which of the following is true regarding anorexia nervosa?

    I. Anorexia nervosa (AN) is characterized by recurrent and inappropriate compensatory behavior in order to prevent weight gain
    II. Patients with AN generally appear to be of normal weight for age and height
    III. AN patients have an intense fear of gaining weight or becoming fat, although they are underweight

18. What *DSM-IV* criteria for AN are diagnostic for this type of eating disorder?

    I. Absence of at least three consecutive menstrual cycles
    II. Sunken eyes with dark circles underneath
    III. Binge eating/purging episode occurs at least once in the past 6 months

19. Which of the following is true regarding bulimia nervosa (BN)?

    I. The individual may consume 5000-20,000 calories in a single binge episode that may last as long as 2-8 hours
    II. The two specific types of bulimic patients are purging type and nonpurging type.
    III. There is an average of two binges/week for 3 consecutive months

20. Patients with AN may demonstrate which of the following characteristics?

  I.   Kleptomania
  II. Laxative/diuretic abuse
 III. Amenorrhea

21. Which of the following is the most appropriate treatment for bulimia nervosa?

  A.   Insight-oriented therapy
  B.   Fluoxetine 20 mg QD
  C.   Fluoxetine 60 mg QAM + CBT
  D.   Olanzapine 10 mg QHS
  E.   Olanzapine 20 mg QHS + Family Therapy

Answers

1. **D.** The patient is on haloperidol 10 mg bid. Therefore, to convert to the decanoate injection, the total oral daily dose is multiplied by 10. The dose would be Haldol-D 200 mg IM every 4 weeks.

2. **B.** The patient is experiencing a dystonic reaction, which can be treated with either benztropine 1-2 mg IM or diphenhydramine 25-50 mg IM every 30 minutes until resolved. The dystonic reaction is thought to occur due to an imbalance in dopamine and acetylcholine in the nigrostriatal region of the brain.

3. **D.** Delusions are false beliefs or wrong judgments held with conviction despite incontrovertible evidence to the contrary. Such symptoms are referred to as "positive" for patients with schizophrenia.

4. **B.** The symptoms that the patient is displaying appear to be the result of neuroleptic malignant syndrome (NMS). All neuroleptics have the propensity to cause this rare but deadly adverse effect. The first steps in treating NMS are to discontinue the offending agent, offer supportive therapy, and prescribe a dopamine agonist and (commonly) a skeletal muscle relaxant.

5. **D.** Initiation of lithium requires several baseline lab tests: pregnancy test (if patient is of childbearing age); ECG and BP to assess CV status; thyroid function tests to rule out euthyroid goiter or hypothyroidism; SCr/BUN (lithium is 100% renally eliminated); and CBC with differential to evaluate for leukocytosis. Electrolytes should also be evaluated (decreased sodium can increase lithium levels).

6. **A.** Common side effects that occur with the initiation of lithium include polyuria, polydipsia, tremor, and GI upset. Common side effects that may occur later in therapy include weight gain and mental dulling. Elevated hepatic enzymes and alopecia are side effects that may occur with divalproex sodium.

7. **C.** Agranulocytosis is a side effect that is monitored weekly with clozapine therapy for 6 months. After 6 months, monitoring can be done every 2 weeks for the duration of therapy.

8. **E.** All of the therapies listed have been used for mood stabilization in bipolar disorder.

9. **C.** SSRIs commonly cause insomnia, GI upset, anxiety, headache, and sexual dysfunction. Phenelzine, amitriptyline, and trazodone cause sedative effects.

10. **D.** Due to fluoxetine's long half-life, 5 weeks should pass before initiating MAOI therapy. If fluoxetine is not cleared from the body by the time the MAOI is started, there is a risk of developing "serotonin syndrome".

11. **A.** Many medications can cause or worsen depression, eg, antihypertensives (reserpine, methyldopa, propranolol, and clonidine), antiparkinsonian agents (levodopa, carbidopa, and amantadine), hormonal agents (estrogens and progesterone), corticosteroids, cycloserine, and the anticancer agents vinblastine and vincristine.

12. **C.** ECT is a safe and effective therapy for pregnant females and patients with COPD. Relative contraindications include increased intracranial pressure, recent MI, recent intracerebral hemorrhage, and cerebral lesions. Memory loss is a common side effect, but usually only on the day of treatment and perhaps the following day. The induced seizure lasts 30-90 seconds and is monitored by EEG. Additionally, ECT does not cause amenorrhea in female patients.

13. **B.** The patient experienced a violent and frightening episode 2 weeks before her symptoms appeared. The symptoms of re-experiencing the event, night terrors, and mood lability are common in patients with PSTD.

14. **C.** The patient is displaying signs and symptoms of OCD (eg, a long time is spent getting ready and there is repeated checking behavior and preoccupation with rearranging items to 90-degree angles). These activities are time consuming and limit his social and occupational functioning.

15. **B.** Because SSRIs can be activating and may initially cause symptoms of anxiety, it is important to "start low and go slow" with these agents when utilized for anxiety disorders.

16. **D.** Buspirone's mechanism of action is agonism of $5-HT_{1A}$ receptors. Buspirone also possesses moderate affinity for D_2 receptors. It does not interact with the BZD-GABA receptor complex like the BZDs. The BZDs cross the blood–brain barrier and are cross-tolerant with alcohol. If BZDs are abruptly discontinued, seizures can result.

17. **C.** Patients with AN refuse to maintain body weight at or above a minimal, normal weight for age and height (less than 15% of expected body weight). Patients with AN may respond to antidepressants, but psychotherapy is usually more effective. AN is most commonly seen in Caucasian, middle- to upper-class females.

18. **A.** *DSM-IV* criteria list the refusal to maintain body weight at or above a minimal, normal weight for age and height (85% or less of expected body weight and an intense fear of gaining weight or becoming fat although underweight), disturbance in self-perception of body weight (ie, size, proportion, and attractiveness), and amenorrhea for at least three consecutive cycles.

19. **E.** All of the answers are correct regarding BN.

20. **D.** Patients with AN commonly reduce weight by reducing food intake. Many patients use other ways to lose weight such as excessive exercise, laxative and/or diuretic use, substance abuse, and self-induced vomiting. Amenorrhea ensues as a result of estrogen deficiency; it may occur before weight loss.

21. **C.** Fluoxetine is approved for treating BN, 60 mg most common dose. Combination of psychotherapy and pharmacotherapy is preferred.

8. References

American Diabetes Association, American Psychiatric Association, American Association of Clinical Endocrinologists, North American Association for the Study of Obesity. Consensus development conference on antipsychotic drugs and obesity and diabetes. *Diabetes Care.* 2004;27:596-601.

American Psychiatric Association. *Diagnostic and Statistical Manual of Mental Disorders,* 4th ed. Text Revision. Washington: American Psychiatric Association; 2000.

American Psychiatric Association. *Practice Guideline for the Treatment of Patients with Eating Disorders,* 3rd ed. www.psych.org/psych_pract/treatg/pg/ EatingDisorders3ePG_04-28-06.pdf (accessed 2007 September 17).

Bennett JA, Dunayevich E, McElroy SL, et al. The new mood stabilizers and the treatment of bipolar disorder. *Drug Benefit Trends.* 2000;12:3-16.

Botts SR, Raskind J. Gabapentin and lamotrigine in bipolar disorder. *Am J Health-Syst Pharm.* 1999;56:1939-1944.

Canales PL, Cates M, Wells BG. Anxiety disorders. In: Herfindal ET, Gourley DR, eds. *Textbook of Therapeutics: Drug and Disease Management,* 7th ed. Philadelphia: Lippincott Williams & Wilkins; 2000:1185-1202.

Cohen LJ, Jermain DM, Clarke SO, et al. Psychiatric Pharmacy Practice Specialty Certification Examination Review Course. Course presented at ASHP Psychiatric Clinical Specialists Meeting, Denver, CO, 2001, March 31-April 1.

DeVane CL. Keeping depression at bay. *Drug Topics.* 2001;15:49-58.

Easson WM, Rock NL. Psychiatry Specialty Board Review. New York: Brunner/Mazel; 1991.

Emsam® [package insert]. Princeton, (NJ): Bristol-Myers Squibb Company; 2006.

Fuller MA, Sajatovic M, eds. *Drug Information for Mental Health,* 1st ed. Cleveland: Lexi-Comp; 2001.

Gutierrez MA, Stimmel GL. Mood Disorders. In: Helms RA, Quan DJ, Herfindal ET, et al. eds. *Textbook of Therapeutics: Drug and Disease Management,* 8th ed. Philadelphia: Lippincott Williams & Wilkins; 2006:1416-1431.

Gutierrez MA, Stimmel GL. Schizophrenia. In: Helms RA, Quan DJ, Herfindal ET, et al., eds. *Textbook of Therapeutics: Drug and Disease Management,* 8th ed. Philadelphia: Lippincott Williams & Wilkins; 2006:1432-1442.

Jacobson JL, Jacobson AM, eds. *Psychiatric Secrets.* Philadelphia: Hanley & Belfus; 1996.

Kane JM. Drug therapy: Schizophrenia. *N Engl J Med.* 1996;334:34-41.

Kane JM, McGlashan TH. Treatment of schizophrenia. *Lancet.* 1995;346:820-825.

Keck PE, Perlis RH, Otto MW, et al. The expert consensus guideline series. Treatment of bipolar disorder 2004. Postgraduate Medicine Special Report. 2004 (December): 1-120.

Lieberman JA, Stroup TS, McEvoy JP, et al. Effectiveness of antipsychotic drugs in patients with chronic schizophrenia. *N Engl J Med.* 2005;353:1209-23.

Mandl DL, Iltz JL. Obesity and eating disorders. In: Herfindal ET, Gourley DR, eds. *Textbook of Therapeutics: Drug and Disease Management,* 7th ed. Philadelphia: Lippincott Williams & Wilkins; 2000:1271-1287.

McElroy SL, Keck PE. Pharmacologic agents for the treatment of acute bipolar mania. *Biol Psychiatry.* 2000;48:539-557.

McElroy SL, Shapira NA, Arnold LM, et al. Topiramate in the long-term treatment of binge-eating disorder associated with obesity. *J Clin Psychiatry.* 2004;65(Suppl 11):1463-1469.

McEvoy JP, Lieberman JA, Stroup TS, et al. Effectiveness of clozapine versus olanzapine, quetiapine, and risperidone in patients with chronic schizophrenia who did not respond to prior atypical antipsychotic treatment. *Am J Psychiatry.* 2006:163:600-610.

McEvoy JP, Scheifler PL, Frances A. The expert consensus guideline series. Treatment of schizophrenia. *J Clin Psychiatry.* 1999;60(Suppl 11):3-80.

National Institute of Mental Health. Anxiety disorders. Bethesda, MD: NIH publication no. 00-3879; 2000.

National Institute of Mental Health. Pamphlet on eating disorders. Washington: U.S. Department of Health and Human Services; NIH publication no. 94-3477; 1994.

Newcomer JW, Nasrallah HA, Loebel AD. The atypical antipsychotic therapy and metabolic issue national survey. *J. Clin. Psychopharmacology.* 2004;24(Suppl 1):S1-S6.

Norton J. Oxcarbazepine in mood disorders. *Hosp Pharm.* 2001;36:1254-1256.

Post RM. Rapid cycling: clinical presentation and treatment approaches. New research presented at the 155th Annual Meeting of the American Psychiatric Association. Philadelphia; May 2002.

Practice guideline for the treatment of patients with bipolar disorder (revision). American Psychiatric Association Practice Guidelines. *Am J Psychiatry.* 2002;159(Suppl):1-50.

Practice guideline for the treatment of patients with major depressive disorder (revision). American Psychiatric Association Practice Guidelines. *Am J Psychiatry.* 2000;157(4 Suppl):1-45.

Practice guideline for the treatment of patients with schizophrenia. American Psychiatric Association Practice Guidelines. *Am J Psychiatry.* 1997;154(Suppl 4):1-63.

Risby E, Donnigan D, Nemeroff CB. Pharmacotherapeutic considerations for psychiatric disorders: Depression. *Formulary.* 1997;32:46-59.

Sachs GS, Printz DJ, Kahn DA, et al. The expert consensus guideline series. Medication treatment of bipolar disorder 2000. *Postgraduate Med.* 2000;4:1-104.

Schneider LS, Tariot PN, Dagerman KS, et al. Effectiveness of atypical Antipsychotic Drugs in Patients with Alzheimer's Disease. M. Engle. *J Med.* 2006;355:1525.38

Stahl SM. *Psychopharmacology of Antidepressants.* London: Martin Dunitz; 1998.

Stahl SM. *Psychopharmacology of Antipsychotics.* London: Martin Dunitz; 1999.

Stroup TS, Lieberman JA, McEvoy JP, et al. Effectiveness of olanzapine, quetiapine, risperidone, and ziprasidone in patients with chronic schizophrenia following discontinuation of a previous atypical antipsychotic. *Am J Psychiatry.* 2006: 163:611-622.

Substance Abuse and Mental Health Services Administration and National Institute of Mental Health. Mental Health: A Report from the Surgeon General. www.surgeongeneral.gov/Library/MentalHealth/home.html (accessed March 12, 2003).

U.S. Food and Drug Administration Department of Health and Human Services Center for Drug Evaluation and Research: FDA Proposes New Warnings About Suicidal Thinking, Behavior in Young Adults Who Take Antidepressant Medications. www.fda.gov/bbs/topics/NEWS/2007/NEW01624.html (accessed 2007 September 17).

U.S. Food and Drug Administration Department of Health and Human Services Center for Drug Evaluation and Research: FDA Public Health Advisory: Deaths with Antipsychotics in Elderly Patients with Behavioral Disturbances. www.fda.gov/Cder/drug/advisory/antipsychotics.htm (accessed 2007 September 16).

26. Common Dermatologic Disorders

James C. Eoff III, PharmD, BSPh
Executive Associate Dean and Professor,
Department of Clinical Pharmacy
University of Tennessee College of Pharmacy

Contents

1. Acne (Acne Vulgaris)

- Acne is an inflammatory disorder of the pilosebaceous glands, which occurs most commonly during the teenage years, at or soon after puberty.
- It may reappear later or begin in adults who had clear skin in their teens, more commonly in women than men.

Classification and Clinical Presentation

Type I (comedonal)
- A mild form, with primarily noninflammatory lesions (open and closed comedones) and relatively few superficial inflammatory lesions with no scarring

Type II (papular)
- A moderate form, with multiple papules on the face and trunk, with minimal scarring

Type III (pustular)
- An advanced form that can lead to moderate scarring

Type IV (nodulocystic)
- The most severe and destructive form with multiple deep inflammatory lesions or nodules (often called cysts) that leads to extensive scarring

Pathophysiology

- Increased sebum production by androgenic hormones at the onset of puberty
- Obstruction of hair follicle opening due to increasing adherence and production of epithelial cells, producing closed comedones (whiteheads) progressing ultimately to open comedones (blackheads)
- Increased growth of a primary microorganism on the skin and in the sebaceous ducts, *Propionibacterium acnes* (*P acnes*), a gram-positive anaerobic rod that produces enzymes, including lipases
- Inflammation due to the enzymatic breakdown of triglycerides into free fatty acids, which causes the influx of polymorphonuclear leukocytes, ultimately resulting in pustule formation

Treatment Principles

Type I (comedonal)
- Topical nonprescription medications
  * Benzoyl peroxide is usually the first line of therapy.

Type II (papular)
- Topical antibiotics and/or topical retinoids

Type III (pustular)
- Oral antibiotics in addition to topical medications

Type IV (nodulocystic)
- Isotretinoin

Topical Therapy

Nonprescription agents
- Benzoyl peroxide (most effective OTC agent)
- Benzoyl peroxide products 2.5, 5, and 10%:
  * Clearasil® maximum strength vanishing cream
  * Exact® vanishing cream
  * Neutrogena® oil-free acne mask
  * Noxzema® anti-acne lotion
  * Oxy-10®
  * Benzac®
  * Panoxyl®
  * Zapzyt® gel

Mechanism of action
- Destroy the anaerobic *P acnes* due to release of oxygen
- Exfoliant effect, causing peeling of the outer layers of the skin
- *P acnes* does not become resistant to benzoyl peroxide; therefore, it can be used concurrently with topical antibiotics to prevent resistance (eg, using BP for one course of therapy, alternating with a course of topical antibiotic therapy).

Patient counseling
- Use with caution with sensitive skin.
- Do not allow contact with eyes, lips, or mouth.
- Avoid unnecessary sun exposure and/or use sunscreen.

Adverse effects
- May cause redness, dryness, burning, itching, peeling, and swelling
- May bleach hair or dyed fabrics

Other products
- Sulfur (3-8%)
  * SAStid® soap: precipitated sulfur 10% (keratolytic and antibacterial action)
- Salicylic acid (0.5-2%)
  * Clearasil Clearstick®, Neutrogena® Oil Free Acne Wash®, Noxzema®, Stridex®: irritant effect, keratolytic, and increases rate of turnover of epithelial cells
- Resorcinol
  * Keratolytic (usually combined with sulfur)

- Combinations:
    * Sulfur and resorcinol: Clearasil®, Acnomel®
- Medicated soaps and cleansers: alcohol, acetone, other degreasing lotions

Topical antimicrobial therapy
- See Table 1.

Clindamycin
Mechanism of action
- Suppresses growth of *P acnes*
- May directly reduce free fatty acid concentrations on the skin

Patient counseling
- Contact physician if no improvement is seen within 6 weeks.
- Discontinue medication and contact physician if severe diarrhea and/or abdominal cramps or pain develop.

Adverse effects
- Contact dermatitis or hypersensitivity
- Dry or scaly skin or peeling
- Rarely: pseudomembranous colitis (severe abdominal cramps, pain, bloating, and severe diarrhea)

Erythromycin
Mechanism of action
- Suppresses growth of *P acnes*

Patient counseling
- Wait at least 1 hour before applying any other topical acne medication.
- Avoid contact with eyes, mouth, nose, and other mucous membranes.
- While improvement is generally expected within 4 weeks, some patients do not respond for 8-12 weeks.

Adverse effects
- More common: dry or scaly skin, irritation, and itching
- Less common: stinging, peeling, and redness

Retinoids
- See Table 2.

Mechanism of action
- Retinoids are chemically related to vitamin A.
- Retinoids normalize follicular keratinization, heal comedones, decrease sebum production, and decrease inflammatory lesions.

Patient counseling
- Do not use astringents, drying agents, abrasive scrubs, or harsh soaps concurrently, and only use mild soap once or twice daily.
- Apply every other night to adjust to drying effect for the first 2 weeks.
- Apply nightly after 2 weeks.
- May take up to 2-3 months before skin improves
- Use sunblock on face before sun exposure due to increased sensitivity.

Adverse drug effects
- May irritate skin and cause redness, dryness and scaling
- Tazarotene is the most irritating retinoid.
- Adapalene appears to be least irritating and is preferred for sensitive skin.

Azelaic acid 20%
- Trade names Azelex® and Finevin®

Mechanism of action
- Suppresses growth of *P acnes*

Table 1

Topical Antimicrobials

Generic name	Trade name	Form
Clindamycin	Cleocin-T®	Liquid
Erythromycin	Theramycin Z®	Liquid
	Benzamycin® 2%	Gel
	Emgel® 2%	Gel

Table 2

Retinolds

Generic name	Trade name	Form and strength
Tretinoin	Retin-A®	0.015%, 0.05%, 0.1% cream; 0.1% gel, 0.05% lotion
	Renova®	0.05% cream
	Avita®	0.025% cream and gel
Adapalene	Differin®	0.1% gel
Tazarotene	Tazorac®	0.05%, 0.1% gel
Alitretinoin	Panretin®	0.1% gel

- Improves inflammatory and noninflammatory lesions.
- Normalization of keratinization leading to anticomedonal effect

Patient counseling
- If sensitivity develops, discontinue use.
- Keep away from mouth, eyes, and mucous membranes.
- Other topical medications must be used at different times during the day.

Adverse drug effects
- Temporary dryness and skin irritation (pruritus and burning) may occur upon initiation of therapy.
- Hypopigmentation (caution in dark skinned individuals)

Systemic Therapy

Antimicrobials
- See Table 3.

General
- Useful for type 2 (papular) acne and type 3 (pustular) acne
- After 6-8 weeks, dosage may be increased if necessary.
- If the first antibiotic was ineffective after increasing the dosage, a second antibiotic is prescribed.
- After 6 months to 1 year of therapy, the antibiotic dose may be tapered if continued at all.

Mechanism of action
- Suppresses growth of *P acnes* in sebaceous ducts
- Possible direct anticomedonal effect

Patient counseling, adverse drug effects, and drug interactions
- See chapter on antimicrobials.

Table 3

Oral Antimicrobials

Generic name	Trade name	Dosage and form
Tetracycline	Achromycin®, Sumycin®	500 mg qd or bid caps
Erythromycin	E.E.S.®, Erythrocin®	250-500 qd or bid tabs
Doxycycline	Vibramycin®	100 mg qd caps/tabs
Minocycline	Minocin®	50 mg bid caps

Isotretinoin
- Trade name Accutane®, Amnesteem®, Claravis™, or Sotret® 10-, 20-, and 40-mg capsules

General
- For patients with severe, nodulocystic, draining acne who have not responded to systemic antibiotic therapy or who have required more than 3 years of systemic antibiotic therapy
- Over 90% effective in producing an acne-free state for years following a 4- to 5-month course of therapy
- Originally held in reserve for severe cases of nodulocystic acne, but may also be indicated as first-line treatment for severe acne that results in scarring

iPLEDGE® program
- The U.S. Food and Drug Administration (FDA) has approved an enhanced risk management program designed to minimize fetal exposure to isotretinoin known as iPLEDGE®, which will replace the S.M.A.R.T. Program (the System to Manage Accutane Related Teratogenicity) on December 30, 2005. iPLEDGE will require mandatory registration of prescribers, patients, wholesalers, and pharmacies to further the public health goal to eliminate fetal exposure to isotretinoin.
- Pharmacies will not be able to dispense isotretinoin to people with severe acne without enrolling in the iPLEDGE program through a physician who is also enrolled. After a pharmacy registers for iPLEDGE at http://www.ipledgeprogram.com, the "Responsible Site Pharmacist" is sent a follow-up mailing, which contains instructions on how to activate their pharmacy. Pharmacies that have not registered and activated by December 30, 2005, will not be eligible to order isotretinoin from their wholesaler and must return all unused product to the manufacturer.
- Patients currently treated with isotretinoin may be registered in the iPLEDGE program or continue in their current program until February 28, 2006. Starting March 1, 2006, all patients taking isotretinoin must be registered in the iPLEDGE program.
- Wholesalers that have not registered by December 30, 2005, will not be eligible to order isotretinoin from the manufacturers, and must return all unused product to the manufacturer.
- Prescribers who have not registered and activated by March 1, 2006, will not be eligible to prescribe isotretinoin for patients.

Mechanism of action
- Reduces sebum production (up to 90% inhibition)
- Decreased production of microcomedones, possibly by decreasing cohesiveness of follicular epithelial cells
- Possible anti-inflammatory effect

Patient counseling

- Should be taken with food and best absorbed with a fatty meal
- Can take the dose divided twice daily or the entire dose with the evening meal
- Effects are gradual, and acne may worsen during the first month of therapy; however, improvement usually begins by the sixth week of therapy.
- Use lip balm to treat cheilitis and moisturizers to treat dry skin.

Adverse drug effects

- *Teratogenic: Absolutely contraindicated in pregnancy*
  * Causes significant birth defects
  * Females of childbearing potential must take measures to avoid pregnancy during the course of isotretinoin therapy.
  * Females should be tested for pregnancy before initiation of therapy and told to use two methods of contraception for at least 1 month prior to initiation of therapy, and 1 month after discontinuation of therapy.

Side effects and toxicity

- Most common (90-100%):
  * Cheilitis (chapped lips)
  * Dry mouth
  * Dry skin
  * Pruritus
- Common (30-40%):
  * Dry nose, leading to nasal crusting and epistaxis
  * Dry eyes, leading to conjunctivitis and problems with contact lenses
  * Muscular soreness or stiffness
- Less common (10-25%):
  * Headaches
  * Hyperlipidemia (primarily elevation of triglycerides, which may lead to attack of pancreatitis)
- Rare (less than 5%):
  * Decreased night vision
  * Thinning of hair
  * Easily injured skin
  * Peeling of palms and soles
  * Skin rash and skin infections
- Very rare (<1%):
  * Acute depression: very rare, but reversible if detected early
  * Pseudotumor cerebri (benign intracranial hypertension with visual disturbances)

- Treatment of most common side effects:
  * Cheilitis: frequent use of lip balm
  * Dry skin: skin lubrication with moisturizers
  * Nosebleeds: lubricate the nostrils with petrolatum
  * Muscular soreness or stiffness: mild OTC analgesic/anti-inflammatory agents

Monitoring parameters

- Lipid panel
- Liver function tests (elevations are common during initiation of therapy, but usually return to normal during treatment).
- Complete blood counts
- Pregnancy testing for women prior to use of drug

Dosing

- 1 mg/kg per day (may start out 0.5 mg/kg per day for the first month before increasing) taken once or twice daily with food; best absorbed with a fatty meal
- Goal: a total dose of 120-150 mg/kg over 4-5 months
- Longer courses of 6-8 months may be required.

Other

- Approximately 20% relapse within 1 year, and up to 40% within 3 years after discontinuation of therapy.
- Repeat therapy for 4-6 months is acceptable and effective

Oral corticosteroids

- Commonly known as "prom pills"
- Can temporarily suppress acne with a 7- to 10-day course of prednisone 20 mg daily
- Rapidly effective when a brief course is necessary to cause prompt improvement (eg, important social event such as wedding, prom, etc)
- Systemic corticosteroids used continuously may actually cause or worsen acne.
- Topical corticosteroids have no value in the treatment of acne, and the high-potency topical corticosteroids will aggravate acne and should never be used on the face of acne patients.

2. Fungal Skin Infections

- Tinea are skin infections known as dermatomycoses caused by the fungi *Trichophyton, Microsporum,* and *Epidermophyton.*

Classification

- Tinea pedis (athlete's foot)
- Tinea capitis (ringworm of the scalp)
- Tinea cruris (jock itch)
- Tinea corporis (ringworm of the skin)
- Tinea unguium (onychomycosis; fungal infection of toenails or fingernails)

Pathophysiology

- The fungi invade dead cells of the stratum corneum of skin, hair, and nails, digesting keratin.
- Unlike *Candida,* they cannot exist on unkeratinized mucous membranes.
- More common in immunosuppressed patients

Treatment Principles and Goals

- Tinea pedis: self-treat topically initially; if ineffective, add orals.
- Tinea capitis: oral systemic therapy
- Tinea cruris: self-treat topically initially; if ineffective, add orals.
- Tinea corporis: self-treat topically initially; if ineffective, add orals.
- Tinea unguium: oral systemic therapy

Drug Therapy

OTC treatment
- Terbinafine 1% (Lamisil AT®) cream and spray
    * Most effective OTC antifungal agent
- Miconazole 2% (Micatin®)
- Clotrimazole 1% (Lotrimin AF®, Desenex AF®)
- Tolnaftate 1% (Tinactin®, Aftate®, Blis-To-Sol®, Dr. Scholl's Fungi Solution®)
- Undecylenic acid 10-25% (Cruex®, Desenex®)

Prescription treatment
- See Table 4.

Topicals
- Newer antifungals are initially applied only once daily, and recurrences can be prevented by once- or twice-weekly applications.

Table 4

Prescription Topical Antifungals

Generic name	Trade name
Econazole	Spectazole® cream, Ecostatin® cream
Naftifine	Naftin® gel, cream
Ciclopirox	Loprox® gel, cream, lotion; Penlac® solution
Butenafine	Mentax® cream

Systemic therapy
- Occasionally topical therapy is not effective for tinea pedis, tinea cruris, and tinea corporis, and systemic therapy is required.
- Systemic antifungal therapy is required for tinea capitis (ringworm of the scalp) and tinea unguium (fungal infections of the fingernails and toenails):
    * Griseofulvin
    * Ketoconazole
    * Fluconazole
    * Itraconazole
    * Terbinafine
- See chapter on antimicrobials for discussion of systemic antifungals.

3. Hair Loss (Alopecia)

- Male pattern baldness (androgenic alopecia) is the gradual and progressive loss of hair in males as they age.

Clinical Presentation

- Onset and progression vary greatly.
- Distinct pattern of progressive hair loss in the frontotemporal areas and crown with sparing of the occiput
- Hair loss limited to scalp
- Miniaturization of hair is seen, where normal thick terminal hairs are converted to very fine vellus hairs.

Pathophysiology

- Alopecia is primarily due to two factors:
  * Heredity (genetic)
  * Testosterone, which promotes growth of hair in the beard, axillae, pubis, and other parts of the body, does not promote the growth of scalp hair, and actually contributes to premature loss because it is converted by the enzyme 5-α-reductase to dihydrotestosterone, which binds preferentially to receptors in the hair follicles on the scalp, causing them to produce progressively thinner hair, until the follicles eventually cease activity altogether.

Treatment Principles and Goals

- Although there is no cure, there are two drugs available for the treatment of androgenic alopecia:
  * Minoxidil (Rogaine®; available OTC)
  * Finasteride (Propecia®; by prescription only)
- In the early stages, topical minoxidil or oral finasteride may reverse the gradually decreasing diameter of the hair shaft.
- Any hair growth stimulation is temporary and only lasts as long as therapy continues; if therapy is discontinued, new hair growth is lost within 1 year.
- Early hair loss occurring recently in younger men is more likely to respond than later hair loss at an older age or when hair loss is not recent.
- Alopecia of the crown in men responds better than hair loss in the frontotemporal area.

Drug Therapy

Minoxidil
- OTC: trade names Rogaine® 2% and Rogaine Extra Strength® 5%

Mechanism of action
- Probably increased cutaneous blood flow directly to hair follicles due to vasodilation
- Possible stimulation of resting hair follicles (telogen phase) into active growth (anagen phase)
- Possible stimulation of hair follicle cells

Patient counseling
- Apply 1 mL twice daily (approximately one 60-mL bottle each month).
- May be applied without shampooing hair
- Use at least 4 hours before bedtime to avoid oil on pillows and bed linens.
- Absorbed over a 4-hour period, so do not swim, shampoo, or walk in rain for 4 hours.
- Wash hands immediately after application to prevent unwanted absorption.
- Do not inhale mist as systemic absorption is possible.
- Do not use on infected, irritated, inflamed, or sunburned skin.
- Discontinue use immediately and contact physician if chest pain, increased heart rate, faintness or dizziness, or swollen hands or feet occur.
- Women should avoid 5% strength (no better results than 2%); women have greater incidence of increased growth of facial hair with 5% solution.
- Generally takes 4-6 months before any benefit occurs.
- No effects within 8 months for women and 12 months for men indicates therapeutic failure and treatment should be discontinued.
- Must continue using to maintain new hair growth

Adverse drug effects
- Scalp dermatitis is common, producing dryness, pruritus, and flaking or scaling.
- Hypertrichosis (excessive hair growth) on areas other than scalp (chest, forearms, ear rim, back, face, arms, etc)
- Some women report unwanted facial hair growth when applied to scalp, primarily with the 5% solution.
- May rarely produce systemic side effects (chest pain, increased heart rate, faintness or dizziness)
- Contraindicated in patients less than age 18 years old
- Contraindicated in women who are pregnant or breastfeeding

Finasteride
- Trade name: Propecia 1 mg
- Originally approved in 1992 for the treatment of enlarged prostate glands (benign prostatic hypertrophy) in a 5-mg dose (Proscar®)

- 1-mg daily dose approved for men only as prescription treatment for androgenic alopecia.
- Effectiveness: over a 2-year period, may halt the progressive hair loss of androgenic alopecia

Mechanism of action
- Inhibits the enzyme 5-α-reductase, which is responsible for the conversion of testosterone to the more powerful dihydrotestosterone (DHT), which is the main androgen responsible for androgenic hair loss

Patient counseling
- May be taken with or without food
- Take for at least 3 months to see if effective
- Improvement lasts only as long as treatment continues (new hair will be lost with 1 year of stopping treatment).

Adverse drug effects
- Gynecomastia (breast enlargement and tenderness) reported from 2 weeks to 2 years following initial therapy; usually reversible when therapy is discontinued.
- Hypersensitivity (skin rash, swelling of lips)
- Decreased libido, erectile dysfunction, and ejaculatory dysfunction, which are reversible when the drug is discontinued
- Contraindicated in women of childbearing age, due to abnormalities of the external genitalia in male fetuses; and also not effective in postmenopausal women

4. Dry Skin

- Refers to lack of moisture or sebum in the stratum corneum
- Most commonly occurring in the winter (also known as "winter rash")
- More common in older adults

Clinical Presentation

- Flaking and scaling
- Xerosis and roughness
- Pruritus
- Loss of skin elasticity

Pathophysiology

- Dry skin is due to inadequate moisture retention in the stratum corneum, which is caused by the following factors:
    * Decreased sebum production and decreasing moisture binding capacity of skin in elderly patients
    * Low humidity causes the skin to lose water, and become dry and hardened.
    * Overexposure to sunlight
    * Excessive cleansing and bathing removes lipids and other skin components.
    * Chronic skin diseases that impair moisture retention of skin (psoriasis, scleroderma, ichthyosis, and contact dermatitis)

Treatment Principles and Goals

- Increasing moisture level of the stratum corneum by increasing cell hydration and binding capacity, which improves skin permeability and restores elasticity

Drug Therapy

Emollients and moisturizing agents (petrolatum; mineral oil [Lubriderm® Bath and Shower Oil])
- Increase relative moisture content of the stratum corneum
- Produce a general soothing effect by reducing frictional heat and perspiration

Humectants (glycerin [Corn Husker's® Lotion], propylene glycol, phospholipids)
- Hygroscopic agents that increase hydration of the stratum corneum

Keratin-softening agents
- Urea (10-30%) (Aquacare®, Carmol®)
    * Improves the skin's moisture-binding capacity
    * Keratolytic at higher concentrations
    * May cause irritation and burning
- Lactic acid (2-5%) (LactiCare®, Lowila Cake®)
    * Increases skin hydration by controlling the rate of keratinization
    * Markedly hygroscopic
- Allantoin (Alphosyl®, Psorex®, Tegrin®)
    * Relieves dry skin by disrupting keratin structure (less effective than urea)
    * Desensitizes many skin-sensitizing drugs as a protectant

Antipruritic agents
- Camphor and menthol provide a cooling sensation.
- Local anesthetics (benzocaine, pramoxine, etc)
- Colloidal oatmeal (Aveeno®)
    * *Caution:* colloidal oatmeal can cause an extremely slippery bathtub.
- Systemic antihistamines (H_1-receptor antagonists): limited effectiveness

Hydrocortisone
- Reduces inflammatory response that accompanies dry skin conditions
- Although HC does not directly increase skin hydration, it does prevent itching associated with dry skin and inhibits dehydration.
- Ointment is better than cream for dry skin.
- Must use sparingly
- Do not use more than 5 to 7 days for dry skin pruritus.

Astringents
- Aluminum acetate 0.1-0.5% (Burow's solution)
- Hamamelis water (witch hazel)

Protectants
- Zinc oxide

Nondrug Recommendations and Therapy

- Bathe less frequently.
- Reduce use of soap to a minimum and only where necessary.
- Lubricate skin immediately after bathing (eg, application of bath oil after bathing and before drying).
- Use extrafatted soaps such as Basis®.

Use combination products to treat dry skin
    * Alpha Keri® Moisture Rich Cleansing Bar: mineral oil, lanolin oil, glycerin
    * Aveeno® Bath Treatment Moisturizing Formula: colloidal oatmeal and mineral oil

* Jergens® Advanced Therapy Dry Skin Care Lotion: dimethicone, lanolin, cetyl alcohol, isopropyl myristate, glycerin
* Keri® Original Dry Skin Lotion: mineral oil, lanolin oil, glyceryl stearate, propylene glycol
* Moisturel® Lotion: petrolatum, dimethicone, cetyl alcohol, glycerin
* Neutrogena® Body Oil: isopropyl myristate, sesame oil
* Pacquin® Plus Dry Skin Hand and Body Cream: lanolin anhydrous, cetyl alcohol, glycerin
* Sardo® Bath Oil: mineral oil, isopropyl palmitate
* Vaseline® Dermatology Formula Lotion: white petrolatum, mineral oil, dimethicone, glyceryl stearate, cetyl alcohol, glycerin

5. Dermatitis

- Nonspecific term to describe a variety of inflammatory dermatologic conditions characterized by erythema
- A general term to describe any eczematous rash of unknown etiology that cannot be classified among the major endogenous dermatoses
- Eczema and dermatitis are often used interchangeably.

Types and Classification

- Several of the major classifications or types of dermatitis are:
    * Atopic dermatitis (atopic eczema)
    * Chronic dermatitis (hand dermatitis)
    * Contact dermatitis (irritant and allergic)

Clinical Presentation

Atopic dermatitis (atopic eczema)
- Occurs primarily in infants and children
- May disappear before adulthood
- Cause unknown; possibly genetic
- Usually seen on face, knees, elbows, and neck
- Frequently seen with asthma, allergic rhinitis, and urticaria
- Exacerbating factors: soaps, detergents, chemicals, temperature changes, molds, allergens

Chronic dermatitis (hand dermatitis or hand eczema)
- Stubborn itchy rash referred to as eczema that occurs in certain persons with sensitive or irritable skin.
- Skin very dry and easily irritated by overuse of soaps, detergents, and/or rough woolen clothing
- Exacerbated by very hot or very cold weather
- Probably genetically determined
- No permanent cure
- Usually can control by enhancing skin hydration with emollients and moisturizers, and using hydrocortisone cream to relieve itching

Contact dermatitis
Irritant contact dermatitis (chemical contact dermatitis)
- Caused by exposure to irritating substances producing mechanical or chemical trauma
- Examples: soap, solvents, paints, abrasive cleansers, cosmetics, lubricants, antiseptics, cacti, rose hips, thorns, peppers, tobacco
- Not a sensitization, but direct toxicity to skin tissue

Allergic contact dermatitis
- Process of sensitization with reaction on elicitation
- Over 50% of all dermatitis is allergic contact dermatitis.
- Examples: benzocaine, zinc pyrithione (ZPT), neomycin, sodium bisulfite, perfumes, many cosmetics, skin lubricants, antiseptic creams, rubber and epoxy glues, poison ivy and oak, and many other common substances

Treatment Principles and Goals

- Treated by applying a corticosteroid:
    * Ointments and creams are more lubricating than solutions, lotions, or gels.
    * Ointments should be recommended if skin is dry.
    * Lotions or gels should be recommended for a weeping, eczematous dermatitis.
    * Lotions, solutions, and gels are also easier to use in hairy areas of the body.
- Patient should apply small amounts of corticosteroid cream or ointment and massage in gently but thoroughly.
- Apply the moderate- and high-strength cortisones only once daily.
- Improvement should begin within 1 week.
- Avoid excess soap, and keep skin lubricated with moisturizers.
- Treat itching with camphor, menthol, phenol, or local anesthetics.
- Occasionally with severe cases (less than 5%) may have to use systemic corticosteroids for 1-2 weeks.

Drug Therapy

Topical corticosteroids (see Table 5).

Adverse effects
- Striae may result in skin folds.
- Thinning of epidermis where subcutaneous vessels become visible
- The more potent types can cause or aggravate acne or rosacea on the face.
- Percutaneous absorption leading to systemic effects: (see chapter on endocrine diseases for complete list of systemic adverse effects).
    * Hyperglycemia
    * Glycosuria
    * Hypothalamic-pituitary-adrenal (HPA) axis suppression which could pose a threat in case of surgery, systemic illness, or trauma/injury
- Percutaneous absorption leading to systemic effects most likely with:
    * The higher potency (HP) types of agents
    * Inflamed skin, and also in infants and children

Table 5

Topical Corticosteroids Classified by Relative Potency

Relative potency	Generic name	Trade name	Strength
Low	Hydrocortisone (OTC)	Cortaid®, Cortizone®	1% = OTC
		Allercort®, Hytone®, Synacort®, Emo-Cort®	2.5% = Rx only
Medium	Desonide	Tridesilon Des Owen®	0.05%
	Fluocinolone acetonide	Synalar®	0.01-0.025%
	Flurandrenolide	Cordran®	0.025-0.05%
	Hydrocortisone butyrate	Locoid®	0.1%
	Hydrocortisone valerate	Westcort®	0.2%
	Triamcinolone acetonide	Aristocort®	0.025%
High	Betamethasone valerate	Valisone®, Dermabet®	0.1%
	Fluocinolone	Synalar®, Synemol®	0.025%
	Triamcinolone acetonide	Aristocort®	0.1%
Very high	Desoximetasone	Topicort®	0.25%
	Diflorasone diacetate	Maxiflor®	0.05%
	Fluocinonide	Lidex®	0.01-0.05%
	Halcinonide	Halog®	0.1%
Ultra-high	Betamethasone dipropionate	Diprosone®, Maxivate®	0.05%
	Betamethasone dipropionate (in optimized vehicle)	Diprolene AF®	0.05%
	Clobetasol propionate	Temovate®	0.05%
	Diflorasone diacetate	Psorcon®	0.05%
	Halobetasol propionate	Ultravate®	0.05%

* Long-term use and/or use over a large area of the skin
* Occlusion markedly increases absorption of topical corticosteroids and should therefore be used cautiously in limited areas and reserved for severe, resistant lesions.

Topical antipruritics
* Local anesthetics (benzocaine up to 20% and pramoxine 1%)
* Benzyl alcohol
* Colloidal oatmeal (Aveeno®)
* Others (camphor, menthol, phenol)

Emollients
* Petrolatum
* Lanolin
* Mineral oil

Topical immunomodulators
* Approved for atopic dermatitis
* Inhibits activation of T cells and release of certain inflammatory mediators (cytokines)
* Applied bid with onset in 1 to 3 weeks

* Side effects: stinging, burning, pruritus, rare flu-like symptoms
* *Caution:* Use sunscreen.

Immunomodulator products
* Tacrolimus (Protopic®) 0.03% and 0.1% ointment
* Pimecrolimus (Elidel®) 1% cream

Oral corticosteroids
* Corticosteroids are the only systemic anti-inflammatory agents that are effective.

Oral antihistamines
* Very limited effectiveness, possibly antipruritic

6. Poison Ivy, Poison Oak, and Poison Sumac Allergy (Rhus Dermatitis)

- Allergic reaction to sap (urushiol) of some plants of the genus *Rhus* (poison ivy, poison oak, and poison sumac)
- The most common form of allergic contact dermatitis
- Direct contact with leaves, roots, or branches is not required to get a rash; sap can reach skin indirectly from clothing, a pet, or burning (volatilization).
- *Rhus* allergy is acquired; individuals are not born with it.
- Most persons are sensitized to *Rhus* because it is such a common plant; however, some people are never allergic to it
- No effective way to desensitize a person with allergy to rhus plants.

Types and Classification

Mild
- Localized patches of pruritus and erythema, followed by appearance of vesicles and papules on the upper and/or lower extremities

Moderate
- Extensive pruritus and irritation, with severe vesicles and appearance of bullae and edematous swelling

Severe
- Extreme pruritus, irritation, severe vesicle and bullae formation
- Extensive involvement, widespread over the body and/or face
- Extensive edema of extremities and/or face
- Eye, genitalia, or mucous membrane involvement

Clinical Presentation

- Not contagious
- Fluid in blisters does not spread rash.
- Rash appears after a latent period that varies from 4 hours to 10 days, depending on an individual's sensitivity and the amount of plant contact.
- When more rash appears after treatment has begun, these are areas with a longer latent period.
- Symptoms may last from 5-21 days following initial rash.
- Secondary infections can occur if scratching excoriates the skin and the abrasion become infected.

Treatment Principles and Goals

- Self-limited: mild cases will clear without treatment within 7-14 days.
- Prevent itching and excessive scratching and possible secondary skin infections.

Treatment options
- Mild cases: topical antipruritics, such as calamine, camphor, menthol, phenol, or local anesthetics to prevent itching and topical HC cream or ointment
- Moderate cases: topical high-potency corticosteroids for small areas
- Severe cases: systemic corticosteroids daily up to 2 weeks
    * Severe rash needs systemic corticosteroids to ease the misery and disability.
    * Usually needed during early severe stages because remedies applied to skin may not penetrate deeply enough

Therapy

OTC topical therapy
- Astringents/protectants: compresses, soaks, or wet dressings will dry the oozing, reduce the weeping, aid in removal of crusts, and soothe the skin.
    * Aluminum acetate solution 1:40 ratio (Burow's solution)
    * Aluminum sulfate (Domeboro® powder)
    * Calamine lotion
    * Others: aluminum hydroxide gel, kaolin, zinc acetate, zinc carbonate, zinc oxide
- Local anesthetics (benzocaine up to 20% and pramoxine 1%, benzyl alcohol)
    * Caladryl® lotion: calamine and pramoxine 1%
    * Ruli® calamine spray: calamine, benzocaine, and camphor
    * Ivarest® 8-Hour Medicated Cream: calamine and diphenhydramine 2%
    * Ivy Dry® Cream: benzyl alcohol, camphor, menthol, zinc acetate
- 1% Hydrocortisone products
- Colloidal oatmeal (Aveeno) provides temporary skin protection from exposures.
- Cool compresses

Prescription topical therapy
- Topical medium- to high-potency corticosteroids (see section on allergic contact dermatitis).

Prescription systemic corticosteroid therapy
- See section on allergic contact dermatitis and the chapter on endocrine disorders for complete details.

- Use of systemic corticosteroids is the only therapy that will actually reduce the severity and duration of the allergic response.
- Effects of oral corticosteroids are dramatic (can take up to 40-100 mg prednisone for 2 or 3 weeks if necessary); however, many patients clear up quickly with a corticosteroid "dosepak" (eg, Aristocort®, Decadron®, or Medrol®).
- Extremely severe cases or large-scale rash may require parenteral dose of corticosteroid (100 mg prednisone equivalent).

Other recommendations
Prevention
- Avoidance: "leaves of three, let it be."
- Removal: washing with soap and water within 15 minutes of exposure may reduce the extent and duration of dermatitis.
- Bentoquatam 5% solution: Ivy Block® lotion
    * An organoclay
    * Only barrier product approved by the FDA
    * Patient instructions: apply 15 minutes before possible plant contact; reapply every 4 hours.

7. Scaly Dermatoses

- There are three common forms of scaly dermatoses: dandruff, seborrhea, and psoriasis.

Dandruff

- Dandruff is a chronic, noninflammatory scalp condition resulting in excessive scaling of the scalp epidermis.
- It is a common condition affecting 20% of the population.
- It is not a serious disorder, but can be cosmetically unsightly.

Clinical presentation
- Scaling and pruritus, causing white flakes to accumulate on the scalp

Pathophysiology
- Increased epidermal cell turnover rate of approximately twice normal (time reduced from 25-30 days to 13-15 days) prevents complete keratinization of desquamated cells due to unknown processes.
- May be related to increased *Pityrosporum ovale*, a fungal scalp organism

Treatment
- Routine shampooing with mild hypoallergenic shampoo is essential.

Cytostatic agents
- Cytostatic agents suppress cell turnover; goal is to reduce epidermal rate of turnover of scalp cells.
    * Zinc pyrithione (ZPT) (0.3-2%) (Head and Shoulders®, X-Seb®, Zincon®); mechanism of action: antifungal effect and/or reducing cell turnover rate
    * Selenium sulfide 1% (Selsun Blue® 1%; Selsun® 2.5%); mechanism of action: reduce the cell rate turnover and/or inhibit growth of *P ovale*
    * Coal tar (Balnetar®, Denorex®, Estar®, Ionil T®, Polytar®, Tegrin®); mechanism of action: coal tar reduces the number and size of epidermal cells.
    * Patient instructions: contact time with cytostatic agents is very important for effectiveness; advise patients to rub shampoo in well and leave in up to 5 minutes before rinsing out.

Keratolytics

- Salicylic acid (1.8-3%) (Ionil®, Sebucare®)
    * Ability to lower the pH of tissues, increasing the water concentration of epidermal cells, which softens and destroys the stratum corneum; causes upper skin layer to become inflamed and soft, followed by desquamation; this keratolytic action removes the scales of dandruff.
- Sulfur (2-5%) (Sulfoam®, Sulray®, Exsel®)
    * Possibly exerts an antifungal effect
    * Usually found in combinations with salicylic acid
- Combination sulfur and salicylic acid: Meted® and Sebulex®

Antifungals

- Ketoconazole (1%) shampoo (Nizoral AD®)
- Ciclopirox 1% shampoo (Loprox®)
    * Active against *P ovale*
    * Use twice weekly, or every 3 or 4 days
    * Stress adequate contact time for a minimum of 3 minutes.
    * Adverse effects include itching, stinging, or irritation

Seborrhea (Seborrheic Dermatitis)

- Seborrhea is a chronic inflammatory skin disease in areas of greatest sebaceous gland activity: on the scalp and other hairy areas such as the face, trunk, armpits, and groin.

Clinical presentation

- Scaling rash accompanied by pruritus
- Yellowish, greasy scales unlike the dry scale of dandruff
- Inflammatory, often accompanied by erythema
- Fluctuates in severity and characterized by exacerbations and remissions
- Most commonly occurs on the face, eyebrows, and eyelashes, but not on the extremities
- Aggravated and worsened by nervous stress and poor health
- Not contagious
- Persists for life; no cure, but can control

Pathophysiology

- Accelerated cell turnover rate of approximately 3 times normal rate, probably as few as 9-10 days
- Higher cell turnover rate than dandruff, but less than psoriasis
- *Pityrosporum ovale* may be causative, but this is not universally accepted.

Treatment

- Similar to treatment for dandruff, but more difficult to treat (overuse of selenium can make scalp oily and actually exacerbate seborrhea).
- Topical corticosteroids are used to control itching and inflammation (up to 7 days) (Cortaid®, others).
- Add the topical antifungal ketoconazole 1% shampoo (Nizoral AD) or ciclopirox 1% shampoo (Loprox)
    * Active against *Pityrosporum ovale*
    * Use twice weekly, every 3 or 4 days
    * Stress adequate contact time; leave in for at least 3 minutes.
    * Adverse effects include itching, stinging, or irritation.

"Cradle cap" (infantile seborrheic dermatitis)

- Seborrhea of the scalp in newborns or infants
- Most common in the first few months of life
- Most common on top of head; may be due to poor washing
- Probably not related to fungal infection
- Treatment:
    * Massage with oils
    * Nonmedicated shampoos
    * Use milder keratolytics (Meted, Sebulex) 2 or 3 times per week

Psoriasis

- Psoriasis is a chronic inflammatory papulosquamous erythematous skin disease.
- It is marked by the presence of silvery scales with sharply delineated edges.
- Lesions are usually localized, but can gradually grow to cover large areas.
- It can have significant physiological and psychological effects.
- It affects 1-3% of the population, 98% Caucasian.

Classification

Type I
- Early age of onset, family history, increased frequency of human lymphocyte antigen

Type II
- Develops later in life, no family history

Pathophysiology

- Hyperproliferative skin condition resulting from skin cell turnover rate of approximately 10-20 times normal; skin cells of psoriatic plaque reach the outermost layer in 3-4 days.
- Genetic predisposition, as well as exposure of skin to trauma or triggering factors such as stressful incidents

Clinical presentation

- Plaque most common and known as *psoriasis vulgaris*
- Plaque known also as scales; silvery on top and pink to red beneath
- May be found anywhere on the body, but more likely on scalp, sacral area, extensor surfaces of knees and elbows (less common on face)
- Borders of plaque are sharp with inflammation surrounding the plaque
- Chronic condition; varies from mild forms of the disease to very severe with such extensive coverage that it hinders social and work life
- Marked by spontaneous exacerbations and remissions

Treatment
Topicals

- Topical corticosteroids
- Coal tar: contained in Denorex, DHS®, Ionil T, MG217®, Neutrogena T®, Pantene Pro-V®, Polytar®, Tegrin, X-Seb T Plus®
- Keratolytics: salicylic acid and sulfur
- Combinations: Sebutone (salicylic acid, sulfur, and coal tar)
- Retinoids: tretinoin, adapalene, tazarotene, alitretinoin
- Anthralin: Anthraforte®, Anthranol®, Dritho-Scalp®
- Calcipotriene: Dovonex® ointment, cream, solution (a vitamin D_3 analog)
    * *Caution:* If used in conjugation with PUVA therapy (psoralens with UV-A), apply after light treatment, as PUVA inactivates this product.

Systemic treatment

- Oral corticosteroids
- Antimetabolites (eg, methotrexate and cyclosporine)
- Psoralens (combined with UV light therapy)
- Immunosuppressants: alefacept (Amevive®); efalizumab, (Raptiva®); etanercept, (Enbrel®)
- Retinoids: acitretin (Soriatane®), etretinate: (Tegison®)
- Vitamin A analogs are reserved for severe and extensive psoriasis.
- Approaches effectiveness of methotrexate or cyclosporine when combined with UV light therapy.
- Adverse effects: dry lips, skin, nail changes, dry eyes, hair loss, hyperlipidemia, pancreatitis, hepatotoxicity, myalgias, arthralgias, teratogenic

Other therapy

- Ultraviolet light therapy
    * Following coal tar applications
    * Concurrent with oral psoralens

8. Pediculosis

- Head lice is the primary or most common form.
- Very common, especially in schoolchildren
- Lice are transmitted by direct contact with the head of an infected individual or through fomites (inanimate objects capable of transmitting disease, eg, sharing combs, brushes, or headwear).
- Most common in August and September, after long holidays and/or summer camps
- Body lice is a less common form that usually occurs in individuals who do not change clothing often (eg, the homeless).
- Pubic lice (crab lice) is transferred through sexual contact and is found primarily in pubic areas, but also can affect armpits.

Classification

- There are three types of human pediculosis:
    * Head lice: *Pediculus humanus* capitis
    * Body lice: *Pediculus humanus corporis* (same species as head lice)
    * Pubic lice: *Pthirus pubis* (crab louse is a different species)

Clinical Presentation

- Pruritus is the most common symptom.
- Often symptomatic, diagnosis is made visually by seeing live lice.
- Difficult to locate or visualize the flat, gray-brown adult lice; the nits (larvae) firmly attached to hair shafts may be more visible.

Drug Therapy

Synergized pyrethrins (0.17-0.33%; A-200®, Barc®, End-Lice®, Lice-Enz®, Pronto®, R&C® shampoo, Rid®, Triple X®)
- Natural chemical derived from chrysanthemums which is synergized by addition of 2-4% piperonyl butoxide (petroleum derivative)

Mechanism of action
- Blocks transmission of nerve cell impulses in lice, causing paralysis

Patient counseling
- Wash and dry hair and apply for 10 minutes.
- Use lice/nit comb to remove dead lice and nits following rinsing.
- Treat all family members.
- Avoid contact with the eyes, mouth, and nose
- Do not use on irritated or inflamed scalp.

- Treatment should be repeated in 1 week to 10 days.

Adverse drug effects
- Irritation, erythema, itching

Permethrin 1% (Nix® Cream Rinse); permethrin 5%, prescription-only strength (Acticin®, Elimite® Cream)
- Synthetic chemical derivative of pyrethrin
- 1% OTC-strength approved only for head lice; however, it is effective against pubic lice.
- 5% prescription-strength is approved for scabies (mites) infestation.
- Patients prefer these because of single-application effectiveness.

Mechanism of action
- Blocks transmission of nerve cell impulses in lice, causing paralysis

Patient information
- Applied to washed hair and scalp
- Leave on hair for 10 minutes, then rinse
- After rinsing, comb with lice comb to remove lice and nits.
- One-time treatment (do not repeat in 10 days).
- Recommend that all family members be treated.

Adverse effects
- Scalp irritation, pruritus, and stinging
- Contraindicated in patients allergic to chrysanthemums
- Contraindicated in children under 2 years of age

Lindane (Kwell® shampoo, cream, lotion; prescription only)
- Former name was gamma benzene hexachloride
- Effective against pediculosis capitis and pubis and scabies (caused by *Sarcoptes scabiei*)
- The drug is currently unavailable for use in the U.S.

Adverse effects
- Lindane is absorbed significantly through the skin and has been reported to have significant neurotoxic effects, especially in infants and children.
- CNS effects reported: convulsions, dizziness, incoordination, restlessness, irritability
- Other effects: rapid heartbeat, muscle cramps, vomiting
- The OTC medications are considered much safer, especially in children.

Nondrug recommendations
- Change clothing daily.
- Treat infested clothes and shower daily.
- All household contacts should be inspected and treated if necessary.
- All bed linens and clothes should be dry cleaned or washed in the hot water cycle and dried on the heated air cycle for at least 20 minutes.
- Wash hairbrushes, combs, and toys in hot water for at least 10 minutes.
- Treat surrounding environment (bedding, pillows, carpets, draperies, furniture) with A-200® Control Spray or Rid® Control Spray.

9. Warts

- Warts (verrucae) are harmless skin growths resulting from an infectious disease caused by the human papillomavirus (HPV).

Classification

- Common warts (verruca vulgaris) on fingers, hands, knees
- Common flat warts (verruca plana) on face, hands, legs
- Plantar warts (verruca plantaris) on the soles of the feet
- Anogenital warts (verruca genitalia) on the anogenital area

Clinical Presentation

- Warts are contagious, and may spread on the body.
- Warts are more common in children and immuno-compromised patients.
- Warts on the face or hands protrude.
- Warts occurring on pressure areas such as the bottom of the feet (plantar warts) grow inward from the pressure of standing and walking, are often painful, and may be confused with corns.

Treatment Principles and Goals

- Warts can be eliminated by:
    * Direct application of the following caustics: salicylic acid, formalin, lactic acid, trichloroacetic acid, podophyllin
    * Freezing (cryotherapy)with liquid nitrogen or Dimethyl ether and propane (DMEP)
    * Surgery

OTC drug therapy
Salicylic acid
- Use topical salicylic acid preparations on a daily basis until the wart is removed.
- Since warts are contagious, use special care in washing hands before and after treatment, and use a separate towel for drying other parts of the body.
- Do not use salicylic acid on irritated, broken, or infected skin.
- If the wart remains after 12 weeks of continuous treatment, see a dermatologist or podiatrist.
- Salicylic acid products are contraindicated in patients with diabetes and other patients with poor circulation because reduced sensation in the foot delays awareness of skin breakdown, allowing possible development of infection that can lead to sepsis.

- Refer diabetics to a physician or podiatrist for removal of warts.

OTC salicylic acid products
- Salicylic acid 17% in flexible collodion vehicle:
    * Compound W®, Duofilm®, Wart-Off®,Off-Ezy® Wart Remover Kit
- Salicylic acid 40% embedded in pads or discs:
    * Clear Away® discs, Dr. Scholl's Clear Away®, Compound W® One Step Pads

OTC cryotherapy products
- Dimethyl ether and propane: Wartner Wart Removal System®; approved for removal of common warts
- Dimethyl ether, propane, and isobutane: Compound W Freeze Off®: approved for removal of common warts and plantar warts
- Dimethyl ether and propane (DMEP) is FDA approved for OTC removal of common warts and plantar warts.

Mechanism of action
- Cryotherapy irritation leads the host to produce an immune response against the causative virus (similar to liquid nitrogen, which can only be administered by a primary care provider). As a result of freezing, a blister will form under the wart. After about 10 days, the frozen skin and wart fall off, revealing newly formed skin underneath.

Patient instructions
- Place the applicator in the spray can, which becomes very cold (–55°C)
- After the applicator is saturated, the patient holds it on the wart for a product-specific time period to freeze the wart (20 seconds for Wartner; 40 seconds for Compound W).
- The process may be repeated after 10 days as many as 3 or 4 times for persistent warts.
- *Caution:* Do not use in children under 4 years old; diabetics; if pregnant or breastfeeding; on the face, armpits, breasts, buttocks or genitals; on irritated skin; or on mucous membranes (eg, mouth, nose, anus).

10. Corns and Calluses

- Corns and calluses are excessive growth of the upper keratinized layer of the skin.
- They are more common in women than men.
- Diabetics have an increased incidence of calluses on their feet due to the loss of sensation, preventing them from noticing the pressure that would otherwise be uncomfortable.

Classification

- Hard corns (heloma durum): corns overlying a bony prominence such as the toes or bottom of the heel
- Soft corns (heloma molle; interdigital corns): corns between the toes (especially the fourth and fifth)
- Calluses (callosities): superficial patches of hornified epidermis; flattened, but thickened with no central core

Clinical Presentation and Pathophysiology

- Caused by excessive growth of the upper keratinized layer of the skin (hyperkeratoses), due to friction or pressure, usually from improper or tight-fitting shoes

Treatment

- The only FDA-approved OTC medication is salicylic acid formulated in flexible collodion, plasters, disks, or pads.

Mechanism of action
- Salicylic acid produces a keratolytic action, increasing hydration and lowering the pH of the outer skin, which initially softens, then destroys the outer layer of skin.

Patient counseling
- Do not apply to irritated, infected, or reddened skin.
- If discomfort persists after using for 14 days, see a physician or podiatrist.
- Contraindicated in diabetics

Adverse drug effects
- Salicylic acid products are contraindicated in patients with diabetes and other patients with poor circulation because reduced sensation in the foot delays awareness of skin breakdown, allowing possible development of infection that can lead to sepsis.
- Refer diabetics to a physician or podiatrist for removal of corns or calluses.

OTC salicylic acid (SA) corn and callus products
- Freezone® Corn and Callus Remover 13.6% SA
- Freezone® One Step Corn Remover 40% SA
- Mediplast® 40% SA plaster, cut to size
- Mosco® Corn and Callus Remover 17.6% SA
- Off Ezy® Corn and Callus Remover 17% SA
- One Step® Callus Remover 40% SA
- Dr. Scholl's® Corn and Callus Remover Liquid 12.6% SA
- Dr. Scholl's® Corn or Callus Cushion Gel 40% SA
- Dr. Scholl's® One Step Corn or Callus Remover Disc 40% SA

11. Key Points

Acne
- Acne occurs primarily in the teenage years due to the increase of androgens during puberty that produces increased activity of the sebaceous glands.
- Isotretinoin (Accutane) is the drug of choice for nodulocystic acne (type IV acne), which if left untreated will lead to extensive scarring.
- Isotretinoin (Accutane) is contraindicated in pregnancy due to the high incidence of serious birth defects.
- The most common side effects of isotretinoin (Accutane) are cheilitis (dry, chapped lips), dry skin, and dry eyes.

Fungal infections of the skin
- The most efficacious nonprescription topical antifungal is terbinafine (Lamisil).
- Systemic antifungal therapy is required for treatment of tinea capitis (ringworm of the scalp) and tinea unguium (fungal infection of the toenails).

Hair loss
- Androgenic alopecia, predominantly seen in males, is due to the conversion of testosterone to dihydrotestosterone, which binds to the hair follicles causing them to produce progressively thinner hair.
- In the treatment of androgenic alopecia, minoxidil (Rogaine) should be applied and left on the scalp for 4 hours for maximum effects.
- Finasteride (Propecia) decreases the effect of androgens on hair follicles by inhibiting 5-α-reductase, which prevents the conversion of testosterone to dihydrotestosterone.

Dry skin
- Dry skin occurs primarily in older adults due to decreased sebum production and decreased moisture binding capacity of the skin.
- Products containing urea and lactic acid improve the skin's moisture binding capacity, thereby increasing skin hydration.

Dermatitis
- Contact dermatitis, whether irritant or allergic, is initially treated with topical corticosteroid products.
- The absorption and subsequent adverse systemic effects of topical corticosteroids is increased with (1) occlusion, (2) in infant skin, (3) with the use of high-potency agents, and (4) with long-term use.

Poison ivy and oak
- Poison ivy, poison oak, and poison sumac are examples of causes of allergic contact dermatitis, and are the result of contact with the sap of plants of the genus *Rhus*.
- Severe cases of poison ivy, poison oak, or poison sumac require systemic corticosteroids to relieve symptoms, decrease the severity of the rash, and shorten the course of the disorder.

Scaly dermatoses
- The cytostatic agents that suppress cell rate turnover, zinc pyrithione (ZPT; Head and Shoulders) and selenium sulfide (Selsun Blue), are the primary agents of choice for treatment of dandruff.
- Seborrhea usually requires topical corticosteroids and/or the topical antifungal ketoconazole for effective treatment.
- Psoriasis is a chronic inflammatory disease characterized by inflammation and silvery scales (known as plaques) with sharp delineated edges.
- Treatment of advanced psoriasis may require systemic corticosteroids and/or antimetabolites in addition to topical treatments in order to effectively manage the disease.

Pediculosis
- Head lice (*Pediculus humanus capitis*) occur most commonly in elementary schoolchildren in the months of August and September.
- Permethrin (Nix) is the nonprescription agent of choice for treatment of head lice (*Pediculus humanus capitis*) because it usually does not have to be repeated in 7-10 days as do other available nonprescription pediculicidal agents (synergized pyrethrins).

Corns and warts
- Nonprescription products for the treatment of corns and warts contain salicylic acid.
- Self treatment for corns or warts with OTC agents is not recommended for diabetic patients due to reduced sensation in their feet which delays awareness of possible development of infections, and can lead to sepsis.
- Warts result from an infection of the human papilloma virus, and therefore are contagious and may spread on the body.
- Warts may be eliminated by surgery, freezing with liquid nitrogen (cryotherapy), or the direct application of caustics (eg, salicylic acid, formalin, lactic acid, trichloroacetic acid, or podophyllin).

12. Questions and Answers

1. Initial treatment of mild to moderate acne would include which of the following?

   I. Topical antimicrobials
   II. Topical retinoids
   III. Isotretinoin

   A. I only
   B. II only
   C. III only
   D. I and II
   E. I, II, and III

2. Acne is due to

   I. increased sebum production
   II. obstruction of hair follicle openings
   III. inflammation

   A. I only
   B. II only
   C. III only
   D. I and II
   E. I, II, and III

3. Patients using topical retinoids such as tretinoin (Retin-A) should be counseled

   I. to use sunblock before exposure to sunlight
   II. not to use it with astringents, drying agents, or abrasive soaps
   III. that rapid improvement occurs within 2 or 3 days of starting therapy

   A. I only
   B. II only
   C. III only
   D. I and II
   E. I, II, and III

4. The most common side effects of isotretinoin (Accutane) include which of the following?

   I. Cheilitis (dry chapped lips)
   II. Acute depression
   III. Decreased night vision

   A. I only
   B. II only
   C. III only
   D. I and II
   E. I, II, and III

5. Which of the following is an important contraindication and precaution to the use of isotretinoin (Accutane)?

   A. Hypertension
   B. Migraines
   C. Allergic rhinitis
   D. Pregnancy
   E. Streptococcal infections

6. Which of the following is the most efficacious nonprescription topical antifungal?

   A. Tolnaftate (Tinactin)
   B. Terbinafine (Lamisil)
   C. Miconazole (Micatin)
   D. Undecylenic acid (Cruex)
   E. Clotrimazole (Lotrimin AF)

7. Which of these fungal infections may be treated effectively with the use of topical antifungal agents?

   I. Tinea capitis (ringworm of the scalp)
   II. Tinea unguium (fungal infection of the nails)
   III. Tinea corporis (ringworm of the skin)

   A. I only
   B. II only
   C. III only
   D. I and II
   E. I, II, and III

8. Tinea pedis is also known as

   A. athlete's foot
   B. jock itch
   C. onychomycosis
   D. ringworm of the scalp
   E. ringworm of the skin

9. The treatment of choice for tinea unguium (fungal infection of the nails) would be

   A. clotrimazole
   B. miconazole
   C. undecylenic acid
   D. griseofulvin
   E. tolnaftate

10. All of the following are true regarding androgenic alopecia EXCEPT:

A. It is predominantly seen in males.
B. It is due to the conversion of testosterone to dihydrotestosterone, which binds to the hair follicles, causing them to produce progressively thinner hair
C. Hair growth stimulation is temporary and only lasts as long as therapy
D. Hair loss in the frontotemporal area responds to treatment better than hair loss on the crown.
E. Early hair loss occurring recently in young males is more likely to respond than later hair loss at an older age.

11. All of the following are true regarding the patient instructions for the proper use of minoxidil EXCEPT:

A. It should be applied and left on the scalp for 4 hours for maximum effect
B. The patient should not swim, shampoo, or walk in rain soon after the application of minoxidil
C. Do not use on infected, irritated, inflamed, or sunburned skin
D. The patient must continue therapy to maintain effectiveness
E. Women with alopecia should use the 5% strength of minoxidil rather than the 2% strength

12. Adverse effects of minoxidil include which of the following?

I. Hypertrichosis
II. Dermatitis and pruritus of the scalp
III. Hepatic damage

A. I only
B. II only
C. III only
D. I and II
E. I, II, and III

13. The mechanism of action of finasteride (Propecia) to reduce male baldness is

A. a direct effect on hair follicles to deepen hair roots
B. inhibition of the enzyme 5-α-reductase, which blocks the conversion of testosterone to dihydrotestosterone

C. increased cutaneous blood flow to the hair follicles on the scalp due to vasodilation
D. increased cutaneous blood flow to the hair follicles on the scalp due to opening the potassium channel
E. increased development of new hair follicles on the scalp

14. All of the following are true regarding finasteride EXCEPT:

A. It is contraindicated in females of childbearing age
B. It was originally approved for treatment of benign prostatic hypertrophy
C. Improvement lasts only as long as treatment continues (new hair will be lost within 1 year of stopping treatment)
D. It must be taken on an empty stomach for complete absorption
E. Two percent of men report reversible sexual dysfunction while taking it

15. All of the following regarding dry skin are true EXCEPT:

A. It occurs primarily in older adults
B. It occurs most commonly in the summer months
C. It is caused by decreasing sebum production and decreased moisture binding capacity of the skin
D. Flaking, scaling, xerosis, and pruritus are common manifestations of dry skin
E. Excessive cleansing and bathing removes lipids and worsens dry skin

16. All of the following statements are true regarding the treatment of dry skin EXCEPT:

A. Hydrocortisone should only be used for short-term therapy of dry skin to relieve itching
B. Urea-containing products improve the skin's moisture-binding capacity
C. Lactic acid is a keratolytic agent which removes the upper epidermal skin cells and relieves the itching of dry skin
D. Emollients and moisturizers are helpful in the treatment of dry skin, especially when applied immediately after bathing
E. While colloidal oatmeal may be helpful in the treatment of dry skin, patients should be cautioned about prevention of falls due to slippery bathtubs

17. The agent of choice for the initial treatment of contact dermatitis, whether irritant or allergic, is

    A. topical antihistamines
    B. oral antihistamines
    C. topical corticosteroids
    D. local anesthetics
    E. coal tar products

18. An increase in topical corticosteroid systemic absorption with subsequent systemic side effects may be seen in which of the following?

    I. Occlusion
    II. Infant's skin
    III. Long-term use of high-potency agents

    A. I only
    B. II only
    C. III only
    D. I and II
    E. I, II, and III

19. All of the following are true regarding poison ivy EXCEPT:

    A. It is an example of allergic contact dermatitis
    B. It is the result of contact with the sap of plants of the genus *Rhus*
    C. The treatment of choice is desensitization
    D. It may be caused by direct or indirect contact (eg, with clothing or pets)
    E. Skin eruptions may occur from several hours up to 10 days following contact with the plants

20. The treatment of choice for severe or extensive cases of poison ivy or poison oak is

    A. local anesthetics such as benzocaine
    B. bentoquatam (Ivy Block®)
    C. camphor and menthol antipruritics
    D. colloidal oatmeal
    E. systemic corticosteroids

21. Which of the following agents for treatment of dandruff are cytostatic agents that suppress cell rate turnover?

    I. Zinc pyrithione (Head and Shoulders)
    II. Selenium sulfide (Selsun Blue)
    III. Salicylic acid (Ionil)

    A. I only
    B. II only
    C. III only
    D. I and II
    E. I, II, and III

22. All of the following statements are true regarding seborrhea EXCEPT:

    A. It is a chronic inflammatory skin disease seen in areas of greatest sebaceous gland activity
    B. It fluctuates in severity and is worsened by stress and poor health
    C. Moderate to severe cases require topical corticosteroids and/or the topical antifungal ketoconazole for effective treatment
    D. It is called "cradle cap" when it occurs in infants
    E. It most commonly occurs on the legs and arms

23. Which of the following are characteristic of psoriasis?

    I. Chronic inflammation
    II. Silvery scales (known as plaques) with sharply delineated edges
    III. Spontaneous exacerbations and remissions

    A. I only
    B. II only
    C. III only
    D. I and II
    E. I, II, and III

24. Treatment of advanced psoriasis may require topical therapy combined with which of the following systemic agents?

    I. Corticosteroids
    II. Antimetabolites such as methotrexate
    III. Anthralin

    A. I only
    B. II only
    C. III only
    D. I and II
    E. I, II, and III

25. All of the following are true statements regarding head lice (*Pediculus humanus capitis*) EXCEPT:

    A. It occurs most commonly in elementary schoolchildren
    B. It occurs most commonly in the springtime months of April and May
    C. It is transmitted by direct contact
    D. Pruritus is the most common symptom
    E. Head lice is the most common type of pediculosis infestation

26. All of the following statements are true regarding treatment of pediculosis with synergized pyrethrins (piperonyl butoxide and pyrethrins) EXCEPT:

    A. All family contacts should be inspected and treated if necessary
    B. Apply after washing and drying the hair and leave on overnight
    C. Remove dead lice and nits after treatment with a lice/nit comb
    D. Treatment should be repeated in 7-10 days
    E. Avoid contact with the eyes, nose, and mouth

27. The most effective nonprescription agent for treatment of head lice (*Pediculus humanus capitis*) is which of the following agents?

    A. Permethrin (Nix®)
    B. Synergized pyrethrins (A-200)
    C. Lindane (Kwell)
    D. Ketoconazole
    E. Salicylic acid

28. Nonprescription products for the treatment of corns and warts contain which of the following agents?

    A. Salicylic acid
    B. Ketoconazole
    C. Lactic acid
    D. Acetylsalicylic acid
    E. Hydrocortisone

29. All of following are true statements regarding corns EXCEPT:

    A. They are excess growth of the upper keratinized layer of skin
    B. Salicylic acid is available in pads, disks, or flexible collodion for removal of corns
    C. Self treatment for corns or warts with OTC agents is not recommended for diabetic

patients due to their reduced sensation in the feet, which delays awareness of development of infections and may lead to sepsis
    D. They are contagious and may spread on the body
    E. They are usually caused by pressure or friction from improper or tight-fitting shoes

30. All of the following are true regarding warts EXCEPT:

    A. They result from infection with the human papillomavirus
    B. They are contagious
    C. They may spread on the body
    D. Plantar warts are located on the fingers, hands, and knees
    E. They are more common in children and immunocompromised patients

31. Warts may be eliminated by which of the following procedures?

    I.   Surgery
    II. Freezing with liquid nitrogen (cryotherapy)
    III. The direct application of caustics (eg, salicylic acid)

    A. I only
    B. II only
    C. III only
    D. I and II
    E. I, II, and III

Answers

1. **D.** Topical antimicrobials and/or topical retinoids are the agents of choice for mild to moderate acne. Isotretinoin (Accutane) is reserved for nodulocystic acne (type IV acne), which if left untreated will lead to extensive scarring.

2. **E.** Acne is primarily due to hormonal changes occurring at or near puberty which increase sebum production and obstruct the hair follicle opening, and the breaking down of triglycerides to free fatty acids due to enzymes from *P acnes* which causes inflammation.

3. **D.** Topical retinoid therapy will sensitize skin to ultraviolet light rays; therefore, patients should use sunblock prior to sun exposure. Patients using topical retinoids should use only mild soaps for cleansing the face, and avoid astringents, drying agents, and abrasive soaps. Improvement will usually occur within 2-3 weeks after initiation of therapy.

4. **A.** Cheilitis (dry chapped lips), along with dry skin and dry eyes, are the most common side effects of isotretinoin therapy.

5. **D.** Isotretinoin (Accutane) is contraindicated in pregnancy due to the high incidence of serious birth defects.

6. **B.** Terbinafine (Lamisil) is the most effective nonprescription topical antifungal.

7. **C.** Topical antifungal agents are the first line of therapy against tinea corporis (ringworm of the skin). However, systemic antifungal therapy is usually required for treatment of tinea capitis (ringworm of the scalp) and tinea unguium (fungal infection of the nails).

8. **A.** Tinea pedis is also known as athlete's foot.

9. **D.** The treatment of choice for tinea unguium (fungal infection of the nails) is a systemic antifungal agent such as griseofulvin. Topical therapy is generally not effective for fungal infections of the nails.

10. **D.** Hair loss in the crown responds to treatment better than hair loss of the frontotemporal areas.

11. **E.** Women with alopecia should only use the 2% strength of minoxidil. Studies indicate that there is no greater degree of effectiveness with the 5% strength and the incidence of adverse effects including increased growth of facial hair is much greater in women using the 5% preparation.

12. **D.** Common adverse effects of minoxidil include hypertrichosis (increased hair growth in areas other than the scalp) and dermatitis and pruritus of the scalp. Systemic side effects with topical minoxidil are rare and do not include hepatic damage.

13. **B.** The mechanism of action of finasteride to reduce male baldness is blocking the conversion of testosterone to dihydrotestosterone by inhibiting the enzyme 5-α-reductase.

14. **D.** Finasteride does **not** have to be taken on an empty stomach. It may be taken with or without food. Finasteride was originally approved for treatment of benign prostatic hypertrophy. Improvement of alopecia lasts only as long as treatment continues, is contraindicated in females of childbearing age, and 2% of men report reversible sexual dysfunction.

15. **B.** Dry skin occurs most commonly in the winter months and is often referred to as "winter rash."

16. **C.** Lactic acid is used in the treatment of dry skin, not as a keratolytic agent, but as an agent which increases skin hydration.

17. **C.** Topical corticosteroids are the agents of choice for the initial treatment of irritant or allergic contact dermatitis. If the condition is severe or widespread, oral corticosteroids may be useful. Oral or topical antihistamines have minimal effect in the course of the treatment of contact dermatitis, possibly producing some antipruritic effect, but not affecting the course of the disorder.

18. **E.** Topical corticosteroid systemic absorption is increased with occlusion, long-term use, use of high-potency agents, and on an infant's skin. Systemic corticosteroid adverse effects may be severe and include adrenocortical suppression.

19. **C.** Desensitization has no place in the treatment of poison ivy, and most studies indicate desensitization is not an effective method to prevent poison ivy.

20. **E.** The treatment of choice for severe or extensive cases of poison ivy or poison oak is systemic corticosteroids. Topical agents are limited in effectiveness and do not alter the course of the disease.

21. **D.** Zinc pyrithione (Head and Shoulders) and selenium sulfide (Selsun Blue) are cytostatic agents used in the treatment of dandruff that suppress cell rate turnover. Salicylic acid is a keratolytic agent.

22. **E.** Seborrhea most commonly occurs on the face, especially eyebrows and eyelashes, but not on the extremities.

23. **E.** Psoriasis is a chronic inflammatory disease marked by silvery scales (known as plaques) with sharp delineated edges and is marked by spontaneous exacerbations and remissions.

24. **D.** Treatment of advanced psoriasis may require both topical therapy combined with either oral corticosteroids or antimetabolites such as methotrexate.

25. **B.** Head lice (*Pediculus humanus capitis*) occurs most commonly in the months of August and September.

26. **B.** Synergized pyrethrins should be applied after washing and drying the hair and left on for 10 minutes, *not* overnight.

27. **A.** Permethrin (Nix) does not have to be repeated in 7-10 days like the other available nonprescription pediculicidal agent, synergized pyrethrins (A-200). Lindane (Kwell) is not available over the counter and significant neurologic toxicities have been reported with its use.

28. **A.** Nonprescription products for the treatment of corns and warts contain salicylic acid as the active therapeutic agent.

29. **D.** Corns are not contagious and may not spread on the body. Corns are an excess growth of the upper keratinized layer of skin, usually caused by pressure or friction from improper or tight-fitting shoes. Salicylic acid is available OTC for removal of corns in pads, disks, or flexible collodion. Self treatment for corns or warts with OTC agents is not recommended for diabetic patients due to their reduced sensation in the feet, which delays awareness of the development of infections which could lead to sepsis.

30. **D.** Plantar warts are not located on the fingers, hands, or knees. Plantar warts are located on the soles of the feet.

31. **E.** Warts may be eliminated by surgery, freezing with liquid nitrogen (cryotherapy), or the direct application of caustics (eg, salicylic acid).

13. References

Arndt KA. *Manual of Dermatologic Therapeutics,* 5th ed. Boston: Little, Brown; 1995.

Arndt KA, Wintroub BU, Robinson JK, et al, eds. *Primary Care Dermatology.* Philadelphia: WB Saunders; 1997.

Berardi RR, et al, eds. *The Handbook of Nonprescription Drugs,* 14th ed. Washington: American Pharmaceutical Association; 2004.

Burnham TH, ed. *Drug Facts and Comparisons.* St. Louis: Facts and Comparisons, Inc; 2005.

Champion RH, Burton JL, Burns DA, eds. *Textbook of Dermatology,* 6th ed. Oxford, England: Blackwell Scientific Publications; 1998.

DiPiro JT, et al, eds. *Pharmacotherapy: A Pathophysiologic Approach,* 5th ed. Stamford, CT: Appleton & Lange; 2004.

Epstein E. *Common Skin Disorders,* 5th ed. Philadelphia: WB Saunders; 2001.

Freedberg IM, Eisen AZ, Wolff K, et al. *Dermatology in General Medicine,* 5th ed. New York: McGraw-Hill; 1999.

Fitzpatrick JE. *Dermatology Secrets in Color,* 2nd ed. Philadelphia: Hanley and Belfus; 2001.

Habif TP, Campbell JL, Quitadamo MJ. *Skin Disease: Diagnosis and Treatment.* St. Louis: Mosby; 2001.

Herfindal T, Gourley D, eds. *Textbook of Therapeutics,* 6th ed. Baltimore: Williams & Wilkins; 2000.

Nonprescription drug therapy; guiding patient self-care. St. Louis: Facts and Comparisons, Inc; 2003.

Odom RB, James WD, Berger TG, eds. *Andrew's Diseases of the Skin: Clinical Dermatology.* Philadelphia: WB Saunders; 2000.

Pray WS. *Nonprescription Product Therapeutics.* Hagerstown, MD: Lippincott Williams & Wilkins; 1999.

Top OTC/HBC Brands in 2002. *Drug Topics.* 2003;145:33-34.

Wolverton SE, ed. *Comprehensive Dermatologic Drug Therapy.* Philadelphia: WB Saunders; 2001.

27. Nonprescription Medications

Andrea Franks, PharmD, BCPS
Associate Professor
Departments of Clinical Pharmacy and Family Medicine
University of Tennessee College of Pharmacy

Contents

1. **Cough, Cold and Allergy**

2. **Constipation**

3. **Diarrhea**

4. **Nausea and Vomiting**

5. **Pain and Fever**

6. **Ophthalmic Disorders**

7. **Otic Disorders**

8. **Home Monitoring and Testing Devices**

9. **Smoking Cessation**

10. **Natural and Herbal Products**

11. **Sleep Aids and Stimulants**

12. **Key Points**

13. **Questions and Answers**

14. **References**

1. Cough, Cold, and Allergy

The Common Cold

Etiology
- Usually viral, most commonly rhinoviruses
- Transmitted via hand-to-hand contact followed by touching eyes or nasal mucosa

Pathophysiology
- Release of numerous inflammatory mediators, primarily cytokines

Clinical presentation
- Sore throat, nasal symptoms, watery eyes, sneezing, cough, malaise, low-grade fever
- High fever and myalgias more characteristic of influenza
- Gradual onset with slow progression
- Duration: 1-2 weeks

Treatment
- Nonprescription drug treatment (symptomatic):
  * Decongestants for nasal congestion
  * Antihistamines for excess nasal discharge
  * Analgesics for related pain or headaches
  * Local anesthetic lozenges/sprays for sore throat (pharyngitis)
- Nondrug therapy:
  * Humidifiers
  * Increase fluid intake
  * Rest

Allergic Rhinitis

Etiology
- Exposure to allergens and development of nasal symptoms
  * Perennial
  * Seasonal

Pathophysiology
- Complex, involving numerous mediators (primarily histamine) and cell types (mast cells)

Clinical presentation
- Nasal: congestion, rhinorrhea, nasal pruritus, sneezing, post-nasal drip
- Ocular: itching, lacrimation, redness, irritation
- General: headache, malaise, mood swings, irritability

Treatment
- Avoidance: avoid offending allergens
  * Limit outside exposure during periods of high pollen
  * Avoid indoor and outdoor mold
  * Avoid dust, especially in the bedroom
  * Avoid pet dander, especially cats

Pharmacotherapy for allergic rhinitis
- Mild allergies
  * Antihistamines as needed
- Moderate allergies
  * Nasal congestion: antihistamine plus decongestant
  * Ocular symptoms: ophthalmic antihistamine
- Chronic allergies
  * Cromolyn sodium (Nasalcrom) nasal spray
  * Scheduled nonsedating antihistamine
- Severe allergies
  * Nasal corticosteroids: prescription only
- Very severe allergies
  * Systemic corticosteroids: prescription only
  * Adverse effects with chronic use

Immunotherapy (allergy shots)
- If pharmacotherapy fails to relieve symptoms, resort to immunotherapy.

Drug Therapy for Treatment of the Common Cold and Allergies

Antihistamines (Table 1)
Pharmacology
- H_1-receptor antagonists
- First-generation: nonselective, sedating
- Second-generation: peripherally selective, nonsedating

Table 1

Selected Nonprescription Antihistamine Products

Generic name (trade name)	Adult dosage/max in 24 h
Chlorpheniramine (Chlor-Trimeton)	4 mg q4-6h/24 mg
Brompheniramine (Dimetane)	4 mg q4-6h/24 mg
Diphenhydramine (Benadryl)	25-50 mg q6h/200 mg
Clemastine (Tavist)	1.34 mg bid/2.68 mg
Triprolidine (in Actifed)	2.5 mg q6h/10 mg
Loratadine (Claritin, Alavert)	10 mg qd

Side effects
- Sedation
- Anticholinergic effects (primarily with first-generation antihistamines)
- Dry mouth
- Dry eyes
- Urinary retention
- Constipation
- Paradoxical stimulation in some children and elderly patients

Precautions and contraindications
- Counsel patients not to drive or operate heavy machinery.
- Avoid use with alcohol.
- Prostatic hyperplasia
- Narrow-angle glaucoma

Prescription products
- Second-generation antihistamines: low incidence of sedation; no anticholinergic effects
    * Azatadine (Optimine 1 mg bid)
    * Cetirizine (Zyrtec 5-10 mg qd)
    * Desloratadine (Clarinex 5 mg qd)
    * Fexofenadine (Allegra 60 mg bid or 180 mg qd)

Oral decongestants (Table 2)
Pharmacology
- α-Adrenergic agonists, vasoconstrictors
- Constrict blood vessels to decrease blood supply to nasal mucosa and decrease mucosal edema.
- No effect on histamine or allergy-mediated reaction.

Side effects
- Products relatively safe with no dependence
- Can be used long term
- Most common side effects:
    * Nervousness
    * Irritability
    * Restlessness
    * Insomnia
- Less common side effects:
    * Increased heart rate
    * Increased blood pressure
    * Irregular heartbeat
    * Palpitations

Precautions and contraindications
- Hypertension: generally accepted with mild or well-controlled hypertension; should not use with uncontrolled hypertension
- Heart disease (arrhythmias, ischemic heart disease): increase heart rate
- Diabetes: minimal effect on blood sugar level
- Hyperthyroidism: more sensitive to sympathomimetics
- Enlarged prostrate: exacerbates BPH by constricting smooth muscle of the bladder neck
- Narrow-angle glaucoma: dilation increases intraocular pressure
- MAO inhibitors interact with decongestants to increase blood pressure.

Topical decongestants
Pharmacology
- α-Adrenergic agonists act locally as vasoconstrictors.
- Constrict blood vessels, decrease blood supply to nose, decrease mucosal edema
- No effect on histamine or allergy-mediated reaction

Side effects
- Minimal systemic absorption results in few side effects.
- Local effects may include burning, nasal irritation, and sneezing.

Table 2

Selected Nonprescription Oral Decongestant Products

Generic name	Products	Comments	Side effects	Adult dosage (maximum daily dose)
Phenylephrine	Combination products	Weakest oral decongestant	+	10 mg q4h (60 mg)
Pseudoephedrine	Sudafed	Less CNS stimulation	++	60 mg q6h (240 mg)
Phenylpropanolamine	Withdrawn 11/2000	Increased risk of hemorrhagic stroke	+++	25 mg q4h (150 mg)
Ephedrine	Combination products for asthma	Used as bronchodilator due to β agonist activity	++++	12.5-25 mg q4h (150 mg)

Precautions and contraindications
- Rhinitis medicamentosa (rebound congestion) may occur if duration of use is >3-5 days.

Topical decongestant dosage forms
- Sprays
    * Simplest dosage delivery
    * Large surface area covered
    * Imprecise dosing, contamination of bottle possible
- Drops
    * Preferred for use in small children
    * Cover small surface area
    * They pass to the larynx, where they may be swallowed and result in systemic effects.
- Nasal inhaler
    * Requires an unobstructed airway to deliver drug to the nasal mucosa.
    * Sympathomimetic amines; also contain camphor and menthol
    * Loses efficacy after 2-3 months
    * Propylhexedrine (Benzedrex inhaler)
    * Levodesoxyephedrine (Vicks inhaler)

Select products
- Short-acting: phenylephrine (Neo-Synephrine, Vicks Sinex)
- Intermediate-acting: naphazoline (Privine)
- Long-acting: xylometazoline (Otrivin)
- Longest-acting: oxymetazoline (Afrin, Neo-Synephrine 12-hour)

Nasal saline solution
- Very safe
- Good for use in infants and children
- Can be used with oral decongestants
- Saline drops (Ayr, NaSal)
- Saline sprays (Ayr, NaSal, Ocean Nasal Spray, HuMist)

Cromolyn (Nasalcrom)
- Role in therapy: prevention and treatment of allergic symptoms
- Pharmacology: mast cell stabilizer; prevents the mast cells from releasing inflammatory mediators
- Dosage: one spray each nostril q4-6h up to 4-6 times daily
- Onset of action: approximately 1 week, 2-3 weeks for maximal effect
- Not efficacious if taken prn; must be taken on a scheduled basis
- Side effects: nasal irritation, nasal burning, stinging, sneezing, cough, unpleasant taste

Analgesics
- Role in therapy: pain, fever, and headaches associated with cold, flu, or allergies
- Aspirin (mostly replaced now by acetaminophen and NSAIDs)
- Acetaminophen (APAP)
- Nonsteroidal anti-inflammatory drugs (NSAIDs)
    * Ibuprofen
    * Ketoprofen
    * Naproxen

Selected cold, allergy, and sinus products
Decongestant/analgesic
- Advil Cold & Sinus (pseudoephedrine 30 mg, ibuprofen 200 mg)
- Tylenol Sinus, Maximum Strength Day Nondrowsy (pseudoephedrine 30 mg, APAP 500 mg)
- Sinutab Sinus (pseudoephedrine 30 mg, APAP 500 mg)

Antihistamine/decongestant/analgesic
- Alka-Seltzer Plus Cold Medicine (APAP 250 mg, chlorpheniramine 2 mg, phenylephrine 5 mg)
- Tylenol Allergy Sinus (APAP 500 mg, chlorpheniramine 2 mg, pseudoephedrine 30 mg)

Antihistamine/decongestant (short-acting)
- Actifed Cold and Allergy Tablets (triprolidine 2.5 mg, pseudoephedrine 60 mg)
- Benadryl Allergy and Sinus Tablets (diphenhydramine 25 mg, pseudoephedrine 60 mg)

Antihistamine/decongestant (long-acting)
- Drixoral Cold and Allergy 12 Hour Relief (pseudoephedrine 120 mg, dexbrompheniramine 6 mg)
- Claritin D 12 Hour (loratadine 5 mg, pseudoephedrine 120 mg)
- Claritin D 24 Hour (loratadine 10 mg, pseudoephedrine 240 mg)

Cough

Pathophysiology
- Important defense mechanism to rid the airways of mucus, foreign bodies
- May be acute (<3 weeks duration) or chronic (>3 weeks duration)

Causes
- Upper respiratory infection (viral or bacterial)
- Sinusitis
- Rhinitis
- Asthma, chronic obstructive pulmonary disease (COPD)
- Gastroesophageal reflux disease (GERD)
- Congestive heart failure

- Drug-induced cough
  * ACE inhibitors
  * β-Blockers

Cough characteristics
- Productive
- Nonproductive

Treatment
Antitussives/cough suppressants
Narcotic
- Codeine
  * Gold standard antitussive
  * Available in some states without prescription
  * Mechanism of action: centrally-mediated suppression of cough
  * Adult dose: 10-20 mg q4h (120 mg/d maximum)
  * Role in therapy: used primarily for night cough
  * Side effects: sedation, nausea, constipation

Nonnarcotic
- Dextromethorphan (DM)
  * Only category 1 OTC nonnarcotic antitussive
  * Mechanism of action: centrally-mediated suppression of cough
  * Adult dosage: 10-30 mg q4-8h (120 mg/d maximum)
  * Role in therapy: nonproductive cough
  * Side effects: drowsiness, gastrointestinal effects
  * Drug interactions: MAO inhibitors
- Diphenhydramine
  * Category II antitussive
  * Mechanism of action: centrally-mediated suppression of cough center, anticholinergic
  * Adult dosage: 25 mg q4h (75 mg/d maximum)
- Benzonatate (Tessalon Perles)
  * Prescription only
  * Anesthetizes stretch receptors in respiratory passages, lungs
  * Adult dose: 100-200 mg tid
  * Side effects: sedation, bronchospasm

Expectorant
Guaifenesin (Robitussin, Mucinex, Humibid)
- Only category I OTC expectorant
- Mechanism of action: thins mucus to enhance clearance
- Adult dosage:
  * Immediate-release 200-400 mg q4h (maximum 2400 mg/d)
  * Extended-release: 600-1200 mg q12h (maximum 2400 mg/d)
- Role in therapy: productive cough
- Side effects: gastrointestinal discomfort
- Patient education: increase fluid intake

Topical antitussives
Volatile oils
- Only camphor and menthol are FDA-approved.
- Mechanism of action: local anesthetic effect in nasal mucosa
- Product availability: lozenge, ointment, steam inhalation
- Patient education: ointment and solution toxic if ingested

Selected cough products
- Expectorant: guaifenesin
  * Immediate-release: Robitussin Syrup (100 mg/5 mL)
  * Extended-release: Mucinex (600 mg or 1200 mg); Humibid Sprinkle (30 mg)
- Cough suppressant: dextromethorphan
  * Benylin Adult Cough Formula Liquid (15 mg/5 mL)
  * Delsym Extended Release Suspension (30 mg/5 mL)
- Expectorant/cough suppressant:
  * Robitussin DM (guaifenesin 100 mg, dextromethorphan 10 mg/5 mL)
- Expectorant/decongestant:
  * Robitussin PE (guaifenesin 100 mg, pseudoephedrine 30 mg/5 mL)

Sore Throat Remedies

- Saline gargle
- Sprays, lozenges:
  * Benzocaine: Chloraseptic lozenges, Cepacol lozenges
  * Dyclonine: Cepacol Spray
  * Phenol: Chloraseptic Gargle
  * Menthol: Halls

2. Constipation

Clinical Presentation

- Difficult or infrequent passage of stools
- Patient may complain of abdominal or rectal fullness.

Etiology

- Inadequate fluid intake
- Inadequate fiber intake
- Lack of physical exercise
- Diseases:
  - * Neurologic disease
    - Parkinson's disease
    - Multiple sclerosis
    - Cerebrovascular disease
  - * Gastrointestinal disease
    - Irritable bowel syndrome
    - Hemorrhoids
    - Masses (polyps, tumors)
    - Diabetes
    - Hypothyroidism
- Drug-induced constipation:
  - * Antacids containing aluminum or calcium
  - * Anticholinergics
  - * Phenothiazines
  - * Tricyclic antidepressants
  - * Opiates (codeine, morphine)
  - * Antihistamines, especially in children
  - * ACE inhibitors
  - * Calcium channel blockers (especially verapamil)
  - * Sucralfate
  - * Iron

Treatment

Nondrug therapy
- Increase fluid intake
- Increase dietary fiber
- Exercise
- Establish good bowel habits

Drug therapy
Bulk-forming laxatives
Pharmacology
- Mechanism of action
  - * Natural or semisynthetic hydrophilic polysaccharide derivatives
  - * Absorb water to soften stool, increase bulk, facilitate peristalsis and elimination
  - * Effects may not be seen for 2-3 days

- Role in therapy:
  - * Safest, most natural therapy for constipation
  - * Most often recommended for chronic use
- Drug interactions:
  - * May bind digoxin, warfarin, and other drugs
  - * Calcium complexes may bind with tetracycline, inhibiting its absorption
  - * Recommend separating doses from other medications
- Side effects:
  - * Potential for allergic reaction/anaphylaxis
  - * Inhalation of powder reported to cause bronchospasm
  - * Caution diabetics about sugar content of some products

Selected bulk forming laxative products
- Psyllium seed (plantago seed): Metamucil, Perdiem
- Methylcellulose: Citrucel
  - * Synthetic cellulose derivative
- Carboxymethyl cellulose sodium
- Calcium polycarbophil: Fibercon
- Malt soup extract: Maltsupex

Emollient laxatives (stool softeners)
Pharmacology
- Act as surfactants, absorbing water into the stool
- Effects may take 2-3 days
- May cause systemic absorption of mineral oil, therefore concurrent use contraindicated
- Often used in combination products
- Useful for patients who should avoid straining
  - * Rectal surgery
  - * Postpartum
  - * Recent myocardial infarction

Selected emollient laxative products
- Docusate sodium: Colace
- Docusate calcium: Surfak
- Docusate potassium: Dialose

Stimulant laxatives
- Stimulate bowel motility via localized mucosal irritation
- Increase secretion of fluids into bowel
- Can cause cramping
- Impaired colon function with chronic use

Anthraquinones
- Pharmacology:
  - * Absorbed into bloodstream with action on large intestines
  - * Onset of effects: 6-12 hours
  - * Dose at bedtime
- Side effects:

* Discoloration of urine
* Stimulant habituation
* Melanosis coli: dark pigmentation of colonic mucosa
- Precautions and contraindications:
  * Contraindicated in breastfeeding
- Select anthraquinone products:
  * Senna (Senokot, Ex-Lax)
    - Anthraquinone drug of choice
- FDA recently banned substances (2002):
  * Aloe
  * Cascara sagrada
  * Casanthranol

Diphenylmethanes
- Bisacodyl (Dulcolax tablets or suppositories, Correctol Stimulant Laxative)
  * Minimal systemic absorption
  * Only stimulant compatible with breastfeeding
  * Enteric coated: do not crush or take with antacids
  * Onset of effects varies with route of administration
    - Rectal: 15-60 minutes
    - Oral: 6-8 hours
  * Also available in suppository form

Phenolphthalein (removed from market 1998)

Stimulant oils (castor oil)
* Acts on small intestine
* Strong cathartic: may induce fluid/electrolyte disturbances
* Rapid onset: 2-6 hours
* Contraindicated in pregnancy (may induce labor)

Dangers of chronic stimulant laxative use
- Laxative habit
- Cathartic colon
- Melanosis coli
- Loss of fluids on electrolytes
- Cramping pains

Hyperosmotic laxative (glycerin)
Pharmacology
- Osmotic effect and local irritant stimulates bowel movement.
- Onset of action usually within 30 minutes
- Glycerin suppositories safe for infants

Selected products
- Glycerin suppositories
- Fleet Babylax

Saline and osmotic laxatives
Pharmacology
- Nonabsorbable cations create osmotic gradient to pull water into intestine
- Onset varies with route of administration:
  * Rectal: 5-30 minutes
  * Oral: 30 minutes to 4 hours
- 20% of magnesium may be absorbed systemically
- Contraindicated in patients with impaired renal function (magnesium- or phosphate-containing), congestive heart failure, or hypertension (sodium-containing)

Selected saline and osmotic laxative products
- Magnesium hydroxide (milk of magnesia)
- Magnesium citrate (citrate of magnesia)
- Magnesium sulfate (epsom salts)
- Sodium phosphate (Fleet Phospho-Soda)

Lubricant laxatives
Pharmacology
- Soften the feces by emulsifying contents of intestinal tract
- Onset of action: 6-8 hours
- May decrease absorption of fat-soluble vitamins and some drugs
- Contraindicated in children and elderly patients due to risk of aspiration and lipid pneumonitis
- Do not administer with stool softeners.

Selected lubricant laxative products
- Mineral oil: liquid petrolatum
- Olive oil: "sweet oil"
- Combination products:
  * Softener-stimulants
    - Senokot-S: docusate sodium and senna

Enemas
- Fleet Enema (monobasic and dibasic sodium phosphates)
- Oil retention
- Soap suds
- Warm tap water

Lactulose
- Chronulac, Duphalac, Cephulac
- Prescription only
- Nonabsorbed disaccharide, metabolized by bacteria in gastrointestinal tract to produce acetic and formic acid; it then exerts osmotic effect.

Special patient populations
Pregnancy
- Hormonal changes cause smooth muscle relaxation early in pregnancy.
- Enlarged uterus compresses colon.
- Recommend only bulk-forming laxatives or stool softeners.

3. Diarrhea

Clinical Presentation

- Abnormal increase in frequency of stools and stool looseness
- May be acute (<14 days) or chronic (>4 weeks)

Etiology

Acute infectious diarrhea
Viral
- Norwalk virus (adults and children)
- Rotaviruses (young children)

Bacterial
- Food-borne illness
- Contaminated water
- Traveler's diarrhea

Protozoal

Drug-induced diarrhea
- Antibiotics
- Laxatives
- Antacids
- Cytotoxic agents

Diet-induced diarrhea
- Allergies
- Spicy foods
- High carbohydrate load
- Lactose intolerance

Complications
- Dehydration (especially in infants, elderly)
- Electrolyte abnormalities

Nondrug Treatment

- Oral rehydration therapy (ORT; eg, Pedialyte)
  * Rehydration
  * Maintenance
- Avoid fatty foods, spicy foods, high sugar content

Drug Therapy

Loperamide (Imodium AD)
- Pharmacology: synthetic opioid agonist slows gastrointestinal motility
- Dosage: 4 mg initially, then 2 mg after each loose stool; <16 mg/d. (For OTC use, maximum dose is 8 mg/day, but can increase to 16 mg/day with medical supervision.)

Side effects
- Well-tolerated
- Constipation
- Dizziness
- Dry mouth

Precautions and contraindications
- Not recommended for children under 6 years old without medical supervision.
- Should not be used if patient has bloody or black stool; consult physician before use if patient has fever, mucus in stool, or a history of liver disease.
- Antiperistaltic action could worsen effects of invasive or inflammatory bacterial infection.

Adsorbents
- Pharmacology: nonselective absorption of toxins, bacteria, water

Side effects
- Constipation
- Bloating

Precautions and contraindications
- Do not use in children age <12 years.

Drug interactions
- May absorb other drugs from gastrointestinal tract (digoxin, antibiotics)
- Separate doses to avoid drug interactions.
- In the 2003 Final Monograph, the FDA required that products containing the adsorbents pectin and attapulgite be reformulated or withdrawn.

Selected adsorbent products
- Kaolin
  * The only monograph adsorbent, but no single-ingredient products are currently available.

Bismuth subsalicylate (BSS)
Pharmacology
- Reacts with stomach acid to form salicylic acid and bismuth oxychloride
- Reduces frequency of diarrhea.
- Improves stool consistency
- Direct antimicrobial effect, therefore effective in traveler's diarrhea

Side effects
- Salicylate toxicity (tinnitus)
- Bismuth toxicity (neurotoxicity)
- Gray-black discoloration of tongue and/or stool

Precautions and contraindications
- Contraindicated in aspirin allergy
- Contraindicated in children/teens with viral illness (Reye's syndrome)
- Contraindicated if history of GI bleeding, or on warfarin
- New labeling recommends that patients younger than 12 years old consult a physician prior to use.

Selected bismuth subsalicylate products
- Pepto-Bismol
- Kaopectate Liquid

Polycarbophil and Calcium polycarbophil
- The bulk forming laxatives polycarbophil and calcium polycarbophil were previously used for diarrhea. The 2003 Final Monograph reclassified these agents to nonmonograph status.

4. Nausea and Vomiting

Definitions

- Nausea: the sensation that one is about to vomit
- Vomiting: forceful expulsion of gastric contents through the mouth

Physiology

- Vomiting is coordinated by the vomiting center in the medulla.
- Stimuli from the peripheral nervous system and within the central nervous system act on the vomiting center.
- Responding to these impulses, the vomiting center stimulates the abdominal muscles, stomach, and esophagus to induce vomiting.

Etiology

Irritation of chemoreceptor trigger zone (CTZ)
- Drug-induced:
    * Cancer chemotherapy
    * Narcotics
    * Theophylline
    * Digoxin
    * Antibiotics
    * Drug withdrawal (opiates, sedatives)
- Systemic disorders:
    * Ketoacidosis (diabetes)
    * Uremia due to renal disease
    * Pregnancy
    * Electrolyte imbalances

Vestibular disorders
- Motion sickness
- Vestibular inflammation
    * Otitis interna
    * Meniere's syndrome

Central nervous system disorders
- Psychogenic vomiting
- Migraine headache
- Increased intracranial pressure

Gastrointestinal tract disorders
- Obstruction
- Gastroparesis
- Gastroenteritis
- Viral or bacterial infection
- Locally irritating drugs
    * Alcohol
    * NSAIDs
    * Antibiotics

Complications

- Dehydration
- Electrolyte imbalance
- Aspiration
- Malnutrition
- Acid-base disturbances

Treatment

Nonprescription antiemetics (Table 3)
Antihistamines
- Cross the blood-brain barrier to depress vestibular excitability

Phosphorated carbohydrate solution (Emetrol)
- Hyperosmolar solution
- Mixture of levulose (fructose), dextrose (glucose), and phosphoric acid
- Buffered to a pH of 1.5
- Reduces gastric muscle contraction through an unknown direct effect
- Must not be diluted (raises the pH)

Bismuth salts (Pepto-Bismol)
- Available as nonprescription suspension, caplet, and chewable tablet
- See diarrhea section for additional information.

Histamine$_2$-receptor antagonists (H$_2$-antagonists)
- May provide symptomatic relief by inhibiting gastric acid secretion
- Potential drug interactions with cimetidine
- Side effects:
  - * Headache
  - * Constipation
  - * Diarrhea
- See peptic ulcer disease section for additional information on H$_2$-antagonists.

Antacids
- May treat nausea, dyspepsia, and stomach upset associated with excessive intake of food or drink
- Combinations of magnesium hydroxide, sodium salts, aluminum hydroxide, calcium carbonate, and magnesium carbonate
- Usual adult dosage: 15 mL 30 minutes after meals and at bedtime
- Side effects:
  - * Constipation
  - * Diarrhea
  - * Sodium overload
- Drug interactions:
  - * May decrease absorption of some medications
  - * Administer other medications 1-2 hours before or after antacids

Special patient populations
Pregnancy
- Nausea may be associated with pregnancy, especially during the first trimester.
- Recommend nonpharmacologic therapy initially:
  - * Small, frequent meals
  - * Avoid rich, fatty foods
  - * Snack on salty crackers or pretzels
- Refer to primary care provider if considering pharmacologic therapy
  - * Pyridoxine 25 mg tid
  - * Antihistamines
  - * Prescription antiemetics

Table 3

Nonprescription Drugs of Choice for Prevention of Motion Sickness

Generic name (trade name)	Adult dosage (max daily dose)	Children age 6-12 (max daily dose)	Children age 2-6 (max daily dose)
Dimenhydrinate (Dramamine)	50-100 mg q4-6h (400 mg)	25-50 mg q6-8h (150 mg)	12.5-25 mg q6-8h (75 mg)
Diphenhydramine	25-50 mg q4-6h (300 mg)	12.5-25 mg q4-6h (150 mg)	6.25 mg q4-6h (37.5 mg)
Cyclizine	50 mg q4-6h (200 mg)	25 mg q6-8h (75 mg)	Not recommended
Meclizine (Bonine)	25-50 mg qd (50 mg)	Not recommended	Not recommended

5. Pain and Fever

Pathophysiology of Pain

- Nociceptors are peripheral pain receptors.
- Nociceptors send pain stimuli to the spinal cord via afferent, nociceptive nerves.
- Impulses then pass to the brain via dorsal root ganglia.

Pathophysiology of Fever

- Core temperature is the temperature of the blood surrounding the hypothalamus.
- The thermoregulatory center in the anterior hypothalamus controls body temperature via physiologic and behavioral mechanisms.
- Pyrogens, fever-producing substances, increase the thermoregulatory set point, raising the body temperature.

Treatment

Acetaminophen (Table 4)
Pharmacology
- Exerts analgesic and antipyretic activity via central inhibition of prostaglandin synthesis
- Does not have peripheral anti-inflammatory activity

Side effects
- Generally well tolerated
- Hepatotoxicity

Drug interactions
- Alcohol: increases risk of hepatotoxicity
- Warfarin: higher doses may enhance hypoprothrombinemic effect of warfarin

Precautions and contraindications
- Increased risk of hepatotoxicity
- Dose >4 g/day
- Pre-existing liver disease
- Alcohol use
- Fasting

Special patient populations
- Accepted in pregnancy and breastfeeding

Salicylates
Pharmacology
- Inhibit peripheral prostaglandin synthesis
- Reduce pain, inflammation, and fever
- Acetylated salicylates (eg, aspirin) inhibit platelet aggregation
- Nonacetylated salicylates (eg, prescription salsalate, choline magnesium salicylate) do not have significant antiplatelet activity

Side effects
- Gastritis
- Gastric ulcers/bleeding
- Allergy and hypersensitivity:
    * Rare (<1 %) in the general population
    * Higher risk in individuals with asthma, nasal polyps
- Reye's syndrome:
    * Potentially fatal illness associated with salicylate use in children/teens with concurrent viral illness (influenza, varicella-zoster)

Drug interactions
- Alcohol: enhances gastrointestinal toxicity
- Methotrexate: salicylates displace methotrexate from protein-binding sites
- Warfarin: salicylates enhance hypoprothrombinemic effects of warfarin

Table 4

Selected Analgesic/Antipyretic Products

Generic name (trade name)	Adult dosage (max daily dosage)	Pediatric dosage (max daily dosage)
Acetaminophen (Tylenol, Tempra)	650-1000 mg q4-6h (4000 mg)	10-15 mg/kg q4-6h (5 doses/day)
Aspirin (Bayer)	650-1000 mg q4-6h (4000 mg)	10-15 mg/kg q4-6h (80 mg/kg per day)
Ibuprofen (Motrin, Advil)	200-400 mg q4-6h (1200 mg OTC)	5-10 mg/kg q6-8h (40 mg/kg per day)
Naproxen (Aleve)	220-440 mg q8-12h (660 mg)	Not recommended <12 years old; >12 years old: use adult dosage
Ketoprofen (Orudis)	12.5-25 mg q6-8h (75 mg)	Not recommended <16 years old; >16 years old: use adult dosage

Precautions and contraindications
- Bleeding disorders
- Hemophilia
- Peptic ulcer disease
- Children/teenagers with viral illness (Reye's syndrome)
- Gout

Special patient populations
- Avoid in third trimester of pregnancy

Nonsteroidal anti-inflammatory drugs (NSAIDs)
Pharmacology
- Peripheral inhibition of prostaglandin synthesis
- Analgesic, antipyretic, anti-inflammatory activity

Side effects
- Gastrointestinal effects, including bleeding
- Rash
- Photosensitivity
- High incidence of cross-reactivity in individuals with aspirin allergy

Drug interactions
- Warfarin: increased bleeding risk
- Alcohol: increased risk of gastrointestinal bleeding
- Methotrexate: decreased methotrexate clearance
- Antihypertensives:
    * ACE inhibitors: decreased hypotensive effects, hyperkalemia
    * β-Blockers: decreased hypotensive effects
    * Potassium-sparing diuretics: hyperkalemia
- Digoxin: decreased renal clearance, risk of digoxin toxicity

Precautions and contraindications
- Alcohol: increased risk of GI bleeding
- Renal impairment
- Congestive heart failure

Special patient populations
- Ibuprofen, naproxen compatible with breastfeeding
- Avoid NSAIDs in third trimester of pregnancy

6. Ophthalmic Disorders

Dry Eye

- Definition: tear film instability caused by a deficiency of any component of the tear film
- Clinical presentation: ocular discomfort, blurred vision, desire to rub the eyes, burning or redness

Etiology

- Aqueous tear deficiency
- Exposure to dry air
- Keratoconjunctivitis sicca
- Sjögren's syndrome
- Blepharitis
- Vitamin A deficiency
- Allergic conjunctivitis
- Contact lenses
- Drug-induced (anticholinergic agents, antihistamines)

Nonpharmacologic treatment
- Avoid known irritants
- Use cool-mist humidifier/warm-steam vaporizer

Pharmacologic treatment
- See Table 5

Loose Foreign Material in the Eye

- Symptoms: irritation, inflammation, involuntary tearing, uncontrollable blinking, discomfort
- Etiology: dirt, an eyelash, or particles suspended by the tears

Treatment
Eyewashes
- Isotonic, buffered solutions of sterile water

Key points
- Eyewashes should not be used if the patient has open wounds near the eye.
- Contact lens wearers should remove their lenses prior to using eyewashes, if possible.
- Use of eye cups should generally be avoided.

Redness Caused by Minor Irritation

- Common causes: airborne pollutants (gases or smoke), chlorinated water, infectious diseases, glaucoma

Table 5

Pharmacologic Treatment of Dry Eyes

Product	Common preparations	Comments
Artificial tears: act as demulcents to mimic mucin; use twice daily as suggested		
Cellulose derivatives (carboxymethylcellulose)	Bion Tears , Celluvisc , Clear Eyes CLR	Enhanced duration compared to other products; tend to form dry crusts which may be easily washed off with warm water
Polyvinyl alcohol (glycerin, propylene glycol, polyethylene glycols, polysorbate 80)	Moisture Eyes , Hypo Tears , Murine Tears , Tears Plus	Shorter duration; no crust formation
Povidone and dextran 70	AquaSite	Can cause transient stinging/burning
Ocular emollients: ointments have longer contact; more likely to cause blurred vision		
Lanolin, mineral oil, petrolatum, white ointment, white wax or yellow wax	Moisture Eyes PM , Lacri-Lube SOP , Refresh PM , Stye	

Treatment
Ophthalmic vasoconstrictors (see Table 6)
- Constrict blood vessels of the conjunctiva
- 1-2 drops in the affected eye up to four times daily
- Contraindicated in patients with narrow-angle glaucoma (causes mydriasis)
- Avoid use in contact lens wearers
- Can cause a rebound hyperemia, especially with overuse
- Can cause tachycardia and aggravate arrhythmias if absorbed systemically
- Minimize systemic absorption by closing the eye after instillation, and occluding the tear duct with a finger (punctual occlusion).
- *Warnings:* ocular decongestants should be avoided in patients with heart disease, high blood pressure, an enlarged prostate, or narrow-angle glaucoma

Allergic Conjunctivitis

- *Symptoms:* chronic, recurring itching; eyes that are slightly red, tearing, burning, with little discharge
- *Etiology:* animal hair, pollen, ragweed, or other plants
- *Treatment:* combination products containing ophthalmic vasoconstrictor and ocular antihistamine
- Naphazoline + pheniramine or antazoline (Naphcon A , Visine A , Opcon-A , Vasocon-A)
- 1-2 drops in affected eye(s) up to four times daily
- *Warnings:* combination products containing ocular decongestants should be avoided in patients with heart disease, high blood pressure, enlarged prostate, or narrow-angle glaucoma

Table 6

Ophthalmic Vasoconstrictors

Product	Common preparations	Key points
Phenylephrine	Prefrin Liquifilm Relief	Can precipitate angle-closure glaucoma
Naphazoline	Clear Eyes , Clear Eyes ACR , Bausch & Lomb Sensitive Eyes	Ocular decongestant of choice
Tetrahydrozoline	Visine , Visine AC , Visine Advanced Relief	Less likely to alter pupil size; may cause stinging upon instillation
Oxymetazoline	Visine LR	Relatively free of ocular or systemic side effects

Conditions Requiring Referral to a Physician or Eye Care Specialist

Corneal edema
- *Symptoms:* foggy vision, haloes around lights, photophobia, irritation, foreign-body sensation, extreme pain
- *Causes:* prolonged contact lens wearing, infection, glaucoma, iritis

Treatment
- Referral to an eye care specialist
- Sodium chloride (2-5%)
- 1-2 drops in affected eye(s) every 3-4 hours

Foreign body in the eye
- Metal shavings, wood splinters, or dust
- Improper removal may lead to permanent damage.

Ocular trauma
- Automobile accidents, sports injuries

Chemical exposure
- Remove contact lenses
- Flush immediately with lukewarm water for at least 15 minutes.
- Do not place drops in the eyes.

7. Otic Disorders

Impacted Cerumen

Cerumen-softening agents
- Instill in ear
- Follow with warm water irrigation using otic syringe
    * Carbamide peroxide in anhydrous glycerin + alcohol
        - Debrox®, Murine® Earwax Removal System
        - Softens ear wax and facilitates removal
    * Hydrogen peroxide/water
        - 1:1 solution of warm water:3% hydrogen peroxide
        - Not effective drying agent
    * Olive oil (sweet oil)
    * Glycerin
        - Emollient and humectant

Water-Clogged Ears

- 95% isopropyl alcohol in 5% anhydrous glycerin
    * Swim Ear® Drops
    * Only FDA-approved ear drying aid
- Compounded 50:50 acetic acid (5%) + isopropyl alcohol (95%)
    * Recommended by American Academy of Otolaryngology

Boils

- Infected hair follicles in the ear canal
- Usually self-limiting
- Apply warm compress

8. Home Monitoring and Testing Devices

Diabetes

* See diabetes chapter

Fertility Prediction Tests

Basal thermometry
* Temperatures taken orally, rectally, and vaginally
* Taken every morning before arising
* Results are plotted graphically.
* Resting temperatures are usually below normal for first part of the reproductive cycle.
* Temps closer to normal after ovulation.
* Temp results plotted against time to assess spikes (ovulation).
* Very user-dependent

Bioself®, Fertility Indicator
* Digital temp readings
* Must input first day of menses into device.
* Calculates user's average cycle length.
* Predicts user's most fertile period.
* Each morning indicator displays prediction (90% effective).
* Indicates if nonfertile phase, conception possible, or most fertile
* Can obtain printout via modem download

Ovulation prediction kits
* Test contains antibodies that bind to LH in urine.
* LH surge is detected by difference in color or color intensity from one day to the next.
* Early morning urine collection is recommended.
* User must know the length of the last three cycles before using.
* Testing usually begins 2-4 days prior to ovulation (based on the average of the last three cycles).

Clear Plan Easy, Fertility Monitor
* Measures both LH and E3G (estrogen component)
* Tests 20 consecutive days to establish baseline in the first month
* Tests 10-20 days per month
* Peak time identified by meter.

Fertility microscopes
* Reusable microscope that analyzes saliva changes to predict ovulation
* OVU-Tec Fertility Detector, Cycle View
* Do not use within 2 hours of smoking, drinking, or eating.

Male fertility testing
* FertilMARQ®
* Determines if sperm concentration is adequate
* Two tests needed to confirm
* Test sample color is compared to known control color sample

Pregnancy detection
* Early testing is very important.
* Detects levels of hCG in urine (within 1-2 weeks after conception)
* Antibodies designed to react with hCG in shape of straight line, check, or plus sign.
* If pregnant, color is produced
* Pregnancy tests are 98-100% accurate; however, human error decreases that rate to 50-75% (Table 7)

Important tips for patients using pregnancy tests
* Encourage use of first morning urine to test (hCG is more concentrated)
* If not first morning urine sample, restrict fluids 4-6 hours before urine collection.
* Use only supplied collection devices.
* Try to test sample immediately after collection (if not, allow refrigerated samples to come to room temperature).
* If negative, wait 1 week and retest if no cycle yet.
* If positive, contact ob/gyn immediately and start prenatal vitamins.

Urinary Tract Infection Tests

* Tests for nitrites in urine
* Specific for gram-negative organisms only
* AZO, Test Strips, First Response, Urinary Tract Infection Kit: test for both nitrites and leukocyte esterase
* False-negative: vegetarian diet, vitamin C, tetracycline
* False-positive: phenazopyridine

Table 7

Causes of Error in Home Pregnancy Testing

False positives	False negatives
Miscarriage within previous 8 weeks	Test performed first day of a missed cycle
Childbirth within previous 8 weeks	Refrigerated urine not allowed to come to room temperature
Use of fertility medications (Pergonal , Profasi)	Use of wax cups or soap residues in household containers

Colorectal Cancer

- ColoCARE , Stool Blood Test
- EZ-Detect™, Hidden Blood in the Stool
- Colorimetric assay for hemoglobin
- Blue-green color indicates positive test.
- More likely to detect lower GI problems
- Uses biodegradable paper that is placed in the toilet bowl after bowel movement
- Ingestion of red meat or vitamin C may cause false-positive test.

Hypercholesterolemia

CholesTrak Home Cholesterol Test
- Tests for total cholesterol only
- Results available without the need for a lab.

Biosafe Cholesterol Collection Kit
- Fingerstick blood placed on small collection card
- Sample mailed to Biosafe Lab
- Results for whole lipid profile given
- Results are reviewed by licensed MD before being sent to the patient.

Home Access Instant Cholesterol Test
- Fingerstick blood sample sent to Home Access lab
- Results reviewed by "professionals" and patient given counseling
- May be the least expensive versus other tests

BioScanner
- Potential to test full lipid panel, glucose, and ketones
- Stores results
- Reusable

Hypertension

Mercury column devices
- Blood pressure reference standard
- Routine home discouraged because they are cumbersome; risk of mercury poisoning
- Requires good eyesight and hearing

Aneroid devices
- Most accurate and reliable (except mercury column)
- Light, portable, affordable
- Many come with an attached stethoscope
- Requires good eyesight and hearing for effective use (large-print devices available)

Digital devices
- Less accurate than aneroid devices
- Semiautomatic (manually inflated)
- Fully automatic (autoinflating)

Acquired Immunodeficiency Syndrome (AIDS)

Home Access and Home Access Express
- Tests for antibodies to HIV virus
- Can take 3 weeks to 6 months before antibodies are detectable
- Fingerstick blood sample placed on the specimen card
- Mailed to lab within 10 days
- Home Access: results in 7 days
- Home Access Express: results in 3 days

Illicit Drug Use Testing

PDT-90 (hair testing)
- Not subject to tampering like urine
- Subject must have used drugs for longer periods
- Collect as close to the scalp as possible (from the crown).
- Results reported as low, medium, high (not THC)
- Do not collect from hairbrush.
- Samples mailed from home to independent lab
- Results obtained anonymously by phone
- Tests for marijuana, cocaine, opiates, methamphetamine, PCP

Urine testing
- Is subject to tampering
- Detects use of drugs from several hours to 2-3 days prior to test
- Results reported as positive or negative; not quantified
- Results available within 2-3 business days.
- Products: Dr. Brown's, Parent's Alert

Hepatitis C

Home Access, Hepatitis C Check
- Apply blood to card, allow to dry for 30 minutes prior to mailing.
- Results are available in 4-10 business days.

9. Smoking Cessation

- Unless the patient has contraindications, pharmacotherapy should be offered to all patients attempting to quit smoking (Table 8).
- First-line agents (double long-term smoking abstinence rates):
    * Nicotine replacement therapy (NRT)
        - Nicotine gum (Nicorette®, generic) OTC
        - Nicotine patch (Nicotrol®, Nicoderm CQ®, generic) OTC
        - Nicotine inhaler (Nicotrol® inhaler) (Rx only)
        - Nicotine nasal spray (Nicotrol NS®) (Rx only)
    * Bupropion SR (Zyban®) (Rx only)
- Second-line agents (if fail/cannot tolerate first-line):
    * Clonidine
    * Nortriptyline

Combination nicotine replacement therapy

- Combining the nicotine patch with a self-administered form of nicotine replacement therapy (either the nicotine gum or nicotine nasal spray) may be more efficacious than a single form of nicotine replacement. Combined treatment should be recommended if the patient is unable to quit using a single type of first-line pharmacotherapy.

Side effects of nicotine replacement therapy (NRT)

- Insomnia/sleep disturbances
    * Can be minimized by using the 16-hour patch or removing patch at night
- Patch: local irritation
    * 50% of patients
    * Usually resolves by rotating site
    * Treat with hydrocortisone cream or triamcinolone cream
- Nasal spray
    * Nasal irritation

Contraindications and precautions for nicotine replacement therapy (NRT)

- Cardiovascular disease
    * <2 weeks post-MI
    * Serious arrhythmias
    * Serious/worsening angina
- Esophagitis, peptic ulcer disease (gum)
- Seek medical advice if pregnant or breastfeeding
- Do not smoke while using NRT.
- Allergies, asthma, sinus conditions (nasal spray)

Table 8

The "5 A's" Clinicians Should Use to Assist Patients in Smoking Cessation

Ask about tobacco use.	Identify and document tobacco use status for every patient at every visit.
Advise to quit.	In a clear, strong, and personalized manner urge every tobacco user to quit.
Assess willingness to make a quit attempt.	Is the tobacco user willing to make a quit attempt at this time?
Assist in quit attempt.	For the patient willing to make a quit attempt, use counseling and pharmacotherapy to help him or her quit.
Arrange follow-up.	Schedule follow-up contact, preferably within the first week after the quit date.

10. Natural and Herbal Products

- Complementary and alternative medicine (CAM) definitions:
  * *Conventional treatment:* medical practices widely accepted and practiced by the mainstream medical community
  * *Complementary therapy:* therapy used in addition to conventional treatment(s)
  * *Alternative:* therapy used instead of conventional treatment(s)

Dietary Supplement and Health Education Act of 1994 (DSHEA)

- Definition of a dietary supplement: "A product intended to supplement the diet that . . . contains one or more of the following dietary ingredients: a vitamin, mineral, herb or other botanical, amino acid; a dietary substance for use by man to supplement the diet by increasing the total daily intake, or a concentrate, metabolite, constituent, extract, or combination of these ingredients" (Table 9).

- Regulation of dietary supplements:
  * FDA: regulates labeling, safety, and manufacturing
  * FTC: regulates advertising

Herbal Natural Products

Ginkgo biloba
- Common uses:
  * Enhance memory and concentration
  * Intermittent claudication
  * Vertigo and tinnitus
  * Impotence (in combination with papaverine)

Table 9

Drugs versus Dietary Supplements

Drug	Dietary supplement
Active ingredient identified	May not identify active ingredient
Safety and efficacy proven by manufacturer	No proof of efficacy required; FDA must provide proof if unsafe
Purity and contents regulated	No standards for quality or purity
Claims to treat/cure/prevent disease	No claims to treat/cure/prevent specific disease

- Proposed mechanisms:
  * Increases blood flow
  * Antioxidant
  * Inhibits platelet aggregation

Dosage
- Recommend standardized product, 120-240 mg/d divided bid or tid

Side effects
- Mild: GI distress, headache, dizziness
- Serious: spontaneous bleeding has been reported (eg, subdural hematomas, subarachnoid hemorrhage)

Drug interactions
- Drugs (aspirin, ticlopidine, clopidogrel, dipyridamole, warfarin) or herbs (garlic, ginseng) with antiplatelet or anticoagulant activity

Contraindications
- Ginkgo should be discontinued prior to surgery to avoid potential bleeding complications.

St. John's wort (*Hypericum perforatum*)
- Common uses:
  * Depression
  * Anxiety
- Proposed mechanism:
  * Inhibition of dopamine, serotonin, and norepinephrine reuptake
  * Decreased IL-6 concentrations

Dose
- Product standardized to 0.3% hypericin, 300 mg tid

Side effects
- Mild GI distress, dizziness, fatigue, insomnia, itching, dry mouth, hypertension
- Photosensitivity: recommend sun avoidance or sunscreen

Drug interactions
- Numerous, potentially serious
- Antidepressants (SSRIs, TCAs):
  * Similar mechanisms
  * Serotonin syndrome
- CYP450-3A4 inducer significantly decreases levels of:
  * Cyclosporine
  * Indinavir
- Decreases levels of digoxin
- Oral contraceptives (increases metabolism of estradiols)

Asian ginseng
- Common uses:
  * Fatigue
  * Enhance concentration
- Proposed mechanism:
  * Suppresses and stimulates CNS
  * Corticosteroid activity
  * Hypoglycemic activity

Dosage
- 1-2 g of crude root or 100-300 mg of ginseng extract tid

Side effects
- Hypertension
- Euphoria, restlessness, nervousness, insomnia
- Rash
- Edema
- Diarrhea

Contraindications
- Hypertension
- Antipsychotic drugs
- Ginseng should be discontinued prior to surgery to avoid potential bleeding complications.

Precautions
- Heart disease
- Diabetes
- Hypotension

Drug interactions
- Risk with anticoagulants and antiplatelet agents (aspirin, ticlopidine, clopidogrel, dipyridamole, warfarin), other herbs (ginkgo, garlic)
- Stimulants (including caffeine)
- Antipsychotics
- Diabetes drugs

Garlic (*Allium sativum L.*)
- Common uses:
  * Lower cholesterol
  * Prevent atherosclerosis
- Proposed mechanisms:
  * Inhibits platelet aggregation
  * Free radical scavenger
  * Stimulates fibrinolysis
  * Lowers cholesterol and lipid levels by inhibition of HMG-CoA reductase

Dosage
- 4 g of fresh minced garlic bulb, 600-900 mg/d (100-mg garlic powder tablets); or 2-5 mg allicin daily

Side effects
- Malodorous breath, smell of garlic may permeate the skin
- GI discomfort, heartburn, gas
- Dermatitis, allergic reactions

Drug interactions
- Anticoagulants and antiplatelet agents (aspirin, ticlopidine, clopidogrel, dipyridamole, warfarin, ginkgo, ginseng)
- Saquinavir AUC decreased by 50% in healthy volunteers

Contraindication
- Garlic should be discontinued prior to surgery to avoid potential bleeding complications.

Echinacea purpurea
- Common uses:
  * Colds and other respiratory tract infections
  * Topical use for poorly healing wounds and chronic ulcerations
- Proposed mechanisms:
  * Stimulates the immune system
  * Increases white blood cells

Dosage
- One capsule (contains 900-1000 mg powdered herb) tid
- Dosing should begin at the onset of viral symptoms.
- Continue treatment until 24-48 hours after symptoms abate.

Side effects
- Allergic reactions can occur.
- Tolerance: limit use to 6-8 weeks at a time.

Disease interactions
- Autoimmune disorders (immune system stimulation)
- Potentially severe allergic response, including anaphylaxis, in individuals with asthma or allergies to members of the daisy family (ragweed, daisies, chrysanthemums, marigolds)

Drug interactions
- Immunosuppressive agents

Saw palmetto (*Serenoa repens*)
- Common uses:
  * Benign prostatic hyperplasia

Proposed mechanism
- Inhibits 5α-reductase and dihydrotestosterone (DHT) binding to androgen receptors
- Antiandrogenic

Dosage

- Fluid extracts 1:1 = 1-2 mL bid; 1:2 = 2-4 mL bid
- Dry extract 4:1 (w/w) (~25% fatty acids) = 400 mg bid
- Product with 80-90% fatty acids, dose of 160 mg bid
- Take with morning and evening meals to decrease GI upset
- Treatment usually lasts for 3 months.

Side effects

- Rarely: GI upset, headache, hypertension
- Urinary tract symptoms (urine retention, dysuria)
- Impotence

Precautions

- Recommend thorough prostate exam and discussion with physician before starting treatment.

Kava-kava (root)

- Common uses:
    * Anxiety/stress

Proposed mechanism

- Possibly binds at GABA receptors
- Possibly dopamine antagonist

Dosage

- 100 mg 2-3 times a day

Side effects

- Similar to alcohol (adversely affects motor reflexes and judgment for driving and/or operating heavy machinery) but does not act as a CNS depressant
- Mydriasis

- Extrapyramidal symptoms
- Kava dermopathy: yellow, flaking, scaly skin, eye redness
- Liver failure leading to transplantation or death (Table 10)

Drug interactions

- L-dopa: decreased effectiveness
- Barbiturates, benzodiazepines, alcohol: additive sedative effects

Contraindications

- Pre-existing liver disease
- Regular alcohol ingestion

Precautions

- Do not take for >4 weeks.
- Discontinue immediately if jaundice occurs.

Ma huang (ephedra)

- In 2004, the FDA ruled to withdraw all ephedrine alkaloid products from the market due to risk of myocardial infarction, stroke, and death.

Nonbotanical Natural Products

S-adenosylmethionine (SAMe)

- Common uses:
    * Depression
    * Osteoarthritis

Proposed mechanisms:

- Depression: methyl donor to catecholamines (increased norepinephrine, dopamine)

Table 10

Natural Products Associated with Serious Toxicity

Common name	Promoted for	Associated with
Blue cohosh	Uterotonic, diuretic	Vasoconstriction, GI spasms
Comfrey	Gout, arthritis, infections	Obstruction of blood flow to the liver possibly resulting in death
Chinese weight loss preparations (*Aristolochia fangchi* mistaken for *Stephania tetrandra*)	Primarily weight loss	Kidney cancer, referred to as "Chinese-herb nephropathy"
Ephedra/ma huang	Weight loss, energy, decongestion	Hypertension, arrhythmias, seizures, stroke, myocardial infarction, ***death***
Kava-kava	Stress reduction	Liver failure
Licorice root	Peptic ulcers, expectorant	Pseudoaldosteronism
Yohimbe	Aphrodisiac	Weakness, paralysis, anxiety, ***death*** (overdose)

- Anti-inflammatory: enhances the synthesis of proteoglycans in chondrocytes

Dosing
- Depression: 800-1600 mg/d divided tid-qid
- Arthritis: 200 mg tid (range 400-1200 mg/d)

Side effects
- Generally mild: gas, vomiting, diarrhea, nausea
- Patients with bipolar disorder may experience switch to mania.

Melatonin
- Common uses:
    * Sleep disorders
    * Reset sleep-wake cycle (jet lag)

Proposed mechanism:
- Mimics endogenous release of melatonin from the pineal gland
- Concentrations increase significantly 1-2 hours before sleep.

Dosage
- Insomnia: 0.1-1 mg at bedtime
- Jet lag: 3-5 mg for 3 days before and after departure

Side effects
- Infertility
- Headache
- Confusion
- Possible immune stimulant

Drug interactions
- Benzodiazepines: enhanced anxiolytic effects

Dehydroepiandrosterone (DHEA)
- Common uses:
    * Depression
    * General anti-aging effects
    * Osteoporosis
    * Antidiabetogenic

Proposed mechanisms:
- Adult concentrations of DHEA fall to about 20% of maximum by 70 years of age.
- Sex hormone precursor
- Increased secretion of IL-2
- Inhibits platelet aggregation
- Enhanced fibrinolysis

Dosage
- ~50 mg/d is average

Side effects
- Oily skin, acne, hirsutism

- Abnormal menses
- Headache
- Abnormal aggressiveness

Contraindications
- Patients with hormone-sensitive tumors (eg, breast cancer, prostate cancer)

Glucosamine
- Common uses:
    * Osteoarthritis

Proposed mechanism:
- Serves as a precursor to glycosaminoglycans, which make up cartilage and synovial fluid
- May help regenerate cartilage and replete synovial fluid

Dosage
- 500 mg tid (with meals) glucosamine sulfate for 6-8 weeks

Side effects
- Mild GI effects: nausea, heartburn
- Little is known about long-term use.
- Diabetes: may worsen insulin resistance (case reports)

11. Sleep Aids and Stimulants

Insomnia

Nonpharmacologic treatment of insomnia
- Establish regular waking and sleeping schedule.
- Exercise regularly.
- Do not nap during the daytime.
- Avoid caffeine, especially after noon.
- Avoid large meals close to bedtime.
- Participate in a relaxing activity at bedtime (eg, reading, hot bath)

Pharmacologic treatment of insomnia: nonprescription products (Table 11)
Antihistamines
- Diphenhydramine
- Doxylamine

Pharmacology
- Block histamine$_1$ and muscarinic receptors

Role in therapy
- Antihistamines should be used for short-term management of occasional insomnia in conjunction with good sleep hygiene.

Dosage
- Diphenhydramine 25-50 mg 30-60 minutes before bedtime (elderly, 25 mg)
- Do not exceed 7-10 days of therapy (to avoid tolerance).

Side effects
- Sedation, especially the next morning
- Anticholinergic effects
    * Dry mouth/eyes
    * Constipation
    * Urinary retention
    * Confusion (elderly)

Contraindications and precautions
- Benign prostatic hyperplasia (BPH)
- Dementia
- Narrow-angle glaucoma

Drowsiness

Nonpharmacologic treatment of drowsiness
- Good sleep hygiene preferable to drug therapy (see insomnia section, above).

Pharmacologic treatment of drowsiness
Caffeine
- The only FDA-approved nonprescription stimulant
- Acts as a CNS stimulant
- Physical dependence can develop.
- 50-200 mg: increased alertness, decreased fatigue
- >200 mg: nervousness, insomnia, irritability

Precautions
- Peptic ulcer disease
- Cardiac dysrhythmias
- Anxiety disorders

Special patient populations
- Pregnancy: restrict to <300 mg caffeine per day to minimize risk of low birth weight
- Breastfeeding: 1% of caffeine crosses into breast milk; peak effect 1 hour after consumption; minimize caffeine use in breastfeeding, especially in infants.

Table 11

Selected Nonprescription Products for Insomnia

Drug or combination	Trade name
Doxylamine	Unisom Nighttime Sleep Aid Tablets
Diphenhydramine	Nytol, Sominex
Diphenhydramine + acetaminophen	Tylenol PM, Unisom Pain Relief
Diphenhydramine + aspirin	Bayer PM

12. Key Points

Cough, cold, and allergy
- Nonprescription drug therapy for the common cold includes symptomatic management using decongestants (nasal congestion), antihistamines (excess nasal discharge), analgesics (headache), and local anesthetic lozenges or sprays (pharyngitis).
- Nonprescription treatment of allergies includes systemic antihistamines (sedating or nonsedating), ocular antihistamines, decongestants (if nasal congestion), and cromolyn (scheduled, not as needed).
- Cough can be relieved by a product containing a cough suppressant (dextromethorphan). An expectorant (guaifenesin) should be recommended to enhance clearance of mucus.

Constipation
- Diet and lifestyle changes should always be recommended to prevent or treat constipation (increase in fiber and fluid intake, exercise).
- Bulk-forming laxatives and stool softeners are the safest products to prevent and treat constipation, and can be used chronically.
- Stimulant laxatives should be used only occasionally to avoid laxative dependence or other complications.

Diarrhea
- Loperamide or bismuth subsalicylate may be recommended to treat diarrhea.
- Maintaining adequate hydration is very important, especially in young children and the elderly.

Nausea and vomiting
- Nonprescription treatment options for nausea and vomiting include antihistamines (meclizine, dimenhydrinate) and phosphorated carbohydrate solution (Emetrol®).
- Histamine$_2$-receptor antagonists (cimetidine, ranitidine), antacids, or bismuth salts (Pepto-Bismol) may relieve gastric discomfort or indigestion.

Pain and fever
- Pain and fever may be treated with aspirin and other salicylates, nonsteroidal anti-inflammatory drugs (NSAIDs), or acetaminophen.
- Aspirin and NSAIDs inhibit platelet aggregation. Nonacetylated salicylates and acetaminophen do not have antiplatelet activity.
- Salicylates and NSAIDs can cause gastropathy, including gastritis, gastric ulcers, and gastric bleeding. They may decrease the effectiveness of some antihypertensives, and may have deleterious effects on kidney function.
- Acetaminophen does not have anti-inflammatory activity, and can be hepatotoxic in excessive doses (>4 g/d), or when used concurrently with alcohol.

Ophthalmic products
- Dry eyes can be treated with artificial tears or ocular emollients.
- Ophthalmic vasoconstrictors (ocular decongestants) cause vasoconstriction in the conjunctiva to treat redness. Naphazoline is the ocular decongestant of choice. Ocular decongestants are contraindicated in narrow-angle glaucoma, due to the potential to cause rebound.
- Combination products containing an ophthalmic vasoconstrictor and ocular antihistamine should be recommended for allergic conjunctivitis (naphazoline + pheniramine or antazoline).

Otic products
- Impacted cerumen can be treated with cerumen-softening agents (carbamide peroxide in anhydrous glycerin + alcohol; hydrogen peroxide + water).
- Water-clogged ears may be managed with the commercial preparation of isopropyl alcohol + anhydrous glycerin, or compounded acetic acid + isopropyl alcohol.

Home monitoring and testing devices
- Home tests are available for:
  * Blood glucose monitoring (diabetes)
  * Fertility and ovulation
  * Pregnancy
  * Urinary tract infection
  * Colorectal cancer
  * Blood pressure monitoring
  * Acquired immunodeficiency syndrome (AIDS)
  * Illicit drug use
  * Hepatitis C

Smoking cessation
- First-line agents for pharmacotherapy in smoking cessation:
  * Nicotine gum (Nicorette, generic) OTC
  * Nicotine patch (Nicotrol, Nicoderm CQ) OTC
  * Nicotine inhaler (Nicotrol inhaler)
  * Nicotine nasal spray (Nicotrol NS)
  * Bupropion SR (Zyban)
- Contraindications/precautions for nicotine replacement therapy:
  * Cardiovascular disease
    - <2 weeks post-MI
    - Serious arrhythmias
    - Serious/worsening angina
  * Esophagitis, peptic ulcer disease (gum)
  * Seek medical advice if pregnant or breastfeeding
  * Do not smoke while using NRT.
  * Allergies, asthma, sinus conditions (nasal spray)

Natural and herbal products

- Herbal products that should be discontinued prior to surgery: ginkgo, garlic, ginseng
- St. John's wort: takes several weeks to see effect; potential for serious drug interactions.

Sleeping aids

- Ethanolamine antihistamines (diphenhydramine, doxylamine) should be used for short-term management of occasional insomnia in conjunction with good sleep hygiene.

Stimulants

- Caffeine, a CNS stimulant, is the only FDA-approved nonprescription stimulant.
- The recommended dosage of 50-200 mg may increase alertness and decrease fatigue.
- Doses exceeding 200 mg may cause nervousness, insomnia, and/or irritability.

13. Questions and Answers

1. The primary advantage of recommending dextromethorphan instead of codeine is:

    A. It is twice as effective as codeine in suppression of cough
    B. It has less dependence potential
    C. It has peripheral rather than central action
    D. It is less expensive
    E. It is much longer acting than codeine

2. All of the following statements regarding guaifenesin are correct EXCEPT:

    A. It is the only FDA-approved OTC expectorant
    B. It requires large amounts of water to be effective
    C. It is available OTC as Robitussin
    D. It may cause an decrease in platelet aggregation and an increase in bleeding time
    E. It is available in some prescription cough and cold formulations

3. All of the following statements regarding diphenhydramine are true EXCEPT:

    A. It is less likely to cause drowsiness compared to other OTC antihistamines
    B. It is the active ingredient in some OTC products for insomnia
    C. It is available OTC under the trade name of Benadryl
    D. A small percentage of children may exhibit a paradoxical CNS stimulant effect
    E. Elderly patients may experience delirium or confusion with diphenhydramine

4. All of the following statements about the routine use of oral decongestants in treating the common cold are true EXCEPT:

    A. Phenylpropanolamine has been removed from all OTC cold and allergy products
    B. They are relatively safe with no dependence
    C. They are absolutely contraindicated in patients with controlled diabetes and mild hypertension
    D. The most common side effects are nervousness and insomnia
    E. They cannot be used in patients on MAO inhibitor antidepressants

5. All of the following are correct generic and trade name combinations EXCEPT:

   A. Chlor-Trimeton® = chlorpheniramine
   B. Dimetane® = diphenhydramine
   C. Claritin = loratadine
   D. Nasalcrom = cromolyn
   E. Zyrtec = cetirizine

6. Which of the following is not a side effect of loperamide?

   A. Sedation
   B. Dizziness
   C. Dry mouth
   D. Drowsiness
   E. Insomnia

7. Which of the following is not an adverse effect of Pepto-Bismol?

   A. Anticholinergic effects, dry mouth, and dry eyes
   B. Tinnitus
   C. Cross-sensitivity to aspirin allergy
   D. Grayish-black tongue
   E. Dark stools

8. Which of the following drugs exhibits analgesic and antipyretic properties, but not peripheral anti-inflammatory properties?

   A. Ibuprofen
   B. Sodium salicylate
   C. Acetaminophen
   D. Magnesium salicylate
   E. Naproxen

9. Which drug does not interact with NSAIDs?

   A. Methotrexate
   B. Warfarin
   C. Antihypertensive agents
   D. Diphenhydramine
   E. None of the above

10. Mary is a 32-year-old female with asthma and serious aspirin sensitivity. She comes to the pharmacist seeking assistance selecting a nonprescription product for aches and pains. Which of the following should the pharmacist recommend for Mary?

    A. Ibuprofen
    B. Naproxen
    C. Acetaminophen
    D. A and B only
    E. All of the above

11. Nonprescription antiemetics are primarily useful for preventing which type of nausea?

    A. Nausea due to alterations in the vestibular apparatus
    B. Nausea due to drugs acting centrally on the chemoreceptor trigger zone
    C. Nausea due to visceral pain
    D. Nausea due to cortical stimulation from smells or sight
    E. Nausea due to afferent impulses from the gastrointestinal tract

12. A mother requests advice for her 6-month-old who has been constipated the last 2 days after beginning cereal feedings. Which of the following agents would be the best laxative agent to recommend?

    A. Dulcolax
    B. Fletcher's Castoria
    C. Mineral oil
    D. Glycerin suppositories
    E. Milk of magnesia

13. All of the following statements about stool softeners are true EXCEPT:

    A. They are not safe to use in pregnancy
    B. The onset of action is usually between 1 and 2 days
    C. They are useful in patients with constipation who have hemorrhoids
    D. Extra water helps their effectiveness
    E. They are often combined with mild stimulant laxatives

14. All of the following statements about bisacodyl are true EXCEPT:

    A. It should not be taken concurrently with antacids
    B. It can be crushed or chewed if needed
    C. It should not be recommended in pregnancy
    D. It is available in oral tablet and suppository dosage forms
    E. It is the active ingredient in Doxidan

15. Which of the following ethanolamine anti-histamines are available in OTC products for insomnia?

    A. Diphenhydramine
    B. Doxylamine
    C. Loratadine
    D. A and B
    E. All of the above

16. Baby Matthew is 1 year old and weighs 24 lb. He has a fever of 102°F, is irritable, seems uncomfortable, and isn't sleeping well. His mother is confused by the assortment of fever relief products. You recommend acetaminophen. Which product and dosage do you recommend?

    A. Tylenol Infant Drops 80 mg/0.8 mL; give 1.6 mL q4-6h
    B. Tylenol Children's Liquid 160 mg/5 mL; give 2 tsp. q6-8h
    C. Advil Infant Drops 50 mg/1.25 mL; give 1.25 mL q4-6h
    D. Motrin Children's Suspension 100 mg/5 mL; give 2.5 mL q6-8h
    E. Tylenol Infant Drops 80 mg/0.8 mL; give 3.2 mL q4-6h

17. The next morning, baby Matthew's mother comes back to your pharmacy. Her pediatrician recommended alternating the maximum dose of ibuprofen with the acetaminophen, and she is asking for help selecting an ibuprofen product and dosage. Which do you recommend?

    A. Advil Infant Drops 50 mg/1.25 mL; give 0.625 mL q8h
    B. Motrin Children's Suspension 100 mg/5 mL; give 2 tsp. q4h
    C. Motrin Infant Drops 50 mg/1.25 mL; give 2.5 mL q6h
    D. Advil Children's Chewable Tablet 50 mg; give one tablet q8h
    E. Advil Children's Chewable Tablet 50 mg; $^1/_2$ tablet q4h

18. Which of the following tests does not require a blood sample?

    A. Cholesterol test
    B. Ovulation prediction tests
    C. HIV tests
    D. Hepatitis C test
    E. Accu-Chek Advantage

19. B.R. is a 62-year-old obese male who has been diagnosed by his physician with benign prostatic hyperplasia (BPH). Which of the following herbal remedies might be used to treat his symptoms?

    A. Ginseng
    B. Echinacea
    C. DHEA
    D. Garlic
    E. Saw palmetto

20. Which of the following products should be discontinued prior to surgery?

    A. Ginkgo biloba
    B. Gentian root
    C. Glutamine
    D. Glucosamine
    E. Folic acid

Answers

1. **B.** Although there have been reports of limited recreational abuse of dextromethorphan, its potential for dependence/addition is significantly less than that of codeine.

2. **D.** Guaifenesin does not have any effects on platelet aggregation or bleeding time. It is the only FDA-approved OTC expectorant, works better with increased fluid intake, and is included in Robitussin products.

3. **A.** Diphenhydramine, an ethanolamine, is the most sedating OTC antihistamine.

4. **C.** Systemic decongestants are not recommended in individuals with uncontrolled diabetes or hypertension due to their sympathomimetic effects. They are contraindicated with MAOIs, and can commonly cause nervousness or insomnia. Phenylpropanolamine was removed from the market in 2000.

5. **B.** Dimetane contains brompheniramine.

6. **E.** Dizziness, dry mouth, and drowsiness are common side effects of loperamide.

7. **A.** Common adverse effects of Pepto-Bismol include tinnitus and grayish-black tongue or stools. It does contain a salicylate, and therefore should not be used in individuals with aspirin allergy.

8. **C.** Acetaminophen is a centrally-acting antipyretic and analgesic, but does not exhibit peripheral anti-inflammatory activity. Salicylates and other NSAIDs do.

9. **D.** NSAIDs can significantly decrease methotrexate clearance, enhance the effect of warfarin, and blunt the hypotensive effect of hypertensive medications. There is no known interaction with diphenhydramine.

10. **C.** All NSAIDs and aspirin-containing products should be avoided in individuals with aspirin sensitivity. Acetaminophen can be recommended in this setting.

11. **A.** Nonprescription antiemetics are antihistamines that exert their effect by inhibiting histamine in neural centers controlling vomiting, salivation, and vestibular excitability, making them especially well suited for motion sickness.

12. **D.** Glycerin suppositories are safe for infants. The other agents should not be used in this patient population.

13. **A.** Stool softeners are safe to use in pregnancy, and usually exert their effect within 1-2 days. Stool softeners are recommended for individuals in whom hard stools or straining could cause pain or complications (eg, hemorrhoids, postoperatively, postpartum, post-MI). Increased fluid intake enhances their effectiveness. They are frequently used in combination products containing stimulant laxatives.

14. **B.** Because bisacodyl is an enteric-coated product, it should not be taken with antacids, or be crushed, chewed, or broken. It should not be used in pregnancy. It is available in both oral tablets and rectal suppositories.

15. **D.** Both diphenhydramine and doxylamine are ethanolamines used in sleeping aids. Loratadine is a nonsedating antihistamine.

16. **A.** The pediatric dosage of acetaminophen is 10-15 mg/kg q4-6h.

$$24 \text{ lb} \times \text{kg}/2.2 \text{ lb} = 10.9 \text{ kg} \times 10\text{-}15 \text{ mg/kg}$$
$$= 109 - 163.5 \text{ mg}$$

Tylenol Infant Drops 80 mg/0.8 mL;
1.6 mL = 160 mg acetaminophen

17. **C.** The pediatric dosage of ibuprofen is 5-10 mg/kg q6-8h.

$$24 \text{ lb} \times \text{kg}/2.2 \text{ lb} = 10.9 \text{ kg} \times 5\text{-}10 \text{ mg/kg}$$
$$= 54.5 - 109 \text{ mg}$$

Motrin Infant Drops 50 mg/1.25 mL;
2.5 mL = 100 mg ibuprofen

18. **B.** Cholesterol, HIV, hepatitis C, and blood glucose tests all require a blood sample. Most ovulation prediction tests use urine.

19. **E.** Saw palmetto may have some efficacy in treating BPH, although the patient should be evaluated by a physician to rule out prostate cancer.

20. **A.** Ginkgo biloba has antiplatelet activity, and should therefore be withheld prior to surgical procedures.

14. References

Berardi RR, ed. *Handbook of Nonprescription Drugs: An Interactive Approach to Self Care,* 15th ed. Washington: American Pharmacists Association; 2006.

Pray WS. *Nonprescription Product Therapeutics,* 2nd ed. Baltimore: Lippincott Williams & Wilkins; 2006.

Fiore MC, Bailey WC, Cohen SJ, et al. Treating Tobacco Use and Dependence. Clinical Practice Guideline. Rockville, MD: U.S. Department of Health and Human Services; Public Health Service: June 2000.

Robbers JE, Tyler VE. *Tyler's Herbs of Choice: The Therapeutic Use of Phytomedicinals.* New York: The Hayworth Herbal Press; 1999.

Scott GN, Elmer GW. Update on natural product-drug interactions. *Am J Health-Syst Pharm.* 2002;59:339-347.

28. Asthma and Chronic Obstructive Pulmonary Disease

Timothy H. Self, PharmD
Professor, Department of Clinical Pharmacy
University of Tennessee College of Pharmacy

Contents

1. Asthma

2. Chronic Obstructive Pulmonary Disease (COPD)

3. Key Points

4. Questions and Answers

5. References

1. Asthma

- Asthma is a chronic inflammatory disorder of the airways in which many cells and cellular elements play a role, in particular mast cells, eosinophils, T lymphocytes, neutrophils, and epithelial cells. In susceptible individuals, this inflammation causes recurrent episodes of wheezing, breathlessness, chest tightness, and cough, particularly at night and in the early morning. Asthma affects over 15 million Americans, and is the most common cause of missed school days for children. Mortality due to asthma is increasing; death rates are greatest in inner city African-Americans and Hispanics.

Types and Classifications

- Childhood-onset (atopic): positive family history of asthma, allergy to tree or grass pollen, house dust mites, household pets, and molds (extrinsic asthma)
- Adult-onset: usually a negative family history and negative skin tests to common aeroallergens (intrinsic asthma)
- Classification of severity is shown in Figure 1 (this classification is extremely important in defining treatment options; see Figure 2).

Clinical Presentation

- Episodic wheezing, coughing, chest tightness, shortness of breath; worse at night, early morning, and with exercise

Pathophysiology

- Inflammatory airway disease; also a disease with bronchospasm
- Common triggers of symptoms include aeroallergens, respiratory viral illness, exercise (especially in cold, dry air), environmental smoke, fumes, and cats.
- Drug-induced asthma includes that due to aspirin, NSAIDs, and β-blockers (low-dose β_1-selective agents okay if concurrent post MI or CHF and do not have severe asthma; COX-2 inhibitors may be okay in aspirin-sensitive asthma)
- Complex interaction among inflammatory cells (eg, mast cells, eosinophils, lymphocytes), mediators (eg, leukotrienes), and cytokines (eg, IL-4, IL-5)
- The result is airway inflammation (mucus and swelling in the lining of the airways) and airway hyperreactivity.
- *Early phase* response to inhaling an aeroallergen occurs immediately; *late phase* response occurs 4-12 hours later.

- Asthma is commonly worsened by poorly controlled concurrent allergic rhinitis, sinusitis, and GERD; it may also worsen in the premenstrual or perimenstrual period.

Diagnostic Criteria

- The main basis for diagnosis is a detailed history of episodic symptoms that are typically worse at nighttime/early morning and associated with common triggers.
- Reversible airway obstruction (improvement in pulmonary function tests [FEV_1] of >12% after inhaling a short-acting β_2 agonist)
- Exclude alternate diagnoses.

Treatment Principles and Goals

- Optimal long-term management of asthma includes four major areas, including objective assessment and monitoring, environmental control, pharmacologic therapy, and patient education as a partnership.
- Treatment goals are shown in Figure 1; a stepwise approach to managing asthma is shown in Figures 2 and 3. See Table 1 for long-term control medications.
- Inhaled corticosteroids are the most efficacious drugs for long-term management of persistent asthma. Addition of a long-acting inhaled β_2 agonist is recommended for patients with moderate or severe persistent asthma.
- Omalizumab (Xolair®) was released in the U.S. in 2003 after the NIH Asthma Guidelines were last updated. This anti-IgE therapy is primarily indicated for severe persistent asthma patients who have frequent emergency department visits and hospitalizations despite optimal therapy. It is given SC every 2-4 weeks.

Drug therapy for acute exacerbations of asthma
- See Table 2 for quick-relief medications, and Figure 4 for management of asthma exacerbations.

Monitoring

- Optimal management for the great majority of patients will result in a dramatic reduction in symptoms (including nocturnal and early morning symptoms), as well as reduced acute care visits, lost work or school days, and the need for quick-relief medications.
- Monitoring peak expiratory flow (PEF) using a peak flow meter at home is required ("green zone" is 80-100% of personal best value; "yellow zone" is 50-79% of personal best, and indicates consultation with a health care professional is advisable; and "red

Figure 1.

Classification of asthma severity.

Goals of Asthma Treatment

- Prevent chronic and troublesome symptoms (e.g., coughing or breathlessness in the night, in the early morning, or after exertion)
- Maintain (near) "normal" pulmonary function
- Maintain normal activity levels (including exercise and other physical activity)
- Prevent recurrent exacerbations of asthma and minimize the need for emergency department visits or hospitalizations
- Provide optimal pharmacotherapy with minimal or no adverse effects
- Meet patients' and families' expectations of and satisfaction with asthma care

Classify Severity of Asthma

Clinical Features Before Treatment*

	Symptoms**	Nighttime Symptoms	Lung Function
STEP 4 Severe Persistent	■ Continual symptoms ■ Limited physical activity ■ Frequent exacerbations	Frequent	■ FEV_1 or PEF ≤60% predicted ■ PEF variability >30%
STEP 3 Moderate Persistent	■ Daily symptoms ■ Daily use of inhaled short-acting beta$_2$-agonist ■ Exacerbations affect activity ■ Exacerbations ≥2 times a week; may last days	>1 time a week	■ FEV_1 or PEF >60% –<80% predicted ■ PEF variability >30%
STEP 2 Mild Persistent	■ Symptoms >2 times a week but <1 time a day ■ Exacerbations may affect activity	>2 times a month	■ FEV_1 or PEF ≥80% predicted ■ PEF variability 20–30%
STEP 1 Mild Intermittent	■ Symptoms ≤2 times a week ■ Asymptomatic and normal PEF between exacerbations ■ Exacerbations brief (from a few hours to a few days); intensity may vary	≤2 times a month	■ FEV_1 or PEF ≥80% predicted ■ PEF variability <20%

* The presence of one of the features of severity is sufficient to place a patient in that category. An individual should be assigned to the most severe grade in which any feature occurs. The characteristics noted in this figure are general and may overlap because asthma is highly variable. Furthermore, an individual's classification may change over time.

** Patients at any level of severity can have mild, moderate, or severe exacerbations. Some patients with intermittent asthma experience severe and life-threatening exacerbations separated by long periods of normal lung function and no symptoms.

PEF, peak expiratory flow; FEV_1, forced expiratory volume in 1 second.
Reproduced from NIH Expert Panel Report 2.

Figure 2.

Stepwise approach for managing infants and young children (≤5 years of age) with acute or chronic asthma.

Classify Severity: Clinical Features Before Treatment or Adequate Control	Symptoms/Day Symptoms/Night	Medications Required To Maintain Long-Term Control
		Daily Medications
Step 4 Severe Persistent	Continual Frequent	■ **Preferred treatment:** – **High-dose inhaled corticosteroids** **AND** – **Long-acting inhaled beta₂-agonists** **AND,** if needed, – Corticosteroid tablets or syrup long term (2 mg/kg/day, generally do not exceed 60 mg per day). (Make repeat attempts to reduce systemic corticosteroids and maintain control with high-dose inhaled corticosteroids.)
Step 3 Moderate Persistent	Daily > 1 night/week	■ **Preferred treatments:** – **Low-dose inhaled corticosteroids and long-acting inhaled beta₂-agonists** **OR** – **Medium-dose inhaled corticosteroids.** ■ Alternative treatment: – Low-dose inhaled corticosteroids and either leukotriene receptor antagonist or theophylline. If needed (particularly in patients with recurring severe exacerbations): ■ **Preferred treatment:** – Medium-dose inhaled corticosteroids and long-acting beta₂-agonists. ■ Alternative treatment: – Medium-dose inhaled corticosteroids and either leukotriene receptor antagonist or theophylline.
Step 2 Mild Persistent	> 2/week but < 1x/day > 2 nights/month	■ **Preferred treatment:** – **Low-dose inhaled corticosteroid (with nebulizer or MDI with holding chamber with or without face mask or DPI).** ■ Alternative treatment (listed alphabetically): – Cromolyn (nebulizer is preferred or MDI with holding chamber) OR leukotriene receptor antagonist.
Step 1 Mild Intermittent	≤ 2 days/week ≤ 2 nights/month	■ No daily medication needed.

Quick Relief All Patients	■ Bronchodilator as needed for symptoms. Intensity of treatment will depend upon severity of exacerbation. – Preferred treatment: **Short-acting inhaled beta₂-agonists** by nebulizer or face mask and space/holding chamber – Alternative treatment: Oral beta₂-agonist ■ With viral respiratory infection – Bronchodilator q 4–6 hours up to 24 hours (longer with physician consult); in general, repeat no more than once every 6 weeks – Consider systemic corticosteroid if exacerbation is severe or patient has history of previous severe exacerbations ■ Use of short-acting beta₂-agonists >2 times a week in intermittent asthma (daily, or increasing use in persistent asthma) may indicate the need to initiate (increase) long-term control therapy.

 Step down
Review treatment every 1 to 6 months; a gradual stepwise reduction in treatment may be possible.

 Step up
If control is not maintained, consider step up. First, review patient medication technique, adherence, and environmental control.

Note
■ The stepwise approach is intended to assist, not replace, the clinical decisionmaking required to meet individual patient needs.
■ Classify severity: assign patient to most severe step in which any feature occurs.
■ There are very few studies on asthma therapy for infants.
■ Gain control as quickly as possible (a course of short systemic corticosteroids may be required); then step down to the least medication necessary to maintain control.
■ Provide parent education on asthma management and controlling environmental factors that make asthma worse (e.g., allergies and irritants).
■ Consultation with an asthma specialist is recommended for patients with moderate or severe persistent asthma. Consider consultation for patients with mild persistent asthma.

Goals of Therapy: Asthma Control

■ Minimal or no chronic symptoms day or night
■ Minimal or no exacerbations
■ No limitations on activities; no school/parent's work missed

■ Minimal use of short-acting inhaled beta₂-agonist (< 1x per day, < 1 canister/month)
■ Minimal or no adverse effects from medications

Reproduced from National Institutes of Health 2002, Guidelines for the Diagnosis and Management of Asthma.

Figure 3.

Stepwise approach for managing asthma in adults and children >5 years of age: Treatment.

Classify Severity: Clinical Features Before Treatment or Adequate Control			Medications Required To Maintain Long-Term Control
	Symptoms/Day **Symptoms/Night**	**PEF or FEV₁** **PEF Variability**	**Daily Medications**
Step 4 **Severe Persistent**	Continual ——— Frequent	≤ 60% ——— > 30%	■ **Preferred treatment:** – **High-dose inhaled corticosteroids** **AND** – **Long-acting inhaled beta₂-agonists** AND, if needed, – Corticosteroid tablets or syrup long term (2 mg/kg/day, generally do not exceed 60 mg per day). (Make repeat attempts to reduce systemic corticosteroids and maintain control with high-dose inhaled corticosteroids.)
Step 3 **Moderate Persistent**	Daily ——— > 1 night/week	> 60% – < 80% ——— > 30%	■ **Preferred treatment:** – **Low-to-medium dose inhaled corticosteroids and long-acting inhaled beta₂-agonists.** ■ Alternative treatment (listed alphabetically): – Increase inhaled corticosteroids within medium-dose range OR – Low-to-medium dose inhaled corticosteroids and either leukotriene modifier or theophylline.
			If needed (particularly in patients with recurring severe exacerbations): ■ **Preferred treatment:** – **Increase inhaled corticosteroids within medium-dose range and add long-acting inhaled beta₂-agonists.** ■ Alternative treatment: – Increase inhaled corticosteroids within medium-dose range and add either leukotriene modifier or theophylline.
Step 2 **Mild Persistent**	> 2/week but < 1x/day ——— > 2 nights/month	≥ 80% ——— 20–30%	■ **Preferred treatment:** – **Low-dose inhaled corticosteroids.** ■ Alternative treatment (listed alphabetically): cromolyn, leukotriene modifier, nedocromil, OR sustained release theophylline to serum concentration of 5–15 mcg/mL.
Step 1 **Mild Intermittent**	≤ 2 days/week ——— ≤ 2 nights/month	≥ 80% ——— < 20%	■ **No daily medication needed.** ■ Severe exacerbations may occur, separated by long periods of normal lung function and no symptoms. A course of systemic corticosteroids is recommended.

Quick Relief **All Patients**	■ Short-acting bronchodilator: 2–4 puffs **short-acting inhaled beta₂-agonists** as needed for symptoms. ■ Intensity of treatment will depend on severity of exacerbation; up to 3 treatments at 20-minute intervals or a single nebulizer treatment as needed. Course of systemic corticosteroids may be needed. ■ Use of short-acting beta₂-agonists >2 times a week in intermittent asthma (daily, or increasing use in persistent asthma) may indicate the need to initiate (increase) long-term control therapy.

Step down
Review treatment every 1 to 6 months; a gradual stepwise reduction in treatment may be possible.

Step up
If control is not maintained, consider step up. First, review patient medication technique, adherence, and environmental control.

Note
■ The stepwise approach is meant to assist, not replace, the clinical decisionmaking required to meet individual patient needs.
■ Classify severity: assign patient to most severe step in which any feature occurs (PEF is % of personal best; FEV₁ is % predicted).
■ Gain control as quickly as possible (consider a short course of systemic corticosteroids); then step down to the least medication necessary to maintain control.
■ Provide education on self-management and controlling environmental factors that make asthma worse (e.g., allergens and irritants).
■ Refer to an asthma specialist if there are difficulties controlling asthma or if step 4 care is required. Referral may be considered if step 3 care is required.

Goals of Therapy: Asthma Control

■ Minimal or no chronic symptoms day or night
■ Minimal or no exacerbations
■ No limitations on activities; no school/work missed
■ Maintain (near) normal pulmonary function
■ Minimal use of short-acting inhaled beta₂-agonist (< 1x per day, < 1 canister/month)
■ Minimal or no adverse effects from medications

Table 1

Long-Term Asthma Control Medications

Generic name	Trade name	Usual dosage range	Dosage form	Schedule[1]
Inhaled corticosteroids				
Beclomethasone HFA 40 mcg/puff; 80 mcg/puff	QVAR®	80-480 mcg/day	MDI	bid
Budesonide 200 mcg/inhalation	Pulmicort®	1-3 inhalations/day	Turbuhaler	bid
Budesonide 0.25 & 0.5 mg	Respules®	0.5-2.0 mg/day	Nebulized	bid
Flunisolide 250 mcg/puff	Aerobid®	1-8 puffs/day	MDI	bid
Fluticasone 44, 110, 220 mcg/puff	Flovent®	88-660 mcg/day	MDI	bid
Fluticasone	Flovent Rotadisk®	100-500 mcg/day	DPI	bid
Fluticasone-salmeterol combination (each dose: 50 mcg salmeterol + 100, 250, or 500 mcg fluticasone)	Advair Diskus® (Advair 100, 250, 500)	1 inhalation	DPI	bid
Mometasone 220 mcg/inhalation	Asmanex® Twisthaler	1-2 inhalations/day	DPI	hs
Triamcinolone 100 mcg/puff	Azmacort®	4-20 puffs/day	MDI/spacer	bid
Leukotriene modifiers				
Montelukast	Singulair®	4 mg (12-23 months)	Oral granules	qhs
		4 mg (age 2-5 y)	Chewable tab	qhs
		5 mg (age 6-14 y)	Chewable tab	qhs
		10 mg (adult) tablet	Tablet	qhs
Zafirlukast	Accolate®	20-40 mg/day tablet	Tablet	bid
Zileuton	Zyflo®	2400 mg/day tablet	Tablet	qid
Mast cell stabilizers				
Cromolyn	Intal®	1-4 puffs MDI	MDI	qid
	Intal®	20 mg	Nebulizer solution	qid
Nedocromil	Tilade®	1-4 puffs MDI	MDI	qid
Long-acting inhaled β_2 agonists				
Formoterol	Foradil Aerolizer®	1 inhalation DPI	DPI	bid
Salmeterol	Serevent Diskus®	1 inhalation DPI	DPI	bid
Methylxanthines				
Theophylline (numerous products)	Uniphyl®	10 mg/kg per day[2] up to 300 mg max in adults to start; aim for 5-15 mcg/mL steady state	Tablet	Daily; 5 or 6 pm

MDI, metered dose inhaler; DPI, dry powder inhaler (breath-activated).

[1]Usual schedule (some patients do well on once-daily dosing).

[2]Complex, high-risk drug to dose; see references cited for details; do not use unless competent in dosing and monitoring serum theophylline concentrations.

zone," or <50% of personal best, indicates a written action plan should be implemented, and if there is no quick response, immediate medical attention should be sought).

- Spirometry in the physician's office

Mechanism of Action

(For more details, see the section on mechanism of action from the NIH Expert Panel Report 2.)

Long-term control medications

Corticosteroids

- Anti-inflammatory: block late reaction to allergen

Table 2

Quick-Relief Asthma Medications

Generic name	Trade name	Usual dosage[1]	Dosage form	Schedule
Short-acting inhaled β_2 agonists[2]				
Albuterol	Proventil®, Ventolin®	2 puffs	MDI	q4h prn
		2.5 mg	Nebulizer solution	q4h prn
Pirbuterol	Maxair Autohaler®	2 puffs	MDI	q4h prn
Anticholinergics				
Ipratropium	Atrovent®	2 puffs	MDI	q6h
		0.25 mg	Nebulizer solution	q6h
Ipratropium with albuterol	Combivent®	2 puffs	MDI	q6h
		3 mL	Nebulizer solution	q6h
Systemic corticosteroids[3]				
Methylprednisolone	Medrol®	1 mg/kg per day	Tablets	Daily
Prednisone		1 mg/kg per day	Tablets/liquid	Daily
Prednisolone		1 mg/kg per day	Tablets	Daily

[1]Usual dosage for routine home use (dose in emergency department is higher/more frequent).

[2]For prevention of exercise-induced asthma, inhale 2 puffs 5-15 minutes before exercise. Increasing use indicates poor asthma control; increase anti-inflammatory therapy and reassess environmental control (good asthma control is indicated by infrequent need for quick-relief therapy).

[3]Short courses are used for <2 weeks.

and reduce airway hyperresponsiveness; inhibit cytokine production, adhesion protein activation, and inflammatory cell migration and activation
- Reverse β_2-receptor downregulation: inhibit microvascular leakage

Cromolyn and nedocromil
- Anti-inflammatory: block early and late reaction to allergen; interfere with chloride channel function; stabilize mast cell membranes and inhibit activation and release of mediators from eosinophils and epithelial cells
- Inhibit acute response to exercise, cold dry air, and SO_2

Long-acting β_2 agonists
- Bronchodilation: smooth muscle relaxation following adenylate cyclase activation and increase in cyclic AMP, producing functional antagonism of bronchoconstriction
- In vitro, inhibit mast cell mediator release, decrease vascular permeability, and increase mucociliary clearance
- Compared to short-acting inhaled β_2 agonist, salmeterol (but not formoterol) has a slower onset of action (15-30 minutes) but longer duration (>12 hours).

Methylxanthines
- Bronchodilation: smooth muscle relaxation from phosphodiesterase inhibition and possibly adenosine antagonism
- May affect eosinophilic infiltration into bronchial mucosa as well as decrease T-lymphocyte numbers in epithelium
- Increases diaphragm contractility and mucociliary clearance

Leukotriene modifiers
- Leukotriene receptor antagonist; selective competitive inhibitor of LTD_4 and LTE_4 receptors
- 5-Lipoxygenase inhibitor

Anti-IgE therapy
- Omalizumab (Xolair) is a humanized monoclonal anti-IgE antibody that binds circulating IgE, thus inhibiting the allergic inflammatory cascade that results when aeroallergens bind to IgE on mast cells.

Quick-relief medications
Short-acting inhaled β_2 agonists
- Bronchodilation: smooth muscle relaxation following adenylate cyclase activation and increase in

Figure 4.

Management of asthma exacerbations: Emergency department and hospital-based care.

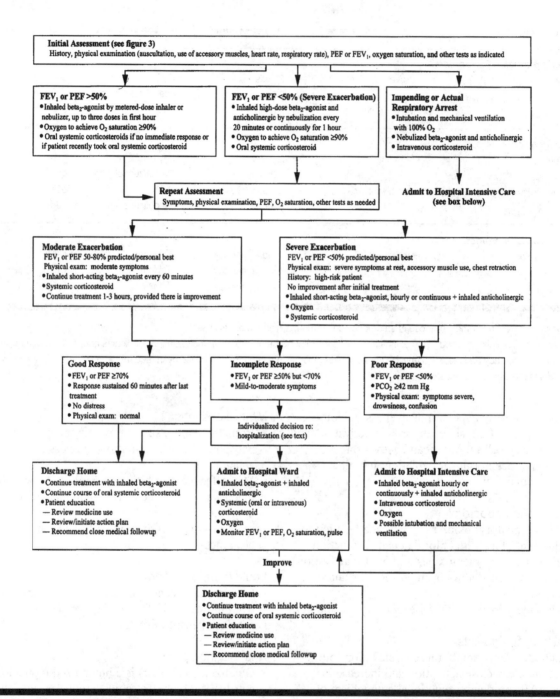

PCO₂, partial pressure of carbon dioxide; PEF, peak expiratory flow; FEV₁, forced expiratory volume in 1 second.
Reproduced from NIH Expert Panel Report 2.

cyclic AMP, producing functional antagonism of bronchoconstriction

Anticholinergics
- Bronchodilation: competitive inhibition of muscarinic cholinergic receptors
- Reduce intrinsic vagal tone to the airways; may block reflex bronchoconstriction secondary to irritants or to reflux esophagus
- May decrease mucus gland secretion

Patient Instructions and Counseling

- Patient education is absolutely essential for optimal asthma management.
- Emphasize the necessity to take controller/preventer medications *EVERY DAY,* even when the patient feels well and is having no breathing problems.
- Instruct the patient regarding the dangers of overuse of short-acting inhaled β_2 agonists (if inflammation is worsening, see a physician if the usual dose does not give quick relief).
- Demonstrate the correct use of the MDI, the MDI plus spacer, and dry powder inhalers (DPI), and then OBSERVE the patient using the devices (most patients do not perform well initially; the devices can be difficult to use at first; see Figure 5 for MDI or MDI spacer use). For DPIs, remember to stress that inhalation must be RAPID and deep.
- Demonstrate correct use of peak flow meters and OBSERVE the patient using them (Table 3); explain about the green, yellow, and red zones (including the written action plan).
- Teach how to prevent exercise-induced asthma.
- Be sure patients receive an influenza vaccination every fall.

Adverse Drug Effects

(For more details, see the section on adverse drug effects from NIH Expert Panel Report 2.)
Long-term control medications
Inhaled corticosteroids
- Cough, dysphonia, oral thrush (candidiasis)
- In high doses, systemic effects may occur, although studies are not conclusive, and the clinical significance of these effects (eg, adrenal suppression, osteoporosis, growth suppression, skin thinning, and easy bruising) has not been established.

Cromolyn and nedocromil
- Fifteen to twenty percent of patients complain of an unpleasant taste from nedocromil.

Table 3

Directions for Use of Peak Flow Meter[1]

1. Stand while using the meter.
2. Position the indicator at the bottom of the scale.
3. Hold the peak flow meter so your fingers do not block the opening.
4. Inhale as deeply as possible, place mouthpiece well into your mouth, and make sure your lips form a tight seal around it.
5. Blow out as fast and as hard as possible![2] BLAST! Emphasize to the patient that the maneuver is highly effort-dependent.
6. Repeat steps 2-5 two more times, and record the highest of the three readings along with the date and time.

[1]If a short-acting inhaled β_2 agonist is required in the early morning, remember to check the peak expiratory flow before using the drug, and record the value; then repeat PEF testing 15 minutes later.
[2]Do not accelerate air with your tongue (ie, use a spitting motion). This incorrect maneuver will give false elevation in PEF.

Long-acting β_2 agonists
- Tachycardia, skeletal muscle tremor, hypokalemia, prolongation of QTc interval in overdose
- A diminished bronchoprotective effect may occur within 1 week of chronic therapy. Clinical significance has not been established.

Methylxanthines
- Dose-related acute toxicities include tachycardia, nausea and vomiting, tachyarrhythmias (SVT), central nervous system stimulation, headache, seizures, hematemesis, hyperglycemia, and hypokalemia.
- Adverse effects at usual therapeutic doses include insomnia, gastric upset, aggravation of ulcer or reflux, increase in hyperactivity in some children, and difficulty in urination in elderly males with prostatism.

Leukotriene modifiers
(updated from 1997 NIH Guidelines)
- Montelukast and zafirlukast are usually well tolerated.
- Zileuton can cause liver dysfunction.

Figure 5.

Steps for using an inhaler.

<u>P</u>lease demonstrate your inhaler technique at every visit.

1. Remove the cap and hold inhaler upright.
2. Shake the inhaler.
3. Tilt your head back slightly and breathe out slowly.
4. Position the inhaler in one of the following ways (A or B is optimal, but C is acceptable for those who have difficulty with A or B. C is required for breath-activated inhalers):

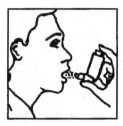 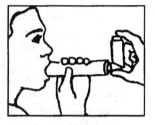 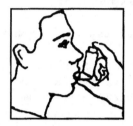 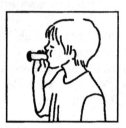

A. Open mouth with inhaler 1 to 2 inches away.

B. Use spacer/holding chamber (that is recommended especially for young children and for people using corticosteroids).

C. In the mouth. Do not use for corticosteroids.

D. NOTE: Inhaled dry powder capsules require a different inhalation technique. To use a dry powder inhaler, it is important to close the mouth tightly around the mouthpiece of the inhaler and to inhale rapidly.

5. Press down on the inhaler to release medication as you start to breathe in slowly.
6. Breathe in slowly (3 to 5 seconds).
7. Hold your breath for 10 seconds to allow the medicine to reach deeply into your lungs.
8. Repeat puff as directed. Waiting 1 minute between puffs may permit second puff to penetrate your lungs better.
9. Spacers/holding chambers are useful for all patients. They are particularly recommended for young children and older adults and for use with inhaled corticosteroids.

Avoid common inhaler mistakes. Follow these inhaler tips:

- Breathe out *before* pressing your inhaler.
- Inhale *slowly.*
- Breathe in through your mouth, not your nose.
- Press down on your inhaler at the *start* of inhalation (or within the first second of inhalation).
- Keep inhaling as you press down on inhaler.
- Press your inhaler only *once* while you are inhaling (one breath for each puff).
- Make sure you breathe in evenly and deeply.

NOTE: Other inhalers are becoming available in addition to those illustrated above. Different types of inhalers may require different techniques.

Reproduced from NIH Expert Panel Report 2.

Quick-relief medications

Short-acting inhaled β₂ agonists

- Tachycardia, skeletal muscle tremor, hypokalemia, increased lactic acid, headache, hyperglycemia; in general the inhaled route causes few systemic adverse effects; patients with preexisting cardiovascular disease, especially the elderly, may have adverse cardiovascular reactions with inhaled therapy

Anticholinergics

- Drying of mouth and respiratory secretions, increased wheezing in some individuals, blurred vision if sprayed in eyes

Systemic corticosteroids

- Short-term use: reversible abnormalities in glucose metabolism, increased appetite, fluid retention, weight gain, mood alteration, hypertension, peptic ulcer, and rarely aseptic necrosis of the femur
- Consideration should be given to coexisting conditions that could be worsened by systemic corticosteroids, such as herpes virus infections, varicella, tuberculosis, hypertension, peptic ulcer disease, and strongyloidiasis.

Drug-Drug and Drug-Disease Interactions

- For zafirlukast, administration with meals decreases bioavailability; take at least 1 hour before or 2 hours after meals.
- Zileuton and zafirlukast may increase the effect of warfarin and increase theophylline levels.
- Well known inducers of cytochrome P450 (carbamazepine, phenobarbital, phenytoin, and rifampin) are documented to decrease the effect of systemic corticosteroids.
- Examples of drugs that may increase the effect of systemic corticosteroids include erythromycin, clarithromycin, itraconazole, oral contraceptives, and conjugated estrogen.

Parameters to Monitor

- Refill record for daily controller/preventer meds and quick-relief meds
- Reduction in symptoms (including nocturnal and early morning symptoms)
- ED visits and hospitalizations; unscheduled office visits
- Need for "bursts" of systemic corticosteroids
- Lost work or school days, and the need for quick-relief medications
- Peak expiratory flow (PEF) using a peak flow meter at home

- If the patient also has rhinitis or GERD, monitor refills to ensure optimal control (if rhinitis and GERD are not well controlled, asthma control will likely suffer).

Kinetics

- Theophylline is no longer used extensively in asthma, but when it is used, knowledge of its kinetics is essential due to its high risk.
- Other drugs, disease states, smoking, age, and diet can all affect theophylline kinetics and dose requirements.
- Therapeutic serum theophylline concentrations are 5-15 mcg/mL (**NOT** the old recommendation of 10-20 mcg/mL; see latest NIH Guidelines [1997 and 2002]).
- Elimination half-life in an otherwise healthy non-smoking adult is about 8 hours, but in a smoker about 4 hours, and in a small child (>1 year) about 4 hours.
- Neonates have greatly prolonged elimination half-life.
- Elimination half-life in decompensated heart failure or cirrhosis is about 24 hours.
- Volume of distribution is about 0.5 L/kg.
- High-fat meals may cause "dose dumping" for some products (check product literature).

Other

- MDIs should be stored at room temperature, between 59 and 86°F; if left in a car in freezing or near-freezing temperatures, aerosol particles will be too large to inhale into the lungs.
- MDIs should be "primed" (release one dose) only with first use, or if it is a prn agent used only once every few weeks (frequent priming is unnecessary and wastes expensive medications).
- MDI dust cap should be left on inhaler when not in use! Check mouthpiece for foreign objects before inhaling!

Non-Drug Therapy

- An essential component of optimal asthma management is environmental control.
- Without good control of the environment at home, school, and work, drug therapy will often be inadequate.
- Have the patient identify known asthma triggers, and help the patient identify potential triggers not yet realized (do not forget someone smoking at home or work!).

Table 4.

Factors Affecting Serum Theophylline Levels

Factor	Decreases Theophylline Concentrations	Increases Theophylline Concentrations	Recommended Action
Food	↓ or delays absorption of some sustained-release theophylline (SRT) products	↑ rate of absorption (fatty foods) products	Select theophylline preparation that is not affected by food.
Diet	↑ metabolism (high protein)	↓ metabolism (high carbohydrate)	Inform patients that major changes in diet are not recommended while taking theophylline.
Systemic, febrile viral illness (e.g., influenza)		↓ metabolism	Decrease theophylline dose according to serum concentration level. Decrease dose by 50 percent if serum concentration measurement is not available.
Hypoxia, cor pulmonale, and decompensated congestive heart failure, cirrhosis		↓ metabolism	Decrease dose according to serum concentration level.
Age	↑ metabolism (1 to 9 years)	↓ metabolism (<6 months, elderly)	Adjust dose according to serum concentration level.
Phenobarbital, phenytoin, carbamazepine	↑ metabolism		Increase dose according to serum concentration level.
Cimetidine		↓ metabolism	Use alternative H_2 blocker (e.g., famotidine or ranitidine).
Macrolides: TAO, erythromycin, clarithromycin		↓ metabolism	Use alternative antibiotic or adjust theophylline dose.
Quinolones: ciprofloxacin, enoxacin, pefloxacin		↓ metabolism	Use alternative antibiotic or adjust theophylline dose. Circumvent with ofloxacin if quinolone therapy is required.
Rifampin	↑ metabolism		Increase dose according to serum concentration level.
Ticlopidine		↓ metabolism	Decrease dose according to serum concentration level.
Smoking	↑ metabolism		Advise patient to stop smoking; increase dose according to serum concentration level.

* This list is not all-inclusive; for discussion of other factors, see package inserts.

Reproduced from NIH Expert Panel Report 2.
TAO, triacetyloleandomycin.

2. Chronic Obstructive Pulmonary Disease (COPD)

- COPD is characterized by airflow limitation that is not fully reversible. The airflow limitation is usually both progressive and associated with an abnormal inflammatory response of the lungs to noxious particles or gases. COPD is a major cause of death and suffering in the U.S. and around the world. It is the fourth leading cause of chronic morbidity and mortality in the U.S.

Types and Classifications (Table 5)

- Some clinicians still refer to chronic bronchitis and emphysema in characterizing different levels of COPD (eg, emphysema patients have destructive damage to the alveolar walls, whereas chronic bronchitis is associated with chronic productive cough).

Clinical Presentation

- Shortness of breath
- Cough and sputum production
- Usually a history of cigarette smoking for several years
- In the more severe form, respiratory failure and heart failure

Pathophysiology

- Usually caused by long-term smoking (may also be caused by exposure to other noxious particles and gases)
- Chronic inflammation throughout the airways but via different inflammatory cells and mediators than those that cause asthma (thus the response to inhaled corticosteroids is much less than that seen with asthma)
- Imbalance of proteinases and antiproteinases in the lung
- A rare hereditary cause of emphysema is α_1-antitrypsin deficiency.
- Pathologic changes are found in the central and peripheral airways as well as the alveoli and pulmonary vasculature.
- Mucus hypersecretion
- Ciliary dysfunction
- Airflow limitation
- Lung hyperinflation
- Gas exchange abnormalities
- Secondary pulmonary hypertension
- Cor pulmonale

Diagnostic Criteria

- History of cigarette smoking or exposure to other noxious particles or fumes
- Chronic cough and sputum production
- Spirometry (reduced FEV_1; see Table 5 for classification of severity)
- Rule out other lung diseases.

Table 5

Classification of COPD by Severity

Stage	Characteristics
0: At Risk	• Normal spirometry • Chronic symptoms (cough, sputum, production)
I: Mild COPD	• FEV_1/FVC <70% • FEV_1 ≥80% predicted • With or without chronic symptoms (cough, sputum production)

II: Moderate COPD	• FEV_1/FVC <70%
	• 50% ≤ FEV_1 <80% predicted
	  (IIA: 50% FEV_1 <80% predicted)
	  (IIB: 30% FEV_1 <50% predicted)
	• With or without chronic symptoms (cough, sputum production, dyspnea)

III: Severe COPD	• FEV_1/FVC <70% • 30% ≤ FEV_1 < predicted or FEV_1 <50% predicted plus respiratory failure or clinical signs of right heart failure
IV: Very severe COPD	FEV_1/FVC <70% FEV_1 <30% predicted or FEV_1 <50% predicted plus chronic respiratory failure

FEV_1, forced expiratory volume in 1 second, FVC, forced vital capacity.
Respiratory failure defined as arterial partial pressure of oxygen (PaO_2) less than 8.0 kPa (60 mm Hg) with or without arterial partial pressure of CO_2 ($PaCO_2$) greater than 6.7 kPa (50 mm Hg) while breathing air at sea level.
From Pauwels et al, 2001.

Treatment Principles and Goals

- Prevent disease progression.
- Relieve symptoms.
- Improve exercise tolerance.
- Improve health status.
- Prevent and treat complications.
- Prevent and treat exacerbations.
- Reduce mortality.
- Bronchodilators are central to the symptomatic treatment of COPD; these agents will increase exercise capacity without necessarily improving the FEV_1.
- Inhaled bronchodilators are preferred to oral bronchodilators for initial therapy; the specific choice of agent depends on patient response.
- Long-acting inhaled bronchodilators are more effective and convenient but more expensive.
- One of the long-acting anticholinergic bronchodilators (tiotropium, Spiriva®) is a logical first choice for maintenance therapy of moderate to severe COPD.
- Short-acting inhaled β_2 agonists are preferred for prn use in patients already receiving long-acting β_2 agonists and anticholinergics.
- Theophylline is a logical step 3 agent for maintenance therapy in patients who are not optimally controlled with β_2 agonists and anticholinergics.

Therapy at each stage
(per Global Initiative for Chronic Obstructive Lung Disease [GOLD] Workshop Summary 2004 Update)
- For each stage, avoid risk factors (eg, smoking cessation) and receive influenza vaccine each autumn. Also, consider pneumococcal vaccine per current guidelines.

Stage 0: At risk
- No recommended drug treatment

Stage I: Mild COPD
- As-needed short-acting bronchodilator

Stage II: Moderate COPD
- Add regular treatment with one or more long-acting bronchodilators and rehabilitation

Stage III: Severe COPD
- Regular treatment with one or more long-acting bronchodilators
- Add inhaled corticosteroids if significant symptoms and lung function responses or if repeated exacerbations occur.

Stage IV: Very severe COPD
- Same treatments as for stage III and consider surgical treatment
- Long-term O_2 therapy if chronic respiratory failure

Drug therapy for acute exacerbations of COPD
- Inhaled albuterol and/or ipratropium
- Systemic corticosteroids (eg, prednisone 40 mg daily for 10 days)
- Oral antibiotics for purulent sputum (typically trimethoprim-sulfamethoxazole, amoxicillin, or doxycyline)
- O_2

Monitoring
- Spirometry: FEV_1
- Symptoms of dyspnea, cough, sputum production, change in sputum color and volume
- Pao_2
- Exercise tolerance/fatigue

Long-term drug therapy
- See content under asthma for specific drugs.
- Tiotropium is a once-daily anticholinergic bronchodilator that is arguably step one treatment of moderate to severe COPD. It is administered by a DPI (Handihaler®). Each dose must be loaded, and deep inhalation does not have to be forceful, but must be sufficient to hear the capsule vibrate.

Nondrug therapy
- The most important nondrug therapy is smoking cessation (ie, nicotine replacement therapy, bupropion, support groups, and counseling).
- Oxygen therapy
- Nutritional support
- Psychosocial support
- Pulmonary rehabilitation

3. Key Points

Asthma
- Asthma is primarily an inflammatory airway disease.
- It is undertreated, resulting in much unnecessary suffering and economic loss.
- Managing patients via the principles of the NIH Guidelines has been clearly shown to reduce ED visits and hospitalizations and improve patient quality of life.
- Optimal long-term management includes objective assessment, environmental control, drug therapy, and patient education working in a partnership.
- Patients with persistent asthma need daily controller therapy (anti-inflammatory agents).
- Inhaled corticosteroids are the most efficacious agents to control asthma.
- Inhaled long-acting inhaled β_2 agonists are indicated with inhaled corticosteroids for patients with moderate persistent or severe persistent asthma.
- Short-acting inhaled β_2 agonists are the agents of choice for quick relief of symptoms.
- Pharmacists should teach patients how to use inhalers (MDI, MDI-spacer, and DPI) by demonstrations and *OBSERVATION* of the patient.
- Pharmacists should instruct patients on how to use peak flow meters, including color-coded zone management with a written action plan.
- Patients must clearly understand the purpose of daily controller/preventer meds vs. quick-relief meds.

Chronic obstructive pulmonary disease
(Taken from GOLD Workshop Summary 2004 Update)
- The overall approach to managing stable COPD should be characterized by a stepwise increase in treatment, depending on the severity of the disease.
- For patients with COPD, health education can play a role in improving skills, ability to cope with the illness, and health status. It is effective in accomplishing certain goals, including smoking cessation.
- None of the existing medications for COPD has been shown to modify the long-term decline in lung function that is the hallmark of this disease. Therefore, pharmacotherapy for COPD is used to improve symptoms and/or decrease complications.
- Bronchodilator medications are central to the symptomatic management of COPD.
- The principal bronchodilator treatments are β_2 agonists, anticholinergics, theophylline, and a combination of one or more of these drugs. Inhaled therapy with long-acting agents is preferred.
- Combining bronchodilators may improve efficacy and decrease the risk of side effects compared to increasing the dose of a single bronchodilator.
- Regular treatment with inhaled glucocorticosteroids should only be prescribed for symptomatic COPD patients with a documented spirometric response to glucocorticosteroids or for those with an FEV_1 <50% predicted and repeated exacerbations requiring treatment with antibiotics and/or oral glucocorticosteroids.
- Chronic treatment with systemic glucocorticosteroids should be avoided because of an unfavorable benefit:risk ratio.
- All COPD patients benefit from exercise training programs, improving with respect to both exercise tolerance and symptoms of dyspnea and fatigue.
- The long-term administration of oxygen (>15 hours per day) to patients with chronic respiratory failure has been shown to increase survival.

4. Questions and Answers

1. Asthma is primarily due to which underlying problem?

   A. Pulmonary fibrosis
   B. Infection
   C. Inflammation
   D. Bronchospasm
   E. Granulomas

2. Which objective measure for routine monitoring of asthma is available at home?

   A. PEF
   B. FEV_1
   C. FVC
   D. O_2 saturation
   E. PD20

3. Which device requires slow inhalation?

   A. Diskus
   B. Turbuhaler
   C. Aerolizer
   D. MDI
   E. Rotadisk

4. How many seconds is optimal for breath holding after inhaling from an MDI?

   A. 4
   B. 5
   C. 15
   D. 2
   E. 10

5. When using a peak flow meter, what percentage of the personal best value is the yellow zone?

   A. <50
   B. <60
   C. 50-79
   D. 60-89
   E. 40-60

6. What are the trade names for long-acting inhaled β_2 agonists?

   A. Foradil and Serevent
   B. Pulmicort and Flovent
   C. Aerobid and Combivent
   D. Maxair and Atrovent
   E. Flovent and Ventolin

7. Which disease states decrease theophylline elimination and often result in reduced dosage requirements?

   A. Hepatitis
   B. Heart failure (decompensated)
   C. Hypertension
   D. A, B, and C
   E. A and B

8. Which drug(s) are preferred for long-term treatment of moderate persistent asthma?

   A. Budesonide + formoterol
   B. Fluticasone + salmeterol
   C. Beclomethasone + ipratropium
   D. A or B
   E. B or C

9. Which drug is a once-daily anticholinergic bronchodilator?

   A. Atrovent
   B. Serevent
   C. Foradil
   D. Spiriva
   E. Proventil

10. For patients with asthma or COPD exacerbations not responding adequately to inhaled broncho-dilators, what is the agent of choice to add to manage the acute exacerbation?

    A. Fluticasone
    B. Budesonide
    C. Cromolyn
    D. Theophylline
    E. Prednisone

11. Which drug may increase serum theophylline concentrations?

    A. Clarithromycin
    B. Hydrochlorothiazide
    C. Carbamazepine
    D. Rifampin
    E. Phenytoin

12. Which side effect of inhaled corticosteroids is reduced by spacer devices?

    A. Hoarseness
    B. Decreased bone density
    C. Thinning of skin
    D. Oropharyngeal candidiasis
    E. Cataracts

Case Study 1: Medication Profile

Patient Name:	Thomas Johnson			
Address:	5689 Washington St.			
DOB:	9-15-55			
Drug Allergies:	aspirin sensitivity			
Height:	5'10"	Weight:	75 kg	
Diagnosis:	(1) asthma (childhood onset, moderate persistent)			
	(2) allergic rhinitis			
	(3) hypertension			

Medications:

Date	Rx #	MD	Drug & Strength	Quantity	Sig	Refills
3/16	94385	Betts	Accolate 20 mg	60	1 bid	3
3/16	94386	Betts	albuterol MDI	1	2 puffs q4h	6
3/16	94387	Betts	Flonase	1	bid as dir.	3
3/25	95523	T. Jones	Lopressor 50 mg	60	1 bid	6
3/27	95734	Betts	albuterol MDI	1	2 puffs q4h	5

Pharmacist Notes: 3/16—discussed proper use of MDI and observed patient use. Coached Mr. Johnson to inhale slowly (he was inhaling fast); he used the MDI correctly for the other steps.

13. The therapeutic range for theophylline per the NIH Guidelines for asthma management is:

    A. 5-15 mcg/mL
    B. 8-12 mcg/mL
    C. 10-20 mcg/mL
    D. 15-25 mcg/mL
    E. 10-15 mcg/mL

14. Which asthma controller drug is given qhs?

    A. Accolate
    B. Singulair
    C. Zyflo
    D. Intal
    E. Tilade

15. When it is not well controlled, which disease state may worsen asthma?

    A. Coronary artery disease
    B. GERD
    C. Diabetes
    D. Hypertension
    E. Arthritis

16. Which class of drugs is only indicated in COPD patients who have frequent exacerbations?

    A. Long-acting inhaled β_2 agonists
    B. Anticholinergics
    C. Short-acting inhaled β_2 agonists
    D. Inhaled corticosteroids
    E. Methylxanthines

The next two questions relate to Case Study 1.

17. Which class of drugs is preferred in Mr. Johnson for optimal control of asthma?

    A. Anticholinergics
    B. Inhaled corticosteroids
    C. Methylxanthines
    D. Mast cell stabilizers
    E. Oral corticosteroids

18. What is an appropriate alternative to Lopressor in Mr. Johnson?

    A. An ACE inhibitor
    B. Propranolol 40 mg bid
    C. Clonidine
    D. Hydralazine
    E. Atenolol 200 mg daily

The next two questions relate to Case Study 2.

19. What concerns should the pharmacist have in this situation regarding theophylline?

    A. Cirrhosis is well documented to decrease elimination of theophylline
    B. The milligrams per kilogram dose is too low
    C. Mrs. Adams should be on a q12h product
    D. Theophylline SR should be dosed in the morning, not evening
    E. Long-acting inhaled β_2 agonists increase theophylline clearance

Case Study 2: Medication Profile

Patient Name:	Mrs. S.T. Adams		
Address:	7129 James Ave.		
DOB:	1-6-37		
Drug Allergies:	sulfonamides		
Height:	5'3"	Weight:	55 kg
Diagnosis:	(1) COPD—53 pack-year Hx smoking		
	(quit 2 years ago)		
	(2) cirrhosis		

Medications:

Date	Rx #	MD	Drug & Strength	Quantity	Sig	Refills
2/18	84389	Jones	Serevent Diskus	1	1 bid	6
2/18	84390	Jones	albuterol MDI	1	2 puffs q4h prn	6
2/18	84391	Jones	Atrovent MDI	1	2 puffs q6h	6
2/18	84392	Jones	Uniphyl 600 mg	30	1 qd 6 PM	2

Pharmacist Notes: 2/18—discussed proper use of Diskus and observed patient use; taught Mrs. Adams to inhale deeply and rapidly (she was inhaling slowly for only <2 seconds). Also observed use of MDI (she forgot to exhale gently before pressing down on MDI).

20. The patient has a friend who has COPD and has told her about Spiriva. Mrs. Adams wants to know the opinion of the pharmacist. You would say:

    A. I'll call your doctor and suggest a new prescription for Spiriva
    B. Spiriva is a third-line drug for COPD; I would not use it now
    C. Spiriva is a good drug, but I want to talk to your doctor about starting a medicine called Flovent
    D. Since you have a prescription for Atrovent, I will call your doctor and suggest changing from Atrovent to Spiriva
    E. I think Foradil Aerolizer would be better for you

21. Which drug is best for long-term management of mild persistent asthma?

    A. Cromolyn
    B. Montelukast
    C. Nedocromil
    D. Theophylline
    E. Budesonide

22. Which total daily dose of prednisone is best for home management of an acute exacerbation of asthma in a 60-kg adult?

    A. 5 mg
    B. 60 mg
    C. 10 mg
    D. 20 mg
    E. 7.5 mg

23. Which drug is most likely to cause an asthma exacerbation in a patient sensitive to aspirin?

    A. Ibuprofen
    B. Acetaminophen
    C. Celecoxib
    D. Salsalate
    E. Sodium salicylate

24. Which type of inhaler does not work well in very cold temperatures?

    A. Diskus
    B. Turbuhaler
    C. Aerolizer
    D. MDI
    E. Rotahaler

Answers

1. **C.** Although asthma certainly does have a bronchospastic component, it is primarily due to inflammation, so good control of inflammation dramatically reduces bronchospasm. A good indicator of disease control is the rare need for short-acting inhaled β_2 agonists.

2. **A.** Peak flow meters are inexpensive and relatively easy to use. Good measurement of peak expiratory flow (PEF) requires appropriate technique, and if good technique is used, patients have valuable objective evidence of asthma control (or exacerbation).

3. **D.** Dry powder inhalers currently available require rapid inhalation. MDIs require slow inhalation to minimize impaction of aerosol in the mouth and throat.

4. **E.** Ten seconds is best; there is no need to hold longer. Four to five seconds is okay if 10 seconds is uncomfortable.

5. **C.** The yellow zone is 50-79%, which indicates suboptimal control (the red zone is <50%, which indicates to start the crisis action plan and seek medical attention).

6. **A.** Foradil (formoterol) and Serevent (salmeterol).

7. **E.** Hepatitis and decompensated heart failure both can dramatically reduce theophylline clearance.

8. **D.** (A. budesonide + formoterol *or* B. fluticasone + salmeterol). See Figures 2 and 3.

9. **D.** Atrovent is also a quick-relief agent, but it is not as efficacious in asthma and has a slower onset than albuterol and other short-acting inhaled β_2 agonists.

10. **E.** Prednisone or other systemic corticosteroids (eg, methylprednisolone) are well documented to be efficacious in asthma and acute exacerbations of COPD.

11. **A.** Clarithromycin is documented to increase serum concentrations. Hydrochlorothiazide does not affect serum theophylline concentrations and the remaining choices are all documented to decrease serum theophylline concentrations.

12. **D.** Oropharyngeal candidiasis or thrush is correct. The other side effects are not reduced by spacers.

13. **A.** The currently accepted range for asthma is 5-15 mcg/mL (*NOT* the old range of 10-20 mcg/mL). There is no benefit in exceeding 15 mcg/mL, and many patients receive benefit at lower doses.

14. **B.** Since asthma is a disease of circadian rhythm and is worse between 2 AM and 6 AM, it is best to give this once-daily drug at bedtime.

15. **B.** GERD can worsen asthma if it is not properly treated. The exact mechanisms are debated, but there is excellent documentation that asthma improves if this condition is well managed.

16. **D.** This class of drugs should *NOT* be used routinely in COPD patients with mild disease. In moderate disease, inhaled corticosteroids are only indicated if there are frequent exacerbations. Remember: In asthma, inhaled corticosteroids are the best agents for long-term control, but in COPD their role is limited.

17. **B.** Inhaled corticosteroids is correct (see Figures 2 and 3 for treatment choices). The pharmacist should share the NIH Guidelines with Mr. Johnson's prescriber to help ensure optimal care. In addition, the pharmacist should educate the patient regarding the purpose of the meds and proper use of inhalers (eg, should observe the patient using the device).

18. **A.** An ACE inhibitor should be efficacious with few side effects (monitor for cough). β-Blockers should be avoided in Mr. Johnson unless he is post MI or had CHF (in which case use a low dose of a β_1-selective blocker and monitor carefully).

19. **A.** Cirrhosis is well documented to decrease elimination of theophylline. Ensure a check of a steady-state theophylline level (peak) and anticipate dose reduction (usually 50% dose reduction in liver disease).

20. **D.** Since the patient has prescriptions for Atrovent and Serevent, a logicial change here would be to discontinue the short-acting anticholinergic Atrovent, and add the long-acting once-daily anticholinergic tiotropium (Spiriva).

21. **E.** Budesonide is an inhaled corticosteroid, the class of drugs recommended to treat even mild persistent asthma.

22. **B.** Sixty milligrams is an appropriate dose. If it is started as soon as the patient is in the red zone and not responding quickly to short-acting inhaled β_2 agonists, usually only a few days of treatment will be required (usually <1 week).

23. **A.** Ibuprofen has the same mechanism of action as aspirin and will predictably trigger symptoms in an aspirin-sensitive patient (ie, increased production of leukotrienes). COX-2 inhibitors are likely to be safe (rofecoxib was proven safe in one excellent study). Acetaminophen is the choice agent for minor pain in these patients.

24. **D.** MDIs release large aerosol particles that do not penetrate deeply into the lungs in cold temperatures. Dry powder inhalers are okay.

5. References

Asthma

Berger WE, Qaquandah PV, Blake K, et al. Safety of budesonide inhalation suspension in infants aged six to twelve months with mild to moderate persistent asthma or recurrent wheeze. *J Pediatr*. 2005;146:91-95.

Bousquet J, Cabrera P, Berkman P, et al. The effect of treatment with omalizumab, an anti-IgE antibody, on asthma exacerbations and emergency medical visits in patients with severe persistent asthma. *Allergy*. 2005;l60:302-308.

Busse WW, Lemanske RF. Asthma. *N Engl J Med*. 2001;344:350-362.

Dolovich MB, Ahrens RC, Hess DR, et al. Device selection and outcomes of aerosol therapy: Evidence-based guidelines: American College of Chest Physicians/American College of Asthma, Allergy, and Immunology. *Chest*. 2005;127:335-371.

Hendeles L, Jenkins J, Temple R. Revised FDA labeling guideline for theophylline oral dosage forms. *Pharmacotherapy*. 1995;15:409.

Knorr B, Matz J, Bernstein JA, et al. Montelukast for chronic asthma in 6- to 14-year-old children. *JAMA*. 1998;279:1181-1186.

National Institutes of Health. Expert Panel Report 2. Guidelines for the Diagnosis and Management of Asthma, 1997. NIH publication no. 97-4051.

National Institutes of Health. Guidelines for the Diagnosis and Management of Asthma—Update on Selected Topics 2002. NIH publication no. 02-5075. Also published in *J Allergy Clin Immunol*. 2002;110:S141-S219; available online at www.nhlbi.nih.gov/guidelines/asthma/asthsumm.htm

Pauwels R, Lofdahl CG, Postma DS, et al. Effect of inhaled formoterol and budesonide on exacerbations of asthma. Formoterol and Corticosteroids Establishing Therapy (FACET) International Study Group. *N Engl J Med*. 1997;337:1405; erratum in *N Engl J Med*. 1998;338:139.

Self TH, Finch CK. Studies demonstrating improved outcomes in patients with asthma: A 10 year review. *Am J Manag Care*. 2001;7:187-196.

Shannon M. Life threatening events after theophylline overdose: a 10-year prospective analysis. *Arch Intern Med.* 1999;159:989.

Shapiro G, Lumry W, Wolfe J, et al. Combined salmeterol 50 mcg and fluticasone propionate 250 mcg in the Diskus device for the treatment of asthma. *Am J Respir Crit Care Med.* 2000;161:527.

Weiss KB, Sullivan SD. The health economics of asthma and rhinitis. I. Assessing the economic impact. *J Allergy Clin Immunol.* 2001;107:3.

Chronic obstructive pulmonary disease
Calverley P, et al. Combined salmeterol and fluticasone in the treatment of COPD: a randomized controlled trial. *Lancet.* 2003;361:449-456.

Gross NJ. Tiotropium bromide. *Chest.* 2004;126:1946-1953.

Dahl R, Greefhorst LA, Nowak D, et al. Inhaled formoterol dry powder versus ipratropium bromide in COPD. *Am J Respir Crit Care Med.* 2001;164:778-784.

Mahler D, Donohue JF, Barbee RA, et al. Efficacy of salmeterol xinafoate in the treatment of COPD. *Chest.* 1999;115:957-965.

Pauwels RA, Buist AS, Calverley PM, et al and the GOLD Scientific Committee. Global strategy for the diagnosis, management, and prevention of chronic obstructive pulmonary disease. NHLBI/WHO Global Initiative for Chronic Obstructive Lung Disease (GOLD) Workshop summary. *Am J Respir Crit Care Med.* 2001;163:1256-1276; website: www.goldcopd.com. (2004 Updated Guidelines accessed 3-7-05)

Pauwels R, Lofdahl CG, Laitinen LA, et al. Long term treatment with inhaled budesonide in persons with mild COPD who continue smoking. European Respiratory Society Study on Chronic Obstructive Pulmonary Disease. *N Engl J Med.* 1999;340:1948-1953.

Rigotti NA. Treatment of tobacco use and dependence. *N Engl J Med.* 2002;346:506-512.

29. Infectious Disease

Joyce E. Broyles, PharmD, BCNSP
Associate Professor, Department of Clinical Pharmacy
University of Tennessee College of Pharmacy

Contents

1. General Principles of Infectious Disease

Note: Several infectious disease topics are addressed in other chapters of this review. They are: HIV/AIDS in Chapter 31, common colds in Chapter 27, and otitis media in Chapter 33. For additional information about specific anti-infective agents, please see Chapter 30.

Diagnosis

- Diagnosis of most infectious diseases consists of: (1) isolation and identification of microorganisms; (2) assessment of patient signs and symptoms; and (3) analysis of other laboratory data.

Isolation of organisms
- To identify the causative agent of the disease, samples should be taken from appropriate body sites prior to the initiation of anti-infective therapy. Higher predictive value comes from organisms isolated from normally sterile body sites (blood, urine, and spinal fluid), than from normally bacteriologically colonized areas such as skin or fecal material.

Identification of organisms
- Organisms should be Gram stained as soon as it is practical to determine cell morphology and guide empiric therapy. After the species of organism is determined, standardized concentrations of antibiotics are exposed to the isolated organism to determine what concentrations inhibit growth. The lowest concentration that prevents microbial growth after 18-24 hours is called the minimum inhibitory concentration (MIC). Breakpoint concentrations of antibiotics are defined as susceptible, intermediate, or resistant. These concentrations are determined by considering tissue concentrations with normal dosing and population distribution of the organism and determine if the antibiotic can be used for therapy.
- Physical signs and symptoms of infection such as fever, redness, swelling, pain, and cough must be considered both for initial diagnosis and assessment of antibiotic effectiveness.

Laboratory tests
- White blood cell (WBC) count. In the initial stage of infection, the neutrophil count may increase above normal, and immature neutrophil forms (bands) may appear.
- Inflammatory markers such as C-reactive protein, erythrocyte sedimentation rate, and tumor necrosis factor may increase during infection.
- Laboratory tests may not be reliable in patients who are elderly, malnourished, neonatal, or severely infected.

Treatment Strategies

- Anti-infective agents should only be used when a significant infection has been diagnosed, is strongly suspected, or where indication for prophylactic therapy exists.

Prophylactic therapy
- Anti-infective therapy is directed to prevent infection. Common uses of prophylactic therapy are after exposure to infection, such as tuberculosis, or before surgical intervention in areas of high bacterial inoculum, such as bowel surgery.
- *Empiric therapy,* usually broad-spectrum in nature, is therapy that is directed toward all common pathogens associated with a disease state.
- *Culture-guided therapy* is characterized by a narrower spectrum than empiric therapy; therapy covers only the specific organism isolated that is sensitive to the therapy. This approach is preferred due to increased cost-effectiveness and decreased bacterial resistance from unnecessary antibiotic exposure.

Choice of Anti-Infective Agent

- The clinician must answer several questions to determine optimal anti-infective therapy, or to review the appropriateness of other decisions. These include:
  * Is an antibiotic indicated on the basis of the clinical findings?
  * Have appropriate specimens been obtained, examined, and sent for culture?
  * What organisms are most likely to be causing the infection?
  * If several antibiotics are available to treat this likely or known organism, which agent is best for the patient? Patient allergies and concurrent disease states will be of consideration.
  * Is an antibiotic combination appropriate? A combination of drugs should be given only when clinical experience has shown such therapy to be more effective than single-agent therapy in a particular setting. Such multiple-agent regimens can increase the risk of toxic drug effects, and occasionally may result in drug antagonism and loss of effectiveness. However, some combinations of anti-infective agents have demonstrated increased effectiveness that is greater than their individual effectiveness combined, a phenomenon known as *synergy.* An example of this is the combination of aminoglycosides with cell wall inhibitors

such as penicillin in many gram-positive organisms.

* What is the best route of administration? This will depend on the overall plan for the patient. Oral therapy is preferred for outpatient therapy, and many intravenous anti-infectives have oral forms with similar pharmacokinetic profiles.
* What is the appropriate dose and dose interval? Regimen design should take into account patient size, renal/hepatic function, the disease state to be treated, and pharmacodynamic considerations of the agents used.
* Will initial therapy need modification after culture data are returned?
* What is the optimal duration of therapy, and is the development of resistance during prolonged therapy likely to occur?

Lack of Therapeutic Effectiveness

- When anti-infective therapy fails, careful analysis of possible causes should be made prior to changing the regimen. Factors associated with therapeutic failure include: misdiagnosis of the infection, improper drug regimen, inappropriate choice of antibiotic agent, microbial resistance, and situations in which antibiotic therapy may not be effective without additional interventions, such as surgical drainage.

2. Common Bacterial, Fungal, and Viral Infections

Meningitis

- Meningitis is defined as an inflammation of the meninges that is identified by an abnormal number of white blood cells in the cerebrospinal fluid.

Causative agents
- A wide variety of organisms are associated with this disease, including many gram-positives and gram-negatives.

Clinical presentation
- Patients may present with fever, headache, photophobia, neck rigidity, diarrhea, vomiting, and altered mental status. Infants may present with a bulging anterior fontanelle.

Diagnostic criteria
- Analysis of the cerebrospinal fluid may be diagnostic of the infective agent. Bacterial agents are associated with a large increase in WBCs, increased CSF protein, and decreased CSF glucose. Fungal and viral agents exhibit smaller increases in CSF WBCs, smaller increases in CSF protein, and limited decreases in CSF glucose.

Treatment
- Empiric treatment is usually determined by the age of the patient. Due to limited antibiotic penetration by many agents, the highest safe antibiotic doses are generally used. Table 1 summarizes empiric therapy for meningitis.

Endocarditis

- Endocarditis is an infection of the endocardium, the membrane lining the heart chamber and valves.

Causative agents
- Most patients have previous damage to the heart, such as artificial valve placement, prior to infection. The most common organisms are *Streptococcus* and *Staphylococcus* species.

Clinical presentation
- Patients present with low-grade fever, fatigue, and weakness. A diagnostic finding is the presence of splinter hemorrhages and petechiae.

Diagnostic criteria
- There are no specific laboratory tests for this infection; most present with elevated ESR or CRP.

Table 1

Empiric Treatment of Meningitis

Age of patient	Most likely organism(s)	Empiric treatment
Newborn to 1 month	Gram negative enterics (E coli) Group B streptococci *Listeria monocytogenes*	Ampicillin and aminoglycoside **or** Cefotaxime **or** Ceftriaxone
1 month to 4 years	*Haemophilus influenzae* *Neisseria meningitidis* *Streptococcus pneumoniae*	Cefotaxime or ceftriaxone **and** Vancomycin
5-29 years	*Neisseria meningitidis* *Streptococcus pneumoniae* *Haemophilus influenzae*	Cefotaxime or ceftriaxone **and** Vancomycin
30-60 years	*Streptococcus pneumoniae* *Neisseria meningitidis*	Cefotaxime or ceftriaxone **and** Vancomycin
>60 years	*Streptococcus pneumoniae* Gram-negative enterics (*E coli*) *Listeria monocytogenes*	Ampicillin and aminoglycoside/vancomycin **or** Cefotaxime **or** Ceftriaxone

Visualization of the vegetations on the surface of the heart is often diagnostic of the disease.

Treatment
- According to American Heart Association guidelines, treatment varies by causative organism and the presence of prosthetic devices (which requires longer therapy) (Table 2).

Acute/Chronic Bronchitis

- Bronchitis is an inflammation of the bronchioles, often associated with bronchopneumonia. Chronic bronchitis is largely associated with heavy smoking.

Causative agents
- Viral infections account for half of all cases. *Mycoplasma pneumoniae, Streptococcus pneumoniae, Haemophilus influenzae, Moraxella catarrhalis,* and *Chlamydia pneumoniae* are common bacterial pathogens.

Clinical presentation
- Patients present with a history of acute productive cough, low-grade fever, and a clear chest x-ray.

Diagnostic criteria
- Sputum cultures are usually not useful in diagnosis due to multiple etiologies, and most physicians prescribe from physical findings.

Treatment
- Treatment is controversial for most acute illnesses due to the large percentage of viral cases. Chronic cases are treated, but due to multiple antibiotic treatments, bacterial resistance can easily develop (Table 3).

Pneumonia

- Pneumonia is an inflammation of the lung parenchyma characterized by consolidation of the affected part, filling of the alveolar air spaces with exudates, inflammatory cells, and fibrin. Distribution may be lobar, segmental, or lobular. If associated with bronchitis (see above), it is termed bronchopneumonia.

Causative agents
- Multiple bacterial etiologies are possible, depending on predisposing conditions (Table 4).

Table 2

Therapy for Endocarditis

Organism	Therapy	Duration (wk)
Penicillin-susceptible streptococci	Penicillin G alone **or**	4
	Penicillin G with gentamicin **or**	2
	Ceftriaxone alone **or**	4
	Vancomycin (if allergic to penicillin)	4
Streptococci relatively resistant to penicillin	Penicillin G alone **or**	4
	Penicillin G with gentamicin **or**	2
	Vancomycin (if allergic to penicillin)	4
Staphylococcus without prosthetic material (methicillin-sensitive)	Nafcillin or oxacillin	4-6
	(3-5 days of gentamicin may be added)	4-6
	Cefazolin (with or without gentamicin)	4-6
	Vancomycin (if allergic to penicillin)	4-6
Staphylococcus without prosthetic material (methicillin-resistant)	Vancomycin (if allergic to penicillin)	4-6

Clinical presentation

- Typically, the onset of illness is abrupt or subacute, with fever, chills, dyspnea, and productive cough predominating. On physical examination, the patient is tachypneic and tachycardic, frequently with chest wall retractions and grunting respirations. The complete blood count usually reflects a leukocytosis with a predominance of polymorphonuclear cells.

Diagnostic criteria

- Sputum culture may be useful in identification of some pathogens. However, difficulty in obtaining deep sputum cultures, and problems in culturing some organisms (such as *Legionella*) makes positive identification of the organism difficult.

Table 3

Treatment for Acute and Chronic Bronchitis

Illness	Treatment (7-10 days usual duration)
Acute (rare; for severe disease only)	Erythromycin, clarithromycin, azithromycin (drugs used for treatment of chronic disease may be used; see below)
Chronic	Amoxicillin, amoxicillin-clavulanate, trimethoprim-sulfamethoxazole (TMP-SMX), erythromycin, clarithromycin, azithromycin, doxycycline, cefuroxime, cefaclor, cefprozil

Macrolides [handwritten annotation]

Treatment

- Varies by age groups

Tuberculosis

- Tuberculosis is a communicable infectious disease caused by *Mycobacterium tuberculosis*. It can produce silent, latent infection as well as active infection. Although infection of any tissue or organ with *Mycobacterium tuberculosis* is possible, the usual site of infection is pulmonary.

Clinical presentation

- Tuberculosis can present with generalized symptoms of weight loss, fever, and night sweats with persistent cough productive of sputum. Latent disease is defined by a positive PPD test, in absence of other symptoms.

Diagnostic criteria

- Diagnosis is often made by a combination of chest x-ray, which often shows patchy or nodular infiltrates in the apical areas of the upper lobes or the superior segment of the lower lobes, and positive PPD skin test. Patients with severe HIV disease may not react to the standard PPD skin test. Sputum or lung biopsy may be acid-fast stained to reveal the organism. Due to the extended time period needed to grow the organism, sensitivities to anti-infective agents may take weeks to months to determine.

Treatment

- See Table 5.

Table 4

Empiric Treatment for Pneumonia

Age or type	Usual organisms	Empiric treatment(s)
Neonatal	Group B streptococci, *Listeria monocytogenes, Escherichia coli*	Ampicillin **and** gentamicin **or** cefotaxime **and** gentamicin
1-3 months	*Chlamydia trachomatis, Bordetella*	Erythromycin, clarithromycin, cefuroxime
3 months to 5 years	*Streptococcus pneumoniae, C trachomatis*	Clarithromycin, cefuroxime, cefotaxime
5-18 years	*Mycoplasma pneumoniae, S pneumoniae, Chlamydia pneumoniae*	Clarithromycin, erythromycin, cefuroxime
Adult, community acquired	*S pneumoniae, Haemophilus influenzae, Klebsiella pneumoniae, M pneumoniae*	***Ambulatory:*** oral macrolide (azithromycin, clarithromycin, erythromycin) or fluoroquinolone (levofloxacin, gatifloxacin or moxifloxacin) *Resp.* ***Hospitalized:*** cefotaxime or ceftriaxone with or without macrolide, or fluoroquinolone alone (levofloxacin, gatifloxacin or moxifloxacin)
Adult, hospitalized acquired	*K pneumoniae, Enterobacter aerogenes, Serratia* spp, *Acinetobacter* spp, *Pseudomonas aeruginosa, Staphylococcus aureus*	Aminoglycoside (tobramycin, amikacin or gentamicin) plus one of the following: cefotaxime, ceftriaxone, cefepime, ticarcillin/-clavulanic acid, piperacillin-tazobactam, meropenem, or imipenem; vancomycin to be added if MRSA suspected
Adult, aspiration	Mouth anaerobes	***Uncomplicated:*** penicillin G, clindamycin ***Hospital-acquired:*** ticarcillin-clavulanic acid, *Timentin* piperacillin-tazobactam *Zosyn*

Infectious Diarrhea

- Diarrhea is defined as an increase in frequency and/or liquidity of stool compared with a patient's normal stool.

Causative agents
- Many disease states, drugs, and infectious organisms have been associated with diarrhea.

Clinical presentation
- The patient may present with several of the following symptoms: fever, chills, nausea, vomiting, and abdominal cramping.

Diagnostic criteria
- Etiology is often determined by patient history and physical examination. Due to the nature of the disease, cultures are not often diagnostic, except for determination of carrier states.

Table 5

Treatment of Tuberculosis

Disease stage	Treatment	Duration
Latent (probably isoniazid sensitive)	Isoniazid	9 months (6 months possible except for children and HIV+ persons)
Latent (probably isoniazid resistant)	Rifampin + pyrazinamide	2 months
Active disease	Isoniazid + rifampin + pyrazinamide	2-4 months

Treatment (Table 6)

- Supportive care (hydration, antipyretics, and antiemetics) is useful. Antimotility agents are discouraged due to the potential to cause toxic megacolon. Antibacterial therapy is reserved for severe presentations or patients with risk factors.

Skin and Soft Tissue Infections

- Bacterial infection of the skin can be classified as direct infection of the skin (cellulitis) or secondary infection of a wound or incision.

Causative agents

- Cellulitis is usually infection by a single organism. The most common organisms are *Streptococcus pyogenes* and *Staphylococcus aureus*. Secondary infections may be polymicrobial, including both anaerobic and aerobic organisms.

Clinical presentation

- These infections are characterized by erythema and edema of the skin.

Diagnostic criteria

- Diagnosis is usually made from physical examination. Cultures are not usually diagnostic.

Treatment

- Treatment is empiric, based on likely organisms (Table 7).

Urinary Tract Infections

- Infections of the urinary tract represent a wide variety of clinical syndromes, including urethritis, cystitis, prostatitis, and pyelonephritis.

Causative agents   *E. coli*

- The most common agents are gram-negative facultatively anaerobic rods (coliforms). Hospitalized catheterized patients may also acquire *Pseudomonas* and *Staphylococcus* species.

Clinical presentation

- Lower urinary tract infections tend to present with dysuria, urgency, frequency, nocturia, and suprapu-

Table 6

Treatment of Infectious Diarrhea

Symptoms	Organism	Treatment
Violent presentation 1-6 hours after eating high-protein foods (eggs)	*Staphylococcus aureus*	Supportive
Indolent presentation with mild fever after eating meat, vegetables, or eggs	*Bacillus cereus*	Supportive
Mild to severe presentation 8-16 hours after eating canned products	*Clostridium perfringens*	Supportive
Mild to severe presentation with mild fever; may be associated with meat/egg contamination or contamination of other foods with contaminated water	*Escherichia coli*	Supportive, if outpatient; if hospitalized, fluoro- *Cipro* quinolones or trimethoprim-sulfamethoxazole (TMP-SMX)
Mild to severe presentation with mild fever, chills, and cramping; associated with contamination of other foods with contaminated water; carrier state possible	*Salmonella* spp	Treatment only if febrile (fluoroquinolones or TMP-SMX)
Bloody mucoid diarrhea with fever and cramps	*Shigella* spp	TMP-SMX
Mild indolent presentation, often thought to be "flu"; transmitted by contaminated water	*Campylobacter*	Macrolides or fluoroquinolones
Severe presentation with fever and abdominal pain associated with seafood ingestion	*Yersinia enterocolitica*	Fluoroquinolones
Mild presentation with fever and abdominal pain associated with seafood ingestion	*Vibrio parahaemolyticus*	Tetracycline or fluoroquinolones
Severe, explosive presentation associated with contaminated water	*Vibrio cholerae*	Tetracycline or fluoroquinolones
Mild to severe presentation associated with travel, 6-10 days after exposure, with cramping and low-grade fever	*Escherichia coli*	Mostly supportive; severe prophylactic regimens

Xifaxan

(Rifaximin)

Table 7

Treatment of Infections of the Skin and Soft Tissues

Infection	Organisms	Treatments
Cellulitis	Group A streptococcus; *Staphylococcus aureus*	***Outpatient:*** dicloxacillin, cefadroxil, cephalexin, erythromycin ***Inpatient:*** cefazolin, erythromycin ***Severe cases:*** vancomycin
Diabetic foot infections	*Proteus* spp, *Escherichia coli, S aureus, Bacteroides fragilis,* anaerobic streptococci	Clindamycin or cephalexin ***Severe cases:*** ticarcillin-clavulanic acid or other beta-lactamase inhibitor; vancomycin may be needed if MRSA
Decubitus ulcers	Gram-negative bacilli, *Pseudomonas aeruginosa,* anaerobes	As for diabetic foot infections, above

bic heaviness or pain. Fever is rare. Upper urinary tract infections tend to present with flank pain and fever.

Diagnostic criteria
• Key to the diagnosis of urinary tract infections is the ability to demonstrate significant numbers of organisms present in an appropriately drawn urine sample. In general, higher numbers of organisms ($>10^5$ cells/mL) are needed to diagnose UTIs in females than males ($>10^3$ cells/mL), due to the fact that more organisms are able to ascend the shorter female urethra. In addition, the presence of WBCs in the urine sample may be a significant clue for infection.

Treatment
• A variety of antibacterials may be useful for the treatment of urinary tract infections (Table 8). These include: fluoroquinolones, cephalosporins, TMP-

SMX, and doxycycline. Fluoroquinolones are especially useful for treatment of prostatitis. Length of therapy varies according to the severity of disease.

Bacterial Venereal Diseases (Gonorrhea and Syphilis)

• Venereal diseases are diseases that can be transmitted via sexual intercourse. This section covers only the major bacterial venereal diseases, gonorrhea and syphilis. Additional viral venereal diseases will be covered in sections below (ie, herpes and hepatitis), or in other chapters (HIV, Chapter 31).

Causative agents
• Syphilis is caused by an infection with the spirochete *Treponema pallidum,* while gonorrhea is caused by the gram-negative coccus *Neisseria gonorrhoeae.*

Table 8

Treatment of Urinary Tract Infections

Diagnosis	Organisms	Treatments
Acute uncomplicated cystitis	*E coli, Staphylococcus saprophyticus*	TMP-SMX x 3 days **or** Quinolone x 3 days Cipro, Levo
Acute pyelonephritis	*E coli, Proteus mirabilis, Klebsiella pneumoniae, Enterococcus*	Quinolone x 14 days **or** TMP-SMX x 14 days; if severe, parenteral therapy with quinolone, extended-spectrum penicillin plus aminoglycoside should be used
Prostatitis	*E coli, Proteus* spp, *K pneumoniae*	Quinolone x 4-6 weeks **or** TMP-SMX x 4-6 weeks

Clinical presentation

- Primary syphilis presents as a painless lesion or chancre appearing at the site of infection around 21 days after exposure. These lesions persist for about 8 weeks before spontaneously disappearing. Secondary syphilis develops 2-6 weeks after the onset of the primary stage. It is characterized by a variety of rashes and flu-like symptoms. These symptoms disappear without treatment within 4-10 weeks. Untreated patients will develop symptoms of tertiary syphilis within 2-25 years after infection. These include general paresis, nerve deafness, progressive dementia, and aortic insufficiency.
- Gonorrhea, in contrast, presents as a urethritis within 2-3 days of exposure. Dysuria, urinary frequency, and purulent discharge are common. The majority of infected patients become asymptomatic without treatment within 6 months. About 15% of infected women will develop pelvic inflammatory disease, which can be an indirect cause of infertility.

Diagnostic criteria

- Since *T pallidum* cannot be grown in culture, dark-field or indirect fluorescent antibody microscopic examination is used in conjunction with serologic testing for diagnosis. The most common tests are the Venereal Disease Research Laboratory (VDRL) and the rapid plasma reagin (RPR) tests. Gonorrhea is diagnosed by Gram stain and culture of infected secretions. Alternative methods of diagnosis include enzyme immunoassay and DNA probes. Patients should be screened for the presence of other venereal diseases.

Treatment

- Due to the potential of both diseases to cause significant morbidity to infants born to infected mothers, diagnosis and treatment of pregnant women is of concern. The two organisms differ sharply in resistance to anti-infective agents. *Treponema pallidum* is sensitive to penicillin and has not developed any significant resistance. *Neisseria gonorrhoeae* has not only developed significant resistance to penicillin, but fluoroquinolones as well, leaving third-generation cephalosporins as the major treatment modality (Table 9). Patients diagnosed with gonorrhea should also receive therapy against chlamydial infection (usually doxycycline 100 mg bid for 7 days or azithromycin 1 g once). All sexual partners must also be treated.

Sepsis

- Sepsis has been defined by the American College of Chest Physicians as the systemic inflammatory response syndrome (SIRS) produced in response to infection. SIRS has been defined as requiring two of the following criteria: T >38°C or <36°C; HR >90 bpm; RR >20 breaths/min or $PaCo_2$ <32 torr; WBC >12,000 cells/mm^3 or <4000 cells/mm^3, or >10% immature (band) forms.

Causative agents

- Sepsis may be caused by a variety of organisms, including gram-negative and gram-positive organisms, as well as fungi. Most cases occur in the setting of hospitalized patients and reflect the organisms and resistance pattern of the institution.

Clinical presentation

- In the early phase, the patient may have fever or hypothermia, rigors, chills, tachycardia, tachypnea, hyperglycemia, and lethargy, progressing to hypotension, hypoglycemia, myocardial depression, oliguria, leukopenia, and pulmonary edema leading to multisystem organ failure.

Table 9

Treatment for Syphilis and Gonorrhea

Type	Syphilis	Gonorrhea
Uncomplicated adult presentation	Benzathine penicillin G 2.4 million units IM x 1	Ceftriaxone 125 mg IM x 1 **or** Spectinomycin 2 g IM q12h x 2
Infant born of untreated mother	Penicillin G 50,000-75,000 U/kg q12h x 10-21 days	Cefotaxime 25 mg/kg q12h x 7 days
Disseminated infections	***Secondary/latent disease:*** benzathine penicillin G 2.4 million units IM q week x 3 ***Tertiary disease:*** penicillin G 2-4 million units q4h for 10-14 days	Ceftriaxone 1 g qd x 10 days

Diagnostic criteria
- In addition to physical signs and symptoms, cultures of blood, urine, and sputum may yield clues for antibacterial therapy.

Treatment
- Local organisms and sensitivities will determine anti-infective therapy. Initial therapy should be broad, covering all likely organisms, until culture results are obtained. The *Medical Letter* suggests the following regimens for life-threatening sepsis in adults: cefotaxime, ceftriaxone, cefepime, ticarcillin-clavulanic acid, piperacillin-tazobactam, meropenem, or imipenem with an aminoglycoside (tobramycin, gentamicin, or amikacin). If gram-positive organisms are suspected, vancomycin may be added to the regimen.

Tick-Borne Systemic Febrile Syndromes (Lyme Disease, Rocky Mountain Spotted Fever, Ehrlichiosis, and Tularemia)

- These diseases are similar in transmission and natural history. The organisms responsible for these infections are *Rickettsia,* known for their intracellular growth in host cells. As such, they cannot be grown in culture media, and serologic tests are used for diagnosis. Patients present with fever, rash, and flu-like symptoms, with a history of tick exposure.

Treatment
- See Table 10.

Systemic Fungal Infections

- Fungal infections fall into two categories: primary, able to cause infection in both healthy and immuno-compromised patients; and opportunistic, able to cause infection only in immunocompromised patients. Many fungal infections have a pulmonary focus, due to the aerosol spread of mold spores. Due to increasing use of antibacterial agents and the increase in immunocompromised patients, the incidence of fungal infection is rising.

Clinical presentation
- Patients present with a gradual onset of general malaise, fever, and weakness, unrelieved by antibacterial therapy. Pulmonary infection presents with pneumonia-like symptoms.

Diagnostic criteria
- Diagnosis is made from patient history, cultures (usually blood, sputum, and biopsy of lesions), and serologic tests.

Treatment
- Treatment is often empiric until the organism is isolated (Table 11). Due to the relatively slow culture of most fungi, and the lack of commercial testing against antifungal agents, patient response is used to determine resistance to therapy.

Viral Infections (Hepatitis, Influenza, and the Herpes Simplex Family)

Note: Antiviral therapy is not curative, but decreases the level of virus so that a patient's immune system can handle the infection.

Hepatitis
- Hepatitis is a general term referring to a generalized inflammation of the liver. Etiologies may be viral or chemical.

Causative agents
- Five viruses (hepatitis types A through E) have been identified as causative agents for hepatitis. Syndromes may be either acute or chronic.

Clinical presentation
- Patients present with a history of anorexia, nausea, fatigue, and malaise. This usually progresses to

Table 10

Treatment of Tick-Borne Diseases

Disease	Causative agent	Primary treatment	Alternative treatment
Lyme disease	*Borrelia burgdorferi*	Doxycycline	Cefuroxime
Rocky Mountain spotted fever	*Rickettsia rickettsii*	Doxycycline	Chloramphenicol
Ehrlichiosis	*Ehrlichia phagocytophila*	Doxycycline	Tetracycline
Tularemia	*Francisella tularensis*	Gentamicin or tobramycin	Chloramphenicol; possibly ciprofloxacin

Table 11

Treatment of Systemic Fungal Infections

Disease	Organism	Treatment(s)
Invasive pulmonary disease	*Aspergillosis* spp	Amphotericin B, itraconazole, caspofungin, voriconazole
Cutaneous, pulmonary or extrapulmonary	*Blastomyces dermatitidis*	Itraconazole, amphotericin B, fluconazole
Bloodstream infection	*Candida albicans*	Fluconazole, amphotericin B
Primary pulmonary disease	*Coccidioides immitis*	Itraconazole, fluconazole
Meningitis	*Cryptococcus neoformans*	Amphotericin B + flucytosine, fluconazole
Pulmonary, disseminated, or localized	*Histoplasma capsulatum*	Itraconazole (moderate disease); amphotericin B (severe disease)

fever, right upper quadrant pain, dark urine, light colored stools, and worsening of systemic symptoms. Some patients have no symptoms and little hepatic damage.

Diagnostic criteria
- In addition to physical signs, laboratory tests are remarkable for elevations in AST, ALT, and serum bilirubin.

Treatment
- Treatment is dependent upon the viral strain and type of presentation (Table 12). Standard therapies have not been established for hepatitis A, D, or E.

Influenza
- Influenza is an acute respiratory viral infection.

Causative agents
- Three viruses, influenza A, B, and C, are responsible for most infections.

Clinical presentation
- Patients present with sudden onset of chills, fever, severe prostration, headache, muscle aches, and a cough that usually is dry and may be followed by secondary bacterial infections.

Diagnostic criteria
- Diagnosis is from patient physical signs and symptoms.

Therapy
- Therapy may be either prophylactic or treatment and is determined by viral strain in the community (Table 13). Currently, no therapies exist for influenza C infections.

Herpes simplex family (herpes, cytomegalovirus [CMV], chickenpox/shingles)
- The herpes simplex family is responsible for three serious viral infections: herpes genital infections, cytomegalovirus infections in the immunocompromised, and varicella-zoster infections (chickenpox/shingles).

Table 12

Treatment for Hepatitis

Organism	Presentation	Therapy
Hepatitis B	Chronic	Lamivudine + interferon alfa-2b
Hepatitis C	Chronic	Interferon alfa-2b + ribavirin
Hepatitis C	Acute	Interferon alfa-2b

Table 13

Treatment for Influenza

Organism	Treatment type	Therapy
Influenza A	Prophylaxis	Oseltamivir, rimantadine, amantadine
Influenza A	Treatment	Zanamivir, oseltamivir, rimantadine, amantadine
Influenza B	Prophylaxis	Oseltamivir
Influenza B	Prophylaxis	Zanamivir, oseltamivir

Causative agents
- Each disease is caused by a slightly different herpes virus.

Clinical presentation
- Varies by disease:
  * Genital herpes presents with flu-like symptoms of fever, headache, malaise, and myalgias, in addition to development of painful pustular or ulcerative lesions on the external genitalia.
  * CMV usually presents as retinitis, colitis, or esophagitis.
  * Varicella zoster presents with flu-like symptoms with a pustular rash located on body dermatomes.

Diagnostic criteria
- Mostly from signs and symptoms, although tissue samples may be examined for the presence of the virus by immunofluorescence.

Treatment
- Depends upon viral and disease state; treatment is summarized in Table 14.

3. Key Points

- The hallmark of initial anti-infective therapy is to target the specific organisms associated with the disease.
- Conversely, after the identification of the organism causing the disease, anti-infective therapy should be narrowed to cover that specific organism.
- Therapy should reflect not only the best anti-infective agent for the organism, but also should reflect aspects of the patient's condition (eg, renal function and concurrent disease states).
- Combination anti-infective therapy should be reserved for documented clinical efficacy, therapeutic failure of monotherapy, and polymicrobial infection.
- Clinical signs of infection should be followed to determine patient response to therapy.
- Empiric therapy of meningitis is age-specific, reflecting the age-specific nature of the common pathogens.
- Endocarditis therapy is specific to the organism isolated. The presence of a prosthetic valve increases the time of therapy.
- Many cases of bronchitis are viral in etiology, making routine antibiotic therapy controversial.
- Empiric pneumonia therapy reflects both coverage of age-related organisms and organisms associated with patient-specific risk factors.
- Diarrhea therapy should be mainly supportive, with careful use of anti-infectives and antimotility agents.
- Diagnosis of urinary tract infections varies by numbers of organisms found in the urine. Higher numbers ($>10^5$ cells/mL) are needed to diagnose UTIs in females than are needed in males ($>10^3$ cells/mL), due to the higher numbers of organisms able to ascend the shorter female urethra.

Table 14

Treatment of Herpes Virus Infections

Organism	Disease	Treatment
Herpes simplex	Initial episode	Acyclovir
	Reoccurrence	Famciclovir
	Chronic suppression	Valacyclovir
	Immunocompromised	Acyclovir
	Resistant to acyclovir	Foscarnet
Cytomegalovirus	Retinitis, colitis, esophagitis	Ganciclovir, valganciclovir, foscarnet, cidofovir, fomivirsen
Varicella zoster	Chickenpox, shingles	Acyclovir
Varicella zoster	Immunocompromised, resistant to acyclovir	Foscarnet

- A frequently overlooked aspect of treatment of bacterial venereal disease is treatment of sexual partners.
- Initial therapy of sepsis should be broad in scope, covering all likely organisms, until results of cultures are obtained.
- Due to the long doubling time of most fungi, and the difficulty in obtaining sensitivity to specific antifungal agents, patient response is used to determine resistance to therapy.
- Antiviral therapy is not curative, but decreases the level of virus so that a patient's immune system can handle the infection.

4. Questions and Answers

1. The lowest concentration of anti-infective that prevents microbial growth is called the

   A. minimum bactericidal concentration
   B. minimum bacteriostatic concentration
   C. minimum inhibitory concentration
   D. minimum inhibiting concentration
   E. minimum Schillings concentration

2. Laboratory markers of infections, such as C-reactive protein, white blood cell count, and erythrocyte sedimentation rate may not be accurate in which patient populations?

   I. Elderly patients
   II. Patients with chronic obstructive pulmonary disease
   III. Malnourished patients

   A. I only
   B. II only
   C. I and III only
   D. II and III only
   E. I, II, and III

3. The hallmark of empiric therapy is

   A. coverage of the most common pathogen associated with the infection
   B. coverage of the common pathogens associated with the infection
   C. coverage of all possible pathogens associated with the infection
   D. coverage of polymicrobial pathogens associated with the infection
   E. coverage of all viral organisms associated with the infection

4. When two anti-infective therapies together produce a greater effect than the effects of each added together, this is termed

   A. commensalism
   B. synergy
   C. antagonism
   D. additive
   E. interacting

5. Analysis of the cerebrospinal fluid may give valuable clues to the identity of the pathogen in meningitis. Given the following results, what would be indicative of a fungal infection?

I.   Increase in WBCs
II. Decreased glucose
III Increased protein

    A. I only
    B. II only
    C. I and III only
    D. II and III only
    E. I, II, and III

6.   Empiric therapy for meningitis for patients up to 1 month of age includes

    A. vancomycin and ampicillin
    B. aminoglycoside and ampicillin
    C. ceftriaxone and vancomycin
    D. vancomycin and aminoglycoside
    E. ampicillin and ceftriaxone

7.   When treating penicillin-allergic patients for endocarditis, _____ may be used for therapy.

    A. vancomycin
    B. erythromycin
    C. cefazolin
    D. meropenem
    E. nafcillin

8.   Patients presenting with acute bronchitis without risk factors should be treated empirically with

    A. supportive care
    B. clarithromycin
    C. cefuroxime
    D. ciprofloxacin
    E. erythromycin

9.   The most common organism(s) associated with community-acquired pneumonia in adults are

    A. *Chlamydia pneumoniae, Mycoplasma pneumoniae, Haemophilus influenzae*
    B. *Streptococcus pneumoniae, Haemophilus influenzae, Chlamydia pneumoniae*
    C. *Mycoplasma pneumoniae, Chlamydia pneumoniae, Streptococcus pneumoniae*
    D. *Mycoplasma pneumoniae, Streptococcus pneumoniae, Haemophilus influenzae*
    E. *Chlamydia pneumoniae, Staphylococcus aureus, Haemophilus influenzae*

10. Empiric therapy for patients with hospital-acquired pneumonia should include

    A. tobramycin and gentamicin
    B. cefotaxime and cefepime
    C. vancomycin and gentamicin
    D. gentamicin and cefepime
    E. cefepime and vancomycin

11. Treatment of latent tuberculosis infections where isoniazid-resistant strains of *Mycobacterium tuberculosis* are predominant should include

    A. rifabutin and pyrazinamide
    B. rifampin and pyrazinamide
    C. isoniazid, rifampin, and pyrazinamide
    D. isoniazid, rifabutin, and pyrazinamide
    E. ethambutol and rifampin

12. The use of antimotility agents in infectious diarrhea is

    A. discouraged, due to the potential to cause toxic megacolon
    B. encouraged, due to increased cure rates
    C. discouraged, due to increased reinfections
    D. encouraged, due to decreased reinfections
    E. discouraged, due to lack of efficacy

13. Cellulitis is usually associated with

    A. *Staphylococcus aureus*
    B. *Streptococcus bovis*
    C. *Peptostreptococcus boydii*
    D. *Escherichia coli*
    E. *Klebsiella pneumoniae*

14. The best empiric regimen to treat prostate infection is

    A. ciprofloxacin for 10 days
    B. TMP-SMX for 10 days
    C. ciprofloxacin and TMP-SMX for 10 days
    D. ciprofloxacin for 4-6 weeks
    E. TMP-SMX for 4-6 weeks

15. Tertiary syphilis in adults should be treated with

    A. benzathine penicillin 2.4 million units x 1
    B. penicillin 50,000 U/kg q12h x 10-21 days
    C. penicillin 4 million units q4h x 10-14 days
    D. benzathine penicillin 2.4 million units q week x 3
    E. penicillin 150,000 U/kg q12h x 10-21 days

16. *Candida albicans* infections may be treated with

    A. itraconazole
    B. amphotericin B

C. voriconazole
D. caspofungin
E. ketoconazole

17. The antiviral agent with the widest spectrum of activity against influenza is

A. zanamivir
B. rimantadine
C. amantadine
D. oseltamivir
E. amantadine

18. Herpes infections resistant to acyclovir may be treated with

A. famciclovir
B. valacyclovir
C. foscarnet
D. ganciclovir
E. high-dose acyclovir

19. The only organism below that can be easily cultured is

A. *Treponema pallidum*
B. *Mycobacterium tuberculosis*
C. *Rickettsia rickettsii*
D. *Ehrlichia phagocytophila*
E. *Francisella tularensis*

20. Anti-infective therapy should always be used with infectious diarrhea caused by which organism?

A. *Escherichia coli*
B. *Vibrio cholerae*
C. *Staphylococcus aureus*
D. *Salmonella*
E. *Bacillus cereus*

21. J.B. is an 18-year-old white female who just gave birth to her first child. Since she presented without any prenatal care or history, a full prenatal panel of tests including a vaginal swab was taken. Two days after birth, she complained of a purulent vaginal discharge and low-grade fever. Blood cultures were negative, but the vaginal swab revealed the presence of gram-negative cocci. WBCs are elevated at 13,000 cells/mm^3. What is the probable infection that J.B. has?

A. Herpes simplex
B. Gonorrhea
C. Syphilis

D. Urinary tract infection
E. Food poisoning

22. What should be done for J.B. and her baby?

A. Both mother and child should be treated
B. Neither mother nor child should be treated
C. The child should be treated, but the mother should not
D. The mother should be treated, but the child should not
E. Mother, child, and partner should be treated

23. L.B. is a 45-year-old white female presenting to the emergency department with a fever of 103°F, flank pain, dysuria, urgency, and frequency. Her laboratory tests are significant for an increased WBC of 18,000 cells/mm^3 and 3% immature forms (bands). Her urinalysis revealed >105 cells/mL of gram-negative rods. What does L.B. have?

A. Herpes simplex
B. Gonorrhea
C. Syphilis
D. Urinary tract infection
E. Food poisoning

24. What therapy would be useful for L.B.?

A. Oral quinolone
B. IV quinolone
C. Oral penicillin
D. IV carbapenem
E. IV vancomycin

Answers

1. **C.** The minimum inhibitory concentration determines the level of anti-infective to which dosing regimens may be set.

2. **C.** Each of these groups of patients may not be able to respond with appropriate laboratory markers of infections, due to limited reserves or deletion of inflammatory factors.

3. **B.** Coverage of common pathogens associated with the infection increases the probability of curing the infection without increasing anti-infective exposure to other organisms, which increases the possibility of resistance.

4. **B.**

5. **E.** Although fungal CNS infections show relatively slight changes in WBCs, protein, and glucose compared to bacterial infections, the trend is similar.

6. **B.** This regimen covers the most likely organism(s) for meningitis in this age group: gram-negative enterics, such as *E coli,* group B streptococci, and *Listeria monocytogenes.*

7. **A.** Vancomycin covers all gram-positive organisms associated with endocarditis, with no cross-sensitivity to penicillin.

8. **A.** Since half of bronchitis infections are caused by a viral etiology, antibacterial therapy for low-risk patients should not be attempted, with the exception of severe presentation.

9. **D.** *Chlamydia pneumoniae* is not a pathogen associated with adult pneumonia.

10. **D.** Empiric therapy for hospital-acquired pneumonia should have an aminoglycoside and one other gram-negative agent, such as cefepime. Vancomycin can be added if MRSA is suspected.

11. **B.** Latent infections are usually treated with isoniazid alone. In the case of isoniazid-resistant TB, rifampin and pyrazinamide are effective at treating latent infections. The three-drug regimens are used to treat active disease.

12. **A.** Use of such agents increases the chance of intestinal perforation and increases the length of symptoms.

13. **A.** Most cellulitis infections are associated with *Staphylococcus aureus* and *Streptococcus pyogenes.*

14. **D.** Prostate infections are difficult to treat, requiring 4-6 weeks of therapy. Although TMP-SMX is a reasonable choice to treat most prostate infections, ciprofloxacin is preferred due to its ability to concentrate in prostatic fluid.

15. **C.** Due to the organism load of tertiary syphilis, high doses of penicillin G are needed for clinical cure. B and E are congenital syphilis doses for neonates.

16. **B.** Voriconazole and caspofungin have activity against *Candida,* but have not yet been tested in a variety of settings. Ketoconazole and itraconazole should not be used for serious *Candida* infections. Amphotericin B and fluconazole are currently recommended for *Candida.*

17. **D.** Oseltamivir may be used for either treatment or prophylaxis against both influenza A and B.

18. **C.** Foscarnet has activity against acyclovir-resistant herpes.

19. **B.** *Mycobacterium tuberculosis,* although very slow growing, can be grown on culture media. The remaining organisms cannot be grown without use of cell culture techniques, forcing the clinician to rely on serum testing and direct staining for identification of the organism.

20. **B.** *Staphylococcus* and *Bacillus* diarrhea is an intoxication, not caused by a living organism. Both *Salmonella* and *E coli* diarrheas should not be treated unless severe, or signs of systemic infection are present. *Vibrio cholerae* causes a severe diarrhea requiring anti-infective treatment.

21. **B.** Given the lack of prenatal care, physical signs and symptoms, and presence of gram-negative cocci, J.B. most likely has gonorrhea.

22. **E.** Mother, partner, and child should be treated. J.B. and her partner should receive ceftriaxone 125 mg IM x 1 and treatment for concurrent chlamydial infection (doxycycline 100 mg bid x 7 days). The child should receive cefotaxime 25 mg/kg q12h x 7 days. Both mother and child should be screened for additional sexually transmitted diseases.

23. **D.** Given the clinical presentation and laboratory test results, L.B. has a severe urinary tract infection. The presence of systemic symptoms (fever and chills) suggests an upper urinary tract infection or pyelonephritis.

24. **B.** Given the severity of disease, parenteral therapy would be reasonable for initial therapy. Since the Gram stain of the urine revealed gram-negative rods, either a quinolone or extended-spectrum penicillin in combination with an aminoglycoside would be reasonable empiric therapy until the organism was identified and sensitivities obtained.

5. References

Many general references will provide basic information concerning anti-infective therapy. A good brief yearly review of antibacterial and antiviral therapies is published by *The Medical Letter* (www.medletter.com). Listed here are recent practice guidelines in areas of infectious disease.

Endocarditis
Wilson WR, Karchmer AW, Dajani AS, et al. Antibiotic treatment of adults with infective endocarditis due to streptococci, enterococci, and staphylococci, and HACEK microorganisms. *JAMA*. 1995;274:1706-1713.

Pneumonia
Bartlett JG, Dowell SF, Mandell LA, et al. Practice guidelines for the management of community-acquired pneumonia in adults. Infectious Diseases Society of America. *Clin Infect Dis*. 2000;31:347-382.

Guidelines for the management of adults with hospital-acquired, ventilator-associated, and healthcare-associated pneumonia. American Thoracic Society and the Infectious Diseases Society of America. *Am J Respir Crit Care Med*. 2004;171:388-416.

Tuberculosis
Horsburgh CR, Feldman S, Ridzon R. Practice guidelines for the treatment of tuberculosis. *Clin Infect Dis*. 2000;31:633-639.

Infectious diarrhea
Diagnosis and management of food borne illnesses: a primer for physicians. *MMWR Recomm Rep*. 2001;50(RR-2):1-69.

Guerrant RL, Van Gilder T, Steiner TS, et al. Practice guidelines for the management of infectious diarrhea. *Clin Infect Dis*. 2001;32:331-351.

Soft tissue infections
Lipsky BA, Berendt BA, Deery HG, et al. Diagnosis and treatment of diabetic foot infections. *Clin Infect Dis*. 2004;39:885-910.

Urinary tract infections
Warren JW, Abrutyn E, Hebel JR, et al. Guidelines for antimicrobial treatment of uncomplicated acute bacterial cystitis and acute pyelonephritis in women. Infectious Diseases Society of America (IDSA). *Clin Infect Dis*. 1999;29:745-758.

Sexually transmitted diseases
Centers for Disease Control and Prevention. Diseases characterized by genital ulcers. Sexually transmitted diseases treatment guidelines. *MMWR Recomm Rep*. 2002;51(RR-6):11-25.

Centers for Disease Control and Prevention. Diseases characterized by urethritis and cervicitis. Sexually transmitted diseases treatment guidelines. *MMWR Recomm Rep*. 2002;51(RR-6):30-42.

Centers for Disease Control and Prevention. Vaccine preventable STDs. Sexually transmitted diseases treatment guidelines. *MMWR Recomm Rep*. 2002;51(RR-6):59-64.

Sepsis
American College of Chest Physicians/Society of Critical Care Medicine Consensus Conference. Definitions for sepsis and organ failure and guideline for the use of innovative therapies in sepsis. *Crit Care Med*. 1992;20:864-874.

Practice guidelines for evaluating new fever in critically ill adult patients. *Crit Care Med*. 1998;26:392-408.

Tick-borne disease
Wormser GP, Nadelman RB, Dattwyler RJ, et al. Practice guidelines for the treatment of Lyme disease. *Clin Infect Dis*. 2000;31(Suppl 1):1-14.

Fungal infections
Chapman SW, Bradsher RW, Campbell GD, Pappas PG, Kauffman CA. Practice guidelines for the management of patients with blastomycosis. Infectious Diseases Society of America. *Clin Infect Dis*. 2000;30:679-683.

Pappas PG, Rex JH, Sobel JD, et al. Guidelines for the treatment of candidiasis. *Clin Infect Dis*. 2004;38:161-89.

Saag MS, Graybill RJ, Larsen RA, et al. Practice guidelines for the management of cryptococcal disease. Infectious Diseases Society of America. *Clin Infect Dis*. 2000;30:710-718.

Stevens DA, Kan VL, Judson MA, et al. Practice guidelines for diseases caused by *Aspergillus*. Infectious Diseases Society of America. *Clin Infect Dis*. 2000;30:696-709.

Viral infections

Association for Genitourinary Medicine (AGUM), Medical Society for the Study of Venereal Disease (MSSVD). 2002 National guideline for the management of genital herpes. London: AGUM, MSSVD; 2002.

Association for Genitourinary Medicine (AGUM), Medical Society for the Study of Venereal Disease (MSSVD). 2002 National guideline on the management of the viral hepatitides A, B, and C. London: AGUM, MSSVD; 2002.

Bridges CB, Fukuda K, Uyeki TM, Cox NJ, Singleton JA. Prevention and control of influenza. Recommendations of the Advisory Committee on Immunization Practices (ACIP). *MMWR Recomm Rep.* 2002;51(RR-03):1-31.

30. Anti-Infective Agents

Ronald L. Braden, PharmD
Associate Professor, Department of Clinical Pharmacy
University of Tennessee College of Pharmacy

Contents

1. Aminoglycosides

Aminoglycosides are antibiotics active against most aerobic gram-negative bacteria and select aerobic gram-positive bacteria, but they are not effective against most anaerobic bacteria. Aminoglycosides are primarily used in serious infections due to their significant toxicity. The most commonly used aminoglycosides include amikacin, kanamycin, gentamicin, neomycin, netilmicin, streptomycin, and tobramycin.

Mechanism of Action

• Aminoglycosides inhibit bacterial protein synthesis through binding to the 30S ribosomal subunit, thereby irreversibly inhibiting bacterial RNA synthesis. Aminoglycosides are bactericidal.

Spectrum of Activity

• Amikacin is a semisynthetic parenteral aminoglycoside with the broadest antimicrobial activity of the class, and it frequently possesses activity against bacteria resistant to other aminoglycosides.
• Kanamycin is a minimally absorbed oral aminoglycoside used to decrease bacterial content of the bowel. Kanamycin has been used for preoperative bowel preparation and as an adjunct in hepatic encephalopathy.
• Gentamicin is a parenteral aminoglycoside that is more active against *Acinetobacter, Serratia,* and enterococci than tobramycin.
• Neomycin: see kanamycin.
• Netilmicin is a parenteral aminoglycoside that may be the least ototoxic aminoglycoside.
• Streptomycin is a parenteral aminoglycoside active against enterococci, streptococci, mycobacteria, and some gram-negative anaerobes. Streptomycin is used as an adjunct agent only because many bacterial isolates are resistant to streptomycin monotherapy. Streptomycin should only be administered by IM injection.
• Tobramycin is a parenteral aminoglycoside that is more active against *Pseudomonas* than gentamicin.

Adverse Drug Events

• Nephrotoxicity is demonstrated by an increase in blood urea nitrogen (BUN) and serum creatinine. The nephrotoxicity is usually manifest as non-oliguric renal failure and may cause potassium, calcium, and magnesium wasting. Nephrotoxicity may occur in 10-25% of patients receiving aminoglycosides and is usually reversible upon discontinuation of the agent. Risk factors include:

  * Pre-existing renal dysfunction
  * Prolonged duration of therapy
  * Concomitant use of other nephrotoxic agents
  * Possibly elevated trough concentrations:
    • Gentamicin and tobramycin >2 mcg/mL
    • Amikacin >8 mcg/mL
• Neuromuscular blockade is an uncommon but potentially serious toxicity. Risk factors include:
  * Concomitant use of neuromuscular blocking agents
  * Myasthenia gravis
  * Hypocalcemia
  * Elevated peak serum concentrations
• Ototoxicity is due to eighth cranial nerve damage demonstrated by auditory and vestibular symptoms. Auditory symptoms include tinnitus and loss of high-frequency hearing. Vestibular toxicity is demonstrated by dizziness, nystagmus, vertigo, and ataxia. The incidence of ototoxicity is not clearly known since profound high-frequency hearing loss can occur prior to detection.

Pharmacokinetics
• Aminoglycosides are renally eliminated.
  * $t_{1/2}$ = 2.5-2.7 hours (normal renal function)
  * $t_{1/2}$ = ~69 hours (anephric clearance)
  * Vd = 0.27-0.3 L/kg (IBW)

Target serum concentrations (traditional dosing; Table 1)
  * Amikacin peak = 15-30 mcg/mL
  * Amikacin trough = <5 mcg/mL
  * Gentamicin and tobramycin peak = 4-10 mcg/mL
  * Gentamicin and tobramycin trough = <2 mcg/mL

Extended interval dosing
  * Amikacin trough = <3 mcg/mL
  * Gentamicin and tobramycin = <1 mcg/mL

Table 1

Aminoglycosides

Generic name	Trade name	Dosage forms	Normal dose	Elimination
Amikacin	Amikin®	IV, IM	15 mg/kg per day	Renal
Gentamicin	Garamycin®	IV, IM	3 mg/kg per day conventional dose, 7 mg/kg per day extended interval	Renal
Kanamycin		IV, PO	15 mg/kg per day	Renal
Neomycin		PO	50-100 mg/kg per day	Renal
Netilmicin		IV, IM	3-6 mg/kg per day	Renal
Streptomycin		IM	15 mg/kg per day	Renal
Tobramycin		IV, IM	3 mg/kg per day conventional dose, 7 mg/kg per day extended interval	Renal

Note: Use ideal body weight for all aminoglycoside dosing.

2. Penicillins

Mechanism of Action

- Penicillin binding proteins (PBPs) make up the cell wall. When penicillin binds to these PBPs, it is able to inhibit cell wall synthesis in the bacteria, causing cell wall lysis and ultimately cell death.
- Bactericidal (they inhibit bacterial cell wall synthesis).
- They are known as β-lactam antibiotics because their chemical structure consists of a β-lactam ring adjoined to a thiazolidine ring.
- Penicillinase-resistant penicillins: substitutions to the β-lactam ring sterically inhibit penicillinase.

Spectrum of Activity and Dosing

- See Tables 2 and 3.

Adverse Drug Events

- Allergic/hypersensitivity reaction occurs in 3-10% of patients. Rash (4-8%) to anaphylaxis (0.01-0.05%) can occur within 10-20 minutes; IV > PO.
- GI: nausea and vomiting with PO use

- Neurologic reactions (seizures) are seen with high doses of penicillin given to patients with renal insufficiency.
- Hypokalemia, hypernatremia (carboxypenicillins; carbenicillin > ticarcillin)
- Increased transaminases: oxacillin, nafcillin, carbenicillin
- Cholestatic jaundice: ureidopenicillins
- Hematologic reactions (hemolytic anemia)
- Interstitial nephritis

Drug-Drug Interactions

- Probenecid increases blood levels of natural penicillins and may be given with them for this purpose.
- Aminoglycosides: either incompatible or synergistic
- Oral contraceptives: concomitant use may decrease the effectiveness of oral contraceptives and increase incidence of breakthrough bleeding.

Other Characteristics

- Nafcillin and oxacillin: primarily biliary excretion, therefore do not have to adjust for renal dysfunction
- Penicillin G benzathine: repository drug formulation; given IM, insoluble salt allows slow drug absorption from the injection site, and therefore it has a longer duration of action (12-24 h).

Table 2

Spectrum of Activity of the Penicillins

Category	Spectrum
Natural penicillins	Effective against all viridans streptococci, *S pyogenes*, and 60% of *S pneumoniae*, mouth anaerobes, and *Clostridium perfringens* (gas gangrene) Because natural penicillins are readily hydrolyzed by penicillinases (β-lactamases), they are ineffective against *S aureus* and other organisms that resist penicillin Penicillin G is 5-10 times more active than penicillin V against gram-negative organisms and some anaerobic organisms
Penicillinase-resistant penicillins	Methicillin-sensitive staphylococci, streptococci (not enterococci species)
Aminopenicillins	Greater penetration of outer membrane of gram-negative rods and higher affinity for PBPs Cover most enterococci, *Listeria, Proteus mirabilis* Cover 60% of *Streptococcus pneumoniae, Haemophilus influenzae, Escherichia coli*, some *Salmonella* and *Shigella*
Carboxypenicillins and ureidopenicillins	Spectrum like ampicillin, but less gram-positive coverage; covers *Proteus* (including *P vulgaris*), *Klebsiella* (not ticarcillin), *Enterobacter, Pseudomonas* (piperacillin > ticarcillin); add an aminoglycoside for synergy for serious gram-negative infections Ureidopenicillins possess better in vitro activity against *Pseudomonas* and other gram-negative organisms Ureidopenicillins have in vitro activity against streptococci, enterococci, most Enterobacteriaceae, *Pseudomonas*, and many anaerobes, including *Bacteroides fragilis, Fusobacterium, Clostridium,* and peptostreptococci; β-lactamase–producing staphylococci and *H influenzae* are resistant to the ureidopenicillins
β-Lactamase inhibitors (clavulanic acid, sulbactam, and tazobactam)	Active against some chromosomally produced β-lactamases of *S aureus, H influenzae, Moraxella catarrhalis, Bacteroides, E coli*, and other Enterobacteriaceae Not active against the chromosomally produced β-lactamases of *Enterobacter, Citrobacter, Serratia,* and *Pseudomonas*
Amoxicillin-clavulanic acid	*H influenzae, M catarrhalis, Klebsiella pneumoniae*, methicillin-sensitive *S aureus* (MSSA), anaerobes
Ticarcillin-clavulanic acid	More activity against *H influenzae, M catarrhalis, Klebsiella pneumoniae*, MSSA, anaerobes
Piperacillin-tazobactam	More gram-positive, gram-negative, and anaerobic coverage than ticarcillin-clavulanic acid; monotherapy treatment failures against *Pseudomonas*

3. Cephalosporins

Cephalosporins are β-lactam antibiotics that are structurally and pharmacologically similar to penicillins.

Mechanism of Action

- Cephalosporins are bactericidal agents. Antimicrobial activity is achieved via inhibition of mucopeptide synthesis in the bacterial cell wall, which results in the formation of defective cell walls and subsequent cell lysis and cell death.

Spectrum of Activity

- Cephalosporins are broad-spectrum antimicrobial agents; however, the spectrum of activity varies greatly among the individual agents. Thus, cephalosporins are grouped into four broad classes, or generations, according to their antimicrobial coverage (Table 4).

Table 3

Dosing of Penicillins

Type and generic name	Trade name	Elimination route	Administration route	Common doses
Natural penicillins				
Penicillin G	Pfizerpen®	Renal	IV, IM, PO	2-4 million units IV q4h
Penicillin G procaine	Wycillin®	Renal	IM	300,000-600,000 U/d
Penicillin G benzathine	Bicillin LA®	Renal	IM	Strep throat: 1.2 million units; syphilis: 2.4 million units
Penicillin V (phenoxymethyl penicillin)	Pen-Vee K®; Veetids®	Renal	PO	250-500 mg PO bid-qid (250 mg bid for prophylaxis)
Penicillinase-resistant penicillins				
Methicillin[1]	Staphcillin®	Renal	IV, IM	1-2 g IV q4-6h
Oxacillin	Prostaphilin®, Bactocill®[1]	Hepatic	PO, IV, IM	1-2 g IV q4-6h
Nafcillin	Nafcil®, Unipen®	Hepatic	IV, IM	1-2 g IV q4-6h
Cloxacillin	Cloxapen®	Renal	PO	200-500 mg q6h
Dicloxacillin	Dynapen®, Dycill®	Renal	PO	250-500 mg PO q6h
Aminopenicillins				
Ampicillin	Omnipen®, Principen®	Renal	PO, IM, IV	1-2 g IV q6h
Amoxicillin	Amoxil®, Trimox®	Renal	PO	250-500 mg PO q8h
Bacampicillin	Spectrobid®	Renal	PO	400-800 mg q12h
Carboxypenicillins				
Carbenicillin	Geopen®	Renal	IM, IV	1-5 g q4-6h
Ticarcillin	Ticar®	Renal	IV, IM	3-4 g IV q4-6h
Ureidopenicillins				
Azlocillin	Azlin®	Renal	IV, IM	2-4 g IV q4-6h
Mezlocillin	Mezlin®	Renal	IV, IM	1-3 g q4-6h
Piperacillin	Pipracil®	Renal	IV, IM	3-4 g IV q4-6h
Penicillin plus β-lactamase inhibitors				
Amoxicillin-clavulanic acid	Augmentin®	Renal	PO	250-500 mg PO tid, 500-875 mg PO bid
Ampicillin-sulbactam	Unasyn®	Renal	IV, IM	1.5 or 3 g IV q6-8h
Piperacillin-tazobactam	Zosyn®	Renal	IV	3.375 g IV q6h
Ticarcillin-clavulanic acid	Timentin®	Renal	IV	3.1 g IV q4-6h

[1]Discontinued in the United States.

First-generation agents (cefadroxil, cefazolin, cephalexin)

- Gram-positive activity is extensive, including many strains of *Staphylococcus aureus* and *S epidermidis* in addition to *Streptococcus pyogenes* (group A beta-hemolytic streptococci), *S agalactiae* (group B strep-tococci), and *S pneumoniae*. First-generation agents are inactive against enterococci, methicillin-resistant staphylococci (MRSA/MRSE), and *Listeria monocytogenes*.

Table 4

Cephalosporins

Generic name	Trade name	Dosage forms	Dose	Elimination	Notes
First-generation (more gram-positive than gram-negative activity)					
Cefadroxil	Duricef®, Ultracef®	PO	1-2 g/d	Renal	
Cefazolin	Ancef®, Kefzol	IV	250-1000 mg q8h	Renal	
Cephalexin	Keflex®	PO	250-500 mg q6h	Renal	
Cephapirin	Cefadyl®	IV, IM	500-2000 mg q4-6h	Renal	
Cephradine	Anspor®, Velosef®	PO, IV	250-500 mg q6h	Renal	
Second-generation (enhanced gram-negative activity vs. first-generation drugs)					
Cefaclor	Ceclor®	PO	250-500 mg q8h	Renal	
Cefmetazole	Zefazone®	IV	2 g q6-12h	Renal	NMTT side-chain
Cefonicid	Monocid®	IV	1-2 g/d	Renal	
Cefotetan	Cefotan®	IV, IM	1-2 g q12h	Renal	Anaerobic activity, NMTT side-chain
Cefoxitin	Mefoxin®	IV	1-2 g q6-8h	Renal	Anaerobic activity
Cefprozil	Cefzil®	PO	250-500 mg q12-24h	Renal	Anaerobic activity
Cefuroxime	Ceftin®, Zinacef®	IV, IM	750-1500 mg q8h	Renal	
Cefamandole	Mandole®	IV	500-1000 mg q4-8h	Renal	NMTT side-chain
Loracarbef	Lorabid®	PO	200 mg q12h	Renal	Anaerobic activity
Third-generation (more gram-negative than gram-positive activity; CSF penetration)					
Cefixime	Suprax®	PO	400 mg/d	Renal	
Cefdinir	Omnicef®	PO	300 mg q12h	Renal	
Cefoperazone	Cefobid®	IV	2-4 g q12h	Hepatic	NMTT side-chain
Cefotaxime	Claforan®	IV	1-2 g q6-8h	Renal	
Cefpodoxime	Vantin®	PO	100-400 mg q12h	Renal	Anaerobic activity
Ceftazidime	Fortaz®, Tazicef®	IV, IM	1-2 g q8-12h	Renal	Antipseudomonal activity
Ceftibuten	Cedax®	PO	400 mg/d	Renal	
Ceftizoxime	Cefizox®	IV	1-2 g q8-12h	Renal	
Ceftriaxone	Rocephin®	IV, IM	1-2 g/d	Renal	
Fourth-generation (gram-positive and gram-negative activity)					
Cefepime	Maxipime®	IV, IM	1-2 g q12h	Renal	Antipseudomonal activity

[1]Discontinued in the United States.

- Gram-negative activity is limited, although some strains of *Escherichia coli, Klebsiella pneumoniae, Proteus mirabilis,* and *Shigella* may display susceptibility. First-generation agents are inactive against *Haemophilus influenzae, Pseudomonas, Entero-* *bacter, Citrobacter, Serratia,* other *Proteus* spp, and anaerobes such as *Bacteroides fragilis.*

Second-generation agents (cefaclor, cefamandole, cefotetan, cefoxitin, cefprozil, cefuroxime, cefmetazole, loracarbef)

- Gram-positive activity is similar to that of first-generation agents.
- Gram-negative activity of second-generation agents is generally more extensive than that of first-generation agents, including some strains of *Acinetobacter, Citrobacter, Enterobacter, Neisseria, Proteus,* and *Serratia,* in addition to *E coli* and *Klebsiella.* Second-generation agents are active against *Haemophilus influenzae,* and some (cefotetan, cefoxitin, cefamandole) also have anaerobic activity. Second-generation agents are inactive against *Pseudomonas.*

Third-generation agents (cefixime, cefoperazone, cefotaxime, ceftizoxime, ceftriaxone)

- Gram-positive activity is decreased versus first- and second-generation agents.
- Gram-negative activity is extensive, including *Enterobacter, Citrobacter, Serratia, Neisseria,* and *Haemophilus.* Some third-generation agents are active against *Pseudomonas* (ceftazidime, cefoperazone). Anaerobic coverage varies among individual agents.

Fourth-generation (cefepime)

- Gram-positive activity is increased versus third-generation agents. Cefepime is inactive against MRSA, enterococci, and *Listeria.*
- Gram-negative activity is extensive, including enhanced activity against *Pseudomonas* and Enterobacteriaceae that produce inducible β-lactamases.
- The extended spectrum of activity of cefepime is attributed to a more rapid penetration of the outer membrane of gram-negative bacteria. Cefepime is also more resistant to inactivation by β-lactamases.

Adverse Drug Events

- Hypersensitivity: fever, rash, pruritus, urticaria, anaphylaxis, hemolytic anemia
- Gastrointestinal effects: nausea, vomiting, diarrhea
- Nephrotoxicity (rare)
- Seizures: potential risk with high doses in patients with renal impairment
- *Clostridium difficile* colitis
- Bleeding/hypoprothrombinemia (cefoperazone, cefmetazole, cefotetan): this is due to the presence of an N-methylthiotetrazole (NMTT) side chain in the structure of these agents and can be prevented or reversed with administration of vitamin K.
- Blood dyscrasias (rare)

Drug-Drug Interactions

- Disulfiram-like reactions have been reported with ingestion of alcohol during treatment with cephalosporin antibiotics.
- Probenecid competitively inhibits tubular secretion of cephalosporins, resulting in higher serum concentrations.

Drug-Disease Interactions

- All cephalosporins (except cefoperazone) require dosage adjustments in patients with renal insufficiency.

Monitoring Parameters

- Serum concentration monitoring is not necessary.
- Patients should be monitored for clinical response and resolution of infection.

Patient Instructions and Counseling

- Verify that the patient is not allergic to penicillins. Cross-sensitivity with penicillins has been reported in up to 10% of patients receiving cephalosporins. A thorough history should be obtained in any patient with a previous hypersensitivity reaction to any β-lactam antibiotic. In general, cephalosporins should be avoided in these patients.

Other

- Bacterial resistance to cephalosporins may result via production of β-lactamases.

4. Gram-Positive Antibiotics

Linezolid

- Linezolid is a synthetic oxazolidine antibiotic (Table 5).

Mechanism of action
- Linezolid binds to the 23S ribosomal subunit of the 50S RNA subunit which inhibits bacterial translation.

Spectrum of activity
- Linezolid is bacteriostatic against enterococci and staphylococci and bactericidal against streptococci. Linezolid is active against *Enterococcus faecium* isolates, including VRE, while most *E faecalis* isolates are resistant.

Adverse drug effects
- Hematologic effects including myelosuppression (anemia, leukopenia, pancytopenia, and thrombocytopenia) have been reported. Hematologic effects appear to be reversible upon discontinuation of the agent.
- Monoamine oxidase inhibition: linezolid is a weak MAO inhibitor, but caution should be exercised in patients receiving vasopressors.

Quinupristin-Dalfopristin

- Quinupristin-dalfopristin is a semisynthetic streptogramin antibiotic. The combination acts synergistically against gram-positive bacteria.

Mechanism of action
- Quinupristin inhibits late phase protein synthesis, while dalfopristin inhibits early phase protein synthesis through binding to the 50S subunit of bacterial RNA.

Spectrum of activity
- Quinupristin-dalfopristin is bactericidal against staphylococci and streptococci and bacteriostatic against *Enterococcus faecium,* including VRE. Quinupristin-dalfopristin is not active against *E faecalis.*

Adverse drug effects
- Thrombophlebitis and severe injection site reactions are common, and some sources recommend administration via a central venous catheter only.
- Hyperbilirubinemia has been reported in up to 25% of patients receiving the agent.
- Arthralgias and myalgias are common, some requiring discontinuation of the agent.

Vancomycin

- Vancomycin is a glycopeptide antibiotic.

Mechanism of action
- Vancomycin binds to the bacterial cell wall, inhibiting peptidoglycan synthesis. This binding occurs at a site different from that of the penicillins. Vancomycin may also inhibit RNA synthesis.

Spectrum of activity
- Vancomycin is active against most gram-positive bacteria including staphylococci (including MRSA), streptococci, enterococci, *Corynebacterium,* and *Clostridium* (including *C difficile*). Vancomycin is bactericidal against all susceptible isolates except enterococci (bacteriostatic). Vancomycin acts synergistically with aminoglycosides against enterococci.

Adverse drug effects
- Nephrotoxicity is manifested by an increase in serum creatinine and BUN. The incidence of nephrotoxicity is not well described, but appears to be low in the absence of concomitant nephrotoxic agents. Renal dysfunction is normally reversible upon discontinuation of the agent, but may be irreversible.

Table 5

Gram-Positive Antibiotics

Generic name	Trade name	Dosage forms	Dose	Elimination	Notes
Linezolid	Zyvox®	IV, PO	600 mg q12h	Renal	
Quinupristin-dalfopristin	Synercid®	IV	7.5 mg/kg q8h	Hepatic	
Vancomycin	Vancocin®	IV, PO	500 mg q6h or 1 g q12h IV; 125-250 mg PO q6h	Renal	Adjust dose per serum concentrations

- Ototoxicity is induced by eighth cranial nerve damage and has been reported to cause permanent hearing loss. Vancomycin rarely causes vestibular toxicity. The incidence of ototoxicity appears to be low in the absence of concomitant ototoxic agents.
- Thrombophlebitis is common and requires frequent IV site rotation.
- Histamine release or "red-man syndrome" is a reaction most commonly associated with rapid IV infusion. Histamine reactions can be minimized by slow IV infusion, not to exceed 500 mg/30 min.

Monitoring
- Vancomycin trough concentrations should be monitored in patients with pre-existing renal dysfunction or patients with increased serum creatinine or BUN during therapy. Vancomycin peak concentrations are not routinely required, but may be monitored in patients with serious infections, central nervous system infections, or those patients not responding to therapy.

Pharmacokinetics
- Vancomycin is renally eliminated.
  * $t_{1/2}$ = 6 hours (normal renal function)
  * $t_{1/2}$ = 7-10 days (anephric patients)
  * Vd = 0.7 L/kg (TBW)
  * Peak concentration = 20-40 mcg/mL
  * Trough concentration = 5-10 mcg/mL

5. Fluoroquinolones

- Quinolones are broad-spectrum antibacterial agents (Table 6).

Mechanism of Action

- Fluoroquinolones are bactericidal agents. The mechanism of action of these agents is not understood entirely, but antimicrobial activity is known to involve inhibition of bacterial DNA topoisomerase and subsequent disruption of bacterial DNA replication.

Spectrum of Activity

- Gram-positive activity includes many strains of staphylococci. Streptococcal activity is variable, and streptococcal resistance to quinolones is increasingly common. Newer fluoroquinolones (sparfloxacin, gatifloxacin, clinafloxacin, moxifloxacin) generally demonstrate superior gram-positive coverage versus older agents (ciprofloxacin, ofloxacin, levofloxacin). Fluoroquinolones have limited enterococcal activity and are inactive against MRSA.
- Gram-negative activity is extensive, including *Escherichia coli, Klebsiella, Enterobacter, Citrobacter, Proteus, Salmonella,* and *Shigella,* in addition to *Moraxella catarrhalis* and *Haemophilus influenzae.* Activity against *Pseudomonas aeruginosa* and *Stenotrophomonas maltophilia* varies among individual agents.
- Anaerobic coverage is poor.
- Atypical coverage varies among individual agents. All fluoroquinolones are highly active against *Legionella.* Newer agents have more reliable coverage of *Mycoplasma pneumoniae* and *Chlamydia pneumoniae.*

Adverse Drug Events

- GI: nausea, dyspepsia
- CNS: headache, dizziness, insomnia
- CV: QT prolongation (avoid use in patients with pre-existing QT prolongation)
- Endocrine: hypoglycemia or hyperglycemia
- GU: crystalluria (at high doses with alkaline pH)
- Other: arthropathy, tendinitis, photosensitivity
- Rare: rash, urticaria, leukopenia, hepatotoxicity (trovafloxacin)

Table 6

Fluoroquinolones and Nonfluorinated Quinolones

Generic name	Trade name	Dosage forms	Normal dose	Elimination	Notes
Fluoroquinolones					
Ciprofloxacin	Cipro®	IV	400 mg q12h	Renal	Less gram-positive activity, enhanced
		PO	500 mg q12h		antipseudomonal activity versus
					other fluoroquinolones
Enoxacin	Penetrex®	PO	200-400 mg q12h	Renal	
Gatifloxacin	Tequin®	IV, PO	400 mg q24h	Renal	
Levofloxacin	Levaquin®	IV, PO	500 mg q24h	Renal	
Lomefloxacin	Maxaquin®	PO	400 mg qd	Renal	
Moxifloxacin	Avelox®	PO	400 mg qd	Hepatic	
Norfloxacin	Noroxin®	PO	400 mg bid	Hepatic	
Ofloxacin	Floxin®	PO, IV	100-400 mg/d	Renal	
Sparfloxacin	Zagam®	PO	200 mg q24h	Renal	Enhanced anaerobic activity
Trovafloxacin	Trovan®	IV alatrofloxacin	300 mg q24h	Hepatic/fecal	Gram-negative, gram-positive,
		PO	200 mg q24h		atypicals, anaerobes; rarely used
					due to hepatotoxicity
Nonfluorinated quinolones					No gram-positive activity; effective only in GU and GI tracts
Cinoxacin	Cinoxacin®/Cinobac®	PO	500 mg bid	Renal	
Nalidixic acid	NegGram®	PO	1 g q6h	Renal	

Drug-Drug Interactions

- Ciprofloxacin increases theophylline levels. Concomitant use should be avoided, or theophylline levels should be monitored during treatment. The risk of theophylline toxicity is less with other fluoroquinolones.
- Antacids, sucralfate, and divalent or trivalent cations (Ca, Mg, Fe) significantly decrease the absorption of fluoroquinolones. These agents should not be administered for at least 2 hours after each dose of a fluoroquinolone.
- Fluoroquinolones may enhance the effects of oral anticoagulants. PT and INR should be monitored if concomitant therapy cannot be avoided.
- Agents that increase the QT interval (cisapride, class IA or III antiarrhythmics) increase the risk of torsades de pointes. Concomitant use of fluoroquinolones with these agents should be avoided.

Drug-Disease Interactions

- Dosage adjustments should be made for renally-cleared fluoroquinolones when CrCl is <40 mL/min.

Monitoring Parameters

- Serum concentrations are not monitored.
- The patient should be monitored for clinical response/resolution of infection.

Kinetics

- Quinolones display concentration-dependent activity and have a post-antibiotic effect against most susceptible organisms.
- Fluoroquinolones have a large volume of distribution and achieve high tissue concentrations in the lung, gallbladder, kidney, prostate, and genital tract.

Patient Instructions and Counseling

- Fluoroquinolones should be avoided in children or pregnant or nursing women due to the risk of cartilage erosion in growing bone tissue.
- Do *NOT* take antacids, multivitamins, or other calcium, magnesium, or iron supplements for at least 2 hours after each dose.

6. Macrolides

Mechanism of Action

- Macrolides are bacteriostatic against susceptible organisms (Table 7). The agents bind to the 50S RNA subunit, thereby inhibiting RNA synthesis.
- Ketolides are similar to the macrolides. Telithromycin is a derivative of 14-membered ring macrolides and is the first ketolide antibiotic.

Spectrum of Activity

- Macrolides, or erythromycins, are active principally against gram-positive organisms including penicillin-resistant streptococci. The macrolides are also effective against *Chlamydia, Mycoplasma, Ureaplasma,* spirochetes, and mycobacteria.
- Telithromycin possesses greater in vitro activity against multidrug-resistant gram-positive organisms and *Haemophilus influenzae* compared to the erythromycins.

Adverse Drug Events

- Gastrointestinal effects: erythromycins stimulate GI motility, leading to abdominal pain and cramping, nausea, vomiting, and diarrhea. Clarithromycin appears to be the least stimulating to the GI tract.
- Local effects: erythromycin lactobionate is reported to cause venous irritation and thrombophlebitis. The agent should be diluted in at least 250 mL and infused over 30-60 minutes to decrease the venous irritation.

- Cardiac effects: QT interval prolongation and torsades de pointes have been rarely reported with erythromycins. Adequate dilution and slow IV infusion appear to decrease this reaction.
- Ototoxicity: erythromycin has been rarely reported to be ototoxic in doses of 4 g/d or more.
- Telithromycin appears comparable to the macrolides.

Table 7

Macrolides and Ketolide

Generic name	Trade name	Dosage forms	Normal dose	Elimination	Notes
Macrolides					
Azithromycin	Zithromax®	PO, IV	250 mg/d	Hepatic	PO dose = IV dose
Clarithromycin	Biaxin®, Biaxin XL®	PO	250 mg bid	Renal	XL = qd dosing
Erythromycin	Various	PO	250-500 mg q6h	Hepatic	Erythromycin base, ethyl succinate, and stearate
		IV	500-1000 mg q6h	Hepatic	Erythromycin lactobionate
Ketolide					
Telithromycin	Ketek®	PO	800 mg/d	Hepatic	Treatment duration: 5 days for bronchitis, 7-10 days for community-acquired pneumonia

7. Tetracyclines

Mechanism of Action

- Bacteriostatic: they inhibit bacterial protein synthesis by reversible binding on the 30S ribosomal subunit and blocking the attachment of transfer RNA to an acceptor site on the messenger RNA ribosomal complex (Table 8).

Spectrum of Activity

- Tetracyclines are the drugs of choice for infections caused by the following organisms:
    * Respiratory infections: atypical pneumonia (*Mycoplasma pneumoniae, Chlamydia pneumoniae*)
    * Genital infections: *Chlamydia trachomatis,* granuloma inguinale
    * Systemic infections: relapsing fever (*Borrelia recurrentis*), *Vibrio* (*V cholerae, V vulnificus,* and *V parahaemolyticus*)
    * Other infections: methicillin-resistant *Staphylococcus aureus* and *S epidermidis* (minocycline) when vancomycin or other agents are not considered appropriate; *Pasteurella multocida, Mycobacterium marinum, Yersinia pestis, Helicobacter pylori* (in combination with bismuth subsalicylate and metronidazole or clarithromycin)
    * Prophylaxis: mefloquine-resistant *Plasmodium falciparum* malaria
- Doxycycline:
    * *Mycobacterium fortuitum* and *M chelonae*
    * *Streptococcus pneumoniae*

- *Pseudomonas* and *Proteus* organisms are now resistant to tetracyclines.
- Used in the treatment of *Propionibacterium acnes*

Patient Instructions and Counseling

- Administering the drug with food can minimize GI distress.

Adverse Drug Events

- Photosensitivity reactions (may be less frequent with doxycycline and minocycline)
- Generally contraindicated during pregnancy, breastfeeding, and in children younger than 8 years old because of their association with tooth discoloration and interference with bone growth
- Hepatotoxicity, specifically acute fatty necrosis, may occur in pregnant women and in patients with renal impairment.
- Minocycline use:
    * Vestibular side effects (dizziness, ataxia, nausea, and vertigo)
    * Skin and mucous membrane pigmentation
    * Lupus-like symptoms
- GI intolerance (diarrhea, nausea, anorexia)
- Cross-sensitivity within the tetracycline group is common.
- IV tetracyclines may cause phlebitis.

Drug-Drug and Drug-Disease Interactions

- Milk, antacids, iron supplements, and probably other substances with calcium, magnesium, aluminum, and iron decrease tetracycline GI absorption considerably and should be ingested at least several hours before or after administration of tetracycline.

Table 8

Tetracyclines

Generic name	Trade name	Dosage forms	Common doses	Primary mode of elimination
Demeclocycline	Declomycin®	PO	300-1000 mg/d	Renal
Doxycycline	Vibramycin® and others	PO	100-200 mg q12h	Renal
Methacycline		PO, IV	150 mg q6h to 300 mg q12h	Hepatic
Minocycline	Minocin®	PO, IV	100-200 mg q12h	Hepatic
Oxytetracycline	Terramycin®	PO, IM	250-500 mg q6h, 250-500 mg qid, or 300 mg/d in 1 or 2 divided doses	Renal
Tetracycline	Achromycin V®, Sumycin®, Tetracyn®, and others	PO, IV, IM	1-2 g/d	Renal

- Although doxycycline and minocycline absorption may be less affected by these divalent and trivalent cations, avoiding administration within 1 to 2 hours after ingestion of interfering foods is wise.
- Anticonvulsants (eg, barbiturates, carbamazepine, and phenytoin) induce hepatic microsomal metabolism of tetracyclines and therefore decrease tetracycline serum concentrations.
- If given with cholestyramine or colestipol, may bind tetracycline and reduce GI absorption.
- Oral contraceptive efficacy may be decreased with concurrent use of tetracyclines.
- May potentiate warfarin-induced anticoagulation; therefore monitor PT and INR.
- Demeclocycline antagonizes the action of antidiuretic hormone.

8. Sulfonamides

Sulfonamides are synthetic derivatives of sulfanilamide (Table 9). Sulfonamide utility has decreased over time due to the development of resistance.

Mechanism of Action

- Sulfonamides interfere with bacterial folic acid synthesis by competitively inhibiting p-aminobenzoic acid utilization. Sulfonamides are bacteriostatic.

Spectrum of Activity

Gram-positive bacteria
- Staphylococci (MSSA and MRSA); streptococci (not enterococci); *Bacillus anthracis; Clostridium perfringens; Nocardia*

Gram-negative bacteria
- *Enterobacter; E coli; Klebsiella; Proteus; Salmonella; Shigella*

Other organisms
- *Chlamydia trachomatis; Toxoplasma gondii; Plasmodium*

Adverse Drug Effects

- Hypersensitivity reactions appear to be cross-reactive with other sulfonamides, diuretics (including acetazolamide and thiazides), and sulfonylurea antidiabetic agents.
- Dermatologic reactions include rash, urticaria, and Stevens-Johnson syndrome.

Table 9

Sulfonamides

Generic name	Trade name	Dosage forms	Dose	Elimination	Notes
Sulfadiazine		IV, PO	2-4 g/d	Renal	
Sulfamethizole	Urobiotic®	PO	0.5-1 g q6h	Renal	
Sulfamethoxazole	Septra®	IV, PO	1-3 g/d	Hepatic	Combined with trimethoprim (Septra)
Sulfisoxazole	Gantrisin®	IV, PO	2-8 g/d	Renal	

9. Miscellaneous Antibiotics

Clindamycin

Clindamycin is a semisynthetic antibiotic derived from lincomycin (Table 10).

Mechanism of action
- Clindamycin inhibits the 50S subunit, thereby inhibiting RNA synthesis. Clindamycin is either bacteriostatic or bactericidal depending on the serum concentration of the agent and the MIC of the organism.

Spectrum of activity
- Clindamycin is active against most aerobic gram-positive and most anaerobic gram-negative bacteria. Clindamycin has no activity against aerobic gram-negative bacteria.

Adverse drug effects
- Adverse GI effects occur frequently with all forms of clindamycin, and include nausea, vomiting, diarrhea, abdominal pain, and tenesmus. Clindamycin has induced *C difficile* enterocolitis.
- IV administration can lead to thrombophlebitis, erythema, and pain and swelling at the IV site. IM administration has caused pain, induration, and sterile abscesses.
- Clindamycin has caused transient leukopenia, neutropenia, eosinophilia, thrombocytopenia, and agranulocytosis. These effects are usually reversible upon discontinuation of the drug.

Imipenem-Cilastatin

Imipenem is a semisynthetic carbapenem β-lactam antibiotic. Cilastatin prevents renal metabolism of imipenem by dehydropeptidases.

Mechanism of action
- Imipenem binds to penicillin-binding proteins similarly to β-lactams, thereby inhibiting peptidoglycan synthesis. Imipenem is bactericidal in susceptible isolates. Cilastatin competitively inhibits dehydropeptidase, an enzyme present on the brush border of the proximal renal tubule, which hydrolyzes imipenem. Cilastatin has no antibacterial activity.

Spectrum of activity
- Imipenem is a very broad-spectrum antibiotic with activity against most gram-positive and gram-negative aerobes and anaerobes, as well as activity against some *Mycobacterium* and *Chlamydia* spp.

Adverse drug effects
- GI adverse effects are the most common ADRs reported with imipenem. The effects include nausea, vomiting, diarrhea (including *C difficile* enterocolitis), gastroenteritis, abdominal pain, glossitis, papillary hypertrophy, staining of the teeth, heartburn, pharyngeal pain, and taste abnormalities.
- Eosinophilia, leukopenia, neutropenia, agranulocytosis, hemolytic anemia, and thrombocytopenia have been reported.
- Seizures have been reported in approximately 0.4% of patients receiving imipenem. Risk factors include:
  * History of seizures or head trauma
  * High doses
  * Renal dysfunction

Meropenem

- Similar to imipenem with the following differences:
  * Decreased CNS toxicity
  * No hydrolysis by dehydropeptidases

Table 10

Miscellaneous Antibiotics

Generic name	Trade name	Dosage forms	Dose	Elimination	Notes
Clindamycin	Cleocin®	IV, PO	300 mg q6h PO; 600-900 mg q8h IV	Hepatic	PO only for *C difficile*
Imipenem-cilastatin	Primaxin®	IV, IM	250 mg q6h; 500 mg or 1 g q6h or q8h depending on whether the organism is fully or moderately susceptible	Renal	
Meropenem	Merrem®	IV	500-2000 mg q8h	Renal	

10. Antifungal Agents

Amphotericin B

Amphotericin B is a polyene antifungal agent used in the treatment of potentially life-threatening systemic fungal infections (Table 11).

Mechanism of action
- Amphotericin B binds to ergosterol in the fungal cell wall, leading to increased permeability and cell death. Amphotericin B is fungistatic.

Spectrum of activity
- *Aspergillus, Coccidioides, Cryptococcus, Histoplasma, Mucor*
- *Candida,* including *C albicans, C dubliniensis, C glabrata, C krusei, C parapsilosis,* and *C tropicalis; C lusitaniae* exhibits variable sensitivity

Adverse drug effects
- Infusion reactions: fever, chills, hypotension, rigors, pain, thrombophlebitis, anaphylaxis
- Renal and electrolyte effects: nephrotoxicity is the major dose-limiting toxicity.
  * Hypokalemia, hypocalcemia, hypomagnesemia
  * Usually reversible upon discontinuation of the agent
  * Renal tubular acidosis and nephrocalcinosis are possible.
- Hematologic effects: normocytic, normochromic anemia secondary to decreased erythropoietin production

- Hepatic effects: increased AST, ALT, alkaline phosphatase, bilirubin

Amphotericin B lipid formulations
- Amphotericin B cholesterol sulfate complex (Amphotec®), amphotericin B lipid complex (Abelcet®), and amphotericin B liposomal (AmBisome®) formulations are available for the treatment of severe fungal infections in patients who fail or are intolerant of conventional amphotericin B. The lipid formulations may decrease toxicity ~20-30%.

Caspofungin

Caspofungin is approved for the treatment of aspergillosis in patients refractory to or intolerant of other therapies.

Adverse drug effects
- Hepatic effects: increased AST, ALT
- Sensitivity reactions: histamine-release reactions such as rash, pruritus, and anaphylaxis
- Infusion reactions: fever, thrombophlebitis, nausea, vomiting, myalgias

Fluconazole

Fluconazole is a synthetic triazole antifungal and is fungistatic.

Table 11

Antifungal Agents

Generic name	Trade name	Dosage forms	Normal dose	Elimination	Notes
Amphotericin B	Fungizone®	IV	0.5-1 mg/kg per day	Unknown	Dose should not exceed 1.5 mg/kg/d
Caspofungin	Cancidas®	IV	50 mg/d	Hepatic	
Fluconazole	Diflucan®	IV, PO	100-800 mg/d	Renal	
Flucytosine	Ancobon®	PO	50-150 mg/kg per day	Renal	
Griseofulvin	Fulvicin P/G®	PO	500 mg	Hepatic	
Itraconazole	Sporanox®	IV, PO	200-600 mg/d	Hepatic	
Ketoconazole	Nizoral®	PO, topical	200-400 mg bid	Hepatic	Requires acid environment for dissolution and absorption
Nystatin	Mycostatin®	Topical		Fecal	
Terbinafine	Lamisal®	PO	250 mg/d	Hepatic	Pulse therapy also effective
Voriconazole	Vfend®	IV, PO	200 mg q12h PO; 4-6 mg/kg q12h IV	Renal	

Mechanism of action

- The azole antifungals appear to inhibit fungal cytochrome P450 14-α-demethylase, thereby decreasing ergosterol concentrations in susceptible fungi.

Spectrum of activity

- *Candida krusei, C glabrata, C lusitaniae,* and *C tropicalis* are commonly resistant.

Adverse drug effects

- GI effects: nausea, vomiting, abdominal pain, and diarrhea
- Hepatic effects: cholestasis, increased AST, ALT, and GGTP, hepatic necrosis, and rarely severe hepatic dysfunction
- Hemolytic effects: eosinophilia, anemia, leukopenia, neutropenia, and thrombocytopenia
- Nervous system effects: dizziness, headache, somnolence, coma, and seizures are rare.

Flucytosine

Mechanism of action

- Flucytosine appears to enter fungal cells, where it is converted to 5-fluorouracil. Flucytosine is either fungistatic or fungicidal depending on the concentration of the agent.

Spectrum of activity

- Active against most strains of *Candida* and *Cryptococcus*

Adverse drug effects

- GI effects: GI hemorrhage, ulcerative colitis due to the antiproliferative effects, anorexia, abdominal pain, nausea, vomiting, and diarrhea
- Hepatic effects: increased AST, ALT, and bilirubin
- Renal effects: increased serum creatinine, BUN, and crystalluria
- Nervous system effects: confusion, hallucinations, psychosis, headache, parkinsonism, paresthesias, peripheral neuropathy, hearing loss, and vertigo
- Sensitivity reactions: erythema, pruritus, urticaria, rash, and toxic epidermal necrolysis

Griseofulvin

Mechanism of action

- Griseofulvin disrupts the fungal cell's mitotic spindle structure, thereby inhibiting the metaphase of cell division. Griseofulvin is fungistatic.

Spectrum of activity

- *Trichophyton, Microsporum,* and *Epidermophyton*

Adverse drug effects

- Nervous system effects: headache, fatigue, dizziness, paresthesias of the hands and feet after prolonged therapy
- GI effects: epigastric pain, nausea, vomiting, flatulence, and diarrhea
- Renal effects: proteinuria and nephrosis
- Sensitivity reactions: rash, urticaria, erythema multiforme, angioedema, serum sickness, photosensitivity, and lupus-like reactions

Itraconazole

Itraconazole is a synthetic triazole antifungal.

Spectrum of activity

- Effective in aspergillosis, blastomycosis, histoplasmosis, oropharyngeal and esophageal candidiasis, sporotrichosis, onychomycosis, coccidioidomycosis, and cryptococcosis

Adverse drug effects

- GI effects: nausea, vomiting, diarrhea, abdominal pain, dyspepsia, dysphagia, flatulence, gastritis, ulcerative stomatitis
- Dermatologic and sensitivity reactions: rash, pruritus, urticaria, angioedema, Stevens-Johnson syndrome
- Nervous system reactions: headache, dizziness, tremor, neuropathy
- Cardiovascular effects: congestive heart failure, peripheral edema, pulmonary edema, prolonged QT interval, ventricular dysrhythmias, and death
- Hepatic effects: increased AST, ALT
- Electrolyte and metabolic effects: hypokalemia, adrenal insufficiency, gynecomastia

Ketoconazole

Ketoconazole is a synthetic imidazole antifungal.

Spectrum of activity

- Blastomycosis, candidiasis, coccidioidomycosis, histoplasmosis, dermatophytosis

Adverse drug effects

- GI effects: nausea, vomiting, abdominal pain, GI bleeding
- Hepatic effects: increased AST, ALT, alkaline phosphatase
- Endocrine and metabolic effects: gynecomastia, decreased cortisol production
- Dermatologic and sensitivity reactions: pruritus, rash, dermatitis, purpura
- Nervous system effects: headache, dizziness, lethargy, photophobia, abnormal dreams

Nystatin

Mechanism of action
- Nystatin binds to fungal sterols. Nystatin is fungistatic.

Spectrum of activity
- Cutaneous and mucocutaneous candidiasis

Adverse drug effects
- Mild nausea and diarrhea

Terbinafine

Terbinafine is a synthetic allylamine antifungal.

Mechanism of action
- Interferes with sterol biosynthesis

Spectrum of activity
- *Trichophyton, Microsporum, Epidermophyton, Aspergillus,* blastomycosis, and yeasts

Adverse drug effects
- Hepatic effects: hepatitis, hepatic failure
- Dermatologic and sensitivity reactions: anaphylactoid reactions, Stevens-Johnson syndrome, and erythema multiforme

Voriconazole

Voriconazole is a synthetic triazole antifungal.

Spectrum of activity
- Aspergillosis

Adverse drug effects
- Hepatic effects: hepatitis, cholestasis, fulminant hepatic failure
- Dermatologic and sensitivity reactions: anaphylactoid reactions, pruritus, rash, Stevens-Johnson syndrome, and photosensitivity

11. Antitubercular Agents

Aminosalicylic Acid

Mechanism of action

- Aminosalicylic acid (PAS; para aminosalicylate) inhibits folic acid synthesis similarly to the sulfonamides and is bacteriostatic (Table 12).

Spectrum of activity
- Aminosalicylic acid is active against *Mycobacterium tuberculosis* only.

Adverse drug events
- Gastrointestinal effects: nausea, vomiting, abdominal pain, diarrhea, and anorexia
- Vitamin and mineral absorption: vitamin B_{12}, folic acid, and iron malabsorption have been rarely reported.
- Hypersensitivity reactions: fever, skin eruptions, joint pain, and leukopenia have been reported.

Capreomycin

Mechanism of action
- The exact mechanism of action of capreomycin is unknown. The agent is bacteriostatic against susceptible isolates.

Spectrum of activity
- Capreomycin is active against the following *Mycobacterium* species: *M tuberculosis, M bovis, M kansasii,* and *M avium.*

Adverse drug events
- Renal effects: Nephrotoxicity is exhibited in up to 30% of patients receiving the agent. It is manifest as acute tubular necrosis which is usually reversible upon discontinuation of the agent.
- Ototoxicity: experienced by up to 30% of patients; caused by eighth cranial nerve damage which can produce irreversible hearing loss
- Hepatic effects: elevated liver function tests have been noted when used in conjunction with other hepatotoxins
- Hypersensitivity reactions: fever, urticaria, and skin eruptions have been noted.

Cycloserine

Mechanism of action
- Cycloserine is structurally similar to d-alanine and inhibits cell wall synthesis by competing for incorporation into the bacterial cell wall.

Table 12

Antitubercular Agents

Generic name	Trade name	Dosage forms	Normal dose	Elimination	Notes
Aminosalicylic acid	Paser®	PO	150 mg/kg per day	Renal	Max dose 12 g/d
Capreomycin	Capastat®	IM	15 mg/kg per day	Renal	Max dose 1 g/d
Cycloserine	Seromycin®	PO	15-20 mg/kg per day	Renal	Max dose 1 g/d
Ethambutol	Myambutol®	PO	15-25 mg/kg per day	Hepatic	
Ethionamide	Trecator-SC®	PO	500-1000 mg per day	Hepatic	
Isoniazid	Various	PO	5-10 mg/kg per day	Hepatic	Max dose 300 mg/d
Pyrazinamide	Various	PO	15-30 mg/kg per day	Hepatic	Max dose 2 g/d
Rifampin	Various	PO, IV	10-20 mg/kg per day	Hepatic	Max dose 600 mg/d

Spectrum of activity
- Cycloserine is active against the following *Mycobacterium* species: *M tuberculosis, M bovis, M avium,* and some *M kansasii* isolates.

Adverse drug events
- CNS effects: headache, vertigo, confusion, psychosis, and seizures

Ethambutol

Mechanism of action
- Ethambutol appears to inhibit bacterial cellular metabolism and is bacteriostatic.

Spectrum of activity
- Ethambutol is active against the following *Mycobacterium* species: *M tuberculosis, M bovis,* and some isolates of *M kansasii* and *M avium.*

Adverse drug events
- Ocular effects: optic neuritis with decreased visual acuity, central and peripheral scotomas, and loss of red-green color discrimination have been noted. These effects are usually reversible upon discontinuation of the agent.

Ethionamide

Mechanism of action
- Ethionamide appears to inhibit cell wall synthesis by an unidentified mechanism. Ethionamide is bacteriocidal or bacteriostatic depending on tissue concentrations of the agent.

Spectrum of activity
- Ethionamide is active against the following *Mycobacterium* species: *M tuberculosis, M bovis, M kansasii,* and some *M avium* isolates.

Adverse drug events
- Hepatic effects: hepatitis is a rare complication.

Isoniazid (INH)

Mechanism of action
- INH appears to inhibit the bacterial cell wall of susceptible isolates and is therefore active against actively dividing cells only. INH is bacteriocidal or bacteriostatic depending on tissue concentrations of the agent.

Spectrum of activity
- INH is active against the following *Mycobacterium* species: *M tuberculosis, M bovis,* and some strains of *M kansasii.*

Adverse drug events
- CNS effects: peripheral neuritis and rarely seizures, encephalopathy, and psychosis have been reported.
- Hepatic effects: increases in bilirubin, AST, and ALT are noted in up to 20% of patients receiving this agent. INH has lead to fulminant hepatitis and death.
- Hematologic effects: agranulocytosis, eosinophilia, thrombocytopenia, and hemolytic anemia have been reported.

Pyrazinamide (PZA)

Mechanism of action
- *Mycobacterium tuberculosis* converts PZA to pyrazinoic acid which possesses antitubercular activity.

Spectrum of activity

• PZA is active against *Mycobacterium tuberculosis* only.

Adverse drug events

• Hepatic effects: increased liver enzymes are common, and fulminant hepatitis has been reported.
• Gout: PZA inhibits renal excretion of uric acid and may induce or worsen gout.

Rifampin

Mechanism of action

• Rifampin inhibits RNA synthesis in susceptible isolates.

Spectrum of activity

• Rifampin is active against the following *Mycobacterium* species: *M tuberculosis, M bovis, M kansasii,* and some *M avium* isolates.
• Rifampin also has activity against many gram-positive and gram-negative organisms.

Adverse drug events

• GI effects: nausea, vomiting, diarrhea, and abdominal pain may require discontinuation of the agent. *C difficile* colitis has been reported with rifampin.
• CNS effects: headache, dizziness, mental confusion, and psychosis have been reported.
• Hepatic effects: increased bilirubin, AST, and ALT are common. Fulminant hepatitis has been reported.
• Hematologic effects: thrombocytopenia, leukopenia, and hemolytic anemia have been reported rarely.
• Renal effects: renal insufficiency and interstitial nephritis have been reported.

12. Key Points

Aminoglycosides

• Aminoglycoside antibiotics exhibit concentration-dependent bacterial killing.
• Aminoglycoside antibiotics are reserved for severe infections or for use against multidrug-resistant bacteria.
• Aminoglycoside antibiotic dosing should be pharmacokinetically tailored for each patient to optimize the therapeutic effect and minimize toxicity.

Antifungal anti-infectives

• Amphotericin B, caspofungin, fluconazole, itraconazole, and voriconazole are effective against systemic fungal infections.
• Imidazole antifungal antibiotics are potent inhibitors of hepatic metabolism, thereby decreasing the elimination of numerous agents.

Gram-positive antibiotics

• Linezolid and quinupristin-dalfopristin are clinically effective against MRSA, MRSE, and VRE.
• Vancomycin is a broad-spectrum gram-positive antibiotic that should be pharmacokinetically tailored for each patient to maximize therapeutic benefit and minimize toxicity.

Miscellaneous antibiotics

• Clindamycin is an effective anaerobic antibiotic as well as an effective gram-positive aerobic antibiotic with activity against many MRSA isolates.
• The carbapenem antibiotics possess a very broad spectrum of activity and should be restricted to appropriate indications to minimize development of resistance.

Penicillins NO renal

• Penicillin antibiotics exhibit time-above-MIC-dependent bacterial killing.
• All penicillins, except nafcillin and oxacillin, are renally eliminated and require dosage adjustments in renal dysfunction.

Cephalosporins

• Cephalosporin antibiotics exhibit time-above-MIC-dependent bacterial killing.
• First-generation cephalosporins: gram-positive activity is extensive, but gram-negative activity is limited.
• Second-generation cephalosporins: gram-positive activity is similar to that of first-generation agents, but gram-negative activity is generally more extensive than that of first-generation agents.

- Third-generation cephalosporins: gram-positive activity is decreased versus first- and second-generation agents, but gram-negative activity is extensive.

Fluoroquinolones
- Quinolone antibiotics exhibit concentration-dependent bacterial killing similar to the aminoglycosides.
- The later-generation quinolones possess improved gram-positive activity, including resistant streptococci.

Sulfonamides
- Sulfonamides are primarily urinary anti-infectives whose utility has decreased due to the development of resistance.

Tetracyclines
- Tetracyclines are drugs of choice for atypical pneumonias.

Macrolides
- Erythromycins are primarily active against gram-positive bacteria including penicillin-resistant streptococci.
- Telithromycin possesses greater in vitro activity against multidrug-resistant gram-positive organisms and *Haemophilus influenzae* compared to the erythromycins.

Antitubercular agents
- Isoniazid, rifampin, and streptomycin exhibit the lowest incidence of resistance.
- Isoniazid, rifampin, and pyrazinamide are the agents of first choice.

13. Questions and Answers

1. Which of the following statements regarding aminoglycoside antibiotics is/are true?

   I. Aminoglycoside antibiotics are bactericidal against most susceptible isolates
   II. Aminoglycoside antibiotics exhibit concentration-dependent bacterial killing
   III. Aminoglycoside antibiotics should be reserved for serious infections

   A. I only
   B. I and II
   C. I and III
   D. II and III
   E. I, II, and III

2. Which of the following statements most accurately characterizes aminoglycoside toxicity?

   I. Ototoxicity due to eighth cranial nerve damage
   II. Nephrotoxicity exhibited as acute tubular necrosis
   III. Bone marrow suppression

   A. I only
   B. II only
   C. III only
   D. I and II
   E. II and III

3. Which of the following statements best characterizes aminoglycoside antimicrobial activity?

   I. Active against most aerobic gram-negative bacteria
   II. Active against most anaerobic gram-negative bacteria
   III. Active against most fungal isolates

   A. I only
   B. II only
   C. II only
   D. I and II
   E. II and III

4. Which of the following antifungals is/are effective against systemic infections?

   I. Amphotericin B
   II. Fluconazole
   III. Nystatin

A. I only
B. II only
C. III only
D. I and II
E. I and III

5. Which of the following statements is/are true about amphotericin B–induced nephrotoxicity?

I. Nephrotoxicity is the major dose-limiting toxicity
II. Nephrotoxicity is usually reversible upon discontinuation of the drug
III. Amphotericin B lipid formulations decrease nephrotoxicity by 20-30%

    A. I only
    B. II only
    C. I and II
    D. II and III
    E. I, II, and III

6. Which of the following statements best describe the drug interactions noted with the imidazole antifungals?

I. Increased elimination of warfarin
II. Decreased elimination of warfarin
III. Increased metabolism of the oral contraceptives

    A. I only
    B. II only
    C. III only
    D. II and III
    E. I, II, and II

7. Linezolid is best described by which of the following statements?

I. Linezolid is bacteriostatic against staphylococci
II. Linezolid is bactericidal against staphylococci
III. Linezolid is a weak MAO inhibitor

    A. I only
    B. II only
    C. I and III
    D. II and III
    E. I, II, and III

8. Linezolid possesses activity against which of the following bacteria?

I. MRSA
II. *Enterococcus faecium*
III. *Enterococcus faecalis*

A. I only
B. II only
C. III only
D. I and II
E. I and III

9. Quinupristin-dalfopristin is best described by which of the following statements?

I. Exhibits activity against MSSA
II. Exhibits activity against MRSA
III. Exhibits activity against streptococci

    A. I only
    B. II only
    C. III only
    D. I and II
    E. I, II, and III

10. Vancomycin is best described by which of the following statements?

I. Exhibits activity against MRSA
II. Exhibits activity against *Enterobacter*
III. Exhibits activity against *Clostridium difficile*

    A. I only
    B. II only
    C. III only
    D. I and II
    E. I and III

11. Vancomycin toxicity is best described by which of the following statements?

I. Nephrotoxicity exhibited as acute tubular necrosis that is seldom reversible
II. Ototoxicity that is commonly exhibited as vestibular toxicity
III. Histamine release or "red-man syndrome," which is associated with rapid IV infusion

    A. I only
    B. II only
    C. III only
    D. I and II
    E. II and III

12. Which of the following statements best describes appropriate vancomycin monitoring?

I. Trough serum concentrations should be routinely monitored in patients with pre-existing renal dysfunction.

II. Peak serum concentrations should be routinely monitored in patients with pre-existing renal dysfunction.
III. Serum concentration monitoring is of no benefit in vancomycin monitoring.

A. I only
B. II only
C. III only
D. I and II
E. II and III

13. Clindamycin exhibits antibacterial activity against which of the following micro-organisms?

I. Aerobic gram-positive bacteria
II. Anaerobic gram-negative bacteria
III. Aerobic gram-negative bacteria

A. I only
B. II only
C. III only
D. I and II
E. I and III

14. Which statements best describes the carbapenem antibiotics?

I. Exhibit activity against most gram-positive and gram-negative aerobes and anaerobes
II. Meropenem induces seizures more commonly than imipenem
III. Cilastatin exhibits activity against most gram-positive aerobes

A. I only
B. II only
C. III only
D. I and II
E. II and III

15. Which of the following statements best describes the penicillins?

I. Exhibit concentration-dependent bacterial killing
II. Exhibit time-above-MIC-dependent bacterial killing
III. Exhibit excellent MRSA activity

A. I only
B. II only
C. III only
D. I and II
E. II and III

16. Which of the following penicillins require dosage adjustment in renal dysfunction?

I. Ampicillin
II. Nafcillin
III. Oxacillin

A. I only
B. II only
C. III only
D. I and II
E. II and III

17. Which of the following statements best describes the cephalosporins?

I. Exhibit concentration-dependent bacterial killing
II. Exhibit time-above-MIC-dependent bacterial killing
III. Exhibit excellent MRSA activity

A. I only
B. II only
C. III only
D. I and II
E. II and III

18. Which of the following statements best describes the antibacterial activity of the cephalosporins?

I. First-generation cephalosporins: gram-positive activity is extensive, but gram-negative activity is limited
II. Second-generation cephalosporins: gram-positive activity is similar to that of first-generation agents, but gram-negative activity is generally more extensive than that of first-generation agents
III. Third-generation cephalosporins: gram-positive activity is decreased versus first- and second-generation agents, but gram-negative activity is extensive

A. I only
B. II only
C. III only
D. All of the above
E. None of the above

19. Which of the following statements best describes the antibacterial activity of the quinolones?

I. Exhibit concentration-dependent bacterial killing
II. Exhibit time-above-MIC-dependent bacterial killing
III. Exhibit extensive anaerobic activity

A. I only
B. II only
C. III only
D. I and III
E. II and III

20. Which of the following statements best describes the important patient counseling points for the quinolones?

I. Avoid use in children and pregnant or nursing women due to the risk of cartilage erosion in growing bone tissue
II. Do not take within 2 hours of antacids, multivitamins, calcium, magnesium, or iron supplements
III. Take with a full glass of water and remain sitting or upright for 2 hours to avoid esophageal irritation

   A. I only
   B. II only
   C. III only
   D. I and II
   E. II and III

21. Which of the following statements best describes the sulfonamides?

I. Interfere with vitamin B_{12} synthesis by competitively inhibiting PABA utilization
II. Drugs of choice for *C difficile* colitis
III. Primarily urinary anti-infectives whose utility has decreased due to the development of resistance

   A. I only
   B. II only
   C. III only
   D. I and II
   E. I, II, and III

22. Which of the following statements best describes the tetracyclines?

I. Exhibit bacteriostatic activity
II. Are the drugs of choice for atypical pneumonia
III. Tetracycline is contraindicated in children less than 8 years old

   A. I only
   B. II only
   C. III only
   D. I and II
   E. I, II, and III

23. Which of the following statements best describes the macrolides?

I. Primarily effective against gram-positive aerobic bacteria
II. Effective against penicillin-resistant streptococci
III. Ineffective against penicillin-resistant streptococci

   A. I only
   B. II only
   C. III only
   D. I and II
   E. I and III

24. Which antitubercular agent(s) exhibits the lowest incidence of resistance?

I. Isoniazid
II. Rifampin
III. Streptomycin

   A. I only
   B. II only
   C. III only
   D. I and II
   E. I, II, and III

25. Which of the following drug combination regimens are considered the agents of first choice for empiric treatment of TB?

I. Isoniazid, rifampin, and streptomycin
II. Isoniazid, rifampin, and pyrazinamide
III. Isoniazid, ethambutol, and cycloserine

   A. I only
   B. II only
   C. III only
   D. All of the above
   E. None of the above

Answers

1. **E.** Aminoglycoside antibiotics are bacteriocidal against most susceptible isolates, exhibit concentration-dependent bacterial killing, and are usually reserved for serious infections due to toxicity.

2. **D.** Ototoxicity is due to eighth cranial nerve damage and may be irreversible. Nephrotoxicity is exhibited as an acute tubular necrosis that is usually reversible and seldom requires dialysis. Neuromuscular blockade is the third most

common toxicity noted with the aminoglycosides.

3. **A.** Aminoglycosides are active against most aerobic gram-negative and selected aerobic gram-positive bacteria. They have no activity against anaerobic bacteria or fungi.

4. **D.** Amphotericin B, caspofungin, fluconazole, itraconazole, and voriconazole are effective against systemic fungal infections.

5. **E.** Acute renal dysfunction is the most common dose-limiting amphotericin B toxicity, the renal dysfunction is usually reversible and seldom requires dialysis, and lipid formulations decrease toxicity by ~20-30%.

6. **B.** The imidazole antifungals decrease hepatic clearance of numerous hepatically metabolized medications, thereby increasing their activity and risk for toxicity.

7. **C.** Linezolid is bacteriostatic against staphylococci and enterococci. It is bacteriocidal against *Streptococcus* species only. The agent is a weak MAO inhibitor.

8. **D.** Linezolid is active against MSSA, MRSA, and *Enterococcus faecium* (VRE). *Enterococcus faecalis* isolates are resistant.

9. **E.** Quinupristin-dalfopristin is active against MSSA, MRSA, streptococci, and *Enterococcus faecium* (VRE). *Enterococcus faecalis* isolates are commonly resistant.

10. **E.** Vancomycin is active against aerobic gram-positive bacteria only; it has no clinically significant gram-negative activity. Vancomycin is the second-line drug of choice for *C difficile* colitis.

11. **C.** Vancomycin nephrotoxicity is uncommon and is exhibited as acute tubular necrosis, which is commonly reversible and seldom requires dialysis. Ototoxicity is due to eighth cranial nerve damage which is manifest as high-frequency hearing loss, seldom affecting the vestibular system. The histamine or "red-man syndrome" reaction is most commonly infusion rate–related.

12. **A.** Vancomycin serum concentration monitoring is not required in patients responding well to therapy and with normal renal function. Vancomycin trough concentrations should be assessed in patients with pre-existing renal dysfunction, worsening renal function, or those not responding to therapy.

13. **D.** Clindamycin exhibits activity against aerobic gram-positive bacteria and anaerobic gram-positive and gram-negative bacteria. It has no clinically significant aerobic gram-negative activity.

14. **A.** Carbapenems are active against most aerobic and anaerobic gram-positive and gram-negative bacteria. Imipenem is more likely to induce seizures, and cilastatin inhibits the metabolism of imipenem but has no antibacterial activity.

15. **B.** Penicillins exhibit time-dependent bacterial killing and have no activity against MRSA.

16. **A.** All penicillins with the exception of nafcillin and oxacillin require dosage adjustment in renal dysfunction.

17. **B.** Cephalosporins exhibit time-dependent bacterial killing and have no activity against MRSA.

18. **D.** First-generation cephalosporins exhibit extensive gram-positive activity but limited gram-negative activity. Second-generation cephalosporins maintain gram-positive activity similar to the first-generation agents, but their gram-negative activity is generally improved. Third-generation cephalosporins exhibit decreased gram-positive activity, but gram-negative activity is significantly improved.

19. **A.** Quinolones exhibit concentration-dependent bacterial killing similar to the aminoglycosides. They possess good aerobic gram-positive and gram-negative activity, but have limited anaerobic activity.

20. **D.** Quinolones have been shown to decrease cartilage formation in beagle pups, but this effect in humans is somewhat controversial. Their use in children should be reserved for serious infections to avoid the risk. Quinolones are bound to divalent cations and should not be coadministered. They do not cause significant esophageal irritation.

21. **C.** Sulfonamides interfere with folic acid metabolism by inhibiting PABA utilization. They have no activity against *C difficile* colitis, and are primarily relegated to urinary anti-infectives due to resistance.

22. **E.** Tetracyclines are bacteriostatic. They are drugs of choice for atypical pulmonary pathogens, and should not be administered to children less than 8 years old to avoid permanent tooth staining and potential deposition into bone.

23. **D.** Erythromycins are primarily gram-positive aerobic antibiotics with good activity against most penicillin-resistant *Streptococcus* isolates.

24. **E.** Isoniazid, rifampin, and streptomycin exhibit the lowest incidence of MTB resistance.

25. **B.** Isoniazid, rifampin, and pyrazinamide are considered agents of first choice for empiric treatment of TB due to a low incidence of resistance and acceptable tolerability profile. Ethambutol is commonly added to the regimen in areas of increased resistance.

14. References

Alvarez-Elcoro S, Enzler MJ. The macrolides: Erythromycin, clarithromycin, and azithromycin. *Mayo Clin Proc.* 1999;74:613-634.

Cunha BA, ed. *Antibiotic Therapy,* Part I. The Medical Clinics of North America. Philadelphia: WB Saunders; 2000.

Cunha BA, ed. *Antibiotic Therapy,* Part II. The Medical Clinics of North America. Philadelphia: WB Saunders; 2001.

Edson RS, Terrell CL. The aminoglycosides. *Mayo Clin Proc.* 1999;74:519-528.

Hardman JG, Limbird LE, Molinoff PB, et al, eds. Goodman and Gilman's *The Pharmacological Basis of Therapeutics,* 9th ed. New York: McGraw-Hill; 1996.

Hellinger WC, Brewer NS. Carbapenems and monobactams: Imipenem, meropenem, and aztreonam. *Mayo Clin Proc.* 1999;74:420-434.

Kucers A, Bennett NM, eds. *Use of Antibiotics: A Comprehensive Review with Clinical Emphasis,* 4th ed. Philadelphia: Lippincott Williams & Wilkins; 1998.

Kasten MJ. Clindamycin, metronidazole, and chloramphenicol. *Mayo Clin Proc.* 1999;74:825-834.

Mandell GL, Bennett JE, Dolin R, eds. *Principles and Practice of Infectious Diseases,* 5th ed. Philadelphia: Churchill Livingstone; 2000.

Marshall WF, Blair JE. The cephalosporins. *Mayo Clin Proc.* 1999;74:187-195.

Patel R. Antifungal agents. Part I. Amphotericin B preparations and flucytosine. *Mayo Clin Proc.* 1998;73:1205-1225.

Reese RE, Betts RF, eds. *A Practical Approach to Infectious Diseases,* 4th ed. Boston: Little, Brown and Company; 1996.

Shain CS. Telithromycin: The first of the ketolides. *Ann Pharmacother.* 2002;36:452-464.

Smilack JD. The tetracyclines. *Mayo Clin Proc.* 1999;74:727-730.

Smilack, JD. Trimethoprim-sulfamethoxazole. *Mayo Clin Proc.* 1999;74:730-734.

Terrrell CL. Antifungal agents. Part II. The azoles. *Mayo Clin Proc.* 1999;74:78-100.

Van Scoy RE, Wilkowske CJ. Antimycobacterial therapy. *Mayo Clin Proc.* 1999;74:1038-1048.

Walker RC. The fluoroquinolones. *Mayo Clin Proc.* 1999;74:1030-1037.

Wilhelm MP. Vancomycin. *Mayo Clin Proc.* 1999;74: 928-935.

Wright AJ. The penicillins. *Mayo Clin Proc.* 1999;74: 290-308.

31. Human Immunodeficiency Virus and the Acquired Immunodeficiency Syndrome

Camille W. Thornton, PharmD, BCPS
Assistant Professor, Department of Clinical Pharmacy
University of Tennessee College of Pharmacy

Contents

1. **Overview**

2. **Drug Therapy**

3. **Prevention**

4. **Hematologic Complications**

5. **Key Points**

6. **Questions and Answers**

7. **References**

1. Overview

- Human immunodeficiency virus (HIV) is a retrovirus that depletes the helper T lymphocytes (CD4 cells), resulting in continued destruction of the immune system and subsequent gradual development of opportunistic infections and malignancies.
- Acquired immunodeficiency syndrome (AIDS) is HIV with a CD4 count less than 200 cells/mm³ or a history of opportunistic infection (eg, unexplained fever for more than 2 weeks, thrush, *Pneumocystis carinii* pneumonia, toxoplasmosis, cryptococcal meningitis, histoplasmosis, and *Mycobacterium avium*).

Epidemiology

- At the end of 2004, these were the global estimates of children and adults with HIV/AIDS:
  - * People living with HIV/AIDS: 39.4 million
  - * New HIV infections in 2004: 2.9 million
  - * Deaths due to HIV/AIDS in 2004: 3.1 million
  - * Cumulative number of deaths due to HIV/AIDS: 31 million
- Complete current world epidemiology can be found at www.unaids.org.
- At the end of 2003, these were the estimates of children and adults with HIV/AIDS in the U.S.:
  - * People living with HIV/AIDS: 850,000-950,000
  - * New HIV infections in 2003: 43,171
  - * Deaths due to HIV/AIDS in 2003: 18,017
  - * Cumulative number of deaths due to HIV/AIDS: 524,060
  - * 180,000-280,000 don't know they are infected with HIV
- Complete current United States epidemiology can be found at: www.cdc.gov/hiv/stats/hasrlink.htm.

Subtypes
- HIV-1: most commonly found in the U.S.
- HIV-2: most commonly found in Africa

Clinical Presentation

- Opportunistic infection
- Patient not ill but has tested as HIV-positive
- Acute retroviral syndrome:
  - * 50-90% of patients acutely infected with HIV experience some of the symptoms.
  - * Symptoms generally appear 2-4 weeks after virus exposure.
  - * Duration of the clinical syndrome is ~14 days (the range is a few days to >10 weeks).

- * The disease is not readily recognized in the primary care setting because its symptoms are similar to those of the flu, mononucleosis, and other common illnesses.

Pathophysiology

- A retrovirus that replicates in and destroys CD4 cells
- The result is a chronically deteriorating immune system leading to opportunistic infections and eventual death.
- Seroconversion typically occurs ~3 weeks after the acute infection (the range is from 2 weeks to 6 months).
- Antibodies generally appear within 3 months of infection (the range is from 2 weeks to 6 months).
- Transmission is via infected blood or hazardous body fluids:
  - * Unprotected sexual contact with an infected person
    - Multiple partners increase risk.
    - Ongoing or past medical history of sexually transmitted disease increases risk.
  - * Sharing needles and/or syringes with an infected person
  - * Transfusions of infected blood or blood clotting factors (the U.S. began screening the blood supply in 1985).
  - * Vertical transmission (infected mother to infant)
  - * Breastfeeding
  - * Occupational exposure is rare.
  - * Household contact is rare.

Diagnostic Criteria

- Enzyme-linked immunosorbent assay (ELISA):
  - * Initial screening test for detection of anti-HIV antibodies
  - * False-positive results can occur in patients with:
    - Collagen vascular diseases
    - Chronic hepatitis
    - Other chronic diseases
- Western blot:
  - * All positive ELISA tests must be confirmed by a Western blot.
  - * Specificity and sensitivity of the Western blot is >99%.
  - * Western blot tests for anti-HIV antibodies.
- Other diagnostic tests are available (all should be confirmed by Western blot).
  - * Rapid tests can give results from a fingerstick or swab of oral fluid in 20 minutes.

Monitoring Tools

Viral load
- Measures amount of virus in blood
- Can assess disease progression and evaluate the efficacy of antiretroviral therapy
- Lower limit of detection is less than 50 copies/mL for ultrasensitive assays (less than 400 copies/mL for non-ultrasensitive assays).
- A minimally significant change in viral load is considered to be a threefold or $0.5 \log_{10}$ increase or decrease.
- Acute illness and immunizations can cause increases in viral load for 2-4 weeks; testing should not be performed during this time.
- Baseline viral loads are established by averaging two viral loads (that do not differ by $>0.5 \log_{10}$) taken 2-4 weeks apart.
- Monitoring of viral load in patients not on antiretroviral therapy should occur every 3-4 months.
- Monitoring of viral load in patients starting a new regimen should occur 2-8 weeks after treatment initiation and then every 3-4 months.

CD4 cell count
- Indicates extent of immune system damage and risk of developing opportunistic infections
- Normal $CD4^+$ cell counts are 800-1200 cell/mm^3.
- $CD4^+$ cell counts should be measured every 3-4 months in patients on or off antiretroviral therapy.
- A significant change in $CD4^+$ cells is considered to be a 30% increase or decrease from baseline.

Treatment Principles and Goals

Goals of therapy
- Maximal and durable suppression of viral load
- Restoration and/or preservation of immunologic function
- Improvement in quality of life
- Reduction of HIV-related morbidity and mortality
- Factors involved in achieving goals of therapy:
  - * Adherence to the antiretroviral regimen
  - * Rational sequencing of drugs
  - * Preservation of future treatment options
  - * Use of resistance testing in selected clinical settings
- See Table 1 for indications for the initiation of antiretroviral therapy in the chronically HIV-1 infected patient.
- See Table 2 for antiretroviral agents recommended by DHHS for initial treatment of established HIV infection.

Indications for Consideration of Changing Antiretroviral Therapy

- Failure to suppress plasma HIV RNA to undetectable levels (<50 copies/mL) within 4-6 months of initiating a therapy
- Repeated detection of virus in plasma following initial suppression to undetectable levels
- Consider genotyping and/or phenotyping to assist in identifying drugs for the next regimen if:
  - * Adherent to failing regimen for at least the previous 4-6 weeks or within 4 weeks after regimen discontinuation

Table 1

Indications for the Initiation of Antiretroviral Therapy in the Chronically HIV-1 Infected Patient

Clinical category	CD4$^+$ cell count	Plasma HIV RNA	Recommendation
Symptomatic (AIDS, severe symptoms)	Any value	Any value	Treat
Asymptomatic, AIDS	<200/mm^3	Any value	Treat
Asymptomatic	>200/mm^3 but <350/mm^3	Any value	Treatment should generally be offered though controversy exists
Asymptomatic	>350/mm^3	Viral load >100,000 copies/mL	Some experts would recommend initiating therapy, recognizing that the 3-year risk of developing AIDS in untreated patients is >30%, and some would defer therapy and monitor CD4+ cell counts more frequently
Asymptomatic	>350/mm^3	Viral load <100,000 copies/mL	Many experts would defer therapy and observe, recognizing that the 3-year risk of developing AIDS in untreated patients is <15%

Table 2

Antiretroviral Regimens for Treatment of HIV Infection in Antiretroviral-Naïve Patients

NNRTI-based regimens

Preferred regimens	Efavirenz[1] + (lamivudine *or* emtricitabine) + (zidovudine *or* tenofovir)
Alternative regimens	Efavirenz[1] + (lamivudine *or* emtricitabine) + (didanosine *or* abacavir *or* stavudine)
	Nevirapine[2] + (lamivudine *or* emtricitabine) + (zidovudine + *or* stavudine or didanosine *or* abacavir *or* tenofovir)

PI-based regimens

Preferred regimens	Lopinavir + ritonavir (co-formulation) + (lamivudine *or* emtricitabine) + zidovudine		

Alternative regimens (use one medication from each column)	**Column A**	**ColumnB**	**Column C**
	Atazanavir[3]	Lamivudine	Zidovudine
	Fosamprenavir	Emtricitabine	Stavudine
	Fosamprenavir/r[4]		Abacavir
	Indinavir/r[4]		Tenofovir
	Lopinavir/r[4]		Didanosine
	Nelfinavir		
	Saquinavir[5]/r[4]		

3 NRTI-based	Abacavir + zidovudine + lamivudine: only when a preferred or an alternative NNRTI- or PI-based regimen cannot or should not be used

NNRTI, non-nucleoside reverse transcriptase inhibitor; NRTI, nucleoside reverse transcriptase inhibitor; PI, protease inhibitor.

[1]Efavirenz is not recommended for use in first-trimester pregnancy or in women with a high pregnancy potential.

[2]Use caution in women with CD4 cell counts >250 cells/mm^3 and men with CD4 cell counts >400 cells/mm^3 due to increased risk of nevirapine-associated toxicity.

[3]Must boost atazanavir with low-dose ritonavir if used with tenofovir.

[4]Low-dose 100-400 mg ritonavir.

[5]Saquinavir is currently available in 3 formulations: soft gel caps, hard gel caps, and the mesylate tablet formulation, which is preferred.

IAS-USA guidelines differ slightly from DHHS guidelines above. Preferred PI regimens include atazanavir/r, saquinavir/r, and indinvir/r as well as lopinavir/r. Nucleoside reverse transcriptase inhibitor (NRTI) pairs are (zidovudine or tenofovir) plus (lamivudine or emtricitabine) for both PI- and NNRTI-based regmiens.

       * Viral load above 1000 copies/mL
- Persistently declining CD4$^+$ T cell numbers as measured on at least two separate occasions
- Clinical deterioration
- Never change just one medication in a failing regimen (ie, use at least two new drugs, and preferably an entirely new regimen).
- Changing one medication in a successful regimen can be done if a patient is experiencing intolerable side effects or if there is overlapping toxicity with other medications (Table 3).
- Use the treatment history and past and current resistance test results to identify active agents (preferably two or more) to design a new regimen.

2. Drug Therapy

Nucleoside Reverse Transcriptase Inhibitors (NRTIs) (Table 4)

Mechanism of action
- Interfere with HIV viral RNA-dependent DNA polymerase, resulting in chain termination and inhibition of viral replication

Class toxicities (monitor for signs and symptoms)
- Lactic acidosis
- Severe hepatomegaly with steatosis
- Most patients should be dose-adjusted for renal impairment (exception: abacavir).

Table 3

HIV-Related Drugs with Overlapping Toxicities

Bone marrow suppression	Peripheral neuropathy	Pancreatitis	Nephrotoxicity	Hepatotoxicity	Rash	Diarrhea	Ocular effects
Amphotericin B	Didanosine	Cotrimoxazole	Acyclovir	Azithromycin	Abacavir	Atovaquone	Cidofovir
Cidofovir	Isoniazid	Didanosine	(IV, high-dose)	Clarithromycin	Amprenavir	Clindamycin	Didanosine
Cotrimoxazole	Linezolid	Lamivudine	Adefovir	Delavirdine	Atazanavir	Darunavir	Ethambutol
Cytotoxic	Stavudine	(children)	Aminogylcosides	Efavirenz	Atovaquone	Didanosine	Linezolid
chemotherapy	Zalcitabine	Pentamidine	Amphotericin B	Fluconazole	Cotrimoxazole	(buffered	Rifabutin
Dapsone		Ritonavir	Cidofovir	Isoniazid	Dapsone	formulations)	Voriconazole
Flucytosine		Stavudine	Foscarnet	Itraconazole	Darunavir	Fosamprenavir	
Ganciclovir		Zalcitabine	Indinavir	Ketoconazole	Delavirdine	Lopinavir/	
Hydroxyurea			Pentamidine	Neviraprine	Efavirenz	ritonavir	
Interferon alfa			Tenofovir	NRTIs	Fosamprenavir	Nelfinavir	
Linezolid				PIs – especially	Nevirapine	Ritonavir	
Peginterferon alfa				tipranavir	Sulfadiazine	Tipranavir	
Primaquine				Rifabutin	Voriconazole		
Pyrimethamine				Rifampin			
Ribavirin				Voriconazole			
Rifabutin							
Sulfadiazine							
Trimetrexate							
Valganciclovir							
Zidovudine							

- Didanosine, stavudine, and lamivudine are dosed based on weight.
- Lamivudine and emtricitabine are chemically similar and should not be used in the same regimen.
- Most are not affected by food (except didanosine).
- Low pill burden as a class; few drug interactions.
- All are prodrugs requiring 2-3 phosphorylations for activation.
- Do not use zidovudine with stavudine due to antagonism (both require thymidine for activation).
- Do not use didanosine with stavudine during pregnancy due to increased risk of lactic acidosis and liver damage.
- Tenofovir increases didanosine levels and decreases atazanavir levels; dosage adjustments are required.
- Four combination products are available:
  * Combivir® (zidovudine 300 mg + lamivudine 150 mg) every 12 hours
  * Trizivir® (zidovudine 300 mg + lamivudine 150 mg + abacavir 300 mg) every 12 hours
  * Truvada® (tenofovir 300 mg + emtricitabine 200 mg) every 24 hours
  * Epzicom® (lamivudine 300 mg + abacavir 600 mg) every 24 hours

- No special storage requirements are necessary for drugs in this class.
- The "D" drugs (ddI [didanosine], d4T [stavudine], and ddC [zalcitabine]) can cause pancreatitis and peripheral neuropathy; when used together, this effect can be additive.
- The "D" drugs are more closely associated with lactic acidosis.
- Therapy with zalcitabine has the highest incidence of peripheral neuropathy and is contraindicated with didanosine, stavudine, and lamivudine.
- Usually use two NRTIs in combination with 1 NNRTI or 1 PI

Non-Nucleoside Reverse Transcriptase Inhibitors (NNRTIs) (Table 5)

Mechanism of action
- Bind to reverse transcriptase at a different site than the NRTIs, resulting in inhibition of HIV replication
- Class toxicities include rash and hepatic toxicity.
- One-step mutation confers class resistance.
- All should be dose-adjusted for hepatic impairment.
- Most are not affected by food (except efavirenz).

Table 4

Characteristics of Nucleoside Reverse Transcriptase Inhibitors (NRTIs)

Generic name [trade name]	Zidovudine (AZT, ZDV) [Retrovir®]	Lamivudine (3TC) [Epivir®]	Abacavir (ABC) [Ziagen®]	Didanosine (ddI) [Videx EC®, Videx®]
Form	100 mg caps; 300 mg tabs; also available in combination products[1]; available as generic	150, 300 mg tabs; 10 mg/mL oral solution; also available in combination products[1]	300 mg tabs; 20 mg/mL oral solution; also available in combination products[1]	Videx EC® caps: 125, 200, 250, 400 mg; Videx® buffered tabs: 25, 50, 100, 150, 200 mg; Videx® buffered powders: 100, 167, 250 mg; available as generic: Didanosine DR
Dosing recommendations	**300 mg q12h;** 200 mg q8h	**150 mg q12h; 300 mg q24h** (dosage based on weight for pediatrics)	**300 mg q12h; 600 mg q24h**	>60 kg: **400 mg q24h;** with TDF ↓ddI to 250 mg; <60 kg: 250 mg q24h; with TDF: appropriate ddI dose not known
Food effect	Take without regard to meals	Take without regard to meals	Take without regard to meals	Take $1/_2$ h before or 2 h after meals
Adverse events	**Bone marrow suppression (macrocytic anemia or neutropenia); GI intolerance,** headache, insomnia, asthenia	Minimal toxicity	**Hypersensitivity reaction can be fatal; symptoms include rash, fever,** nausea/vomiting, malaise or fatigue, loss of appetite; respiratory symptoms include sore throat, cough, shortness of breath	**Pancreatitis, peripheral neuropathy,** nausea, diarrhea
Drug interactions	Ribavirin, stavudine, methadone; with high dose: ganciclovir, TMP-SMX, other medications that can cause bone marrow suppression	No clinically significant drug interactions	Alcohol increases abacavir levels by 41%	Methadone, ribavirin, tenofovir, ganciclovir, alcohol; medications that need acidic environment for absorption—buffered forms; use caution with other meds that can cause peripheral neuropathy
Monitoring[2]	CBC, LFTs	None necessary	Signs and symptoms of hypersensitivity reaction	CBC, LFTs, amylase, uric acid; signs and symptoms of above side effects

(continued)

Bold type highlights the most common dosing and important side effects.

1 Combivir: zidovudine 300 mg + lamivudine 150 mg; 1 tablet q12h

   Trizivir: zidovudine 300 mg + lamivudine 150 mg + abacavir 300 mg; 1 tablet q12h

   Epzicom: abacavir 600 mg + lamivudine 300 mg; 1 tablet q24h

2 Monitor all for signs and symptoms of NRTI class toxicities, lactic acidosis, and hepatic steatosis.

- Efavirenz is contraindicated in pregnancy.
- Usually use one NNRTI in combination with two NRTIs.
- No special storage requirements are necessary for drugs in this class.
- Drug interactions: all are cytochrome P450 (CYP450)-3A4 inducers and/or inhibitors; see Tables 6 and 7.

Protease Inhibitors (PIs) (Table 8)

Mechanism of action

- PIs inhibit protease, which then prevents the cleavage of HIV polyproteins and subsequently induces the formation of immature noninfectious viral particles.
- All should be dose-adjusted for hepatic impairment.
- Most should be taken with food (except amprenavir and indinavir).

Table 4

Characteristics of Nucleoside Reverse Transcriptase Inhibitors (NRTIs) (continued)

Generic name [trade name]	Stavudine (d4T) [Zerit®]	Zalcitabine (ddC) [Hivid®]	Tenofovir (TDF) [Viread®]	Emtricitabine (FTC) [Emtriva®]
Form	15, 20, 30, 40 mg caps	0.375, 0.75 mg tabs; will no longer be manufactured by the end of 2006	300 mg tabs; also available in combination products[1]	200 mg tabs; also available in combination products[1]
Dosing recommendations	>60 kg: **40 mg q12h**; <60 kg: 30 mg q12h	**0.75 mg q8h**	**300 mg q24h**	**200 mg q24h**
Food effect	Take without regard to meals	Take without regard to meals	Take without regard to meals	Take without regard to meals
Adverse events	**Pancreatitis; peripheral neuropathy;** lipodystrophy, hyperlipidemia; rapidly progressive ascending neusomuscular weakness (rare)	**Pancreatitis, peripheral neuropathy,** stomatitis	**Renal insufficiency,** asthenia, headache, diarrhea, nausea/vomiting, flatulence	Minimal toxicity; hyperpigmentation of palms of hands and soles of feet (rare)
Drug interactions	Use with caution with other medications that can cause peripheral neuropathy	Use with caution with other medications that can cause peripheral neuropathy	Didanosine, atazanavir, cidofovir, ganciclovir, valganciclovir	No clinically significant drug interactions
Monitoring	Signs and symptoms of above side effects	Signs and symptoms of above side effects	Renal function	None necessary

Bold type highlights the most common dosing and important side effects.

1 Truvada: tenofovir 300 mg + emtricitabine 200 mg; 1 tablet q24h

  Atripla – Tenofovir 300 mg + emtricitabine 200 mg + efavirenz 600 mg; 1 tablet q24h at bedtime

2 Monitor all for signs and symptoms of NRTI class toxicities, lactic acidosis, and hepatic steatosis; higher incidence with stavudine than with other NRTIs.

- Amprenavir and fosamprenavir are chemically similar and should not be used in the same regimen
- Atazanavir and indinavir require normal acid levels in the stomach for absorption.
- Ritonavir is the most potent inhibitor in the class and is primarily used for intensification of other PIs.
- Lopinavir/ritonavir, ritonavir, and saquinavir soft gel caps require refrigeration.
- Goals of intensification:
  * Decrease pill burden
  * Decrease frequency of doses (ie, decrease from q8h to q12h)
- Class toxicities:
  * Lipodystrophy
  * Hyperglycemia
  * Hyperlipidemia
  * Hypertriglyceridemia
  * Bleeding in hemophiliacs
  * Osteonecrosis and avascular necrosis of the hips
  * Ostcopenia and ostcoporosis
- PI monitoring (baseline is 4-6 weeks after starting PI and every 3-6 months thereafter):
  * Glucose
  * LFTs
  * Total cholesterol panel (particularly triglycerides)
  * GI side effects
  * Signs and symptoms of bone pain (particularly hip pain)
  * Signs and symptoms of fat redistribution
- Usually use one PI in combination with two NRTIs
- All are CYP450-3A4 inhibitors (ie, drug interactions are typical of CYP450-3A4 inhibitors); see Tables 9 and 10.

Table 5

Characteristics of Non-Nucleoside Reverse Transcriptase Inhibitors (NNRTIs)

Generic name [trade name]	Efavirenz (EFV) [Sustiva®]	Nevirapine (NVP) [Viramune®]	Delavirdine (DLV) [Rescriptor®]
Form	50, 100, 200 mg caps; 600 mg tabs; Also available in combination product[1]	200 mg tab; 10 mg/mL oral suspension	100, 200 mg tabs
Dosing recommendations	**600 mg q24hs at bedtime**	**200 mg q24h x 14 d, then 200 mg q12h (note CD4 cell count)[2]**	**400 mg q8h**
Food effect	Take on an empty stomach	Take without regard to meals	Take without regard to meals
Adverse events	**CNS side effects[3]**; rash[4], ↑LFTs, false-positive cannabinoid test, teratogenic in monkeys	**Rash[4], symptomatic hepatitis, including fatal hepatic necrosis have been reported**	**Rash[4]**, ↑ **LFTs,** headaches
Drug interactions	CYP450-3A4, -2C19 inhibitor and -3A4 inducer (see Tables 6 and 7)	CYP450-3A4 inducer (see Tables 6 and 7)	CYP450-3A4 and -2D6 inhibitor (see Tables 6 and 7); separate dosing with buffered ddI or antacids by 1 hour
Monitoring[5]	CNS side effects, LFTs, rash	LFTs 2, 4, and 6 weeks, and then monthly for the first 18 weeks	LFTs, rash

Bold type highlights the most common dosing and important side effects.

[1] Atripla - tenofovir 300 mg + emtricitabine 200 mg + efavarenz 600 mg - one tablet q24h at bedtime

[2] Due to the increased risk of symptomatic hepatic events, nevirapine should not be started in women with baseline CD4 cell counts of greater than 250 cells/mm^3 or men with baseline CD4 cell counts greater than 400 cells/mm^3

[3] CNS side effects include: dizziness, somnolence, insomnia, abnormal dreams, confusion, abnormal thinking, impaired concentration, amnesia, agitation, depersonalization, hallucinations and euphoria. Use caution in patients with a psychiatric history or previous addictions.

[4] Rare cases of Stevens-Johnson syndrome have been reported with the use of NNRTIs, the highest incidence seen with nevirapine use.

[5] Monitor all for signs and symptoms of NNRTI class toxicities, rash and hepatic toxicity

Table 6

Drugs That Should Not Be Used with NNRTIs

Drug category	Nevirapine	Delavirdine	Efavirenz
Calcium channel blockers	None	None	None
Cardiac	None	None	None
Lipid-lowering agents	None	Simvastatin, lovastatin	None
Antimycobacterial	Rifampin, rifapentine	Rifampin, rifapentine, rifabutin	Rifapentine
Antihistamine	None	Astemizole, terfenadine	Astemizole, terfenadine
Gastrointestinal drugs	None	Cisapride, H$_2$-blockers, proton pump inhibitors	Cisapride
Psychotropics	None	Alprazolam, midazolam, triazolam	Midazolam, triazolam
Ergot alkaloids (vasoconstrictor)	None	Ergotamine derivatives	Ergotamine derivatives
Herbs	St. John's wort	St. John's wort	St. John's wort
Other		Amprenavir, fosamprenavir, carbamazepine, phenobarbital, phenytoin	Voriconazole

Table 7

Drug Interactions with NNRTIs Requiring Dose Modifications or Cautious Use

Drugs affected	Nevirapine (NVP)	Delavirdine (DLV)	Efavirenz (EFV)
Antifungals			
Ketoconazole (keto)	Levels: keto ↓63%; NVP ↑15-30%; dose: not recommended	DLV C_{min} ↑50%; keto levels: no data; dose: standard	No data
Voriconazole (vori)	Metabolism of vori may be induced by NVP; vori may inhibit NNRTI metabolism; frequently monitor for NNRTI toxicity and antifungal outcome	Metabolism of vori may be inhibited by DLV; vori may inhibit NNRTI metabolism; frequently monitor for NNRTI toxicity and antifungal outcome	Levels: EFV ↑44%; vori: ↓77%; dose: not recommended
Fluconazole (flu)	Levels: NVP ↑100%; flu: no change; risk of hepatotoxicity may increase with this combination; if concomitant use is necessary, recommend monitoring of NVP toxicity	No clinically significant changes in DLV or flu concentrations	No clinically significant changes in DLV or flu concentrations
Antimycobacterials			
Rifampin	Levels: NVP ↓20-58%; virologic consequences are uncertain; the potential for additive hepatotoxicity exists; use of this combination is not recommended; however, if used, coadministration should be done with careful monitoring	Levels: DLV ↓96%; contraindicated	Levels: EFV ↓25%; dose: consider ↑EFV to 800 mg q24h
Rifabutin	Levels: NVP ↓16%; no dose adjustments[1]	Levels: DLV ↓80%; rifabutin ↑100%; dose: not recommended	Levels: EFV unchanged; rifabutin ↓35%; dose: ↑ rifabutin dose to 450-600 mg qd or 600 mg 3 x per wk; EFV dose standard
Clarithromycin (clarithro)	Levels: NVP ↑26%; clarithro ↓30%; monitor for efficacy or use alternative agent	Levels: DLV ↓44% clarithro ↑100%; dose adjust for renal failure	Levels: clarithro ↓39%; monitor for efficacy or use alternative agent
Oral contraceptives	Levels: ethinyl estradiol (EE) ↓20%; use alternative or additional birth control methods	Levels: EE may increase; clinical significance unknown	Levels: EE ↑37%; no data on other component; use alternative or additional birth control methods
Lipid-lowering agents			
Simvastatin (simva), lovastatin	No data	Potential for large increase in statin levels; avoid concomitant use	Levels: simva AUC ↓ 58%; EFV unchanged; dose: adjust simva dose according to lipid responses, not to exceed the maximum simva dose
Atorvastatin (atorva)	No data	Potential for inhibition of atorva metabolism; use lowest dose and monitor for toxicity	Levels: atorva AUC ↓ 58%; EFV unchanged; adjust atorva dose according to lipid responses, not to exceed the maximum atorva dose

(continued)

[1]These recommendations apply to regimens that do not include PIs, which can substantially increase rifabutin levels.

Table 7

Drug Interactions with NNRTIs Requiring Dose Modifications or Cautious Use (continued)

Drugs affected	Nevirapine (NVP)	Delavirdine (DLV)	Efavirenz (EFV)
Anticonvulsants			
Phenobarbital, phenytoin, carbamazepine	Unknown; use with caution; monitor anticonvulsant levels	Levels: DLV C_{min} ↓90%; contraindicated	Use with caution; monitor anticonvulsant levels
Methadone	Levels: NVP unchanged, methadone ↓ significantly; ↑ methadone dose often necessary	Levels: DLV unchanged; methadone: no data; potential for ↑ methadone levels; monitor for toxicity; may require dose reduction	Levels: methadone ↓60%; ↑ methadone dose often necessary; titrate methadone dose to effect
Miscellaneous	No data	May ↑ levels of dapsone, warfarin, quinidine; sildenafil: vardenafil, tadalafil	Monitor warfarin when used concomitantly

Table 8

Characteristics of Protease Inhibitors (PIs)

Generic name [trade name]	Lopinavir + ritonavir (LPV/r) [Kaletra®]	Nelfinavir (NFV) [Viracept®]	Atazanavir (ATV) [Reyataz®]
Form	200 mg lopinavir + 100 mg ritonavir tabs; 400 mg lopinavir + 100 mg ritonavir per 5 mL oral solution500 mg q 12h with ritonavir 200 mg q 12h	250, 625 mg tabs; 50 mg/g oral powder	100, 150, 200 mg caps
Dosing recommendations	400 mg lopinavir + 100 mg ritonavir q 12h; 800 mg lopinavir + 200 mg ritonavir q 24h	1250 mg q 12h; 750 mg q 8h	400 mg q day; ATV 300 mg + RTV 100 mg q 24h
Food effect	Tab – No food effect Liquid - Take with food	Take with food	Take with food
Adverse events[1]	GI intolerance, asthenia, ↑ LFTs	Diarrhea	Increased indirect hyperbilirubinemia, prolonged PR interval-some patients experienced asymptomatic 1st degree AV block, use with caution in patients with underlying conduction defects or on concomitant medications that can cause PR prolongation
Drug interactions	CYP450 3A4 inhibitor and substrate, see tables 10 and 11	CYP450 3A4 inhibitor and substrate, see tables 10 and 11	CYP450 3A4 inhibitor and substrate, see tables 10 and 11
Storage	Tabs – Room temperature Refrigerated liquid stable until date on label; stable for 2 months at room temperature	Room temperature	Room temperature
Additional information	Oral solution contains 42% alcohol	Needs 500 kcal of food for absorption; take after eating; boosting with RTV not effective	Reduced incidence of hyperlipidemia, must use boosted regimen with tenofovir or efavirenz, needs normal GI acid concentrations for absorption

Bold type highlights the most common dosing and important side effects.

1 PI class side effects: lipodystrophy, hyperglycemia, hyperlipidemia, hypertriglyceridemia, bleeding in hemophiliacs, osteonecrosis and avascular necrosis of the hips, osteopenia and osteoporosis

Table 8

Characteristics of Protease Inhibitors (PIs)

Generic name [trade name]	Fosamprenavir (f-APV) [Lexiva®]	Amprenavir (APV) [Agenerase®]	Saquinavir (SQV) SQV-hard gel cap (HGC) [Invirase®]	Darunavir (TMC-114) [Prezista®]
Form	700 mg tab	50 mg cap, 15 mg/mL oral solution	200 mg cap, 500 mg tab	300 mg tabs
Dosing recommendations	ART naïve patients: f-APV 1,400 mg q 12h; or **f-APV 1,400 mg + RTV 200 mg q day**; or f-APV 700 mg + RTV 100 mg q 12h PI experienced patients: **f-APV 700 mg + RTV 100 mg q 12h**	1,400 mg q 12h (oral solution) – Do not take with RTV oral solution	**SQV 1,000 mg + RTV 100 mg q 12 h** – Invirase is not recommended as a single PI	600 mg q 12h with ritonavir 100 mg q 12h
Food effect	With or without food	With or without food, avoid high fat meal	Take with food	Take with food
Adverse events[1]	**Skin rash**, GI intolerance, headache	**GI intolerance, skin rash**, oral paresthesias, ↑LFTs	**GI intolerance**, headache, ↑LFTs	Diarrhea, nausea, headache nasopharyngitis, rash, ↑pancreatic amylase (significance unknown)
Drug interactions	CYP450 3A4 inhibitor, inducer and substrate, see Tables 10 and 11	CYP450 3A4 inhibitor, inducer and substrate, see Tables 10 and 11	CYP450 3A4 inhibitor, and substrate, see Tables 10 and 11	CYP 450 3A4 inhibitor and substrate
Storage	Room temperature	Room temperature	Room temperature	Room temperature
Additional information	Sulfonamide, caution in patients with history of sulfa allergy, caps and solution are not equivalent, oral solution contains propylene glycol[2]	Sulfonamide, caution in patients with history of sulfa allergy	Invirase is not recommended as a single PI, always boost Fortovase will no longer be manufactured by the end of 2006.	TMC-114 has a sulfonamide moiety, use with caution in patients with known sulfonamide allergy

---

Bold type highlights the most common dosing and important side effects.

[1] PI class side effects: lipodystrophy, hyperglycemia, hyperlipidemia, hypertriglyceridemia, bleeding in hemophiliacs, osteonecrosis and avascular necrosis of the hips, osteopenia and osteoporosis.   [2] Contraindicated in pregnant women, children <4 years old, patients with hepatic or renal failure, and patients treated with disulfiram or metronidazole.

(continued)

Table 8

Characteristics of Protease Inhibitors (PIs) (continued)

Generic name [trade name]	Tipranavir (TPV) [Aptivus®]	Ritonavir (RTV) [Norvir®]	Indinavir (IDV) [Crixivan®]
Form	250 mg caps	100 mg caps; 600 mg/7.5 mL oral solution	200, 333, 400 mg caps
Dosing recommendations	500 mg q 12h with ritonavir 200 mg q 12h	100-400 mg with other PIs for intensification; 600 mg q 12h as single PI	800 mg q 8h or 800 mg IDV + 100-200 mg RTV q 12h
Food effect	Take with food	Take with food	Take 1 h before or 2 h after meals; may take with skim milk or low fat meal, when boosting can take with or without food
Adverse events[1]	**Hepatotoxicity, skin rash,** intracranial hemorrhage (rare), inhibits human platelet aggregation, ↑PT and pTT in rodents	**GI intolerance,** paresthesias, hepatitis, pancreatitis, asthenia, taste perversion	**Nephrolithiasis,** GI intolerance, ↑bilirubinemia, headache, asthenia, blurred vision, dizziness, rash, metallic taste, thrombocytopenia, alopecia, hemolytic anemia
Drug interactions	CYP450 3A4 inducer and substrate Net effect when combined with RTV – CYP 3A4 and 2D6 inhibitor	CYP450 3A4, 2D6 inhibitor	CYP450 3A4 inhibitor
Storage	Refrigerated caps stable until date on label; stable for 60 days at room temperature	Refrigerated caps stable until date on label; stable for 1 month at room temperature	Room temperature
Additional information	Clinical hepatitis including hepatic decompensation has been reported, monitor closely, esp. in patients with underlying liver diseases. TPV has a sulfonamide moiety, use with caution in patients with known sulfonamide allergy Fourteen intracrainial hemorrhage (ICH) events including 8 fatalities have been reported. Many ICH patients had other medical conditions increasing risk.	Primary role is in intensification of other PIs, most potent CYP450 inhibitor in the class, when used as a single PI dose should be titrated to above target dose	Patients should drink ≥ 48 oz of H₂O daily to reduce incidence of kidney stones; boosted indinavir increases incidence of kidney stones, requires additional monitoring for signs and symptoms of kidney stones, indirect bilirubin and platelets

Bold type highlights the most common dosing and important side effects.

[1]PI class side effects: lipodystrophy, hyperglycemia, hyperlipidemia, hypertriglyceridemia, bleeding in hemophiliacs, osteonecrosis and avascular necrosis of the hips, osteopenia and osteoporosis

- Entry inhibitors include enfuvirtide (T20), Fuzeon®
  * Mechanism of action: binds to gp41 on HIV surface, which inhibits HIV binding to CD4 cell
  * Dose: 90 mg SC q12h
  * Side effects: injection-site reactions, increased rate of bacterial pneumonia, hypersensitivity
- Generally reserved for deep salvage regimens
- Preferably should be used with at least two other active drugs
- Resistance develops quickly with less potent regimens and in cases of poor adherence.

- No known significant drug interactions seen to date.
- Take without regard to meals.
- Store at room temperature; reconstituted form should be stored in the refrigerator, where it will be stable for 24 hours.

Counseling
- All patients should be counseled on the importance of adherence.
  * >95% adherence is necessary to decrease the incidence of resistance.

Table 9

Drugs That Should Not Be Used with PIs

Drug category	Indinavir	Ritonavir	Saquinavir	Darunavir	Tipranavir
Calcium channel blockers	None	Bepridil	None	None	Bepridil
Cardiac	Amiodarone	Amiodarone, flecainide, propafenone, quinidine	None	None	Amiodarone, flecainide, propafenone, quinidine
Lipid-lowering agents	Simvastatin, lovastatin	Simvastatin, lovastatin	Simvastatin, lovastatin	Simvastatin, lovastatin	Simvastatin, lovastatin
Antimycobacterial	Rifampin, rifapentine	Rifapentine	Rifampin, rifabutin, rifapentine	Rifampin	Rifampin, rifapentine
Antihistamine	Astemizole, terfenadine	Astemizole, terfenadine	Astemizole, terfenadine	Astemizole, terfenadine	Astemizole, terfenadine
Gastrointestinal drugs	Cisapride	Cisapride	Cisapride	Cisapride	Cisapride
Neuroleptic	Pimozide	Pimozide	Pimozide	Pimozide	Pimozide
Psychotropic	Midazolam, triazolam	Midazolam, triazolam	Midazolam, triazolam	Midazolam, triazolam	Midazolam, triazolam
Ergot alkaloids (vasoconstrictor)	Ergot derivatives	Ergot derivatives	Ergot derivatives	Ergot derivatives	Ergot derivatives
Herbs	St. John's wort	St. John's wort	St. John's wort	St. John's wort	St. John's wort
Other	Atazanavir	Voriconazole (with RTV ≥400 mg bid), fluticasone, alfuzosin		Carbamazepine, phenobarbital, phenytoin	Fluticasone

(continued)

Antiretroviral Therapy in the HIV-Infected Pregnant Woman

- Highly active antiretroviral therapy (HAART) should be offered if the patient is not already receiving treatment.
    * Efavirenz should be avoided.
    * Avoid combining stavudine and didanosine.
    * Consider starting treatment after the first trimester.
- Continue current combination regimens (preferably with zidovudine) if the patient is already receiving therapy (decreases the risk of transmission from 30 to 2.5%).
- Zidovudine alone can decrease risk of transmission when taken during pregnancy. The mother should also receive IV zidovudine during labor; the infant should receive 6 weeks of zidovudine (Table 11).
- Single-dose nevirapine at onset of labor in women who have had no prior antiretroviral therapy and given once to the infant between 48 and 72 hours of age, has been shown to decrease the transmission rate. This can also result in resistance to nevirapine if used in future regimens.

Postexposure Prophylaxis (PEP) (Table 12)

- Use universal precautions.
- The most common infectious exposure is needle-sticks or cuts (1 in 300 risk).
- The risk with mucous membrane exposure is much lower (1 in 1000 risk).
- There have been 52 documented cases of occupationally-acquired HIV infection.
- Postexposure prophylaxis can reduce HIV infection by about 80%.
- Start therapy within 1-2 hours of exposure.
- Length of therapy is 4 weeks.

Postexposure Prophylaxis After Sexual, Injection-Drug Use, or Other Nonoccupational Exposure to HIV (nPEP)

- Patients with exposure to HIV from a known positive source should receive nPEP.
- nPEP should be started within 72 hours of the exposure.

- Patients should be given tools to facilitate adherence to complicated regimens (eg, pill boxes, calendars, pagers, etc).
- Patients should be counseled on class side effects, especially any that are unique or potentially serious.

Table 9

Drugs That Should Not Be Used with PIs (continued)

Drug category	Nelfinavir	Amprenavir Fosamprenavir	Lopinavir/ ritonavir	Atazanavir
Calcium channel blockers	None	Bepridil	None	Bepridil
Cardiac	None	None	Flecainide, propafenone	None
Lipid-lowering agents	Simvastatin, lovastatin	Simvastatin, lovastatin	Simvastatin, lovastatin	Simvastatin, lovastatin
Antimycobacterial	Rifampin, rifapentine	Rifampin, rifapentine	Rifampin, rifapentine	Rifampin, rifapentine
Antihistamine	Astemizole, terfenadine	Astemizole, terfenadine	Astemizole, terfenadine	Astemizole, terfenadine
Gastrointestinal drugs	Cisapride	Cisapride	Cisapride	Cisapride, proton pump inhibitors
Neuroleptic	Pimozide	Pimozide	Pimozide	Pimozide
Psychotropic	Midazolam, triazolam	Midazolam, triazolam	Midazolam, triazolam	Midazolam, triazolam
Ergot alkaloids (vasoconstrictor)	Ergot derivatives	Ergot derivatives	Ergot derivatives	Ergot derivatives
Herbs	St. John's Wort	St. John's Wort	St. John's Wort	St. John's Wort
Other		Delavirdine, oral contraceptives	Fluticasone	Indinavir, irinotecan

- The length of therapy is 28 days.
- Treatment options are the same as those listed on the DHHS guidelines for initial regimens (see Table 2).

Opportunistic Infections

- Only two opportunistic infections require primary prophylaxis:
  - * *Pneumocystis carinii* pneumonia (PCP)
    - When CD4$^+$ cells fall below 200/mm^3
    - The treatment of choice is trimethoprim-sulfamethoxazole (TMP-SMX) DS PO qd (see Table 13 for alternatives).
  - * *Mycobacterium avium* complex bacteremia (MAC)
    - When CD4$^+$ cells fall below 50/mm^3
    - Treatment of choice is azithromycin 1200 mg PO every week
- All other primary prophylaxis occurs only if the patient is antigen-positive and at high risk of exposure to the causative factor.
- All other opportunistic infections are treated when the patient is diagnosed.
- After treatment, patients receive suppressive therapy.
- Some primary and secondary prophylaxis could possibly be discontinued with immune reconstitution (undetectable viral load and an increase in CD4 cells in response to HAART therapy; see Table 13).

3. Prevention

- Abstain from sex with an infected person.
- Ask about the sexual history of current and future sex partners.
- Reduce the number of sex partners to minimize the risk of HIV infection.
- Always use a latex condom from start to finish during any type of sex (vaginal, anal, or oral).
- Use only water-based lubricants.
- Avoid alcohol, illicit drugs, and sharing of needles (or syringes, cookers, or other drug paraphernalia).
- Do not share personal items such as toothbrushes, razors, or any devices used during sex. Such items may be contaminated by blood, semen, or vaginal secretions.
- Do not donate blood, plasma, sperm, body organs, or tissues if you are infected with HIV or have engaged in sex or needle-sharing behaviors that are risk factors for infection with HIV.

Table 10

Drug Interactions with PIs Requiring Dose Modifications or Cautious Use

Drugs affected	Indinavir (IDV)	Ritonavir (RTV)	Saquinavir (SQV)
Antifungals			
Itraconazole (itra)	Levels: IDV ↑	No data, but potential for bi-directional inhibition between itra and RTV; monitor for toxicities	Bi-directional interaction between itra and SQV has been observed
Ketoconazole (keto)	Levels: IDV ↑68%	Levels: keto ↓ 3x	Levels: SQV ↑ 3x
Voriconazole (vori)	No changes in levels of either drug	Levels: vori AUC ↓ 82% when coadministered with 400 mg bid of RTV; concomitant therapy contraindicated	No data, but potential for bi-directional inhibition between vori and PIs; monitor for toxicities
Antimycobacterials			
Rifampin	Contraindicated	Levels: RTV ↓35%; dose: no change; ↑ liver toxicity possible	Levels: SQV ↓84%; contraindicated
Rifabutin	Levels: IDV ↓ 32%; rifabutin ↑ 2x; dose: ↓ rifabutin to 150 mg qd or 300 mg 3 x per week; IDV 1000 mg q8h	Levels: rifabutin ↑ 4x; dose: ↓ rifabutin to 150 mg qd or 300 mg 3x/week	Levels: SQV ↓40%; contraindicated unless using SQV/RTV; dose: ↓ rifabutin to 150 mg qd or 300 mg 3x/week
Clarithromycin (clarithro)	Levels: clarithro ↑53%; no dose adjustment	Levels: clarithro ↑77%; dose: adjust dose for moderate and severe renal impairment	Levels: clarithro ↑45%; SQV ↑177%; no dose adjustment
Oral contraceptives	Levels: norethindrone ↑26%, ethinyl estradiol ↑24%; no dose adjustment	Levels: ethinyl estradiol ↓40%; use alternative or additional method	No data
Lipid-lowering agents			
Simvastatin, lovastatin	Levels: potential for large increase in statin levels; avoid concomitant use	Levels: potential for large increase in statin levels; avoid concomitant use	Levels: potential for large increase in statin levels; avoid concomitant use
Atorvastatin (atorva)	Use lowest possible starting dose of atorva with careful monitoring	Use lowest possible starting dose of atorva with careful monitoring	Use lowest possible starting dose of atorva with careful monitoring
Pravastatin (prava)	No data	Adjust prava dose based on lipid response	Levels: ↓50% when administered with SQV/RTV
Anticonvulsants			
Phenobarbital, phenytoin, carbamazepine	Carbamazepine ↓ IDV	↑ Carbamazepine levels	All may ↓ SQV levels
Methadone	No change in methadone levels	↓ Methadone levels	↓ Methadone levels
Erectile dysfunction agents			
Sildenafil	Sildenafil AUC ↑ 3-fold; use with caution and lowest dose	Sildenafil AUC ↑ 11-fold; use with caution and lowest dose	Sildenafil AUC ↑ 2-fold; use with caution and lowest dose
Vardenafil	Vardenafil AUC ↑ 16-fold; use with caution and lowest dose	Vardenafil AUC ↑ 49-fold; use with caution and lowest dose	No data but same interaction as with other PIs is suspected; use with caution and lowest dose
Tadalafil	Tadalafil AUC ↑ substantially; use with caution and lowest dose	Tadalafil AUC ↑ 124%; use with caution and lowest dose	Tadalafil AUC ↑ substantially; use with caution and lowest dose
Miscellaneous	Grapefruit juice ↓ IDV levels 26%; vitamin C ≥1 g/d ↓ IDV levels; amlodipine AUC ↑ 90%	Many possible interactions; desipramine ↑145%; trazodone AUC ↑ 2.4-fold; theophylline ↓47%; ↑ oral or nasal fluticasone	Grapefruit juice ↑ SQV levels; dexamethasone ↓ SQV levels

(continued)

Table 10

Drug Interactions with PIs Requiring Dose Modifications or Cautious Use (continued)

Drugs affected	Nelfinavir (NFV)	Amprenavir (APV)	Fosamprenavir (f-APV)
Antifungals			
Itraconazole (itra)	No data, but potential for bi-directional inhibition between itra and PIs; monitor for toxicities	No data, but potential for bi-directional inhibition between itra and PIs; monitor for toxicities	No data, but potential for bi-directional inhibition between itra and PIs; monitor for toxicities
Ketoconazole (keto)	No dose adjustment necessary	Levels: keto ↑44%; APV ↑31%	Presumably similar interactions as with APV
Voriconazole (vori)	No data, but potential for bi-directional inhibition between vora and PIs; monitor for toxicities	No data, but potential for bi-directional inhibition between vora and PIs; monitor for toxicities	No data, but potential for bi-directional inhibition between vora and PIs; monitor for toxicities
Antimycobacterials			
Rifampin	Contraindicated	Contraindicated	Contraindicated
Rifabutin	Rifabutin ↑ 2x; dose: ↓ rifabutin to 150 mg qd or 300 mg 3x/week; NFV 1250 mg q12h	Levels: rifabutin ↑193%; dose: ↓ rifabutin to 150 mg qd or 300 mg 3x/week	Presumably similar interactions as with APV
Clarithromycin (clarithro)	No data	No dose adjustment	Presumably similar interactions as with APV
Oral contraceptives	Levels: norethindrone ↓18%, ethinyl estradiol ↓47%; use alternative or additional method	Levels: ↑ levels of ethinyl estradiol and norethindrone; APV levels ↓20%; use alternative method	Presumably similar interactions as with APV
Lipid-lowering agents			
Simvastatin, lovastatin	Levels: potential for large increase in statin level; avoid concomitant use	Levels: potential for large increase in statin level; avoid concomitant use	Levels: potential for large increase in statin level; avoid concomitant use
Atorvastatin (atorva)	Use lowest possible starting dose of atorva with careful monitoring	Use lowest possible starting dose of atorva with careful monitoring	Use lowest possible starting dose of atorva with careful monitoring
Pravastatin (prava)	No data	No data	No data
Anticonvulsants			
Phenobarbital, phenytoin, carbamazepine	Unknown, but may ↓ NFV levels substantially	Unknown, but may ↓ APV levels substantially	Unknown, but may ↓ f-APV levels substantially
Methadone	↓ Methadone levels	↓ Methadone levels	↓ Methadone levels
Erectile dysfunction agents			
Sildenafil	Sildenafil AUC ↑ 2- to 11-fold; use with caution and lowest dose	Sildenafil AUC ↑ 2- to 11-fold; use with caution and lowest dose	Presumably similar interactions as with APV
Vardenafil	No data, but vardenafil AUC may be substantially ↑ ; use with caution and lowest dose	No data, but vardenafil AUC may be substantially ↑ ; use with caution and lowest dose	Presumably similar interactions as with APV
Tadalafil	Tadalafil AUC ↑ substantially; use with caution and lowest dose	Tadalafil AUC ↑ substantially; use with caution and lowest dose	Presumably similar interactions as with APV

(continued)

Table 10

Drug Interactions with PIs Requiring Dose Modifications or Cautious Use (continued)

Drugs affected	Atazanavir (ATV)	Lopinavir (LPV)
Antifungals		
Itraconazole (itra)	No data, but potential for bi-directional inhibition between itra and PIs; monitor for toxicities	Levels: ↑ itra
Ketoconazole (keto)	No dose adjustment necessary	Levels: keto ↑ 3-fold; LPV AUC ↓ 13%
Voriconazole (vori)	No data, but potential for bi-directional inhibition between vori and PIs; monitor for toxicities	No data, but potential for bi-directional inhibition between vora and PIs; monitor for toxicities
Antimycobacterials		
Rifampin	Contraindicated	Contraindicated
Rifabutin	Rifabutin AUC ↑ 2.5-fold; dose: ↓ rifabutin to 150 mg qd or 300 mg 3x/week; NFV 1250 mg q12h	Levels: rifabutin AUC ↑ 3-fold; dose: ↓ rifabutin to 150 mg qd or 300 mg 3x/week
Clarithromycin (clarithro)	Clarithro AUC ↑94%; may cause QT prolongation; ↓ dose 50%	Clarithro AUC ↑ 77%; adjust clarithro dose for moderate to severe renal impairment
Oral contraceptives	Levels: norethindrone AUC ↑110%, ethinyl estradiol ↑48%; use alternative or additional method	Levels: ↑ ethinyl estradiol 42%; use alternative or additional method
Lipid-lowering agents		
Simvastatin, lovastatin	Levels: potential for large increase in statin level; avoid concomitant use	Levels: potential for large increase in statin level; avoid concomitant use
Atorvastatin (atorva)	Use lowest possible starting dose of atorva with careful monitoring	Use lowest possible starting dose of atorva with careful monitoring
Pravastatin (prava)	No data	No dosage adjustment necessary
Anticonvulsants		
Phenobarbital, phenytoin, carbamazepine	Unknown, but may ↓ ATV levels substantially	Avoid concomitatnt use or monitor LPV level
Methadone	No change in methadone levels	↓ Methadone levels
Erectile dysfunction agents		
Sildenafil	Sildenafil levels ↑; use with caution and lowest dose	Sildenafil AUC ↑ 11-fold; use with caution and lowest dose
Vardenafil	No data, but vardenafil AUC may be substantially ↑; use with caution and lowest dose	No data, but vardenafil AUC may be substantially ↑; use with caution and lowest dose
Tadalafil	Tadalafil AUC ↑ substantially; use with caution and lowest dose	Tadalafil AUC ↑ substantially; use with caution and lowest dose
Miscellaneous	Diltiazem AUC ↑ 125%; caution with other calcium channel blockers; contraindicated with irinotecan; separate from H_2-blockers by 12 hours; separate from antacids (give ATV 2 hours before or 1 hour after antacids)	

(continued)

Table 10

Drug Interactions with PIs Requiring Dose Modifications or Cautious Use (continued)

Drugs affected	Tipranavir (TPV)
Antifungals	
Itraconazole (itra)	No data. Use with caution; do not exceed 200 mg itraconazole daily.
Ketoconazole (keto)	No data. Use with caution; do not exceed 200 mg ketoconazole daily.
Voriconazole (vori)	Potential for bi-directional inhibition between voriconazole and PIs exists. Voriconazole AUC ↓ 39% with RTV 100 mg BID; interaction between TPV and voriconazole unknown. Co-administration is not recommended unless the benefit outweighs the risk.
Antimycobacterials	
Rifampin	No data; should not be coadministered
Rifabutin	Levels: Rifabutin AUC ↑ 2.9 fold
	Dose: ↓ rifabutin to 150 mg qod or 3x/week
Clarithromycin (clarithro)	Levels: TPV ↑ 66%, clarithromycin ↑ 19%, 14-hydroxy-clarithromycin metabolite ↓ 97%.
	Dose: No adjustment for patients with normal renal function; reduce clarithromycin dose by 50% for CrCl 30-60 mL/min; reduce clarithromycin dose by 75% for CrCl < 30 mL/min.
Oral contraceptives	Levels: ↓ ethinyl estradiol Cmax and ↓ AUC 50%.
	Use alternative or additional method. Women on estrogen may have ↑ risk of non-serious rash.
Lipid-lowering agents	
Simvastatin, lovastatin	Levels: Potential for large increase in statin level. Avoid concomitant use.
Atorvastatin (atorva)	Levels: atorvastatin AUC ↑ 9 fold. Use lowest possible starting dose of atorvastatin with careful monitoring.
Pravastatin (prava)	No data
Anticonvulsants	
Phenobarbital, phenytoin, carbamazepine	No data. Consider alternative anticonvulsant. Monitor anticonvulsant levels and consider obtaining TPV levels.
Methadone	No data. Dosage of methadone may need to be increased when co-administered with TPV/r.
Erectile dysfunction agents	
Sildenafil	No data. Starting dose should not exceed 25 mg sildenafil within 48 hours.
Vardenafil	No data. Starting dose should not exceed 2.5 mg vardenafil every 72 hours.
Tadalafil	No data. Starting dose should not exceed 10 mg tadalafil every 72 hours.
Miscellaneous	Abacavir ↓ 35-44%. Appropriate doses for combination of ABC and TPV/r have not been established.
	Zidovudine ↓ 31-43%. Appropriate doses for the combination of ZDV and TPV/r have not been established.
	Loperamide ↓ 51%. TPV Cmin ↓ 26% with loperamide
	Antacids ↓ TPV ~30%, TPV should be administered 2 hrs before or 1 hour after antacids.
	Fluconazole: Doses > 200 mg/day are not recommended to be given with TPV.
	TPV capsules contain alcohol. Avoid use of disulfiram and metronidazole.

(continued)

Table 10

Drug Interactions with PIs Requiring Dose Modifications or Cautious Use (continued)

Drugs affected	Darunavir (TMC-114)
Antifungals	
Itraconazole (itra)	No data. Use with caution; do not exceed 200 mg itraconazole daily.
Ketoconazole (keto)	Use with caution; do not exceed 200 mg ketoconazole daily.
Voriconazole (vori)	Potential for bi-directional inhibition between voriconazole and PIs exists. Voriconazole AUC ↓ 39% with RTV 100 mg BID; interaction between TMC-114 and voriconazole unknown. Co-administration is not recommended unless the benefit outweighs the risk.
Antimycobacterials	
Rifampin	
Rifabutin	Levels: ↑ rifabutin; ↓ TMC-114 Dose: ↓ rifabutin to 150 mg qod or 3x/week
Clarithromycin (clarithro)	↑ Clarithromycin – no dose adjustment of TMC-114 or clarithromycin is required for patients with normal renal function. Reduce clarithromycin dose by 50% for CrCl 30-60 mL/min; reduce clarithromycin dose by 75% for CrCl <30 mL/min.
Oral contraceptives	↓ ethinyl estradiol; ↓ norethindrone Use alternative or additional method.
Lipid-lowering agents	
Simvastatin, lovastatin	Levels: Potential for large increase in statin level. Avoid concomitant use.
Atorvastatin (atorva)	Levels: ↑ atorvastatin. Use lowest possible starting dose of atorvastatin with careful monitoring.
Pravastatin (prava)	Levels: ↑ pravastatin AUC 81% - 5 fold. Use lowest possible starting dose of pravastatin with careful monitoring.
Anticonvulsants	
Phenobarbital, phenytoin, carbamazepine	Contraindicated
Methadone	↓ methadone
Erectile dysfunction agents	
Sildenafil	↑ sildenafil. Starting dose should not exceed 25 mg sildenafil within 48 hours.
Vardenafil	↑ vardenafil. Starting dose should not exceed 2.5 mg vardenafil every 72 hours.
Tadalafil	↑ tadalafil. Starting dose should not exceed 10 mg tadalafil every 72 hours.
Miscellaneous	Concentrations of bepridil, lidocaine, quinidine and amiodarone may be ↑ when co-administered with TMC-114. Caution is warranted and therapeutic monitoring is recommended. ↑ levels of trazadone – use with caution Concentrations of felodipine, nifedipine, and nicardipine may be ↑ when co-administered with TMC-114. Caution is warranted and therapeutic monitoring is recommended. ↓ TMC-114; ↑ fluticasone, dexamethasone (theoretical) – consider alternatives ↓ sertraline, ↓ paroxeitine – monitor carefully

Table 11

ACTG 076 Guidelines: Dosing of AZT for Prevention of Vertical Transmission

Antepartum	Initiation at 14-34 weeks' gestation and continued throughout pregnancy
	A. PACTG 076 regimen: AZT 100 mg 5 times daily
	B. Acceptable alternative regimens:
	AZT 200 mg 3 times daily
	or
	AZT 300 mg 2 times daily
Intrapartum	During labor, AZT 2 mg/kg IV over 1 hour, followed by a continuous infusion of 1 mg/kg/h IV until delivery
Postpartum	Oral administration of AZT to the newborn: AZT syrup 2 mg/kg every 6 hours for the first 6 weeks of life, beginning 8-12 hours after birth

---

Table 12

Prevention or Postexposure Prophylaxis Treatment Options

Small volume, short duration *and* high HIV titer exposure *or* Large volume or less severe percutaneous *and* low HIV titer exposure	AZT 200 mg PO q8h or 300 mg PO q12h *plus* 3TC (lamivudine) 150 mg PO q12h
Large volume or less severe percutaneous *and* high HIV titer exposure *or* More severe percutaneous *and* low or high HIV titer exposure	AZT 200 mg PO q8h or 300 mg PO q12h + 3TC (lamivudine) 150 mg PO q12h + Indinavir 800 mg q8h *or* Nelfinavir 750 mg PO q8h or 1250 mg q12h

---

4. Hematologic Complications

Anemia

Causes
- HIV infection of marrow progenitor cells
- Drug-induced marrow suppression (AZT, ganciclovir, amphotericin, ribavirin, pyrimethamine, interferon, TMP-SMX)

Treatment

- See Figure 1.

5. Key Points

- Human immunodeficiency virus (HIV) is a virus that destroys the immune system.
- Acquired immunodeficiency syndrome (AIDS) is caused by HIV and is defined as a CD4$^+$ cell count less than 200/mm^3 or the presence of an opportunistic infection.
- Acute retroviral syndrome occurs in 50%-90% of patients within the first 2-4 weeks of infection with HIV.
- The viral load indicates the amount of virus in the body and is an indication of how well antiretroviral medications are working.
- The CD4$^+$ cell count refers to the status of the immune system and how at-risk a patient is for developing an opportunistic infection.
- Nucleoside reverse transcriptase inhibitors (NRTIs),

Table 13

Opportunistic Infections

Pathogen	Indication	First choice	Alternative regimens	Comments
Pneumocystis jiroveci pneumonia (PCP)	**Prophylaxis**: CD4+ <200/mm³; thrush; unexplained fever ≥2 weeks; history of PCP	TMP-SMX DS qd; TMP-SMX SS PO qd	Dapsone 100 mg PO qd; atovaquone 1500 mg qd; aerosolized pentamidine 300 mg q mo; TMP-SMX DS q MWF; others	Primary and secondary prophylaxis can possibly be stopped for PCP upon immune reconstitution (patients on HAART with CD4+ greater than 200/mm³ for >3 mo)
Pneumocystis jiroveci pneumonia (PCP)	**Acute infection**	TMP 15-20 mg/kg/d + SMX 75-100 mg/kg/d PO or IV x 21 d in 3-4 divided doses (typical oral dosage is TMP-SMX DS 2 tabs q8h)	TMP 15 mg/kg/d PO + dapsone 100 mg PO qd x 21 d; atovaquone 750 mg suspension PO with meal bid 21 days; pentamidine 4 mg/kg/d IV x 21 d (severe cases); clindamycin 600-900 mg IV q8h or 300-450 mg PO q6h + primaquine 15-30 mg base PO/d x 21 d; trimetrexate 45 mg/m² IV/d + folinic acid 20 mg/m² PO or IV q6h	Patients with Po₂ <70 mm Hg or A-a gradient >35 mm Hg should receive a corticosteroid taper; treatment is for 21 d
Candida	**Treatment**	**Oropharyngeal (thrush)**: fluconazole 100 mg qd x 7-14 days; itraconazole solution 200 mg qd x 7-14 days; clotrimazole oral troches 10 mg 5 x/d for 7-14 d; nystatin 500,000 U gargled qid for 7-14 d; **esophagitis**: fluconazole 100-400 mg qd x 2-3 wk; itraconazole solution 200 mg qd x 2-3 wk; voriconazole 200 mg bid x 2-3 wk; caspofungin 50 mg IV qd x 2-3 wk	**Thrush**: fluconazole 100 mg qd; amphotericin B 0.3-.05 mg/kg/d IV; itraconazole solution 7200 mg PO qd; **esophagitis**: ketoconazole 200 mg qd; itraconazole 200 mg qd (caps) or 100 mg qd (susp)	**Thrush**: treat for 10-14 d; CD4+ <500/mm³ increases risk; **esophagitis**: treat for 2-3 wk; CD4+ <500/mm³ increases risk

(continued)

non-nucleoside reverse transcriptase inhibitors (NNRTIs), protease inhibitors (PIs), and entry inhibitors are the currently available classes of medications used to treat HIV.

- Prevention of vertical transmission occurs by treating the mother with highly active antiretroviral therapy (HAART; preferred) or zidovudine alone.

- *Pneumocystis carinii* pneumonia (PCP) requires primary prophylaxis at CD4+ cell counts <200/mm³. TMP-SMX is the preferred treatment.
- *Mycobacterium avium* complex (MAC) requires primary prophylaxis at CD4+ cell counts <50/mm³. Azithromycin is the preferred drug.
- All other opportunistic infections require treatment followed by secondary prophylaxis.

Table 13

Opportunistic Infections (continued)

Pathogen	Indication	First choice	Alternative regimens	Comments
Candida	**Maintenance**	**Thrush**: fluconazole 100 mg qd; **esophagitis**: fluconazole 100-200 mg qd	**Thrush**: itraconazole solution 200 mg qd; **esophagitis**: itraconazole solution 200 mg qd	**Thrush**: most patients relapse within 3 mo in absence of immune reconstitution; options are treatment of each episode or maintenance: **esophagitis**: maintenance therapy is generally needed to prevent relapse
Candida	**Primary prophylaxis**	Not recommended; efficacy of fluconazole is established for AIDS patients with CD4 counts <100/mm^3; not done because no survival benefit was found, the cost was high, and there is risk of azole-resistant infections		
Cryptococcal meningitis	**Treatment**	Amphotericin B 0.7 mg/kg/d IV with or w/o flucytosine 100 mg/kg/d x 14 d, **then** fluconazole 400 mg/d for 8-10 wk; liposomal amphotericin B 4 mg/kg IV qd +/– flucytosine	Fluconazole 400-800 mg/d PO with or w/o flucytosine 100 mg/kg/d PO x 4-6 wk	CD4$^+$ <100/mm^3 increases risk; spread through inhalation of soil contaminated with bird droppings; fluconazole is superior to itraconazole
Cryptococcal meningitis	**Maintenance**	Fluconazole 200 mg qd	Amphotericin B 0.6-1 mg/kg 1-3x/wk; fluconazole 400 mg qd; itraconazole 400 mg qd (caps) or 200 mg oral susp qd	Primary and secondary prophylaxis can possibly be stopped for cryptococcosis upon immune reconstitution (patients on HAART with CD4$^+$ >100-200/mm^3 for >6 mo)
Cryptococcal meningitis	**Primary prophylaxis**	Not generally recommended	Fluconazole 200 mg qd; itraconazole 200 mg PO or 100 mg oral susp qd	**Indications for primary prophylaxis**: antigen-positive high-risk patients (CD4$^+$ <100/mm^3 and work with soil)
Toxoplasmosis	**Treatment**	Pyrimethamine PO 200 mg loading dose then 50-75 mg + folinic acid PO 10-20 mg/d + sulfadiazine PO 1-2 g q6h for at least 6 wk	Pyrimethamine + folinic acid + clinda-mycin 650 mg IV or PO q6h or q6h; pyrimethamine + folinic acid + azithromycin 900-1200 mg/d or atovaquone 1500 mg with food bid	Spread through raw or under-cooked meat (lamb, beef, and pork) and by contact with infected cat feces; may require dexamethasone if significant cerebral edema is present
Toxoplasmosis	**Suppressive therapy**	Pyrimethamine PO 25-50 mg/d + folinic acid PO 10-25 mg/d + sulfadiazine PO 0.5-1 g q6h	Pyrimethamine + folinic acid + clinda-mycin ot atovaquone	May be able to discontinue when CD4 >200/mm^3 for >6 mo and free of signs and symptoms
Toxoplasmosis	**Primary prophylaxis**	Not generally recommended	TMP-SMX DS qd	**Indications for primary prophylaxis**: positive IgG serology plus CD4+ <100/mm^3

(continued)

Table 13

Opportunistic Infections (continued)

Pathogen	Indication	First choice	Alternative regimens	Comments
Histoplasmosis	**Treatment**	Amphotericin B 0.7 mg/kg/d IV for 3-10 d; liposomal amphotericin B 4 mg/kg IV qd; itraconazole 200 mg PO tid x 3 d, then 200 mg PO bid x 12 weeks	Fluconazole 800 mg/d; itraconazole 400 mg IV qod	Spread through inhalation of dust particles; found in soils heavily contaminated by avian or bat feces; the Ohio and Mississippi River valleys are endemic areas in the U.S.
Histoplasmosis	**Maintenance therapy**	After amphotericin: itraconazole 200 mg bid x 12 weeks, then 200-400 mg qd indefinitely	Amphotericin B 1.0 mg/kg weekly; fluconazole 800 mg/d	Itraconazole is superior to fluconazole; No data for discontinuation
Histoplasmosis	**Primary prophylaxis**	Not generally recommended	Itraconazole 200 mg PO qd; fluconazole 200 mg PO qd	**Indications for primary prophylaxis**: antigen positive and live in endemic area or if at high risk (CD4+ <100/mm^3 and work with soil)
Mycobacterium avium complex (MAC)	**Treatment**	Clarithromycin 500 mg PO bid + ethambutol 15 mg/kg/d PO with or w/o rifabutin 300 mg PO qd	Azithromycin + ethambutol with or w/o rifabutin	Treatment is indefinite without immune reconstitution; may be discontinued when MAC treatment is >1 y, CD4 >100/mm^3 for 6 months, and patient is asymptomatic
Mycobacterium avium complex (MAC)	**Primary prophylaxis**: generally recommended at CD4 counts <50/mm^3	Azithromycin 1200 mg PO q week; clarithromycin 500 mg PO bid	Rifabutin; azithromycin + rifabutin	May be able to discontinue when CD4 >100/mm^3 for >6 mo with substantial suppression of viral load
Cytomegalovirus retinitis	**Treatment**	Intraocular ganciclovir release device[1] (Vitrasert®) q 6 months + valganciclovir 900 mg PO bid x 21 d; foscarnet IV x 14-21 d; ganciclovir IV x 14-21 d; cidofovir IV q wk x 2 wk	Intraocular injections of foscarnet; fomivirsen intravitreal injection	Oral ganciclovir should not be used as sole induction therapy
Cytomegalovirus retinitis	**Maintenance**	Valganciclovir 900 mg PO qd; ganciclovir IV q 5-7 d/wk; foscarnet IV/d; cidovovir IV q 2 wk; intraocular ganciclovir release device (Vitrasert) q 6 mo + oral ganciclovir 1.0-1.5 g PO tid	Ganciclovir PO 1 g tid	Lifelong maintenance therapy is required for retinitis in patients without immune recovery (CD4 >100-150/mm^3 for greater than 6 mo)
Cytomegalovirus retinitis	**Primary prophylaxis**	Not generally recommended unless positive serology and CD4 count <50/mm^3		

[1]Intraocular device does not protect contralateral eye and does not protect against systemic infection with cytomegalovirus.

Figure 1.

Guidelines for the treatment of anemia in the HIV patient.

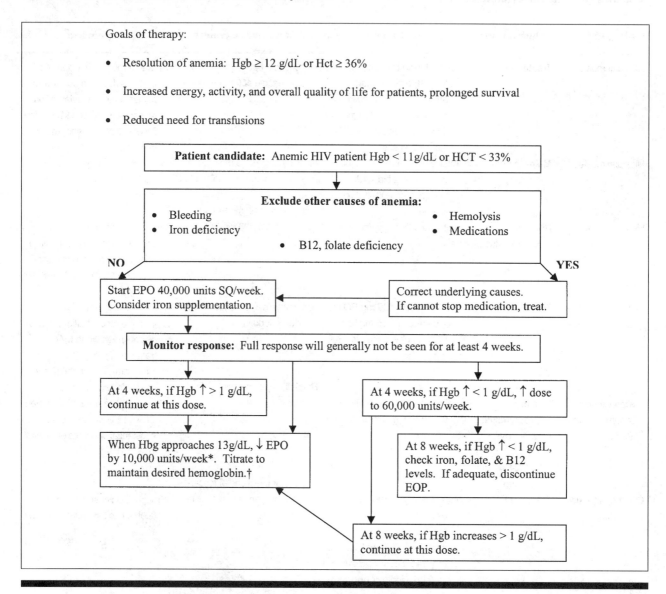

Goals of therapy:

- Resolution of anemia: Hgb ≥ 12 g/dL or Hct ≥ 36%

- Increased energy, activity, and overall quality of life for patients, prolonged survival

- Reduced need for transfusions

Patient candidate: Anemic HIV patient Hgb < 11g/dL or HCT < 33%

Exclude other causes of anemia:
- Bleeding
- Iron deficiency
- Hemolysis
- Medications
- B12, folate deficiency

NO   **YES**

Start EPO 40,000 units SQ/week. Consider iron supplementation.

Correct underlying causes. If cannot stop medication, treat.

Monitor response: Full response will generally not be seen for at least 4 weeks.

At 4 weeks, if Hgb ↑ > 1 g/dL, continue at this dose.

At 4 weeks, if Hgb ↑ < 1 g/dL, ↑ dose to 60,000 units/week.

When Hbg approaches 13g/dL, ↓ EPO by 10,000 units/week*. Titrate to maintain desired hemoglobin.†

At 8 weeks, if Hgb ↑ < 1 g/dL, check iron, folate, & B12 levels. If adequate, discontinue EOP.

At 8 weeks, if Hgb increases > 1 g/dL, continue at this dose.

EPO, erythropoietin.

*If Hgb >15 g/dL at any point, hold EPO and restart when Hgb <12 g/dL, using dose reduced by 10,000 U/week.

†During the dose adjustment phase, Hgb should be monitored every 2-4 weeks. Allow at least 4 weeks to assess response to dose changes.

6. Questions and Answers

1.   C.T. is a 23-year-old HIV-positive female who presents to the emergency department with shortness of breath and a fever. Physical exam reveals a temperature of 102°F, HR of 100 bpm, and decreased breath sounds in the left lower lobe of lungs. Chest x-ray is positive for infiltrates in the left lung. She is diagnosed with PCP pneumonia. She has no previous history of opportunistic infections and is not on any medications at this time (she has not been seen by a health care provider in over a year). Her CD4+ count is 13 cells/mm^3 and viral load is 170,198 copies/mL. What is the treatment of choice for C.T.'s PCP?

A. TMP-SMX DS 2 tabs PO q8h for 21 days, then 1 tab PO qd

B. Azithromycin 500 mg PO on day one, then 250 mg PO qd indefinitely

C. Doxycycline 100 mg PO bid for 7 days, then 100 mg PO qd

D. Clarithromycin 500 mg PO bid for 10 days, then 250 mg PO qd

E. Vancomycin 1 g IV q12h for 10 days, then TMP-SMX DS PO qd

2. Should C.T. receive any other prophylaxis against opportunistic infections?

A. Yes, against MAC: Zithromax® 1200 mg PO q week

B. Yes, against thrush: Diflucan® 100 mg PO qd

C. Yes, against toxoplasmosis: Bactrim DS® 1 tab PO q M, W, and F

D. Yes, against CMV: Valcyte® 450 mg PO q M, W, and F

E. No

3. Six weeks later C.T. presents to the HIV clinic for follow-up. Her CD4$^+$ count is 12 cells/mm^3 and viral load is 140,202 copies/mL. Should C.T. be started on HIV therapy?

A. Yes; her CD4$^+$ cell count is <200 cells/mm^3 and she has had an opportunistic infection

B. Yes; her viral load is greater than 100,000 copies/mL

C. Yes; her Western blot was positive for HIV

D. Yes; all patients with HIV should be treated as soon as the diagnosis is made

E. No

4. C.T. wishes to be started on HIV therapy. Which of the following would be an appropriate regimen?

A. Zidovudine + efavirenz + nelfinavir

B. Zidovudine + stavudine + indinavir

C. Zalcitabine + didanosine + amprenavir

D. Zidovudine + lamivudine + lopinavir/ritonavir

E. Nelfinavir + indinavir + amprenavir

5. HIV can be transmitted by:

A. Unprotected sexual contact with an infected person

B. Sharing needles or syringes with an infected person

C. Infected mother to infant (vertical transmission)

D. Transfusion of blood (before 1985)

E. All of the above

6. M.J. is 13 weeks pregnant and just tested positive for HIV. Her viral load is 22,434 copies/mL and her CD4$^+$ cell count is 425 cells/mm^3. M.J. wishes to receive treatment for her HIV. Which of the following would be an appropriate regimen for M.J.?

A. Zidovudine + stavudine + indinavir

B. Zidovudine + lamivudine + nelfinavir

C. Zidovudine + lamivudine + efavirenz

D. Stavudine + didanosine + nevirapine

E. No treatment is necessary

7. Which of the following antiretroviral medications has shown efficacy as monotherapy in decreasing the vertical transmission of HIV?

A. Efavirenz

B. Nelfinavir

C. Zidovudine

D. Zalcitabine

E. Stavudine

8. R.C. is a nurse in the emergency department. She has just been stuck with a needle that was used for an HIV-positive patient with a known high viral load. Which of the following is true concerning postexposure prophylaxis?

I. The regimen should be started within 2 hours of exposure

II. R.C. will only need to be treated with zidovudine

III. R.C. will need to be treated with a combination of zidovudine + lamivudine + nelfinavir *Viracept-NFV*

IV. Treatment will continue for 4 weeks

A. I, III, and IV

B. II only

C. II, III, and IV

D. I, IV

E. I, II, and IV

9. The CD4$^+$ cell count relates to

I. the activity of the virus

II. the status of the immune system

III. how at-risk a patient is for acquiring an opportunistic infection

IV. when the patient was infected

V. time to death in treated patients

A. IV, V

B. I, II, and III

C. II, III

D. II, III, and IV
E. I, II, V

10. The viral load relates to

   A. the activity of the virus and efficacy of antiretroviral therapy
   B. the status of the immune system
   C. when the patient was infected
   D. how at-risk a patient is for acquiring an opportunistic infection
   E. time to death in a treated patient

11. S.J. presents to the emergency department with extreme flank pain with nausea and vomiting. He is diagnosed with a kidney stone. His past medical history is positive for HIV and diabetes. His medications include indinavir, stavudine, didanosine, dapsone, and metformin. Which of his medications might have caused his kidney stone?

   A. Indinavir
   B. Stavudine
   C. Didanosine
   D. Metformin
   E. Dapsone

12. L.L. comes to the clinic today with a chief complaint of burning and tingling in his feet that started about 1 month ago. His current medications include nelfinavir, stavudine, lamivudine, sertraline, and gemfibrozil. Which medication(s) might be causing this problem?

   A. Nelfinavir
   B. Stavudine
   C. Lamivudine
   D. Sertraline
   E. Gemfibrozil

13. S.E. presents to the emergency department with a 2-day history of extreme nausea, vomiting, and abdominal pain. Labs reveal elevations in amylase and lipase and a diagnosis of pancreatitis is made. His medications include nevirapine, tenofovir, didanosine, and amitriptyline. Which of his medications could have caused his pancreatitis?

   A. Nevirapine
   B. Tenofovir
   C. Didanosine
   D. Amitriptyline
   E. All of the above

14. Which of the following HIV medications has a 5% incidence of a hypersensitivity reaction?

   A. Efavirenz
   B. Ritonavir
   C. Zidovudine
   D. Abacavir
   E. Lamivudine

15. C.J. is starting efavirenz, zidovudine, lamivudine, and TMP-SMX today. What should C.J. be counseled about concerning efavirenz?

   A. Anemia
   B. CNS side effects
   C. Neutropenia
   D. Renal toxicity
   E. Kidney stones

16. Which of the following can cause hepatotoxicity and requires monitoring of liver enzymes at baseline, 2 weeks, 4 weeks, 6 weeks, and then monthly for the first 18 weeks of therapy? *NNRTI*

   A. Zidovudine
   B. Zalcitabine
   C. Lopinavir
   D. Amprenavir
   E. Nevirapine

17. Which of the following can cause hyperglycemia, hyperlipidemia (particularly elevations in triglycerides), and lipodystrophy? *PIs*

   A. Amprenavir
   B. Delavirdine
   C. Didanosine
   D. Abacavir
   E. Lamivudine

18. Lactic acidosis and hepatic steatosis have been reported with which of these antiretroviral medications?

   A. Nevirapine
   B. Efavirenz
   C. Stavudine
   D. Saquinavir
   E. Nelfinavir

19. The mechanism of action of nucleoside reverse transcriptase inhibitors is to *NRTI*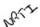

   A. directly inhibit reverse transciptase
   B. prevent entry of the proviral DNA into the nucleus of the CD4$^+$ cell

C. cause chain termination, resulting in a defective copy of proviral DNA

D. prevent entry of HIV into the CD4⁺ cell

E. prevent cleavage of the newly formed polypeptide chains into a viable HIV

20. The mechanism of action of non-nucleoside reverse transcriptase inhibitors is to

A. prevent cleavage of the newly formed polypeptide chains into viable HIV

B. prevent entry of HIV into the CD4⁺ cell

C. prevent entry of the proviral DNA into the nucleus of the CD4⁺ cell

D. directly inhibit reverse transcriptase

E. cause chain termination, resulting in a defective copy of proviral DNA

21. The mechanism of action of protease inhibitors is to

A. cause a defective copy of proviral DNA to be made

B. prevent entry of the proviral DNA into the nucleus of the CD4⁺ cell

C. prevent cleavage of the newly formed polypeptide chains into a viable HIV

D. prevent entry of HIV into the CD4⁺ cell

E. directly inhibit reverse transcriptase

22. Which of the following nucleoside reverse transcriptase inhibitor combinations is acceptable?

A. Stavudine + zidovudine

B. Zalcitabine + stavudine

C. Tenofovir + emtricitabine

D. Zalcitabine + didanosine

E. Zalcitabine + delavirdine

23. Which of the following opportunistic infections are the only ones requiring primary prophylaxis?

A. PCP and MAC

B. PCP and toxoplasmosis

C. MAC and histoplasmosis

D. MAC and CMV

E. PCP and thrush

24. The antifungal of first choice for maintenance therapy after treatment of cryptococcal meningitis is

A. itraconazole

B. fluconazole

C. ketoconazole

D. amphotericin B — Initiate

E. terbinafine

25. The first-choice antifungal for treatment of histoplasmosis is

A. itraconazole

B. fluconazole

C. ketoconazole

D. caspofungin

E. terbinafine

Answers

1. **A.** The treatment of choice for PCP is TMP-SMX in patients who are not allergic to sulfa medications. Duration of treatment is for 21 days. Since this patient's CD4⁺ cell count is below 200 cells/mm³ and she has had PCP, she will require secondary prophylaxis once treatment is completed. Preferred prophylaxis is once-daily TMP-SMX DS.

2. **A.** This patient's CD4⁺ cell count is below 50 cells/mm³; therefore she requires primary prophylaxis against MAC. Zithromax is the drug of choice. Prophylaxis against other opportunistic infections is generally not required.

3. **A.** Current guidelines state that any patient who has had an opportunistic infection or a CD4⁺ cell count less than 200 cells/mm³ should start treatment for HIV. This patient has had both.

4. **D.** Most regimens contain two NRTIs and either one PI or one NNRTI. A includes one NRTI, one NNRTI and one PI. E includes three PIs. Zidovudine and stavudine competitively inhibit each other and would not be used in the same regimen (thus B is incorrect). Zalcitabine is contraindicated with didanosine, stavudine, and lamivudine, due to increased toxicity (which makes C incorrect).

5. **E.** All items are important risk factors for transmission of HIV. Breastfeeding, history of STDs, occupational exposure to HIV-infected fluids (rare), and household exposure to HIV-infected fluids (rare) are also risk factors.

6. **B.** All HIV-positive pregnant women should receive treatment for HIV to decrease the risk of transmission to their offspring. Zidovudine and stavudine competitively inhibit each other and should not be used together. Efavirenz is

teratogenic and should not be used in pregnancy. Stavudine and didanosine together are contraindicated in pregnancy due to increased risk of lactic acidosis and liver damage.

7. **C.** Zidovudine and neviripine are the only HIV medications that can reduce vertical transmission when used as monotherapy. Most practitioners treat with combination therapy due to the increased risk of resistance with monotherapy, which has an impact on future choices of drug regimen.

8. **A.** The approved regimens for postexposure prophylaxis are zidovudine and lamivudine with or without nelfinavir or indinavir. Treatment should continue for 4 weeks and should start within 2 hours of exposure.

9. **C.** CD4$^+$ cell count describes the status of the immune system (ie, how at-risk a patient is for acquiring an opportunistic infection).

10. **A.** Viral load relates to the activity of the virus and efficacy of antiretroviral therapy. The goal of therapy is an undetectable viral load (<50 copies/mL).

11. **A.** Indinavir can cause kidney stones. Patients should drink at least 48 ounces of water a day to decrease the risk of developing a kidney stone.

12. **B.** All the "D" drugs, d4T (stavudine), ddI (didanosine), and ddC (zalcitabine), can cause peripheral neuropathy and pancreatitis.

13. **C.** All the "D" drugs, d4T (stavudine), ddI (didanosine), and ddC (zalcitabine), can cause peripheral neuropathy and pancreatitis.

14. **D.** Abacavir has a 5% incidence of hypersensitivity. Symptoms can include rash, fever, stomach symptoms, throat symptoms, or flu-like symptoms.

15. **B.** Efavirenz can cause CNS side effects such as dizziness, trouble sleeping, drowsiness, trouble concentrating, and/or unusual dreams during the first 2-4 weeks of treatment.

16. **E.** All NNRTIs can cause hepatotoxicity. There have been rare reports of hepatotoxicity after just one dose of nevirapine. Liver enzymes should be monitored at baseline, 2 weeks, 4 weeks, 6 weeks, and monthly for the first 18 weeks of therapy.

17. **A.** Class side effects of PIs include hyperglycemia, hyperlipidemia, lipodystrophy, increased bleeding in hemophiliacs, and possibly osteoporosis or osteopenia.

18. **C.** Class side effects of NRTIs include lactic acidosis and hepatic steatosis.

19. **C.** NRTIs affect reverse transcriptase by causing chain termination, resulting in a defective copy of proviral DNA.

20. **D.** NNRTIs affect reverse transcriptase by directly inhibiting reverse transcriptase, resulting in less proviral DNA being made.

21. **C.** PIs prevent cleavage of the newly formed polypeptide chains into viable HIV, resulting in an immature virus that is unable to infect other CD4$^+$ cells.

22. **C.** Stavudine is contraindicated with zidovudine due to competitive inhibition. Zalcitabine is contraindicated with other NRTIs that may cause peripheral neuropathy (eg, stavudine and didanosine). Delavirdine is an NNRTI.

23. **A.** PCP requires primary prophylaxis when the CD4$^+$ cell count falls below 200 cells/mm^3. The preferred medication is TMP-SMX. MAC requires primary prophylaxis when the CD4$^+$ cell count falls below 50 cells/mm^3. The preferred medication is azithromycin.

24. **B.** Generally, cryptococcal meningitis is initially treated with amphotericin B during the induction phase, and then fluconazole for the consolidation phase and maintenance therapy.

25. **A.** Histoplasmosis is generally initially treated with amphotericin B or itraconazole for induction therapy, and then itraconazole for maintenance therapy.

7. References

Bartlett JG, Gallant JE. 2003 *Medical Management of HIV Infection.* Baltimore: Johns Hopkins University Press; 2000:357-360.

Carr A, Miller J, Law M, Cooper DA. A syndrome of lipoatrophy, lactic acidaemia, and liver dysfunction associated with HIV nucleoside analog therapy: Contribution to protease inhibitor–related lipodystrophy syndrome. *AIDS.* 2000;14:F25-F32.

Carr A, Samars K, Thorisdottir A, et al. Diagnosis, prediction, and natural course of HIV-1 protease inhibitor associated lipodystrophy, hyperlipidaemia, and diabetes mellitus: a cohort study. *Lancet.* 1999;353:2093-2099.

Centers for Disease Control and Prevention, Perinatal HIV Guidelines Working Group. Public Health Service Task Force recommendations for the use of antiretroviral drugs in pregnant women infected with HIV-1 for maternal health and for reducing perinatal HIV-1 transmission in the United States. *MMWR Morb Mortal Wkly Rep.* 1998;47:1-30.

Centers for Disease Control and Prevention. 1993 revised classification system for HIV infection and expanded surveillance case definition for AIDS among adolescents and adults. *MMWR Morb Mortal Wkly Rep.* 1992;41:1-19.

Chaisson RE, Keruly JC, Moore RD. Association of initial CD4 cell count and viral load with response to highly active antiretroviral therapy. *JAMA.* 2000;284:3128-3129.

Chesney MA. Factors affecting adherence to antiretroviral therapy. *Clin Infect Dis.* 2000;30(suppl 2):S171-176.

Current United States epidemiology figures can be located at www.cdc.gov/hiv/stats/hasrlink.htm.

Current world epidemiology figures can be found at www.unaids.org.

Finzi D, Hermankova M, Pierson T, et al. Identification of a reservoir for HIV-1 in patients on highly active antiretroviral therapy. *Science.* 1997;278:1295-1300.

Furret H, Egger M, Opravil M, et al. Discontinuation of primary prophylaxis against *Pneumocystis carinii* pneumonia in HIV-1 infected adults treated with combination antiretroviral therapy. Swiss HIV Cohort Study. *N Engl J Med.* 1999;340:1301-1306.

Guidelines for postexposure prophylaxis can be located as a living document on the web at www.aidsinfo.nih.gov, which is updated 3-4 times a year.

Guidelines for prevention and treatment and medications used for the treatment of HIV can be located as a living document at www.aidsinfo.nih.gov, which is updated 3-4 times a year.

Guidelines for prophylaxis and treatment of opportunistic infections can be located as a living document at www.aidsinfo.nih.gov, which is updated 3-4 times a year.

Guidelines for prevention of vertical transmission can be located as a living document at www.aidsinfo.nih.gov, which is updated 3-4 times a year.

Yeni PG, Hammer SM, Hirsch MS, et al. Treatment for adult HIV infection: 2004 recommendations of the International AIDS Society-USA Panel. *JAMA.* 2004;292:250-265.

Hoen B, Dumon B, Harzic M, et al. Highly active antiretroviral treatment initiated early in the course of symptomatic primary HIV-1 infections: Results of the ANRS 053 trial. *J Infect Dis.* 1999;180:1342-1346.

Mellors JW, Munoz A, Giorgi JV, et al. Plasma viral load and CD4[+] lymphocytes as prognostic markers of HIV-1 infections. *Ann Intern Med.* 1997;126:946-954.

Report of the NIH panel to define principles of therapy of HIV infection. *MMWR Morb Mortal Wkly Rep.* 1998;47(RR-5):1-41.

1999 USPHS/IDSA guidelines for the prevention of opportunistic infections in persons infected with human immunodeficiency virus. *MMWR Morb Mortal Wkly Rep.* 1999;48(RR-10):1-67.

Sperling RS, Shapiro DE, Coombs RW, et al. Maternal viral load, zidovudine treatment, and the risk of transmission of human immunodeficiency virus type 1 from mother to infant. Pediatric AIDS Clinical Trials Group Protocol 076 Study Group. *N Engl J Med.* 1996;335:1621-1629.

Update: Provisional Public Health Service recommendations for chemoprophylaxis after occupational exposure to HIV. *MMWR Morb Mortal Wkly Rep.* 1996;45:468-480.

Vittinghoff E, Scheer S, O'Malley P, et al. Combination antiretroviral therapy and recent declines in AIDS incidence and mortality. *J Infect Dis.* 1999;179:717-720.

32. Immunization

Stephan L. Foster, PharmD
Associate Professor, Department of Clinical Pharmacy
University of Tennessee College of Pharmacy

Contents

1. Introduction

Definitions

Immunity: a naturally or artificially acquired state resulting in an individual being resistant or relatively resistant to the occurrence or effects of a foreign substance; this is the mechanism the body develops for protection from infectious disease. This is usually very specific to a single organism or to a group of closely related organisms.

Antigen: a live or inactivated substance capable of evoking antibody production; antigens can be a live organism, such as bacteria or viruses, or an inactivated or killed organism or portion of an organism. A live organism generally evokes the most effective immune response.

Antibody: a protein evoked by an antigen which acts to eliminate that antigen

Mechanisms for Acquiring Immunity

Active immunity: protection produced by an individual's own immune system; immunity acquired in this manner has a delayed onset and is usually permanent. Active immunity may be acquired by having an active disease or by vaccination. B lymphocytes (B cells) circulate in the blood and bone marrow for many years. Re-exposure to the antigen causes the cells to replicate and to produce antibody. These cells are also called memory B cells.

Passive immunity: protection produced by an animal or human and transferred to another; immunity acquired in this manner has a rapid onset and usually has a brief duration. This is the type of immunity an infant receives from his or her mother. All types of blood products contain varying amounts of antibody. Immune globulins and hyperimmune globulins are also used to induce passive immunity. One source of passive immunity is antitoxins, which contain antibodies against a known toxin.

2. Vaccines

Vaccination is the process of producing active immunity via use of vaccines. The immunological response is similar to natural infection, with a lower risk than that of the disease itself.

Classification of Vaccines

Live, attenuated vaccines: These are vaccines produced by modifying a virus or bacteria to produce immunity. These vaccines usually do not produce disease, however they may. When this occurs the disease is usually much milder than the natural disease. These vaccines must replicate to be effective. These vaccines also require special handling, such as protection from heat and light, to keep them alive. Circulating antibody from another source may destroy the vaccine virus and cause vaccine failure (Table 1).

Inactivated vaccines: These are vaccines composed of all or a fraction of a virus or bacterium. These fractions include subunits (subvirions), bacterial cell-wall polysaccharides, conjugated (attached to a protein carrier) bacteria cell-wall polysaccharides, or inactivated toxins (toxoids). The bacteria or virus is inactivated using heat and/or chemicals. Inactivated vaccines are not alive and cannot replicate, therefore they are unable to induce disease. Inactivated antigens are not affected by circulating antibody (Table 2).

Table 1

Live Vaccines Available in the United States, 2005

Herpes zoster

Influenza (live-attenuated)

Measles

Mumps

Rotavirus

Rubella

Typhoid oral

Varicella

Vaccinia (smallpox)

Yellow fever

Table 2

Inactivated Vaccines Available in the United States, 2005

Anthrax

Diphtheria

Haemophilus influenzae type b

Hepatitis A

Hepatitis B

Human papillomavirus

Influenza

Japanese encephalitis

Meningococcal A, C, Y, W-135 polysaccharide

Meningococcal A, C, Y, W-135 conjugate

Pertussis, acellular

Pneumococcal polysaccharide

Pneumococcal conjugate

Polio

Rabies

Tetanus toxoid

Typhoid injectable

Vaccination Schedules

- Vaccination schedules are available for children, adolescents, and adults (Figures 1 and 2). The schedules indicate the most ideal times to administer vaccines. Additional catch-up schedules are available for children and adolescents who are behind in their vaccinations.
- Intervals between doses of the same vaccine in a series are described in the tables.
- The minimum interval in a series for most vaccines is 4 weeks. Decreasing the interval may interfere with antibody response and protection.
- Usually the last dose in a series is separated from the previous dose by 4-6 months.
- Increasing the interval does not affect vaccine effectiveness. You never need to restart a series except for oral typhoid vaccine.

Administration of Multiple Vaccines

- There are no contraindications to the simultaneous administration of any vaccines. Inactivated and live vaccines may be given in any combination at the same time.
- Live vaccines must be separated from the administration of antibodies, such as blood products and immune globulins. Inactivated vaccines are not affected by circulating antibody.
- If two live vaccines are not given at the same time, a 4-week minimal interval must be observed. This is not true for two inactivated vaccines or an inactivated plus a live vaccine.

Vaccine Adverse Reactions

- Vaccine adverse reactions are any untoward side effects caused by a vaccine.
- Local reactions are the most common type of adverse reaction. These include pain, swelling, and redness at the site of injection. These usually occur within minutes to hours of the injection and are usually mild and self-limiting. Occasionally, severe local reactions occur and are known as hypersensitivity reactions.
- Systemic adverse reactions include fever, malaise, myalgias, and headache. Systemic adverse reactions are more common following live vaccines, and are similar to a mild case of the disease.
- Allergic reactions are reactions to the vaccine antigens or some component of the vaccine. While rare, these reactions may be life threatening.
- Vaccine Adverse Events Reporting System (VAERS) is a CDC-monitored surveillance system, which should be notified within 30 days of an adverse event that requires medical attention.

Contraindications and Precautions

- A contraindication is a condition that increases the risk of an adverse reaction or decreases the effect of a vaccine.
- A precaution is a condition that might possibly increase the risk of an adverse event or decrease the effect of a vaccine.

Contraindications include:
- An anaphylactic reaction to any previous dose of vaccine or to any of its components
- Pregnancy for live vaccines and selected inactivated vaccines
- Immunosuppression for live vaccines and selected inactivated vaccines
- Active, untreated tuberculosis and live vaccines

Figure 1.

Recommended adult immunization schedule by vaccine and age group—United States, October 2005-September 2006.

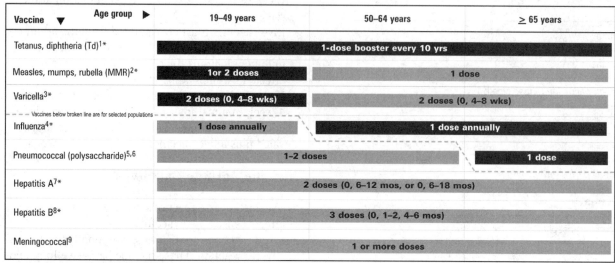

NOTE: These recommendations must be read along with the footnotes.
*Covered by the Vaccine Injury Compensation Program.

Footnotes to Figure 1.

1. Tetanus and Diphtheria (Td) vaccination. Adults with uncertain histories of a complete primary vaccination series with diphtheria and tetanus toxoid-containing vaccines should receive a primary series using combined Td toxoid. A primary series for adults is 3 doses; administer the first 2 doses at least 4 weeks apart and the third dose 6-12 months after the second. Administer 1 dose if the person received the primary series and if the last vaccination was received ≥10 years previously. Consult ACIP statement for recommendations for administering Td as prophylaxis in wound management (www.cdc.gov/mmwr/preview/mmwrhtml/0041645.htm). The American College of Physicians Task Force on Adult Immunization supports a second option for Td use in adults: a single Td booster at age 50 years for persons who have completed the full pediatric series, including the teenage/young adult booster. A newly licensed tetanus-diphtheria-acellular pertussis vaccine is available for adults. ACIP recommendations for its use will be published.

2. Measles, Mumps, Rubella (MMR) vaccination. *Measles component:* adults born before 1957 can be considered immune to measles. Adults born during or after 1957 should receive ≥1 dose of MMR unless they have a medical contraindication, documentation of ≥1 dose, history of measles based on health care provider diagnosis, or laboratory evidence of immunity. A second dose of MMR is recommended for adults who (1) were recently exposed to measles or in an outbreak setting, (2) were previously vaccinated with killed measles vaccine, (3) were vaccinated with an unknown type of measles vaccine during 1963-1967, (4) are students in post-secondary educational institutions, (5) work in a health care facility, or (6) plan to travel internationally. Withhold MMR or other measles-containing vaccines from HIV-infected persons with severe immunosuppression. *Mumps component:* 1 dose of MMR vaccine should be adequate for protection for those born during or after 1957 who lack a history of mumps based on health care provider diagnosis or who lack laboratory evidence of immunity. Rubella component: administer 1 dose of MMR vaccine to women whose rubella vaccination history is unreliable or who lack laboratory evidence of immunity. For women of childbearing age, regardless of birth year, routinely determine rubella immunity and counsel women regarding congenital rubella syndrome. Do not vaccinate women who are pregnant or might become pregnant within 4 weeks of receiving the vaccine. Women who do not have evidence of immunity should receive MMR vaccine upon completion or termination of pregnancy and before discharge from the health care facility.

3. Varicella vaccination. Varicella vaccination is recommended for all adults without evidence of immunity to varicella. Special consideration should be given to those who (1) have close contact with persons at high risk for severe disease (health care workers and family contacts of immunocompromised persons) or (2) are at high risk for exposure or transmission (eg, teachers of young children; child care employees; residents and staff members of institutional settings, including correctional institutions; college students; military personnel; adolescents and adults living in households with children; nonpregnant women of childbearing age; and international travelers). Evidence of immunity to varicella in adults includes any of the following: (1) documented age-appropriate varicella vaccination (ie, receipt of 1 dose before age 13 years or receipt of 2 doses [administered at least 4 weeks apart] after age 13 years); (2) born in the United States before 1966; (3) history of varicella disease based on health care provider diagnosis or self- or parental-report of typical varicella disease for non-U.S.-born persons born before 1966 and all persons born during 1966-1997 (for a patient reporting a history of an atypical, mild case, health care providers should seek either an epidemiologic link with a typical varicella case or evidence of laboratory confirmation, if it was performed at the time of acute disease); (4) history of herpes zoster based on health care provider diagnosis; or (5) laboratory evidence of immunity. Do not vaccinate women who are pregnant or might become pregnant within 4 weeks of receiving the vaccine. Assess pregnant women for evidence of varicella immunity. Women who do not have evidence of immunity should receive dose 1 of varicella vaccine upon completion or termination of pregnancy and before discharge from the health care facility. Dose 2 should be given 4-8 weeks after dose 1.

4. Influenza vaccination. *Medical indications:* chronic disorders of the cardiovascular or pulmonary systems, including asthma; chronic metabolic diseases, including diabetes mellitus, renal dysfunction, hemoglobinopathies, or immunosuppression (including immunosuppression caused by medications or by HIV); any condition (eg, cognitive dysfunction, spinal cord injury, seizure disorder or other neuromuscular disorder) that compromises respiratory function or the handling of respiratory secretions or that can increase the risk of aspiration; and pregnancy during the influenza season. No data exist on the risk for severe or complicated influenza disease among persons with asplenia; however, influenza is a risk factor for secondary bacterial infections that can cause severe disease among persons with asplenia. *Occupational indications:* health care workers and employees of long-term care and assisted living facilities. *Other indications:* residents of nursing homes and other long-term care and assisted living facilities; persons likely to transmit influenza to persons at high risk (ie, in-home household contacts and caregivers of children birth through 23 months of age, or persons of all ages with high-risk conditions); and anyone who wishes to be vaccinated.

For healthy nonpregnant persons aged 5-49 years without high-risk conditions who are not contacts of severely immunocompromised persons in special care units, intranasally administered influenza vaccine (FluMist) may be administered in lieu of inactivated vaccine.

5. Pneumococcal polysaccharide vaccination. *Medical indications:* chronic disorders of the pulmonary system (excluding asthma); cardiovascular diseases; diabetes mellitus; chronic liver diseases, including liver disease as a result of alcohol abuse (eg, cirrhosis); chronic renal failure or nephrotic syndrome; functional or anatomic asplenia (eg, sickle cell disease or splenectomy [if elective splenectomy is planned, vaccinate at least 2 weeks before surgery]); immunosuppressive conditions (eg, congenital immunodeficiency, HIV infection [vaccinate as close to diagnosis as possible when CD4 cell counts are highest], leukemia, lymphoma, multiple myeloma, Hodgkin's disease, generalized malignancy, organ or bone marrow transplantation); chemotherapy with alkylating agents, antimetabolites, or high-dose, long-term corticosteroids; and cochlear implants. *Other indications:* Alaska Natives and certain American Indian populations; residents of nursing homes and other long-term care facilities.

6. Revaccination with pneumococcal polysaccharide vaccine. One-time revaccination after 5 years for persons with chronic renal failure or nephrotic syndrome; functional or anatomic asplenia (eg, sickle cell disease or splenectomy); immunosuppressive conditions (eg, congenital immunodeficiency, HIV infection, leukemia, lymphoma, multiple myeloma, Hodgkin's disease, generalized malignancy, organ or bone marrow transplantation); or chemotherapy with alkylating agents, antimetabolites, or high-dose, long-term corticosteroids. For persons aged ≥65 years, one-time revaccination if they were vaccinated ≥5 years previously and were aged <65 years at the time of primary vaccination.

7. Hepatitis A vaccination. *Medical indications:* persons with clotting factor disorders or chronic liver disease. Behavioral indications: men who have sex with men or users of illegal drugs. *Occupational indications:* persons working with hepatitis A virus (HAV)-infected primates or with HAV in a research laboratory setting. *Other indications:* persons traveling to or working in countries that have high or intermediate endemicity of hepatitis A (for list of countries, visit www.cdc.gov/travel/diseases.htm#hepa) as well as any person wishing to obtain immunity. Current vaccines should be given in a 2-dose series at either 0 and 6-12 months, or 0 and 6-18 months. If the combined hepatitis A and hepatitis B vaccine is used, administer 3 doses at 0, 1, and 6 months.

8. Hepatitis B vaccination. *Medical indications:* hemodialysis patients (use special formulation [40 mcg/mL] or two 20-mcg/mL doses) or patients who receive clotting factor concentrates. *Occupational indications:* health care workers and public safety workers who have exposure to blood in the workplace; and persons in training in schools of medicine, dentistry, nursing, laboratory technology, and other allied health professions. Behavioral indications: injection-drug users; persons with more than one sex partner in the previous 6 months; persons with a recently acquired sexually transmitted disease (STD); and men who have sex with men. *Other indications:* household contacts and sex partners of persons with chronic hepatitis B virus (HBV) infection; clients and staff of institutions for the developmentally disabled; all clients of STD clinics; inmates of correctional facilities; or international travelers who will be in countries with high or intermediate prevalence of chronic HBV infection for >6 months (for list of countries, visit www.cdc.gov/travel/diseases.htm#hepa).

9. Meningococcal vaccination. *Medical indications:* adults with anatomic or functional asplenia, or terminal complement component deficiencies; first-year college students living in dormitories; microbiologists who are routinely exposed to isolates of *Neisseria meningitidis;* military recruits; and persons who travel to or reside in countries in which meningococcal disease is hyperendemic or epidemic (eg, the "meningitis belt" of sub-Saharan Africa during the dry season [Dec-June]), particularly if contact with the local populations will be prolonged. Vaccination is required by the government of Saudi Arabia for all travelers to Mecca during the annual Hajj. Meningococcal conjugate vaccine is preferred for adults meeting any of the above indications who are aged ≤55 years, although meningococcal polysaccharide vaccine (MPSV4) is an acceptable alternative. Revaccination after 5 years may be indicated for adults previously vaccinated with MPSV4 who remain at high risk for infection (eg, persons residing in areas in which disease is epidemic).

Figure 2.

Recommended childhood and adolescent immunization schedule—United States, 2006.

Vaccine ▼ Age ▶	Birth	1 month	2 months	4 months	6 months	12 months	15 months	18 months	24 months	4–6 years	11–12 years	13–14 years	15 years	16–18 years
Hepatitis B[1]	HepB	HepB	HepB[1]		HepB					HepB Series				
Diphtheria, Tetanus, Pertussis[2]			DTaP	DTaP	DTaP	DTaP				DTaP	Tdap	Tdap		
Haemophilus influenzae type b[3]			Hib	Hib	Hib[3]	Hib								
Inactivated Poliovirus			IPV	IPV	IPV					IPV				
Measles, Mumps, Rubella[4]						MMR				MMR	MMR			
Varicella[5]						Varicella					Varicella			
Meningococcal[6]						Vaccines within broken line are for selected populations				MPSV4	MCV4	MCV4 / MCV4		
Pneumococcal[7]			PCV	PCV	PCV	PCV				PCV	PPV			
Influenza[8]					Influenza (Yearly)					Influenza (Yearly)				
Hepatitis A[9]						HepA Series								

This schedule indicates the recommended ages for routine administration of currently licensed childhood vaccines, as of December 1, 2005, for children through age 18 years. Any dose not administered at the recommended age should be administered at any subsequent visit when indicated and feasible. ▇ Indicates age groups that warrant special effort to administer those vaccines not previously administered. Additional vaccines may be licensed and recommended during the year. Licensed combination vaccines may be used whenever any components of the combination are indicated and other components of the vaccine are not contraindicated and if approved by the Food and Drug Administration for that dose of the series. Providers should consult the respective ACIP statement for detailed recommendations. Clinically significant adverse events that follow immunization should be reported to the Vaccine Adverse Event Reporting System (VAERS). Guidance about how to obtain and complete a VAERS form is available at **www.vaers.hhs.gov** or by telephone, **800-822-7967**.

▇ Range of recommended ages   ▇ Catch-up immunization   ▇ 11–12 year old assessment

1. **Hepatitis B vaccine (HepB).** *AT BIRTH:* **All newborns** should receive monovalent HepB soon after birth and before hospital discharge. **Infants born to mothers who are HBsAg-positive** should receive HepB and 0.5 mL of hepatitis B immune globulin (HBIG) within 12 hours of birth. **Infants born to mothers whose HBsAg status is unknown** should receive HepB within 12 hours of birth. The mother should have blood drawn as soon as possible to determine her HBsAg status; if HBsAg-positive, the infant should receive HBIG as soon as possible (no later than age 1 week). **For infants born to HBsAg-negative mothers**, the birth dose can be delayed in rare circumstances but only if a physician's order to withhold the vaccine and a copy of the mother's original HBsAg-negative laboratory report are documented in the infant's medical record. *FOLLOWING THE BIRTHDOSE:* The HepB series should be completed with either monovalent HepB or a combination vaccine containing HepB. The second dose should be administered at age 1–2 months. The final dose should be administered at age ≥ 24 weeks. It is permissible to administer 4 doses of HepB (e.g., when combination vaccines are given after the birth dose); however, if monovalent HepB is used, a dose at age 4 months is not needed. **Infants born to HBsAg-positive mothers** should be tested for HBsAg and antibody to HBsAg after completion of the HepB series, at age 9–18 months (generally at the next well-child visit after completion of the vaccine series).

2. **Diphtheria and tetanus toxoids and acellular pertussis vaccine (DTaP).** The fourth dose of DTaP may be administered as early as age 12 months, provided 6 months have elapsed since the third dose and the child is unlikely to return at age 15–18 months. The final dose in the series should be given at age ≥ 4 years.
   Tetanus and diphtheria toxoids and acellular pertussis vaccine (Tdap – adolescent preparation) is recommended at age 11–12 years for those who have completed the recommended childhood DTP/DTaP vaccination series and have not received a Td booster dose. Adolescents 13–18 years who missed the 11–12-year Td/Tdap booster dose should also receive a single dose of Tdap if they have completed the recommended childhood DTP/DTaP vaccination series. Subsequent **tetanus and diphtheria toxoids (Td)** are recommended every 10 years.

3. *Haemophilus influenzae* **type b conjugate vaccine (Hib).** Three Hib conjugate vaccines are licensed for infant use. If PRP-OMP (PedvaxHIB® or ComVax® [Merck]) is administered at ages 2 and 4 months, a dose at age 6 months is not required. DTaP/Hib combination products should not be used for primary immunization in infants at ages 2, 4 or 6 months but can be used as boosters after any Hib vaccine. The final dose in the series should be administered at age ≥ 12 months.

4. **Measles, mumps, and rubella vaccine (MMR).** The second dose of MMR is recommended routinely at age 4–6 years but may be administered during any visit, provided at least 4 weeks have elapsed since the first dose and both doses are administered beginning at or after age 12 months. Those who have not previously received the second dose should complete the schedule by age 11–12 years.

5. **Varicella vaccine.** Varicella vaccine is recommended at any visit at or after age 12 months for susceptible children (i.e., those who lack a reliable history of chickenpox). Susceptible persons aged ≥ 13 years should receive 2 doses administered at least 4 weeks apart.

6. **Meningococcal vaccine (MCV4).** Meningococcal conjugate vaccine (MCV4) should be given to all children at the 11–12 year old visit as well as to unvaccinated adolescents at high school entry (15 years of age). Other adolescents who wish to decrease their risk for meningococcal disease may also be vaccinated. All college freshmen living in dormitories should also be vaccinated, preferably with MCV4, although **meningococcal polysaccharide vaccine (MPSV4)** is an acceptable alternative. Vaccination against invasive meningococcal disease is recommended for children and adolescents aged ≥ 2 years with terminal complement deficiencies or anatomic or functional asplenia and certain other high risk groups (see *MMWR* 2005;54 [RR-7]:1-21); use MPSV4 for children aged 2–10 years and MCV4 for older children, although MPSV4 is an acceptable alternative.

7. **Pneumococcal vaccine.** The heptavalent **pneumococcal conjugate vaccine (PCV)** is recommended for all children aged 2–23 months and for certain children aged 24–59 months. The final dose in the series should be given at age ≥ 12 months. **Pneumococcal polysaccharide vaccine (PPV)** is recommended in addition to PCV for certain high-risk groups. See *MMWR* 2000; 49(RR-9):1-35.

8. **Influenza vaccine.** Influenza vaccine is recommended annually for children aged ≥ 6 months with certain risk factors (including, but not limited to, asthma, cardiac disease, sickle cell disease, human immunodeficiency virus [HIV], diabetes, and conditions that can compromise respiratory function or handling of respiratory secretions or that can increase the risk for aspiration), healthcare workers, and other persons (including household members) in close contact with persons in groups at high risk (see *MMWR* 2005;54[RR-8]:1-55). In addition, healthy children aged 6–23 months and close contacts of healthy children aged 0–5 months are recommended to receive influenza vaccine because children in this age group are at substantially increased risk for influenza-related hospitalizations. For healthy persons aged 5–49 years, the intranasally administered, live, attenuated influenza vaccine (LAIV) is an acceptable alternative to the intramuscular trivalent inactivated influenza vaccine (TIV). See *MMWR* 2005;54(RR-8):1-55. Children receiving TIV should be administered a dosage appropriate for their age (0.25 mL if aged 6–35 months or 0.5 mL if aged ≥ 3 years). Children aged ≤ 8 years who are receiving influenza vaccine for the first time should receive 2 doses (separated by at least 4 weeks for TIV and at least 6 weeks for LAIV).

9. **Hepatitis A vaccine (HepA).** HepA is recommended for all children at 1 year of age (i.e., 12–23 months). The 2 doses in the series should be administered at least 6 months apart. States, counties, and communities with existing HepA vaccination programs for children 2–18 years of age are encouraged to maintain these programs. In these areas, new efforts focused on routine vaccination of 1-year-old children should enhance, not replace, ongoing programs directed at a broader population of children. HepA is also recommended for certain high risk groups (see *MMWR* 1999; 48[RR-12]1-37).

- DTaP or Tdap: Encephalopathy within 7 days of previous DTaP or DTP

Precautions include:
- Acute moderate to severe illness
- Recent administration of an antibody-containing blood products and live vaccines
- DTP or DTaP: unstable or evolving neurological disorder
- MMR: history of thrombocytopenia or thrombocy-topenic purpura
- High fever, shock, persistent crying, seizure, or Guillain-Barré syndrome due to previous dose of DTP or DTaP

Vaccine Management

- Maintain cold-chain during shipping.
- Follow manufacturers' recommendation for shipping.
- Nonfrozen vaccines must not freeze during transport.
- Refrigerate or freeze depending upon vaccine imme-diately upon arrival
- Utilize proper refrigerators.
  - * Monitor temperatures daily.
  - * Do not store vaccines in refrigerator door.
  - * Store in the middle of the refrigerator.
  - * Keep temperature log.

- Inventory management
  - * Maintain inventory log.
  - * Rotate stock.
  - * Follow manufacturers' guidelines for shelf life.
  - * Check expiration dates.
  - * Designate a person to be responsible for vaccines.
  - * Train all staff to recognize vaccine shipment arrivals.
- Follow manufacturers' directions for reconstitution.

3. Diseases and Vaccines

Pneumococcal Disease

- *Streptococcal pneumonia:* 90 known serotypes of gram-positive bacteria with a polysaccharide capsule
- Primary serious diseases include pneumonia, sepsis, and meningitis.

Rates of disease
- Highest rates seen in children less than 2 years of age
- Other children at high risk include those with asplenia, patients with HIV, American Indian-Alaskan Natives, African Americans, and day-care attendees.
- The elderly have fatality rates of 30-60% (those over the age of 50).
- Pneumococcal disease is one of the leading causes of vaccine-preventable diseases, with 20,000 to 40,000 cases of invasive disease every year.
- Pneumococcal bacteria are common respiratory tract inhabitants, with estimated asymptomatic carriage rates varying from 5-70%.
- Transmission is through direct person-to-person droplet contamination or autoinoculation by carriers.
- Clinical features include abrupt onset, fever, otitis media, shaking chills, productive cough, pleuritic chest pain, dyspnea, hypoxia, tachypnea, headaches, lethargy, vomiting, irritability, nuchal rigidity, seizures, coma, and death.
- Resistance to antibiotics is up to 35% in certain areas of the country and rising.

23-Valent polysaccharide vaccine (Pneumovax-23® by Merck)
- Ineffective in children less than 2 years old
- Effective against 88% of serotypes causing bacteremic disease

Indications
- Adults over the age of 65
- Everyone over age 2 years with chronic disease

Dose
- 0.5 mL IM or SC
- Revaccination (2-dose maximum)
  * Patients at high risk of disease if >5 years since previous dose
  * Everyone 65 years and older who received initial dose under the age of 65 and if >5 years since previous dose

Adverse reactions
- Adverse reactions include pain, swelling, and redness at the injection site and slight to moderate systemic reactions such as fever and myalgias.

7-Valent conjugated polysaccharide vaccine (Prevnar® by Wyeth)
- Effective against 86% of serotypes causing bacteremic disease, 83% of serotypes against meningitis, and 65% of serotypes causing otitis media

Indications
- Routine vaccination for all children less than 2 years of age
- Children 24-59 months of age with high-risk medical conditions

Dose
- 0.5 mL IM at 2, 4, 6, and 12-15 months of age (see schedules for catch-up recommendations)
- Revaccination not recommended but high-risk children should receive 23-valent polysaccharide vaccine after 2 years of age.

Adverse reactions
- Adverse reactions include pain, swelling, and redness at injection site, difficulty in moving the limb (rare), and slight to moderate systemic reactions such as fever and myalgias.

Influenza

- RNA virus of orthomyxovirus family
- Antigenic drift: frequent minor changes in the antigenic structure of the virus; this can reach epidemic proportions, but not every year. This is why yearly adjustments in vaccine formulations are required. All three types (A, B, and C) can undergo drifts.
- Antigenic shift: major changes in one or both of the major antigens in influenza A, resulting in a different subtype; this can result in major pandemics in all ages.

Influenza A
- Subtypes are based upon two surface antigens: hemagglutinin and neuraminidase.
- Six types of hemagglutinin (H1, H2, H3, H5, H7, and H9) cause disease in humans and cause virus attachment to cells.
- Two types of neuraminidase cause disease in humans (N1 and N2) and have a role in viral penetration of cells.
- Causes moderate to severe disease in all ages and can be transmitted in other animals

Influenza B
- No subgroups
- Causes milder disease and affects primarily children
- Only affects humans

Influenza C
- Rarely reported and many cases are subclinical

Influenza disease
- Major serious complications in all types include pneumonia, Reye's syndrome (progressive neurological symptoms associated with aspirin use in children), myocarditis, worsening of chronic bronchitis, and death.
- Rates of disease are highest in the elderly (>65), children less than 2 years of age, and persons of any age with medical conditions.
- Influenza is one of the leading causes of vaccine-preventable disease, with 20,000-40,000 deaths during epidemics. Pandemics could result in the deaths of over 400,000 people.
- Influenza virus penetrates the respiratory epithelial cells and destroys the host.
- Virus is shed in respiratory secretions for 5-10 days and transmission is through direct person-to-person droplet contamination or contact. The incubation period is approximately 2 days (range 1-5 days).
- Clinical features include abrupt onset, fever, myalgias, sore throat, nonproductive cough, and headache.
- Disease peaks between December and March in the Northern Hemisphere, but may occur earlier or later. Year-round cases may be seen in tropical climates.

Influenza vaccine (Fluvirin® by Novartis, Fluzone® by sanofi pasteur, Fluarix® by GSK)
- Inactivated, split-virus vaccine
- Contains 3 vaccine components (2 type A viruses and 1 type B virus)
- Vaccines are named according to the virus' type/geographic origin/strain sequence number/year of isolation (hemagglutinin neuraminidase for type A only): for example, A/Panama/2007/99(H3N2) or B/Hong Kong/330/2001.
- Effective in up to 90% of healthy adults, 50-60% of the elderly, and 30-40% of the frail elderly

Indications
- All children 6-59 months of age
- Close contacts of children 6-59 months of age
- Adults over the age of 50
- Adults and children over age 23 months with certain chronic diseases
- Residents of nursing homes or long-term care facilities
- People who may infect others, including contacts of patients with diseases, and health care workers
- Pregnancy in all trimesters or women who will become pregnant during the influenza season
- Patients 6 months to 18 years of age on chronic aspirin therapy
- Patients with neurological or neuromuscular disorders
- Anyone who wishes to decrease the likelihood of influenza disease

Dose
- 6-35 months: 0.25 mL IM (repeat in 1 month if first time); 3-8 years: 0.5 mL (repeat in 1 month if first time); >8 years: 0.5 mL
- Fluvirin by Novartis is indicated for those ≥4 years of age
- Fluarix is indicated for those ≥18 years of age
- Revaccination yearly

Contraindications
- Contraindications include severe allergic reactions to previous dose and egg allergy.

Adverse reactions
- Adverse reactions include pain, swelling, and redness at injection site and slight to moderate systemic reactions such as fever, myalgias, chills, and malaise. Severe neurologic reactions are rare.

Live attenuated influenza vaccine (LAIV) (FluMist® by MedImmune)
- Attenuated, cold-adapted live influenza vaccine
- Same vaccine antigens as in inactivated influenza vaccine
- Efficacy 86-93%
- Must be kept frozen (15°C or lower)

Indications
- Similar to inactivated vaccine unless contraindications exist
- Healthy persons age 5-49 years
- Contacts with high-risk patients, except the severely immunocompromised.

Contraindications (use inactivated influenza vaccine)
- Persons with chronic medical diseases
- Close contacts of severely immunocompromised persons
- Pregnancy
- Children receiving aspirin therapy
- Persons with a history of Guillain-Barré syndrome

Dose
- 0.25 mL sprayed in each nostril (0.5 mL total)
- Children age 5-8 who receive influenza vaccine for the first time need 2 doses 6-8 weeks apart.

Adverse reactions
- Similar to inactivated vaccine
- Nasal congestion
- Headache
- Vomiting

Tetanus

- Exotoxin produced by *Clostridium tetani,* a gram-positive anaerobic rod that may develop a highly resistant spore; these spores are widely spread in soil, animal intestines and feces, skin surfaces, and infected plants.
- The disease is characterized by generalized rigidity and convulsive spasms of skeletal muscles; usually involves muscles of the face (lockjaw) and neck. Spasms may last 3-4 weeks and complete recovery may take months.
- Enters the body through contamination of a wound. Spores germinate in an anaerobic environment. Toxins are released and transported through the body.
- Incubation period is usually 8 days (range, 3-21 days).
- Transmission risk factors include puncture wounds, surgery, burns, minor wounds, dental infections, animal bites, injection drug use, diabetes, and approximately 10% of cases are due to an unknown cause.
- Tetanus is not contagious person to person.
- Tetanus occurs in the U.S. at a rate of 0.02-0.05 per 100,000 per year. The case fatality rate is approximately 10%.
- Complications include: laryngospasm, fractures, hypertension, nosocomial infections, pulmonary embolism, aspiration, and death.
- Wound management recommendations may include tetanus immune globulin (Table 3).

Table 3

CDC Guidelines for Tetanus Wound Management

Vaccination history	Clean minor wounds		All other wounds	
	Td[1] or Tdap[2]	TIG[3]	Td[1] or Tdap[2]	TIG
Unknown or <3	Yes	No	Yes	Yes
Three or more	No[4]	No	No[5]	No

[1]Td, tetanus-diphtheria vaccine.
[2]Tdap, tetanus-diphtheria-pertussis vaccine.
[3]TIG, tetanus immune globulin.
[4]Yes, if >10 years since last dose.
[5]Yes, if >5 years since last dose.

Tetanus toxoid vaccine
- Usually combined with diphtheria toxoid pertussis vaccine
- Toxoid is formaldehyde-inactivated toxin adsorbed to aluminum.

Dose
- Pediatric dose: 0.5 mL IM of DT or DTaP given at 2, 4, 6, and 15-18 months of age; booster dose should be given at 4-6 years.
- Adolescent dose: 0.5 mL Tdap at 11-12 years
- Adult dose: 0.5 mL of Tdap if tetanus-containing vaccine is indicated
- Revaccination with Td every 10 years

Adverse reactions
- Adverse reactions include pain, swelling (nodule may form), and redness at injection site and systemic reactions are uncommon. An exaggerated (Arthus-type) reaction with extensive painful swelling from shoulder to elbow can occur at injection site and is thought to be caused by too-frequent injections.

Diphtheria

- Toxin produced by *Corynebacterium diphtheriae,* an aerobic gram-positive bacterium; this bacterium must be infected by a virus that carries a genetic code for toxin production.
- The most common presentation of diphtheria is characterized by early, nonspecific URI symptoms that develop into pharyngitis. Two to three days later, a bluish-white membrane starts to form that can cover the entire soft palate. The membrane can turn dark if bleeding occurs and manipulation of the membrane can result in bleeding. Airway obstruction may occur.
- Other sites of infection may include the larynx or the skin.
- Other complications may include myocarditis, neuritis with paralysis, respiratory failure, and death (overall case fatality rate of 5-10%).
- Asymptomatic human carriers are the source of most infections.
- The incubation period is usually 2-5 days (range, 1-10 days).
- Treatment of acute disease is with antitoxin and antibiotics.

Diphtheria toxoid vaccine
- Combined with tetanus toxoid pertussis vaccine; single toxoid antigen is not available.
- Toxoid is formaldehyde-inactivated toxin adsorbed to aluminum.
- Pediatric version of the combination (DT or DTaP)

contains 3-4 times as much antigen as the adult version (Td).

Dose

- Pediatric dose: 0.5 mL IM of DT or DTaP given at 2, 4, 6, and 15-18 months of age; booster dose should be given at 4-6 years.
- Adolescent dose: 0.5 mL Tdap at 11-12 years
- Adult dose: 0.5 mL of Tdap if tetanus-containing vaccine is indicated
- Revaccination with Td every 10 years

Adverse reactions

- Adverse reactions include pain, swelling (nodule may form), and redness at injection site; systemic reactions are uncommon. An exaggerated (Arthus-type) reaction with extensive painful swelling from shoulder to elbow can occur at the injection site and is thought to be caused by too-frequent injections of the tetanus antigen component of the combination vaccines.

Pertussis

- Pertussis, or whooping cough, is caused by *Bordetella pertussis,* an aerobic, gram-negative rod. The bacteria produces multiple antigenic products that are responsible for the clinical disease. The bacteria produces toxin that paralyzes the respiratory cilia and causes inflammation of the respiratory tract.
- The presentation of pertussis is in three stages. The first stage is a catarrhal stage with nonspecific URI symptoms. After 1-2 weeks the paroxysmal stage with the characteristic cough and inspiratory whoop begins and lasts up to 6 weeks. Recovery is gradual and the cough usually resolves in 2-3 weeks.
- The presentation in older children and adults may be much milder and present with a persistent mild cough that lasts up to 7 days and may appear to be similar to other upper respiratory infections.
- Complications may include pneumonia, encephalopathy, seizures, and death (overall case fatality rate of 0.2%).
- Asymptomatic human carriers are the source of most infections.
- The incubation period is usually 7-10 days (range, 14-21 days).
- Treatment of acute disease includes supportive care, antibiotics, and prophylaxis of contacts.
- Transmission is human-to-human by the respiratory route. Pertussis is highly contagious with attack rates of 80% in susceptible contacts.

Pertussis vaccine

- Combined with tetanus toxoid and diphtheria toxoid for children; single toxoid antigen is not available.
- Whole cell vaccine was developed in the 1930s, but is no longer available in the United States.
- Acellular pertussis vaccine was first licensed in 1991 and has fewer side effects than the whole cell vaccine.

Dose

- Pediatric dose: 0.5 mL IM of DTaP given at 2, 4, 6, and 15-18 months of age; booster dose should be given at 4-6 years.
- Adolescent dose: 0.5 mL of Tdap
- Adult dose: 0.5 mL of Tdap (one-time dose only)

Adverse reactions

- Adverse reactions include pain, swelling (nodule may form), and redness at the injection site and systemic reactions are uncommon. An exaggerated (Arthus-type) reaction with extensive painful swelling from shoulder to elbow can occur at the injection site and is thought to be caused by too-frequent injections of the tetanus antigen component of the combination vaccines.

Hepatitis B

- Hepatitis B is caused by a DNA virus and causes one of the most common infections worldwide. There are an estimated 200-300 million chronic carriers of hepatitis B worldwide.
- The clinical course is similar to that of all other types of viral hepatitis, with symptoms of malaise, weakness, anorexia, nausea, jaundice, abdominal pain, headache, and dark urine. Malaise and fatigue may last for weeks to months after all other symptoms disappear.
- Fulminant hepatitis occurs in 1-2% of all cases, with mortality rates of 60-90%.
- Complications are usually related to chronic infections with hepatitis B virus, and include chronic hepatitis, cirrhosis, liver failure, and hepatocellular carcinoma. Twenty-five percent of all carriers develop chronic, active hepatitis.
- The risk of becoming a carrier following infection ranges from 6-50%.
- The incubation period is usually 7-10 days (range, 14-21 days).
- Transmission is human-to-human by exposure of body fluids by parenteral or mucosal contact. Hepatitis B is a common sexually transmitted disease. Perinatal transmission is a significant mode of infection.

Hepatitis B vaccine

- The first vaccine was a plasma-derived vaccine released in 1981 and removed from the market in 1992.
- The current vaccine is hepatitis B surface antigen (HBsAg) produced using recombinant DNA technology; it was first released in 1986. Two products are currently marketed: Recombivax HB® (Merck) and Engerix-B® (GlaxoSmithKline). Although the antigen contents are different, the two vaccines are interchangeable.

Dose

- Pediatric dose: the usual dose is 0.5 mL IM given at birth, 2 months, and 6 months.
- Indications include all infants, all adolescents, and high-risk adults (eg, multiple sex partners, STDs, injection drug use, dialysis, hemophilia, others).
- The usual adult dose is 1.0 mL given at 0, 2, and 6 months.
- Adolescents aged 11-15 years may be given a two-dose series separated by 4 months. This is only approved for Recombivax HB.
- Booster doses should not be given.

Adverse reactions

- Adverse reactions include pain, swelling (nodule may form), and redness at the injection site; systemic reactions are uncommon.

Haemophilus influenzae Type b (Hib)

- *Haemophilus influenzae* is a gram-negative coccobacillus, whose outer shell consists of a polyribosyl-ribitol phosphate (PRP) polysaccharide capsule. There are six distinctly different types of *H influenzae,* labeled a-f; however, type b is responsible for 95% of human disease.
- The organism enters through the nasopharynx and may cause disease or may colonize the nasopharynx, creating an asymptomatic carrier.
- The most common clinical infections caused by Hib are meningitis, epiglottitis, pneumonia, arthritis, and cellulitis. Meningitis accounts for 50-65% of all clinical disease and results in a mortality of 2-5% and neurological sequelae in 15-30% of cases. Other diseases caused by *Haemophilus influenzae* include otitis, sinusitis, and bronchitis; however, these are usually due to nontypable (unencapsulated) strains.
- Hib is primarily a disease of children, with a peak at age 6-7 months and rarely attacks after the age of 5 years.
- Treatment of acute disease includes hospitalization, intravenous antibiotics, and prophylaxis of contacts.
- Transmission is human-to-human by respiratory droplet spread to susceptible individuals.

Haemophilus influenzae vaccine

- The incidence of Hib disease has decreased by more than 99% since the introduction of vaccine.
- The first vaccine licensed (1985-1988) was a pure polysaccharide vaccine that was ineffective in children less than 18 months of age.
- Current vaccines are polysaccharide vaccine conjugated to protein carriers. The specific carriers vary by manufacturer (Table 4).
- HbOC (HibTITER), PRP-T (ActHIB or OmniHIB), and PRP-OMB (PedvaxHIB) are indicated for infants ≥6 weeks of age.
- Doses given before 6 weeks of age may inhibit the production of antibodies to subsequent doses; therefore the vaccines are contraindicated in children less than 6 weeks of age.

Dose

- The usual dose for the vaccines approved for infants is 0.5 mL IM given at 2 months, 4 months, and 6 months. A booster dose is recommended for children

Table 4

Haemophilus influenzae **Type B Vaccines**

Vaccine	Protein carrier	Manufacturer	Age indications
HbOC (HibTITER®)	Mutant diphtheria toxoid	Lederle-Praxis	≥6 weeks
PRP-T (ActHIB® or OmniHIB®)	Tetanus toxoid	Aventis Pasteur	≥6 weeks
PRP-OMB (PedvaxHIB®)	Meningococcal group B outer membrane protein	Merck & Co	≥6 weeks

12-15 months of age. If PRP-OMB (PedvaxHIB) is used for the pediatric series, the 6-month dose should be omitted.
- The catch-up series for Hib vaccine varies by age and manufacturer. Consult the package insert for complete dosing information.
- Vaccination of children >59 months of age is not indicated unless there are certain medical indications. These include persons with asplenia, immunodeficiency conditions, and those undergoing immunosuppressive therapy.
- Combination vaccines of Hib vaccine and hepatitis B vaccine (COMVAX® by Merck) and Hib vaccine and DTaP (TriHIBit® by sanofi pasteur) are available. TriHIBit is not approved for the initial pediatric series (2, 4, and 6 months) and can only be used for a dose at ≥12 months of age when a previous dose of Hib was given ≥2 months earlier, and TriHIBit will be the last dose in the Hib series. COMVAX must not be administered before 6 weeks of age.

Adverse reactions
- Adverse reactions include pain, swelling, and redness at the injection site; systemic reactions are uncommon.

Hepatitis A

- Hepatitis A is caused by an RNA virus and is the most common hepatitis infection in the United States.
- The clinical course is similar to that of all other types of viral hepatitis, with symptoms of malaise, weakness, anorexia, nausea, jaundice, abdominal pain, headache, and dark urine. Malaise and fatigue usually lasts for 2 weeks; however, symptoms may last or recur for up to 6 months.
- Fulminant hepatitis A is rare, but can occur. The incidence increases with age >40 years. Not indicated for children <1 year of age
- While serious complications are not as common as with hepatitis B, morbidity and its associated costs (health care costs and lost work days) are significant.
- There is no risk of becoming a chronic carrier.
- The incubation period averages 28 days (range, 15-50 days).
- Treatment of acute disease is supportive.
- Transmission is human-to-human by the fecal-oral route of exposure.
- Exposure of an unimmunized person to hepatitis A requires the administration of immune globulin intramuscular (IGIM) as well as beginning the hepatitis A vaccine series.

Hepatitis A vaccine: Havrix® by GlaxoSmithKline and VAQTA® by Merck and Co.)
- Inactivated whole virus vaccines
- Both vaccines are available in pediatric and adult formulations.
- Hepatitis A vaccine is not indicated for children <1 year of age.
- The two vaccines use different potency measurements, but the volume and schedule of the dose is the same.

Dose
- Children and adolescents over 1 year of age are given 0.5 mL and repeated in 6-12 months (Havrix) or 6-18 months (VAQTA), for a total of 2 doses.
- Adults over 18 years old are given 1.0 mL and repeated in 6-12 months, for a total of 2 doses.

Combination vaccine (Twinrix® by GlaxoSmithKline)
- A combination product with hepatitis B (adult dose) and hepatitis A (pediatric dose)
- Given at 0, 1, and 6-12 months
- Indicated for persons ≥18 years of age

Adverse reactions
- Adverse reactions include pain, redness, and swelling at the injection site. Mild systemic reactions are rare.

Meningococcal

- Meningococcal disease is caused by *Neisseria meningitidis,* a gram-negative bacteria with a polysaccharide capsule.
- The clinical diseases caused by *Neisseria meningitidis* include meningitis, sepsis, pneumonia, myocarditis, and urethritis. It is one of the leading causes of meningitis in the United States.
- The types of *Neisseria meningiditis* that cause over 95% of disease are serogroups A, B, C, W-135, and Y.
- There are approximately 2500-3000 cases per year with an incidence rate of 2 cases per 100,000 people. The incidence in college freshmen that live in dormitories is approximately 4 cases/100,000.
- There is a carrier state that increases in incidence during epidemics.
- Parts of the world, including parts of Africa and Asia, have a high rate of disease.
- Treatment of acute disease is with antibiotics.

Polysaccharide meningococcal vaccine (Menomune® by Sanofi Pasteur)
- This is a polysaccharide vaccine effective against serogroups A, C, W-135, and Y. The vaccine does

not protect against serogroup B, a common cause of infection.
- Indicated for persons over the age of 2 years.
- Those who should be vaccinated include military personnel, freshmen college students living in dormitories, those with anatomic or functional asplenia, and travelers to the "meningitis belt" of sub-Saharan Africa. Evidence of immunization is required for religious pilgrimages to Saudi Arabia for the Islamic Hajj. Vaccine may also be useful during an outbreak.

Dose
- The dose is 0.5 mL given subcutaneously.
- A booster dose after 3-5 years may be needed.

Adverse reactions
- Adverse reactions include pain, swelling (nodule may form), and redness at the injection site and mild systemic reactions, such as fever, headaches, and malaise.

Conjugated polysaccharide meningococcal vaccine (Menactra® by sanofi pasteur)
- This is a polysaccharide vaccine that is conjugated to diphtheria toxoid.
- It is effective against serogroups A, C, W-135, and Y. The vaccine does not protect against serogroup B, a common cause of infection.
- Approved for ages 11-55
- The Advisory Committee on Immunization Practices (ACIP) recommends vaccination for those aged 11-12 and college freshmen living in dormitories.
- Indications are the same as for the polysaccharide vaccine.

Dose
- The dose is 0.5 mL given intramuscularly.
- It is unknown if a booster dose will be needed.

Polio

- There are three poliovirus types identified as P1, P2, and P3.
- The virus enters the mouth and replicates in the gastrointestinal tract. From the GI tract, the virus enters the bloodstream and infects the cells of the central nervous system.
- Up to 95% of all infections are asymptomatic; however, these persons may transmit the infection to others.
- Approximately 4-8% of infections are mild with nonspecific symptoms of upper respiratory infection, gastroenteritis, and influenza-like symptoms.
- One to two percent of infections present as nonparalytic aseptic meningitis, which typically resolves in 2-10 days.

- Flaccid paralysis occurs in less than 1% of those infected.
- The incubation period is usually 6-20 days (range, 3-35 days).
- Treatment of acute disease includes supportive care.
- Transmission is person to person by the fecal-oral route.

Polio vaccine (IPOL® by sanofi pasteur)
- The current vaccine available in the United States is an inactivated, trivalent injectable vaccine (IPV).
- Use of oral polio vaccine (OPV) was discontinued in the United States due to the elimination of wild-type polio disease and because yearly cases of vaccine-associated paralytic poliomyelitis (VAPP) were reported.

Dose
- Pediatric dose: 0.5 mL IM given at 2, 4, 6-18 months, and 4-6 years of age
- Routine vaccine or booster doses for adults are not recommended.

Adverse reactions
- Adverse reactions include minor pain, swelling, and redness at the injection site; systemic reactions are uncommon.

Measles, Mumps, and Rubella

Measles
- Measles is a viral infection whose main presentation is a maculopapular rash.
- The virus is shed through the nasopharynx.
- Ten to twelve days after exposure, the prodrome phase begins, with progressive fever, cough, coryza, and conjunctivitis.
- Two to four days after the prodrome begins, a maculopapular rash begins on the face and head and gradually spreads throughout the body.
- The rash lasts 3-5 days then gradually fades.
- The incubation period is 10-12 days.
- Transmission is person to person through large respiratory droplets.
- Measles is highly contagious.
- Complications may include pneumonia, otitis, encephalitis, and death.

Mumps
- Mumps is a viral infection with a presentation of parotitis in 30-40% of cases.
- The virus is shed through the nasopharynx.
- Fourteen to eighteen days after exposure, the prodrome phase begins, with headache, malaise, myalgias, and low-grade fever.

- Two days after the prodrome begins is when the parotitis begins.
- Symptoms start to decrease after 1 week and disappear after 10 days.
- The incubation period is 14-18 days (range, 14-25 days).
- Transmission is person to person through large respiratory droplets.
- Complications can include orchitis, oophoritis, pancreatitis, and deafness.

Rubella

- Rubella is a viral infection with up to 20-50% of cases subclinical and inapparent.
- The virus is shed through the nasopharynx.
- A 1-5 day prodrome phase begins after incubation, with headache, malaise, myalgias, lymphadenopathy, low-grade fever, and URI symptoms. This phase is rare in children.
- Fourteen to seventeen days after exposure, a maculopapular rash appears, first on the face, and then descending to cover the rest of the body.
- The rash disappears after about 3 days.
- The incubation period is 14 days (range, 12-23 days).
- Transmission is person to person through large respiratory droplets.
- Complications may include arthritis, arthralgias, encephalitis, and hemorrhaging.
- The major complication is congenital rubella syndrome, which occurs in the offspring of a woman who had rubella during pregnancy. Babies born with CRS have major birth defects that can affect many organs.

Measles-mumps-rubella vaccine (MMRII® by Merck)

- The current vaccine available in the United States is a live, attenuated vaccine against all three diseases.

Dose

- Pediatric dose: 0.5 mL IM given at 12 months of age
- A second dose is recommended at 4-6 years of age to produce immunity in those who did not respond to the first dose.
- This vaccine is contraindicated in pregnancy. Pregnancy should be avoided for 4 weeks following vaccination.
- Serologic testing may be necessary to document immunity to rubella.
- Vaccination with the combination product should be used when one or more of the vaccines are needed unless a contraindication exists for an antigen component of the vaccine.

Adverse reactions

- Adverse reactions include minor pain, swelling, and redness at the injection site, and systemic reactions that mimic a mild case of the diseases.

Varicella (Chickenpox)

- Chickenpox is a viral infection caused by the herpes zoster virus.
- The primary infection is called chickenpox and the recurrent disease is herpes zoster (called shingles).
- The virus enters through the respiratory tract and replicates in the nasopharynx and regional lymph glands.
- The incubation period is 14-16 days (range, 10-21 days).
- A prodromal phase may precede the rash with a slight fever and malaise.
- The rash progresses from a macule to a papule to a vesicle before it crusts over.
- The rash appears in several waves that last 2-3 days each.
- The rash first appears on the face and then the trunk (where most of the rash occurs), and the extremities.
- Recurrent disease (herpes zoster) appears to be related to aging and immunosuppression.
- Recurrent disease usually presents as an outbreak of lesions along a dermatome and is usually unilateral. Neuralgia and intense pain may be present.
- Transmission is person to person by infected respiratory secretions.
- Complications may include pneumonia, secondary bacterial infections, CNS infections and symptoms, and Reye's syndrome if a child is taking aspirin.

Varicella vaccine (Varivax® by Merck)

- The current vaccine available in the United States is a live, attenuated vaccine.

Dose

- Pediatric dose: 0.5 mL IM given at 12-18 months of age
- A second dose is recommended at 4-6 years of age
- The adult dose (age >13 years) is 2 doses of 0.5 mL each separated by 4-8 weeks.
- This vaccine is contraindicated in pregnancy and pregnancy should be avoided for 4 weeks following vaccination.
- Other contraindications include immunosuppressive disease or patients receiving immunosuppressive therapy, and those receiving antibody-containing blood products.
- Adverse reactions include minor pain, swelling and redness at the injection site, and systemic reactions that mimic a mild case of the disease, including a mild generalized rash.

- The vaccine must be stored frozen at +5°F (−15°C). The diluent used to reconstitute the vaccine should be stored at room temperature.

Combination Vaccines

- As mentioned in several sections previously, there are several vaccination combinations on the market.
- Tetanus, diphtheria, and pertussis combinations (various manufacturers): DTaP, DT, Td, Tdap
- Twinrix by GlaxoSmithKline: a combination product with hepatitis B (adult dose) and hepatitis A (pediatric dose)
- Hib vaccine and hepatitis B vaccine: COMVAX by Merck
- Hib vaccine and DTaP: TriHIBit by sanofi pasteur
- Pediarix® (GlaxoSmithKline)
  * DTaP + hepatitis B + inactivated polio
  * Indicated when all vaccine components are indicated
  * Not approved for <6 weeks or >7 years of age
  * Efficacy, contraindications, and adverse reactions are similar to those of the vaccine components given separately.
  * Dose: 0.5 mL IM given at 2, 4, and 6 months of age
  * Must be shaken vigorously prior to drawing up in syringe
  * Can be given even if infant receives birth dose of hepatitis B vaccine
- ProQuad® by Merck: a combination vaccine of measles, mumps, rubella, and varicella vaccine

4. Key Points

- The two types of vaccine antigens include live viruses and inactivated viruses or bacterial components.
- There are two types of immunity: active and passive.
- Adverse effects of inactivated vaccines include pain at the injection site and mild systemic symptoms (mild fever). Adverse effects of live vaccines mimic a mild case of the disease.
- Live vaccines should be avoided during pregnancy.
- Influenza viruses undergo shifts and drifts, which accounts for the need for yearly vaccine changes.
- Wound management must include evaluation for the need for tetanus toxoid and tetanus immune globulin.
- Diphtheria toxoid and tetanus toxoid should always be given together, unless there is a contraindication to one of the components. If there is a need for one, then there is a need for both.
- A new combination vaccine of tetanus, diphtheria, and pertussis is available for use in adolescents and adults (Tdap). It is recommended one time for persons 11-64 years of age. Children under the age of 7 years receive DTaP or DT (if unable to tolerate pertussis vaccine). All other ages should receive Td if vaccination is indicated.
- Hepatitis B vaccine is now recommended for all infants, starting at birth, as well as all adolescents. Other indications include adults with high-risk occupations or behaviors.
- Hepatitis A vaccine is recommended for travel to most parts of the world.
- Inactivated polio vaccine (IPV) is the only polio vaccine recommended for use in the U.S. Oral polio vaccine (OPV) is not recommended due to the high incidence of vaccine-associated paralytic poliomyelitis (VAPP).
- A second dose of MMR vaccine and varicella vaccine is recommended at 4-6 years of age.
- Combination vaccines are available to decrease the number of injections.

5. Questions and Answers

1. A 62-year-old patient presents to your pharmacy for a refill of his insulin. It is October and he asks you to review his immunization status with him. About which adult vaccine do you need to ask his status?

   I. Influenza vaccine
   II. Pneumococcal vaccine
   III. Meningococcal vaccine
   IV. Hepatitis A vaccine
   V. Diphtheria-tetanus (Td) vaccine

   A. I only
   B. I and II only
   C. III and IV only
   D. I, III, and V only
   E. I, II, and V only

2. The patient in question 1 states that he received his pneumococcal vaccine 2 years ago. When should he receive another?

   A. Never
   B. Every year
   C. In 5 years
   D. When he reaches the age of 67
   E. When he reaches the age of 65

3. Which of the following describes the current injectable influenza vaccine used in the United States?

   A. Inactivated virus
   B. Live attenuated virus
   C. Conjugated vaccine
   D. Toxoid
   E. Toxin

4. Indications for meningococcal conjugate vaccine include

   I. all adolescents aged 11-12
   II. travel to the "meningitis belt" of sub-Saharan Africa
   III. asplenia
   IV. pilgrimage to Saudi Arabia for the Islamic Hajj
   V. college freshmen living in dormitories

   A. I only
   B. II, III, and V only
   C. I, II, and III only
   D. II, III, IV, and V only
   E. All of the above

5. At what age does one switch from DTaP to Td?

   A. 2 years
   B. 5 years
   C. 7 years
   D. 10 years
   E. DTaP can be used in all age groups

6. Which of the following vaccines has BOTH a polysaccharide and a conjugated vaccine on the U.S. market?

   I. Influenza
   II. Meningococcal vaccine
   III. *Haemophilus influenzae* type B vaccine
   IV. Hepatitis vaccine
   V. Pneumococcal vaccine

   A. IV only
   B. II and V only
   C. I, II, and III only
   D. II, III, and V only
   E. All of the above

7. Which polio vaccine schedule is recommended in the United States?

   A. Four doses of IPV
   B. Four doses of OPV
   C. Four doses of IPV plus a booster at 18 years of age
   D. Two doses of OPV and 2 doses of IPV
   E. Polio vaccine is no longer recommended in the United States.

8. Hepatitis B vaccine is a

   A. polysaccharide vaccine
   B. recombinant hepatitis B surface antigen vaccine
   C. live vaccine
   D. conjugate vaccine
   E. a toxoid

9. An 18-year-old, healthy student is told that she needs to come to the pharmacy for her routine vaccinations prior to starting college. She will be living in the dormitory at school. She has not received any vaccines since grade school. Which of the following vaccines are indicated?

   I. MMR if she has not received a second dose
   II. Varicella if she has not had previous vaccination or varicella vaccination
   III. Meningococcal vaccine
   IV. Pneumococcal vaccine

V.   Tdap if she has not received one for 10 years

    A. All of the above
    B. I and II only
    C. I, II, III, and IV only
    D. I, III, and V only
    E. I, II, III, and V only

10. The patient in question 9 is exposed to a patient with hepatitis A 1 month later. She should receive the following vaccines.

    A. Hepatitis A vaccine series only
    B. Hepatitis B vaccine series only
    C. Hepatitis A vaccine series plus IGIM
    D. Hepatitis A vaccine plus hepatitis B vaccine series
    E. IGIM only

11. Which of the following are high-risk groups that should be targeted for annual influenza vaccination?

    A. Persons aged 5-49 years
    B. Persons with diabetes
    C. Patients aged 21-49 with hypertension
    D. Construction workers
    E. Healthy teenagers

12. Which complication of rubella infection is the most significant health problem?

    A. Congenital rubella syndrome
    B. Secondary infection
    C. Patent ductus arteriosus
    D. Diarrhea
    E. Arthritis

13. Which of the following is a valid contraindication to the receipt of a live-virus vaccine?

    A. Taking antibiotics
    B. Recent administration of antibody-containing blood products
    C. Age over 12 months
    D. Allergies to penicillin
    E. A parent or sibling with a cold who is living in the same household

14. The most common adverse reaction to an inactivated vaccine is

    A. Rash
    B. Severe headache
    C. Injection site reactions

    D. Rhinorrhea
    E. Stomach pain

15. The only vaccine recommended at birth is

    A. DTaP
    B. IPV
    C. Hib
    D. pneumococcal conjugate vaccine
    E. hepatitis B

16. A 32-year-old female is injured in an automobile accident and her spleen is removed. Which of the following vaccines is NOT routinely recommended for asplenic adult patients?

    A. Pneumococcal vaccine
    B. Meningococcal vaccine
    C. IPV
    D. *Haemophilus influenzae* type B vaccine
    E. Yearly influenza vaccines

17. If a second dose of a vaccine were given too soon (before the minimal interval time period has passed), the correct course of action would be

    A. Restarting the entire series
    B. Do not count that dose and repeat it after the minimal time period has passed since the incorrect dose
    C. Do not worry about it and continue with the next dose as scheduled
    D. Draw antibody titers to confirm immunity
    E. Double the next dose

18. Which of the following groups of children are NOT at increased risk for pneumococcal disease?

    A. Children with mild asthma
    B. Children of Native Alaskan descent
    C. Children of African-American descent
    D. Children with sickle cell disease
    E. Children infected with HIV

19. Which of the following statements are true concerning *Haemophilus influenzae* type b vaccine (Hib)?

  I.   Hib is recommended for all infants without contraindications
  II. Standard dosing for Hib vaccine is 2, 4, 6, and 12-18 months of age
  III. The 6-month dose is omitted if PedvaxHIB is used for the first 2 doses

IV. Hib vaccine is not routinely recommended for children aged 5 years and older

A. Only I is correct
B. Only I, II, and III are correct
C. Only II, III, and IV are correct
D. Only II and III are correct
E. All are correct

20. Which of the following vaccines available in the United States is a live, attenuated virus vaccine?

A. Polio (IPV)
B. *Haemophilus influenzae* vaccine (Hib)
C. DTaP
D. Varicella vaccine
E. Pneumococcal vaccine

Answers

1. **E.** Routine vaccinations in the adult are a yearly influenza vaccine, Td vaccine every 10 years, and a single pneumococcal vaccine for patients with select chronic illnesses (such as diabetes). Meningococcal and hepatitis vaccines are recommended only for certain indications.

2. **D.** Routine revaccination with pneumococcal vaccine is not recommended. Revaccination is recommended for select high-risk groups and everyone 65 years and older who received an initial dose under the age of 65 and if >5 years have elapsed since the previous dose.

3. **A.** Influenza vaccine is an attenuated, split virus vaccine. The LAIV is administered intranasally.

4. **E.** With the recent availability of a conjugate meningococcal vaccine, the ACIP recommended including all adolescecents aged 11-12 among the other recommendations.

5. **C.** DTaP is indicated for children under the age of 7. Due to adverse effects of DTaP in children aged 7 and older, Td is used.

6. **B.** Polysaccharide pneumococcal vaccine (23-valent) is indicated for those over the age of 2 years and conjugated polysaccharide vaccine (7-valent) is approved for ages 2 months to 7 years. There is a recently approved meningococcal conjugate vaccine; however, the polysaccharide vaccine will be removed from the market once supplies of the conjugate vaccine are adequate.

7. **A.** OPV is no longer recommended in the United States and vaccination with IPV will continue until poliovirus is eradicated worldwide.

8. **B.**

9. **E.** Pneumococcal vaccine is not recommended for a healthy individual until the age of 65.

10. **C.** The hepatitis A vaccine will not protect an individual who has previously been exposed to the virus. IGIM, a source of antibodies (short-term protection), will help to protect immediately, and the vaccine will protect against future exposures (long-term protection).

11. **B.** High-risk groups targeted for influenza vaccination beginning in October include persons aged 6-23 months, persons >50 years old, persons at increased risk (age >24 months with chronic pulmonary disease [eg, emphysema, COPD], cardiovascular disease [eg, CHF, post-MI, heart anomalies], metabolic disease [eg, diabetes], renal dysfunction, hemoglobinopathies [eg, sickle cell], and immunosuppression [eg, HIV infection, chemotherapy]), residents of long-term care facilities, people 24 months to 18 years old on aspirin chronically, pregnant women in all trimesters, hospital and outpatient employees, nursing home employees with patient contact, home health care providers working with high-risk persons, household members of high-risk persons, and persons desiring to avoid influenza infection.

12. **A.** Complications of rubella may include arthritis, arthralgias, encephalitis, and hemorrhaging; however, the major complication is congenital rubella syndrome, which occurs in the offspring of a woman who had rubella during pregnancy. Babies born with CRS have major birth defects that can affect many organs.

13. **B.** Live virus vaccines will be killed if there has been recent administration of antibodies. The length of time that must separate these two products depends on the dose and type of antibody-containing blood product being used.

14. **C.** Local reactions are the most common type of adverse reaction, and include pain, swelling, and redness at the site of injection. These usually occur within minutes to hours of the injection and are usually mild and self-limiting. Systemic adverse reactions include fever, malaise,

myalgias, and headache, and are more common following live vaccines.

15. **E.** All of the other listed vaccines are first given at 2 months of age. Hepatitis B vaccine is recommended at birth to decrease the incidence of hepatitis B in infants of hepatitis B–infected mothers.

16. **C.** Asplenic patients require protection against the encapsulated bacteria (pneumococcus, meningococcus, and *Haemophilus*), as well as common viral infections. Previous series completions of routine vaccines, such as measles, varicella, and polio, are adequate for protection. Td vaccines should be repeated every 10 years.

17. **B.** The minimal interval in a series for most vaccines is 4 weeks. Decreasing the interval may interfere with antibody response and protection. Usually the last dose in a series is separated from the previous dose by 4-6 months. Increasing the interval does not affect vaccine effectiveness. You never need to restart a series except for oral typhoid vaccine.

18. **A.** Rates of pneumococcal disease are highest in children <2 years of age, those with asplenia, patients with HIV, American Indian-Alaskan Natives, African-Americans, and day care attendees. Mild asthma is not considered a high-risk disease for pneumococcal infection.

19. **E.** While all of the answers are correct, HIB vaccine may be indicated for children over the age of 5 with certain chronic conditions. This vaccine is relatively complicated to use since recommendations vary among manufacturers. Please consult package inserts before administering.

20. **D.** Varicella, live attenuated influenza vaccine (LAIV), and measles-mumps-rubella vaccines are the only routinely administered live vaccines in the U.S. Other non-routinely administered live vaccines include oral typhoid vaccine, vaccinia (smallpox) vaccine, and yellow fever vaccine. The majority of vaccines are inactivated or killed vaccines.

6. References

Advisory Committee on Immunization Practices. General recommendations on immunizations. *MMWR Morb Mortal Wkly Rep.* 2000;49(RR-2):1-36.

Advisory Committee on Immunization Practices. Poliomyelitis prevention in the United States: updated recommendations. *MMWR Morb Mortal Wkly Rep.* 2000;49(RR-5):1-22.

Advisory Committee on Immunization Practices. Prevention and control of influenza. *MMWR Morb Mortal Wkly Rep.* 2005;54(RR-8):1-40.

Advisory Committee on Immunization Practices. Prevention and control of meningococcal disease and meningococcal disease and college students. *MMWR Morb Mortal Wkly Rep.* 2000;49(RR-5):1-20.

Advisory Committee on Immunization Practices. Prevention of hepatitis A through active or passive immunization. *MMWR Morb Mortal Wkly Rep.* 1999;48(RR-12):1-37.

Advisory Committee on Immunization Practices. Prevention of pneumococcal disease. *MMWR Morb Mortal Wkly Rep.* 1997;46:1-24.

Advisory Committee on Immunization Practices. Preventing pneumococcal disease among infants and young children. *MMWR Morb Mortal Wkly Rep.* 2000;49(RR-9):1-38.

Advisory Committee on Immunization Practices. Prevention of varicella. *MMWR Morb Mortal Wkly Rep.* 1996;45(RR-11):1-36.

Advisory Committee on Immunization Practices. Prevention of varicella: updated recommendations of the ACIP. *MMWR Morb Mortal Wkly Rep.* 1999;48(RR-6):1-5.

Advisory Committee on Immunization Practices. Revised ACIP recommendation for avoiding pregnancy after receiving a rubella-containing vaccine. *MMWR Morb Mortal Wkly Rep.* 2001;50:1117.

Advisory Committee on Immunization Practices. Update: recommendations to prevent hepatitis B virus transmission—United States. *MMWR Morb Mortal Wkly Rep.* 1999;48(RR-12):1-37.

Advisory Committee on Immunization Practices. Update: vaccine side effects, adverse reactions, contraindications, and precautions. *MMWR Morb Mortal Wkly Rep.* 1996;45(RR-12):1-35, errata *MMWR Morb Mortal Wkly Rep.* 1997;46:227.

Advisory Committee on Immunization Practices. Use of diphtheria toxoid-tetanus toxoid-acellular pertussis vaccine as a five dose series. *MMWR Morb Mortal Wkly Rep.* 2000;49(RR-13):1-8; erratum *MMWR Morb Mortal Wkly Rep.* 2000;49(47):1074.

Centers for Disease Control and Prevention. *Epidemiology and Prevention of Vaccine-Preventable Diseases,* 7th ed. CDC; 2003.

Centers for Disease Control and Prevention. National Immunization Website: http://www.cdc.gov/nip

Grabenstein JD. Immunofacts: Vaccines and Immunologic Drugs, Revision 26. St. Louis: Facts and Comparisons; May 2002.

Plotkin SA, Orenstein WA, ed. *Vaccines,* 3rd ed. Philadelphia: WB Saunders; 1999.

33. Pediatrics

Catherine M. Crill, PharmD, BCPS, BCNSP
Assistant Professor,
Departments of Clinical Pharmacy and Pediatrics
University of Tennessee College of Pharmacy

Contents

1. Special Drug Therapy Considerations in Pediatric Patients

Pediatric Age Definitions

Preterm: <36 weeks gestation
Term: ≥36 weeks gestation
Neonate: <1 month
Infant: 1 month to 1 year
Child: 1 to 11 years
Adolescent: 12 to 16 years

Absorption

Gastric pH

- Infants may be considered to be in a relative state of achlorhydria (due to decreased basal acid secretion and total volume of secretions); however, they are capable of producing sufficient gastric acid with stimuli (eg, in response to histamine or pentagastrin challenge, enteral feeding, or stress).
- Gastric acid production reaches adult values by approximately 3 years of age.

Implications for drug therapy
- * Increased bioavailability of basic drugs
- * Decreased bioavailability of acidic drugs
- * Increased bioavailability of acid-labile drugs (eg, penicillin G)

Gastric emptying time in pediatric patients

- Gastric emptying time (GET) is longer than it is for adults.
   - * GET is inversely related to postconceptional age.
- Irregular and unpredictable peristalsis
- Decreased motility
- Premature neonates have longer GET than term neonates and have a greater incidence of gastroesophageal reflux (GER)
- Related to type of feeding (formula-fed infants exhibit longer transit time than breast-fed infants)
- Approaches adult function by 7 to 9 months
   - * Stomach muscles are mature at 7 months.
   - * Stomach muscles are completely innervated at 9 months.

Implications for drug therapy
- * Erratic absorption of sustained-release products (eg, theophylline)
- * The rate of absorption in small intestine, where most drugs are absorbed, is slower; peak drug concentrations are lower than for adults.

Pancreatic enzymes and bile salts
- Low levels of amylase and lipase
- Low intraluminal bile acid concentrations and synthesis
- Decreased proteolytic ability

Implications for drug therapy
- Erratic absorption of drugs requiring pancreatic enzymes for hydrolysis (eg, chloramphenicol)
- Decreased absorption of lipid-soluble drugs
- Decreased fat absorption from enteral feedings
- Decreased absorption of fat-soluble vitamins

GI mucosa
- Decreased functional integrity of intestinal mucosa
- The surface area of the gastric mucosa is small compared to that of intestinal mucosa (most drugs are absorbed from the small intestine).
- Changes in splanchnic blood flow in the neonatal period may alter the concentration gradient across the intestinal mucosa.

Other absorption routes
Skin
- * Absorption via skin is inversely related to the thickness of the stratum corneum and directly related to hydration of the skin.
- * Neonates (particularly premature) have increased skin hydration.
- * The stratum corneum of preterm infants is immature and ineffective as an epidermal barrier.
- * Premature neonates may develop drug toxicity if a drug is administered via the dermal route.

Buccal route
- Not typically used in pediatric patients

Intramuscular route
- * Drug delivery is restricted by volume of medication and the pain associated with administration. Results are variable in premature neonates due to (1) blood flow and vasomotor instabilities; and (2) insufficient muscle mass and tone, contraction, and oxygenation.

Rectal administration
- Effective for drug delivery in older infants and children

Administration via intraosseous route (IO route)
- * This vessel-rich marrow (up to 5 years of age) is a great site for drug delivery to the systemic circulation. It may be an acceptable route in emergency situations for children over 5 years

of age (vessel-rich marrow is then replaced by yellow marrow).

Distribution

Protein binding
- Decreased albumin and α_1-acid glycoprotein concentrations
- Lower binding capacity
- Qualitative differences in neonatal plasma proteins
- Competitive binding by endogenous substances (unconjugated bilirubin, free fatty acids)
- Risk of kernicterus (hypoalbuminemia, unconjugated hyperbilirubinemia, displacement by highly protein-bound drugs or free fatty acids)
- Exhibit adult-like binding by 3 to 6 months of age; adult concentrations of albumin and α_1-acid glycoprotein are achieved at 10 to 12 months.

Differences in body composition
- Altered vascular and tissue perfusion
- The brain and liver are the largest organs in children.
- Total body water is greater in neonates and infants.
- Extracellular fluid volume is greater in neonates and infants.
- Relative lack of adipose tissue in neonates and infants (adipose level increases into adulthood)

Implications for drug therapy in neonates and infants
- Increased free fraction of drugs
- Increased potential of drug displacement by endogenous substances
- Potential risk of kernicterus with physiologic jaundice (unconjugated hyperbilirubinemia)
- Hydrophilic drugs, which parallel water in the body (eg, aminoglycosides), exhibit greater volume of distribution.
- Lipophilic drugs (eg, diazepam) parallel body fat and will exhibit a smaller volume of distribution.

Liver Metabolism

Phase I reactions (nonsynthetic): Oxidation, reduction, hydrolysis, and hydroxylation
  * The hepatic cytochrome P450 (CYP450) enzyme system is responsible for most phase I reactions.
  * The capacity of isoenzymes in the CYP450 system at birth is 20-70% of adult capacity and increases with postnatal age.
  * Full capacity for reduction at birth
  * Hydrolysis is most developed at birth, followed by the processes of oxidation and hydroxylation.

  * Benzyl alcohol, a preservative present in certain medications, can accumulate in neonates due to underdeveloped alcohol dehydrogenase. Gasping syndrome (ie, metabolic acidosis, respiratory failure, seizures, neurologic deterioration and CV collapse) can result.

Phase II reactions (synthetic): Conjugation with glycine or glutathione, glucuronidation, sulfation, methylation, and acetylation
  * The sulfation pathway is the most developed pathway at birth.
  * Glucuronidation begins around 2 months of age (it reaches adult capacity by 3 years of age).
  * Assumptions about substances primarily metabolized by glucuronidation (ie, morphine, bilirubin, chloramphenicol):
    - Potentially toxic in neonates
    - May exhibit long half-lives (eg, toxicity with chloramphenicol)
    - May require greater dosing in infants (eg, morphine conjugated to its more active metabolite)
    - May be metabolized by another pathway in infants (eg, acetaminophen is primarily metabolized via sulfation in infants).
  * Methylation is functional in infants but not significantly expressed in adults. (Methylation is responsible for the conversion of theophylline to caffeine.)

Implications for drug therapy
- For drugs undergoing phase I and II reactions, metabolism is reduced and half-life prolonged in infants and neonates.
- Insufficiency of one pathway may lead to metabolism via another.
- Drug metabolism, slower in the neonate, increases between 1 and 5 years of age and is similar to drug metabolism in adults after puberty.

Renal Elimination

- Renal blood flow is only 5-6% of cardiac output at birth, compared to 15-25% in adults (12 mL/min versus 140 mL/min).
- Glomerular filtration rate is lower at birth and reaches adult values by 1 to 5 months of age in term infants.
- Tubular secretion is low at birth and reaches adult values by 7 months of age in term infants.
- Renal elimination is affected by prematurity and postconceptional age; it increases with maturity.

Estimation of creatinine clearance in pediatric patients

- Altered by differences in renal blood flow, glomerular filtration, tubular secretion, and muscle mass
- May be affected by the presence of maternal serum creatinine over the first week of life (ie, false underestimation of creatinine clearance)
- The Schwartz equation may be used for calculation of creatinine clearance:

$$CrCl \ (mL/min/1.73 \ m^2) = k \times (length \ in \ cm)/SCr$$

k = proportionality constant that changes with age and sex (Table 1)

Other Pediatric Drug Issues

- Digoxin-like immunoreactive substance (DLIS) is produced in infants and may interfere with digoxin assays and falsely elevate concentrations.
- Di(2-ethylhexyl)phthalate (DEHP), a plasticizer contained in IV bags, is shown to have an effect on the male reproductive system. Pediatric patients at highest risk of DEHP exposure are neonates on ECMO, those receiving parenteral and enteral nutrition, and those receiving plasma exchange transfusions.
- Polyethylene glycol (PEG), an additive used to promote stability in certain IV medications, can cause hyperosmolarity in infants.

Table 1

Proportionality Constant for Calculation of Creatinine Clearance Using the Schwartz Equation[1]

Age	k
Low birth weight ≤1 year	0.33
Full term ≤1 year	0.45
1-12 years	0.55
14-21 years (female)	0.55
14-21 years (male)	0.70

[1]From Schwartz et al, 1987.

2. Specific Infections and Disease States in the Pediatric Population

Otitis Media

Otitis media is an inflammatory process of the middle ear.

Classification
- Acute otitis media is an inflammation of the area behind the eardrum (tympanic membrane) in the chamber called the middle ear. It is accompanied by the presence of fluid in the middle ear (effusion) and by the rapid onset of signs or symptoms of ear infection (also see AAP/AAFP definition in section on diagnostic criteria).
- Recurrent otitis media is the diagnosis of three episodes of acute otitis media within a 6-month period or four episodes within a year.
- Otitis media with effusion is fluid in the middle ear (effusion) without the associated signs or symptoms of acute infection.

Clinical presentation
- Signs and symptoms include fever, otalgia (often manifested as ear tugging or pulling), otorrhea (discharge from the ear), changes in balance or hearing, irritability, difficulty sleeping, lethargy, anorexia, vomiting, and diarrhea.
- Associated findings may be runny nose, congestion, and/or cough.

Pathophysiology
Eustachian tube dysfunction
  * The infant's eustachian tube is shorter and more horizontal than that of the adult.
  * This prevents drainage of middle ear secretions into the nasopharynx and promotes pooling of secretions in the middle ear.
- Anatomic abnormalities increase risk (eg, cleft palate, adenoid hypertrophy).
- Immature immune system or altered host defenses increase risk.
- Viral infections and allergies increase risk.
- Risk factors include male gender; Native American, Canadian Eskimo, or Alaskan descent; family history of acute otitis media or respiratory tract infection; early age of first episode (earlier age is associated with greater severity and recurrence); day care environment; parental smoking; children not breastfed; and pacifier use.
- Complications include mastoiditis, meningitis, subdural empyema, hearing loss, and delayed speech and language development.

Microbial pathogens

Viral

- Up to 50% of cases of acute otitis media may be viral in origin.

Bacterial

- *Streptococcus pneumoniae* is responsible for 40-50% of bacterial otitis media. Resistance is becoming an increasing problem; bacterial resistance occurs primarily through alteration in penicillin-binding protein (decreased affinity for binding sites).
- *Haemophilus influenzae* (primarily nonencapsulated/nontypable strains) is responsible for 20-30% of bacterial otitis media cases. Bacterial resistance occurs via β-lactamase production.
- *Moraxella catarrhalis* is responsible for 10-15% of bacterial otitis media; almost all strains are β-lactamase–producing.

Diagnostic criteria

- Clinical presentation (ie, signs and symptoms consistent with infection)
- The American Academy of Pediatrics (AAP) and American Academy of Family Physicians (AAFP) Clinical Practice Guideline on the Diagnosis and Management of Acute Otitis Media was published in 2004 and presented a revised definition of acute otitis media as follows:
    * Diagnosis requires: (1) a history of acute onset of signs and symptoms, (2) the presence of middle ear fluid (by a bulging tympanic membrane, limited/absent mobility of or air-fluid level behind the tympanic membrane, or otorrhea), and (3) signs and symptoms of middle ear inflammation (distinct erythema of the tympanic membrane or distinct otalgia referable to the middle ear that interferes with normal sleep/activity).
- The presence of middle ear disease:
    * Otoscopic examination determines color, translucency, and position.
        • Redness or opacity of membrane, absence of light reflection, or bulging membrane
    * Pneumatic otoscopic examination determines mobility of tympanic membrane (ie, presence or absence of effusion).
        • Membrane will not move briskly with positive and negative pressure if effusion is present.
    * Tympanocentesis (ie, a needle is inserted through the tympanic membrane to withdraw fluid) allows for culture and identification of the pathogen.

Treatment principles and goals

- Assess and control pain.
- Eradicate infection.
- Prevent complications.
- Avoid unnecessary antibiotic therapy.
- Improve compliance.
- Eliminate presence of effusion.
- Prevent recurrence.

Drug therapy

- Many episodes of otitis media will have spontaneous resolution; however, since there is a risk of developing complications from untreated otitis media, antimicrobials remain the mainstay of therapy. Observation therapy may be appropriate in certain patients based on age, diagnostic certainty, and severity of illness, and when follow-up can be ensured.

First-line therapy

- Amoxicillin is the drug of choice for uncomplicated acute otitis media.
    * Excellent in vitro activity against *S pneumoniae* and most *H influenzae*
    * Optimal pharmacodynamic profile of available agents; reaches good concentrations in middle ear fluid
    * Excellent safety and efficacy profile with narrow spectrum of activity
    * Palatable and inexpensive
    * May overcome drug-resistant *S pneumoniae* with higher doses (ie, achieves greater concentrations in middle ear fluid)
    * Does not eradicate β-lactamase–producing organisms
- For penicillin-allergic patients (non–type I hypersensitivity, ie, urticaria or anaphylaxis), cefdinir, cefpodoxime, or cefuroxime may be used. In patients with type I reactions, azithromycin, clarithromycin, trimethoprim-sulfamethoxazole (6-10 mg/kg/day of trimethoprim), or erythromycin-sulfisoxazole (50 mg/kg/day of erythromycin) may be substituted; however, resistance appears to be increasing with these agents. Based on severity of illness, ceftriaxone therapy may be initiated. Clindamycin may be used when drug-resistant *S pneumoniae* is suspected.
- Amoxicillin-clavulanate may be used as first-line therapy based on severity of illness.
- Other effective antimicrobial agents include other cephalosporins (cefprozil, cefaclor, loracarbef, ceftibuten). Fluoroquinolones (ciprofloxacin, ofloxacin, levofloxacin) are thought to be effective, but they are not approved for use in pediatric patients.

Dosing issues and drug resistance (Table 2)
- Amoxicillin
  * Standard dose: 40-45 mg/kg per day (no longer recommended)
  * High dose: 80-90 mg/kg per day (recommended)
- Amoxicillin-clavulanate
  * Standard dose (no longer recommended) versus high dose (recommended) while maintaining clavulanate dose of <10 mg/kg/day (to prevent diarrhea)
  * If using a high dose, use a formulation with higher ratio of amoxicillin to clavulanate (7:1 formulation). Alternatively, additional amoxicillin may be added to standard amoxicillin-clavulanate (4:1 formulation); however, this approach complicates therapy.
- IM ceftriaxone
  * Single dose versus three daily doses

Duration of therapy
- Standard 10-day course
- Shorter course (1-7 days)
  * Advantages are improved compliance, decreased adverse effects of drug therapy, decreased risk of bacterial resistance, and lower costs.
  * Disadvantages are delayed or no cure, increased risk of complications from untreated acute otitis media, and greater risk of recurrence.
  * Not appropriate for:
    - Children <2 years of age (AAP/AAFP states <6 years of age)
    - Children with severe disease
    - Those in day care
    - Those with underlying diseases
    - Those with a history of recurrent otitis media

Table 2

Treatment Options for Otitis Media

	First line	Penicillin allergy
***Non-severe illness:* At diagnosis (initial antibiotic therapy)**	Amoxicillin (80-90 mg/kg/day)	Non type I: Cefdinir (14 mg/kg/day in 1 or 2 doses) **OR** cefuroxime (30 mg/kg/day in 2 doses) **OR** cefpodoxime (10 mg/kg/day once daily)
		Type I: Azithromycin (10 mg/kg day 1, 5 mg/kg days 2-5 OR clarithromycin (15 mg/kg/day in 2 doses)
***Severe illness:* At diagnosis (initial antibiotic therapy)**	Amoxicillin-clavulanate (90 mg/kg/day amoxicillin, 6.4 mg/kg/day clavulanate)	Ceftriaxone (50 mg/kg daily for 1 or 3 days)
***Non-severe illness:* Treatment failure at 48-72 hours (initial observation option)**	Amoxicillin (80-90 mg/kg/day)	Non type I: Cefdinir (14 mg/kg/day in 1 or 2 doses) **OR** cefuroxime (30 mg/kg/day in 2 doses) **OR** cefpodoxime (10 mg/kg/day once daily)
		Type I: Azithromycin (10 mg/kg day 1, 5 mg/kg days on 2-5 **OR** clarithromycin (15 mg/kg/day in 2 doses)
***Severe illness:* Treatment failure at 48-72 hours (initial observation option)**	Amoxicillin-clavulanate (90 mg/kg/day amoxicillin, 6.4 mg/kg/day clavulanate)	Ceftriaxone (50 mg/kg daily for 1 or 3 days)
***Non-severe illness:* Treatment failure at 48-72 hours (initial antibiotic therapy)**	Amoxicillin-clavulanate (90 mg/kg/day amoxicillin, 6.4 mg/kg/day clavulanate)	Non-type I: Cefriaxone (50 mg/kg daily for 3 days) Type I: Clindamycin (30-40 mg/kg/day in 3 doses)
***Severe illness:* Treatment failure at 48-72 hours (initial antibiotic therapy)**	Ceftriaxone (50 mg/kg daily for 3 days)	Tympanocentesis; clindamycin (30-40 mg/kg/day in 3 doses)

Observation option: must have follow-up at 48-72 hours; access to antibiotics if symptoms persist or worsen.

Non-severe illness: mild otalgia and fever <39°C.

Severe illness: moderate to severe otalgia or fever of 39°C.

From AAP/AAFP Clinical Practice Guideline, 2004.

Other therapy

- Antipyretics (acetaminophen, ibuprofen)/analgesics
    * Use acetaminophen with caution in high doses (hepatotoxicity).
    * Use ibuprofen with caution in patients with vomiting, diarrhea, and poor fluid intake (dehydration predisposes to ibuprofen-induced renal insufficiency).
    * Avoid alternating antipyretic therapy. Encourage parents to choose one agent, inform them of any adverse effects, and educate them about symptoms of these effects (ie, hepatotoxicity or renal insufficiency).
- Narcotic analgesics may be used for moderate to severe pain not controlled with acetaminophen or ibuprofen.
- Topical analgesics include otic solutions, such as antipyrine-benzocaine (Auralgan®, Americaine Otic®) and naturopathic agents (Otikon Otic Solution®).
- Topical antimicrobials may have a place in therapy, particularly with ruptured membranes (fluoroquinolone or fluoroquinolone/steroid combination otic suspensions [Floxin®, Cipro HC®, Ciprodex®]).
- Antihistamines/decongestants are ineffective at eliminating effusion or relieving symptoms. Use them only if indicated for other signs or symptoms.

Patient instructions and counseling

- Complete the entire course of prescribed antibiotics.
- Shake bottle well before administering dose. Follow labeling regarding temperature for storage of medication.
- Contact the physician if patient develops a rash, has difficulty breathing, or if symptoms persist after 72 hours of initiating therapy.

Adverse drug events

- Gastrointestinal: nausea and diarrhea
- Hypersensitivity: rash, anaphylaxis

Drug interactions

- Macrolides, particularly erythromycin and clarithromycin

Nondrug therapy

- Local heat or cold therapy may be used (counsel the caregiver on appropriate use and technique to prevent burn injury).
- Tympanostomy tubes decrease recurrent episodes, restore hearing, and relieve discomfort. Risks include anesthesia and permanent tympanic membrane scarring.

Observation therapy

- Appropriate only when follow-up at 48-72 hours can be ensured and antimicrobials initiated if symptoms persist or worsen
- Not appropriate for:
    * Infants <6 months of age
    * Infants and children between 6 months and 2 years old with a certain diagnosis (nonsevere or severe illness) or an uncertain diagnosis (severe illness)
    * Children ≥2 years of age with a certain diagnosis and severe illness
- Nonsevere illness: mild otalgia and fever <39.0°C
- Severe illness: moderate to severe otalgia or fever ≥39.0°C

Immunization and immunoprophylaxis

- Pneumococcal conjugate vaccination should provide some protection against strains responsible for a majority of bacterial otitis media.
- *Haemophilus influenzae* type B vaccination is of no benefit in otitis media (note that most strains causing otitis media are nontypable and not prevented by vaccination).
- Killed and live-attenuated intranasal influenza vaccine may decrease episodes of acute otitis media during the respiratory season (most children studied were >2 years of age).

Risk reduction

- Alter day care attendance (when possible).
- Exclusive breastfeeding for 6 months
- Avoid supine bottle feeding.
- Reduce or eliminate pacifier use after 6 months of age.
- Eliminate passive exposure to tobacco smoke.

Recurrent otitis media

- Prophylaxis with half therapeutic dosing of amoxicillin or sulfisoxazole has been initiated in high-risk patients; however, this practice is no longer recommended due to concerns over emergence of drug-resistant organisms

Otitis media with effusion

- The AAP, AAFP, and the American Academy of Otolaryngology-Head and Neck Surgery published a clinical practice guideline on otitis media with effusion in 2004.
- It applies to infants and children (2 months to 12 years of age) with or without developmental disabilities or underlying conditions that predispose patients to otitis media with effusion.
- Recommendations include:
    * Pneumatic otoscopy as the primary diagnostic method

* Distinguish otitis media with effusion from acute otitis media.
* Determine the risk of speech, language, and learning problems.
  • At-risk children: more rapid evaluation and intervention
  • Children not at risk: watchful waiting for 3 months from date of onset or diagnosis
* No role for antihistamines, decongestants, antimicrobials or corticosteroids
* Hearing testing: recommended with effusion ≥3 months or when language delay, learning problems, or hearing loss exists
* Persistent otitis media with effusion (not at risk): perform evaluations every 3 to 6 months until resolution of effusion, hearing loss is identified, structural abnormalities are suspected, or when the child becomes a surgical candidate (tympanostomy tube insertion preferred).

Otitis Externa

Otitis externa is an inflammation of the outer ear canal, also referred to as swimmer's ear.

Clinical presentation
• Itching, pain, otic exudate, and hearing impairment

Pathophysiology
• Presence of moisture in the ear canal
• Disruption of the integrity of the ear canal
• Most common organisms are *Pseudomonas aeruginosa* and *Staphylococcus aureus.*
• Other pathogens include fungi and *Bacillus* and *Proteus* species.
• Therapy consists of antibiotic/steroid otic preparations: neomycin/polymyxin/hydrocortisone (Cortisporin Otic®), neomycin/colistin/hydrocortisone (Coly-Mycin S Otic®), fluoroquinolone otic preparations (ciprofloxacin; Cipro HC; ofloxacin; Floxin), acetic acid and hydrocortisone otic preparations (VoSol HC Otic®), or oral analgesics.
• Preventive measures include drying ears after exposure to moisture, using drops containing isopropyl alcohol with or without acetic acid to reduce pH, and avoiding cotton swabs.
• Application of otic drops (see APhA Special Report, 1994):
1. Wash hands before and after administration.
2. Warm otic drops to room temperature by holding bottle in hands for several minutes. Avoid instilling cold or hot drops into the ear canal.
3. Shake the bottle if indicated on the label.
4. Tilt the child's head to the side or have the child lie down.

5. Pull the child's ear backward and upward and instill the drops in the ear canal. Do not put the dropper bottle inside the ear canal (to remain free from contamination it should not come into contact with the ear).
6. Press gently on the small flap over the ear to push the drops into the canal.
7. Have the child remain in the same position for the period of time indicated in the labeling. If this is not possible, place a cotton ball gently into the ear to prevent the drops from draining out of the ear canal.
8. Wipe excess medication from the outside of the ear.

Cystic Fibrosis

Cystic fibrosis is an autosomal recessive disease of exocrine gland function resulting in abnormal mucus production.

Genetic classification
• Cystic fibrosis is the result of a gene mutation on the long arm of chromosome 7. The protein encoded by this gene, the cystic fibrosis transmembrane regulator (CFTR), is a channel involved in the transport of water and electrolytes.

Defects in processing
• The most common genetic mutation involves a 3-base-pair deletion at position 508 (ΔF508).
• Patients homozygous for ΔF508 are pancreatic insufficient.
• Prognosis is not as good as for those who are pancreatic sufficient.
• Defects in protein production, regulation, and conduction

Clinical presentation
Pulmonary complications
• Initial manifestations include chronic cough, wheezing, hyperinflation of lungs, or lower respiratory tract infections.
• Patients present with hypoxia, clubbing, labored breathing, acute respiratory exacerbations (fever, sputum production, and increased oxygen requirements, and dyspnea); changes in forced vital capacity (FVC), forced expiratory volume in 1 second (FEV_1), and residual volume; and the development of a chronic obstructive picture as the disease progresses.

Gastrointestinal complications
• Poor digestion of proteins and fats, resulting in foul-smelling steatorrhea; distal intestinal obstruction

(commonly manifested as vomiting of bilious material, abdominal distension, and pain)
- Infants may have meconium ileus and gastro-esophageal reflux.

Other
- Cirrhosis and cholelithiasis
- Pancreatic function
- Insulin insufficiency, diabetes mellitus
- Malnutrition
- Nasal polyps and sinusitis, anemia, arthritis, osteopenia, and osteoporosis

Pathophysiology
- Defect in the chloride transport channel in secretory epithelial cells

Normal physiology
- Chloride is transported out of blood followed by sodium and water.

Cystic fibrosis
- Decreased chloride and water secretion and increased sodium absorption leads to thick, dehydrated secretions and mucus.
- Exocrine gland involvement: pancreas, hepatobiliary ducts, gastrointestinal tract, and the lungs (secretions build up and block airways and pancreatic and hepatobiliary exocrine flow)

Pulmonary system
- Initial obstruction of small airways with mucus plugging results in bronchiolitis and persistence of bacteria.
- Early bacterial pathogens: *Staphylococcus aureus* and *Haemophilus influenzae* present in younger patients.
- Later bacterial pathogens: *Pseudomonas aeruginosa* is the primary pathogen in late childhood.
- Other bacterial pathogens: *Proteus* and *Klebsiella* species, *Stenotrophomonas maltophilia,* and *Burkholderia cepacia*
- Possible viral pathogens
- Chronic pulmonary infection and inflammation progress to large airway and eventual chronic obstructive disease

Pancreatic system
- Pancreatic enzyme insufficiency (trypsin, chymotrypsin, lipases, and amylase) and decreased bicarbonate secretion (necessary for optimal pancreatic enzyme activity)
    - * Maldigestion of fats and proteins and fat-soluble vitamin deficiency
- Insulin insufficiency (resistance and decreased secretion) leads to glucose intolerance and the devel-

opment of diabetes mellitus (occurs later in the disease process and may be associated with increased morbidity and mortality).

Biliary system
- Biliary cirrhosis or fatty infiltration may lead to portal hypertension, development of bleeding varices, hypersplenism, and cholelithiasis.

Sweat glands
- High concentration of sodium and chloride in sweat (representing the failure of sweat glands to reabsorb sodium and chloride)

Reproductive system
- Male infertility is common due to bilateral absence of vas deferens.
- Female infertility due to abnormal cervical mucus

Diagnostic criteria
- Laboratory confirmation of CFTR dysfunction via sweat chloride analysis (ie, administration of pilocarpine)
1. Sweat is collected and electrolytes are measured.
2. Chloride of 60 mEq/L or more is diagnostic (values of up to 80 mEq/L have been seen in non-CF patients)
3. Levels of 50-60 mEq/L are indeterminate and tests may need to be repeated.
- Presence of clinical characteristics of cystic fibrosis

Treatment goals
- Halt or decrease disease progression.
- Maintain normal growth and development and nutrition status.
- Maintain pulmonary function.
- Optimize drug therapy for pharmacokinetic differences in cystic fibrosis patients.

Drug therapy (Table 3)
Antibiotic therapy in acute exacerbations
Antibiotic selection
- Empiric therapy initially and then treat based on sputum culture and sensitivity
- IV administration of two antibiotics for 14-21 days in combination with aggressive therapy for clearance of secretions
- Coverage for *Staphylococcus aureus, Haemophilus influenzae,* and *Pseudomonas aeruginosa*
- Double coverage of antibiotics when *Pseudomonas* species are suspected, with antipseudomonal penicillin (piperacillin, mezlocillin, piperacillin-tazobactam, ticarcillin-clavulanate, ticarcillin, aztreonam, meropenem, or imipenem) or a cephalosporin (ceftazidime) and an aminoglycoside
    - * Tobramycin plus ticarcillin or piperacillin (*P aeruginosa*)

Table 3

Drug Therapy for Cystic Fibrosis

Therapeutic category	Indication and mechanism of action	Comments
Pancreatic enzymes Capsule (Cotazym®, Ku-Zyme®) Microencapsulated (Cotazym-S®, Creon®, Pancrease®, Pancrelipase®, Protilase®, Ultrase®, Zymase®) Tablet (Ilozyme®, Viokase®) Powder (Viokase®)	Supplementation or replacement of pancreatic enzymes (treatment of malabsorption syndrome) Aids in digestion of proteins, carbohydrates, and fats	Products differ by enzyme content (units of lipase, protease, amylase) and dosage form Primary enzyme component is lipase Dose is typically whole dose with meals; half dose with snacks Adequate replacement decreases bowel movements and improves stool consistency
Fat-soluble vitamins	Supplementation of fat-soluble vitamins A, D, E, and K	May be dosed individually, through the use of 1 or 2 multivitamins daily, or with a water-miscible combination preparation
Nebulization therapy	Liquefaction of pulmonary secretions	Can be accomplished with normal saline or sterile water with or without other therapies[1]
N-acetylcysteine (Mucomyst®)	Lowers mucus viscosity through sulfhydryl group, which opens the disulfide bond in mucoproteins	Bad taste and odor; significant efficacy has not been documented
Recombinant human DNase (dornase alfa, Pulmozyme®)	DNA in mucus contributes to viscosity; mechanism of action is through cleavage of DNA (thereby decreasing mucus viscosity)	Expensive; reduces viscosity, improves pulmonary function; may decrease respiratory exacerbations
Ursodeoxycholic acid (ursodiol, Actigall®)	Bile acid that suppresses hepatic synthesis and secretion of cholesterol; inhibits intestinal cholesterol absorption; solubilizes cholesterol	Aids in dissolution of stones with cholelithiasis
Bronchodilators (β_2-agonists, theophylline)	Bronchodilator in reversible or obstructive airway disease	May be of benefit for patients with component of reactive airway disease; should use β_2-agonist before theophylline because of pharmacokinetic issues Response (improvement in FEV_1) should be documented before initiating long-term therapy
Antibiotics	Treat infection	Altered pharmacokinetics may affect and complicate therapy
Ibuprofen	Nonsteroidal anti-inflammatory; controls airway inflammation	Not used routinely; may have an effect on slowing pulmonary disease High dosages needed to achieve good concentrations (requires therapeutic drug monitoring)
Corticosteroids	Anti-inflammatory	Not used routinely; positive effects on pulmonary function but negative effects on growth and development, glucose sensitivity, and bone health

[1]Other therapies include N-acetylcysteine and recombinant human DNase.

* Tobramycin plus ceftazidime (*P aeruginosa*)
* Oxacillin or nafcillin (methicillin-sensitive *S aureus*)
* Vancomycin (methicillin-resistant *S aureus*)
- *Burkholderia* and *Stenotrophomonas* species are commonly resistant. Follow culture and sensitivity results. Antibiotics that may be effective include trimethoprim-sulfamethoxazole, chloramphenicol, ceftazidime (*B cepacia*), doxycycline, and piperacillin (*S maltophilia*)
- Other agents: ciprofloxacin

Antibiotic therapy and chronic suppression
Chronic inhaled antibiotic therapy with tobramycin (TOB)
- Significant improvement in FEV_1, decreased hospitalizations, and decreased need for IV antibiotics
- Decreased systemic concentrations (ie, less resistance) and high pulmonary concentrations
- Therapy is expensive.

Oral antibiotic therapy
- Fluoroquinolones are the only oral antibiotics with good coverage against *Pseudomonas*.

Patient instructions and counseling
- Compliance with therapeutic regimens

Pancreatic enzyme supplementation
- Give immediately before or during snacks and meals.
- Capsule may be opened and contents sprinkled on applesauce or other acidic carrier; contents should not be crushed or chewed.

Aminoglycosides
- Monitor urine output.
- Use ibuprofen with caution if dehydration, diarrhea, and/or decreased oral intake is present.

Adverse drug events
Aminoglycosides
- Nephrotoxicity and ototoxicity

Ibuprofen
- Renal insufficiency

Fluoroquinolones
- Arthropathy

Drug interactions
- Pancreatic enzymes and acid suppression therapy may decrease inactivation of enzymes by gastric acid, thereby reducing dose requirement.

Parameters to monitor
Clinical status
- Fever, activity level
- Pulmonary function (as indicated by FEV_1, FVC, residual volume, and chest radiography)

Pharmacokinetic considerations
Aminoglycosides
- Increased clearance and larger Vd (necessitating greater dosing); concentration-dependent killing and postantibiotic effect against gram-negative organisms
- Higher doses (10 mg/kg per day)
- Peak concentrations from 8-12 mcg/mL
- Trough concentrations of less than 2 mcg/mL

β-Lactams
- No change or increased clearance
- No change or increased Vd
- No postantibiotic effect or concentration-dependent killing

Fluoroquinolones
- Concentration-dependent killing
- Postantibiotic effect against gram-negative organisms

Nondrug therapy
Pulmonary percussion therapy and postural drainage
- The purpose is to clear mucus and secretions from the pulmonary system.
- Conducted once or twice per day and up to five times daily or more
- Percussion usually conducted after nebulization therapy with or without bronchodilator or mucolytic
- Therapy with hand-held devices or oscillatory vests

Transplantation
- Lung transplantation
- Liver-lung transplantation if there is liver involvement

Attention-Deficit/Hyperactivity Disorder

According to *DSM-IV*, ADHD is a behavioral disorder of childhood onset (by the age of 7 years) characterized by symptoms of inattentiveness and impulsive or hyperactive behavior.

Classification (*DSM-IV*)
- Combined type: criteria for inattention, hyperactivity, and impulsivity are met.
- Predominantly inattentive type: criteria for inattention are met, but not for hyperactivity and impulsivity

- Predominantly hyperactive, impulsive type: criteria for inattention are not met and criteria for hyperactivity and impulsivity are met.
- ADHD not otherwise specified

Clinical presentation

Inattention
- The child has difficulty paying attention, daydreams frequently, is easily distracted and disorganized, and loses things frequently.

Hyperactivity
- The child has difficulty staying seated and talks too much.

Impulsivity
- The child acts and speaks out without thinking; the child also interrupts others frequently.

Pathophysiology
- Imbalance in catecholamine neurotransmission (specifically between dopamine and norepinephrine)

Genetic basis
- Genetic studies have primarily evaluated genes involved in neurotransmission.
- Likely to be due to interaction of many genes
- Most evidence currently indicates that dopamine transmitter (DAT-1) and dopamine D_2 and D_4 receptors are responsible (dopamine and norepinephrine are potent agonists of the D_4 receptor).

Diagnostic criteria must be met for accurate diagnosis
- Diagnosis is based on *DSM-IV* criteria of six or more of the criteria for inattention and/or hyperactivity and impulsivity are met for at least 6 months "to a degree that is maladaptive and inconsistent with developmental level."
- Some impairment was present before 7 years of age
- Impairment is present in at least two settings (eg, home and school).
- Evidence of clinically significant impairment in functioning
- Symptoms are not related to another illness (eg, schizophrenia or mood disorder).

Treatment goals
- Educate the patient and family.
- Improve functioning and behavior.
- Achieve effective drug therapy with minimal side effects.

Drug therapy (Table 4)

Patient counseling
- Advise patients and caregivers of the need to store medications away from other children or siblings due to the potential for lethal overdose (tricyclic antidepressants) and potential for abuse (stimulants).

Adverse drug effects
- Stimulants cause anorexia, abdominal pain, headache, insomnia, jitteriness, social withdrawal, transient motor tics, and weight loss (not height-dependent).
- Methylphenidate is contraindicated in seizure disorder according to the package insert (ie, it lowers the seizure threshold). Canada has suspended marketing of Adderall XR® due to concern over reports of sudden death and stroke in patients taking Adderall® or Adderall XR.
- Tricyclics carry cardiotoxicity risk (sudden death). Patients should undergo ECG testing prior to initiation of therapy and periodically throughout therapy.
- Bupropion may lower the seizure threshold. Seizures are associated with high doses and previous history of seizure disorders. Minimize risk by dividing the daily dose or by using the extended-release formulation.
- Atomoxetine labeling has recently been revised to include warnings of an increased risk of suicidal ideation in children and adolescents and for the potential for severe liver injury.

Drug interactions

Methylphenidate
- MAO inhibitors (severe hypertension)
- Caffeine may enhance stimulant effects.
- Methylphenidate may inhibit metabolism of phenytoin, phenobarbital, warfarin, and tricyclics.

Tricyclics
- Multiple pharmacodynamic and pharmacokinetic drug interactions
- Increased plasma concentrations of tricyclics; potential toxicity when certain antidepressants are added to the regimen (fluoxetine, sertraline, fluvoxamine, paroxetine) as well as with cimetidine, methylphenidate, diltiazem, quinidine, and verapamil
- Decreased concentrations of tricyclics may be seen with concomitant administration of carbamazepine and phenytoin.
- Increased therapeutic effect and potential toxicity with MAO inhibitors
- Increased CNS depressant effects with alcohol and sedatives

Table 4

Drug Therapy for Attention-Deficit/Hyperactivity Disorder

Therapeutic category	Mechanism of action	Comments
Stimulants (first-line therapy)		
Short-acting: Methylphenidate (Ritalin®, Methylin®), Intermediate-acting: Methylphenidate (Ritalin SR®, Metadate ER®, Methylin ER®) Long-acting methylphenidate (Concerta®, Metadate CD®, Ritalin LA®, Daytrana®) Short-acting amphetamine (Dexedrine®, Dextrostat®) Intermediate-acting amphetamine (Adderall®, Dexedrine® Spansule) Long-acting amphetamine (Adderall-XR®)	Reuptake blockade of catecholamines (norepinephrine and dopamine) in presynaptic nerve endings	Due to concern of sudden death and stroke, methylphenidate should not be used in children or adults with structural cardiac abnormalities Do not give after 4 PM; may cause insomnia Spansules may be opened and contents sprinkled on applesauce Methylphenidate is not labeled for use in children <6 years of age Daytrana is a transdermal patch and should be applied every morning to alternating hips and worn for 9 hours Amphetamines are not labeled for use in children <3 years of age Adderall can be crushed Drug holidays (eg, summer is a good time to see if patient is outgrowing disease) Not addictive in children with ADHD, but some parents or siblings may abuse child's medications
Antidepressants (second-line therapy)		
Tricyclics (imipramine, desipramine)	Reuptake blockade of norepinephrine and serotonin presynaptically	May use tricyclics in patients who fail to respond or are intolerant to stimulants Drug of choice in ADHD with depression Longer duration of action No rebound or wearing off effect Rapid onset in ADHD; effect can be noticed in 3-4 days Taper patient off over 2 to 3 weeks Baseline and follow-up ECGs
Bupropion (Wellbutrin®, Wellbutrin SR®, Wellbutrin XL®)	Indirect dopamine agonist and noradrenergic effects	May induce seizures
Other agents (not currently supported by most recent AAP Guidelines, 2001)		
D-threo-enantiomer of racemic methylphenidate, dexmethylphenidate (Focalin®)	Blockade of dopamine and norepinephrine in presynaptic nerve endings	D-enantiomer thought to be the more active enantiomer
Atomoxetine (Strattera®)	Noradrenergic-specific reuptake inhibitor	New nonstimulant agent; discontinue in patients who develop jaundice or laboratory evidence of liver injury
Clonidine	α_2 Noradrenergic agonist	Good drug to use with ADHD and coexisting conditions such as sleep disturbances
Pemoline (Cylert®)	Blockade of dopamine and norepinephrine in presynaptic nerve endings	Recently withdrawn by manufacturer; previously, was rarely used secondary to association with fatal hepatic failure (not dose- or time-related)

Recommendations for therapy and monitoring
Efficacy of therapy
- Assess behavior changes and evaluate feedback from teachers and parents.

Stimulants
- Begin with a low dose and titrate upward to optimal functioning ability.
- May need to decrease dose due to side effects or if no further improvement is seen with larger dose
- No therapeutic drug monitoring or ECG monitoring
- If one stimulant fails, the patient should be tried on another stimulant; children who fail two stimulants can be tried on a third type of stimulant.

Tricyclics
- Initial and periodic ECGs

Pharmacokinetic considerations
- Methylphenidate does not distribute well into adipose tissue (dose on milligram basis instead of milligrams per kilogram).

Nondrug therapy
- Behavioral techniques (ie, positive reinforcement, time-out, response cost, token economy)
- Environmental modifications
- Classroom management

Conjunctivitis

Conjunctivitis is an inflammation of the conjunctiva of the eye.

Classification
- Bacterial, viral, or allergic

Clinical presentation
- Conjunctivitis is characterized by redness of the eye, itching, ocular discharge, foreign body sensation, and crusting of the eye and eyelid. Patient may have alteration in vision due to the presence of discharge.

Pathophysiology
Conjunctivitis of the newborn
- Inflammation of the conjunctiva within the first month of life (causative agents include topical antimicrobial agents; bacteria, primarily *Neisseria gonorrhoeae, Chlamydia trachomatis, Staphylococcus aureus, S epidermidis, Streptococcus pneumoniae, Escherichia coli* and other gram-negative bacteria; viruses, primarily herpes simplex)

Bacterial (outside of first month of life)
- Most commonly *S aureus, S epidermidis, S pneumoniae,* and *Haemophilus influenzae* (also gonococcal and chlamydial)
- Treated with antibiotic therapy

Viral
- "Pink eye" is contagious. Adenovirus is the most common causative agent.
- Commonly preceded by a cold or sore throat or exposure to another person with viral conjunctivitis
- May also see herpes simplex (corneal involvement may yield permanent visual damage)

Allergic
- Caused by exposure to dander, pollen, or topical eye preparation
- Most patients will exhibit itching of the eye.

Diagnostic criteria
- Based on patient's symptoms

Treatment goals
- Eliminate or avoid the allergen (allergic conjunctivitis).
- Treat the underlying infection (bacterial conjunctivitis).
- Decrease severity and provide symptomatic relief (all forms).

Drug therapy
Neonatal
- Preventive medicine includes prophylaxis after delivery with antibacterial ophthalmic ointment (erythromycin, tetracycline, silver nitrate, povidone-iodine)
- Onset day 1: no treatment (secondary to prophylaxis after delivery)
- Onset days 2-4 (*N gonorrhoeae*): penicillin G or ceftriaxone for 7 days
- Onset days 3-10 (*C trachomatis*): oral + erythromycin ointment for 14 days
- Onset days 2-16 (herpes simplex): consider IV acyclovir.

Bacterial (outside of first month of life)
- Topical antibiotic therapy (bacitracin-polymyxin B, trimethoprim-polymyxin B, erythromycin, fluoroquinolone [ciprofloxacin, gentamicin, tobramycin]) in combination with antibiotic ointment [erythromycin or bacitracin] at bedtime for 5-7 days

Gonococcal
- Ceftriaxone for one dose (with corneal ulceration, systemic IV ceftriaxone therapy); also treat for *Chlamydia* species as below.

Chlamydial
- Oral tetracycline or doxycycline for 2-3 weeks (adults); azithromycin single dose (children)

Viral
- Ocular lubricant (artificial tears) every 3-4 hours while awake

Allergic
- Remove allergen; use ocular lubricant (artificial tears), ocular decongestants (phenylephrine, naphazoline, tetrahydrozoline, oxymetazoline: α-adrenergic activity), antihistamines (levocabastine [Livostin®], olopatadine [Patanol®], pheniramine maleate), antihistamine/decongestant combination products, topical mast cell stabilizer (cromolyn sodium), combination mast cell stabilizer and antihistamine, or oral antihistamine therapy.

Adverse drug effects
- Ocular decongestants can cause rebound congestion of the conjunctiva (this is less common with naphazoline and tetrahydrozoline).

Instilling eye drops and ointment
- Wash hands before and after administration. Tilt head back, grasp lower eyelid and pull away from eye, place dropper or ointment tube over eye and have the child look up immediately before instilling the drop. For ointment, use a sweeping motion and instill $1/4$ to $1/2$ inch of ointment inside eyelid. Close eye after instillation and wait 1-2 minutes. Blot excess ointment or solution away from around the eye. Vision may be temporarily blurred with ointment administration. Wait 5 minutes between drops for multiple drop therapy. If using suspension, place that drop in eye last. If using both ointment and drops, instill drops first and wait 10 minutes before applying ointment.

Patient instructions and counseling
- Stress the importance of handwashing and not sharing towels or linens.
- Store products according to labeling instructions.

Nondrug therapy
- Cold compresses

Recent Pediatric Medication Issues and Labeling Changes

- In October 2004, the FDA mandated "black box" warnings for all antidepressants regarding the potential for increased suicidal behavior in children.
- In January 2005, the FDA sent out a letter warning health care professionals that the use of promethazine is contraindicated in children <2 years of age due to the risk of respiratory depression and death.
- In January 2006, the FDA requested the addition of boxed warnings to the labeling for Elidel® Cream (pimecrolimus) and Protopic® Ointment (tacrolimus) to warn about the possible risk of cancer. Use of these drugs in children under 2 years of age is not recommended.
- In May 2006, the FDA requested labeling changes for Serevent Diskus® (salmeterol xinafoate inhalation powder), Advair Diskus® (fluticasone propionate and salmeterol inhalation powder), and Foradil Aerolizer® (formoterol fumarate inhalation powder) to include a warning that these medicines may increase the risk of severe asthma attacks and death when these attacks occur.

3. Key Points

- The pharmacokinetics and pharmacodynamics of medications are altered by developmental differences in absorption, distribution, metabolism, and elimination in pediatric patients.
- Pharmacotherapy should be adjusted according to the developmental differences in order to optimize therapeutic efficacy while minimizing the risk of toxicity.
- Although spontaneous resolution does occur in many cases of acute otitis media, antibiotic therapy is initiated to prevent complications such as meningitis and mastoiditis. The observation option is an acceptable initial treatment for select patients based on age, certainty of diagnosis, and disease severity.
- The incidence of drug-resistant *S pneumoniae* is increasing. Due to its safety profile, cost, and excellent pharmacodynamic profile against sensitive and drug-resistant *S pneumoniae,* amoxicillin remains the drug of choice for uncomplicated acute otitis media. Higher doses should routinely be used.
- Therapy for cystic fibrosis should focus on halting the progression of the disease and maintaining pulmonary function. Appropriate therapies decrease mucus viscosity and increase clearance of secretions, manage acute infectious exacerbations, and by using appropriate pancreatic enzyme supplementation, maintain normal growth and development.
- Pharmacokinetics of medications in cystic fibrosis patients may be altered; therapeutic drug monitoring and dose alterations should be conducted to ensure efficacy and decrease toxicity.
- An accurate diagnosis of attention-deficit/hyperactivity disorder, a behavioral disorder of childhood onset characterized by inattentiveness, hyperactivity, and impulsivity, should be obtained prior to initiating drug therapy.
- Pharmacotherapy for attention-deficit/hyperactivity disorder is with stimulants (first-line) and antidepressants (second-line).
- ADHD pharmacotherapy should be titrated to the desired functional effect without increasing the risk of side effects.
- ADHD therapy should include behavioral modification. Monitoring of drug and nondrug therapy should include input from different environments (ie, parents and teachers).
- Bacterial and viral conjunctivitis may occur in the first month of life; antimicrobial ointment administration should be instituted after delivery for prophylaxis.
- Bacterial, viral, and allergic conjunctivitis should be treated with antimicrobial therapy (bacterial), symptomatic therapy (bacterial, viral, and allergic), and ocular antihistamines, decongestants, mast cell stabilizers, or combination products (allergic).

4. Questions and Answers

1. J.S., a 4-day-old infant (37 weeks' gestation, birth weight 3.2 kg, length 52 cm), has been admitted to the hospital secondary to spiking temperatures. J.S. has demonstrated decreased oral intake and irritability since being discharged home from the newborn nursery 2 days ago. J.S. is started on IV fluid at maintenance volume and antimicrobial therapy with ampicillin 165 mg IV q6h and gentamicin 8 mg IV q8h. Cultures have been obtained and are pending from blood, urine, and CSF. Laboratory assessment includes the following: Na 142 mEq/L, K 3.5 mEq/L, Cl 108 mEq/L, HCO_3 22 mEq/L, BUN 15 mg/dL, SCr 0.9 mg/dL, and Glc 88 mg/dL. What is J.S.'s estimated creatinine clearance (in milliliters per minute)?

   A. 100
   B. 80
   C. 60
   D. 50
   E. 25

2. Which of the following may affect the creatinine clearance estimate in this patient?

   I. The presence of maternal serum creatinine
   II. Decreased glomerular filtration rate
   III. Increased tubular secretion rate

   A. I only
   B. III only
   C. I and II only
   D. II and III only
   E. I, II, and III

3. Aminoglycosides are hydrophilic compounds. Which of the following statements regarding aminoglycoside pharmacokinetic parameters in premature neonates compared to adults is true?

   A. Increased clearance
   B. Increased Vd
   C. Decreased half-life
   D. Unchanged elimination
   E. Increased liver metabolism

4. Which of the following may complicate phenytoin therapy in a 2-day-old infant with new-onset seizures?

   I. Hypoalbuminemia
   II. Physiologic jaundice

III. IV lipid therapy

    A. I only
    B. III only
    C. I and II only
    D. II and III only
    E. I, II, and III

5. A drug metabolized via which of the following reactions is a concern in the neonatal population?

    A. Hydrolysis
    B. Reduction
    C. Sulfation
    D. Glucuronidation
    E. Methylation

6. M.J., a 7-month-old female, is brought to your pharmacy by her mother who describes the infant as having new onset of fever (102.5°F) and increased irritability in the last 24 hours. The mother states that she stayed home with M.J. today instead of sending her to day care. M.J. has been bottle-fed since birth. Family history is significant for an older sibling with a recent upper respiratory tract infection. Examination of her ear canal using a pneumatic otoscope reveals a bulging, red tympanic membrane with no mobility upon negative or positive pressure. Computer records reveal she has been treated for acute otitis media twice since birth (at 3 and 5 months of age). Decisions for antimicrobial therapy in this patient should be based on coverage for which of the following pathogens?

    A. *S epidermidis, S pneumoniae, P aeruginosa*
    B. *S pneumoniae, H influenzae, M catarrhalis*
    C. *H influenzae, S pyogenes, P aeruginosa*
    D. *S pneumoniae, S aureus, M catarrhalis*
    E. *S epidermidis, P aeruginosa, B cepacia*

7. The drug of choice for M.J.'s current episode of acute otitis media is

    A. amoxicillin
    B. amoxicillin-clavulanate
    C. IM ceftriaxone
    D. cefixime
    E. trimethoprim-sulfamethoxazole

8. When counseling M.J.'s mother about the antibiotic suspension prescribed by M.J.'s physician, which of the following should be discussed?

   I. Risks factors for otitis media
   II. Whether or not the suspension should be refrigerated
   III. The need to shake the suspension vigorously prior to administration

    A. I only
    B. III only
    C. I and II only
    D. II and III only
    E. I, II, and III

9. Which of the following is a common side effect of amoxicillin-clavulanate therapy?

    A. Hemolytic anemia
    B. Liver function test abnormalities
    C. Pancreatitis
    D. Diarrhea
    E. Headache

10. Which of the following is a side effect that should be a concern in a child with acute otitis media and nausea and vomiting who is receiving ibuprofen for fever?

    A. Stevens-Johnson syndrome
    B. Renal insufficiency
    C. Hyponatremia
    D. Oral candidiasis
    E. Liver failure

11. Otitis externa or "swimmer's ear" may be treated with

    A. application of an antimicrobial and steroid solution into the ear canal
    B. application of antimicrobial ointment into the ear canal with a cotton swab
    C. application of an antihistamine solution into the ear canal
    D. increase pH of the ear canal with administration of Burow's solution
    E. decrease pH of ear canal with administration of dilute HCl solution

12. R.E., age 15, weighs 40 kg and has cystic fibrosis. R.E. is admitted to the hospital secondary to an acute pulmonary exacerbation. Home medications include Ultrase as directed, TOBI nebulization, ADEK qd, and dornase alfa (qd nebulization). She is started on ceftazidime 2 g IV q8h and tobramycin 130 mg IV q8h. Which of the following should be ordered in this patient?

A. Serum tobramycin peak concentration
B. Serum tobramycin trough concentration
C. Serum tobramycin peak and trough concentrations
D. Sputum ceftazidime concentration
E. Sputum ceftazidime and tobramycin concentrations

13. Sputum cultures taken from R.E. shortly after hospital admission are positive for *S aureus* (non–methicillin sensitive). Which of the following agents should be initiated at this time?

A. Oxacillin
B. Ticarcillin
C. Piperacillin
D. Vancomycin
E. Amikacin

14. Which of the following is a pancreatic enzyme supplement?

A. Actigall
B. Beractant
C. Creon®
D. Diabinese®
E. Pulmozyme

15. Which of the following products can be used to decrease the viscosity of pulmonary secretions?

A. Exosurf®
B. Mucomyst
C. Protilase
D. Liquaemin
E. Serevent®

16. Counseling a patient on the use of pancreatic enzyme supplementation should include which of the following statements?

A. Capsules may be opened and sprinkled over any food
B. Capsule contents should not be crushed or chewed
C. The total daily dose may be given at one time in the evening
D. Adequate supplementation will increase bowel movement frequency
E. The supplementation dose should not change with diet changes

17. N.G., age 8, has newly diagnosed attention-deficit/hyperactivity disorder. Which of the following is not considered first-line therapy for N.G.?

A. Ritalin
B. Dexedrine
C. Wellbutrin
D. Adderall
E. Methylin

18. Atomoxetine is associated with which of the following serious adverse effects?

A. Hepatic injury
B. Renal failure
C. Cardiovascular collapse
D. Anaphylaxis
E. Toxic epidermal necrolysis

19. T.S., age 9, is being started on imipramine therapy after failing therapy for attention-deficit/hyperactivity disorder with several different stimulants. T.S. has two other siblings, a 15-year-old brother and a 3-year-old sister. The pharmacist instructs T.S.'s parents to keep the medicine away and in a safe place. What is the most likely reason for the pharmacist's concern?

I. Toxicity of imipramine with overdose
II. Abuse potential of imipramine
III. Stability of imipramine product

A. I only
B. III only
C. I and II only
D. II and III only
E. I, II, and III

20. A decrease in seizure threshold is a side effect of which of the following agents used for ADHD?

I. Methylphenidate
II. Bupropion
III. Clonidine

A. I only
B. III only
C. I and II only
D. II and III only
E. I, II, and III

21. Every spring, M.S. develops itchy, red eyes that are often swollen and draining. Which of the following is the most likely cause of this ocular disorder?

A. Viral conjunctivitis
B. Bacterial conjunctivitis
C. Allergic conjunctivitis

D. Blepharitis

E. Episcleritis

22. Which of the following therapies is not an appropriate recommendation for M.S.'s symptoms?

    A. Ocular lubricant

    B. Ocular decongestant

    C. Ocular antihistamine

    D. Ocular mast cell stabilizer

    E. Ocular antimicrobial

23. Which of the following is not commonly associated with conjunctivitis?

    A. *Chlamydia*

    B. *Neisseria*

    C. *Staphylococcus*

    D. *Streptococcus*

    E. *Clostridium*

24. Which of the following is a side effect of the prolonged use of ocular decongestants?

    A. Peripheral vasodilation

    B. Rebound conjunctival congestion

    C. Development of arrhythmias

    D. Development of tolerance

    E. Development of allergy to product

Answers

1. **E.** Using the Schwartz equation, J.S.'s estimated creatinine clearance is 26 mL/min (CrCl = 0.45 x 52/0.9).

2. **C.** The presence of maternal serum creatinine that decreases in neonates over the first week of life may falsely underestimate a creatinine clearance estimate calculated during this time. Assuming that by the end of the first week of life, J.S.'s SCr has decreased to within the normal infant range to 0.4 mg/dL, the estimated creatinine clearance would be 59 mL/min (CrCl = 0.45 x 52/0.4). Other factors that affect creatinine clearance in the neonate and infant include a decreased glomerular filtration rate and a decreased tubular secretion rate. Therefore, only I and II are correct answers.

3. **B.** Aminoglycosides are hydrophilic compounds; they will exhibit larger volumes of distribution in patients with greater total body water. Neonates and infants have greater total body water, greater extracellular fluid volume, and a relative lack of adipose tissue.

4. **E.** Phenytoin is highly plasma protein-bound. The total and free concentrations of highly protein-bound drugs may be altered due to developmental differences in protein binding (decreased protein concentrations and altered binding capacity) and displacement by endogenous substances (eg, free fatty acids and unconjugated bilirubin). Physiologic jaundice, as exhibited by increasing total and unconjugated bilirubin concentrations, may occur in the neonatal period. Unconjugated bilirubin may displace drugs from albumin binding sites. Additionally, one of the by-products of lipid metabolism, free fatty acids, may also displace drug from albumin binding sites (thereby increasing the free drug concentration). Kernicterus ("yellow brain") may occur when unconjugated bilirubin displaced by drugs or other endogenous substances (ie, free fatty acids) crosses the blood-brain barrier, where it can deposit in the brain and cause neurologic complications. Therefore, albumin concentration, physiologic jaundice, and the use of IV lipid therapy may complicate therapy with highly protein-bound agents.

5. **D.** UDPG-glucuronyl transferase is responsible for conjugation of endogenous substances (bilirubin) and medications (morphine, chloramphenicol). The capacity for glucuronidation metabolism does not begin until around 2 months of age and reaches adult capacity by 3 years of age. Medications metabolized through this system are potential toxins in the neonatal population. An example would be the use of chloramphenicol in neonates and the development of "gray-baby syndrome" due to drug accumulation. Hydrolysis, reduction, sulfation, and methylation are functional in the neonatal period and should not pose drug therapy complications in this population.

6. **B.** The most common pathogens in acute otitis media are *S pneumoniae* (40-50%), *H influenzae* (20-30 %), and *M catarrhalis* (10-15%).

7. **A.** Despite the emergence of drug resistant *S pneumoniae,* amoxicillin, due to its excellent pharmacodynamic profile, side-effect profile, and cost, remains the drug of choice in uncomplicated acute otitis media. This patient is considered to be in the high-risk group (age <2

years, attending day care, recurrent otitis media). High-dose therapy (80-90 mg/kg per day) is now the accepted dosing regimen for acute otitis media.

8. **E.** Counseling should include specific information about the antibiotic, its side-effect profile, storage information, how to administer the medicine, dosage instructions, importance of taking the full course, and the need to shake the bottle prior to administering the dose. In addition, a discussion of risk factors for acute otitis media and preventive measures (pneumococcal and flu immunization) is appropriate in a counseling session.

9. **D.** The most common side effects with amoxicillin-clavulanate therapy include rash, urticaria, nausea, vomiting, and diarrhea. Although the other listed side effects may be seen with other antibiotic therapies, they do not typically occur with amoxicillin-clavulanate therapy.

10. **B.** Dehydration, which may develop in a vomiting child, is a risk factor for ibuprofen-induced renal insufficiency. If ibuprofen is used as an antipyretic or analgesic in pediatric patients, the parents and/or caregivers should be counseled regarding this risk and the need to follow intakes and outputs during the period of acute illness (ie, gastroenteritis) when the child may be receiving ibuprofen therapy.

11. **A.** The treatment of otitis externa includes the instillation of an antibiotic and steroid otic solution into the ear canal. Cotton swabs should be avoided to prevent otitis externa. Anti-histamine solutions are not indicated in the treatment of otitis externa. Otic solutions containing acetic acid may also be of benefit in otitis externa by decreasing (not increasing) the pH of the ear canal and lowering its bacteria-harboring potential. Hydrochloric acid in any form should not be used in the ear canal.

12. **C.** Therapeutic drug monitoring is a critical part of the overall therapeutic plan in patients with cystic fibrosis. Patients with cystic fibrosis exhibit altered pharmacokinetic parameters of aminoglycosides, primarily increased clearance and greater volumes of distribution. Tobramycin peak concentrations should be obtained to make sure the dose being given is sufficient to reach concentrations of 8-12 mcg/mL and trough concentrations should be obtained to ensure

adequate renal clearance (CF patients receive higher milligram per kilogram doses).

13. **D.** *S aureus* is a common pathogen in cystic fibrosis patients. Methicillin-sensitive *S aureus* may be treated with a number of agents (eg, oxacillin); however, methicillin-resistant *S aureus* (MRSA) should be treated with vancomycin.

14. **C.** Creon is the brand name for a pancreatic enzyme supplement. Creon is available as a microencapsulated formulation.

15. **B.** Mucomyst is the brand name for N-acetlycysteine, which lowers mucus viscosity (the sulfhydryl group opens the disulfide bond in mucoproteins).

16. **B.** Pancreatic enzyme products are available in powder, capsule, tablet, and microencapsulated formulations. The microencapsulated formulations may be opened and the contents sprinkled over acidic foods (ie, applesauce). Contents should not be crushed or chewed. Additionally, the dose should be based on the amount and type of food (ie, full doses with meals, half-doses with snacks and light meals). Adequate replacement will actually decrease bowel movements and improve stool consistency (ie, decrease steatorrhea).

17. **C.** All of the listed products are stimulants, with the exception of Wellbutrin. Stimulants are considered first-line therapy for attention-deficit/hyperactivity disorder; antidepressants may be considered second-line agents.

18. **A.** Atomoxetine's labeling has most recently been updated with a bolded warning about the potential for severe liver injury. Atomoxetine should be discontinued in any patient who develops jaundice or laboratory evidence of liver injury.

19. **A.** Overdose of tricyclic antidepressants may be fatal due to the development of arrhythmias. Since T.S. has a younger sibling in the house, there is a potential for the child to get into her older brother's medicine. Stimulants may have the potential for abuse in patients that do not have ADHD (ie, the 15-year-old brother), but tricyclic antidepressants are not associated with a high abuse potential. There are no stability issues with imipramine.

20. **C.** Both bupropion and methylphenidate may lower the seizure threshold. Clonidine is not associated with seizure occurrence.

21. **C.** Allergic conjunctivitis occurs after exposure to allergens, primarily dander or pollen. Patients suffering from allergic conjunctivitis will typically complain of eye itching.

22. **E.** Antimicrobial therapy has no place in therapy for allergic conjunctivitis. Ocular lubricants, decongestants, antihistamines, mast cell stabilizers, or combinations of these products are appropriate options for allergic conjunctivitis.

23. **E.** The most common pathogens in neonatal bacterial conjunctivitis are *N gonorrhoeae, C trachomatis, S aureus, S epidermidis, S pneumoniae,* and *E coli.* Bacterial conjunctivitis outside of the first month of life is most commonly caused by *S aureus, S epidermidis, S pneumoniae,* and *H influenzae. Clostridium,* an anaerobe, is not a common bacterial pathogen in conjunctivitis.

24. **B.** Not unlike reactions from prolonged use of nasal decongestants, prolonged use of ocular decongestants may cause rebound congestion of the conjunctiva. This effect is less pronounced with naphazoline and tetrahydrozoline.

5. References

American Academy of Child and Adolescent Psychiatry. Practice parameter for the use of stimulant medication in the treatment of children, adolescents, and adults. *J Am Acad Child Adolesc Psychiatry.* 2002;41(Suppl 2):26S-49S.

American Academy of Family Physicians; American Academy of Otolaryngology-Head and Neck Surgery; American Academy of Pediatrics Subcommittee on Otitis Media with Effusion. Otitis media with effusion. *Pediatrics.* 2004;113:1412-1429.

American Academy of Pediatrics, Committee on Quality Improvement and Subcommittee on Attention-Deficit/Hyperactivity Disorder. Clinical Practice Guideline: Treatment of the School-Aged Child with Attention-Deficit/Hyperactivity Disorder. *Pediatrics.* 2001;108:1033-1044.

American Academy of Pediatrics, Committee on Quality Improvement and Subcommittee on Attention-Deficit/Hyperactivity Disorder. Diagnosis and evaluation of the child with attention-deficit/hyperactivity disorder. *Pediatrics.* 2000;105:1158-1170.

American Academy of Pediatrics Subcommittee on Management of Acute Otitis Media. Diagnosis and management of acute otitis media. *Pediatrics.* 2004;113:1451-1465.

American Psychiatric Association. *Diagnostic and Statistical Manual of Mental Disorders (DSM-IV),* 4th ed. Washington: American Psychiatric Association; 1994:78-85.

APhA Special Report: Medication Administration Problem-Solving in Ambulatory Care. Washington: American Pharmaceutical Association; 1994:9.

Beringer P. Cystic fibrosis. In: Herfindal ET, Gourley DR, eds. *Textbook of Therapeutics. Drug and Disease Management,* 7th ed. Baltimore: Lippincott Williams & Wilkins; 2000:781-794.

Bosso JA, Milavetz G. Cystic fibrosis. In: Dipiro JT, Talbert RL, Yee GC, et al, eds. *Pharmacotherapy. A Pathophysiologic Approach,* 5th ed. New York: McGraw-Hill; 2002:563-574.

Clinical Practice Guidelines for Cystic Fibrosis Committee. Clinical Practice Guidelines for Cystic Fibrosis. Bethesda, MD: Cystic Fibrosis Foundation; 1997.

Dowell SF, Butler JC, Giebink GS, et al. Acute otitis media: management and surveillance in an era of pneumococcal resistance—a report from the Drug-resistant *Streptococcus pneumoniae* Therapeutic Working Group. *Pediatr Infect Dis J.* 1999;18:1-9.

Dowell SF, Marcy SM, Phillips WR, Gerber MA, Schwartz B. Otitis media—principles of judicious use of antimicrobial agents. *Pediatrics.* 1998;101:165-171.

Faden H, Duffy L, Boeve M. Otitis media: back to basics. *Pediatr Infect Dis J.* 1998;17:1105-1113.

Fiscella RG, Jensen MK. Ophthalmic disorders. In: Berardi RR, McDermott JH, Newton GD, et al, eds. *Handbook of Nonprescription Drugs. An Interactive Approach to Self-Care,* 13th ed. Washington: American Pharmaceutical Association; 2004:659-689.

Kearns GL, Abdel-Rahman SM, Alander SW, Blowey DL, Leeder JS, Kauffman RE. Developmental pharmacology—drug disposition, action, and therapy in infants and children. *N Engl J Med.* 2003;349:1157-1167.

Krypel L. Otic disorders. In: Berardi RR, McDermott JH, Newton GD, et al, eds. *Handbook of Nonprescription Drugs. An Interactive Approach to Self-Care,* 14th ed. Washington: American Pharmaceutical Association; 2004:723-738.

Leeder JS, Kearns GL. Pharmacogenetics in pediatrics: implications for practice. *Pediatr Clin North Am.* 1998;44:55-77.

Oszko MA. Common ear disorders. In: Herfindal ET, Gourley DR, eds. *Textbook of Therapeutics. Drug and Disease Management,* 7th ed. Baltimore: Lippincott Williams & Wilkins; 2000:1049-1056.

Rappley MD. Attention deficit-hyperactivity disorder. *N Engl J Med.* 2005;352:165-173.

Schwartz GJ, Brion LP, Spitzer A. The use of plasma creatinine concentration for estimating glomerular filtration rate in infants, children, and adolescents. *Pediatr Clin North Am.* 1987;34:571-590.

Solomon SD. Common eye disorders. In: Herfindal ET, Gourley DR, eds. *Textbook of Therapeutics. Drug and Disease Management,* 7th ed. Baltimore: Lippincott Williams & Wilkins; 2000:1037-1048.

Stewart CF, Hampton EM. Effects of maturation on drug disposition in pediatric patients. *Clin Pharmacol.* 1987;6:584-564.

Yaffe SJ, Aranda JV. *Pediatric Pharmacology: Therapeutic Principles in Practice,* 2nd ed. Philadelphia: WB Saunders; 1992.

34. Geriatrics and Gerontology

William Nathan Rawls, PharmD
Professor, Department of Clinical Pharmacy
University of Tennessee College of Pharmacy

Contents

1. Overview

- Gerontology is the study of the problems of aging and all its aspects. Geriatrics focuses on the diseases associated with aging and the treatments for those conditions. Geriatrics is of particular concern for pharmacists.
- Over 12% of the United States population is older than 65 years of age. By the year 2050, it is expected that the percentage will increase to over 20%.
- Persons over 65 years of age have more chronic illnesses and take more prescription and nonprescription drugs than persons in younger age groups.
- Age-related physiologic changes and increased medication use contribute to a greater risk of adverse drug events.
- Changes in vision, hearing, and mental functioning can result in increased problems with medication compliance.

Changes in Pharmacokinetics Associated with Aging

- Decreased absorption of various drugs secondary to decreased stomach acidity and changes in blood flow to the stomach (the least altered by aging)
- Altered drug distribution caused by a decrease in total body water, increased lipid storage, and decreased serum albumin in malnourished elderly persons; these factors can contribute to increased serum levels of drugs
- Decreased hepatic blood flow and reduced hepatic enzyme activity cause slower drug metabolism. Increased levels of drugs require increased metabolism by the liver.
- Elimination of drugs by the kidneys is slowed due to decreased renal blood flow and lowered glomerular filtration; thus, drug accumulation develops.
- By using the Cockcroft-Gault formula for estimation of creatinine clearance, renal function can be predicted in the elderly:

$$\text{CrCl (mL/min)} = \frac{(140 - \text{age}) \times \text{weight in kg}}{72 \times \text{Cr}}$$

Note: Use ideal body weight. The equation above is for males. For females, multiply the result by .85.

- In dosing the elderly the general rule is to start with lower doses than used in younger patients and increase doses at a slower rate.

2. Drugs of Concern

- Drugs that can cause psychiatric symptoms:
  - * Anticholinergics
  - * Narcotics
  - * Tricyclic antidepressants
  - * CNS stimulants
  - * Antiparkinson drugs
- Drugs that can produce anxiety symptoms:
  - * Theophylline
  - * Nasal decongestants
  - * β-Agonists
  - * Antiparkinson drugs
  - * Appetite suppressants
- Drugs that can contribute to nutritional deficiencies:
  - * Diuretics
  - * Digoxin, digitalis
  - * Laxatives (overuse)
  - * Sedatives (overuse)
- Specific drugs with risk to geriatric patients:
  - * Long-acting benzodiazepines (eg, chlordiazepoxide [Librium®] and diazepam [Valium®]) should be avoided due to the risk of prolonged sedation and increased risks of falls and fractures.
  - * Amitriptyline (Elavil®) has potent anticholinergic and sedating effects with risk to older patients.
  - * Digoxin (Lanoxin®) at higher doses (>0.125 mg daily) has an increased risk of toxicity without greater benefits.
  - * Meperidine (Demerol®) taken orally has an increased risk of respiratory and circulatory depression.
  - * Antipsychotic use may result in the increased risk of heart events and infections.

3. Medication Compliance and the Older Adult

- Types of noncompliant behavior in the elderly:
    * Failure to take medications
    * Premature discontinuation of a medication
    * Excessive consumption of a medication
    * Use of medications not currently prescribed
- Strategies to improve patient medication compliance:
    * Limit the number of different medications and decrease dose frequency.
    * Simplify dosage instructions.
    * Tailor the regimen to the patient's schedule.
    * Use compliance aids and telephone reminders.
    * Enlist the assistance of family members and friends.

4. Basic Components of Evaluating Drug Therapy in Older Adults

- Questions to be answered:
    * Why is the drug being used? (diagnosis or reason)
    * Is the drug being given correctly? (dosage, form, and schedule of administration)
    * Are any symptoms or complaints related to drug therapy?
    * Is there ongoing monitoring of treatment?
    * What is the endpoint of therapy?

5. Alzheimer's Disease and Related Dementias

- Dementia is the decline in intellectual abilities (eg, impairment of memory, judgment, and abstract thinking) coupled with changes in personality.
- Dementia patients tend to be described as cognitively impaired.
- Cognition is the mental process by which we become aware of objects of thought and perception, including all aspects of thinking and remembering.
- Impairment of cognition has a significant impact on the life of the dementia patient, his or her family members, and the community in general.

Types of Dementia

- Alzheimer's disease accounts for approximately 70% of dementias.
- Vascular dementias account for approximately 15% of dementias.
- Patients may have both Alzheimer's disease and vascular dementia.

Other Causes of Dementia

- Vascular disease, cerebrovascular accidents (strokes)
- Neurologic disorders such as Parkinson's disease, frontotemporal dementia, dementia with Lewy bodies, and Huntington's chorea
- Metabolic disorders such as hypothyroidism, alcoholism, and anemia
- Infectious diseases (eg, meningitis, syphilis, AIDS)

Clinical Presentation

- Alzheimer's disease is a progressive neurologic disease that results in impaired memory and intellectual functioning and altered behavior.
- Alzheimer's disease is characterized by the slow onset of symptoms leading to loss of ability to function independently.
- Symptoms may include psychoses with hallucinations, illusions, and delusional thinking.
- As Alzheimer's disease progresses, the brain continues to deteriorate.
- Depression can cause cognitive impairment similar to that of Alzheimer's disease and should be identified and treated.

Pathophysiology

- Hallmark pathologic changes in the brain are linked to Alzheimer's disease (ie, neuritic plaques and neurofibrillary tangles increase).

- Neuritic plaques are composed of amyloid proteins deposited on neurons; neurofibrillary tangles exist within neurons and disrupt normal function.
- Neurotransmitters are also altered in Alzheimer's disease; acetylcholine concentrations decrease significantly.

Diagnostic Criteria

- Diagnosis of Alzheimer's disease requires the presence of memory impairment and one or more of the following:
  * Aphasia (language disturbance)
  * Apraxia (impaired motor abilities)
  * Agnosia (failure to recognize objects)
  * Disturbance of executive function (eg, planning, organizing)

Treatment Principles

- When evaluating a patient for treatment of dementia and Alzheimer's disease, review the patient's medications and consider any that might cause mental confusion or worsen underlying disease states.
- Drugs that block activity of acetylcholine can worsen dementia and decrease the effectiveness of medications used to treat Alzheimer's disease.
- Anticholinergic drugs are used for a variety of conditions ranging from depression to incontinence; indications should be identified before treating Alzheimer's disease.
- Anticholinergic effects can be additive (ie, a combination of anticholinergic drugs can result in toxicity even when each is given at low doses; see Table 1).
- Provide support to caregivers and treat the patient's behavioral and mood symptoms.
- Consider a trial of a cholinesterase inhibitor and monitor for benefits to memory and cognitive functioning.

Monitoring

- Monitor memory and cognitive functions every 6-12 months.
- Routinely assess behaviors and ability to perform activities of daily living (eg, bathing, feeding, toileting, dressing).
- Monitor for focal neurologic signs and symptoms that may suggest other causes of changes in cognitive function.

Drug Therapy

- The pharmacologic approach to treatment falls into two categories:

Table 1

Anticholinergic Drugs That Can Worsen Alzheimer's Disease

Class	Drugs
Antidepressants	Highest effects: amitriptyline, amoxapine, clomipramine, protriptyline
	Moderate effects: bupropion, doxepin, imipramine, maprotiline, trimipramine
Antiparkinsonian agents	Benztropine, trihexyphenidyl
Antipsychotics	Highest effects: clozapine, mesoridazine, olanzapine, promazine, triflupromazine, thioridazine
	Moderate effects: chlorpromazine, chlorprothixene, pimozide
Antispasmodics	Atropine, belladonna alkaloids, dicyclomine, glycopyrrolate, hyoscyamine, methscopolamine, oxyphencyclimine, propantheline, oxybutynin, flavoxate, terodiline
Antihistamines	Highest effects: carbinoxamine, clemastine, diphenhydramine, promethazine
	Moderate effects: azatadine, brompheniramine, chlorpheniramine, cyproheptadine, dexchlorpheniramine, triprolidine, hydroxyzine
Antiemetic/antivertigo agents	Meclizine, scopolamine, dimenhydrinate, trimethobenzamide, prochlorperazine
Other agents with some anticholinergic activity	Paroxetine

* Medications used to control behavioral and emotional symptoms
* Medications used to slow or reverse the disease process

Symptomatic therapy
* Medications used to control behavioral and emotional symptoms are used to provide symptomatic improvement and do not affect the outcome of the disease.
* Anxiolytics are used to decrease anxiety and possibly agitation, motor restlessness, and insomnia; eg, lorazepam (Ativan®), oxazepam (Serax®), and buspirone (Buspar®). The benzodiazepines can increase the risk of falls and injury.
* Antidepressants improve depression that can worsen the cognitive functioning of a patient with Alzheimer's disease; eg, sertraline (Zoloft®), citalopram (Celexa®).
* Antipsychotics are used to decrease psychotic symptoms such as hallucinations and delusions. Antipsychotics may reduce agitation and aggressiveness; eg, haloperidol (Haldol®), risperidone (Risperdal®), and aripiprazole (Abilify®). There is an increased risk of cardiac events and infections associated with the use of antipsychotics in demented elderly patients.
* Sedative-hypnotics are used for short-term treatment of insomnia, but can increase confusion and memory impairment; eg, trazodone (Desyrel®), zolpidem (Ambien®), and temazepam (Restoril®).

Cholinesterase inhibitors
* Medications used to slow or reverse the symptoms of Alzheimer's disease have an impact on acetylcholine activity in the brain.
* Acetylcholine levels may be decreased by as much as 90% in Alzheimer's disease; these levels can be increased by inhibiting the enzyme acetylcholinesterase.
* Acetylcholinesterase inhibitors increase acetylcholine but do not replace lost cholinergic neurons or change the underlying pathology. This class of medications is used to prevent or slow deterioration in cognitive functioning.
* The first cholinesterase inhibitor approved to treat Alzheimer's disease was tacrine (Cognex®), which proved beneficial but may cause the following (Table 2):
    * Potential hepatotoxicity (damage to the liver); requires regular liver function testing
    * Tacrine is rarely prescribed.
* Safer cholinesterase inhibitors include:
    * Donepezil (Aricept®) is selective for acetylcholinesterase in the brain (ie, not in peripheral tissues).
    * Rivastigmine (Exelon®), a nonselective cholinesterase inhibitor, decreases both acetylcholinesterase and butyrylcholinesterase.
    * Galantamine (Razadyne®) is a selective acetylcholinesterase inhibitor that activates nicotinic receptors, which may increase acetylcholine.

Patient instructions and counseling
* Donepezil: given orally, 5 mg daily for 4-6 weeks; increase to 10 mg daily at bedtime; take with or without food.
* Rivastigmine: given with gradual dosage increase; beginning at 1.5 mg twice daily, then 3 mg twice daily, 4.5 mg twice daily, and 6 mg twice daily, with a minimum of 2 weeks between dose increases; if

Table 2

Drugs Used to Treat Alzheimer's Disease

Generic name	Trade name	Usual dosage	Dosage forms	Adverse effects
Tacrine	Cognex®	10-20 mg bid	Capsules	Nausea/vomiting, hepatotoxicity
Donepezil	Aricept®	5-10 mg at bedtime	Tablets	Nausea/vomiting
Rivastigmine	Exelon®	1.5-6 mg bid	Capsules	Nausea/vomiting, anorexia, weight loss
Galantamine	Razadyne®	4-12 mg bid	Capsules, oral solution	Nausea/vomiting

rivastigmine is discontinued because of adverse effects, restart at beginning dose; take with meals in divided doses.

- Galantamine: doses begin with 4 mg twice daily for 4 weeks, 8 mg twice daily for 4 weeks, 12 mg twice daily for 4 weeks, then 16 mg twice daily. If discontinued for more than a few days, restart at beginning dose. In hepatic or renal dysfunction doses should not exceed 16 mg/day. Do not use in instances of severe dysfunction. Take with meals in divided doses.

Adverse drug events

- Donepezil: side effects include nausea/vomiting, GI symptoms; these may be minimized by increasing the dose at 6 weeks
- Rivastigmine: side effects include nausea, vomiting, GI upset, and possible significant weight loss. Adverse effects are dose related and may be lessened by increasing the dose at a slower rate.
- Galantamine: adverse effects include nausea, vomiting, and GI upset. Slow dose titration will decrease side effects.

NMDA-receptor antagonists

- Blocking the excitotoxicity effects of the neurotransmitter glutamate at NMDA receptors has been reported to be beneficial in Alzheimer's disease.
- Memantine (Namenda®) is an NMDA-receptor antagonist used for moderate to severe dementia. Doses begin with 5 mg daily for 1 week, increasing to 5 mg twice daily with weekly increases to 10 mg twice daily.
- Reduce dose to 5 mg twice daily in patients with renal impairment (Cr.Cl less than 30mL/min)
- Side effects include drowsiness, dizziness, headache, blood pressure elevations and motor restlessness.

Drug-drug interactions (Table 1)

- Anticholinergic drugs will reduce the effectiveness of cholinesterase inhibitors and cause dry mouth, blurred vision, constipation, and mental confusion (ie, conditions that are more problematic in the elderly).

- Cytochrome P450 enzyme inhibitors of 2D6 and 3A4 increase levels of galantamine and donepezil by inhibiting their metabolism.
- The use of dextromethorphan (Robitussin DM®), a potent NMDA-receptor antagonist, with memantine should be done with caution. Smoking and nicotine products may alter levels of memantine.

Parameters to monitor

- Cognitive function (eg, poor results on mini-mental state exam, decline in performance of activities of daily living, incidence of behaviors that indicate cognitive decline)
- Signs and symptoms of toxicity
- Active peptic ulcer disease, severe bradycardia, and acute medical illness are reasons to discontinue treatment.
- Periodic complete blood cell count and basic chemistries
- Expected benefits with the use of cholinesterase inhibitors and NMDA-receptor antagonists include improvement in memory, some stabilization of behaviors/mood, and possible slowing of the progression of the disease.

Non-prescription agents

- High-dose vitamin E (2000 U daily) has been recommended as an antioxidant to slow progression of Alzheimer's disease. Vitamin E may interfere with vitamin K absorption and result in increased risk of bleeding. Increased mortality has been reported with high-dose vitamin E. The potential toxicity of high-dose vitamin E may outweigh the benefits.
- Ginkgo biloba, an herb, has been used to treat symptoms of Alzheimer's disease with reports of modest benefits. Ginkgo biloba is associated with increased risk of bleeding and hemorrhage, especially when combined with daily aspirin use.

Nondrug Therapy

- The treatment of Alzheimer's disease includes nonpharmacologic and pharmacologic therapy.

- Patients need to live in an environment that permits safe activities while minimizing risk.
- Caregivers need training and support to deal with the behavioral and functional issues associated with this disease.
- Caregivers are at risk for depression and stress-related medical illnesses. Caregivers may also neglect their own health care needs and should be encouraged to maintain a healthy lifestyle.

6. Parkinson's Disease

- Parkinson's disease (PD) is a chronic progressive neurologic disorder with symptoms that present as a variable combination of rigidity, tremor, bradykinesia, and changes in posture and ambulation.
- An estimated 1 million persons in the U.S. suffer from PD. There are approximately 60,000 new cases diagnosed each year.
- The risk of developing PD increases with age, and there is predicted to be a substantial increase in the U.S. population of persons over 60 years of age.
- Since medications are the primary treatment for PD, pharmacists play an important role in the care of these patients.

Classification

- Primary parkinsonism has no identified cause.
- Secondary parkinsonism can be the result of drug use (eg, reserpine, metoclopramide, antipsychotics), infections, trauma, or toxins.

Clinical Presentation

- Clinical signs and symptoms of PD develop insidiously, progress slowly, may fluctuate, and worsen with time despite pharmacologic therapy.

Symptoms

- Tremors at rest may begin unilaterally and are present in 70% of PD patients.
- Tremors (not during sleep) may worsen with stress.
- Rigidity of limbs, trunk, and face with mask-like expression and difficulty with dressing or standing from a seated position
- Akinesia (the absence of movement) and bradykinesia (slowed movements)
- Postural instability with abnormal gait and an increased risk of falls
- Depression and possible dementia
- Other symptoms include micrographia (small writing), drooling, decreased blinking, constipation, and incontinence.

Pathophysiology

- PD involves a progressive degeneration of the substantia nigra in the brain with a decrease in dopaminergic cells (more than the typical decrease that accompanies normal aging).
- The most significant neurotransmitter in PD is dopamine, but other neurotransmitters may play a

role (eg, acetylcholine, glutamate, GABA, serotonin, norepinephrine).
- The etiology is unknown, but there is a possibility of genetic susceptibility.
- Environmental toxins combined with aging may also be responsible for the development of PD.

Diagnostic Criteria

- Clinical diagnosis based on the presence of bradykinesia and either rest tremor or rigidity.
- The stages of disease (Table 3)

Treatment Principles and Goals

- The goal for treating PD is to relieve symptoms and maintain or improve quality of life for the patient.
- Treatment should be initiated when there is functional impairment and discomfort for the patient and/or caregiver.
- A safe environment and caregiver support programs in addition to medications will often allow patients to remain in the community.

Drug Therapy

Mechanism of action

- Medications increase dopamine or dopamine activity by directly stimulating dopamine receptors or by blocking acetylcholine activity, which results in increased dopamine effects (Table 4).
- Selection of an initial medication to treat PD may vary with the prescriber. Some choose to begin therapy with selegiline (Eldepryl®), which offers possible neuroprotection; others prescribe carbidopa-levodopa (Sinemet®), which has proven benefits.

Table 3

The Stages of Parkinson's Disease

Stage 1	Unilateral involvement only with minimal or no functional impairment
Stage 2	Bilateral involvement without impairment of balance
Stage 3	Mild to moderate bilateral disease, some postural instability, can maintain independence
Stage 4	Severe disability, unable to live alone independently
Stage 5	Unable to walk or stand without assistance

Levodopa

- Levodopa is the most effective drug in the treatment of PD and is converted to dopamine in the body.
- Levodopa is given with carbidopa, a decarboxylase inhibitor that prevents the peripheral conversion of levodopa to dopamine, thereby reducing nausea and vomiting while allowing more drug to pass through the blood-brain barrier.
- Generally, doses are increased gradually to minimize the risk of side effects. Doses are given before meals to facilitate absorption.
- Levodopa provides benefits to all stages of PD, but chronic use is associated with adverse effects.
- Patients may have periods of good mobility alternating with periods of impaired motor function.

Treatment complications and strategies for improving patient response

- No initial response to levodopa (carbidopa-levodopa combination)
  * Gradually increase dose to at least 1000-1500 mg of levodopa.
- Suboptimal response
  * After increasing levodopa, add another drug, eg, a dopamine agonist, selegiline, or a COMT inhibitor.
- The "on and off" phenomenon (associated with advancing disease and loss of benefits from a dose of medication)
  * Remedied by more frequent doses and/or use of sustained-release levodopa
- End of dose or "wearing off," ie, decreased duration of benefit after a dose
  * Levodopa wanes after less than 4 hours; therefore, use combination therapy (two or more drugs), give levodopa more frequently, or use sustained-release levodopa (Sinemet CR®).

Patient instructions and counseling

- Usually take medications on an empty stomach; eat shortly afterward to avoid upset stomach.
- Take a missed dose as soon as possible; skip the missed dose if the next scheduled dose is within 2 hours.
- Dizziness, drowsiness, and stomach upset may occur and make operating equipment dangerous.
- Confusion, mood changes, and uncontrolled movements can result and should be reported to the prescriber as soon as possible.
- If taking a sustained-release product, do not crush.

Adverse effects (see Table 5)

Drug-drug interactions (see Table 6)

Table 4

Drugs for Treating Parkinson's Disease

Generic name (trade name)	Mechanism of action	Dosage and available strengths and forms
Carbidopa-levodopa (Sinemet®)	Levodopa increases DA; carbidopa prevents metabolism	25/100 mg/d at breakfast; increase to 25/100 mg tid; may increase to 25/250 mg qid; available in sustained-release 25/100- and 50/200-mg tablets
Bromocriptine (Parlodel®)	Directly stimulates DA receptors	1.25 mg bid with meals; increase by 2.5 mg/d every day, up to 100 mg/d; 2.5- and 5-mg tablets
Pergolide (Permax®)	Directly stimulates DA receptors	0.05 mg/d for 2 days; increase gradually to 2-3.5 mg/d (divided doses); maximum of 5 mg/d; 0.05-, 0.25-, and 1-mg tablets
Pramipexole (Mirapex®)	Directly stimulates DA receptors	0.125 mg tid increase weekly to 0.5-1.5 mg tid; 0.125-, 0.25-, 1-, and 1.5-mg tablets
Ropinirole (Requip®)	Directly simulates DA receptors	0.25 mg tid; increased gradually to a maximum of 24 mg/d; 0.25-, 0.5-, 1-, 2-, 4-, 5-mg tablets
Selegiline (Eldepryl®, Carbex®, Atapryl®, Selpak®)	Inhibits MAOB, increases DA and serotonin	Initially 5 mg at breakfast; increase to 5 mg at breakfast and lunch; 5-mg capsules, 5-mg tablets
Entacapone (Comtan®)	Inhibits COMT, increasing DA	200 mg with each dose of carbidopa-levodopa; maximum 1600 mg/d; 200-mg tablets
Tolcapone (Tasmar®)	Inhibits COMT, increasing DA	100 mg tid; discontinue if no benefits in 3 weeks; 100-, 200-mg tablets
Amantadine (Symmetrel®)	May increase presynaptic release of DA, blocks reuptake	100 mg bid; maximum dose 400 mg/d; 100-mg tablets, 100-mg capsules, 50 mg/5 mL syrup
Benztropine (Cogentin®)	Blocks acetylcholine, may balance DA	1-2 mg PO or IM or IV at bedtime or 0.5-6 mg/d in divided doses; 0.5-, 1-, 2-mg tablets, 1 mg/mL injection
Trihexyphenidyl (Artane®)	Blocks acetylcholine, may balance DA	1 mg/d up to 5 mg/d (divided doses); 2-, 5-mg tablets, 2 mg/5 mL elixir
Carbidopa/entacapone/levodopa (Stalevo®)	Combined effects of all three agents	Dosage individualized, up to 8 tablets per day; available in 3 dosage combinations

COMT, catecholamine O-methyl transferase; DA, dopamine; MAOB, monoamine oxidase B.

Parameters to monitor
- Liver function, complete blood count, basic chemistries (periodically)
- Blood pressure, pulse, ECG (periodically)
- Reduction of rigidity, tremor, slowed movements
- Examination for mental confusion, mood changes, psychotic thinking

Nondrug Therapy for Parkinson's Disease

- Educate patient and caregiver about the benefits and side effects of PD medications.
- Aids for compliance should be provided to enable the patient to participate in medication use as long as physically possible.
- Physical therapy or occupational therapy may be important in maintaining physical activity and improving safety of work and living quarters.
- As PD progresses, speech therapy may be necessary to maintain communication ability.
- Dietary consultation may assist the patient in nutritional concerns related to swallowing difficulties and food selections.

Table 6

Drug-Drug Interactions with Medications Used to Treat Parkinson's Disease

Medication	Interacting drug	Outcome
Dopamine agonists (eg, bromocriptine, pergolide)	Dopamine antagonists (eg, haloperidol, metoclopramide)	Inhibition of benefits with worsening parkinsonism
Levodopa	Dopamine antagonists	Inhibition of benefits with worsening parkinsonism
Selegiline	Serotonergics, SSRIs, buspirone, mirtazapine	Serotonin syndrome may occur (confusion, agitation, tremor, seizures, coma)
COMT Inhibitors	Nonselective MAO inhibitors: phenelzine	Serotonin syndrome; hypertensive crisis secondary to increased catecholamines

COMT, catecholamine O-methyl transferase; MAO, monoamine oxidase; SSRI, selective serotonin reuptake inhibitor.

Table 5

Adverse Effects of Medications Used to Treat Parkinson's Disease

Drug	Adverse effects
Dopaminergics: levodopa, pergolide, bromocriptine, ropinirole, amantadine	Nausea/vomiting, agitation, confusion, depression, psychoses, orthostatic hypotension, dyskinetic movements
Selegiline	Nausea/vomiting, insomnia, dizziness, agitation, confusion, dyskinetic movements, anorexia
Amantadine	Confusion, dizziness, depression, anxiety, psychoses, insomnia
COMT inhibitors: tolcapone, entacapone	Nausea/vomiting, diarrhea, dyskinesia, urine coloration, liver toxicity (tolcapone)
Anticholinergics: benztropine, trihexyphenidyl	Dry mouth, blurred vision, constipation, urinary retention, confusion, agitation, psychoses

COMT, catecholamine O-methyl transferase.

7. Glaucoma

- Glaucoma is a group of eye diseases characterized by an increase in intraocular pressure, which causes pathologic changes in the optic nerve and typical visual field defects.
- Glaucoma affects over 4 million Americans; there may be as many as 15 million more persons with increased intraocular pressure but without clinical signs and symptoms of glaucoma.
- The prevalence of glaucoma increases with age and it is most often seen in those 65 years of age or older.
- The number of persons with glaucoma is expected to increase with the aging of the American population. With improved screening programs to identify those with increased intraocular pressure (IOP), an increase in the number of those diagnosed with glaucoma is expected.

Classification

- Open-angle glaucoma is a form of primary glaucoma. The angle of the anterior chamber remains open in an eye, but filtration of aqueous humor is gradually diminished because of the tissues of the angle. This accounts for approximately 80-90% of cases of glaucoma.
- Angle-closure (narrow angle) glaucoma is a form of primary glaucoma in an eye characterized by a shallow anterior chamber and a narrow angle. The filtration of aqueous humor is compromised as a result of the iris blocking the angle.
- Congenital glaucoma results from defective development of the structures in and around the anterior

chamber of the eye and results in impairment of aqueous humor.

Clinical Presentation

- Clinical signs and symptoms of glaucoma develop slowly and may present with only minor symptoms such as headache and mild eye pain.
- Optic nerve damage results from chronic elevations in IOP and this emphasizes the importance of early and consistent treatment to avoid loss of vision.
- Acute angle-closure glaucoma presents with blurred vision, severe ocular pain, and possible nausea and vomiting. This should be considered a medical emergency and immediate care should be recommended.
- Chronic angle-closure glaucoma may have symptoms similar to those of open-angle glaucoma.
- Tonometry is used to screen for IOP but direct ophthalmoscopy (slit-lamp examination) is necessary to accurately evaluate the eye for changes in the optic nerve.

Pathophysiology

- The pathogenesis of glaucoma results from changes in aqueous humor (the fluid filling the eye and in front of the lens) outflow that results in increased IOP. This increase in pressure leads to optic nerve atrophy and progressive loss of vision.
- Increased IOP can result from decreased elimination or increased production of aqueous humor.
- Aqueous humor is secreted by the ciliary processes into the posterior chamber of the eye. It then flows through the trabecular meshwork and the canal of Schlemm.
- Open-angle glaucoma is the result of decreased elimination of aqueous humor as it passes through the trabecular meshwork, thereby resulting in elevated IOP.
- Angle-closure glaucoma is caused by papillary blockage of aqueous humor outflow.
  - * This can result when a patient has a narrow anterior chamber in the eye or a dilated pupil where the iris comes into greater contact with the lens.
  - * With the blocking of outflow, aqueous humor accumulates in the posterior chamber, presses the lens forward, and further decreases drainage with possible complete blockage as the outcome.

Diagnostic Criteria

- Elevated IOP as determined by tonometry
- Funduscopic assessment to identify characteristic changes in the optic disc and retina

Treatment Principles (Figure 1)

- Reduce IOP to prevent optic nerve damage and visual field loss.
- Use topical medications as first-line treatment.
- Consider acute angle-closure glaucoma as a medical emergency.

Monitoring

- Periodic screening for increased IOP, with yearly examinations for those over 65 years of age and as part of routine eye examination

Drug Therapy

Mechanism of action
- Medications are considered the mainstay of therapy for the treatment of glaucoma (Table 7).
- β-Adrenergic blocking drugs (β-blockers) are considered first-line treatment for open-angle glaucoma.

Figure 1.

Algorithm for the treatment of open-angle glaucoma.

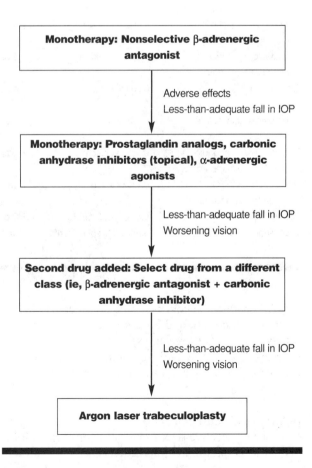

Table 7

Medications for the Treatment of Glaucoma

Generic name (trade name) and type	Form	Usual dosage	Comments
Timolol (Timoptic®), nonselective β antagonist (NSBA)	0.25% and 0.50% solution and gel-forming solution	1 drop twice daily; gel solution used once daily	Nonselective β antagonists are often first choice for open-angle glaucoma
Carteolol (Ocupress®), NSBA	1% ophthalmic solution	1 drop twice daily	
Levobunolol (Betagen®), NSBA	0.25% and 0.50% solution	1-2 drops 1-4 times daily	
Metipranolol (OptiPranolol®), NSBA	0.3% solution	1 drop twice daily	
Betaxolol (Betoptic®), selective β₁ antagonist	0.25% and 0.50% solution	1-2 drops twice daily	Cardioselective; less effect on heart rate and blood pressure
Levobetaxolol (Betaxon®), selective β₁ antagonist	0.50% solution	1 drop twice daily	Cardioselective
Acetazolamide (Diamox®), carbonic anhydrase inhibitor	125-, 250-mg tablets, 500-mg ER capsules	250 mg 1-4 times daily; extended-release 1-2 times daily	Do not use with sulfa allergy
Dorzolamide (Trusopt®) carbonic anhydrase inhibitor	2.0% solution	1 drop three times daily	Do not use with sulfa allergy
Brinzolamide (Azopt®), carbonic anhydrase inhibitor	1.0% solution	1 drop three times daily	Do not use with sulfa allergy
Methazolamide (Neptazane®), carbonic anhydrase inhibitor	25- and 50-mg tablets	15-50 mg 1-3 times daily	Do not use with sulfa allergy
Latanoprost (Xalatan®), prostaglandin analog	0.005% solution; refrigerate	1 drop at bedtime	Can change blue eyes to brown
Bimatoprost (Lumigan®), prostaglandin analog	0.03% solution	1 drop at bedtime	Can cause darkening of eyelids and eyelashes
Travoprost (Travatan®), prostaglandin analog	0.004% solution	1 drop at bedtime	Frequent ocular hyperemia
Unoprostone (Rescula®), prostaglandin analog	0.15% solution	1 drop twice daily	If used with another drop, wait 5 minutes
Brimonidine (Alphagan®), α₂ adrenergic agonist	0.15% solution	1 drop three times daily	Wait at least 15 minutes after using before placing soft contacts
Dipivefrin (Propine®); α-adrenergic agonist	0.1% solution	1 drop twice daily	Prodrug of epinephrine
Pilocarpine (Pilocar®), cholinergic, miotic	0.5%, 1%, 2%, 3%, 4%, 6%, 8% solution, 4% gel	1-2 drops 3-4 times daily; ½ inch gel at bedtime	Once weekly dose form called Ocuserts®

β-Adrenergic antagonists can be nonselective (ie, they block both β₁ and β₂ receptors) or selective (ie, they block only β₁ receptors).

- Drugs that block only β₁ receptors are considered to be cardioselective and cause less decrease in blood pressure and heart rate.

β-Adrenergic antagonists
* Nonselective β antagonists: timolol, carteolol, levobunolol, metipranolol

* β₁-Selective antagonists: betaxolol, levobetaxolol
- Therapy is initiated with a single topical ophthalmic solution, and additional agents are added if there is a less-than-acceptable decrease in IOP.
- The effects of therapy on IOP should be apparent after a week of treatment.
- Prostaglandin analogs are also used as first-line treatment (or in combination with β-blockers).

- Topical carbonic anhydrase inhibitors and α_2 agonists may be used in treatment.
- Medications such as epinephrine, pilocarpine, and oral carbonic anhydrase inhibitors are prescribed less often, but are considered to be effective adjunctive drugs.

Patient instructions and counseling

- Multiple factors present obstacles that can interfere with good compliance.
- Patients are often asymptomatic and do not feel treatment is necessary.
- Since decreased vision is associated with glaucoma, patients may have difficulty with written instructions.
- Adequate glaucoma therapy often requires two or more types of eye drops that may have to be given more than once daily.
- Correct administration of eye drops requires coordination and reasonable cognitive functioning.
- Glaucoma is more common in the elderly, who may have more difficulty complying with prescribed medications.
- Patient guidelines concerning the use of eye drops to treat glaucoma:
  * Wash hands before administering eye drops and avoid touching the dropper tip.
  * Confirm that the medication is not outdated and has been stored properly.
  * Looking upward, pull the lower lid down and instill the correct number of drops.
  * Close the eye to allow the medication to have maximal effect.

  * In most cases wait five or more minutes between different medications.

Adverse drug events (see Table 8)

Drug-drug interactions

- Drug interactions between topical medications and systemic drugs are unlikely.
- Acetazolamide interacts with the following:
  * Aspirin to cause increased aspirin levels and possible toxicity
  * Cyclosporine to cause increased cyclosporine levels
  * Lithium to cause either increased or decreased lithium levels
  * Phenytoin to cause an increased risk of osteomalacia

Parameters to monitor

- Medication use is critical to the successful treatment of glaucoma and should be monitored by the health professional.

Other

- A combination of timolol 0.5% and dorzolamide 2% (Cosopt®) is available. This combination effectively lowers IOP and only requires twice-daily doses. This simplified dosing should improve compliance with treatment. This combination (ie, using two drugs from different categories) represents a sound treatment approach. Poor response to therapy may result in the prescribing of multiple medications, which

Table 8

Classification, Mechanism of Action, and Adverse Effects of Glaucoma Medications

Medication class	Mechanism of action	Adverse effects
β Adrenergic antagonists: timolol, metipranolol, carteolol, levobunolol, etc.	Decrease in aqueous humor formation with slight increase in outflow (β selective)	Adverse cardiac effects, worsening pulmonary disease, depression, dizziness
Miotics (cholinergics): pilocarpine, carbachol	Increase in aqueous humor outflow	Miosis, brow ache, dizziness, nausea, flushing, itching, sweating, confusion
Carbonic anhydrase inhibitors: dorzolamide, brinzolamide	Decrease in aqueous humor formation	Lethargy, decreased appetite, GI upset, urinary frequency
Prostaglandin analogs: latanoprost, travoprost, bimatoprost	Increased uveoscleral outflow without effect on aqueous humor formation	Iris pigmentation, eyelid darkening, macular edema
α_2-Adrenergic agonists: apraclonidine, brimonidine	Decrease in aqueous humor formation	Tachycardia, dry mouth, eyelid elevation, CNS effects in the old and very young
Other α-adrenergic agonists: epinephrine, dipivefrin	Increase in aqueous humor outflow	Tachycardia, increased blood pressure, allergic responses

may negatively impact the patient's ability to successfully use the more complex regimen.

Nondrug Therapy

Laser surgery
- Argon laser trabeculoplasty (ALT) has proven effective as adjunctive therapy that increases the flow of aqueous humor.

Surgery
- The procedure involves creating new means of drainage for aqueous humor to leave the anterior chamber.

8. Key Points

Alzheimer's disease
- Alzheimer's disease is a progressive neurologic disease that results in impaired memory, intellectual functioning, and behavior.
- There is no known cure for Alzheimer's disease, but there are therapies to decrease memory impairment as well as improve behavior and patient functioning.
- Other forms of dementia that are potentially reversible should be identified and treated accordingly.
- New drug therapies may slow the progression of Alzheimer's disease and allow patients to remain in the least restrictive environment possible.
- Caregiver support and education is an important measure to assure patient safety and well-being.

Parkinson's disease
- Parkinson's disease is a chronic, progressive neurologic disease for which there is no cure; medications are available to slow the progression of symptoms.
- The etiology of Parkinson's disease is unknown, but may involve genetic susceptibility combined with environmental toxins and age-related changes in the brain.
- Dopamine, the central neurotransmitter, is decreased in Parkinson's disease and current drug therapy is primarily directed at increasing dopamine levels.
- Drug therapy monitoring in Parkinson's disease requires an understanding of a variety of different medications that may cause significant adverse effects.
- Physical therapy, occupational therapy, dietary considerations, and support counseling for caregivers are necessary components of treating Parkinson's disease.

Glaucoma
- Glaucoma, a group of eye diseases, is characterized by increased intraocular pressure resulting in damage to the optic nerve and possible blindness.
- Open-angle glaucoma is the most common form of this disease; angle-closure glaucoma can be a medical emergency.
- The goal of therapy is to reduce intraocular pressure with the simplest medication regimen possible.
- Drug therapy for glaucoma usually begins with a topical β-adrenergic antagonist; patients often require combination therapy.
- Medication compliance is essential in the control of glaucoma. Education of the patient and caregiver is required to overcome treatment barriers.

9. Questions and Answers

1. Of the following pharmacokinetic processes which is the least altered by aging?

   A. Absorption
   B. Distribution
   C. Metabolism
   D. Elimination
   E. Excretion

2. Which of the following is given as a once-daily dose?

   A. Buspirone
   B. Donepezil
   C. Galantamine
   D. Rivastigmine
   E. Tacrine

3. Galantamine increases levels of which neurotransmitter?

   A. Acetylcholine
   B. Dopamine
   C. Melatonin
   D. Norepinephrine
   E. Serotonin

4. Weight loss is most often associated with which of the following?

   A. Donepezil
   B. Galantamine
   C. Mirtazapine
   D. Rivastigmine
   E. Tacrine

5. What is the correct answer concerning donepezil?

   I. Inhibits acetylcholinesterase but not butyrylcholinesterase
   II. It should be taken with meals in divided doses
   III. Side effects include tachycardia and blood pressure alterations

   A. I only
   B. III only
   C. I and II only
   D. II and III only
   E. I, II, and III

6. All of the following medications are used to treat behavioral and emotional symptoms in Alzheimer's patients EXCEPT

   A. benztropine
   B. buspirone
   C. citalopram
   D. lorazepam
   E. risperidone

7. The maximum daily dose of galantamine in patients with renal impairment is

   A. 8 mg/d
   B. 12 mg/d
   C. 16 mg/d
   D. 24 mg/d
   E. 32 mg/d

8. All of the following could worsen cognition in AD patients EXCEPT

   A. dicyclomine
   B. dimenhydrinate
   C. meclizine
   D. trazodone
   E. trihexyphenidyl

9. Memantine's reported benefits in treating the symptoms of Alzheimer's disease is thought to be the result of

   A. increasing serotonin receptor activity
   B. blocking the effect of glutamate on receptors
   C. direct blocking of acetylcholine receptors
   D. decreasing intracellular dopamine activity
   E. decreasing amyloid deposits in the brain

10. Which works by direct stimulation of dopamine receptors?

    A. Amantadine
    B. Benztropine
    C. Entacapone
    D. Ropinirole
    E. Selegiline

11. In treating parkinsonism the "on and off" phenomenon is most often associated with

    A. benztropine
    B. bromocriptine
    C. carbidopa-levodopa
    D. selegiline
    E. tolcapone

12. What would be the most likely outcome if a Parkinson's patient on levodopa were also prescribed haloperidol?

    A. Excessive nausea and vomiting
    B. Hypertensive crisis
    C. Tachycardia and possible chest pain
    D. Worsening symptoms of Parkinson's disease
    E. Excessive somnolence

13. Which inhibits monoamine oxidase (MAO)?

    A. Benztropine
    B. Bromocriptine
    C. Pramipexole
    D. Selegiline
    E. Tolcapone

14. How does carbidopa affect levodopa?

    A. Slows the release from presynaptic neurons
    B. Prevents the excretion of dopamine
    C. Increases stimulation of dopamine receptors
    D. Decreases tolerance to normal doses
    E. Inhibits the peripheral conversion to dopamine

15. A patient with Parkinson's disease currently taking selegiline has been prescribed mirtazapine (Remeron®). What would be the most likely outcome of this combination?

    A. Inhibition of benefits with worsening parkinsonism
    B. No significant drug interaction
    C. Risk of serotonin syndrome
    D. Increased benefits with improved parkinsonism
    E. Hypertensive episode

16. Which of the following statements are true concerning the treatment of the "on and off" phenomenon that can be associated with PD?

    I. Combine two or more medications with different mechanisms of action
    II. Give more frequent doses of carbidopa-levodopa
    III. Give a sustained-release carbidopa-levodopa product

    A. I only
    B. III only
    C. I and II only
    D. II and III only
    E. I, II, and III

17. Timolol ophthalmic drops would be more likely to cause which adverse effect as compared to levobetaxolol ophthalmic drops?

    A. Agitation and restlessness
    B. Nausea and vomiting
    C. Confusion
    D. Change in heart rate and blood pressure
    E. Altered intraocular pressure

18. Which of the following would not be considered for monotherapy of glaucoma?

    A. Latanoprost
    B. Dorzolamide
    C. Carteolol
    D. Methazolamide
    E. Brimonidine

19. Which of the following can cause iris pigmentation changes?

    A. Acetazolamide
    B. Betaxolol
    C. Brimonidine
    D. Latanoprost
    E. Pilocarpine

20. Which of the following is available as a fixed combination product?

    A. Dorzolamide and timolol
    B. Betaxolol and bimatoprost
    C. Bimatoprost and levobunolol
    D. Latanoprost and timolol
    E. Methazolamide and latanoprost

21. All of the following are available as an ophthalmic solution EXCEPT

    A. Brimonidine
    B. Dipivefrin
    C. Dorzolamide
    D. Methazolamide
    E. Metipranolol

22. Which should not be used if a patient has a sulfa allergy?

    A. Betazolol
    B. Bimatoprost
    C. Brimonidine
    D. Brinzolamide
    E. Unoprostone

23. α_2-Adrenergic agonists cause a(n)

    A. Increase in aqueous humor synthesis
    B. Decrease in aqueous humor formation
    C. Increase in uveoscleral outflow
    D. Increase in aqueous humor outflow
    E. Decreased uveoscleral outflow

24. Which of the following statements concerning glaucoma therapy are correct?

    I. Carteolol is available as an ophthalmic solution and as a gel-forming solution
    II. Latanoprost and metipranolol ophthalmic solutions should be stored in the refrigerator
    III. Prostaglandin analogs, β-adrenergic antagonists, and α-adrenergic agonists can be used as monotherapy

    A. I only
    B. III only
    C. I and II only
    D. II and III only
    E. I, II, and III

Answers

1. **A.** Of all the age-related changes of the pharmacokinetic process, absorption is the least altered. This may relate to the fact that most drugs are passively absorbed.

2. **B.** All cholinesterase inhibitors except donepezil require at least twice-daily dosing. Donepezil has a long half-life, which allows for once-daily doses. None of these agents is available in sustained-release forms. Buspirone is an antianxiety drug that is dosed twice or three times daily.

3. **A.** Galantamine is a cholinesterase inhibitor and all cholinesterase inhibitors increase levels of acetylcholine, the neurotransmitter that appears to be involved with memory function.

4. **D.** Weight loss, probably due to nausea and vomiting, is a warning for rivastigmine. In controlled trials, approximately 26% of women on doses of 9 mg/d or greater had weight loss of equal to or greater than 7% of their baseline weight.

5. **A.** Donepezil is selective for acetylcholinesterase and does not inhibit butyrylcholinesterase. Donepezil does not have to be taken with meals and is given once daily.

Donepezil does not increase heart rate and this class of medications that increase acetylcholine should be used with caution in patients with bradycardia.

6. **A.** Benztropine is an anticholinergic used to treat side effects from antipsychotic medications and is also used to treat incontinence. All other drugs listed can be used to treat specific symptoms associated with AD.

7. **C.** With renal or hepatic dysfunction, galantamine doses should not exceed 16 mg/d. With severe renal or hepatic dysfunction, galantamine should not be used.

8. **D.** All of the drugs listed with the exception of trazodone have anticholinergic activity. Decreasing the activity of acetylcholine could worsen dementia and block benefits of cholinesterase inhibitors. Trazodone is an antidepressant with sedating properties but little anticholinergic activity. It may be given at bedtime to help with sleep. Trazodone does have a side effect of orthostatic hypotension.

9. **B.** Glutamate is the main excitatory neurotransmitter in the CNS and one theory states that blocking the effects of glutamate on NMDA receptors will decrease symptoms of Alzheimer's disease.

10. **D.** Ropinirole directly stimulates dopamine receptors; the other drugs increase dopamine activity by different mechanisms.

11. **C.** The "on and off" phenomenon is associated with advancing disease and loss of benefits from levodopa. It is treated by giving more frequent doses and/or using sustained-release levodopa.

12. **D.** Haloperidol and other antipsychotics block dopamine activity and can worsen PD. They can also block the benefits of PD medications, which increase dopamine activity.

13. **D.** Selegiline is an MAOI that is selective for MAOB, which decreases the potential for drug-drug and drug-food interactions. At doses higher than 10 mg/d this selectivity becomes less.

14. **E.** Carbidopa inhibits the peripheral conversion of levodopa to dopamine, thus allowing more levodopa to cross the blood-brain barrier and decreases adverse effects from dopamine.

15. **C.** The combination of two drugs that increase serotonin levels can result in serotonin syndrome which can cause confusion, agitation, tremor, seizures and coma.

16. **D.** Increasing frequency of drug or using a sustained-release form decreases blood level fluctuations and should improve symptoms.

17. **D.** Timolol is a nonselective β-adrenergic antagonist that causes a reduction in heart rate and blood pressure. There is enough absorption from eye drops to produce these cardiac effects.

18. **D.** All of the other choices could be considered as monotherapy for glaucoma. Methazolamide is an oral carbonic anhydrase inhibitor and is used in conjunction with ophthalmic drops.

19. **D.** Latanoprost, a prostaglandin analog, is known to change iris pigmentation and to darken eyelashes.

20. **A.** Dorzolamide plus timolol (Cosopt) is the only combination ophthalmic solution for treating glaucoma. An advantage for using a combination product would be increased compliance.

21. **D.** Methazolamide and acetazolamide are both available only as oral tablets or capsules. Topical carbonic anhydrase inhibitors are brinzolamide and dorzolamide.

22. **D.** Patients with sulfa allergy should not be given a carbonic anhydrase inhibitor.

23. **B.** α_2-Adrenergic agonists such as brimonidine cause a decrease in aqueous humor formation.

24. **B.** All of these drugs can be used as monotherapy in glaucoma. Timolol and pilocarpine are available as gel forms. Latanoprost (but not metipranolol) should be stored in a refrigerator before dispensing.

10. References

Chen JJ, Shimomua SK. Parkinsonism. In: Herfindal ET, Gourley DR, eds. *Textbook of Therapeutics,* 7th ed. Philadelphia: WB Saunders Co; 2000:1139-1155.

Fujumoto D, Rawls WN. Alzheimer's disease. In: Herfindal ET, Gourley DR, eds. *Textbook of Therapeutics,* 7th ed. Philadelphia: WB Saunders Co; 2000:2063-2076.

Grutzendler J, Morris JC. Cholinesterase inhibitors for Alzheimer's disease. *Drugs.* 2001;61:41-52.

Scarpini E, Scheltens P, Felman H. Treatment of Alzheimer's disease: current status and new perspectives. *Lancet Neurology.* 2003;2:539-547.

Hoyng PF, van Beek LM. Pharmacological therapy for glaucoma. *Drugs.* 2000;59:411-434.

Olanow CW, Watts RL, Koller WC. An algorithm for the management of Parkinson's disease. *Neurology.* 2001;56:872-891.

Wigginton SA, Higginbotham EJ. Glaucoma diagnosis and management. *Ophthalmol Clin North Am.* 2000;12:157-169.

Wurtzbacker JD, Gourt DR, McKenzie C. Glaucoma. In: Herfindal ET, Gourley DR, eds. *Textbook of Therapeutics,* 7th ed. Philadelphia: WB Saunders Co; 2000:1057-1082.

35. Toxicology and Chem-Bioterrorism

Peter A. Chyka, PharmD, FAACT, DABAT
Professor and Vice Chair, Department of Clinical Pharmacy
Associate Dean, Knoxville Campus
University of Tennessee College of Pharmacy

Contents

Acknowledgements

The contributions of Adrianne Y. Butler, PharmD, Billie J. Holliman, PharmD, and C. Renee Adams-McDowell to the first edition of this chapter are acknowledged.

1. Overview of Poisoning and Toxicology

Poisoning in America

- Poisoning exposures and overdoses affect over 2.5 million people annually, and there are over 26,000 deaths yearly (<1% of deaths are in preschool-aged children).
- A great number of poisonings occur in young children, but most fatalities occur in adults.
- Any chemical can become toxic if the exposure is too great in relation to body weight and tolerance.
- Medications are the most common cause of poisoning morbidity and mortality.
- Most poisonings in preschool-aged children are unintentional or accidental.
- Unintentional poisonings can also occur in adolescents and adults; however, intentional (suicide, drug abuse) poisonings and overdoses are common (Table 1).

Table 1

Ranking of Most Frequent Poisonings from U.S. Poison Centers and Emergency Departments During 2004

Cases from poison centers[1]	Cases from emergency departments[2]
Analgesics	Alcohol, alone or in combination
Cleaning substances	Cocaine
Cosmetics and personal care products	Marijuana
Sedative drugs	Opioid analgesic drugs
Foreign bodies	Heroin
Topical drugs	Nonopioid analgesic drugs
Cough and cold drugs	Benzodiazepines
Antidepressant drugs	Amphetamines
Pesticides	Antidepressant drugs
Bites and envenomations	Antipsychotic drugs
Plants	Sedative drugs
Alcohols	Cardiovascular drugs

[1]In decreasing order of frequency and based on 2,438,644 poison exposures. From: Watson WA, Litovitz TL, Rogers GC, et al. 2004 Annual Report of the American Association of Poison Control Centers Toxic Exposure Surveillance System. *Am J Emerg Med.* 2005;23:590-665.

[2]In decreasing order of frequency based on 1,997,993 cases of substance abuse, poisoning, overmedication and attempted suicide. From: Substance Abuse and Mental Health Services Administration, Drug Abuse Warning Network, 2004 national estimates of drug-related emergency department visits. Rockville, MD. Publ. SMA 06-4143.

Poison Prevention Approaches and Pharmacy

Poison Prevention Packaging Act of 1970: "Safety Caps"
- This act was issued to prevent preschool-aged children from opening and ingesting harmful substances or to delay the opening of packaging containing such substances (to limit the amount of harmful substance that may be ingested within a reasonable amount of time).
- Drugs requiring safety caps include aspirin, ibuprofen, acetaminophen, and oral prescription drugs with certain exceptions (eg, birth control pills, nitroglycerin).

Utilization of poison control centers
- Nationwide access is available at 1-800-222-1222 for 24-hour poison center services for the area from which the call is placed in the U.S.

Poison prevention tips for consumers
- Store all drugs and chemicals out of the reach of children.
- Never put chemicals in food containers.
- Choose products with safety caps when there is a choice and use them properly.
- Read and follow all label directions carefully.
- Never call medicine "candy."
- Use safety latches.

Pharmacy Requirements for the Joint Commission on Accreditation of Healthcare Organizations

- Maintain and keep available (for the medical staff) an approved stock of antidotes and other emergency drugs both in the pharmacy and patient care areas.
- Maintain authoritative, current antidote information.
- The phone number of the poison control center should also be readily available in areas outside of the pharmacy where drugs are stored.

Emergency Actions

- First aid, if applicable (Table 2)

Other considerations:
- Avoid wasting time to find an "antidote" at home.
- Do not use home remedies such as saltwater, mustard powder, raw eggs, hydrogen peroxide, cooking grease, or gagging.
- Call 911 or an ambulance if the person is not breathing, has had a seizure, or is unresponsive.
- Contact a poison center immediately to determine first aid or whether a poisoning emergency exists.

Table 2

First Aid for Poisoning Emergencies

Inhaled poison
Immediately get the person to fresh air. Avoid breathing fumes. Open doors and windows wide.

Poison on the skin
Remove any contaminated clothing and flood skin with water for at least 15 minutes.

Poison in the eye
Flood the eye with water. Pour it from a large glass 2-3 inches from the eye. Repeat for a total of 15-30 minutes. Do not force the eyelid open. Remove contact lenses.

Swallowed poison
Unless the victim is unconscious, having convulsions, or cannot swallow, give a small glassful (2-4 ounces) of water immediately. Call a poison center for advice about whether other actions are needed.

Decontamination of the Gastrointestinal Tract

- The practice of using drugs to decrease the absorption of other drugs from the gastrointestinal tract is in a state of change. Drugs such as ipecac syrup are being abandoned by many as a home- or hospital-based therapy. Its use is primarily at the preference of the consulting poison center or health care professional. Current recommendations are described below as well as basic information about the drugs in case they are encountered.

Current recommendations
- Ipecac syrup has questionable effectiveness and its use is generally avoided.
- Gastric lavage involves placing a tube into the stomach through a nostril or the mouth and repetitively washing out the stomach contents with water or a saline solution. This method of gastric decontamination is of questionable effectiveness, particularly if it is performed more than 1 hour after ingestion.
- Cathartics such as magnesium citrate are not routinely used.
- Activated charcoal is often the only treatment necessary if the toxin is adsorbed and it is used within 1-2 hours of ingestion.
- Whole bowel irrigation can be considered if the toxin is poorly or slowly adsorbed and its presence in the gastrointestinal tract is likely.

Ipecac syrup
Indications and dosage
- It was previously used for general prophylaxis of selected poisonings of expected minor or moderate severity in alert patients.
- It has been abandoned by many clinicians as a pre-hospital or hospital treatment. In November 2003 the American Academy of Pediatrics recommended that ipecac syrup no longer be used routinely as a home treatment for poisoning.

Contraindications
- The patient is experiencing pronounced sleepiness, coma, or seizures.
- Ingestion of caustics, aliphatic hydrocarbons, and fast-acting agents that produce coma or seizures (eg, tricyclic antidepressants, clonidine, calcium channel blockers, beta blockers, and hypoglycemic agents)
- Time since ingestion is believed to be 1 hour or more

Adverse effects
- Common: diarrhea, sleepiness, protracted vomiting
- Uncommon: Mallory-Weiss tears, tracheal aspiration into the lungs
- Disadvantages: relative lack of efficacy and emesis complicate administration of other oral therapies

Activated charcoal
Indications and dosage
- Occasionally used to adsorb poisons in an alert or comatose patient
- Administer as a slurry by mouth or through a lavage tube:
  - * Children: 25-50 g
  - * Adults: 25-100 g

Contraindications
- Ingestions of aliphatic hydrocarbons and caustics
- If patient's bowel sounds are absent
- Ingestions of heavy metals (sodium, lithium, iron, or lead) or simple alcohols

Adverse effects
- Uncommon: tracheal aspiration, pneumonitis
- Common: emesis, soiling of clothes and furnishings

Advantages and disadvantages
- Advantages: rapid onset of action, nonspecific action for a wide variety of chemicals, and reasonable effectiveness within 1 hour of ingestion
- Disadvantages: messy and difficult to administer, may also remove beneficial drugs along with the toxin

Cathartics

- Previously used as an adjunct to activated charcoal administration to decrease gastrointestinal transit time
- Efficacy unproved
- Fluid and electrolyte disturbances are possible with repeated doses.
- May contribute to emesis following activated charcoal use
- Agents previously used include magnesium citrate, magnesium sulfate, sodium sulfate, and sorbitol.
- *Note:* Some activated charcoal products contain sorbitol mixed in the preparation. The sorbitol concentration varies from brand to brand.

Whole bowel irrigation

Indications and technique

- Generally used when charcoal may be inappropriate (eg, if iron or lithium was ingested) and the toxin is suspected to be present in the gastrointestinal tract (eg, when drugs are sustained-release formulations or ingested illicit drugs packed in condoms)
- Use larger volumes of polyethylene glycol electrolyte solutions (eg, CoLyte®, GoLYTELY®) than amounts conventionally used for bowel preparation.
- Administer by mouth or through a gastric or duodenal tube for treatment of poisoning:
  * Children: 25 mL/kg per hour (approximately 500 mL/h) up to 2-5 L
  * Adults: 2 L/h up to 5-10 L

Contraindications

- Ingestion of caustics or aliphatic hydrocarbons
- Patients with absent bowel sounds or gastrointestinal tract obstruction

Adverse effects

- Few adverse effects have been reported, but there are limited results available from which to draw conclusions. Some nausea and vomiting has been reported.

Advantages and disadvantages

- Advantages: prompt whole bowel evacuation within 2 hours
- Disadvantages: messy procedure due to rectal effluent

Other hospital-based therapies

- These include supportive and symptomatic care, multiple doses of activated charcoal (to enhance systemic elimination when appropriate), hemodialysis (to enhance systemic elimination when appropriate), and use of antidotes (to antagonize or reverse toxic effects when indicated).

2. Substance Abuse and Toxicology

- Substance abuse often leads to acute and chronic toxicity (Table 3).
- Management of the acute condition generally follows the same guidelines as managing poisonings and overdoses.
- A challenge in treating patients during acute drug overdose is determining the possible agents taken and possible adulterants (eg, talc, strychnine, other drugs) or contaminants.
- Chronic abuse can foster dependence, which often leads to withdrawal symptoms upon stopping use.

3. Antidotes

Role of Antidotes

- An antidote counteracts or changes the nature of a poison.
- There are few antidotes available relative to the large number of potential poisons. Table 4 lists commonly used antidotes for the treatment of a patient with a poisoning or an overdose.
- Many hospitals have an insufficient stock of antidotes; the pharmacy and therapeutics committee of the hospital should regularly review the inventory of antidotes.

Selected Antidotes

Acetylcysteine (Mucomyst® 10%, 20% oral solution; Acetadote® 20% for injection)
Uses
- Treatment of acute acetaminophen overdose
- Unapproved indication: to treat adverse reactions to drugs that may produce free radicals as part of the adverse reaction; the dosage regimen is unique to the application.

Mechanism of action
- It protects the liver from the toxic effects of an acetaminophen metabolite by supplying glutathione to aid in metabolism of the reactive metabolite.
- Other mechanisms are also proposed that include providing sulfate for acetaminophen metabolism and minimizing the formation of free radicals.

Table 3

Selected Drugs of Abuse and Addictive Substances

Substance (slang names)	Methods of abuse	Major or unique health effects
Androgenic anabolic steroids (Roids)	Anabolic steroids are taken orally or injected, typically in cycles of weeks or months ("cycling"); users often combine several different types of steroids ("stacking")	• Synthetic derivatives of testosterone; abuse can lead to serious health problems, some irreversible • Men: shrinking of the testicles, reduced sperm count, infertility, baldness, gynecomastia, increased risk for prostate cancer • Women: growth of facial hair, male-pattern baldness, changes in or cessation of the menstrual cycle, enlargement of the clitoris, deepened voice • Adolescents: stunted growth by premature skeletal maturation and accelerated puberty changes • Other major side effects can include jaundice, fluid retention, high blood pressure, severe acne; extreme mood swings can occur, including manic-like symptoms leading to violence and depression often experienced when drugs are stopped, and such symptoms may contribute to dependence
Barbiturates (barbs, downers)	Ingestion, injection	• CNS depressants that at high doses can become general anesthetics • With high doses, coma, ataxia, depressed reflexes, hypotension, respiratory depression • CNS depressants should not be combined with any medication or substance that causes sedation, including prescription pain medicines, certain over-the-counter cold and allergy medications, or alcoholic drinks. The effects of the drugs can combine to slow breathing, or slow both the heart and respiration, which can be fatal • Discontinuing prolonged use of high doses of barbiturates can lead to withdrawal
Cocaine (snow, crack, rock); crack is the street name given to cocaine that has been processed from cocaine hydrochloride to the free base for smoking	Sniffing or snorting, injecting; smoking of free-base and crack cocaine; poorly absorbed orally	• CNS stimulant that produces euphoric effects and hyperstimulation such as dilated pupils, increased temperature, tachycardia, and hypertension • Prolonged cocaine snorting can result in ulceration of the mucous membranes of the nose and can damage the nasal septum enough to cause it to collapse • Cocaine-related deaths are often a result of cardiac arrest or seizures followed by respiratory arrest • Tolerance to the euphoric effects develops • When addicted individuals stop using cocaine, they often become depressed

(continued)

Table 3

Selected Drugs of Abuse and Addictive Substances (continued)

Substance (slang names)	Methods of abuse	Major or unique health effects
Dextromethorphan (DXM, DM, Robo, Velvet, Rojo)	Orally by drinking dextromethorphan-containing cough syrups; availability of the powdered form has led to repackaging as capsules or tablets and to nasal insufflation (snorting)	• Dextromethorphan (d-3-methoxy-N-methylmorphinan) is the dextro isomer of levomethorphan. It has no analgesic opiate-like dependence-producing properties. A behaviorally-active metabolite, dextrorphan, is structurally related to PCP and ketamine and may contribute to its abuse potential • The typical clinical presentation of intoxication involves hyperexcitability, lethargy, ataxia, slurred speech, sweating, hypertension, and/or nystagmus. The abusers report a heightened sense of perceptual awareness, altered time perception, and visual hallucinations • The majority of abuse occurs among teenagers and young adults who use dextromethorphan alone, or mixed with other drugs. It has been sold as "ecstasy." It has been identified as a filler in confiscated samples of bogus heroin and bogus ketamine. • Procedures are described to extract dextromethorphan from cough syrups on the Internet, which has led to the availability of powdered forms
Ethanol (various names and alcoholic drinks)	Ingestion	• CNS depressant at high doses can lead to hypotension, hypoglycemia, respiratory depression, and death • Acute intoxication leads to ataxia, sedation, emesis, and slurred speech • Chronic abuse leads to many medical complications such as esophageal varices, hepatic failure with ascites, and malnutrition • Tolerance, dependence, and withdrawal develop with chronic abuse
GHB or gamma hydroxybutyrate (liquid ecstasy, soap, easy lay, Georgia home boy, somatomax, scoop, grievous bodily harm)	Ingestion	• CNS depressant abused for euphoric, sedative, and anabolic (body building) effects • Coma and seizures are likely; increased risk of seizures when combined with methamphetamine • Use with alcohol causes nausea and difficulty breathing • GHB and two of its precursors, gamma butyrolactone (GBL) and 1,4 butanediol (BD) have been involved in poisonings, overdoses, date rapes, and deaths; they are produced by illicit laboratories • May produce withdrawal effects
Heroin (smack, H, skag, junk)	Injection, snorting, or smoking	• Abuse associated with fatal overdose, spontaneous abortion, collapsed veins, and infectious diseases, including HIV/AIDS and hepatitis • Euphoria ("rush") followed by an alternately wakeful and drowsy state ("on the nod") • CNS depression, respiratory depression, miosis (pinpoint pupils), pulmonary edema • Street heroin may have additives • With regular use tolerance develops and withdrawal is possible
Inhalants	Inhaled by sniffing and huffing	• A variety of breathable chemical vapors that produce psychoactive effects • Found in industrial or household solvents or solvent-containing products, including paint thinners or solvents, degreasers, dry-cleaning fluids, gasoline, and glues • Nearly all abused inhalants produce short-term intoxicating and CNS depressant effects similar to anesthetics • Intoxication usually lasts only a few minutes; successive inhalations lead to loss of inhibition and control; continued use can lead to coma • In some cases heart failure and death within minutes of a session of prolonged use, called "sudden sniffing death" is seen
Injected drugs (shooting up, mainlining)	Injection	• The injecting drug user is at risk for transmitting or acquiring HIV/AIDS, hepatitis, bacterial infections, and fungal infections if needles or other injection equipment are shared • Chronic users may develop collapsed veins, infection of the heart lining and valves, skin abscesses, cellulitis, and liver disease • Since some abusers dissolve the tablets in water and inject the mixture, emboli can form from the insoluble materials in the tablets

(continued)

Table 3

TOXICOLOGY AND CHEM-BIOTERRORISM **775**

Selected Drugs of Abuse and Addictive Substances (continued)

Substance (slang names)	Methods of abuse	Major or unique health effects
Ketamine (K, special K, cat Valium, vitamin K)	Injected, snorted	• An anesthetic that has been approved for human and veterinary use • Certain doses can cause dream-like states and hallucinations • At high doses, can cause delirium, amnesia, impaired motor function, hypertension, depression, and potentially fatal respiratory depression
LSD, lysergic acid diethylamide (acid, L, blotter, cubes, sugar, dots)	Ingested; often added to absorbent paper, such as blotter paper, and divided into small decorated squares ("blotter acid") or placed on dot-like candy ("dots") or sugar cubes ("cubes," "sugar")	• A hallucinogen sold on the street in tablets, capsules, and liquid form • Effects are unpredictable; physical effects include mydriasis (dilated pupils), elevated temperature, tachycardia, hypertension, sweating, loss of appetite, sleeplessness, dry mouth, and tremors • Sensations and feelings change more dramatically than the physical signs. In sufficient doses, the drug produces delusions and visual hallucinations • Some users experience severe, terrifying thoughts and feelings, fear of losing control, fear of insanity and death, and despair • Fatal accidents have occurred during intoxication • Many users experience flashbacks
Marijuana (pot, herb, weed, grass, widow, ganja, hash, and trademarked varieties of cannabis, such as Bubble Gum, Northern Lights, Juicy Fruit, Afghani #1, and a number of Skunk varieties)	Smoked as a cigarette (joint, nail), in a pipe (bong) or in blunts (cigars that have been emptied of tobacco and refilled with marijuana, often in combination with another drug); also ingested when mixed in food or brewed as a tea	• Main active chemical in marijuana is THC (delta-9-tetrahydrocannabinol) • Delirium, conjunctivitis, food craving are typical • Short-term effects include problems with memory and learning, distorted perception, difficulty in thinking and problem solving, loss of coordination, and tachycardia • Risk of heart attack more than quadruples in the first hour after smoking marijuana • Same respiratory problems as cigarette smokers (see nicotine); burning and stinging of the mouth and throat, often accompanied by a heavy cough • Drug craving and withdrawal
MDMA, 3-4 methylene-dioxymeth-amphetamine (Ecstasy, Adam, XTC, hug, beans, love drug)	Ingestion; some snort or inject it, or use it in suppository form	• A synthetic, psychoactive drug with both stimulant and hallucinogenic properties • Increases pulse and blood pressure • In high doses it can cause malignant hyperthermia leading to rhabdomyolysis (muscle breakdown with kidney and cardiovascular system failure) • Psychological difficulties: confusion, depression, sleep problems, drug craving, severe anxiety, and paranoia, during and sometimes weeks after use • Physical symptoms: muscle tension, involuntary teeth clenching, nausea, blurred vision, nystagmus, faintness, chills, or sweating • Content of the MDMA pills also varies widely, and may include caffeine, dextromethorphan, heroin, and mescaline. In some areas, the MDMA-like substance paramethoxyamphetamine (PMA) has led to death when mistaken for true MDMA; deaths were due to complications from hyperthermia
Methamphetamine (crank, meth, speed, chalk; the clear chunky crystals resembling ice can be smoked and are referred to as ice, crystal, and glass)	Ingestion, snorting the powder, injection, smoking	• An addictive stimulant chemically related to amphetamine • Produces euphoria, irritability, insomnia, confusion, tremors, convulsions, anxiety, paranoia, and aggressiveness; higher doses lead to hypertension, tachycardia, stroke, arrhythmias, cardiovascular collapse, and death • Hyperthermia and convulsions can result in death • Prolonged use leads to extreme anorexia; associated with tooth decay and skin lesions • Made in illegal laboratories and may contain contaminants and by-products • High potential for abuse and dependence
Nicotine (various names and products)	Smoked as cigarettes and other forms of tobacco, such as cigars, pipe tobacco, and chewing tobacco	• Highly addictive CNS stimulant and sedative; stimulation is followed by depression and fatigue leading the user to seek more nicotine • Women who take oral contraceptives are more prone to cardiovascular and cerebrovascular diseases, especially those older than 30 • Pregnant women have an increased risk of having stillborn or premature infants or infants with low birthweight

(continued)

Table 3

Selected Drugs of Abuse and Addictive Substances (continued)

Substance (slang names)	Methods of abuse	Major or unique health effects
Nicotine (various names and products) (cont'd)		• Respiratory problems: daily cough and phlegm production, more frequent acute respiratory illness, a heightened risk of lung infections, and a greater tendency toward obstructed airways, cancer of the respiratory tract and lungs • Tar in cigarettes associated with a higher rate of lung cancer, emphysema, and bronchial disorders • Carbon monoxide in the smoke increases the chance of cardiovascular diseases • Nicotine tolerance, dependence, and withdrawal symptoms occur
Opioids	Ingested, injection	• Includes morphine, codeine, oxycodone (Oxycontin®, MS Contin®), propoxyphene (Darvon®), hydrocodone (Vicodin®), hydromorphone (Dilaudid®), and meperidine (Demerol®) • Cause drowsiness, constipation; large single doses cause coma, hypotension, respiratory depression, and in some cases seizures and death • Mixing with alcohol and other CNS depressants increases the risk of coma and death • Chronic use of opioids produces tolerance, physical dependence, and withdrawal symptoms
Phencyclidine (PCP, angel dust, ozone, wack, rocket fuel; killer joints or crystal supergrass when combined with marijuana)	Snorted, smoked, or eaten; for smoking, often applied to a leafy material such as mint, parsley, oregano, or marijuana	• An addictive hallucinogen and sedative that often leads to psychological dependence, craving, and compulsive PCP-seeking behavior • Users often become violent or suicidal and are very dangerous to themselves and to others • At low to moderate doses, slight tachypnea, more pronounced tachycardia and hypertension, shallow respirations, and profuse sweating; generalized numbness of the extremities and muscular incoordination also may occur • Psychological effects include distinct changes in body awareness, similar to those associated with alcohol intoxication • At high doses, decreased blood pressure, pulse, and respirations; nausea, vomiting; blurred vision, nystagmus; drooling; ataxia; seizures, coma, and death (though death more often results from accidental injury or suicide during PCP intoxication) • Psychological effects at high doses include illusions, hallucinations, and effects that mimic the full range of symptoms of schizophrenia • Interactions with other CNS depressants, such as alcohol and benzodiazepines, can lead to coma • Illegally manufactured in illicit laboratories
Rohypnol (rophie, roofies, roche, roach, rope, the date rape drug, forget-me)	Ingestion	• Rohypnol, a trade name for flunitrazepam, is a benzodiazepine that is not sold in the U.S.; it is smuggled into the U.S. • Produces sedative-hypnotic effects including muscle relaxation and amnesia; it can also produce physical and psychological dependence • When mixed with alcohol, rohypnol can incapacitate victims, prevent them from resisting sexual assault, and can produce anterograde amnesia • May be lethal when mixed with alcohol or other CNS depressants • Abuse of two other similar drugs, clonazepam (Klonopin®) and alprazolam (Xanax®), appears to be replacing rohypnol
Stimulants, amphetamines and related compounds (speed, dexies, uppers)	Ingestion, tablets crushed and snorted	• CNS stimulants increase alertness, attention, and energy as well as increase in blood pressure, pulse, and respiration • High doses: arrhythmias, hypertension, hyperthermia, potential for cardiovascular failure, stroke or lethal seizures; taking high doses of some stimulants repeatedly over a short period of time can lead to hostility or feelings of paranoia in some individuals • Stimulants such as dextroamphetamine (Dexedrine®) and methylphenidate (Ritalin®) when misused can be addictive

Sources: InfoFacts. National Institute on Drug Abuse, National Institutes of Health, Washington, DC.
Available at: http://www.nida.nih.gov/Infofax/Infofaxindex.html. Web page accessed July 21, 2006.
Drugs and Chemicals of Concern. Diversion Control Program, Drug Enforcement Administration, U.S. Department of Justice, Washington, DC.
Available at: http://www.deadiversion.usdoj.gov/drugs_concern. Web page accessed July 21, 2006.

Table 4

Commonly Used Antidotes

Listed below are common antidotes that may need to be used emergently for patients presenting with acute toxic ingestion or dermal or inhalation exposure. Dosages are derived from standard texts and references and are given as convenience references. These should not be considered specific treatment guidelines; consult appropriate resources.

Toxin	Antidote (trade name)	Adult dose	Pediatric dose
Acetaminophen	Acetylcysteine (Mucomyst®)	Oral loading dose: 140 mg/kg; maintenance doses: 70 mg/kg every 4 hours for 17 doses	Same as adult dose regimen
	Acetylcysteine (Acetadote®)	IV infusion: 150 mg/kg in 200 mL D_5W infused over 15 min, then 50 mg/kg in 500 mL D_5W over 4 hours, followed by 100 mg/kg in 1000 mL D_5W over 16 hours	Same as adult dose regimen
Anticholinergic compounds	Physostigmine salicylate (Antilirium®)	1-2 mg slow IV infusion over 3-5 minutes titrated to effect	0.02 mg/kg slow IV infusion over 3-5 minutes titrated to effect
Arsenic	Succimer (Chemet®)	10 mg/kg orally 3 times a day	10 mg/kg orally 3 times a day
	Dimercaprol, also called British anti-lewisite (BAL in Oil®), only if unable to tolerate oral succimer	3-5 mg/kg intramuscular every 4-6 hours	3-5 mg/kg intramuscular every 4-6 hours
Benzodiazepines	Flumazenil[1] (Romazicon®)	0.2 mg IV bolus titrated to effect or total dose of 3 mg	0.01 mg/kg IV bolus titrated to effect or total dose of 1-3 mg
β-Blocker	Glucagon (GlucaGen®)	5-10 mg IV bolus followed by 5-10 mg/h IV infusion titrated to effect	0. 15 mg/kg mg IV bolus followed by 0.1 mg/h IV infusion titrated to effect
Calcium channel blockers	Calcium chloride 10%	10-20 mL IV bolus, repeat doses and IV infusions are common	0.1-0.2 mL/kg IV bolus, repeat doses and IV infusions are common
	Glucagon (GlucaGen)	5-10 mg/ IV bolus followed by 5-10 mg/h IV infusion titrated to effect	0.15 mg/ IV bolus followed by 0. 1 mg/h IV infusion titrated to effect
Carbamates	Atropine	2-4 mg IV bolus, repeat doses titrated to effect	1 mg/kg IV bolus, repeat doses titrated to effect
Cyanide	Cyanide antidote kit:		
	Sodium nitrite 3%	300 mg slow IV infusion	0.15-0. 33 mL/kg to maximum of 300 mg slow IV infusion
	Sodium thiosulfate	12.5 g IV infusion	400 mg/kg up to 12. 5 g IV infusion
Digoxin	Digoxin immune antibody fragment (Digibind®, DigiFab®)	Empiric dosing: 10-20 vials IV bolus for life-threatening toxicity; see package insert for other dosing regimens	Empiric dosing: 10-20 vials IV bolus for life-threatening toxicity; see package insert for other dosing regimens
Ethylene glycol, methanol	Ethanol 10%	Loading dose 10 mL/kg IV or orally followed by maintenance dose 1-2 mL/kg/h IV infusion maintenance dose or orally	Loading dose 10 mL/kg IV or orally followed by 1-2 mL/kg/h IV infusion or orally
	Fomepizole, also called 4-methylpyrazole (Antizol®)	15 mg/kg IV bolus, smaller repeat doses may be necessary	15 mg/kg IV bolus, smaller repeat doses may be necessary
Iron	Deferoxamine (Desferal®)	5-15 mg/kg/h IV infusion titrated to effect	5-15 mg/kg/h IV infusion titrated to effect
Isoniazid	Pyridoxine, also called vitamin B_6	1 g per gram ingested or empiric dosing 5 g IV bolus	1 g per gram ingested or empiric dosing 75 mg/kg IV bolus up to 5 g
Lead	Succimer (Chemet®)	10 mg/kg orally 3 times a day, repeat doses are common	10 mg/kg orally 3 times a day, repeat doses are common

(continued)

Table 4

Commonly Used Antidotes (continued)

Toxin	Antidote (trade name)	Adult dose	Pediatric dose
Lead (continued)	Dimercaprol, also called British anti-lewisite [BAL], only for lead encephalopathy (BAL in Oil)	3-5 mg/kg intramuscularly or 50-75 mg/m² intramuscularly	3-5 mg/kg intramuscularly or 50-75 mg/m² intramuscularly
	Calcium disodium EDTA (Calcium Disodium Versenate®)	20-30 mg/kg diluted in 250 mL IV infusion over 12-24 hours (start 4 hours after BAL administration)	20-30 mg/kg diluted in 250 mL IV infusion over 12-24 hours (start 4 hours after BAL administration)
Methemoglobinemia	Methylene blue	1-2 mg/kg slow IV infusion, repeat doses are common	1-2 mg/kg slow IV infusion, repeat doses are common
Opioids	Naloxone hydrochloride (Narcan®)	0. 4-2 mg IV titrated to effect	0. 4-2 mg IV titrated to effect
Organophosphates	Atropine	2-4 mg IV bolus, repeat doses titrated to effect	0.1 mg/kg IV bolus, repeat doses titrated to effect
	Pralidoxime hydrochloride (Protopam®)	1-2 g slow IV infusion followed by 500 mg/h continuous infusion or 1 g every 4 hours	20-40 mg/kg slow IV infusion followed by 5-10 mg/kg/h continuous infusion or 20 mg/kg every 4 hours
Salicylate	Sodium bicarbonate	150 mEq with 40 mEq KCl in 1 L of D_5W infused to maintain urine output at 1-2 mL/kg/h and a urine pH approximately 7.5	150 mEq with 40 mEq KCl in 1 L of D_5W infused to maintain urine output at 1-2 mL/kg/h and a urine pH approximately 7.5
Tricyclic antidepressants, agents with type 1a antiarrhythmic effects	Sodium bicarbonate	1-2 mEq/kg IV bolus, titrate repeat boluses to QRS duration (do not exceed arterial pH of 7.55)	1-2 mEq/kg IV bolus, titrate boluses to QRS duration (do not exceed arterial pH of 7.55)
Warfarin, superwarfarins	Fresh frozen plasma	Fresh frozen plasma for life-threatening hemorrhage	Fresh frozen plasma for life-threatening hemorrhage
	Vitamin K₁ (Mephyton®, AquaMEPHYTON®)	10-50 mg slow IV infusion, subcutaneous or orally	0.6 mg/kg slow IV infusion, subcutaneous or orally

[1]Potential risks may exceed the benefits due to precipitation of intractable seizures.

Excerpt from: American College of Emergency Physicians: Clinical policy for the initial approach to patients presenting with acute toxic ingestion or dermal or inhalation exposure. *Ann Emerg Med.* 1999;33:735-761.

- It may also be useful to minimize hepatotoxic injury once it has begun and with fulminant hepatic failure.

Indications

- Acute overdoses of acetaminophen produce a reactive metabolite that leads to hepatotoxicity (jaundice, coagulopathy, hypoglycemia, hepatic failure, hepatic encephalopathy, and hepatorenal failure). Symptoms become evident 1-2 days after ingestion.
- N-acetylcysteine can prevent or minimize hepatic injury if given early. For best results, administer within 10 hours of ingestion of acetaminophen overdose. It is minimally effective when started 24 hours after ingestion.
- The need for therapy is determined by a serum concentration of acetaminophen obtained at least 4 hours after ingestion (and within 24 hours) and plotting it on the acetaminophen nomogram to determine whether there is a risk for hepatotoxicity.

Contraindications

- Known hypersensitivity to N-acetylcysteine

Adverse effects

- With oral administration, nausea and vomiting are common.
- With intravenous administration, anaphylactoid reactions (rash, hypotension, wheezing, dyspnea) have

been reported. Acute flushing and erythema may occur during the first hour of infusion and typically resolve spontaneously.

Dosage
- Drug products for oral or intravenous administration are available in the U.S. (Table 4).

Atropine
Indications
- Organophosphate (including chem-bioterrorism nerve agents) and carbamate anticholinesterase insecticide poisoning
- Bradycardia
- Nontoxicologic indications include atropine use for premedication to anesthesia induction (for antisecretory effects) and ophthalmic mydriasis and cycloplegia.

Mechanism of action
- Anticholinergic agent that competitively inhibits acetylcholine at muscarinic receptors. Atropine has little effect on nicotinic receptors.

Indications for use in the treatment of organophosphate or carbamate poisoning
- For control of pulmonary hypersecretion, atropine is given in repeated doses intravenously until secretions have dried. Atropinization may have to be maintained for hours to days.
- For control of bradycardia, atropine is given until the heart rate increases or until a need for alternatives is indicated.

Contraindications
- None for insecticide poisoning

Contraindications for other indications
- Hypersensitivity to atropine or anticholinergics
- Narrow-angle glaucoma
- Reflux esophagitis
- Obstructive gastrointestinal disease
- Ulcerative colitis or toxic megacolon
- Obstructive uropathy
- Unstable cardiovascular status in acute hemorrhage or thyrotoxicosis
- Paralytic ileus or intestinal atony
- Myasthenia gravis

Adverse effects
- Exaggeration of anticholinergic effects (eg, tachycardia, hypertension, sedation, hallucinations, mydriasis, changes in intraocular pressure, warm red skin, dry mouth, urinary retention, ileus, dysrhythmias, and seizures)

- For the use of large doses of atropine, the agent should be preservative-free since agents like benzyl alcohol or chlorobutanol can produce their own toxicity.

Dosage
- For bronchorrhea and bronchospasm from organophosphates or carbamates, the adult dose is 2-5 mg (pediatric dose is 0.05 mg/kg) administered slowly by IV. Dose is repeated at 10- to 30-minute intervals until bronchial hypersecretion is resolved. Severe poisonings may require up to 100 mg over a few hours to several grams over several weeks. If atropinization is required for several days, continuous atropine infusion may be used (rates of 0.02-0.08 mg/kg per hour are recommended).
- For symptomatic bradycardia (for mild poisonings) the adult dose is 1 mg (the pediatric dose is 0.01 mg/kg) intravenously. For moderate to severe poisonings, adult doses increase to 2-5 mg (pediatric doses are 0.02-0.05 mg/kg) and should be repeated every few minutes until heart rate increases.

Digoxin immune Fab (Digibind®, DigiFab®)
Uses
- Treatment of life-threatening acute or chronic digoxin poisoning
- Some cross-reactivity with digitoxin and other digoxin-like compounds (digitalis, foxglove, lily of the valley, bufadienolide from cane frogs)

Mechanism of action
- Digoxin immune Fab binds digoxin in plasma, promotes redistribution from tissues, and enhances elimination in the urine. The digoxin bound to digoxin immune Fab is inactive. Each 40 mg (1 vial) binds 0.6 mg of digoxin.
- Digoxin immune Fab is a monovalent, digoxin-specific, antigen-binding fragment (Fab) that is produced in healthy sheep.

Indications
- Chronic digoxin toxicity typically begins with nausea, vomiting, diarrhea, fatigue, confusion, blurred vision, diplopia, and seeing white borders or halos around dark objects. Deterioration of renal function, hypokalemia, or drug interactions often lead to toxicity.
- Acute digoxin poisoning has early symptoms similar to those of chronic poisoning, but the onset is more abrupt, nausea and vomiting are common, and the serum potassium concentration is typically normal or elevated.
- A wide variety of arrhythmias occur with acute or chronic digoxin poisoning.

- Digoxin immune Fab is reserved for life-threatening symptoms such as bradycardia, second-degree and third-degree heart block unresponsive to atropine, ventricular arrhythmias, and hyperkalemia (typically in excess of 5 mEq/L).

Contraindications
- Hypersensitivity to sheep

Adverse effects
- Common adverse effects include hypokalemia, allergic reactions (1%), and hypotension.
- For patients on maintenance digoxin therapy, the abrupt binding of digoxin will lead to loss of therapeutic effect and a prompt decrease in potassium concentrations.

Dosage
- It is administered by intravenous infusion or rapid intravenous bolus (Table 4).
- Dosage is determined by one of several approaches, depending upon available information, as follows: empiric dosage of 10-20 vials (Table 4), dosing based on the dose of digoxin ingested, or dosing based on the serum digoxin concentration.

Flumazenil (Romazicon®)
Uses
- Benzodiazepine overdose
- Reversal of conscious sedation and general anesthesia from benzodiazepines

Mechanism of action
- Flumazenil is a competitive antagonist of the benzodiazepine receptor in the central nervous system.

Indications
- Flumazenil should be used adjunctively with supportive care. Sedation can reoccur following ingestion of a benzodiazepine with a long half-life, requiring additional doses of flumazenil. In a suicidal overdose, it is rarely used due to the risk of potential co-ingestants. If no response occurs to a 5-mg cumulative dose, it is doubtful if the sedation is related to a benzodiazepine.

Contraindications
- Known hypersensitivity to flumazenil
- Co-ingestion of tricyclic antidepressants may precipitate ventricular dysrhythmias or seizures.
- Other mixed overdoses that can decrease the seizure threshold (ie, haloperidol, bupropion, lithium)
- Abrupt withdrawal in patients on maintenance therapy, such as for treatment of epilepsy, can precipitate seizures.
- Patients with increased intracranial pressure, because

the antidote may potentially alter cerebral blood flow
- It can produce withdrawal in the physically dependent patient.

Adverse effects
- Flumazenil has a wide margin of safety when not contraindicated.
- Side effects include agitation, sweating, headache, abnormal vision, dizziness, and pain at the administration site.
- Rarely reported: bradycardia, tachycardia, hypotension, or hypertension

Dosage
- IV administration (see Table 4)

Naloxone (Narcan)
Uses
- Reversal of opioid anesthesia
- Respiratory or central nervous system depression related to opioid toxicity
- Empiric administration in patients with altered mental status due to unknown etiology

Mechanism of action
- Naloxone is an opioid antagonist. Naloxone competes at three CNS opioid receptors (mu, kappa, and delta) and leads to reversal of the depressive opioid effects.

Indications
- Opioids cause sedation, respiratory depression, hypotension, miosis, and analgesia. Because it has no agonist activity, naloxone will not worsen respiratory depression. The goal of therapy is to restore adequate spontaneous respirations. When administered, a patient should be monitored for respiratory rate changes and for opiate withdrawal symptoms (anxiety, hypertension, tachycardia, diarrhea, and seizure). To avoid withdrawal, use the lowest possible dose that maintains proper ventilation. The patient should be observed for respiratory depression once naloxone therapy is discontinued because the half-life of naloxone may be shorter than that of the opioid. If a patient is not responsive to 10 mg of naloxone, it is doubtful that an opioid is causing the respiratory depression.

Contraindications
- Known hypersensitivity
- Use with caution in the physically-dependent opioid patient.
- Use with caution in patients with preexisting cardiovascular disease or those receiving cardiotoxic drugs.

Adverse effects

- Use in an opiate-dependent patient can precipitate withdrawal.
- Withdrawal convulsions in a neonate can be life threatening.
- Hypertension and dysrhythmias occur more often with opioid reversal in postoperative patients with underlying cardiac and pulmonary complications.

Dosage

- The IV route is preferred in the emergency situation due to rapid onset of action within 1-2 minutes (Table 4).
- Naloxone has poor oral bioavailability.
- The intramuscular and subcutaneous routes have erratic absorption.

Pralidoxime or 2-PAM (Protopam)
Uses

- Severe organophosphate anticholinesterase insecticide or chem-bioterrorism nerve agent poisoning

Mechanism of action

- Pralidoxime dephosphorylates acetylcholinesterase and regenerates acetylcholinesterase activity.

Indications

- Severe organophosphate or nerve agent poisoning, in combination with atropine to resolve nicotinic (muscle and diaphragmatic weakness, fasciculations, muscle cramps) and central (coma, seizures) cholinergic manifestations; it is ineffective for organophosphates without anticholinesterase activity.
- Carbamate poisoning; use is controversial but recommended by some sources for severe cases.

Contraindications

- Hypersensitivity to pralidoxime

Adverse effects

- Tachycardia, dizziness, hyperventilation, and laryngospasm associated with rapid IV infusion
- Nausea, vomiting, diarrhea, bitter aftertaste, and rash after oral doses
- Blurred vision, diplopia
- Possible neuromuscular blockade (weakness) with high levels or in patients with myasthenia gravis

Dosage

- See Table 4 for intravenous doses.

4. Overview of Chem-Bioterrorism

- The world faces the growing threat of attacks with biological, chemical, explosive, and radiological weapons.
- Bioterrorism is the deliberate use of infectious biological agents to cause illness, and is categorized for risk by the Centers for Disease Control and Prevention (CDC).
  * *Category A* agents are high priority agents that can be easily transmitted, result in high mortality rates, and have the potential for major public health impact. They include smallpox, anthrax, plague (*Yersinia pestis*), botulism, tularemia, and viral hemorrhagic fevers (filoviruses [eg, Ebola and Marburg] and arenaviruses [eg, Lassa and Machupo]).
  * *Category B* agents include brucellosis, epsilon toxin of *Clostridium perfringens,* food safety threats (eg, *Salmonella* species, *Escherichia coli* O157:H7, *Shigella*), glanders (*Burkholderia mallei*), melioidosis (*Burkholderia pseudomallei*), psittacosis (*Chlamydia psittaci*), Q fever (*Coxiella burnetii*), ricin, staphylococcal enterotoxin B, typhus fever, viral encephalitis (alphaviruses [eg, Venezuelan equine encephalitis, eastern equine encephalitis, western equine encephalitis]), and water safety threats (eg, *Vibrio cholerae, Cryptosporidium parvum*).
  * *Category C* agents include emerging infectious disease threats such as Nipah virus and hantavirus.
- See Table 5 for clinical features and suggested treatment for the most likely forms of category A diseases, and ricin, a previously weaponized and used category B agent.
- The mode of transmission for biological agents is essentially the same as with all other infectious diseases:
  * Aerosol (most common form for biological weapons)
  * Dermal contact
  * Injection
  * Food-borne
  * Water-borne
- Toxic chemicals that are used in warfare include nerve, blister/vesicant, blood, choking/lung/pulmonary, incapacitating, and riot control/tear- and vomit-inducing agents.
- See Table 6 for descriptions, symptoms, and treatment of the agents most likely to be used.
- Normally they are liquids or solids, often dispersed in the air in aerosols.

Table 5

Biological Agents That May Be Used in a Bioterrorism Attack

Biological agent	Clinical features	Treatment
Smallpox is caused by the variola virus; may be spread by aerosol or direct contact with infected persons/fluids	Early symptoms resemble a mild viral illness, with a 2- to 4-day nonspecific prodrome of fever and myalgias before rash onset. Pustules form, then scabs form and fall off, leaving pitted scars. When all the scabs have fallen off (in about 3 weeks), patients are no longer contagious. Smallpox rash is typically most prominent on the face and extremities, and lesions form at the same time. (By contrast, chickenpox rash is most prominent on the trunk and develops in successive groups of lesions over several days.)	No specific treatment. Vaccine is only preventive. The currently available vaccine (Dryvax® from Wyeth) is a live-virus preparation of vaccinia virus.
Anthrax is caused by *Bacillus anthracis*, a gram-positive spore-forming rod, and has three major forms: cutaneous, inhalation, and gastrointestinal; none are contagious	**Cutaneous:** Begins as a small papule, progresses to a vesicle in 1-2 days, followed by a necrotic, normally painless ulcer. May have fever, malaise, headache, and regional lymphadenopathy. **Inhalation:** Initially resembles a viral illness with sore throat, mild fever, muscle aches, and malaise. Often has minimally productive cough, nausea or vomiting, and chest discomfort that may progress to respiratory failure and shock with meningitis frequently developing. In contrast to influenza, patients rarely have a runny nose and usually have an abnormal chest x-ray and high white blood cell count. **Gastrointestinal:** Causes severe abdominal or oropharyngeal distress followed by fever and signs of septicemia, bloody vomit, and diarrhea.	Ciprofloxacin and doxycycline are FDA-approved for postexposure prophylaxis (PEP). Ciprofloxacin and doxycycline are FDA-approved for treatment. Amoxicillin may be considered if found to be sensitive to its action. Persons at risk for inhalation anthrax need 60 days of prophylactic antibiotics. The CDC recommends anthrax vaccine only for the military and similar high-risk personnel.

(continued)

- The CDC has recently added commonly available agents such as hydrofluoric acid, benzene, ethylene glycol (antifreeze), and metals like arsenic, mercury, and thallium to the threat list, although these are not listed as chemical warfare agents in other sources and are not detailed in Table 6.
- Radiological weapons involve nuclear radiation or radioactive materials with various radionucleotides.
- Radionucleotides can produce topical and systemic effects that may be immediate or delayed, depending upon the agent, route of exposure, and extent of exposure.
- Medical management of radiological emergencies and terrorist attacks is specific for the radionucleotide. Guidance on treatment is available from the Radiation Emergency Assistance Center/Training Site (REAC/TS) at the Oak Ridge Institute for Science and Education. The emergency response phone number is 865-576-1005; ask for REAC/TS.

Program information is available at www.orau.gov/reacts.
- For example, the early use of stable iodine, taken as potassium iodide or sodium iodide tablets, can reduce the uptake of radioiodine by the thyroid. Many individuals near nuclear reactors will maintain a stock of stable iodine tablets in the event of a radioactive accident. Ingestion of stable iodine is of little value for other radionucleotide exposures unless the radioactive constituents are unknown, as in a "dirty bomb."
- Prussian blue 500-mg capsules are approved for the treatment of patients with exposures to radioactive cesium (Cs-137) and thallium (Tl-201). It absorbs the radioactivity that is recirculated in the intestines and thereby enhances its elimination in the stool. The drug is available from the CDC.
- Calcium and zinc salts of diethylene triamine penta-acetic acid for intravenous infusion and aerosol neb-

Table 5

TOXICOLOGY AND CHEM-BIOTERRORISM **783**

Biological Agents That May Be Used in a Bioterrorism Attack (continued)

Biological agent	Clinical features	Treatment
Plague, caused by *Yersinia pestis,* has several forms, with pneumonic plague being the most virulent	Clinical features of aerosolized pneumonic plague include fever, cough with mucopurulent sputum, hemoptysis, and chest pain with signs consistent with severe pneumonia 1-6 days after exposure. Septic shock and high mortality can occur within 2-4 days of symptom onset without early treatment. *Y pestis*–caused bubonic plague is less likely to be weaponized.	Early treatment and PEP with streptomycin, gentamicin, doxycycline, ciprofloxacin, or chloramphenicol is advised. (Vaccine is ineffective for pneumonic plague.)
Botulism, caused by *Clostridium botulinum,* may be food-borne or air-borne	Clinical features include acute symmetric descending paralysis in a proximal to distal pattern, with prominent bulbar palsies such as diplopia, dysarthria, dysphonia, and dysphagia that typically present 12-72 hours postexposure, and respiratory dysfunction from respiratory muscle paralysis or upper airway obstruction without sensory deficits.	A supply of antitoxin is maintained and dispensed by the CDC. Most patients recover after supportive care, often with mechanical ventilation for weeks to months.
Tularemia, caused by *Francisella tularensis,* is one of the most infectious bacteria known	Inhalation exposure causes an abrupt onset of a nonspecific febrile illness beginning 3-5 days postexposure, with incipient pneumonia, pleuritis, and hilar lymphadenopathy. Without treatment, respiratory failure, shock, and death are possible. Like botulism and anthrax, tularemia is not contagious, so patients who have tularemia do not need to be isolated.	Prompt treatment with streptomycin, gentamicin, chloramphenicol, doxycycline, or ciprofloxacin advised, as is early PEP use of doxycycline or ciprofloxacin.
Viral hemorrhagic fevers (VHF): filoviruses and arenaviruses are most virulent, but all listed here are considered serious biological threats; exposure is via all routes, including direct and aerosol	With **filoviruses** (Ebola and Marburg types), an abrupt onset of an undifferentiated febrile illness with high fever occurs 2-21 days after exposure. A maculopapular rash, prominent on the trunk, develops around 5 days later, with progressive bleeding symptoms such as petechiae, ecchymosis, disseminated intravascular coagulation, and hemorrhages. With **arenaviruses** (Lassa and multiple New World arenaviruses, including Machupo that causes Bolivian hemorrhagic fever) symptoms and onset are similar to filoviruses, but with a gradual onset of rash, hemorrhagic diathesis, and shock. **Bunyaviruses** cause Rift Valley fever (<1% develop hemorrhagic fever). **Flaviviruses** cause Yellow fever, Omsk hemorrhagic fever, and Kyasabur Forest disease. (Other VHFs exist, but they are not considered a serious bioterrorism risk.)	The mainstay of treatment is supportive to maintain fluid and electrolyte balance, circulatory volume, and blood pressure. There are no FDA-approved antiviral drugs or vaccines.
Ricin, from castor beans, is cytotoxic via inhibition of protein synthesis; abrin is a similar toxalbumin agent	Within a few hours of inhalation, cough and dyspnea develop, with the lungs rapidly becoming severely inflamed and filled with fluid. Skin might turn blue from cyanosis or flush red. Ingestion causes internal bleeding of the stomach and intestines. Injection kills the closest muscles and lymph nodes before spreading to other organs. Death can occur within 36-48 hours of all types of exposure from multiple organ failure.	No antidote is available. The mainstay of treatment is supportive, varying with the route of exposure. If victims survive more than 5 days, survival is likely.

Table 6

Chemical Agents That May Be Used in a Chem-Bioterrorism Attack

Chemical agents (military name)	Clinical features	Treatment
Nerve agents. G agents: sarin (GB), soman (GD), tabun (GA), cyclohexyl sarin (GF); V agents: VX	These nerve agents are organophosphates that attach to and inhibit acetylcholinesterase at muscarinic and nicotinic receptors, causing cholinergic crisis with miosis, vomiting, diarrhea, excessive secretions (bronchial, lacrimal, dermal, nasal, and salivary), brady- or tachycardia, skeletal muscle fasciculations, paralysis, seizures, and respiratory failure. They are well absorbed through all routes of exposure. Symptoms occur within minutes after significant exposure, and up to 18 hours after liquid exposure.	Rapid, thorough decontamination. Antidotes include atropine to reverse muscarinic symptoms and pralidoxime early to restore acetylcholinesterase before permanent deactivation (aging) of the enzyme. Also give diazepam or lorazepam for seizures.
Blister agents. Mustards: sulfur gas (H), distilled (HD); mustard/T. nitrogen mustards: (HN-1, HN-2, HN-3); sesqui mustard; lewisites: (L, L-1, L-2, L-3); chloroarsines: (ED, MD, PD); mustard/ lewisite combination: (HL); phosgene oxime: (CX)	*Mustards* are vesicants that cause blistering of the skin and mucous membranes on contact, damaging skin, eyes, and lungs. Damage is immediate but symptoms can be delayed 2-24 hours. Liquid forms are more likely to cause burns and scarring than gas. All forms are absorbed through the skin and distributed systemically. Nitrogen mustards cause bone marrow suppression in 3-5 days. Sulfur mustards have garlic, onion, mustard, or no odor. Nitrogen mustards can smell fishy, musty, soapy or fruity. *Lewisites and chloroarsines* are arsenical vesicants that cause immediate pain and damage to the eyes, skin, and respiratory tract, although lesions may take hours to form. After absorption, they cause increased capillary permeability leading to hypovolemia, shock, and organ damage. Lewisite smells like geraniums. Mustard/lewisite is lewisite combined with distilled mustard. *Phosgene oxime* is a readily absorbed urticant or nettle agent, causing immediate, painful corrosive and necrotic tissue damage. Does not cause blisters (but normally classified here). Disagreeable odor.	Sulfur and nitrogen mustards (thought to be alkylating agents that crosslink DNA strands) have no antidote. Avoiding contact or rapid thorough decontamination is only prevention. Treatment is supportive. Not usually fatal (sulfur type <5% fatal in World War I). No mustard in tissue or blister fluids. British anti-lewisite (BAL) is specific antidote for lewisite, used IM for systemic effects or topically as skin or eye ointment. Chloro-arsine treatment is similar, except atropine sulfate ointment is used for eyes. No antidote exists for phosgene oxime. Rapid decontamination and supportive treatment used as for any corrosive agent.

(continued)

ulization (Ca-DTPA and Zn-DTPA) are approved to treat patients who have been exposed to radionucleotides that may be found in a "dirty bomb" such as plutonium, americium, and curium. The drugs form chelates with the radionucleotides that are excreted in the urine. The drugs are available from the CDC.

- Health care professionals should have an awareness of the potential for biological terrorism, an appreciation for epidemiologic clues of a chem-bioterrorist event, and a basic understanding of the classes of agents that can be weaponized and their effects.

- Pharmacists are in a unique position to quickly recognize community-wide patterns of symptoms, illness, and mortality in humans and animals that can be important clues to terrorist events.
- The CDC advises that if citizens believe that they have been exposed to a biological or chemical agent, or if they believe an intentional biological threat will occur or is occurring, they should contact their local health department and/or local police or other law enforcement agency (eg, FBI). These agencies will notify the state health department and other response partners, per a pre-established notification list that channels to the CDC.

Table 6

Chemical Agents That May Be Used in a Chem-Bioterrorism Attack (continued)

Chemical agents (military name)	Clinical features	Treatment
Blood agents. Arsine: (SA); cyanide gases: hydrogen cyanide (AC), cyanogen chloride (CK); cyanide solids: potassium (KCN), and sodium (NaCN) cyanide	*Arsine* is a gas that causes nausea, vomiting, hemolysis, and secondary renal failure in 1-2 hours to 11 days. Garlic-like odor. Inhalation of highly concentrated *cyanide* causes increased rate and depth of breathing in 15 seconds, convulsions within 30 seconds, cessation of respiration in 2-4 minutes, and cessation of heartbeat in 4-8 minutes. Progress and severity of symptoms after ingestion or inhaling lower gas concentrations are slower and dose dependent. May have odor of bitter almonds or peach kernels (AC), with no odor or irritating, lacrimating properties like riot control agents (CK).	Arsines: symptomatic management of hemolysis, normally without chelation. Cyanides bind to cytochrome oxidase. Cyanide antidotes: (1) methemoglobin-forming agents like inhaled amyl nitrite (in civilian kits) and/or IV sodium nitrite free bound cyanide, restoring cellular ATP; (2) IV sodium thiosulfate (sulfur donor to convert cyanide to sodium thiocyanate). Fresh air, oxygen, supportive treatment.
Choking and pulmonary agents. Phosgene (CG), diphosgene (DP); also ammonia, chlorine (CL), hydrogen chloride, nitrogen oxide (NO), Teflon®, perfluroisobutylene (PHIB), others	*Phosgene* gas causes eye, nose, throat, and pulmonary irritation, with serious pulmonary injury and edema delayed up to 48 hours, as it hydrolyzes to hydrochloric acid in moist conditions. New-mown-hay odor. Phosgene is the prototype agent in the group. Other agents cause immediate irritation with potential for more severe delayed effects. *Ammonia* hydrolyzes to caustic ammonium hydroxide. *Chlorine* (pungent, greenish gas) hydrolyzes to hydrochloric acid. *Perfluroisobutylene* is a toxic pyrolysis product of *Teflon*. Nitrogen oxides are components of blast weapons or fire. Others include *red* (RP) and *white phosphorus*, *sulfur trioxide-chlorosulfonic acid* (FS), *titanium tetrachloride* (FM), and *zinc oxide* (HC).	Phosgene has no antidote. Good decontamination and symptomatic treatment needed. Treatment of other agents is similar as all agents in this class are gases with no antidotes (thorough, rapid decontamination with fresh air is best initial management, with thorough flushing of exposed eyes and skin and symptomatic treatment).
Incapacitating agents	Contains a variety of fast-acting central nervous system and respiratory depressants, often with hallucinogenic properties. CDC list includes *BZ/agent 15* (glycolate anticholinergic), *cannabinoids, fentanyls* and other opioids, *LSD,* and *phenothiazines.*	Management is decontamination with supportive treatment and antidotes should be used when they exist (physostigmine for anticholinergics, naloxone for opioids).
Riot control and tear gases	Lacrimators include *chloroacetophenone* (CN) in several solvents, *chloropicrin* (PS), *bromobenzylcyanide* (CA), CR, and CS gases.	Treatment is symptomatic after decontamination. No antidotes are available.
Vomiting agents	Includes *adamsite* (DM), *diphenylchloroarsine* (DA) and *diphenylcyanoarsine* (DC). Rapidly incapacitating, irritant gases.	Symptomatic measures for sneezing, coughing, and vomiting (eg, antiemetics).

- The CDC maintains the Strategic National Stockpile to ensure the availability and rapid deployment of life-saving pharmaceuticals, antidotes, other medical supplies, and equipment necessary to counter nerve agents, biological pathogens, and chemical agents. The SNS program stands ready for immediate deployment to any U.S. location in the event of a terrorist attack using a biological toxin or chemical agent directed against a civilian population. A limited stock of drugs to treat nerve agents (ChemPack) has been deployed to EMS and hospital sites throughout the U.S. and is maintained by the CDC. Further information is available at the CDC website (www.cdc.gov).
- Pharmacists should consider volunteering in their communities to assist with emergency preparedness. Roles in mass dispensing and vaccination clinics, strategic national stockpile deployment, and general disaster medical relief are possible opportunities. Contact the local health department or emergency medical services agency.
- Essential steps to volunteering for emergency preparedness include reaching an understanding with family and employer, registering as a volunteer and identifying skills to contribute, obtaining security credentials, participating in training, and doing whatever it takes when needed.

5. Key Points

- Medications are the most common cause of poisoning morbidity and mortality. Any chemical can become toxic if too much is taken in relation to body weight and tolerance. A great number of poisonings occur in young children, but most fatalities occur in adults.
- Several approaches can minimize the risk of unintentional childhood poisonings (eg, safety latches, proper storage, following label instructions), but the proper use of child-resistant containers ("safety caps") is one of the most effective means. As part of the Poison Prevention Packaging Act of 1970, pharmacists are required to dispense oral prescription drugs (with certain exceptions such as nitroglycerin and oral contraceptives) in child-resistant containers unless the patient or prescriber indicates the desire for a non-safety cap.
- Immediate first aid for a poison exposure can minimize potential toxic effects, and involves water and fresh air, depending on the route of exposure. Contact a poison center immediately through the nationwide access number (1-800-222-1222) to determine first aid or whether a poisoning emergency exists.
- The use of drugs to decrease the absorption of drugs from the gastrointestinal tract after a poisoning or overdose is in a state of change. Ipecac syrup, an orally administered emetic, has questionable effectiveness and its use is generally now avoided. It should not be used (1) when the person exhibits sleepiness, coma, or seizures; (2) when agents such as caustics, aliphatic hydrocarbons, fast-acting agents that produce coma or seizures (eg, tricyclic antidepressants, clonidine, strychnine, and hypoglycemic agents) have been ingested; (3) when the ingestion was greater than 1 hour ago; or (4) there is an obvious need for hospital referral. Cathartics such as magnesium citrate are not routinely used. Activated charcoal, an orally administered adsorbent, is often the only treatment necessary if the toxin can be adsorbed and it is used within 1-2 hours of ingestion. It should be avoided in ingestions of aliphatic hydrocarbons and caustics and in patients with absent bowel sounds, and it is not useful with heavy metals (sodium, lithium, iron, or lead) or simple alcohols. Whole-bowel irrigation, with products such as CoLyte and GoLYTELY, can be considered if the toxin is poorly adsorbed and its presence in the gastrointestinal tract is likely. Other hospital-based therapies include supportive and symptomatic care, multiple doses of activated charcoal (to enhance systemic elimination when appropriate), hemodialysis (to enhance systemic elimination when appropriate),

and use of antidotes (to antagonize or reverse toxic effects when indicated).

- Substance abuse often leads to acute and chronic toxicity from a variety of medications, commercial products, and illicit agents. The management of acute toxicity from substance abuse typically follows the same general approaches as those for poisoning and overdose. A challenge faced in many acute drug overdose episodes is determining the agents taken and possible adulterants or contaminants. Chronic abuse can lead to dependence and withdrawal symptoms upon stopping use.
- There are few antidotes available relative to the large number of potential poisons. The use of an antidote is usually an adjunct to conventional and supportive therapies. Many hospitals have an insufficient stock of antidotes.
- Acetylcysteine (Mucomyst, Acetadote) is a glutathione substitute in the metabolism of the acetaminophen toxic reactive metabolite. It is most effective if given orally within 10 hours of an acetaminophen overdose in preventing hepatotoxicity, and may also help later to minimize hepatic injury once it has begun. Oral (Mucomyst) and intravenous (Acetadote) preparations are available.
- Atropine is used to treat the muscarinic effects (bronchorrhea, bradycardia, etc.) produced by organophosphate and carbamate insecticides and anticholinesterase nerve gas agents by competing with acetylcholine for binding at muscarinic receptors in the nervous system.
- Pralidoxime (Protopam) reactivates the enzyme acetylcholinesterase by dephosphorylation and allows metabolism of accumulated amounts of acetylcholine produced by enzyme inhibition from exposures to anticholinesterase nerve gas agents and organophosphate and carbamate insecticides.
- Digoxin immune Fab (Digibind, DigiFab) is a specific antibody for digoxin, but it exhibits some cross reactivity with other digoxin-like compounds. It is an ovine derived antigen-binding fragment reserved for the treatment of life-threatening symptoms of digoxin overdose (eg, bradycardia, ventricular arrhythmias, second- and third-degree heart block, and hyperkalemia).
- Flumazenil (Romazicon) is a competitive antagonist of benzodiazepines at the benzodiazepine receptor in the central nervous system (CNS). It is used in the treatment of severe CNS and respiratory depression that may occur with benzodiazepines when they are used as an anesthetic or taken as an overdose. Seizures may occur when flumazenil is administered to patients with co-ingestants of tricyclic antidepressants, drugs that lower the seizure threshold, and in patients requiring benzodiazepines for seizure control.

- Administration of naloxone (Narcan), a competitive antagonist of opiate binding at the opioid receptors in the CNS, reverses the CNS and respiratory depression of opiate toxicity. Naloxone may precipitate withdrawal symptoms in opiate-dependent patients.
- Bioterrorism is the deliberate use of infectious biological agents to cause illness. High-priority agents can be easily transmitted, result in high mortality rates, and have the potential for major public health impact. They include smallpox, anthrax, plague (*Yersinia pestis*), botulism, tularemia, and viral hemorrhagic fevers (eg, Ebola, Marburg, Lassa, and Machupo).
- These toxic chemicals are used in warfare and may be used in an attack:
  * Substances that act on nerves (eg, anticholinesterase agents such as sarin)
  * Substances that are blistering/vesicants (eg, mustard agents and lewisites)
  * Substances that act on blood (eg, arsine and cyanide)
  * Substances that act on the pulmonary system (eg, phosgene, chlorine, and ammonia)
  * Substances that are incapacitating (eg, fast-acting CNS depressants or hallucinogens)
  * Substances that can also be used in riot control (eg, various lacrimating agents such as chloroacetophenone [CN]) and vomiting agents (eg, adamsite).
- Health care providers need to have an awareness of the potential for terrorism, an appreciation for epidemiologic clues of a chem-bioterrorist event, and a basic understanding of the classes of agents that can be weaponized and their effects. The Centers for Disease Control and Prevention (CDC) maintains the Strategic National Stockpile that can be rapidly deployed to communities to ensure the availability and rapid deployment of life-saving pharmaceuticals, antidotes, other medical supplies, and equipment necessary to counter nerve agents, biological pathogens, and chemical agents.

6. Questions and Answers

1. Flumazenil is contraindicated in which case?

    A. A patent with QRS widening with a known ingestion of Elavil®
    B. A patient who was previously given flumazenil who complains of abnormal vision and dizziness
    C. A patient with known use of cocaine
    D. A and C
    E. A and B

2. A patient is brought to the emergency department. She is experiencing CNS and respiratory depression due to a suspected ingestion of her sister's MS Contin®. You recommend supportive care and the administration of

    A. flumazenil
    B. naloxone
    C. lorazepam
    D. flumazenil and Narcan
    E. pyridoxine

3. A policeman presents to the emergency room with a rash, fearing he was exposed to a biological weapon several days before the rash appeared. You notice the rash is forming pustules and is most prominent on the face and extremities. The patient says the rash developed all at once. He has possibly contracted

    A. smallpox
    B. chickenpox
    C. anthrax
    D. tularemia
    E. none of the above

4. What is the recommended treatment for the likely disease?

    I.   Supportive; there is no specific treatment
    II. Ciprofloxacin
    III. Doxycycline

    A. II or III
    B. II and III
    C. I only
    D. II only
    E. III only

5. The currently available prevention for smallpox is

    I.   Dryvax® from Wyeth
    II. a live-virus preparation of the vaccinia virus
    III. avoidance of direct contact with infected persons and their body fluids

    A. I only
    B. I and II only
    C. II and III only
    D. I, II, and III
    E. No vaccine is currently available

6. A patient presents with a black, necrotic, painless skin lesion on her arm. She also complains of fever, malaise, headache, and swelling of her underarm lymph nodes. The possible biological agent responsible for these symptoms is

    A. hemorrhagic fever virus
    B. anthrax
    C. botulism
    D. tularemia
    E. arsine

7. The recommended antibiotic treatment of the infection in Question 6 may include

    A. ciprofloxacin
    B. doxycycline
    C. amoxicillin
    D. all of the above
    E. supportive; there is no specific treatment

8. Inhalation exposure to the agent in Question 6 requires:

    A. postexposure prophylaxis with ciprofloxacin, doxycycline, or penicillin G procaine for 60 days
    B. immediate vaccination of civilian personnel
    C. early treatment with streptomycin or gentamicin
    D. early treatment with ribavirin
    E. none of the above

9. A cab driver presents to the emergency department with vomiting, diarrhea, sweating, salivation, moist rales, bradycardia, muscle tremor, and weakness. He reports inhaling a mist dropped from a low-flying plane several hours earlier. You also note that he has miosis and his respiratory difficulty is increasing rapidly. The likely mechanism of toxicity of the poison is

    A. inhibition of protein synthesis
    B. binding of the agent to cytochrome oxidase

C. inhibition of acetylcholinesterase

D. an alkylating agent cross-linking DNA strands

E. none of the above

10. The recommended initial management of the symptoms in Question 9 includes all EXCEPT

A. immediate decontamination of skin and eyes

B. disposal of contaminated clothes

C. British anti-lewisite

D. atropine

E. pralidoxime

11. The patient in Question 9 deteriorates and develops seizures. You recommend:

A. phenytoin

B. diazepam

C. lithium

D. Dryvax

E. all of the above

12. Which one of the following conditions or situations is not a contraindication to the use of ipecac syrup?

A. High blood pressure controlled with drug therapy

B. Seizures shortly before administration

C. Unresponsive to verbal commands

D. A corrosive agent has been ingested

E. A and C

13. Which one of the following is an effect of activated charcoal?

A. Promotes dissolution of tablets

B. Minimizes drug absorption from the gastrointestinal tract

C. Increases urinary flow

D. Enhances systemic elimination of certain drugs

E. B and D

14. Which one of the following drugs is useful in the treatment of acetaminophen poisoning?

A. Acetylcysteine

B. Dimercaprol

C. Pralidoxime

D. Atropine

E. Dryvax

15. Digoxin immune Fab is used to treat which one of the following signs or symptoms of digoxin poisoning?

A. Hypokalemia

B. Diplopia

C. Ventricular tachycardia

D. Second-degree heart block unresponsive to atropine

E. C and D

16. How does crack cocaine differ from pharmaceutical cocaine?

A. Crack is more stable under heat and can be smoked

B. Pharmaceutical cocaine is the hydrochloride salt

C. Crack is the free-base form of cocaine

D. Crack may be contaminated with other substances

E. All of the above

Answers

1. **D.** Flumazenil is contraindicated in all patients who have ingested a tricyclic antidepressant and have cardiac symptoms, as its use could cause ventricular dysrhythmias. It is not recommended in mixed overdose where the co-ingested drug can cause a seizure (ie, cocaine). Answer B is a list of associated adverse effects with its administration; they are not contraindications.

2. **B.** Naloxone is an opioid antagonist.

3. **A.** See Table 5. Smallpox is the most likely agent. The agent causes a pustular rash to form that is typically most prominent on the face and extremities, and lesions form at the same time. Chickenpox rash is most prominent on the trunk and develops in successive groups of lesions over several days. Anthrax forms painless necrotic lesions. Tularemia causes a nonspecific febrile illness that rapidly develops into pneumonia.

4. **C.** See Table 5. Smallpox has no specific treatment. Ciprofloxacin and doxycycline are used in the management of anthrax, plague, and tularemia.

5. **D.** See Table 5. All characteristics are correct.

6. **B.** See Tables 5 and 6. Anthrax forms a painless, necrotic ulcer. Hemorrhagic fever viruses cause

a rash that develops into petechiae, ecchymosis, hemorrhages, and other bleeding symptoms. Botulism causes a symmetric descending paralysis. Tularemia causes a nonspecific febrile illness that rapidly develops into pneumonia. Arsine is a chemical agent that causes nausea, vomiting, hemolysis, and secondary renal failure. Arsine is produced when water comes into contact with metallic arsenide or when acids come into contact with metallic arsenic or arsenical compounds. The mechanism of hemolysis is not specifically known, but the most recent mechanism postulated involves a direct arsine-hemoglobin interaction that forms arsenic metabolites, causing direct alteration of the erythrocyte cell membrane.

7.   **D.** All of the above. See Table 5. Ciprofloxacin, doxycyline, and amoxicillin are FDA-approved for treatment of anthrax. These agents can be used separately or in combination, depending on symptoms and the patient's sensitivity to the agents. Antimicrobial resistance to ciprofloxacin has been growing rapidly due to widespread overuse after the anthrax mail episodes in 2002. At the time of this review, doxycycline is recommended by the CDC (but not by all sources) as the preferred initial treatment unless the patient is intolerant to the agent.

8.   **A.** See Table 5. Persons at risk for inhalational anthrax need 60 days of prophylactic antibiotics. Ciprofloxacin, doxycyline, and penicillin G procaine are FDA-approved for postexposure prophylaxis (PEP). Anthrax vaccine adsorbed (AVA) is currently recommended by the CDC only for high-risk personnel (such as lab personnel working with the agent) and the military, not the civilian population. Strepto-mycin and gentamicin are among the suggested treatments for pneumonic plague. Ribavirin is a potential treatment for some hemorrhagic fever viruses.

9.   **C.** See Table 6. The symptoms exhibited are classically cholinergic and the likely chemical agents causing these symptoms are organophosphates like the nerve agents or possibly organophosphate pesticides. Both can be spread by low-flying planes. Inhibition of protein synthesis is the mechanism of toxicity of ricin or abrin. Cyanides bind to cytochrome oxidase, interrupting normal cellular respiration and causing rapid convulsions. Blister agents like the sulfur and nitrogen mustards are thought to be alkylating agents that cross-link DNA

strands, separating dermal layers in the skin and causing fluid-filled blisters to form.

10.   **C.** British anti-lewisite is a specific antidote for lewisite. See Table 6. It also is used as a chelator for treatment of acute arsenic, inorganic or elemental mercury, gold, and other heavy metal poisonings. See Table 4. The other measures are treatments for organophosphate agents. Good decontamination and disposal of contaminated clothes (especially leather) are needed, because organophosphates are well absorbed across the skin, through the lungs, and via ingestion, essentially all possible routes of exposure. Atropine is used for muscarinic symptoms (miosis, nausea, vomiting, diarrhea, urination, bradycardia, and excessive bronchial, lacrimal, dermal, nasal, and salivary secretions), and pralidoxime is used with atropine to resolve severe organophosphate symptoms (such as those from nerve agents), including nicotinic symptoms of muscle weakness and cramps, fasciculations, tachycardia, and CNS symptoms such as coma and seizures.

11.   **B.** See Table 6. Recommended treatment for seizures due to organophosphate agents is either diazepam or lorazepam. Phenytoin is a seizure medication, but benzodiazepines (then barbiturates if benzodiazepines fail) are generally preferred over phenytoin for the control of overdose- or withdrawal-related seizures. Lithium is not a seizure medicine, and in fact may cause seizures with elevated blood concentrations. Dryvax is a vaccine for smallpox.

12.   **A.** Controlled high blood pressure is not a problem with the use of ipecac syrup, but the other situations are clear contraindications due to potential aspiration (seizures, unrespon-siveness) and additional esophageal burns upon vomiting up gastric contents (corrosive).

13.   **E.** Activated charcoal adsorbs chemicals on contact and prevents their absorption into the bloodstream. For certain drugs (eg, pheno-barbital, theophylline), multiple doses of activated charcoal can promote the back diffusion of drugs across the intestinal capillary bed into the lumen of the gut, trap it there, and promote its elimination. The elimination half-life can be decreased by as much as one-half.

14.   **A.** Acetylcysteine prevents the development of liver injury from acetaminophen if given early

after ingestion and it may help minimize the effects of hepatotoxicity after it has occurred in some cases.

15. **E.** Digoxin immune Fab is reserved for life-threatening symptoms due to its profound effects, scarcity, and high cost. Most serious cases of digoxin poisoning have normal or high potassium concentrations due to the digoxin's interference with the sodium-potassium ATPase pump.

16. **E.** All are differences between the two forms of cocaine.

7. References

General toxicology

American Society of Health-System Pharmacists. AHFS drug information. Bethesda, MD: American Society of Health-System Pharmacists; 2006.

Chyka PA. Clinical toxicology. In: Dipiro JT, Talbert RL, Yee GC, et al, eds. *Pharmacotherapy: A Pathophysiologic Approach,* 6th ed. New York: McGraw-Hill; 2005:125-148.

Dart RC, ed. *Medical Toxicology,* 3rd ed. Philadelphia: Lippincott Williams & Wilkins; 2004.

Ford MD, Delaney KA, Ling LJ, Erickson T. *Clinical Toxicology.* Philadelphia: WB Saunders; 2001.

Goldfrank LR, Flomenbaum NE, Lewin NA, et al. *Goldfrank's Toxicologic Emergencies,* 8th ed. New York: McGraw-Hill; 2006.

Haddad LM, Shannon MW, Winchester JF. *Clinical Management of Poisoning and Drug Overdose,* 3rd ed. Philadelphia: WB Saunders; 1998.

Klasco RK, ed. Poisindex. Greenwood Village, CO: Thomson Micromedex, edition expires July 2006.

Olson KR, ed. *Poisoning & Drug Overdose,* 4th ed. New York: Lange/McGraw-Hill, 2004.

Alsop JA. Managing acute drug toxicity. In: Koda-Kimble MA, Young LY, Kradjan WA, Guglielmo BJ. *Applied Therapeutics,* 8th ed. Philadelphia: Lippincott Williams & Wilkins; 2005:5-1 to 5-22.

Chem-bioterrorism

Abramowicz M, ed. Drugs and vaccines against biological weapons. *Med Letter.* 2001;43:87-9.

Abramowicz M, ed. Prevention and treatment of injury from chemical warfare agents. *Med Letter.* 2002;44: 1-4.

American Society of Health-System Pharmacists, Emergency Preparedness-Counterterrorism Resource Center: http://www.ashp.org/emergency/. Accessed July 21, 2006

Kales SN, Christiani DC. Acute chemical emergencies. *N Engl J Med.* 2004;350:800-8.

Krenzelok EP, ed. *Biological and Chemical Terrorism: A Pharmacy Preparedness Guide.* Bethesda, MD: American Society of Health-System Pharmacists, Inc; 2003.

National Pharmacy Response Team (NPRT), National Disaster Medical Response, U.S. Department of Homeland Security: http://www.oep-ndms.dhhs.gov/nprt.html. Accessed July 21, 2006.

Oak Ridge Institute for Science and Education. Managing radiation emergencies: guidance for hospital medical management. Radiation Emergency Assistance Center/Training Site, Oak Ridge Associated Universities, Oak Ridge, TN. Available at: http://orise.orau.gov/reacts/. Accessed July 21, 2006.

Setlak P. Bioterrorism preparedness and response: Emerging role for health-system pharmacists. *Am J Health-Syst Pharm.* 2004;61:1167-75.

U.S. Centers for Disease Control and Prevention, Emergency Preparedness and Response: http://www.bt.cdc.gov. Accessed July 21, 2006.

U.S. Food and Drug Administration, Drug Preparedness and Response to Bioterrorism: http://www.fda.gov/cder/drugprepare/. Accessed July 21, 2006.

36. Anemias

Ashleigh Thompson, PharmD
Associate Professor, Department of Clinical Pharmacy
University of Tennessee College of Pharmacy

Contents

1. Disease Overview

- Anemia is a reduction in red cell mass that decreases the oxygen-carrying capacity of the blood. The focus of this chapter will be on iron deficiency anemia, megaloblastic anemias, and anemia of renal failure.

Epidemiology

- Approximately 3.4 million Americans have anemia.
- Anemia is more common in women than men.
- 75% of anemias are a result of iron deficiency, anemia of chronic disease, and acute bleeding. Iron deficiency anemia is the most common anemia, accounting for 25% of all cases.
- The remaining 25% of anemias are a result of bone marrow damage, decreased erythropoiesis, and hemolysis.

Classification

- The most common way to classify anemias is by the morphology (shape/structure) of the red blood cells.

Macrocytic (large cell)
- Megaloblastic anemia
- Vitamin B_{12} deficiency
- Pernicious anemia
- Folic acid deficiency

Normochromic, normocytic
- Acute blood loss
- Bone marrow failure
    * *Aplastic anemia:* marrow fails to produce all three types of blood cells, which results in anemia, neutropenia (decreased white blood cells), and thrombocytopenia (decreased platelets). About half of these cases are thought to be caused by drugs or chemicals. Examples of drugs causing aplastic anemia include chloramphenicol, felbamate, and phenytoin.
- Hemolysis
    * Genetically inherited: enzyme deficiencies such as glucose-6-phosphate dehydrogenase (G6PD) deficiency. Red blood cells deficient in G6PD are susceptible to hemolysis when exposed to certain oxidant drugs. Examples of such drugs are dapsone, sulfamethoxazole, and nitrofurantoin.
    * Membrane abnormalities of RBCs such as in hereditary spherocytosis
- Immunologic destruction, such as in autoimmune diseases
    * Anemia of chronic disease

* Renal failure
* Endocrine disorders
* Autoimmune diseases

Hypochromic (low hemoglobin content), microcytic (small cell)
- Iron deficiency anemia
- Genetic anomalies
    * Sickle cell anemia
    * Thalassemia

Clinical Presentation

- The signs and symptoms of anemia depend on the time course over which the anemia developed, and the severity of RBC depletion.
- An anemia developed over a long period of time may be asymptomatic in beginning stages, and then progress to fatigue, malaise, headache, slight exertional dyspnea, angina, pallor, or loss of skin tone.
- A patient with acute anemia, such as from recent blood loss, may present with tachycardia, shortness of breath, or lightheadedness.
- Many of the signs and symptoms of anemia are secondary to tissue hypoxia. In the case of hypoxia, blood supply is shunted to life-sustaining organs (brain, heart, and kidney) and away from non-vital organs, such as extremities or nail beds, which results in pallor of the skin.
- The various types of anemia have additional signs and symptoms which will be discussed in further detail in the diagnosis section.

Pathophysiology

Iron deficiency anemia (IDA)
- IDA is the most common anemia, accounting for a quarter of all anemia cases.
- IDA is caused by iron store depletion resulting from:
    * Inadequate oral intake of iron (especially animal protein)
    * Increased iron demands
        - Pregnancy/lactation
        - Rapid growth: infancy/adolescence
        - Elderly
    * Blood loss
        - Menstruation or postpartum blood loss
        - Trauma
        - GI ulcers
    * Inadequate absorption
        - Medication (eg, tetracyclines)
        - Gastrectomy
        - Enteritis
        - Persistent diarrhea
    * Disease states
        - Carcinomas

- Rheumatoid arthritis
- Hemoglobin is composed of iron (heme) and proteins (globin).
- Lack of iron results in reduced hemoglobin synthesis. The RBCs produced in these conditions are:
  * Hypochromic
    - Decreased concentration of hemoglobin
  * Microcytic
    - RBCs spend longer in marrow awaiting proper hemoglobin synthesis. This results in more cell divisions, which produces a smaller cell.

Megaloblastic anemias

- These anemias are caused by either a deficiency in or an inability to use vitamin B_{12} (cobalamin) or folic acid.
- Vitamin B_{12} deficiency:
  * Decreased intake (strict vegetarians)
  * Decreased absorption
    - Vitamin B_{12} requires gastric intrinsic factor to be absorbed. The lack of intrinsic factor results in *pernicious anemia.* This can be inherited or acquired by gastrectomy.
    - Achlorhydria
  * Inadequate utilization of vitamin B_{12} due to protein deficiencies
- Folic acid deficiency
  * Decreased intake (especially in alcoholics, indigent, elderly)
  * Decreased absorption (Crohn's disease, celiac disease, drugs)
  * Increased demands (pregnancy, growth spurts, malignancy, long-term hemodialysis)
  * Drug induced (methotrexate, phenytoin)
- Vitamin B_{12} and folic acid are both necessary for the RNA and DNA required for cell division during the development of RBCs. Since the RNA and DNA synthesis is impeded, cell divisions are skipped, resulting in an abnormally large cell (macrocytic anemia).

Anemia of renal failure

- The primary reason that patients with renal failure are anemic is due to the lack of production of erythropoietin (EPO). EPO is a hormone produced primarily (90%) in the kidneys that stimulates the synthesis and differentiation of erythroid progenitor cells (precursors to RBCs).
- The uremic environment of chronic renal failure decreases the lifespan of RBCs.
- Folic acid deficiency can also develop due to the increased demands of folic acid during synthesis of RBCs. Additionally, folic acid can be removed during hemodialysis.

- Patients with chronic renal failure can become iron deficient due to loss of iron and blood during dialysis.

Diagnostic Criteria

If anemia is suspected, the following blood tests should be performed:
- Complete blood cell count (CBC) which includes:
  * Hemoglobin (Hgb)
  * Hematocrit (Hct)
  * RBC
  * Red cell indices:
    - Mean corpuscular volume (MCV) is a measure of size of RBCs.
    - Mean corpuscular hemoglobin (MCH) is a measure of weight of hemoglobin in a RBC. MCH will be low in the case of microcytosis or hypochromia.
    - Mean corpuscular hemoglobin concentration (MCHC) is a measure of weight of hemoglobin, but is more useful than MCH because it can distinguish between low hemoglobin and a small cell. MCHC will only be low in the case of hypochromia.
    - Platelets
    - Reticulocyte count (pre-RBCs)
  * Red cell morphology
  * Serum iron, total iron binding capacity (TIBC), transferrin saturation, ferritin
  * Bilirubin (by-product of RBC destruction)

Other tests:
- Test stool for blood
- Peripheral blood smear
- Thorough history and physical examination

Iron deficiency anemia
Blood work
- The first level to decrease will be ferritin (storage form of iron).
- The iron level will be low.
- TIBC increases. This is a measure of the amount of binding space left on transferrin (transport protein of iron). Less iron in the blood translates to more space available on the transferrin molecule.
- As the iron deficiency progresses, there will be a decrease in hemoglobin (iron is a component of hemoglobin). Therefore, this is a hypochromic anemia.
- The hematocrit will also eventually fall.
- MCV will be decreased, which indicates microcytosis.
- MCH and MCHC will be decreased, which indicates decreased hemoglobin.

- Blood smear will show a microcytic, hypochromic cell.

Specific signs and symptoms
- In addition to the general signs and symptoms listed previously for anemia, these additional symptoms may be present in severe IDA:
  * Koilonychias (spoon-shaped nails)
  * Angular stomatitis or glossitis
  * Pica (craving for substances low in iron, such as ice, clay, and cornstarch)

Megaloblastic anemias
Blood work
- Decreased Hct and Hgb
- Decreased RBC
- Elevated MCH, which indicates a macrocytosis
- The iron level, TIBC, and reticulocyte count will be normal.

Vitamin B_{12} deficiency
- The serum B_{12} level will be decreased.
- Positive Schilling test indicates pernicious anemia. (The Schilling test determines absorption of vitamin B_{12} by measuring the amount of radioactive B_{12} excreted in urine.)
- Additional signs and symptoms:
  * Loss of vibratory sensation in lower extremities
  * Ataxia or vertigo
  * Glossitis
  * Muscle weakness
  * Neuropsychiatric abnormalities
    - Irritability or emotional instability
    - Dementia
    - Psychosis

Folic acid deficiency
- Folate level will be decreased.
- Overall, this is very similar to vitamin B_{12} deficiency anemia, except with the absence of neurological symptoms.

Anemia of renal failure
- As the name implies, this anemia occurs in patients with chronic renal failure (CRF).
- Before diagnosis, other causes must be ruled out (eg, blood loss).
- CBC will reveal a normochromic, normocytic anemia.

Treatment Principles and Goals

Iron deficiency anemia
Goals
- To normalize Hgb and Hct
  * 2-g/dL increase in Hgb in 3 weeks
  * 6% increase in Hct in 3 weeks
  * Reticulocytosis will usually occur within 1 week.
  * If these indices do not improve within these time frames, the diagnosis should be re-evaluated.
- Replete iron stores
  * Although Hgb and Hct will return to normal within 1-2 months, iron therapy should continue for 3-6 months after Hgb is normalized to replete total body iron stores.

Megaloblastic anemias
Goals of vitamin B_{12} replacement
- Hgb should rise within 1 week.
- If neurologic symptoms were present, they should improve within 24 hours. However, if vitamin B_{12} deficiency is long-standing, symptoms may not be completely relieved for several months.

Goals of folic acid replacement
- RBC morphology will correct within 1-2 days.
- Hgb starts to normalize within 10 days.
- Hct will return to normal levels within 2 months.
- Maintenance administration of folic acid should continue for as long as nutritional intake of folic acid is a problem.

Anemia of Renal Failure
Goal
- Initial therapy goal is to reach a target Hct of 36% through a slow, steady increase (usually within 2-4 months).
- Medication doses of epoetin should be titrated to maintain Hct in the range of 30%-36%.

2. Drug Therapy

Iron Deficiency Anemia

- Treatment consists of iron supplementation through therapeutic iron preparations (200 mg of elemental iron per day in 2-3 divided doses) (Table 1). Iron is best absorbed in the reduced (ferrous) form. Ferrous sulfate salt is the most common, which is 20% elemental iron. Therefore ferrous sulfate 325 mg tid will adequately treat iron deficiency.
- IV iron preparations should be used only in cases of:
  * Iron malabsorption
  * Oral noncompliance
  * Refusal of blood transfusion
  * IV iron formulations are often used in patients with chronic renal failure who require dialysis along with human recombinant erythropoietin therapy. There are three types of IV products available in the U.S.:
    • Iron dextran (InFeD®)
    • Sodium ferric gluconate (Ferrlecit®)
    • Iron sucrose (Venofer®)
- A fourth IV iron product, ferumoxytol, is currently in phase III clinical trials

Mechanism of action
- Iron supplementation corrects the iron deficiency, and enables Hgb to be synthesized at normal levels.

Patient instructions
- Take 1-2 hours prior to a meal (on an empty stomach)
- If you are not able to tolerate iron on an empty stomach, you may administer with a small snack (crackers), but try to avoid dairy products or tea. (Food can decrease the absorption of iron by 50%.) Take with orange juice if possible (can double absorption).
- Keep out of reach of children. Iron is a major cause of ingestion deaths in children.
- Take iron 1 hour before or 3 hours after any antacids.
- There are medications that interact with iron. Please ask your physician or pharmacist before taking any new medications in combination with iron.
- You may take OTC docusate if constipation occurs.

Adverse drug effects
- The oral formulation has primarily GI effects:
  * Dark colored stools
  * Constipation or diarrhea
  * Nausea and/or vomiting
- IV formulations:
  * Injection site reactions
  * GI: diarrhea, nausea
  * Hypotension
  * Allergic reactions, including anaphylaxis
    • The risk of anaphylaxis is greatest with iron dextran. The patient must be administered a test dose before using this agent.

Drug interactions
- Antibiotics (tetracycline, quinolones): iron binds to these antibiotics, preventing their absorption.
- Antacids: iron needs an acidic environment for optimal absorption.

Monitoring parameters
- Is there an increase in reticulocytes, Hgb, and Hct?
- Tolerability of iron (will influence compliance)
- Is patient symptomatically improving?

Kinetics
- Bioavailability is increased in acidic environment and decreased by food.

Megaloblastic Anemias

- Vitamin B_{12} should be administered orally if absorption is not an issue.
  * Recommended Daily Intake = 2 mcg daily
- Vitamin B_{12} deficiency is usually corrected through IM vitamin B_{12} (cyanocobalamin) supplementation as follows (pernicious anemia):
  * 1000 mcg IM every day for 1 week, then
  * 100-1000 mcg IM every week for 4 weeks, then
  * 100-1000 mcg IM every month thereafter for prevention
  * Although IM B_{12} is still more frequently used, patients with deficiency states may be supple-

Table 1

Drugs Used to Treat Iron Deficiency Anemia

Generic name (trade name)	Elemental Fe (%)	Dose (mg)	Fe content (mg)
Ferrous sulfate (Feosol®, Fer-in-Sol®)	20	325	65
Ferrous gluconate (Fergon®)	12	300	35
Ferrous fumarate (Femiron®, Fumerin®, Feostat®)	33	300	99

mented orally in very high doses, such as 1000-2000 mcg per day.

    * People choosing vegan diets should be supplemented with 1000 mcg (1 mg) B$_{12}$ daily.

Mechanism of action

- Vitamin B$_{12}$ supplementation allows for normal synthesis of the RNA/DNA involved in the synthesis of RBCs.

Patient instructions

- Counsel patient or family member(s) on sterile injection techniques and needle disposal if injections are given at home.

Adverse drug effects

- Increased synthesis of reticulocytes can cause hyperuricemia or hypokalemia.
- Sodium retention
- Increased synthesis of RBCs can produce an expansion of the intravascular volume, which can increase cardiac output causing angina or dyspnea.
- Itching: 1%-10%
- Diarrhea: 1%-10%
- Anaphylaxis: <1%

Monitoring parameters

- Monitor CBC. Is there an increase in Hgb?
- Is the patient symptomatically improving (especially neurologic symptoms, if present)?
- Potassium level

Kinetics

- Absorption: intrinsic factor must be present for vitamin B$_{12}$ to be transported across the GI mucosa.
- Vitamin B$_{12}$ is bound in blood to transcobalamin II and converted in tissues to active coenzymes methylcobalamin and deoxyadenosylcobalamin.

Folic Acid Deficiency Anemia

- Folic acid deficiency anemia is corrected by supplementing folic acid 1 mg daily for 4 months. Once the underlying cause of deficiency is corrected, folic acid may be discontinued. Long-term folate administration is necessary if the cause is not corrected, such as in hemodialysis or alcoholism.

Mechanism of action

- Folic acid supplementation allows for normal synthesis of the RNA and DNA involved in the synthesis of RBCs.

Patient instructions

- Stress compliance with regimen.

- Women of childbearing age should be counseled to take a multivitamin containing folic acid regardless if an anemia is present or not (to prevent neural tube birth defects).

Adverse drug effects

- Less than 1% of patients have allergic reactions to folic acid.

Drug interactions

- Folic acid may increase phenytoin metabolism.
- Phenytoin, primidone, sulfasalazine, para-aminosalicylic acid, and oral contraceptives may decrease folic acid concentrations.
- Chloramphenicol may blunt response to folic acid.

Monitoring parameters

- Is the RBC morphology normalizing?
- Are the Hgb and Hct normalizing?
- Monitor patient compliance.

Kinetics

- Folic acid is a water-soluble B vitamin absorbed in the small intestine with C$_{max}$ at $1/2$-1 hour.

Anemia of Renal Failure

Recombinant human erythropoietin

- Since the primary cause of anemia in renal failure is decreased (EPO) synthesis, the drug of choice for this type of anemia is recombinant human EPO (epoetin alfa, trade names Procrit® or Epogen®).
- Epoetin is indicated in the treatment of anemia associated with chronic renal failure, including dialysis and non-dialysis patients. It is indicated to elevate or maintain the RBCs and to decrease the need for transfusions in these patients. (Non-dialysis patients with symptomatic anemia considered for therapy should have a hematocrit <30%.) The National Kidney Foundation-Kidney Disease Outcomes Quality Initiative Guidelines (NKF-K/DOQI guidelines) recommend that epoetin be administered SC, since this route of administration is as effective (or more effective) than IV. However, epoetin is often administered IV in patients on dialysis, since there is easy access through the dialysis port.

Mechanism of action

- Human recombinant erythropoietin stimulates erythropoiesis (increased RBC production).

Patient instructions

- Do not shake the vial because the epoetin may break down, decreasing effectiveness.
- Store in refrigerator, but do not freeze. Keep out of direct sunlight.

- Make sure that the solution in the vial is clear and free of particulate matter. Do not use if the solution is cloudy or frothy.
- Monitor your blood pressure at home and alert your physician of any significant increases in blood pressure.
- Single-use vials are intended to be used only once. Discard any remaining solution and vial. If the label is marked with an M, it is a multi-dose vial, and it may be stored in the refrigerator for 21 days.
- It is very important that you take your blood pressure medications exactly as prescribed while on this medication, and maintain a sodium-restricted diet.
- Avoid hazardous activity in the first 90 days of therapy (eg, operating heavy machinery).
- Educate the patient about the possibility of allergic reactions:
  * Local reaction (swelling, itching, redness); inform MD if any of these occur.
  * Anaphylactic reaction (shortness of breath, wheezing, low blood pressure, rapid heart rate, sweating). If any of these occur, discontinue use immediately and call 911.
- Patient should be instructed on correct sterile injection technique and needle disposal as described in Figure 1.

Adverse drug effects (Table 2)

- Immunogenicity: pure red cell aplasia (PRCA), in association with neutralizing antibodies to native erythropoietin, has been reported rarely in the literature. If this is suspected, epoetin should be discontinued immediately.
- The most common adverse effect is elevated blood pressure. Epoetin is contraindicated in patients with uncontrolled hypertension.

Drug interactions

- No drug interactions have been reported.

Monitoring parameters

- Prior to initiation of therapy, the patient's iron stores should be evaluated. Transferrin saturation should be at least 20% and ferritin at least 100 ng/mL.
- Monitor Hct very closely. Once Hct approaches 36% or Hct increases more than 4 points in a 2-week period, the dose of epoetin should be decreased. The dose should be increased if Hct has not increased 5-6 points in 8 weeks, and is not in target Hct range of 30%-36%.
- Blood pressure should be adequately controlled prior to initiation of epoetin alfa therapy, and must be closely monitored and controlled during therapy.
- Serum chemistries

Kinetics

- Half life: ~4-13 hours
- There is no apparent difference in half-life between patients not on dialysis with SCr >3 and patients requiring dialysis.

Other

- Initial starting dose IV or SQ is 50-100 U/kg three times weekly. (Use IV in hemodialysis). Thereafter, the maintenance dose is titrated to maintain a Hct of 30%-36% or a Hgb of 10-12 g/dL.

Darbepoetin

Mechanism of action

- Darbepoetin has the same MOA as epoetin.

Patient instructions

- Counseling points are very similar with darbepoetin and epoetin, except that all vials are for single-use only, so dispose of the vial as instructed after each dose.

Adverse drug effects

- The most common adverse effects are:
  * CV: hypertension, hypotension, edema, arrhythmia
  * GI: nausea, vomiting, diarrhea, constipation
  * CNS: fatigue, fever, headache
  * Neuromuscular/skeletal: myalgia, arthralgia, limb pain
  * Respiratory: infection, dyspnea, cough

Drug interactions

- No drug interactions have been reported.

Monitoring parameters

- Iron stores prior to and during therapy
- Blood pressure
- Dose is adjusted by closely monitoring Hgb every week until maintenance dose is established. Target Hgb is 12g/dL.
  * Increase dose if Hgb increase is <1 g/dL over 4 weeks.
  * Decrease dose by 25% if Hgb increase is >1 g/dL over 2 weeks.

Kinetics

- Half-life: IV, 21 hours; SC, 49 hours
- Half-life is approximately three times longer than that of epoetin.

Other

- Initial dose: 0.45 mcg/kg once weekly (IV recommended in hemodialysis patients); thereafter, dose is titrated to maintain Hgb of 12 g/dL. Some patients will require <0.45 mcg/kg, so in these patients, dosing will be only once every 2 weeks. Less frequent dosing is the advantage of darbepoetin over epoetin.

Figure 1.

Instructions for self-administering epoetin alfa.

Preparing the dose

1. Wash your hands thoroughly with soap and water before preparing the medication.

2. Check the date on the epoetin alfa vial to be sure that the drug has not expired.

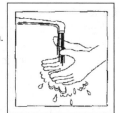

3. Remove the vial of epoetin alfa from the refrigerator and allow it to reach room temperature. **Each epoetin alfa vial is designed to be used only once: do not re-enter the vial.** It is not necessary to shake epoetin alfa. Prolonged vigorous shaking may damage the product. Assemble the other supplies you will need for your injection.

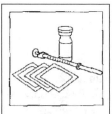

4. Hemodialysis patients should wipe off the venous port of the hemodialysis tubing with an antiseptic swab. Peritoneal dialysis patients should cleanse the skin with an antiseptic swab where the injection is to be made.

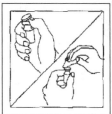

5. Flip off the red protective cap but do not remove the gray rubber stopper. Wipe the top of the gray rubber stopper with an antiseptic swab.

6. Using a syringe and needle designed for subcutaneous injection, draw air into the syringe by pulling back on the plunger. The amount of air should be equal to your epoetin alfa dose.

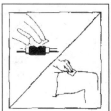

7. Carefully remove the needle cover. Put the needle through the gray rubber stopper of the epoetin alfa vial.

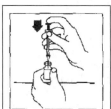

8. Push the plunger in to discharge air into the vial. The air injected into the vial will allow epoetin alfa to be easily withdrawn into the syringe.

9. Turn the vial and syringe upside down in one hand. Be sure the tip of the needle is in the epoetin alfa solution. Your other hand will be free to move the plunger. Draw back on the plunger slowly to draw the correct dose of epoetin alfa into the syringe.

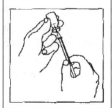

10. Check for air bubbles. The air is harmless, but too large an air bubble will reduce the epoetin alfa dose. To remove air bubbles, gently tap the syringe to move the air bubbles to the top of the syringe, then use the plunger to push the solution and the air back into the vial. Then re-measure your correct dose of epoetin alfa.

11. Double-check your dose. Remove the needle from the vial. Do not lay the syringe down or allow the needle to touch anything.

Injecting the dose
Patients on home hemodialysis using the intravenous injection route:

1. Insert the needle of the syringe into the previously cleansed venous port and inject the epoetin alfa.

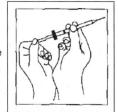

2. Remove the syringe and dispose of the whole unit. Use the disposable syringe only once. Dispose of syringes and needles as directed by your doctor, by following these simple steps:

- Place all used needles and syringes in a hard plastic container with a screw-on cap, or a metal container with a plastic lid, such as a coffee can properly labeled as to contents. If a metal container is used, cut a small hole in the plastic lid and tape the lid to the metal container. If a hard plastic container is used, always screw the cap on tightly after each use. When the container is full, tape around the cap or lid, and dispose of it according to your doctor's instructions.
- Do not use glass or clear plastic containers, or any container that will be recycled or returned to a store.
- Always store the container out of the reach of children.
- Please check with your doctor, nurse, or pharmacist for other suggestions. There may be special state and local laws that they will discuss with you.

(continued)

Figure 1. (continued)

Instructions for self-administering epoetin alfa.

Patients on home peritoneal dialysis or home hemodialysis using the subcutaneous route:

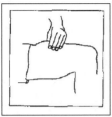

1. With one hand, stabilize the previously cleansed skin by spreading it or by pinching up a large area with your free hand.

2. Hold the syringe with the other hand, as you would a pencil. Double check that the correct amount of epoetin alfa is in the syringe. Insert the needle straight into the skin at a 90° angle. Pull the plunger back slightly. If blood comes into the syringe, do not inject epoetin alfa, as the needle has entered a blood vessel; withdraw the syringe and inject at a different site. Inject the epoetin alfa by pushing the plunger all the way down.

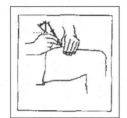

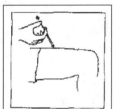

3. Hold an antiseptic swab near the needle and pull the needle straight out of the skin. Press the antiseptic swab over the injection site for several seconds. Use the disposable syringe only once.

4. Use the disposable syringe only once. Dispose of syringes and needles as directed in the instructions at left, under step 2.

5. Always change the site for each injection as directed. Occasionally a problem may develop at the injection site. If you notice a lump, swelling, or bruising that does not go away, contact your doctor. You may wish to record the site you just used so you can keep track.

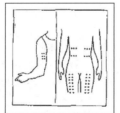

Reproduced with permission from Procrit® package insert. Raritan, NJ: Ortho Biotech Products, LP; 2000.

3. Nondrug Therapy

Iron Deficiency Anemia

Dietary supplementation
- Increase intake of iron-rich foods, such as meat, fish, and poultry.
- Drink orange juice with meals when possible.

Table 2

Percentage of Patients Reporting Adverse Effects of Epoetin Alfa

Event	Patients treated with epoetin alfa (n = 200)	Patients on placebo (n = 135)
Hypertension	24%	19%
Headache	16%	12%
Arthralgias	11%	6%
Nausea	11%	9%
Edema	9%	10%
Fatigue	9%	14%
Vomiting	8%	5%
Chest pain	7%	9%
Skin reaction at site of administration	7%	12%
Asthenia	7%	12%
Dizziness	7%	13%
Clotted access	7%	2%

Significant adverse events of concern in patients with CRF treated in double-blind, placebo-controlled trials occurred in the percentages of patients shown below during the blinded phase of the studies.

Seizure	1.1%	1.1%
CVA/TIA	0.4%	0.6%
MI	0.4%	1.1%
Death	0	1.7%

CRF, chronic renal failure; CVA/TIA, cerebrovascular accident/transient ischemic attack; MI, myocardial infarction.
Reproduced with permission from Procrit® package insert. Raritan, NJ: Ortho Biotech Products, LP; 2000.

- Limit tea or milk with meals. Only use in moderation between meals.

Megaloblastic Anemias

Folic acid deficiency
- In order to get as much dietary folate as possible, do not overcook vegetables. Eat them raw or steamed. Eat a wide variety of properly prepared vegetables, fruits, and mushrooms.

4. Key Points

- Anemia is a reduction in red cell mass, which decreases the oxygen-carrying capacity of the blood.
- Iron deficiency anemia is the most common anemia, accounting for 25% of all cases. IDA presents as a microcytic, hypochromic anemia.
- Iron preparations are best absorbed on an empty stomach.
- Iron preparations are hard to tolerate due to numerous GI effects, and this may necessitate administration with a small snack.
- Megaloblastic anemias are macrocytic and are the result of a folic acid or vitamin B_{12} deficiency.
- Vitamin B_{12} requires intrinsic factor to be absorbed. Patients deficient in intrinsic factor develop pernicious anemia.
- Due to the difficulties with the absorption of vitamin B_{12} in many patients, it is often administered via an IM injection.
- The primary reason that patients with renal failure are anemic is due to the lack of production of erythropoietin (EPO).
- Anemia of renal failure is treated with SC or IV epoetin.
- Patients receiving epoetin must have their hematocrit and blood pressures routinely monitored.
- Darbepoetin has the same mechanism of action as epoetin, but is longer acting, and so can be administered less frequently.

5. Questions and Answers

Patient Profile #1: SuperPrice Drug Store Profile

G.M. McBeavy
1040 Dauberson Avenue
Jesup, IA 50648
319-555-6248

DOB: 7/11/52
Allergies: NKDA
Weight: 193 pounds

Problem List:
Gastroesophageal reflux disease
Iron deficiency anemia
Hypertension

Medication Record:
Ferrous sulfate 325 mg tid
Hydrochlorothiazide 25 mg daily

OTCs Recommended:
Maalox® 1 tbsp q2h prn for "indigestion"
Acetaminophen 325 mg q4-6h prn for headache
Ranitidine 75 mg daily prn for "heartburn"
Docusate 100 mg daily for constipation

Use Patient Profile #1 to answer Questions 1-5.

1. Which OTC medication could present a problem with Mr. McBeevy's iron supplement?

    A. Acetaminophen
    B. Ranitidine
    C. Maalox
    D. Docusate
    E. None of the above

2. Mr. McBeevy admits to you that he is not able to take his iron tablet because it makes him nauseated. What advice can you give him?

    A. Take your iron with some crackers and milk.
    B. Take your iron with some crackers and water.
    C. Don't worry about it. It's only a vitamin.
    D. Start taking your iron with the largest meal of the day.
    E. Take your iron after breakfast.

3. If Mr. McBeevy's IDA progresses to severe stages, what effects may he experience?

    A. Koilonychia (spooning of the nails)
    B. Pica (eg, craving ice, clay, chalk)

C. Glossitis (Sore, beefy red tongue)
D. Extreme fatigue
E. All of the above

4. If you were to examine Mr. McBeevy's blood smear, you would find cells that are:

   A. Microcytic and hypochromic
   B. Macrocytic and hypochromic
   C. Macrocytic and normochromic
   D. Microcytic and normochromic
   E. Any of the above are possible

5. When examining Mr. McBeevy's iron study results, which of the following would be consistent with IDA?

   A. Elevated TIBC
   B. Elevated ferritin
   C. Elevated MCV
   D. Elevated hemoglobin
   E. Elevated hematocrit

6. Which iron preparation is the most likely to cause an anaphylactic reaction?

   A. IV iron dextran
   B. IV iron sucrose
   C. IV sodium ferric gluconate
   D. PO extended-release ferrous sulfate
   E. PO immediate-release ferrous sulfate

7. Why would the sustained-release (SR) preparations of iron not be the ideal formulation?

   A. The incidence of nausea is higher with the SR formulations
   B. They are only dosed once daily, and goal Hct levels are not attained
   C. Since SR preparations are dissolved in the small intestines, the alkaline environment would result in a lower bioavailability than would the acidic environment of the stomach
   D. Dissolution in the small intestines would not be bioavailable, because intrinsic factor is not present in the small intestines
   E. They require dosing with food

8. To optimize iron absorption from meals, which would you advise a patient to drink with his meals?

   A. Orange juice
   B. Coffee
   C. Tea
   D. Milk
   E. Soft drinks

9. The most likely regimen to replace vitamin B_{12} would be:

   A. 1000 mcg PO every month
   B. 1000 mcg IV every month
   C. 1000 mcg IM every month
   D. 1000 mcg IM every day
   E. Any of the above are reasonable regimens

10. Vitamin B_{12} requires the following to be absorbed

    A. Pernicious factor
    B. Transcobalamin II
    C. Intrinsic factor
    D. Vitamin B_{12} absorption factor
    E. All of the above

11. Folic acid deficiency could be found in all of the following EXCEPT

    A. strict vegetarians
    B. alcoholics
    C. the indigent
    D. people who routinely overcook their vegetables
    E. a college student whose diet consists of only burgers and potato chips

12. Folic acid may interact with the following medication:

    A. Propranolol
    B. Propoxyphene
    C. Piroxicam
    D. Phenytoin
    E. Prednisone

13. The two macrocytic anemias are

    A. vitamin B_{12} deficiency and iron deficiency anemias
    B. vitamin B_{12} deficiency and folic acid deficiency anemias
    C. iron deficiency and folic acid deficiency anemias
    D. sickle cell anemia and anemia of renal failure
    E. iron deficiency and pernicious anemias

14. The best regimen to replace folic acid would be

    A. folic acid 1 mg PO every day for 3-4 months

B. folic acid 10 mg PO every day for 3-4 months

C. folic acid 10 mg IV for 2 weeks, then 1 mg PO every day for 2 months

D. folic acid 1 mg PO three times weekly for 3-4 months

E. folic acid 1 mg IM once monthly for 6 months

15. The most common medication given to treat anemia of renal failure is

A. vitamin B$_{12}$
B. solution of citric acid in combination with sodium acetate
C. epoetin
D. PO ferrous sulfate
E. PO folic acid

16. What advantage does darbepoetin have over epoetin?

A. Lower incidence of hypertension
B. Fewer drug interactions
C. Lower cost
D. Longer half-life and less frequent administration
E. Improved tolerability

17. The most common side effect of epoetin is

A. anaphylaxis
B. hypertension
C. pure red cell aplasia
D. injection site reaction
E. weight gain

18. The initial dose of epoetin is

A. 50-100 U/kg three times weekly SC or IV
B. 50-100 U/kg once weekly SC or IV
C. 100 U/kg once weekly SC or IV
D. 50-100 U/kg three times weekly IV
E. 100 U/kg once monthly IV

19. Prior to beginning epoetin therapy, which of the following should be evaluated?

A. Folic acid and vitamin B$_{12}$ levels
B. Transferrin and ferritin levels
C. Erythropoietin receptor level
D. Presence or absence of intrinsic factor
E. All of the above

20. In which of the following patients would it be possible to teach self-administration of epoetin at home?

I. A patient on home hemodialysis taking epoetin via the IV route

II. A patient on home peritoneal dialysis taking epoetin via the SC route

III. A patient on home hemodialysis taking epoetin via the SC route

A. II only
B. II and III only
C. III only
D. I, II, and III
E. I only

Patient Profile #2: Central Dialysis Center

R.S. Wiley
1460 Sawyer Brown Rd
Reidsville, NC 27320
336-555-0001

Allergies: Penicillin (rash)
Weight: 148 pounds
Dialysis schedule: Monday, Wednesday, Friday

Diagnosis:
Hypertension
Diabetes mellitus
End-stage renal disease
Hyperlipidemia

Medications:
Insulin NPH 30 U bid
Simvastatin 20 mg qhs
Atenolol 25 mg after dialysis
Nephrocaps 1 capsule daily

Labs:
ferritin 80ng/ml
transferrin 15%
HCT31
Hemoglobin 11

Use Patient Profile #2 to answer Questions 21-24.

21. Which of the following will be monitored upon starting epoetin therapy in Mrs. Wiley?

A. Blood pressure
B. Hematocrit
C. Serum chemistries
D. Iron profile
E. All of the above

22. The target hematocrit range for Mrs. Wiley is
   A. 30%-36%
   B. 29%-38%
   C. 30%-32%
   D. 26%-34%
   E. 40%-45%

23. Which of Mrs. Wiley's medications will interact with epoetin?

   A. Insulin
   B. Simvastatin
   C. Atenolol
   D. None of the above
   E. All of the above

24. What medication should be added to Mrs. Wiley's regimen?

   A. Oral propranolol
   B. IV iron
   C. Oral levothyroxine
   D. IM vitamin B_{12}
   E. No additional medications are required at this time

Answers

1. **C.** Iron is best absorbed in an acidic environment. Therefore antacids dramatically decrease the absorption of iron. They should be taken 1 hour before or 3 hours after antacids.

2. **B.** Many patients are not able to tolerate iron on an empty stomach. Tell those patients to take iron with a small snack. Milk would not be acceptable in this case, because dairy products decrease the absorption of iron.

3. **E.** Koilonychia, pica, extreme fatigue, and glossitis are all symptoms of severe iron deficiency anemia.

4. **A.** Iron deficiency produces a hypochromic (low-hemoglobin) anemia, given iron is a component of the hemoglobin molecule. The cells are also microcytic (meaning "small cell") because they spend longer in the marrow awaiting proper hemoglobin synthesis, and are therefore smaller.

5. **A.** Total iron-binding capacity, TIBC, is elevated in IDA. TIBC is a measure of the amount of binding space left on transferrin (the transport protein of iron). Less iron in the blood translates into more space available on the transferrin molecule.

6. **A.** IV iron dextran has the highest incidence of anaphylaxis among the three IV iron preparations available.

7. **C.** SR preparations are left intact in the stomach, and are dissolved in the small intestine. The alkaline environment of the small intestine tends to form insoluble iron complexes that cannot be absorbed.

8. **A.** Tea and milk can decrease the absorption of iron from a meal by over 50%. Orange juice, however, can double the absorption of iron from food.

9. **C.** The most common IM dose of vitamin B_{12} is 1000 mcg per month. However, vitamin B_{12} may be supplemented by the oral route if absorption is not impaired. Additionally, it may be supplemented in very high doses, such as 1000-2000 mcg per day in pernicious anemia.

10. **C.** Vitamin B_{12} requires intrinsic factor to be absorbed.

11. **A.** Folic acid deficiency is found in alcoholics, the indigent, and rarely in people who routinely overcook their vegetables. Strict vegetarians do not develop folic acid deficiency because a folate-rich diet includes various types of vegetables.

12. **D.** Phenytoin increases the metabolism of folate, thereby decreasing its effectiveness.

13. **B.** Vitamin B_{12} deficiency and folic acid anemias are both macrocytic (large cell) anemias. Iron deficiency anemia and sickle cell anemia are both microcytic and hypochromic anemias.

14. **A.** Folic acid is administered PO because there is no problem with absorption. The dose of folic acid is 1 mg PO every day, and the deficiency should be corrected in 3-4 months.

15. **C.** Epoetin is the most common medication used to treat anemia of renal failure, because it stimulates erythropoiesis. The lack of erythropoietin production is the primary cause of anemia of renal failure.

16. **D.** Darbepoetin is very similar to epoetin, having the same mechanism of action and similar side effects. It does have a longer half-life and can be administered less frequently.

17. **B.** Hypertension is the most common adverse drug effect from epoetin.

18. **A.** The initial dose of epoetin is 50-100 U/kg three times weekly. This can be given via either the SC or IV route.

19. **B.** Transferrin and ferritin levels should be evaluated prior to epoetin therapy. IDA is a common problem in patients with end-stage renal disease. The transferrin should be at least 20% and ferritin should be at least 100 ng/mL prior to beginning epoetin therapy.

20. **D.** Patients on home peritoneal dialysis or hemodialysis can be taught to self-administer SC injections. Additionally, if patients are receiving home hemodialysis, they can be taught to give their epoetin IV through the dialysis venous port.

21. **E.** Iron profiles need to be monitored prior to epoetin and periodically during therapy, since IDA is very common in dialysis patients. Blood pressure needs to be monitored, given this is the most common adverse effect of epoetin. The hematocrit needs to be checked as a measure of response to epoetin, and needs to be maintained at a level of 30%-36%. Serum chemistries need to be monitored regularly in any patient with end-stage renal disease, since most electrolytes are regulated by the kidney.

22. **A.** The target range of hematocrit for patients receiving epoetin is 30%-36%.

23. **D.** There are no known drug interactions with epoetin.

24. **B.** Mrs. Wiley's ferritin is below 100 ng/mL and her transferrin is below 20%. Most hemodialysis patients receiving epoetin will need iron therapy during their treatment at some point in time.

6. References

Denberg CV, O'Bryant C. Anemias. In: Young LY, Koda-Kimble MA, eds. *Applied Therapeutics: The Clinical Use of Drugs.* Vancouver, WA: Applied Therapeutics, Inc.; 2001:84.1-84.19.

Eschbach JW, Abdulhadi MH, Browne JK, et al. Recombinant human erythropoietin in anemic patients with end-stage renal disease. Results of a phase III multicenter clinical trial. *Ann Intern Med.* 1989;111:992.

Fishbane S. Safety in iron management. *Am J Kid Dis.* 2003;41:S18-S26.

National Kidney Foundation: K/DOQI Clinical Practice Guidelines for Anemia of Chronic Kidney Disease, 2000. *Am J Kidney Dis.* 2001;37(suppl 1):S182-S238.

Parker KP, Mitch WE, Stivelman JC, et al. Safety and efficacy of low-dose subcutaneous erythropoietin in hemodialysis patients. *J Am Soc Nephrol.* 1999;8:288.

Procrit package insert. Raritan, NJ: Ortho Biotech Products, LP; 2000.

Stumpf JL, Townsend KA. Other anemias. In: Herfindal ET, Gourley DR, eds. *Textbook of Therapeutics: Drug and Disease Management.* Baltimore: Lippincott Williams & Wilkins; 2000:237-260.

Teresi M. Iron deficiency and megaloblastic anemias. In: Herfindal ET, Gourley DR, eds. *Textbook of Therapeutics: Drug and Disease Management.* Baltimore: Lippincott Williams & Wilkins; 2000:213-236.

The rationale for treating iron deficiency anemia. *Arch Intern Med.* 1984;144:471.

37. Venous Thromboembolic Disease

Gale Hamann, PharmD, BCPS
Associate Professor, Department of Clinical Pharmacy
University of Tennessee College of Pharmacy

Contents

1. Venous Thromboembolic Disease

Definition and Epidemiology

- Venous thromboembolism (VTE) is a disease process that involves the development of deep vein thrombosis (DVT) and/or a pulmonary embolism (PE).
- Pulmonary embolism is a thrombus or foreign substance from the systemic circulation that lodges in the pulmonary artery or its branches and causes a complete or partial occlusion of pulmonary blood flow.
- Deep vein thrombosis is a thrombus that forms most commonly in the popliteal or femoral veins, veins of the calf, or the iliac veins of the upper leg. Veins of the upper extremities are less commonly involved.
- Approximately two million Americans develop VTE each year; 600,000 people in this group have VTE manifested as a PE, and of these, 200,000 die. It is estimated that one million Americans will develop a clinically silent PE that goes undiagnosed. Complications of VTE are postphlebitic syndrome and pulmonary hypertension. Postphlebitic syndrome is characterized as swelling in the affected lower extremity after a DVT. Pulmonary hypertension is a complication that can occur after a PE.
- The incidence of VTE increases with age and doubles in each decade of life after age 50.
- It is estimated that VTE costs 1.5 billion dollars annually.

Clinical Presentation

- The most common symptoms of a PE are dyspnea, cough, hemoptysis, tachypnea, tachycardia, pleuritic chest pain, diaphoresis, and overwhelming anxiety. The patient may be cyanotic and hypoxemic secondary to having a reduced ability to oxygenate the blood. Patients with a massive PE may present with syncope. The mortality rate of a PE ranges from 2.3 to 17%.
- The most common symptoms of a DVT are pain, tenderness, edema, and erythema of the affected extremity. Other symptoms may include dilation of the superficial veins, a palpable cord, and a positive Homans' sign.

Pathophysiology

- Venous thrombi generally form in areas of the veins where blood flow is slowed or disrupted. Often they begin as small thrombi in the large venous sinuses of a valve cusp pocket in the veins of the calf or thigh. Trauma to the vessel causes the release of tissue fac-

tor. Tissue factor in turn activates the coagulation cascade. This results in the formation of thrombin and ultimately the formation of fibrin to form clots. Other common factors that can precipitate the development of a thrombus include disrupted blood flow from immobility, or hypercoagulability (Table 1).
- A PE is the result of a dislodged thrombus that is embolized from a thrombus in the deep venous structures of the legs, pelvis, or arms. The embolus travels to the lungs where it is trapped in the pulmonary arterial microvasculature. Blood flow is obstructed from the PE, which leads to lung edema and reduced pulmonary compliance. This results in inadequate oxygen exchange leading to hypoxemia. Blood flow in the pulmonary artery increases right ventricular afterload that may lead to right ventricular dilation, dysfunction, and ischemia.

Diagnosis

- A DVT is diagnosed based on a detailed history and clinical symptoms. A duplex ultrasound, which measures both blood flow and compressibility of the affected vessel, confirms the diagnosis.
- A PE is diagnosed based on a detailed history and clinical symptoms. A ventilation-perfusion scan or spiral CT confirms the diagnosis.

Table 1

Risk Factors for VTE

- Age over 40 years
- Prolonged immobility
- Major surgery involving the abdomen, pelvis, and lower extremities
- Trauma, especially fractures of the hips, pelvis, and lower extremities
- Malignancy
- Pregnancy
- Previous venous thromboembolism
- Congestive heart failure or cardiomyopathy
- Stroke
- Acute myocardial infarction
- Indwelling central venous catheter
- Hypercoagulability
- Estrogen therapy
- Varicose veins
- Obesity
- Inflammatory bowel disease
- Nephrotic syndrome
- Myeloproliferative disease

VTE Prophylaxis

- See Table 2.

VTE Treatment

- VTE treatment success with unfractionated heparin (UFH) is related to obtaining therapeutic activated partial thromboplastin time (APTT) levels as rapidly as possible (Table 3). Studies have indicated that the VTE recurrence risk is 20-25% higher if APTT levels are not >1.5 times control, or mean normal. This corresponds to a heparin level of 0.2 international units (IU)/mL.
- The use of low-molecular-weight heparin (LMWH) has enabled the treatment of a DVT to move from a 5- to 7-day hospitalization to either a 1- or 2-day hospital stay, or to the outpatient management of a DVT (Table 4).
- With outpatient DVT treatment the diagnosis may take place in either a physician's office or the emergency department. After the diagnosis of a DVT is confirmed by a Doppler ultrasound, the patient is educated on administration of LMWH, and patients receive their first dose of LMWH at that time. After these steps, administer LMWH and warfarin on an outpatient basis. Warfarin is monitored with an International Normalized Ratio (INR) at 1- to 2-day intervals. After two therapeutic INRs, the LMWH may be discontinued and warfarin continued for 3-6 months, or as indicated (Table 5).

Drug Therapy

Unfractionated heparin (UFH)
Mechanism of action
- UFH binds to antithrombin (AT) and converts it from a slow progressive thrombin inhibitor to a rapid thrombin inhibitor. This in turn catalyzes inactivation of factors XIIa, XIa, IXa, Xa, and IIa (thrombin).

Patient counseling
- Patients need to monitor for signs and symptoms of bleeding or bruising, especially at surgical sites.

Therapeutic use
- Prevention and treatment of VTE
- Prevention of VTE in patients with a previous VTE or a known hypercoagulability
- Prophylaxis for VTE in high-risk populations
- Prevention of a mural thrombosis after myocardial infarction (MI)
- Treatment of patients with unstable angina and MI
- Prevent acute thrombosis after coronary thrombolysis

Parameters to monitor
- Heparin is monitored by an APTT, which is sensitive to the inhibitory effects of heparin on factors IIa (thrombin), Xa, and IXa.
- The College of American Pathologists and the American College of Chest Physicians recommend against the use of a fixed APTT therapeutic range of 1.5 to 2.5 times a control APTT. They do recommend that a therapeutic APTT range is established based on an anti-factor Xa concentration of 0.3-0.7 U/mL.
- An APTT should be measured 6 hours after a bolus dose of heparin or after any dosage change, then every 6 hours until a therapeutic APTT is reached. Once a therapeutic APTT is achieved, an APTT may be evaluated every 24 hours.
- Platelet count and hematocrit should be evaluated at baseline and every 3–5 days.

Pharmacokinetics
- The pharmacokinetics of heparin differs based on an intravenous or subcutaneous route of administration.
- Heparin is cleared from the body by a rapid saturable mechanism that occurs at therapeutic doses. A second slower unsaturable first-order clearance that is largely by renal means occurs at high doses.
- The half-life of heparin varies from approximately 30 minutes after an IV bolus of 25 U/kg to 60 minutes after an IV bolus at 100 U/kg.

Dosing
- Heparin should be dosed using a weight-based nomogram. A therapeutic range for heparin is determined by an anti-factor Xa chromogenic assay of 0.3-0.7 U/mL.
- Weight-based dosing nomograms are effective in achieving a therapeutic APTT, although these are not universally transferable to every hospital. Published nomograms are specific only for the reagent and instrument used to validate that nomogram.
- It may be erroneous to determine a therapeutic range based on the calculation of 1.5-2.5 times the mean control APTT, but this may still be done in some hospital laboratories. Previous weight-based nomograms, which utilize a therapeutic range based on the calculation of 1.5-2.5 times the control APTT, have been recently recognized to be accurate only for that APTT reagent utilized. Table 6 is an example of a weight-based dosing nomogram.
- Each hospital should develop its own nomogram based on their therapeutic range.
- Another approach to heparin therapy is to administer an IV bolus of 5000 IU followed by a continuous infusion of at least 30,000-35,000 IU over 24 hours. The infusion rate is adjusted to maintain a therapeutic APTT.

Table 2

Recommendations for VTE Prophylaxis

Medical Condition	Recommended Therapy
General medical	
• General medical patients with risk factors	LDUH, LMWH
• Acute MI	LDUH, IV UFH
• Ischemic stroke	LDUH, LMWH; if anticoagulation prophylaxis is contraindicated, GSC or IPC
General surgery	
Low-risk	
• Low-risk procedure, <40 years of age	Early ambulation
Moderate-risk	
• General surgery, minor procedure with additional risk factors	LDUH bid, LMWH
• Nonmajor procedure, age 40–60 with no additional risk factors	
• Major surgical procedure, age <40, no additional risk factors	
Higher-risk	
• Nonmajor surgery, age >60, with or with risk factors	LDUH tid, LMWH, IPC; if high risk of bleeding, use mechanical
• Major surgery, age >40, with or with risk factors	prophylaxis with GCS or IPC
Very-high risk	
• General surgery with multiple risk factors	LDUH tid or LMWH combined with ES or IPC
• General surgery with high risk of bleeding	GCS or IPC until bleeding risk resolves
Gynecologic surgery	
• Brief procedure ≤30 minutes with benign disease	Early ambulation
• Major surgery for benign disease without risk factors	LDUH bid, LMWH once daily, or IPC starting just before surgery
• Major surgery for malignancy	LDUH tid, LDUH plus GCS, IPC or higher doses of LMWH
Urologic surgery	
• Transurethral or low-risk procedure	Early ambulation
• Major or open urologic procedure	LDUH, ES, IPC, or LMWH
• Highest-risk patients	ES with or without IPC added to LDUH or LMWH
Elective total hip replacement (THR)	LMWH, fondaparinux, or warfarin for up to 28-35 days
Elective total knee replacement (TKR)	LMWH, fondaparinux, or warfarin for at least 10 days; IPC is alternative option
Hip fracture surgery	LMWH, warfarin, fondaparinux, or LDUH for up to 28-35 days
Neurosurgery	IPC ± GCS, LDUH or LMWH when risk of bleeding resolved
Trauma	LMWH, IPC or GCS if bleeding concerns
Acute spinal cord injury	LMWH ± IPC or ES, convert to warfarin

---

Fondaparinux, 2.5 mg SC q 24 hours; GCS, graduated compression stocking; INR, International Normalized Ratio; IPC, intermittent pneumatic compression device; LDUH, low-dose unfractionated heparin, 5000 U SC q 8–12 hours; UFH, unfractionated heparin; warfarin, target INR 2.5, range 2.0–3.0.

LMWH, low-molecular-weight heparin:

    Enoxaparin 30 mg SC q 12 hours

    Enoxaparin 40 mg SC q 24 hours

    Dalteparin 5000 units SC q 24 hours

The optimal duration of anticoagulation prophylaxis after TKR or THR surgery is unknown, although at least 7–10 days of prophylaxis is recommended, and extended out-of-hospital LMWH prophylaxis may reduce the incidence of clinically significant VTE for high-risk patients.

Adapted with permission from the Seventh ACCP Conference on Antithrombotic and ThrombolyticTherapy. *Chest.* 2004;126:338S–400S.

Table 3

Guidelines for Anticoagulation: IV Unfractionated Heparin[1]

Indication	Guidelines
VTE suspected	• Obtain baseline APTT, PT, and CBC count • Check for contraindications to heparin therapy • Order imaging study; consider giving heparin 5000 IU IV
VTE confirmed	• Rebolus with heparin 80 IU/kg IV and start maintenance infusion at 18 IU/kg • Check APTT at 6 hours to keep APTT in a range that corresponds to a therapeutic blood heparin level • Check platelet count between days 3–5 • Start warfarin therapy on day 1 at 5 mg and adjust subsequent daily dose according to INR • Stop heparin after at least 4–5 days of combined therapy when INR is >2 .0 • Anticoagulate with warfarin for at least 3 months at an INR of 2.5; range 2.0–3.0

[1]For treatment with UFH, give 250 IU/kg SC q 12 hours to obtain a therapeutic APTT at 6–8 hours.
APTT, activated partial thromboplastin time; CBC, complete blood cell count; INR, International Normalized Ratio; PT, prothrombin time.
Adapted with permission from the Seventh ACCP Conference on Antithrombotic and Thrombolytic Therapy. *Chest.* 2004;126:401S–428S.

• UFH may be administered subcutaneously every 12 hours. Initially, the patient should receive a loading dose of 3000-5000 IU IV followed by 17,500 IU or 250 IU/kg SC q12h. The dose should be adjusted to an APTT that corresponds to a plasma heparin level of 0.2 IU/mL. This level should be drawn within 1 hour before the next scheduled dose.

Adverse effects
• The most common adverse effects are minor bleeding in the form of gingival bleeding, epistaxis, and ecchymosis.
• The most common serious adverse effects of heparin are gastrointestinal or urogenital bleeding.
• Fatal or life-threatening adverse effects often result from intracranial or retroperitoneal bleeding.
• Transient thrombocytopenia within the first 2–4 days of therapy
• Heparin-induced thrombocytopenia
• Osteoporosis with chronic use

Table 4

Guidelines for Anticoagulation: Low-Molecular-Weight Heparin or Fondaparinux

Indication	Guidelines
VTE suspected	• Obtain baseline APTT, PT, CBC • Check for contraindications to LMWH therapy • Order imaging study, consider giving heparin 5000 IU IV or LMWH or fondaparinux
VTE confirmed	• Give LMWH or fondaparinux • Check platelet count between days 3–5 • Start warfarin therapy on day 1 at 5 mg and adjust subsequent daily dose according to INR • Stop LMWH after at least 4–5 days of combined therapy when INR is >2 .0 • Anticoagulate with warfarin for at least 3 months at an INR of 2.5; range 2.0–3.0

Dalteparin sodium 200 anti-Xa IU/kg per day SC; single dose should not exceed 18,000 IU.
Enoxaparin 1 mg/kg SC q 12 hours or 1.5 mg/kg SC q 24 hours; single dose should not exceed 180 mg.
Tinzaparin 175 IU/kg SC daily.
Fondaparinux 5 mg for <50 kg; 7.5 mg for 50-100 kg; 10 mg for >100 kg SC q 24 hours.
APTT, activated partial thromboplastin time; CBC, complete blood cell count; INR, International Normalized Ratio; PT, prothrombin time.
Adapted with permission from the Seventh ACCP Conference on Antithrombotic and Thrombolytic Therapy. *Chest.* 2004;126:401S–428S.

Contraindications
• Active bleeding
• Severe uncontrolled hypertension
• History of heparin-induced thrombocytopenia
• Use epidural or spinal anesthesia with caution, as patients are at risk of developing an epidural or spinal hematoma, which can result in long-term or permanent paralysis.

Low-molecular-weight heparins (LMWH) and pentasaccharides (Tables 7 and 8)
Mechanism of action
• LMWHs inhibit factor IIa, and to a much greater extent, factor Xa.
• Fondaparinux is a pentasaccharide. It binds selectively to AT, which potentiates the inactivation of factor Xa in the coagulation cascades. This inhibits the formation of thrombin.

Table 5

Duration of Anticoagulation Therapy

Duration	Indication
3 months	First event with reversible or time-limited risk factors
6-12 months (suggest indefinite therapy)	Idiopathic VTE, first event • Antithrombin deficiency • Deficiency of proteins C or S • Factor V Leiden • Prothrombin 20210 gene mutation • Homocysteinemia • High factor VIII level (>90th percentile of normal)
12 months (suggest indefinite therapy)	Idiopathic VTE, first event • Antithrombin deficiency • Two or more thrombophilias (factor V Leiden and prothrombin 20210 gene mutation)
Indefinite therapy	• Two or more episodes of VTE • Cancer, use LMWH for the first 3-6 months, then warfarin • Atrial fibrillation • Mechanical prosthetic heart valve

Adapted with permission from the Seventh ACCP Conference on Antithrombotic and Thrombolytic Therapy. *Chest.* 2004;126:401S–428S.

Advantages of LMWH over UFH
- LMWHs have fewer interactions with plasma proteins, thus they have a more predictable response at lower doses.
- LMWHs have a much longer half-life, which allows them to be administered SC every 12-24 hours.
- LMWHs have a lower incidence of osteoporosis and heparin-induced thrombocytopenia.

Therapeutic use
- Prevention and treatment of VTE
- Prevention of VTE in patients with a previous VTE or a known hypercoagulability
- Prophylaxis for VTE in high-risk populations
- Arterial embolism prevention in patients with mechanical or tissue prosthetic heart valve replacement
- Arterial embolism prevention in patients with atrial fibrillation or atrial flutter
- Arterial embolism prevention in patients with an acute cardioembolic stroke

Parameters to monitor
- Platelet counts, hematocrit/hemoglobin, and signs and symptoms of bleeding
- Bone mineral density with long-term use

Table 6

Body Weight–Based Dosing of IV Heparin

APTT	Dose
Initial dose	80 U/kg bolus, then 18 U/kg per hour
<35	80 U/kg bolus, then 4 U/kg per hour
35-45	80 U/kg bolus, then 2 U/kg per hour
46-70[1]	No change
72-90	Decrease infusion rate by 2 U/kg per hour
>90	Hold infusion 1 hour, then decrease infusion rate by 3 U/kg per hour

[1]The therapeutic APTT range of 46-70 seconds corresponded to anti-factor Xa activity of 0.3-0.7 U/mL at the time this study was performed. The therapeutic range at any institution should be established by correlation with anti-factor Xa levels in this range.

The table was adapted by Raschke et al. The effectiveness of implementing the weight-based heparin nomogram as a practice guideline. *Arch Intern Med.* 1996;156:1645–1649.

- Anti-Xa heparin levels can be monitored in obese patients or in patients receiving LMWH who have significant renal impairment. Anti-Xa levels should be drawn 4 hours after a dose. Therapeutic levels are 0.6-1.0 IU/mL for twice-daily dosing and 1-2 IU/mL for once-daily dosing.
- PT/INR and APTT are not useful in monitoring LMWH.
- Currently there are no direct monitoring parameters for fondaparinux.

Dosing LMWH and fondaparinux
- See Tables 9 and 10.

Table 7

Low-Molecular-Weight Heparin and Pentasaccharide Dosage Forms

Generic Name	Trade Name	Form and Dose
LMWH		
Dalteparin	Fragmin®	2500 units; 5000-unit syringe
Enoxaparin	Lovenox®	30-, 40-, 60-, 80-, 100-, and 120-mg syringe
Tinzaparin	Innohep®	20,000 anti-Xa IU/mL 2-mL vial
Pentasaccharide		
Fondaparinux	Arixtra®	2.5-, 5-, 7.5-, 10-mg syringe

Table 8

Pharmacokinetics of LMWH and Pentasaccharides

Drug	Bioavailability	Half-life (hours)	Xa:IIa Binding Ratio
Enoxaparin	92%	3–6	1.9:1
Dalteparin	87%	3–5	2.7:1
Tinzaparin	90%	2–6	2:1
Fondaparinux	100%	17–21	Only Xa binding

Patient counseling

- Strict compliance is necessary in order to ensure a consistent level of anticoagulation.
- Notify health care provider if there is an increase in bruising, hematuria, melena, hemoptysis, epistaxis, gingival bleeding, or any other abnormal bleeding.
- Consult a health care provider or pharmacist before taking any over-the-counter medications.
- Avoid aspirin or nonsteroidal anti-inflammatory drugs (NSAIDs).
- The air bubble in the LMWH syringe should be near the plunger prior to injection. This ensures that all of the LMWH is expelled from the syringe and helps to minimize the amount of bleeding from the injection site.

Table 9

Indications and Recommended Doses of Low-Molecular-Weight Heparin and Fondaparinux

Indication	Enoxaparin	Dalteparin	Tinzaparin	Fondaparinux
Total hip replacement	30 mg SC q 12 hours or 40 mg SC q 24 hours	5000 units SC 0–14 hours before surgery, then q 24 hours or 2500 units SC 2 hours before surgery, then 5000 units q 24 hours or 2500 units SC 2 hours before surgery and 4–8 hours after, then 5000 units q 24 hours		2.5 mg SC q 24 hours starting 6–8 hours after surgery
Total knee replacement	30 mg SC q 12 hours			2.5 mg SC q 24 hours starting 6–8 hours after surgery
Abdominal surgery	40 mg SC q 24 hours	2500 units SC 1–2 hours before surgery, then 5000 units q 24 hours		
Hip fracture				2.5 mg SC q 24 hours starting 6–8 hours after surgery
Acute medical illness	40 mg SC q 24 hours	5000 units SC q 24 hours		
Trauma	30 mg SC q 12 hours			
DVT treatment with or without pulmonary embolism	1 mg/kg SC q 12 hours or 1.5 mg/kg SC q 24 hours		175 units/kg SC q 24 hours	
Unstable angina	1 mg/kg SC q 12 hours	120 units/kg SC q 12 hours		

Table 10

Enoxaparin Dosage Regimens for Patients with Severe Renal Impairment (Creatinine Clearance <30 mL/min)

Indication	Dosage Regimen
Prophylaxis in abdominal surgery	30 mg SC once daily
Prophylaxis in hip or knee replacement surgery	30 mg SC once daily
Prophylaxis in medical patients during acute illness	30 mg SC once daily
Prophylaxis of ischemic complications of unstable angina and non–Q-wave myocardial infarction, when concurrently administered with aspirin	1 mg/kg SC once daily
Inpatient treatment of acute deep vein thrombosis with or without pulmonary embolism, when administered in conjunction with warfarin sodium	1 mg/kg SC once daily
Outpatient treatment of acute deep vein thrombosis without pulmonary embolism, when administered in conjunction with warfarin sodium	1 mg/kg SC once daily

Adverse effects

- The most common adverse effects are minor bleeding in the form of gingival bleeding, epistaxis, and ecchymosis.
- The most common serious adverse effects of heparin are gastrointestinal or urogenital bleeding.
- Fatal or life-threatening adverse effects often result from intracranial or retroperitoneal bleeding.
- Heparin-induced thrombocytopenia can occur, but its incidence is greater with UFH.
- Osteoporosis can occur with chronic use.

Direct thrombin inhibitors
Drugs
- Lepirudin (Refludan®)
- Argatroban

Mechanism of action
- Lepirudin is a recombinant DNA–derived polypeptide nearly identical to hirudin. It produces an anticoagulant effect by binding directly to thrombin and does not require AT to produce its effect. Lepirudin does not bind to other plasma proteins as heparin does.

- Argatroban is a synthetic molecule that reversibly binds to thrombin.

Therapeutic use
- Lepirudin is used for the treatment of DVT and heparin-induced thrombocytopenia.
- Argatroban is used for treatment of heparin-induced thrombocytopenia and percutaneous coronary intervention.

Pharmacokinetics
- Lepirudin has a half-life of 1-2 hours. Approximately 45% of lepirudin is eliminated by the kidneys.
- Argatroban is metabolized in the liver to inactive metabolites. The half-life is 0.5-1 hour.

Parameters to monitor
Lepirudin
- CBC and signs and symptoms of bleeding
- The therapeutic effect of lepirudin is monitored by the APTT 4 hours after beginning therapy and after a dosage change. After the APTT is stable within the therapeutic range, daily monitoring is sufficient.

Argatroban
- CBC and signs and symptoms of bleeding; the APTT is used to monitor and adjust argatroban therapy.
- The APTT should be drawn 2 hours after an infusion is started and after each dosage change.
- Argatroban will also elevate a PT/INR. For patients on concomitant warfarin therapy, this may impede monitoring and make proper assessment of the INR difficult. For combination therapy, argatroban may be discontinued after an INR is greater than 4. An INR should be drawn after 4-6 hours. If the INR is in the therapeutic range, continue with warfarin only. If the INR is below the therapeutic range, restart argatroban and increase the dose of warfarin. Repeat this procedure until the INR is within the therapeutic range.

Dosing
Lepirudin
- Administer a bolus dose of 0.4 mg/kg IV with an infusion of 16.5 mg/h. Measure an APTT 4 hours after the infusion. Titrate the infusion to a therapeutic APTT range. If the APTT is below the therapeutic range, increase the infusion by 20%. If the APTT is above the therapeutic range, hold the infusion for 2 hours, and then decrease the infusion by 50%. APTTs should be measured 4 hours after a dosage change.

Argatroban

- Administer a continuous IV infusion at the rate of 2 mcg/kg per minute. Adjust infusion rate to a therapeutic APTT range. The usual dose is 2-10 mcg/kg per minute.
- The dose should be reduced in moderate hepatic insufficiency. A continuous IV infusion should begin at a rate of 0.5 mcg/kg per minute. Draw an APTT 4 hours after initiation or a dosage change due to the prolonged elimination half-life.

Patient counseling

- Monitor symptoms of bruising and bleeding and report it to a health care provider immediately.

Adverse effects

- The most common adverse effects are minor bleeding in the form of gingival bleeding, epistaxis, and ecchymosis.
- The most common serious adverse effects are gastrointestinal or urogenital bleeding.
- Fatal or life-threatening adverse effects often result from intracranial or retroperitoneal bleeding.
- There is no known antidote for lepirudin or argatroban. The anticoagulant effect declines rapidly after discontinuation of the drug.
- Nonhemorrhagic effects such as fever, nausea, vomiting, and allergic reactions rarely occur.

Warfarin (Coumadin®)
Dosage forms

- Tablets: 1 mg (pink), 2 mg (lavender), 2.5 mg (green), 3 mg (tan), 4 mg (blue), 5 mg (peach), 6 mg (teal), 7.5 mg (yellow), and 10 mg (white)
- Injections (intravenous): 5 mg powder for reconstitution (2 mg/mL)

Mechanism of action

- Warfarin is a vitamin K antagonist that produces its pharmacologic effect by interfering with the interconversion of vitamin K and its 2,3 epoxide (vitamin K epoxide). Warfarin leads to the depletion or reduction in activity of vitamin K–dependent coagulation proteins (factors II, VII, IX, and X) produced in the liver. The level and activity of the vitamin K–dependent clotting factors decline over 6-96 hours. At least 4-5 days of warfarin therapy are necessary before a patient is completely anticoagulated.

Therapeutic use

- Prevention and treatment of VTE
- Prevention of VTE in patients with a previous VTE or a known hypercoagulability
- Prophylaxis for VTE in high-risk populations
- Arterial embolism prevention in patients with mechanical or tissue prosthetic heart valve replacement
- Arterial embolism prevention in patients with atrial fibrillation or atrial flutter
- Arterial embolism prevention in patients with a previous cardioembolic stroke
- Prevention of acute myocardial infarction in patients with peripheral arterial disease

Patient counseling

- Warfarin should be taken at the same time every day.
- Strict compliance is necessary in order to ensure a consistent level of anticoagulation.
- Strict compliance with a consistent vitamin K diet is necessary to ensure a consistent level of anticoagulation.
- Notify the health care provider in the event of hematuria, melena, epistaxis, hemoptysis, increased bruising, or any abnormal bleeding.
- Notify all health care providers, including dentists, of warfarin therapy.
- Blood monitoring to determine an adequate level of anticoagulation and compliance is necessary at regular intervals.
- Consult the health care provider or pharmacist before taking any new prescription or over-the-counter medications.
- Avoid aspirin or NSAIDs.
- Women of childbearing age should use an effective form of birth control since warfarin has teratogenic effects.

Parameters to monitor

- Warfarin therapy is monitored by a prothrombin time (PT). The PT responds to a reduction in factors II, VII, and X. The INR is used to standardize the responsiveness of thromboplastin to the anticoagulant effects of warfarin. The INR is calculated by the following equation:
  - $INR = (observed\ PT/mean\ normal\ PT)^{ISI}$
  - ISI is the International Sensitivity Index, which is a measure of thromboplastin sensitivity. The lower the ISI, the more responsive the thromboplastin is to the anticoagulant effects of warfarin
- The Seventh ACCP Conference on Antithrombotic and Thrombolytic Therapy recommends two intensities of anticoagulation: a less intense level with a target INR of 2.5 and a range of 2.0-3.0, and a high-intensity level of anticoagulation with a target INR of 3.0 and a range of 2.5-3.5 (Table 11).
- Upon initiation of warfarin therapy, the INR should be evaluated daily if the patient is in the hospital, and every 2-3 days if the patient is not hospitalized.

Table 11

**Recommended Therapeutic Ranges for
Oral Anticoagulation**

Indication	Target INR (INR Range)
Prophylaxis of VTE (high-risk surgery)	2.5 (2.0–3.0)
Treatment of VTE	2.5 (2.0–3.0)
Prevention of arterial embolism in atrial fibrillation	2.5 (2.0–3.0)
Prevention of arterial embolism with a CarboMedics bileaflet or Medtronic Hall tilting disk mechanical prosthetic heart valve in the aortic position with normal left atrium size and sinus rhythm	2.5 (2.0–3.0)
Prevention of arterial embolism in tilting disk or bileaflet mechanical prosthetic heart valve in the mitral position; caged ball or caged disk mechanical prosthetic valves	3.0 (2.5–3.5)
Mechanical prosthetic valve with additional risk factors such as atrial fibrillation, myocardial infarction, left atrial enlargement or low ejection fraction	3.0 (2.4-3.5) combined with low doses of aspirin 75-100 mg daily
Mechanical prosthetic valve with system embolism despite a therapeutic INR	3.0 (2.4-3.5) combined with low doses of aspirin 75-100 mg daily

INR, International Normalized Ratio.
Reprinted with permission from the Seventh ACCP Conference on Antithrombotic and Thrombolytic Therapy. *Chest.* 2004;126:338S-482S.

Pharmacokinetics

- Warfarin is a racemic mixture of two optically active isomers, warfarin S and warfarin R, in roughly equal amounts. The S isomer is five times more potent than the R isomer.
- Warfarin is rapidly and completely absorbed from the GI tract with peak concentration in approximately 90 minutes. Warfarin is 99% protein-bound with a half-life of 36-42 hours.
- The onset of anticoagulation occurs after 4-5 days of therapy and is due to the depletion of the clotting factors rather than steady-state concentrations of warfarin. Thus the onset of action is based on the half-life of the clotting factors II, VII, IX, and X.

Dosing

- Time in the therapeutic range and intensity of anticoagulation are critical for optimizing the therapeutic efficacy of warfarin and minimizing the risk of hemorrhage.
- Warfarin initiation does not require loading. Loading doses can result in an inappropriate increase in the INR, which is not reflective of an anticoagulant effect.
- Initiating warfarin at 5 mg daily should result in an INR around 2.0 in 4-5 days for most patients. An alternative method is to administer between 5 and 10 mg for the first 1 or 2 days, then adjust the dose based upon the INR response.
- Initiating warfarin at a dose of 2.5-4 mg daily may be appropriate in the elderly, in patients with liver disease, in patients with impaired nutrition, or in patients with a high risk of bleeding.
- Initiating warfarin at a dose of 7.5-10 mg daily may be appropriate for young, healthy, or obese patients.
- If a rapid anticoagulant effect is indicated, IV heparin or LMWH should be administered along with warfarin for at least 4-5 days until a therapeutic INR is reached. Heparin or LMWH may be discontinued when the INR is within the therapeutic range on two consecutive occasions.

Disease state interaction

- Disease states that can increase the response to warfarin are hyperthyroidism, congestive heart failure, liver disease, and fever.
- Disease states that can decrease the response to warfarin are hypothyroidism and genetic warfarin resistance.
- Patient noncompliance can also result in a reduced warfarin response.

Drug-food interactions

- Warfarin is a drug with a narrow therapeutic index. There are numerous drugs that interact with warfarin to potentiate or reduce its anticoagulant effect. Since the S isomer is five times more active than the R isomer, drugs that inhibit or induce the S isomer will have a more significant effect on warfarin than drugs that inhibit or induce the R isomer (Tables 12 and 13).
- Foods that contain high amounts of vitamin K can reduce the anticoagulant effect of warfarin (Table 14). It is important that patients are consistent in their consumption of these foods and that they evenly space out their consumption over a 7-day period. If one suddenly stops eating these foods, the INR may dramatically increase.

Adverse effects

- The most common adverse effect is minor bleeding in the form of gingival bleeding, epistaxis, and ecchymosis.

Table 12

Drugs that Can Potentiate Warfarin's Anticoagulant Effect

Acetaminophen	Alcohol (acute use)	Amiodarone[a]
Anabolic steroids	Cimetidine	Ciprofloxacin[a]
Clofibrate	Dicloxacillin	Disulfiram
Erythromycin	Fluconazole[a]	Isoniazid[a]
Itraconazole[a]	Ketoconazole[a]	Levothyroxine[a]
Metronidazole[a]	Piroxicam	Omeprazole
Phenytoin[a]	Trimethoprim-	Simvastatin
Sulfinpyrazone	sulfamethoxazole[a]	Vitamin E[a]
		(high doses)

[a]Highly significant.

Table 13

Drugs that Can Reduce the Anticoagulant Effect of Warfarin

Alcohol	Barbiturates[a]	Carbamazepine[a]
(chronic use)	Cholestyramine[a]	Enteral feeding[a]
Griseofulvin	Rifampin[a]	Vitamin K–
	Nafcillin[a]	containing foods[a]

[a]Highly significant.

Table 14

Foods High in Vitamin K

Broccoli	Brussels sprouts
Cabbage	Canola oil
Cauliflower	Cole slaw
Collard greens	Endive
Green kale	Lettuce
Mayonnaise	Mustard greens
Soybean oil	Spinach
Turnip greens	

- The most common serious adverse effects of warfarin are either gastrointestinal or urogenital bleeding.
- Fatal or life-threatening adverse effects are related to intracranial or retroperitoneal bleeding. Table 15 outlines the treatment guidelines for the management of elevated INRs or bleeding. Special precautions must be taken for patients undergoing invasive procedures. Table 16 outlines the recommendations for managing anticoagulation in these patients.

Table 15

Management of Elevated INRs or Bleeding in Patients Receiving Vitamin K Antagonists

- INR above therapeutic range but <5.0; no significant bleeding
  * Lower dose or omit dose, monitor more frequently, and resume at lower dose when INR is therapeutic; if only minimally above therapeutic range, no dose reduction may be required.
- INR ≥5.0 but <9.0; no significant bleeding
  * Omit the next one or two doses, monitor more frequently, and resume at a lower dose when the INR is in the therapeutic range.
  * Alternatively, omit dose and give vitamin K_1 (≤5 mg orally), particularly if at increased risk of bleeding. If more rapid reversal is required because the patient requires urgent surgery, vitamin K_1 (2-4 mg orally) can be given with the expectation that a reduction of the INR will occur in 24 hours. If the INR is still high, additional vitamin K_1 (1-2 mg orally) can be given.
- INR ≥9.0; no significant bleeding
  * Hold warfarin therapy and give higher dose of vitamin K_1 (5-10 mg orally) with the expectation that the INR will be reduced substantially in 24-48 hours. Monitor more frequently and use additional vitamin K_1 if necessary. Resume therapy at a lower dose when the INR is therapeutic.
- Serious bleeding at any elevation of INR
  * Hold warfarin therapy and give vitamin K_1 (10 mg by slow IV infusion), supplemented with fresh plasma or prothrombin complex concentrate, depending on the urgency of the situation; recombinant factor VIIa may be considered as an alternative to prothrombin complex concentrate; vitamin K_1 can be repeated every 12 hours.
- Life-threatening bleeding
  * Hold warfarin therapy and give prothrombin complex concentrate supplement with vitamin K_1 (10 mg by slow IV infusion); recombinant factor VIIa may be considered as an alternative to prothrombin complex concentrate; repeat if necessary, depending on INR.

INR, International Normalized Ratio.
Reprinted with permission from the Seventh ACCP Conference on Antithrombotic and Thrombolytic Therapy. *Chest.* 2004;126:204S-233S.

2. Atrial Fibrillation

Definition and Epidemiology

- Atrial fibrillation (AF) is a supraventricular tachy-arrhythmia characterized by uncoordinated atrial activity up to 300-500 beats per minute that is associated with an irregular ventricular response. Uncontrolled AF can result in a rapid ventricular response, which can affect blood circulation. Atrial fibrillation may be chronic or paroxysmal in nature.
- Over 2.5 million Americans have AF, which increases in prevalence after age 45 and greatly accelerates after age 65.
- It is estimated that 10% of Americans over the age of 80 have AF.
- AF is a risk factor for the development of a stroke. It is estimated that 4.5% of patients with nonvalvular AF, if untreated, would experience a stroke. If transient ischemic attack and silent stroke are included, the incidence is around 7%.
- The Framingham Heart Study demonstrated that patients with rheumatic heart disease and AF had a 17-fold increase in the incidence of stroke compared to age-matched controls.

Clinical Presentation

- AF is characterized by an irregularly irregular heartbeat, with the possibility of a rapid ventricular response. Common symptoms are palpitations and fatigue. Patients may complain of their "heart fluttering" and feeling weak.

Drug Therapy

- Warfarin therapy has demonstrated approximately a 68% (50-70%) relative risk reduction in stroke in patients with AF, whereas aspirin therapy has demonstrated only a 21% (0-38%) relative risk reduction. A meta-analysis of five studies reported a 36% relative risk reduction in all strokes, and a 46% reduction in ischemic strokes with warfarin compared to aspirin. Randomized controlled studies have demonstrated that anticoagulation with warfarin, INR 2-3, is highly effective in reducing the risk of stroke. Warfarin therapy with an INR 1.2-1.5 has not been shown to be effective in stroke prevention; in addition, an INR >4 is associated with a higher rate of intracranial hemorrhage. Conversely the risk of bleeding and intracranial hemorrhage is higher with warfarin therapy compared to aspirin. Risk stratifi-

Table 16

Recommendations for Managing Anticoagulation Therapy in Patients Requiring Invasive Procedures

Patients with a low risk of thromboembolism

History of VTE for >3 months

Atrial fibrillation without a history of stroke or other risk factors

Bileaflet mechanical cardiac valve in the aortic position

- Stop warfarin therapy approximately 4 days before surgery, allow the INR to return to near normal, briefly use postoperative prophylaxis (if the intervention itself creates a higher risk of thrombosis) with a low dose of UFH (5000 U SC) or a prophylactic dose of LMWH and simultaneously begin warfarin therapy.
- Alternatively, a low dose of UFH or prophylactic dose of LMWH can also be used preoperatively.

Patients with an intermediate risk of thromboembolism

- Stop warfarin therapy approximately 4 days before surgery, allow the INR to fall, cover the patient beginning 2 days preoperatively with a low dose of UFH (5000 U SC) or a prophylactic dose of LMWH and then commence therapy with low-dose UFH (or LMWH) and warfarin postoperatively; some individuals would recommend a higher dose of UFH or a full dose LMWH in this setting.

Patients with a high risk of thromboembolism

History of VTE for <3 months

Mechanical cardiac valve in mitral position, and old model of cardiac valve (ball/cage)

- Stop warfarin therapy approximately 4 days before surgery, allow the INR to return to normal, begin therapy with a full dose of UFH or LMWH as the INR falls (approximately 2 days preoperatively); UFH can be given as an SC injection as an outpatient, and can then be given as a continuous IV infusion after hospital admission in preparation for surgery and discontinued approximately 5 hours before surgery with the expectation that the anticoagulant effect will have worn off at the time of surgery; it is also possible to continue with SC UFH or LMWH and to stop therapy 12-24 hours before surgery with the expectation that the anticoagulant effect will be very low or have worn off at the time of surgery.

Patients with a low risk of bleeding

- Continue warfarin therapy at a lower dose and operate at an INR of 1.3-1.5, an intensity that has been shown to be safe in randomized trials of gynecologic and orthopedic surgical patients; the dose of warfarin can be lowered 4 or 5 days before surgery; warfarin therapy can then be restarted postoperatively, supplemented with a low dose of UFH (5000 U SC) or a prophylactic dose of LMWH if necessary.

INR, International Normalized Ratio; LMWH, low molecular weight heparin; UFH unfractionated heparin.

Reprinted with permission from the Seventh ACCP Conference on Antithrombotic and Thrombolytic Therapy. *Chest*. 2004;126:204S-233S.

cation for stroke in AF has been developed (Table 17). Treatment guidelines for stroke prevention based upon risk stratifications are shown in Table 18.

Other Therapy

- Elective cardioversion (Table 19).

3. Stroke

Definition and Epidemiology

- Stroke is defined as a sudden onset of focal neurologic deficit lasting longer than 24 hours.
- Transient ischemic attack (TIA) is defined as a focal ischemic neurologic deficit usually lasting 2-5 minutes, that resolves completely in less than 24 hours.
- After heart disease and cancer, stroke is the third leading cause of death in America.
- Approximately 700,000 Americans suffer a stroke each year; 500,000 of these individuals experience their first stroke and 200,000 experience a recurrent stroke.

Table 17

Risk Stratification in AF

High risk

- Previous stroke, transient ischemic attack, or systemic embolism
- Hypertension
- Severe left ventricular systolic dysfunction or congestive heart failure
- Age >75 years
- Diabetes
- Rheumatic mitral valve disease
- Prosthetic heart valve

Moderate risk

- Diabetes
- Age 65–75 years
- Coronary heart disease with preserved left ventricular function

Low risk

- Age <65 years without other risk factors

Adapted with permission from the Seventh ACCP Conference on Antithrombotic and Thrombolytic Therapy. *Chest.* 2004;126:229S–256S.

Table 18

Recommendations for Antithrombotic Therapy in AF

High-risk patients

- Warfarin adjusted to a target INR of 2.5, with a range of 2.0–3.0
- Aspirin 325 mg daily if warfarin is contraindicated or declined by the patient
- For patients with AF and prosthetic heart valves, warfarin adjusted to an INR of 2.5-3.5. The addition of aspirin therapy may be appropriate based on the valve type and position and other risk factors.

Moderate-risk patients

- Either warfarin adjusted to a target INR of 2.5, with a range of 2.0-3.0 or aspirin 325 mg daily

Low-risk patients

- Aspirin 325 mg daily

INR, International Normalized Ratio.
Adapted with permission from the Seventh ACCP Conference on Antithrombotic and Thrombolytic Therapy. *Chest.* 2004;126:229S–256S.

- The incidence of stroke increases with age, and the rate doubles for each decade after age 55.
- Hypertension is a factor in 70% of patients who suffer a stroke (Table 20).
- Risk factors for stroke are outlined in Table 20.
- Cigarette smoking increases the risk of stroke 2-3 times compared to nonsmokers.
- Atrial fibrillation increases the risk of a stroke six times.

Clinical Presentation

- Symptoms of a stroke depend on where the stroke occurred in the brain and the rapidity with which the symptoms develop. It is common for a stroke to be preceded by one or more TIAs. Symptoms range from focal deficits to more significant deficits such as hemiplegia or hemiparesthesia, blindness in one eye, or speech difficulties.

Pathophysiology

- 15% of strokes are hemorrhagic in nature.
- 85% of strokes are ischemic in nature.
  * 20% are cardioembolic
  * 20% are due to atherosclerotic cerebrovascular disease
  * 25% are due to penetrating artery disease or lacunar infarctions
  * 30% are cryptogenic

  * 5% are due to other causes
- Atherosclerosis and plaque formation results in arterial narrowing, which leads to stenosis with reduced blood flow. This may enhance platelet aggregation that can lead to an arterial occlusion. An occlusive clot is present in up to 80% of ischemic strokes.
- The Framingham Study indicates that there is a strong relationship between hypertension and the risk of both hemorrhagic and nonhemorrhagic stroke. Atherothrombotic infarctions occur four times more often in patients with hypertension (blood pressure >165/95 mm Hg) than in patients without hypertension. The treatment of hypertension reduces the incidence of stroke by 35-40%.

- Cardioembolic etiology accounts for one-fifth of all strokes. The most common cause of a cardiac embolism is AF; other factors include valvular heart disease, coronary heart disease, prosthetic heart valves, and dilated cardiomyopathy. A cardioembolic stroke often has an abrupt onset and more commonly involves the middle cerebral artery.

Diagnosis and Prevention

- Diagnosis is based on physical examination, medical history, and diagnostic imaging such as a computed tomography (CT) scan, magnetic resonance imaging (MRI) scan, magnetic resonance angiography (MRA), or cerebral arteriography.

Table 19

Anticoagulation for Elective Cardioversion

- Patients with AF of more than 48 hours, or unknown duration, who are scheduled for elective cardioversion should be anticoagulated with warfarin to a target INR of 2.5 with a range of 2.0-3.0 for 3 weeks prior to direct current (DC) or pharmacologic cardioversion, and for 4 weeks after successful cardioversion. If AF returns, then chronic anticoagulation with warfarin at a target INR of 2.5 (range 2.0-3.0).
- Alternatively, patients with AF ≥48 hours or unknown duration, who are scheduled for elective cardioversion, should be anticoagulated with heparin with a target APTT of 60 seconds (range 50-70 seconds) or at least 5 days of warfarin with a target INR of 2.5 (range 2.0-3.0) at the time of cardioversion, then undergo transesophageal echocardiography (TEE). If no thrombus is seen on TEE and cardioversion is successful, anticoagulation should be continued with a target INR of 2.5 (range of 2.0-3.0) for at least 4 weeks. If a thrombus is seen, then cardioversion should be postponed and anticoagulation should be continued indefinitely. The TEE should be repeated before attempting cardioversion later.
- Although data are limited, the risk of embolism following cardioversion in patients who have been in AF for <48 hours appears to be low. However, the use of anticoagulation during the pericardioversion period is recommended.
- For patients with AF for <48 hours in duration, cardioversion may be performed without anticoagulation. However, if anticoagulation is not contraindicated, suggest beginning IV heparin (target APTT of 60 seconds; range 50-70 seconds) or full dose LMWH at presentation. If the patient has risk factors for stroke, then a TEE-guided approach is a reasonable alternative strategy.
- For emergency cardioversion where a TEE-guided approach is not possible, UFH (target APTT of 50 seconds; range 50-70 seconds) should be started as soon as possible, followed by 4 weeks of anticoagulation with warfarin (target INR 2.5; range 2.0-3.0).
- Oral anticoagulation at the time of cardioversion in patients with atrial flutter is recommended in a manner similar to that used for AF.

APTT, activated partial thromboplastin time; INR, International Normalized Ratio; LMWH, low-molecular-weight heparin; UFH, unfractionated heparin
Adapted with permission from the Seventh ACCP Conference on Antithrombotic and Thrombolytic Therapy. *Chest.* 2004;126:229S–256S.

- Preventive measures are outlined in Table 21.

Drug Therapy

Tissue plasminogen activator (t-PA [Alteplase®])
Mechanism of action
- Since most strokes are due to a thromboembolic occlusion in an intracranial artery, thrombolytic therapy is key to restoring or improving perfusion. t-PA is a plasminogen activator (serine protease) that enhances the conversion of plasminogen to plasmin in the presence of fibrin. t-PA binds to fibrin in a thrombus and converts bound plasminogen to plasmin. Plasmin, an enzyme responsible for clot dissolution, initiates local fibrinolysis.

Table 20

Stroke Risk Factors

- Hypertension
- Smoking
- Heart disease (coronary heart disease, heart failure, left ventricular hypertrophy, and atrial fibrillation)
- Elevated pulse pressure
- Previous transient ischemic attack or stroke
- Diabetes
- Hyperlipidemia
- Obesity

Indications
- Acute treatment of stroke, criteria for use:
  * Onset of symptoms is <3 hours
  * Baseline CT scan of the head does not indicate an intracranial hemorrhage
  * Blood pressure <185/110 mm Hg
  * Platelets >100,000/mm^3
  * No conditions present that would increase the patient's likelihood of bleeding
  * No heparin therapy within 48 hours with an elevated APTT
  * No oral anticoagulants or an INR >1.7 or a PT >15 seconds
  * No suspicion of subarachnoid hemorrhage on pretreatment evaluation

Table 21

Stroke Prevention Therapy

- Maintain blood pressure <140/90 mm Hg or <130/90 mm Hg for patients with diabetes or coronary artery disease
- Hyperlipidemia should be controlled with statin therapy (LDL <100 mg/dL)
- Glycemic control (hemoglobin A$_{1c}$ <7%)
- Smoking cessation
- Weight reduction if overweight
- Exercise (ie, 30 minutes of moderate exercise daily)
- Implement the DASH (Dietary Approaches to Stop Hypertension) diet (low in sodium and saturated fat; high in fruits, vegetables, whole grains, and fiber)

* No gastrointestinal or urinary tract hemorrhage within 3 months
* No stroke or serious head injury within 3 months
* No recent (within 3 months) intracranial or intraspinal surgery
* No seizure at the onset of stroke
* No active internal bleeding
* No intracranial neoplasm, arteriovenous malformation, or aneurysm
* No major surgery or serious trauma within 2 weeks
* No clinical symptoms suggesting post-MI or pericarditis
* Not currently pregnant or lactating
* Specific treatment guidelines are available to evaluate patient characteristics for the use of t-PA in acute stroke.

Dose

* t-PA is administered at a dose of 0.9 mg/kg (maximum dose 90 mg) IV with 10% of the dose given as an initial bolus over 1 minute and the balance infused over 60 minutes.

Parameters to monitor

* Hematocrit, mental status, signs and symptoms of bleeding

Adverse drug reactions

* Bleeding is the most common adverse effect with t-PA. The most common sites of bleeding are gastrointestinal, urogenital, retroperitoneal, and intracranial.

Contraindications

* Intracranial hemorrhage, recent stroke, blood pressure >185/100 mm Hg, active internal hemorrhage, platelets <100,000/mm^3, anticoagulant therapy within 24 hours of t-PA, intracranial neoplasm, arteriovenous malformation, or aneurysm

Antiplatelet drugs

Aspirin

Mechanism of action

* Aspirin produces its antiplatelet effect by irreversibly inactivating the enzyme cyclooxygenase, which prevents the conversion of arachidonic acid to thromboxane A_2. Thromboxane A_2 stimulates platelet aggregation. The effects of aspirin on platelets occur for the life of the platelet (ie, approximately 5-7 days). Aspirin has demonstrated a 27-30% risk reduction of stroke.

Patient counseling

* Notify physician if melena, persistent stomach pain

or discomfort, breathing difficulties, increased bleeding or bruising, or skin rashes develop.
* Avoid NSAIDs or warfarin unless instructed otherwise by a physician.
* Avoid over-the-counter medications that contain aspirin.
* Do not crush or chew enteric-coated aspirin.

Dose

* Within 48 hours of an acute ischemic stroke, patients should receive aspirin 160-325 mg daily. Aspirin is effective for stroke prevention at a dose of 50-325 mg daily.

Monitoring parameters

* Signs and symptoms of bleeding

Adverse drug reactions

* Nausea, vomiting, dyspepsia, gastrointestinal ulceration, gastric erosion, duodenal ulcers, gastrointestinal hemorrhage, rash, urticaria, angioedema, bronchospasm, and asthma exacerbation

Drug-drug interactions

* Warfarin, UFH, LMWH, NSAIDs, fondaparinux, and clopidogrel may increase the risk of bleeding if used in combination with aspirin.

Drug-disease interactions

* Use enteric-coated aspirin after an acute episode of peptic or gastric ulcer disease.
* Avoid aspirin use if there is a risk of aspirin-induced asthma.

Clopidogrel (Plavix®)

Mechanism of action

* Clopidogrel is a selective and irreversible inhibitor of adenosine diphosphate–induced platelet aggregation that does not affect arachidonic acid metabolism. The effects of clopidogrel on platelets occur for the life of the platelet, approximately 5-7 days.
* The CAPRIE Trial demonstrated an 8.7% relative risk reduction of composite outcomes of ischemic stroke, MI, or vascular death with the use of clopidogrel versus aspirin in patients with a recent stroke or MI, or patients with symptomatic peripheral arterial disease. Clopidogrel was most beneficial for patients with peripheral artery disease, and showed a 23.8% relative risk reduction over aspirin.

Dose

* Clopidogrel is effective in stroke prevention at a dose of 75 mg daily.

Patient counseling

* Notify physician for melena, persistent stomach pain

or discomfort, increased bleeding or bruising, or development of a skin rash.
- Avoid NSAIDs or warfarin unless instructed otherwise by a physician.
- Avoid over-the-counter medications that contain aspirin.

Parameters to monitor
- Signs and symptoms of bleeding

Adverse drug reactions
- Nausea, dyspepsia, diarrhea, abdominal pain, increased bruising, and bleeding

Drug-drug interaction
- Warfarin, aspirin, NSAIDs, UFH, fondaparinux, and LMWH can increase the risk of bleeding if combined with clopidogrel.
- Clopidogrel may inhibit cytochrome isoenzyme CYP450-2C9 substrates, thus there is the potential to inhibit the metabolism of fluvastatin, tolbutamide, and torsemide. Close monitoring may be advisable.

Drug-disease interactions
- Use clopidogrel with caution in peptic or gastric ulcer disease.
- It may require dosage reduction in moderate to severe hepatic dysfunction.

Extended-release dipyridamole plus immediate-release aspirin (Aggrenox®)
Mechanism of action
- Dipyridamole is a phosphodiesterase inhibitor that increases cyclic adenosine monophosphate in the platelet, which potentiates the deaggregating effects of prostacyclin on platelets.
- The European Stroke Prevention Study (ESPS)-2 demonstrated that dipyridamole 200 mg/aspirin 25 mg combination bid, demonstrated a 37% stroke risk reduction compared to placebo and reduced the risk of nonfatal and fatal stroke by 23% compared to aspirin.

Patient counseling
- Notify physician of melena, persistent stomach pain or discomfort, breathing difficulties, increased bleeding or bruising, or development of a skin rash.
- Avoid NSAIDs or warfarin unless instructed otherwise by a physician.
- Avoid over-the-counter medications that contain aspirin.
- Take this medication on an empty stomach, 1 hour before or 2 hours after meals. If stomach upset occurs, take it with food or milk.
- Do not crush or chew.

Dose
- A combination of extended-release dipyridamole 200 mg with immediate-release aspirin 25 mg in a capsule that is taken twice daily

Parameters to monitor
- Signs and symptoms of bleeding

Adverse drug reactions
- Headache, nausea, vomiting, dyspepsia, gastrointestinal ulceration, gastric erosion, duodenal ulcers, gastrointestinal hemorrhage, rash, urticaria, angioedema, hypotension, dizziness, flushing, epistaxis, bronchospasm, and asthma exacerbation

Drug-drug interactions
- Warfarin, UFH, LMWH, NSAIDs, fondaparinux, aspirin, and clopidogrel may increase the risk of bleeding if used in combination with this product.

Drug-disease interaction
- Use dipyridamole-aspirin with caution in the presence of peptic or gastric ulcer disease.

4. Key Points

- Appropriate VTE prophylaxis should be used with all patients who have risk factors for its development. The Seventh ACCP Conference on Antithrombotic and Thrombolytic Therapy has developed guidelines for VTE prophylaxis specific for at-risk patient populations.
- UFH should be administered as a bolus of 80 IU/kg IV, then a maintenance infusion of 18 IU/kg per hour. Heparin is monitored by APTT levels. A therapeutic APTT range should be determined for each hospital or laboratory that corresponds to an anti-factor Xa concentration of 0.3-0.7 U/mL
- LMWH offers a more predictable response at lower doses without the need to monitor levels, except in patients with severe renal impairment or in obesity. It has a lower incidence of osteoporosis and heparin-induced thrombocytopenia. It can also be administered once or twice daily by SC injection. This allows care to shift from the hospital to the outpatient arena.
- An acute VTE should be treated with either UFH IV, LMWH or fondaparinux to provide immediate anticoagulation, followed by the initiation of warfarin therapy. Warfarin should be initiated at 5-7.5 mg daily for most patients. Patients with malnutrition, liver disease, a high risk for bleeding, or the elderly, may be started at a lower dose. UFH, LMWH, or fondaparinux should be overlapped with warfarin for at least 4-5 days or until there are two consecutive INRs within the therapeutic range.
- Patients with a single VTE with reversible, time-limited risk factors should be anticoagulated for 3-6 months. Patients with a single idiopathic VTE should be anticoagulated for 6 months or longer. Patients with a recurrent VTE or a VTE with cancer or a known hypercoagulable state should be anticoagulated for 12 months to lifetime.
- Atrial fibrillation is a condition that predisposes a patient to the development of a stroke. Warfarin titrated to a target INR of 2.5 with a range of 2.0-3.0 reduces the risk for stroke by approximately 68% (50-70%). Aspirin is not as effective as warfarin in high-risk patients with AF, with an approximately 21% (0-38%) relative risk reduction.
- Patients with a thromboembolic occlusion in an intracranial artery should receive t-PA, provided the following conditions are met:
  * Onset of symptoms is less than 3 hours
  * CT scan of the head does not indicate an intracranial hemorrhage
  * Blood pressure <185/100 mm Hg
  * Conditions that would increase the patient's likelihood of bleeding are not present

- t-PA is administered at a dose of 0.9 mg/kg (maximum dose 90 mg) IV with 10% of the dose given as an initial bolus over 1 minute and the balance infused over 60 minutes.
- The drugs of choice for a noncardioembolic stroke are:
  * Aspirin 50-325 mg daily
  * Clopidogrel 75 mg daily
  * Aspirin 25 mg/dipyridamole 200 mg bid

5. Questions and Answers

1. A 24-year-old female presents to the emergency department with complaints of severe shortness of breath, dyspnea, and chest pain. She is also experiencing tachycardia and tachypnea. Two days prior she noticed pain and swelling in her left lower extremity. Her past medical history is negative for thrombosis. Her current medications include Tri-Levlen® daily and ibuprofen 600 mg q6h prn for pain. A duplex ultrasound of the left lower extremity revealed a DVT. Her vital signs are: T, 98.4°; P, 124/min; R, 36/min; BP, 162/100 mm Hg; Wt, 100 kg; Ht, 165 cm. The most likely cause of her shortness of breath, dyspnea, and chest pain is

   A. bronchitis
   B. asthma exacerbation
   C. pulmonary embolism
   D. heart failure exacerbation
   E. atrial fibrillation

2. This patient is started on heparin therapy. Which dosage regimen is most appropriate?

   A. IV heparin 20,000 IU bolus, then 5000 IU/h
   B. IV heparin 8000 IU bolus, then 1800 IU/h
   C. IV heparin 5000 IU bolus, then 500 IU/h
   D. IV heparin 5000 IU q12h
   E. SC heparin 5000 IU q12h

3. All of the following are risk factors for a DVT except:

   A. Hip replacement surgery
   B. Knee replacement surgery
   C. Hernia repair surgery
   D. Hip fracture surgery
   E. Abdominal surgery

4. Which diagnostic test would assist with the diagnosis of a pulmonary embolism?

   A. Chest x-ray
   B. Electrocardiogram
   C. Spiral CT of the chest
   D. Bronchoscopy
   E. Echocardiogram

5. A patient is started on warfarin for atrial fibrillation. What is an appropriate starting dose of warfarin?

   A. 1 mg daily
   B. 5 mg daily
   C. 15 mg daily
   D. 20 mg daily
   E. 25 mg daily

6. What laboratory test is used to monitor heparin therapy?

   A. APTT
   B. PT
   C. INR
   D. Clotting time
   E. Factor XIa

7. A 47-year-old patient is diagnosed with a lower extremity DVT. The patient's height is 6 feet and the weight is 220 lb (100 kg). The physician would like to treat this patient on an outpatient basis with warfarin and low-molecular-weight heparin. Which dose below would be the most appropriate?

   A. Enoxaparin 30 mg SC q12h
   B. Enoxaparin 40 mg SC q24h
   C. Enoxaparin 100 mg SC q12h
   D. Enoxaparin 200 mg SC q12h
   E. Enoxaparin 220 mg SC q12h

8. How long should enoxaparin be continued in a patient with an acute DVT?

   A. At least 4-5 days until the INR is >2 on two consecutive occasions
   B. At least 42 days and until the INR is >3.0 on two occasions
   C. At least 24 hours until the INR is >4.0 on two occasions
   D. At least 48 hours and until the INR is >4.0 on two occasions
   E. At least 7-10 days and until the INR is >3.5 on two occasions

9. All of the following statements are important information to communicate to a patient on warfarin therapy except:

   A. Take warfarin every day without missing any doses
   B. Eat a consistent amount of vitamin K–rich foods per week
   C. Report any symptoms of bleeding to your physician
   D. Take warfarin with meals and remain standing for 30 minutes

E. Do not take aspirin-containing products unless directed to do so by your physician

10. Vitamin K–rich foods can affect the anticoagulant effect of warfarin. Which of the following foods can decrease the anticoagulant effects of warfarin?

I. Lima beans
II. Spinach
III. Broccoli

A. Only I is correct
B. Only III is correct
C. I and II are both correct
D. II and III are both correct
E. I, II, and III are correct

11. Drugs can affect the anticoagulant effect of warfarin. Which of the following drugs can increase the effects of warfarin?

I. Ciprofloxacin
II. Trimethoprim-sulfamethoxazole
III. Fluconazole

A. Only I is correct.
B. Only III is correct.
C. I and II are both correct.
D. II and III are both correct.
E. I, II, and III are correct.

12. What is the most appropriate therapy for a patient with atrial fibrillation, cerebrovascular accident, hypertension, and diabetes?

A. Aspirin 325 mg daily
B. Warfarin 5 mg daily
C. Clopidogrel 75 mg daily
D. t-PA 90 mg daily
E. Aspirin 25 mg/dipyridamole 200 bid

13. A patient presents to the emergency department with symptoms of aphasia and dysarthria, which resolved over the course of 3 days. The patient has a history of hyperlipidemia, type 2 diabetes mellitus, and hypertension. An echocardiogram showed an ejection fraction of 55%, normal valve function, and normal chamber size. An electrocardiogram showed normal sinus rhythm. Carotid ultrasound indicated moderate stenosis. A CT of the head showed no hemorrhages. Blood pressure was 178/102 mm Hg. Hemoglobin A_{1c} was 10.2%. A lipid profile was as follows: total cholesterol: 294 mg/dL; HDL: 32 mg/dL; LDL: 218 mg/dL; triglycerides: 200

mg/dL. Medications include glyburide 10 mg daily and hydrochlorothiazide 25 mg daily. Which therapy is indicated in this patient?

A. Aspirin 325 mg PO daily
B. Clopidogrel 75 mg PO bid
C. Aspirin 25 mg/dipyridamole 200 mg PO daily
D. Warfarin 5 mg PO daily
E. t-PA 90 mg PO daily

14. All of the following are other treatment goals for this patient except:

A. Hemoglobin A_{1c} < 7%
B. Blood pressure <130/80 mm Hg
C. LDL <100 mg/dL
D. APTT 70-100 seconds
E. Stop smoking

15. Fondaparinux is an anticoagulant that inhibits which clotting factor?

A. IIa
B. IXa
C. Xa
D. XIa
E. VIIa

16. A 58-year-old male is scheduled for a total knee replacement tomorrow. He has a medical history of hypertension, for which he is treated with amlodipine 5 mg daily. His height is 6 feet 2 inches and his weight is 176 lb (80 kg). What form of DVT prophylaxis is indicated in this patient?

I. Enoxaparin 30 mg SC q12h
II. Fondaparinux 2.5 mg SC q24h
III. Aspirin 325 mg daily

A. Only I is correct
B. Only III is correct
C. I and II are both correct
D. II and III are both correct
E. I, II, and III are correct

17. A 68-year-old male presents to the emergency department with complaints of hematuria and bright red blood per rectum. He has been taking warfarin 8 mg daily. His INR is 10.2. What is the most appropriate therapy to reverse his warfarin toxicity?

A. Hold warfarin for 4 days and restart warfarin at a lower dose when his INR is <3

B. Hold warfarin and administer vitamin K 0.5 mg IV; restart warfarin at a lower dose when his INR is <3.0

C. Hold warfarin and administer tranexamic acid 10 mg I; restart warfarin at a lower dose when his INR is <3.0

D. Hold warfarin and administer vitamin K 5 mg PO; restart warfarin at a lower dose when his INR is <3.0

E. Hold warfarin and administer prothrombin complex 5 mg PO; restart warfarin at a lower dose when his INR is <3.0

18. A 63-year-old is receiving warfarin 7.5 mg daily for atrial fibrillation. What therapeutic INR range is indicated for this patient?

   A. 1.0-2.0
   B. 1.5-2.5
   C. 2.0-3.0
   D. 2.0-3.5
   E. 2.5-3.5

19. A 56-year-old female presents to the emergency department with complaints of flank pain, dysuria, and increased urinary frequency. She is diagnosed with a urinary tract infection. Her past medical history includes type 2 diabetes mellitus, hypertension, and atrial fibrillation. Her medications include metformin 1 g bid, quinapril 40 mg daily, and warfarin 5 mg daily. What would be the most appropriate antibiotic to treat this patient's UTI?

   A. Septra® DS bid
   B. Ciprofloxacin 500 mg bid
   C. Rifampin 300 mg qid
   D. Doxycycline 100 mg bid
   E. Erythromycin 500 mg qid

20. Which of the following drugs produce action by inhibiting platelet activity?

   I. Clopidogrel
   II. Dipyridamole
   III. t-PA

   A. Only I is correct
   B. Only III is correct
   C. I and II are both correct
   D. II and III are both correct
   E. I, II, and III are correct

21. What color is warfarin 7.5 mg?

   A. White
   B. Blue
   C. Yellow
   D. Pink
   E. Green

22. Which of the following is a common side effect associated with unfractionated heparin?

   A. Hypokalemia
   B. Hypoglycemia
   C. Ecchymosis
   D. Nausea
   E. Hyponatremia

23. What is the length of anticoagulation therapy for atrial fibrillation?

   A. 3 months
   B. 6 months
   C. 9 months
   D. 12 months
   E. Long-term

24. Advantages of LMWH over UFH include all of the following except:

   A. SC administration
   B. No dosage adjustment needed with renal insufficiency
   C. Once- or twice-daily dosing
   D. Predictable response at lower doses
   E. Lower incidence of heparin-induced thrombocytopenia

Answers

1. **C.** Symptoms of shortness of breath, dyspnea, chest pain, tachycardia, and tachypnea, along with a recent history of a DVT, are indications of a pulmonary embolism. A ventilation-perfusion scan or a spiral CT of the chest would confirm the diagnosis.

2. **B.** Several studies have indicated that weight-based dosing of heparin is more effective in obtaining therapeutic APTT compared to standard heparin titration. A weight-based protocol with an 80 IU/kg IV bolus followed by an infusion of 18 IU/kg per hour should produce APTTs close to the therapeutic range. The other doses are not appropriate.

3. **C.** High-risk surgeries involve the abdomen and lower extremities; thus hip and knee replacement as well as hip fracture surgery are major risk factors for the development of a VTE. Hernia repair surgery is considered minor surgery, and unless the patient has other risk factors, would not require DVT prophylaxis other than early ambulation.

4. **C.** A spiral CT of the chest or a ventilation-perfusion scan would be necessary to confirm the diagnosis of a PE. Chest x-ray, electrocardiogram, echocardiogram, or bronchoscopy would not assist with the diagnosis.

5. **B.** Warfarin 5 mg daily should result in an INR around 2.0 within 4-5 days. The other doses are either extremely low or high for the majority of patients. Higher doses of warfarin may elevate an INR, but this may not be associated with a level of anticoagulation. A rapid increase in INR is due to depletion of factor VII rather than the anticoagulant effect that is associated with depletion of factor II and X.

6. **A.** An APTT is the laboratory test used to monitor heparin therapy. An APTT should be checked 6 hours after a dosage change and every 24 hours if it is within the therapeutic range. A PT/INR is used to monitor warfarin therapy.

7. **C.** Enoxaparin 100 mg SC q12h or 1 mg/kg SC q12h is the dose for treatment of an acute DVT. Enoxaparin 30 mg SC q12h and 40 mg SC q24h are doses used for DVT prophylaxis. Enoxaparin 200 mg SC q12h and 220 mg SC q12h are extremely high doses.

8. **A.** For the treatment of an active DVT or PE, at least 4-5 days of heparin or LMWH overlap with warfarin is needed before an anticoagulant effect is produced by warfarin. Heparin or LMWH should be discontinued after an INR is >2.0 for two consecutive occasions.

9. **D.** Statements A, B, C, and E are important to discuss with patients on warfarin. Patients should follow strict compliance with warfarin. They should eat vitamin K–rich foods consistently over the course of a week and report any symptoms of bleeding to their physician.

10. **D.** Green, leafy vegetables contain higher amounts of vitamin K; thus spinach and broccoli can reduce an INR. Lima beans, although green, do not have a large amount of vitamin K.

11. **E.** All of these drugs have the potential to produce a major rise in INR. These drugs should not be combined with warfarin if possible.

12. **B.** In a patient with AF with multiple risk factors for a stroke (hypertension, prior cerebrovascular accident, and diabetes), warfarin is the drug of choice, provided that the patient is a good warfarin candidate. Aspirin and clopidogrel are antiplatelet agents and are not as effective as warfarin in stroke risk reduction. t-PT is used for acute stroke treatment and administered intravenously.

13. **A.** Aspirin 325 mg daily is correct. Clopidogrel is dosed at 75 mg daily rather than bid. Aspirin 25 mg/dipyridamole 200 mg is dosed bid rather than daily. Warfarin is not appropriate in this patient because there is no indication that this was a cardioembolic stroke (the echocardiogram and electrocardiogram were normal). t-PA is not utilized orally and is only used for acute treatment of stroke to restore perfusion. Moderate stenosis of the carotid artery indicates atherosclerotic disease is present, and antiplatelet therapy is indicated.

14. **D.** All of the goals are correct except APTT range. Since antiplatelet therapy is indicated in this patient, APTT monitoring is not indicated.

15. **C.** Fondaparinux inhibits factor Xa.

16. **C.** Enoxaparin 30 mg SC q12h or fondaparinux 2.5 mg SC q24h are correct. Enoxaparin 80 mg SC q12h is the dose used for treatment of VTE, and aspirin is not effective for DVT prophylaxis in knee replacement surgery.

17. **D.** Warfarin toxicity with an INR of 10.2 can be effectively reversed by holding the dose of warfarin and administering vitamin K 5 mg orally. Warfarin should be restarted when the INR is <3.0. The IV route is only utilized in emergent situations, since anaphylactic reactions are possible. Prothrombin complex is administered IV only for severe bleeding situations.

18. **C.** The therapeutic range for oral anticoagulation is an INR of 2.0-3.0, with a target of 2.5. Increased bleeding is associated with an INR >4.0 and embolic events are more common with an INR <1.5.

19. **D.** Doxycycline 100 mg bid would be the most appropriate therapy for a UTI. Septra DS, erythromycin, and ciprofloxacin will interact with warfarin to elevate the INR.

20. **C.** Clopidogrel and dipyridamole both inhibit antiplatelet activity. Dalteparin is a low-molecular-weight heparin that has inhibitory effects on factors IIa and Xa, and t-PA is a thrombolytic agent.

21. **C.** Warfarin 7.5 mg is yellow, 1 mg is pink, 10 mg is white, and 4 mg is blue.

22. **C.** Minor bleeding and bruising are common side effects of heparin therapy. Other common areas for bleeding are the urogenital and GI tracts.

23. **E.** The duration of anticoagulation therapy for patients with AF is lifelong. The risk for stroke is present as long as atrial fibrillation is present. Patients who undergo DC cardioversion to normal sinus rhythm require anticoagulation therapy for 4 weeks after conversion because the risk of stroke remains high during this time frame.

24. **B.** Since LMWHs are renally eliminated, they must be dose-adjusted for creatinine clearance <30 mL/min. Guidelines have recently been released for enoxaparin dosing in renal impairment. For DVT prophylaxis, enoxaparin should be administered 30 mg SC q24h rather than q12h. For DVT treatment, enoxaparin should be administered 1 mg/kg SC q24h rather than q12h.

6. References

Adams HP, Adams RJ, Brott T. ASA scientific statement, guidelines for early management of patients with ischemic stroke. *Stroke.* 2003;34:1056-1083.

Albers GW, Easton JD, Sacco RL, et al. Antithrombotic and thrombolytic therapy for ischemic stroke. *Chest.* 2004;126; 429S-456S.

Ansell J, Hirsh J, Dalen JE, Poller L, et al. The pharmacology and management of vitamin K antagonists. *Chest.* 2004;126:204S-233S.

Bradberry JC, Fagan SC. Stroke. In: Dipiro JT, Talbert RL, Yee GC, eds. *Pharmacotherapy: A Pathophysiologic Approach,* 5th ed. New York: McGraw-Hill; 2002.

Buller HR, Giancarla A, Hull RD, et al. Antithrombotic therapy for venous thromboembolic disease. *Chest.* 2004;126:401S-428S.

Deeb SN, Stein PD, Al-Ahmad A, et al. Antithrombotic therapy in valvular heart disease—native and prosthetic. *Chest.* 2004;126:457S-482S.

Fuster V, Ryden LE, Asinger RW, et al. ACC/AHA/ESC Guidelines for the management of atrial fibrillation: Executive summary. *Circulation.* 2001;104:2118-2150.

Geerts WH, Graham F, Heit JA, et al. Prevention of venous thromboembolism. *Chest.* 2004;126:338S-401S.

Goldstein LB, Adams R, Becker K, et al. Primary prevention of ischemic stroke: A statement for healthcare professionals from the stroke council of the American Heart Association. *Circulation.* 2001;103:163-183.

Haines S, Racine E, Zeolla M. Venous thromboembolism. In: Dipiro JT, Talbert RL, Yee GC, eds. *Pharmacotherapy: A Pathophysiologic Approach,* 5th ed. New York: McGraw-Hill; 2002.

Hirst J, Anand SS, Halperin JL, et al. Guide to anticoagulant therapy: Heparin: a statement for healthcare professionals from the American Heart Association. *Circulation.* 2001;103:2994-3018.

Hirsh J, Fuster V, Ansell J, et al. American Heart Association/American College of Cardiology Foundation Guide to warfarin therapy. *Circulation.* 2003;107:1692-1711.

Hirsh J, Raschke R. Heparin and low-molecular-weight heparin. *Chest.* 2004;126:188S-204S.

Singer DE, Alberts GW, Dalen JE, et al. Antithrombotic therapy in atrial fibrillation. *Chest.* 2004;126:483S-512S.

38. 2009 Drug and Data Updates

(New drug approvals, indications, and formulations
from July 2006 through June 2008)

Katie J. Suda, PharmD
Associate Professor and Director, Drug Information Center
Department of Clinical Pharmacy
University of Tennessee College of Pharmacy

Anne M. Hurley, PharmD
Assistant Professor
Department of Clinical Pharmacy
University of Tennessee College of Pharmacy

Trevor McKibbin, PharmD, MSc, BCPS
Assistant Professor
Department of Clinical Pharmacy
University of Tennessee College of Pharmacy

Contents

1. Chapter 8: Hypertension

Drug
Tekturna® (aliskiren)

Class: Direct renin inhibitor

Form: Tablets

Formulations: 150 mg and 300 mg tablets

Dose: The initial dose is 150 mg orally once daily. The dose may be increased up to 300 mg daily. Doses greater than 300 mg did not result in additional lowering of blood pressure.

Mechanism of action: Aliskiren is a direct renin inhibitor. This results in decreases in plasma renin activity and inhibition of the conversion of angiotensinogen to angiotensin I.

FDA-approved indication: The treatment of hypertension alone or in combination with other antihypertensive agents. Use with maximal doses of ACE inhibitors has not been adequately studied.

Adverse reactions: Diarrhea, cough, rash, angioedema, hyperuricemia, gout and kidney stones, headache, dizziness, and fatigue.

Drug interactions: Aliskiren is primarily metabolized by the CYP3A4 enzyme:
- Exposure to furosemide was reduced by co-administration with aliskiren
- Co-administration of atorvastatin resulted in increased exposure to aliskiren
- Co-administration of irbesartan resulted in decreased peak concentrations of aliskiren.

Monitoring parameters: Blood pressure, gastrointestinal symptoms, electrolytes (potassium), and uric acid levels.

Patient counseling: May be taken with or without food. Report dizziness, symptoms of gout, difficulty urinating, and diarrhea. Do not take if you become pregnant.

Drug
Tekturna HCT® (aliskiren/hydrochlorothiazide)

New formulation: Aliskiren and hydrochlorothiazide tablets: 150/12.5 mg, 150/25 mg, 300/12.5 mg, and 300/25 mg

Drug
Lotrel® (amlodipine/benazepril)

New formulation: Amlodipine besylate and benazepril hydrochloride tablets: 5 mg/40 mg and 10 mg/40 mg

Drug
Azor™ (amlodipine/olmesartan medoxomil)

New formulation: Amlodipine and olmesartan combination tablets containing 5/20 mg, 10/20 mg, 5/40 mg, and 10/40 mg

Drug
Exforge® (amlodipine/valsartan)

Class: Calcium channel blocker and angiotensin II receptor blocker

Form: Tablet

Formulations: Amlodipine and valsartan tablets: 5 mg/160 mg, 10 mg/160 mg, 5 mg/320 mg, 10 mg/320 mg

Dose: Amlodipine 2.5 mg to 10 mg and valsartan 80 mg to 320 mg once daily. Titrate to blood pressure control.

Mechanism of action: Amlodipine is a dihydropyridine calcium channel blocker. It inhibits the influx of calcium ions into smooth and cardiac muscles. Valsartan blocks the effects of angiotensin II (vasoconstriction and aldosterone secretion) by blocking the binding of angiotensin II to the AT1 receptor.

FDA-approved indication: Treatment of hypertension. The fixed-dose combination is not indicated for initial therapy.

Adverse reactions: Peripheral edema, nasopharyngitis, upper respiratory tract infection, dizziness, orthostatic hypotension, fatigue, hyperkalemia, and angioedema.

Drug interactions: Concomitant use of potassium-sparing diuretics (e.g., spironolactone, triamterene, amiloride), potassium supplements, or salt substitutes containing potassium may lead to increases in serum potassium.

Monitoring parameters: Blood pressure, heart rate, electrolytes (potassium), serum creatinine, blood urea nitrogen, liver function tests.

Patient counseling: Report dizziness; swelling of the hands, ankles, or feet; nasal congestion; discomfort when swallowing; upper respiratory tract infection.

Drug
Avalide® (irbesartan/hydrochlorothiazide)

New FDA-approved indication: Initial therapy of patients who are likely to need multiple drugs to control blood pressure.

Drug
Dutoprol™ (metoprolol succinate extended release/hydrochlorothiazide)

Class: Beta-blocker and thiazide diuretic

Form: Tablets

Formulations: Metoprolol succinate and hydrochlorothiazide tablets: 25/12.5 mg, 50/12.5 mg, and 100/12.5 mg

Dose: Dosing must be individualized, with attention to baseline and target blood pressure as well as prior response with individual agents. The usual initial dose of metoprolol succinate extended release is 25 to 100 mg in a single dose once daily.

Mechanism of action: Metoprolol is a $beta_1$-selective (cardioselective) adrenergic receptor-blocking agent. At higher concentrations it may also inhibit $beta_2$-adrenoreceptors. Hydrochlorothiazide is a thiazide diuretic, increasing sodium and chloride excretion in the renal tubule and indirectly decreasing plasma volume.

FDA-approved indication: The management of hypertension. The fixed-dose combination is not indicated for initial therapy.

Adverse reactions: Fatigue, dizziness, nausea, bradycardia, shortness of breath, diarrhea, pruritus, rash, electrolyte abnormalities, hyperuricemia, agranulocytosis.

Drug interactions:
Metoprolol:
- Monoamine oxidase (MAO) inhibitors may have an additive effect when given with beta-blocking agents
- Drugs that inhibit CYP2D6, such as quinidine, fluoxetine, paroxetine, and propafenone, are likely to increase metoprolol concentration.
Hydrochlorothiazide:
- May reduce the clearance of lithium
- Dose adjustment of antidiabetic agents may be required

- Barbiturates, narcotics, and alcohol increase the risk for orthostatic hypotension
- Co-administration of nonsteroidal anti-inflammatory drugs may reduce the diuretic effect of hydrochlorothiazide.

Monitoring parameters: Blood pressure, heart rate, electrolytes, blood sugar, serum creatinine, blood urea nitrogen, uric acid, liver function tests, and lipids.

Patient counseling: May be taken with or without food. Report dizziness, shortness of breath, pruritus, and rash. Do not discontinue abruptly.

Drug
Bystolic™ (nebivolol)

Class: Beta-blocker   *β₁ selective @ ↓ doses*

Form: Tablets

Formulations: 2.5 mg, 5 mg, and 10 mg tablets

Dose: The recommended starting dose for most patients is 5 mg daily. The dose may be increased at 2-week intervals up to 40 mg daily. In patients with hepatic or severe renal impairment the recommended starting dose is 2.5 mg daily.

Mechanism of action: Nebivolol is a beta-adrenergic receptor-blocking agent. At doses less than or equal to 10 mg in extensive metabolizers (most of the population), nebivolol is preferentially $beta_1$ selective. At higher doses and in poor metabolizers, nebivolol inhibits both $beta_1$- and $beta_2$-adrenergic receptors.

FDA-approved indication: This medication is indicated for the treatment of hypertension and may be used alone or in combination with other antihypertensive agents.

Adverse reactions: Headache, fatigue, dizziness, nausea, insomnia.

Drug interactions: Nebivolol is predominantly metabolized via direct glucuronidation and to a lesser extent via N-dealkylation and oxidation via cytochrome P450 2D6. Drugs that inhibit cytochrome P450 2D6 can be expected to increase nebivolol plasma levels.

Monitoring parameters: Blood pressure, heart rate, blood sugar, electrolytes, serum creatinine, blood urea nitrogen, and liver function tests.

Patient counseling: May be taken with or without food. Report dizziness and shortness of breath. Do not discontinue abruptly.

Drug
Sular® (nisoldipine extended release)

New formulation: Extended-release tablets: 8.5 mg, 17 mg, 25.5 mg, and 34 mg

Drug
Diovan HCT® (valsartan and hydrochlorothiazide)

New formulation: Valsartan and hydrochlorothiazide tablets: 320 mg/12.5 mg, 320 mg/25 mg

2. Chapter 9: Heart Failure

Drug
Coreg CR™ (carvedilol phosphate extended release)

Class: Beta-blocker

Form: Capsule

Formulations: 10 mg, 20 mg, 40 mg, and 80 mg capsules

Dose: The recommended starting dose is 10 mg once daily. Once initiated, the dose may be adjusted slowly to 20 mg, 40 mg, and 80 mg over succeeding 2-week intervals.

Mechanism of action: Carvedilol possesses nonselective β-adrenoreceptor blocking activity in addition to α_1-adrenergic blocking activity.

FDA-approved indications:
- The treatment of mild to severe heart failure of ischemic or cardiomyopathic origin
- Left ventricular dysfunction following myocardial infarction in clinically stable patients who have survived the acute phase of a myocardial infarction and have a left ventricular ejection fraction of $\leq 40\%$ (with or without symptomatic heart failure)
- Hypertension either alone or in combination with other antihypertensives.

Adverse reactions: Bradycardia, hypotension, dizziness, fatigue, shortness of breath.

Drug interactions: Carvedilol is primarily metabolized by the CYP2D6 and CYP2C9 enzymes.
- Co-administration of rifampin decreased exposure to carvedilol
- Co-administration of cimetidine increased exposure to carvedilol.

Monitoring parameters: Heart rate and blood pressure.

Patient counseling: Do not crush or chew; swallow whole. If unable to swallow, may open capsules and sprinkle beads on cold applesauce. Report dizziness and shortness of breath. Do not discontinue unless under the supervision of a physician.

3. Chapter 11: Ischemic Heart Disease

Drug
Plavix® (clopidogrel)

New FDA-approved indication: Treatment of patients with ST segment elevation acute myocardial infarction.

Drug
Lovenox® (enoxaparin)

New FDA-approved indication: Treatment of patients with acute ST segment elevation myocardial infarction.

Drug
NitroMist™ (nitroglycerin)

Class: Nitrate vasodilator

Form: Oral spray

Formulations: 400 mcg per spray; 230 metered sprays per container

Dose: At onset of an attack, 1 or 2 metered sprays should be administered on or under the tongue. This may be repeated approximately every 5 minutes as needed. A maximum of 3 metered sprays is recommended within a 15-minute period. If chest pain persists after a total of 3 sprays, prompt medical attention is recommended. NitroMist may be used prophylactically 5 to 10 minutes before engaging in activities that might precipitate an acute attack. Excessive use may lead to the development of tolerance.

Mechanism of action: Nitroglycerin is a vasodilator with effects on both arteries and veins, decreasing both preload and afterload.

FDA-approved indications: Acute relief of an attack or acute prophylaxis of angina pectoris due to coronary artery disease.

Adverse reactions: Headache, flushing, drug rash, postural hypotension, dizziness, weakness, and syncope.

Drug interactions: NitroMist is contraindicated in patients who are using a selective inhibitor of phosphodiesterase type 5, including sildenafil, vardenafil, and tadalafil. Patients receiving antihypertensive agents may be at risk for additive hypotensive effects. Patients taking nitroglycerin should avoid ergotamine-related drugs.

Monitoring parameters: Heart rate, blood pressure.

Patient counseling: Container must be primed with 10 sprays prior to use. If container is unused for 6 weeks or longer, it must be re-primed with 2 sprays.

Drug
Ranexa™ (ranolazine extended release)

New formulation: Ranolazine 1000 mg extended-release tablets

4. Chapter 12: Hyperlipidemia

Drug
Lipitor® (atorvastatin calcium)

New FDA-approved indications: To reduce the risk of nonfatal heart attacks, fatal and non-fatal strokes, revascularization procedures, hospitalization for heart failure, and chest pain in patients with heart disease.

Drug
Welchol® (colesevelam hydrochloride)

New FDA-approved indication: Approved as adjunctive therapy to improve glycemic control in adults with type 2 diabetes. Colesevelam can be added to metformin, sulfonylureas, or insulin, either alone or in combination with other antidiabetic agents.

Drug
Zetia® (ezetimibe)

New FDA-approved indications: May be administered in combination with fenofibrate as adjunctive therapy to diet for the reduction of total cholesterol, LDL-C, Apo B, and non-HDL-C in patients with mixed hyperlipidemia.

Drug
Lescol® (fluvastatin sodium)

New FDA-approved indication: Treatment of heterozygous familial hypercholesterolemia in adolescent boys and postmenarchal girls, age 10 to 16 years. Recommended dose range of 20 mg to 40 mg twice daily.

Drug
Lescol XL® (fluvastatin sodium extended release)

New FDA-approved indication: Treatment of heterozygous familial hypercholesterolemia in adolescent boys and postmenarchal girls, age 10 to 16 years. Recommended dose 80 mg once daily.

Drug
Simcor® (niacin extended release/simvastatin)

Class: Combined niacin and HMG-CoA reductase inhibitor

Form: Tablets

Formulations: Niacin extended release and simvastatin: 500/20 mg, 750/20 mg, and 1000/20 mg

Dose: Patients not currently on niacin extended release should start at a single-tablet dose of 500/20 mg daily at bedtime. The dose should not be increased by more than 500 mg of niacin extended release every 4 weeks. The recommended maintenance dose is 1000/20 mg to 2000/40 mg once daily at bedtime, depending on patient tolerability and lipid levels.

Mechanism of action: The effect of niacin on lipid profiles is not completely understood. The mechanism of action may include inhibition of release of free fatty acids from adipose tissue, increased lipoprotein lipase activity, and decreases in synthesis of VLDL-C and LDL-C. Simvastatin is a prodrug, hydrolyzed to the active form after administration. Simvastatin is a specific inhibitor of HMG-CoA reductase. This inhibits an early and rate-limiting step in the biosynthesis of cholesterol.

FDA-approved indications: To reduce total cholesterol, LDL-C, Apo B, non-HDL-C, or triglycerides, or to increase HDL-C in patients with primary hypercholesterolemia and mixed dyslipidemia when treatment with simvastatin monotherapy or niacin extended release monotherapy is inadequate.

Adverse reactions: Flushing, including warmth, redness, itching, or tingling, is the most frequently reported adverse event. Other adverse events include pruritus, headache, and diarrhea. Myopathy and rhabdomyolysis have also been reported with simvastatin.

Drug interactions: Simvastatin is a substrate of cytochrome P450 3A4. Medications and foods that inhibit cytochrome P450 3A4 can be expected to increase the plasma concentration of simvastatin. Co-administration with amiodarone, nefazodone, verapamil, cyclosporine, azole antifungals, and gemfibrozil may increase the risk for myopathy and rhabdomyolysis.

Niacin may potentiate the effect of ganglionic blocking agents and vasoactive drugs. Co-administration of colestipol inhibits absorption of niacin. Nutritional supplements containing high doses of niacin may increase adverse effects of this medication.

Monitoring parameters: Lipid panel, liver function test, serum creatine kinase, uric acid, blood glucose, and platelet count.

Patient counseling: Take before bedtime with a small meal or snack. Tablets should not be broken, crushed, or chewed. If a break in treatment occurs, retitration of the maintenance dose may be needed. Notify physician of any unexplained muscle pain or tenderness. Flushing may be minimized by taking an aspirin 30 minutes prior to dosing. To minimize flushing, avoid alcohol, hot beverages, and spicy foods around the time of dosing.

Drug
Omacor® (omega-3 acid ethyl esters)

Brand name changed to: Lovaza™ (omega-3 acid ethyl esters)

New FDA-approved indication: Treatment as an adjunct to HMG-CoA reductase inhibitor therapy in patients with persistent high triglycerides despite HMG-CoA reductase inhibitor treatment.

Drug
Crestor® (rosuvastatin calcium)

New FDA-approved indication: Approved as an adjunct to diet to slow the progression of atherosclerosis in patients with elevated cholesterol.

5. Chapter 14: Thyroid, Adrenal, and Miscellaneous Endocrine Drugs

Drug
Elaprase™ (idursulfase)

Class: Enzyme replacement

Form: Injection

Formulations: 2 mg/mL solution, in vials containing 3 mL of extractable solution for dilution

Dose: 0.5 mg/kg administered intravenously weekly over 1 to 3 hours (not to exceed 8 hours). The initial infusion rate should be 8 mL/hr for the first 15 minutes. Then, if the infusion is tolerated, the rate may be increased by 8 mL/hr at 15-minute intervals.

Mechanism of action: Hunter syndrome (mucopolysaccharidosis II) is a recessive X-linked genetic disease caused by insufficient levels of the lysosomal enzyme iduronate-2-sulfatase. Idursulfase is a purified form of human iduronate-2-sulfatase, a lysosomal enzyme that hydrolyzes sulfate residues from glycosaminoglycans that would otherwise accumulate.

FDA-approved indication: Indicated for the treatment of patients with Hunter syndrome (mucopolysaccharidosis [MPS] II).

Adverse reactions: Hypoxic episodes, headache, fever, cutaneous reactions, hypersensitivity reactions, and hypertension. Because of the potential for severe infusion-related reactions, appropriate medical support should be readily available.

Drug interactions: No formal drug interaction studies have been conducted.

Monitoring parameters: 6-minute walk test, % of predicted forced vital capacity (FVC), and monitor for allergic and anaphylactic reactions during the infusion.

Patient counseling: Report any dizziness, shortness of breath, swelling, or flushing during or after the infusion.

Drug
Tirosint® (levothyroxine sodium)

Class: Thyroid hormone

Form: Capsule

Formulations: 25 mcg, 50 mcg, 75 mcg, 100 mcg, 125 mcg, and 150 mcg capsules

Dose: Tirosint is administered as a single daily dose, preferably 30 minutes to 1 hour before breakfast. Doses must be individualized and adjusted on the basis of periodic assessment of the patient's clinical response and laboratory parameters.

Mechanism of action: Tirosint capsules contain synthetic levothyroxine (T_4). Levothyroxine is essential in the regulation of multiple metabolic pathways and the growth, development, and maturation of the central nervous system and bone.

FDA-approved indications: Replacement or supplemental therapy in congenital or acquired hypothyroidism of any etiology, except transient hypothyroidism during recovery from subacute thyroiditis. Treatment or prevention of euthyroid goiters, lymphocytic thyroiditis (Hashimoto's thyroiditis), and as an adjunct to surgery and radioiodine therapy in the management of thyrotropin-dependent well-differentiated thyroid cancer.

Adverse reactions: Fatigue, fever, increased appetite, excessive sweating, heat intolerance, headache, hyperactivity, nervousness, tremors, palpitations, tachycardia, arrhythmias, increased blood pressure, shortness of breath, abdominal cramps, diarrhea, vomiting, hair loss, decreased bone mineral density, and menstrual irregularities.

Drug interactions:
- Drugs that may decrease thyroid hormone secretion: aminoglutethimide, amiodarone, iodine, lithium, methimazole, propylthiouracil, sulfonamides, and tolbutamide
- Drugs that may increase thyroid hormone secretion: amiodarone and iodine
- Drugs that decrease T_4 absorption: aluminum and magnesium, simethicone, cholestyramine, colestipol, calcium carbonate, sodium polystyrene sulfonate (Kayexalate), ferrous sulfate, and sucralfate
- Drugs that may increase hepatic metabolism: carbamazepine, hydantoins, phenobarbital, and rifampin
- Thyroid hormones may increase the catabolism of vitamin K-dependent clotting factors, thereby increasing the anticoagulant activity of warfarin
- Concurrent use with antidepressants may increase the toxicity of both drugs

- Careful monitoring of blood sugar is recommended for patients on antidiabetic medications
- Serum digitalis levels may be reduced by levothyroxine.

Monitoring parameters: TSH and T_4, blood pressure, and heart rate.

Patient counseling: Take on an empty stomach at least 30 minutes to 1 hour prior to eating. Do not discontinue or change the amount you are taking without consulting your physician. Notify your physician if you become pregnant or are planning to become pregnant. Report dizziness, palpitations, nausea, vomiting, and diarrhea.

6. Chapter 15: Women's Health

Drug *Vit D3*
Fosamax Plus D™ (alendronate sodium/cholecalciferol)

New formulation: Tablets containing alendronate 70 mg and cholecalciferol 5600 international units

Drug
Yaz® (drospirenone/ethinyl estradiol)

New FDA-approved indication: Treatment of premenstrual dysphoric disorder in women who choose to use an oral contraceptive for birth control.

Drug
Evamist™ (estradiol)

New formulation: Estradiol transdermal spray delivering 1.53 mg estradiol per spray

Drug
Divigel® (estradiol)

Class: Estrogen replacement

Form: Gel

Formulations: Estradiol gel 0.1% in single-dose foil packets containing 0.25 mg, 0.5 mg, and 1 mg doses of estradiol

Dose: Patients should be treated with the lowest effective dose, generally starting at 0.25 g (of Divigel) daily. Dosage adjustments may be made on the basis of individual patient response.

Mechanism of action: Acts as a replacement for diminished estrogen levels in menopause.

FDA-approved indication: Treatment of moderate to severe vasomotor symptoms associated with menopause.

Adverse reactions: Breast pain, headache, impaired glucose tolerance, changes in vaginal bleeding pattern, and abnormal withdrawal bleeding or flow.

Drug interactions: Inhibitors of CYP3A4 may affect estrogen drug metabolism. Inducers of CYP3A4 (St. John's wort, phenobarbital, carbamazepine, and rifampin) may reduce plasma concentrations of estrogens. Inhibitors of CYP3A4 (erythromycin, clarithromycin, ketoconazole, itraconazole, ritonavir, and grapefruit juice) may increase plasma concentrations of estrogens.

Monitoring parameters: Patients should be re-evaluated periodically as clinically appropriate (e.g., 3-month to 6-month intervals) to determine if treatment is still necessary.

Patient counseling: Start at the lowest dose and talk to your health care provider about how well that dose is working for you. Apply to clean, dry, unbroken skin and wash hands with soap and water after application.

Drug
Elestrin™ (estradiol)

Class: Estrogen replacement

Form: Gel

Formulations: Estradiol 0.06% in a metered-dose gel pump. The pump delivers approximately 0.52 mg of estradiol per actuation and is capable of approximately 100 metered doses.

Dose: Patients should be started with the lowest effective dose; one pump per day (0.87 g/day, which contains 0.52 mg of estradiol).

Mechanism of action: Serves as a replacement for diminished estrogen levels in menopause.

FDA-approved indication: Treatment of moderate to severe vasomotor symptoms associated with menopause.

Adverse reactions: Breast pain, headache, impaired glucose tolerance, changes in vaginal bleeding pattern, and abnormal withdrawal bleeding or flow. Women receiving estrogens may be at a higher risk for endometrial cancer, stroke, and deep vein thrombosis.

Drug interactions: Inhibitors of CYP3A4 may affect estrogen drug metabolism. Inducers of CYP3A4 (St. John's wort, phenobarbital, carbamazepine, and rifampin) may reduce plasma concentrations of estrogens. Inhibitors of CYP3A4 (erythromycin, clarithromycin, ketoconazole, itraconazole, ritonavir, and grapefruit juice) may increase plasma concentrations of estrogens.

Monitoring parameters: Patients should be re-evaluated periodically as clinically appropriate (e.g., 3-month to 6-month intervals) to determine if treatment is still necessary.

Patient counseling: The pump must be primed (by depressing the spout 10 times) prior to use. Apply to dry, clean, unbroken skin. Wash hands after application.

Drug
Enjuvia™ (synthetic conjugated estrogens, B)

Class: Estrogen replacement

Form: Tablets

Formulations: 0.3 mg, 0.45 mg, 0.625 mg, 0.9 mg, and 1.25 mg tablets

Dose: Initiate at the lowest dose of 0.3 mg daily. Subsequent dosage adjustment may be made on the basis of individual patient response and indication.

Mechanism of action: Acts as a replacement for diminished estrogen levels in menopause.

FDA-approved indications: Treatment of moderate to severe vasomotor symptoms associated with menopause. Treatment of moderate to severe vaginal dryness and pain with intercourse, symptoms of vulvar and vaginal atrophy associated with menopause (topical products should be considered).

Adverse reactions: Headache, breast pain, irregular vaginal bleeding or spotting, abdominal cramps, and nausea. Women receiving estrogens may be at higher risk for endometrial cancer, stroke, and deep vein thrombosis.

Drug interactions: Inhibitors of CYP3A4 may affect estrogen drug metabolism. Inducers of CYP3A4 (St. John's wort, phenobarbital, carbamazepine, and rifampin) may reduce plasma concentrations of estrogens. Inhibitors of CYP3A4 (erythromycin, clarithromycin, ketoconazole, itraconazole, ritonavir, and grapefruit juice) may increase plasma concentrations of estrogens.

Monitoring parameters: Patients should be re-evaluated periodically as clinically appropriate (e.g., 3-month to 6-month intervals) to determine if treatment is still necessary.

Patient counseling: Estrogens may increase the risk for cancers of the breast and uterus.

Drug
Activella® (estradiol/norethindrone acetate)

New formulation: Tablets containing 0.5 mg of estradiol and 0.1 mg of norethindrone acetate

Drug
Implanon™ (etonogestrel implant)

Class: Steroid contraceptive

Form: Implant

Formulations: Each implant (4 cm length, 2 mm diameter) contains 68 mg of etonogestrel.

Dose: Implant must be removed no later than 3 years after insertion.

Mechanism of action: Etonogestrel suppresses ovulation, increases viscosity of the cervical mucus, and causes alterations in the endometrium.

FDA-approved indication: Indicated in women for the prevention of pregnancy.

Adverse reactions: Headache, weight gain, acne, breast pain, abdominal pain, dizziness, dysmenorrhea, and insertion site pain.

Drug interactions: The effectiveness of contraceptive steroids may be reduced by inducers of hepatic enzymes, including barbiturates, griseofulvin, rifampin, phenylbutazone, phenytoin, carbamazepine, felbamate, oxcarbazepine, topiramate, modafinil, and St. John's wort.

Monitoring parameters: Pregnancy should be excluded prior to insertion of Implanon.

Patient counseling: No contraceptive method is 100% effective. Implanon does not prevent transmission of HIV or other sexually transmitted diseases. Report any chest pain, shortness of breath, sharp pain in the calf, and sudden severe headache. Continue annual exams.

Drug
Lybrel™ (levonorgestrel/ethinyl estradiol)

Class: Combination steroid contraceptive

Form: Tablets

Formulations: Tablets containing levonorgestrel 90 mcg and ethinyl estradiol 20 mcg

Dose: Take one tablet daily. Take all tablets in the pack; there are no placebo tablets.

Mechanism of action: Inhibition of ovulation via the suppression of gonadotropins. Additional actions include changes in cervical mucus and endometrium.

FDA-approved indication: Prevention of pregnancy in women who elect to use oral contraceptives as a method of contraception.

Adverse reactions: Breast pain, abdominal pain, headache.

Drug interactions: Inhibitors of CYP3A4 may affect estrogen drug metabolism. Inducers of CYP3A4 (St. John's wort, phenobarbital, carbamazepine, and rifampin) may reduce plasma concentrations of estrogens. Inhibitors of CYP3A4 (erythromycin, clarithromycin, ketoconazole, itraconazole, ritonavir, and grapefruit juice) may increase plasma concentrations of estrogens.

Monitoring parameters: Report any chest pain, shortness of breath, sharp pain in the calf, or sudden severe headache.

Patient counseling: Regular monthly bleeding does not occur on Lybrel. If you suspect that you may be pregnant, or if you have symptoms of pregnancy such as nausea/vomiting or unusual breast tenderness, you should have a pregnancy test and contact your health care professional.

Drug
Pitocin® (oxytocin)

New formulation: Oxytocin 10 units/mL for injection, in 30 mL vial

Drug
Endometrin® (progesterone)

Class: Fertility agent

Form: Vaginal insert

Formulations: 100 mg vaginal insert

Dose: 100 mg administered vaginally two or three times daily starting at oocyte retrieval and continuing for up to 10 weeks total duration.

Mechanism of action: Progesterone, a naturally occurring steroid hormone, transforms a proliferative endometrium into a secretory endometrium. Progesterone increases endometrial receptivity for embryo implantation and acts to maintain pregnancy.

FDA-approved indication: To support embryo implantation and early pregnancy by supplementation of corpus luteal function as part of an assisted reproductive

technology (ART) treatment program for infertile women.

Adverse reactions: Abdominal pain, nausea, and ovarian hyperstimulation syndrome.

Drug interactions: Inducers of CYP3A4 (such as rifampin and carbamazepine) may increase the elimination of progesterone. Endometrin is not recommended for use with other vaginal products.

Patient counseling: Use only as directed. Contact your health care provider if you
 • Have unusual vaginal bleeding that has not been evaluated by a doctor
 • Currently have or have had liver problems
 • Have or have had blood clots in the legs, lungs, eyes, or elsewhere in your body.

Drug
Evista® (raloxifene hydrochloride)

New FDA-approved indication: To reduce the risk of invasive breast cancer in postmenopausal women at high risk of invasive breast cancer and in postmenopausal women with osteoporosis.

Drug
Actonel® (risedronate sodium)

New formulation: Risedronate 150 mg tablet for once-monthly dosing

Drug
Reclast® (zoledronic acid)

New FDA-approved indication: Reclast is approved for the treatment of osteoporosis in women and the treatment of Paget's disease of bone in men and women. For osteoporosis, the dose is 5 mg zoledronic acid infused over not less than 15 minutes, once yearly. For Paget's disease of bone an initial dose of 5 mg is administered; specific retreatment data are not available. To reduce the risk of hypocalcemia, patients must be adequately supplemented with calcium and vitamin D.

New formulation: Zoledronic acid 5 mg in a 100 mL ready-to-infuse solution

7. Chapter 16: Kidney Disease

Drug
Mircera® (methoxy polyethylene glycol-epoetin beta)

Class: Erythropoiesis-stimulating agent

Form: Prefilled injectable syringes

Formulations: Solution for injection in prefilled syringes containing methoxy polyethylene glycol-epoetin beta 50 mcg, 75 mcg, 100 mcg, 150 mcg, 200 mcg, and 250 mcg

Dose: Starting dose is 0.6 mcg/kg body weight, administered once every 2 weeks intravenously or subcutaneously. The dose may be increased by ~25% of the previous dose if the rate of rise in hemoglobin (Hb) is <1.0 g/dL over 1 month. Further increases of ~25% may be made at monthly intervals until the individual target Hb level is obtained. Dose decreases may be needed if the rate of hemoglobin rise is >2 g/dL in 1 month. Maintenance dosing may be extended to once-monthly intervals.

Mechanism of action: This is a continuous erythropoiesis agonist. Erythropoietin is essential to the regulation of healthy erythropoiesis.

FDA-approved indication: Treatment of anemia associated with chronic kidney disease.

Adverse reactions: The most frequent adverse reaction is hypertension. Less frequent but significant adverse reactions include thrombosis, hypersensitivity, and a slight decrease in platelet count.

Drug interactions: Drug interaction studies have not been performed.

Monitoring parameters: Complete blood count, blood pressure, renal function.

Patient counseling: Inform your physician if you have a history of hypertension or blood clots. Report any pain or swelling in the legs, chest pain, or shortness of breath.

Drug
Renvela® (sevelamer carbonate)

New formulation: Sevelamer carbonate 800 mg tablets. The sevelamer carbonate salt contains the same active moiety as sevelamer hydrochloride (Renagel®). They differ in the counterion, with Renvela using carbonate.

8. Chapter 17: Critical Care, Fluids, and Electrolytes

Drug
DuoDote™ (atropine/pralidoxime chloride)

Class: Nerve agent and insecticide poisoning treatment

Form: Auto-injector

Formulations: Auto-injector delivering 2.1 mg of atropine and 600 mg of pralidoxime

Dose: Administer 1 injection for known or suspected organophosphorous poisoning if the patient experiences two or more mild symptoms (see product information). Repeated dosing is dependent on development of symptoms and response to the first dose. For severe symptoms, immediately administer 3 injections in rapid succession. No more than 3 injections should be administered without definitive medical care.

Mechanism of action: Atropine competitively blocks the effects of acetylcholine at muscarinic cholinergic receptors. Pralidoxime reactivates acetylcholinesterase, which hydrolyzes excess acetylcholine resulting from organophosphorous poisoning.

FDA-approved indications: Treatment of poisoning by organophosphorous nerve agents and organophosphorous insecticides.

Adverse reactions: Muscle tightness and pain at injection site. Additional adverse reactions are related to antimuscarinic effects, including dry eyes, blurred vision, tachycardia, urinary retention, constipation, and anhidrosis.

Drug interactions: No formal drug interaction studies have been conducted.

Monitoring parameters: Wait 10 to 15 minutes after the first injection for effect. If no severe symptoms develop, no additional injections are recommended. Definitive medical care should be sought immediately.

Patient counseling: Treatment with DuoDote should be administered by emergency medical service personnel with adequate training. Do not rely solely on DuoDote for protection from chemical nerve agent and insecticide poisoning.

Drug
Vaprisol® (conivaptan hydrochloride)

New FDA-approved indication: Treatment of hyper-volemic hyponatremia in hospitalized patients.

Drug
Cyanokit® (hydroxocobalamin)

Class: Cyanide poisoning treatment

Form: Injection

Formulations: Two 250 mL glass vials, each containing lyophilized hydroxocobalamin 2.5 g for reconstitution

Dose: The starting dose for adults is 5 g (two 2.5 g vials) of hydroxocobalamin administered by intra-venous infusion over 15 minutes. Depending on the severity of the poisoning and the clinical response, a second dose of 5 g may be administered by intra-venous infusion over 15 minutes to 2 hours for a total dose of 10 g.

Mechanism of action: Each hydroxocobalamin mole-cule can bind one cyanide ion, which is excreted in the urine.

FDA-approved indication: Treatment of known or sus-pected cyanide poisoning.

Adverse reactions: Transient chromaturia, rash, ery-thema, increased blood pressure, nausea, headache, and injection site reactions.

Drug interactions: No formal drug interaction studies have been conducted. The safety of co-administration with other cyanide antidotes has not been established.

Monitoring parameters: Cyanokit should be adminis-tered in conjunction with appropriate airway, ventila-tory, and circulatory support.

Patient counseling: Skin redness may last for up to 2 weeks and urine coloration may last for up to 5 weeks after administration. Patients should avoid direct sun-light during this time.

9. Chapter 18: Nutrition

Drug
Calomist™ (cyanocobalamin USP)

New formulation: Nasal spray supplied in 30 mL plas-tic bottles containing 18 mL of solution. Each actua-tion supplies 25 mcg of cyanocobalamin in 0.1 mL. Each bottle delivers 60 sprays.

Dose: One spray in each nostril daily (25 mcg per nos-tril, total daily dose 50 mcg). Dose may be increased to one spray in each nostril twice daily for patients with an inadequate response to once-daily dosing.

10. Chapter 19: Oncology

Drug
Campath® (alemtuzumab)

New FDA-approved indication: Alemtuzumab is indicated as a single agent for the treatment of B-cell chronic lymphocytic leukemia and is now approved for previously untreated chronic lymphocytic leukemia.

Drug
Emend® (aprepitant; fosaprepitant dimeglumine)

New formulation: Emend is now available in an intravenous formulation (fosaprepitant dimeglumine) supplied in a 115 mg single-dose vial for injection. The oral formulation of Emend (aprepitant) is still available in 80 mg and 125 mg capsules.

Drug
Treanda® (bendamustine hydrochloride)

Class: Alkylating agent

Form: Injection

Formulations: Supplied in individual cartons of 20 mL amber single-use vials containing 100 mg of bendamustine hydrochloride powder

Dose: Initial dose is 100 mg/m^2 infused intravenously over 30 minutes on days 1 and 2 of a 28-day cycle, up to 6 cycles. Dose modifications may be needed for adverse events.

Mechanism of action: The exact mechanism of action of bendamustine is not known. Bendamustine is a bifunctional mechlorethamine derivative. It forms covalent bonds with electron-rich nucleophilic moieties. This bonding may lead to cell death through several pathways.

FDA-approved indication: Treatment of patients with chronic lymphocytic leukemia.

Adverse reactions: Most common adverse reactions (frequency ≥15%) are neutropenia, pyrexia, thrombocytopenia, nausea, anemia, leukopenia, and vomiting. Infusion reactions have been reported with bendamustine. Symptoms include fever, chills, pruritus, and rash. Measures to prevent severe reactions, including antihistamines, antipyretics, and corticosteroids, should be initiated in patients with minor and moderate (Grades 1 and 2) reactions. Discontinuation of bendamustine should be considered in patients with severe (Grade 3 or 4) reactions. Preventive measures for tumor lysis syndrome may be needed, depending on patient risk.

Drug interactions: Bendamustine has active metabolites that are formed via cytochrome P450 1A2. Inhibitors of CYP1A2 (e.g., fluvoxamine, ciprofloxacin) may increase plasma concentrations of bendamustine and decrease plasma concentrations of active metabolites. Inducers of CYP1A2 (e.g., omeprazole, smoking) may decrease plasma concentrations of bendamustine and increase plasma concentrations of active metabolites.

Monitoring parameters: Complete blood count, metabolic panel, renal function, and liver function tests.

Patient counseling: Patients should be informed of the possibility of allergic reactions, myelosuppression, fatigue, nausea and vomiting, diarrhea, and rash.

Drug
Avastin® (bevacizumab)

New FDA-approved indication: Bevacizumab is now approved in combination with paclitaxel for the first-line treatment of metastatic HER2-negative breast cancer.

Drug
Velcade® (bortezomib)

New FDA-approved indication: Bortezomib is now indicated for the treatment of previously untreated multiple myeloma.

Drug
Sprycel® (dasatinib)

New dose: The starting dose of dasatinib is now 100 mg daily for chronic-phase chronic myelogenous leukemia.

Drug
Totect™ (dexrazoxane)

New formulation: The Totect formulation of dexrazoxane is supplied as 500 mg dexrazoxane in a single-use vial and is packaged in a carton containing 10 vials of dexrazoxane for injection and 10 vials of diluent.

New FDA-approved indication: Treatment of extravasation resulting from intravenous anthracycline chemotherapy.

Drug
Taxotere® (docetaxel)

New FDA-approved indication: Docetaxel is now approved in combination with cisplatin and fluorouracil for induction treatment of head and neck cancer; locally advanced squamous cell carcinoma.

Drug
Ixempra™ (ixabepilone)

Class: Microtubule inhibitor

Form: Injection

Formulations: Ixempra kit for injection 15 mg and 45 mg

Dose: The recommended dose of ixabepilone is 40 mg/m^2 infused intravenously over 3 hours every 3 weeks. Dose reductions are required for patients with elevations in AST, ALT, or bilirubin.

Mechanism of action: Ixabepilone binds directly to β-tubulin subunits on microtubules; this interferes with microtubule dynamics. This may lead to a block in the mitotic phase of the cell division cycle, leading to cell death.

FDA-approved indications: Ixabepilone in combination with capecitabine is indicated for treatment of metastatic or locally advanced breast cancer in patients after failure of an anthracycline and a taxane. Ixabepilone as monotherapy is indicated for treatment of metastatic or locally advanced breast cancer in patients after failure of an anthracycline, a taxane, and capecitabine.

Adverse reactions: The most common adverse reactions are peripheral sensory neuropathy, fatigue/asthenia, myalgia/arthralgia, alopecia, nausea, vomiting, stomatitis/mucositis, diarrhea, and musculoskeletal pain. Less common adverse reactions during combination treatment include palmar-plantar erythrodysesthesia syndrome, anorexia, abdominal pain, nail disorders, and constipation. Hematologic abnormalities, including neutropenia, anemia, and thrombocytopenia, are common.

Drug interactions: Strong cytochrome P450 3A4 inhibitors may increase ixabepilone exposure and the risk for adverse events. Concomitant administration should be avoided and dose adjustments may be required. Cytochrome P450 3A4 inducers may lead to reduced exposure and subtherapeutic levels; concomi-tant administration should be avoided. Ixabepilone does not inhibit CYP enzymes at relevant clinical concentrations.

Monitoring parameters: Liver function tests, complete blood count, metabolic panel, peripheral neuropathy, and disease response or progression.

Patient counseling: Ixabepilone should not be used in patients with a history of severe reactions to Cremophor® EL. Severe allergic reactions are most likely to occur during the infusion. Patients should notify their health care provider if any of the following occur: itching; hives; rash; flushed face; sudden swelling of face, throat, or tongue; chest tightness; trouble breathing; and feeling dizzy or faint. Additional counseling points include information regarding adverse events.

Drug
Fusilev™ (levoleucovorin)

Class: Folate analog

Form: Injection

Formulations: Levoleucovorin lyophilized powder 50 mg for solution for intravenous injection

Dose: Rescue recommendations are based on a methotrexate dose of 12 g/m^2 administered by intravenous infusion over 4 hours. Levoleucovorin rescue at a dose of 7.5 mg (approximately 5 mg/m^2) every 6 hours for 10 doses starts 24 hours after the beginning of the methotrexate infusion. Determine serum creatinine and methotrexate levels at least once daily. Continue levoleucovorin administration, hydration, and urinary alkalinization (pH of 7.0 or greater) until the methotrexate level is below 5×10^{-8} M (0.05 micromolar). The dose may need to be adjusted.

Mechanism of action: Levoleucovorin does not require reduction by the enzyme dihydrofolate reductase in order to participate in reactions utilizing folates as a source of "one-carbon" moieties. Administration of levoleucovorin can counteract the effects of methotrexate, which acts by inhibiting dihydrofolate reductase.

FDA-approved indications: Levoleucovorin rescue is indicated after high-dose methotrexate therapy in osteosarcoma. It is also indicated to diminish the toxicity and counteract the effects of impaired methotrexate elimination and of inadvertent overdosage of folic acid antagonists.

Adverse reactions: Allergic reactions to levoleucovorin have been reported. Other adverse events, which may be related to the high-dose methotrexate, include nausea, vomiting, and stomatitis.

Drug interactions: Folic acid in large amounts may counteract the antiepileptic effect of phenobarbital, phenytoin, and primidone and increase the frequency of seizures in susceptible children. Levoleucovorin may share these effects with folic acid. Levoleucovorin may increase the toxicity of fluorouracil.

Monitoring parameters: Renal function, serum electrolytes, metabolic panel, methotrexate level, urine pH, complete blood count.

Patient counseling: Inform your prescriber if you have had an allergic reaction to leucovorin or levoleucovorin, and if you have any kidney problems or difficulty urinating.

Drug
Tasigna® (nilotinib)

Class: Bcr-Abl kinase inhibitor

Form: Capsules

Formulations: 200 mg capsules

Dose: Initial dose 400 mg twice daily. Dose adjustments may be required for adverse events and drug interactions.

Mechanism of action: Nilotinib stabilizes the inactive conformation of Abl protein. This inhibits the function of Bcr-Abl kinase. Nilotinib also has inhibitory activity on PDGFR and c-Kit.

FDA-approved indications: Treatment of chronic-phase and accelerated-phase Philadelphia chromosome-positive chronic myelogenous leukemia in adult patients resistant to or intolerant to prior therapy that included imatinib.

Adverse reactions: Rash, pruritus, nausea, fatigue, diarrhea, constipation, neutropenia, thrombocytopenia, neutropenic fever, elevations in liver function tests, hypophosphatemia, hypomagnesemia, and elevated lipase. Rare but potentially fatal QTc interval prolongation.

Drug interactions: Nilotinib is a competitive inhibitor of cytochrome P450 3A4, cytochrome P450 2C8, cytochrome P450 2C9, cytochrome P450 2D6, and UGT1A1 in vitro, potentially increasing the concentrations of drugs eliminated by these enzymes.

Monitoring parameters: Nilotinib undergoes metabolism by CYP3A4; administration of strong inhibitors or inducers of CYP3A4 can increase or decrease nilotinib concentrations significantly.

Patient counseling: Take on a regular schedule, on an empty stomach with a glass of water, 2 hours after or 1 hour before eating. Inform prescribing physician of all other medications, including over-the-counter products and herbal products.

Drug
Nexavar® (sorafenib)

New FDA-approved indication: Sorafenib is now indicated for the treatment of unresectable hepatocellular carcinoma.

Drug
Hycamtin® (topotecan)

New formulation: Topotecan capsules 0.25 mg and 1 mg

New FDA-approved indication: Treatment of patients with relapsed small-cell lung cancer.

11. Chapter 20: Solid Organ Transplantation

Drug
HepaGam B™ (hepatitis immune globulin intravenous [human])

New FDA-approved indication: To prevent recurrence of hepatitis B following liver transplantation in patients positive for HBsAg. HepaGam B should be administered intravenously for this indication.

Dose: For prevention of hepatitis B recurrence, HepaGam B should be administered intravenously at a dose of 20,000 international units (IU), with the first dose administered during the anhepatic phase of the procedure. Postoperatively, doses are administered daily on days 1 through 7. Weeks 2 through 12 doses are administered every 2 weeks starting at day 14 postoperatively. From month 4 onward, doses are administered monthly. Weekly monitoring of serum anti-HBs is recommended to attain serum anti-HBs >500 IU/L.

Drug
Prograf® (tacrolimus)

New FDA-approved indication: Prophylaxis of organ rejection in patients receiving allogeneic heart transplants.

12. Chapter 21: Gastrointestinal Diseases

Drug
Humira® (adalimumab)

Class: Tumor necrosis factor (TNF) blocker

New FDA-approved indication: Treatment of Crohn's disease. Review the chapter on rheumatoid arthritis, osteoarthritis, gout, and lupus for additional information.

Drug
Entereg® (alvimopan)

Class: Opioid receptor antagonist

Form: Capsule

Formulations: Capsules containing 12 mg alvimopan

Dose: Dosing is initiated with one 12 mg capsule administered 30 minutes to 5 hours prior to surgery, followed by 12 mg twice daily for up to 7 days for a maximum of 15 doses.

Mechanism of action: Alvimopan competitively binds to gastrointestinal tract μ-opioid receptors and antagonizes the peripheral effects of opioids on gastrointestinal motility and secretion. This selective gastrointestinal opioid antagonism occurs without reversing the central analgesic effects of μ-opioid agonists.

FDA-approved indications: Alvimopan is indicated to accelerate the time to upper and lower gastrointestinal recovery following partial large or small bowel resection with primary anastomosis.

Adverse reactions: Urinary retention, back pain, flatulence, and hypokalemia.

Drug interactions: According to in vitro data, alvimopan is not a substrate of CYP enzymes. Alvimopan is unlikely to affect the pharmacokinetics of medications via interaction with CYP enzymes.

Monitoring parameters: Bowel recovery, constipation, diarrhea, serum electrolytes.

Patient counseling: Patients recently exposed to opioids are expected to be more sensitive to the effects of μ-opioid receptor antagonists. Clinical signs of increased sensitivity would likely be limited to the gastrointestinal tract (e.g., abdominal pain, nausea and vomiting, diarrhea).

Drug
Pylera™ (bismuth subcitrate potassium, metronidazole, and tetracycline hydrochloride)

Class: Combination antimicrobial

Form: Capsule

Formulations: Capsules containing 140 mg bismuth subcitrate potassium, 125 mg metronidazole, and 125 mg tetracycline hydrochloride

Dose: 3 capsules 4 times a day, after meals and at bedtime for 10 days.

Mechanism of action: Tetracycline hydrochloride interacts with the 30S subunits of the bacterial ribosome and inhibits protein synthesis. Metronidazole is metabolized through reductive pathways into reactive intermediates that have cytotoxic action. The antibacterial action of bismuth salts is not well understood.

FDA-approved indications: In combination with omeprazole, treatment of patients with *Helicobacter pylori* infection and duodenal ulcer disease to eradicate *H. pylori.*

Adverse reactions: Stool abnormality, diarrhea, dyspepsia, abdominal pain, nausea, headache, flu syndrome, taste perversion, asthenia, and dizziness.

Drug interactions:
Metronidazole:
- May cause elevation of serum lithium concentrations
- Should not be given to patients who have taken disulfiram within the last 2 weeks
- Has been reported to potentiate the anticoagulant effect of warfarin
- Drugs that decrease microsomal liver enzyme activity, such as cimetidine, may prolong the half-life and decrease plasma clearance of metronidazole
- Microsomal liver enzyme inducers, such as phenytoin or phenobarbital, may accelerate the elimination of metronidazole. Impaired phenytoin clearance has also been reported
- Avoid alcohol during therapy and for at least 1 day afterward. Abdominal cramps, nausea, vomiting, headaches, and flushing may occur.

Tetracycline:
- Concurrent use with methoxyflurane has been reported to result in fatal renal toxicity
- Effectiveness of oral contraceptives may be decreased
- Has been shown to depress plasma prothrombin time
- May interfere with the bactericidal action of penicillin.

Monitoring parameters: Serum lithium concentrations and serum creatinine if taking lithium; PT/INR for patients taking anticoagulant therapy.

Patient counseling: One omeprazole 20 mg capsule should be taken twice daily with therapy after the morning and evening meals for 10 days. Alcoholic beverages should be avoided during and for at least 1 day after therapy. Avoid sun exposure. Use a different or additional form of contraception if taking oral contraceptives.

Drug
Cimzia® (certolizumab pegol)

Class: Tumor necrosis factor (TNF) blocker

Form: Injection

Formulations: Supplied in a pack containing 200 mg lyophilized drug with diluent and syringe

Dose: Initial dose 400 mg subcutaneously and at weeks 2 and 4. If response occurs, follow with 400 mg subcutaneously every 4 weeks.

Mechanism of action: Certolizumab binds to human TNF-α, which has a central role in the inflammatory process.

FDA-approved indication: Certolizumab is indicated for reducing signs and symptoms of Crohn's disease and maintaining clinical response in adult patients with moderately to severely active disease who have had an inadequate response to conventional therapy.

Adverse reactions: Immunosuppression leading to increased risk for rare but serious infections, including opportunistic infections such as tuberculosis. Some TNF blockers have been reported to increase the risk of malignancy, including lymphoma. Hypersensitivity reactions have been reported. If such a reaction occurs, discontinue further administration of certolizumab.

Drug interactions: Concurrent administration with an interleukin-1 antagonist may increase the risk for serious infections. Do not administer concomitantly with live vaccines. Certolizumab may cause an erroneously elevated aPTT.

Monitoring parameters: Complete blood count, liver function tests, renal function.

Patient counseling: Most common adverse events include infection and joint pain. Rare but serious adverse events include serious infection, heart failure, allergic reactions, lupus-like syndrome, blood problems, and nervous system problems.

Drug
Nexium® (esomeprazole magnesium)

Class: Proton pump inhibitor

New formulations: Delayed-release oral suspension, 20 mg and 40 mg packets in unit dose packages of 30

Drug
Amitiza® (lubiprostone)

New FDA-approved indication: Treatment of irritable bowel syndrome with constipation in adult women.

Drug
Lialda™ (mesalamine delayed release)

Class: Anti-inflammatory agent

Form: Tablet

Formulations: Delayed-release tablet containing 1.2 g mesalamine

Dose: Two to four 1.2 g tablets once daily with a meal.

Mechanism of action: Mesalamine may diminish inflammation of chronic inflammatory bowel disease by blocking cyclooxygenase and inhibiting prostaglandin production in the colon.

FDA-approved indication: Induction of remission in patients with active, mild to moderate ulcerative colitis.

Adverse reactions: Abdominal pain, constipation, flatulence, and headache. Safety and effectiveness beyond 8 weeks have not been established.

Drug interactions: The concurrent use of mesalamine with known nephrotoxic agents, including NSAIDs, may increase the risk of renal reactions; concurrent treatment with azathioprine or 6-mercaptopurine may increase potential for blood disorders.

Monitoring parameters: Renal function for patients with renal disease.

Patient counseling: Swallow tablets whole. Take care not to break the outer coating, which is designed to protect the active ingredient and ensure its availability throughout the colon.

Drug
Relistor™ (methylnaltrexone bromide)

Class: Opioid receptor antagonist

Form: Subcutaneous injection

Formulations: Vials for injection containing 12 mg methylnaltrexone bromide per 0.6 mL

Dose: The recommended dose is 8 mg for patients weighing 38 to less than 62 kg (84 to less than 136 lb) or 12 mg for patients weighing 62 to 114 kg (136 to 251 lb). Patients whose weight falls outside these ranges should be dosed at 0.15 mg/kg. The usual schedule is one dose every other day as needed, but no more frequently than one dose in a 24-hour period.

Mechanism of action: Methylnaltrexone is a peripherally acting selective antagonist of binding to the μ-opioid receptor. It decreases the constipating effects of opioids without interfering with opioid-mediated analgesic effects.

FDA-approved indications: Treatment of opioid-induced constipation in patients with advanced illness who are receiving palliative care, when response to laxative therapy has not been sufficient.

Adverse reactions: Abdominal pain, nausea, flatulence, dizziness, diarrhea.

Drug interactions: Methylnaltrexone is a weak inhibitor of cytochrome P450 2D6. The clinical relevance of this interaction is not known.

Monitoring parameters: Gastrointestinal function, serum electrolytes.

Patient counseling: In clinical trials, approximately one-third of patients experienced laxation within 30 minutes of dosing. Discontinue if severe or persistent diarrhea develops. Store the medication out of reach of children at 68° to 77° F. Do not freeze.

Drug
Tysabri® (natalizumab)

New FDA-approved indication: Inducing and maintaining clinical response and remission in adult patients with moderately to severely active Crohn's disease with evidence of inflammation who have had an inadequate response to or are unable to tolerate conventional therapies and inhibitors of TNF-α.

Drug
Protonix® (pantoprazole sodium)

New formulation: Delayed-release oral suspension; supplied as pantoprazole sodium enteric-coated granules in a 40 mg unit dose packet. This is intended to be administered in apple juice or applesauce.

Drug
MoviPrep® (PEG-3350, sodium sulfate, sodium chloride, potassium chloride, sodium ascorbate, and ascorbic acid for oral solution)

Class: Colon preparation

Form: Powder for reconstitution

Formulations: 4 pouches (2 of pouch A and 2 of pouch B) containing powder for reconstitution. Each pouch A contains PEG-3350 100 g, sodium sulfate 7.5 g, sodium chloride 2.69 g, and potassium chloride 1.015 g. Each pouch B contains ascorbic acid 4.7 g and sodium ascorbate 5.9 g. One pouch A and 1 pouch B should be dissolved together in 1 L of lukewarm water.

Dose: 2 L of solution (with 1 additional liter of clear fluids) taken orally prior to the colonoscopy, using either split-dose or full-dose method.

Mechanism of action: Produces a watery stool, leading to cleansing of the colon.

FDA-approved indication: Cleansing of the colon as preparation for colonoscopy.

Adverse reactions: Abdominal distention, abdominal pain, thirst, nausea, and vomiting.

Drug interactions: Oral medications administered within 1 hour of the start of treatment may be flushed from the gastrointestinal tract and the medication may not be absorbed.

Monitoring parameters: Consider performing baseline and post-colonoscopy laboratory tests (BUN, calcium, creatinine, potassium, and sodium levels). If a patient experiences severe bloating, abdominal distention, or abdominal pain, administration should be slowed or temporarily discontinued until the symptoms abate.

Patient counseling: Advise patients to adequately hydrate before, during, and after treatment. Patients may have clear soup and/or plain yogurt for dinner, finishing the evening meal at least 1 hour prior to the start of treatment. No solid food should be taken from the start of treatment until after the colonoscopy. The first bowel movement may occur approximately 1 hour after the start of treatment.

13. Chapter 22: Rheumatoid Arthritis, Osteoarthritis, Gout, and Lupus

Drug
Humira® (adalimumab)

Class: Tumor necrosis factor (TNF) blocker

New FDA-approved indication: Treatment of psoriatic arthritis. Also review the chapter on gastrointestinal diseases for additional information.

14. Chapter 23: Pain Management and Migraines

Drug
Soma® (carisoprodol)

Class: Skeletal muscle relaxant

New formulation: 250 mg tablet

Dose: Recommended dose is 250 mg to 350 mg three times a day and at bedtime.

Drug
Flector® Patch (diclofenac epolamine)

Class: Non-opioid analgesic; nonsteroidal anti-inflammatory drug (NSAID)

Form: Topical patch

Formulations: Topical patch containing 1.3% diclofenac epolamine

Dose: Apply one patch to the most painful area twice daily.

Mechanism of action: The exact mechanism of action in unknown, but the anti-inflammatory activity may be attributed to the ability to inhibit prostaglandin synthesis.

FDA-approved indications: Topical treatment of acute pain due to minor strains, sprains, and contusions.

Adverse reactions: Application site reactions (pruritus, dermatitis, burning), nausea, dysgeusia, dyspepsia, headache, paresthesia, and somnolence.

Drug interactions:
- NSAIDs may diminish the antihypertensive effect of ACE inhibitors
- Concomitant administration of diclofenac and aspirin is not recommended because of the potential for increased adverse effects
- NSAID inhibition of prostaglandin synthesis may lead to a reduction of the natriuretic effect of furosemide and thiazides, elevation in plasma lithium levels, and a decrease in renal lithium clearance
- NSAIDs may enhance the toxicity of methotrexate
- The effects of warfarin and NSAIDs on GI bleeding are synergistic.

Monitoring parameters: Signs or symptoms of GI bleeding, signs of renal failure in patients taking diuretics, signs of lithium toxicity in patients taking lithium, and PT/INR.

Patient counseling: Avoid contact of patch with eyes and mucosa. Patch should not be applied to damaged or non-intact skin. Patch should not be worn when bathing or showering.

Drug
Voltaren® Gel (diclofenac sodium)

Class: Nonsteroidal anti-inflammatory drug

New formulation: 20 g tube (physician's sample) and 100 g tube containing 10 mg of diclofenac sodium per gram of gel or 1%

Dose: Total dose should not exceed 32 g per day, over all affected joints.
   • Lower extremities: Apply the gel (4 g) to the affected area 4 times daily. Do not apply more than 16 g daily to any one affected joint of the lower extremities.
   • Upper extremities: Apply the gel (2 g) to the affected area 4 times daily. Do not apply more than 8 g daily to any one affected joint of the upper extremities.

Drug
Fentora™ (fentanyl)

Class: Opioid analgesic

Form: Buccal tablet

Formulations: Fentanyl citrate equivalent to fentanyl base: 100, 200, 300, 400, 600, and 800 mcg buccal tablet

Dose: Initial dose should be 100 mcg. For patients switching from oral transmucosal fentanyl citrate to Fentora, the starting dose should be initiated according to recommendations available in the manufacturer's prescribing information.

Mechanism of action: Precise mechanism of analgesia is unknown; μ-opioid receptor agonist.

FDA-approved indication: Management of breakthrough pain in patients with cancer who are already receiving and are tolerant to opioid therapy for their underlying persistent cancer pain.

Adverse reactions: Nausea, fatigue, dizziness, somnolence, headache, physical dependence and withdrawal, respiratory depression, and application site reactions.

Drug interactions:
   • Ritonavir may decrease the clearance of fentanyl
   • Not recommended for use in patients who have received MAO inhibitors within 14 days
   • Concomitant use of other CNS depressants, potent inhibitors of the CYP3A4 enzyme, and alcoholic beverages may produce increased depressant effects.

Monitoring parameters: Mental and respiratory status and pain reduction.

Patient counseling: Children exposed to fentanyl are at high risk of fatal respiratory depression—keep out of reach of children. Fentanyl is a medication with abuse potential.

Drug
Kadian® (morphine sulfate extended release)

Class: Opioid analgesic

New formulation: 100 mg and 200 mg extended-release capsules

Drug
Opana® ER (oxymorphone hydrochloride)

Class: Opioid analgesic

New formulation: 5 mg, 10 mg, 20 mg, and 40 mg extended-release tablets

Drug
Treximet™ (sumatriptan succinate/naproxen sodium)

Class: Selective 5-hydroxytryptamine$_1$ (5-HT$_1$) receptor subtype agonist and nonsteroidal anti-inflammatory drug

New formulation: Sumatriptan 85 mg/naproxen sodium 500 mg tablets

15. Chapter 24: Seizure Disorders

Drug
Keppra® (levetiracetam)

Class: Antiepileptic

New FDA-approved indications: Adjunctive therapy in the treatment of myoclonic seizures in adults and adolescents 12 years of age and older with juvenile myoclonic epilepsy. Adjunctive therapy in the treatment of primary generalized tonic-clonic seizures in adults and children 6 years of age and older with idiopathic generalized epilepsy.

New formulation: Single-use 500 mg/5 mL injection vial

16. Chapter 25: Psychiatric Disease

Drug
Abilify® (aripiprazole)

Class: Atypical antipsychotic

New FDA-approved indications: Acute and maintenance treatment of schizophrenia in adolescents 10 to 17 years of age. Acute and maintenance treatment of manic and mixed episodes associated with bipolar I disorder with or without psychotic features in pediatric patients 10 to 17 years of age. Adjunctive therapy to either lithium or valproate for the acute treatment of manic and mixed episodes associated with bipolar I disorder with or without psychotic features in adults and pediatric patients 10 to 17 years of age.

Dose:

- Schizophrenia in adolescents: initial dose 2 mg daily, recommended dose 10 mg daily, maximum dose 30 mg daily
- Bipolar mania in pediatrics as monotherapy or as an adjunct to lithium or valproate: initial dose 2 mg daily, recommended dose 10 mg daily, maximum dose 30 mg daily.

Drug
Aplenzin® (bupropion hydrobromide)

Class: Aminoketone antidepressant

New formulation: 174 mg, 348 mg, and 522 mg extended-release tablets

Dose: Starting dose 174 mg. Usual target dose 348 mg daily.

Drug
Pristiq® (desvenlafaxine succinate extended release)

Class: Selective serotonin and norepinephrine reuptake inhibitor (SNRI)

Form: Extended-release tablet

Formulations: 50 mg and 100 mg tablets

Dose: 50 mg once daily with or without food.

Mechanism of action: Potently and selectively inhibits reuptake of serotonin and norepinephrine, thereby potentiating the neurotransmitter activity in the central nervous system.

FDA-approved indication: Treatment of major depressive disorder.

Adverse reactions: Nausea, vomiting, xerostomia, headache, dizziness, insomnia, hyperhidrosis, constipation, somnolence, fatigue, blurred vision, decreased appetite, anxiety, raised serum cholesterol, raised serum triglycerides, and erectile dysfunction.

Drug interactions: Other CNS-active drugs, monoamine oxidase inhibitors (MAOIs), serotonergic drugs, nonsteroidal anti-inflammatory drugs, aspirin, and warfarin. Inhibitors of CYP3A4 and drugs metabolized by CYP2D6 (desipramine) may result in higher concentrations of desvenlafaxine. Coadministration with drugs metabolized by CYP3A4 (midazolam) may result in decreased concentrations of drugs metabolized by CYP3A4.

Monitoring parameters: Serum cholesterol and triglycerides, blood pressure, signs and symptoms of serotonin syndrome, and signs and symptoms of hyponatremia.

Patient counseling: Symptomatic improvement may not be seen for several weeks. Do not take MAOIs within 14 days before or after taking desvenlafaxine. Avoid activities that require mental alertness or coordination until the effects of desvenlafaxine are realized. Report worsening depression, suicidal ideation, or unusual changes in behavior. Sudden discontinuation of desvenlafaxine may precipitate withdrawal symptoms and should therefore be avoided.

Drug
Cymbalta® (duloxetine hydrochloride delayed release)

Class: Selective serotonin and norepinephrine reuptake inhibitor (SSNRI)

New FDA-approved indication: Management of fibromyalgia.

Drug
Luvox® CR (fluvoxamine maleate extended release)

Class: Selective serotonin reuptake inhibitor (SSRI)

New formulation: 100 mg and 150 mg extended-release capsules

Drug
Vyvanse® (lisdexamfetamine dimesylate)

Class: Amphetamine

New FDA-approved indication: Attention-deficit/hyperactivity disorder in adults.

Drug
Concerta® (methylphenidate hydrochloride extended release)

Class: Central nervous system stimulant

New FDA-approved indication: Attention-deficit/hyperactivity disorder in adults.

Dose: Recommended starting dose 18 or 36 mg daily; recommended dosage range 18 mg to 72 mg daily.

Drug
Seroquel® XR (quetiapine fumarate)

Class: Atypical antipsychotic

New FDA-approved indication: Maintenance treatment of schizophrenia in adults.

Drug
Effexor XR® (venlafaxine hydrochloride extended release)

Class: Selective serotonin and norepinephrine reuptake inhibitor

New formulation: 225 mg extended-release tablet

17. Chapter 26: Common Dermatologic Disorders

Drug
Humira® (adalimumab)

Class: Tumor necrosis factor blocker

New FDA-approved indication: Moderate to severe chronic plaque psoriasis.

Dose: Initial dose 80 mg, then 40 mg every other week starting 1 week after the initial dose.

Drug
Differin® (adapalene)

Class: Topical retinoid

New formulation: Gel containing 0.3% adapalene in a 45 g tube

Drug
Taclonex® (calcipotriene/betamethasone dipropionate)

Class: Topical corticosteroid

New formulation: Topical suspension. Calcipotriene 0.005% and betamethasone dipropionate 0.064% in 60 g and 100 g collapsible tubes.

Dose: Apply an adequate layer to the affected area(s) once daily for up to 4 weeks. Maximum weekly dose should not exceed 100 g.

Drug
Ziana™ (clindamycin phosphate/tretinoin)

Class: Topical lincosamide antibiotic and retinoid combination

Form: Gel

Formulations: Clindamycin phosphate 1.2% and tretinoin 0.025% gel in 30 and 60 g tubes

Dose: Apply a pea-sized amount to the entire face once daily at bedtime. Do not apply to eyes, mouth, angles of the nose, or mucous membranes.

Mechanism of action: Clindamycin binds to the 50S ribosomal subunits of susceptible bacteria and prevents elongation of peptide chains by interfering with peptidyl transfer, thereby suppressing bacterial protein synthesis. Current evidence suggests that topical tretinoin decreases cohesiveness of follicular epithelial cells with decreased microcomedo formation. Tretinoin also stimulates mitotic activity and increased turnover of follicular epithelial cells, causing extrusion of comedones.

FDA-approved indication: Topical treatment of acne vulgaris in patients 12 years of age or older.

Adverse reactions: Erythema, scaling, itching, burning, stinging, and dry skin.

Drug interactions: Concomitant topical medication and/or products may cause increased skin irritation and should be used with caution. Erythromycin-containing products and neuromuscular blocking agents should not be used concomitantly.

Monitoring parameters: Signs of skin irritation.

Patient counseling: Avoid excessive exposure to the sun, cold, and wind. If your face becomes sunburned, stop treatment until your skin has healed. Do not apply more than once a day.

Drug
Olux® (clobetasol propionate)

Class: Corticosteroid

New formulation: Topical foam, 0.05%

Drug
Desonate™ (desonide)

Class: Topical corticosteroid

New formulation: Gel containing 0.05% desonide in 15, 30, and 60 g tubes

Drug
Verdeso™ (desonide)

Class: Topical corticosteroid

Form: Emulsion aerosol foam

Formulations: Foam containing 0.05% desonide in 50 g and 100 g aluminum cans

Dose: Apply a thin layer to the affected area(s) twice daily. Treatment should not exceed 4 consecutive weeks.

Mechanism of action: Desonide's exact mechanism of action is unknown, but it is thought to stimulate phospholipase A2-inhibitory proteins, thus blocking the release of arachidonic acid, a precursor of leukotrienes and prostaglandins, which are potent mediators of inflammation.

FDA-approved indication: Treatment of mild to moderate atopic dermatitis in patients 3 months of age and older.

Adverse reactions: Application site reactions, infections, headache, and cough.

Drug interactions: A theoretical interaction between bupropion and systemic steroids, which lower the seizure threshold.

Monitoring parameters: Reduced inflammation and pruritus and hypothalamic-pituitary-adrenal (HPA) axis suppression tests.

Patient counseling: Prior to use, shake the can and dispense the foam by inverting the can. Apply the smallest amount of foam necessary to cover the affected area(s). Use for the minimum amount of time necessary to achieve desired results, because of the potential to suppress the HPA axis. The treated skin area should not be bandaged.

Drug
Yaz® (drospirenone/ethinyl estradiol)

Class: Oral contraceptive

New FDA-approved indication: Treatment of moderate acne vulgaris in women at least 14 years of age who have achieved menarche. Please also see "Women's Health" chapter for additional information.

Drug
Locoid® (hydrocortisone butyrate)

Class: Corticosteroid

New formulation: Lotion containing 0.1% hydrocortisone butyrate

Drug
Extina® (ketoconazole)

Class: Antifungal

Form: Foam

Formulations: Foam containing 2% ketoconazole in 50 and 100 g tubes

Dose: Apply to affected area(s) twice daily for 4 weeks.

Mechanism of action: The mechanism of action of ketoconazole in the treatment of seborrheic dermatitis is not known.

FDA-approved indication: Topical treatment of seborrheic dermatitis in immunocompetent patients 12 years of age and older.

Adverse reactions: Application site reactions.

Drug interactions: Drug interaction studies have not been conducted.

Monitoring parameters: Contact sensitization, including photoallergenicity.

Patient counseling: Do not apply foam directly to hands. Spray foam directly into the cap of the can or other cool surface. Apply to affected areas using fingertips. Wash hands after application.

Drug
Xolegel™ (ketoconazole USP)

Class: Topical antifungal

Form: Gel

Formulations: Gel containing 2% ketoconazole in a 15 g tube

Dose: Apply to the affected area once daily for 2 weeks.

Mechanism of action: It is postulated that the therapeutic effect of ketoconazole in seborrheic dermatitis is due to the reduction of *Malassezia furfur* (also known as *Pityrosporum ovale*), which leads to death of the organism.

FDA-approved indication: Topical treatment of seborrheic dermatitis in immunocompetent adults and children 12 years of age and older.

Adverse reactions: Headache and application site burning.

Drug interactions: Drug interaction studies have not been conducted.

Monitoring parameters: Severe skin irritation, pruritus, stinging, and contact dermatitis.

Patient counseling: Do not wash the area where you applied the medication for at least 3 hours. Wait at least 20 minutes after application to apply makeup or sunscreens to the affected areas.

Drug
Altabax™ (retapamulin)

Class: Topical antibacterial

Form: Ointment

Formulations: 1% ointment in 5, 10, and 50 g tubes

Dose: Apply a thin layer to the affected area (up to 100 cm^2 in total area in adults or 2% of total body surface area in pediatric patients 9 months of age or older) twice daily for 5 days.

Mechanism of action: Selectively inhibits bacterial protein synthesis by interacting at a site on the 50S subunit of the bacterial ribosome through an interaction that is different from that of other antibiotics.

FDA-approved indications: Treatment of impetigo due to *Staphylococcus aureus* (methicillin-susceptible isolates only) or *Streptococcus pyogenes* in patients 9 months of age or older.

Adverse reactions: Application site irritation.

Drug interactions: Because of low systemic exposure following topical application, dosage adjustments are unnecessary when retapamulin is co-administered with CYP3A4 inhibitors such as ketoconazole. Retapamulin is unlikely to affect the metabolism of other P450 substrates. The effect of concurrent application of other topical products to the same area of skin has not been studied.

Monitoring parameters: Signs and symptoms of sensitization or severe local irritation.

Patient counseling: Wash hands after application if the hands are not the affected area. The treated area may be covered with a sterile bandage or gauze dressing if desired. Use for the full duration recommended; even though symptoms may have improved.

Drug
Veregen™ (sinecatechins)

Class: Topical botanical

Form: Ointment

Formulations: Ointment containing 15% sinecatechins available in a 15 g tube

Dose: Apply three times per day to all external genital and perianal warts.

Mechanism of action: The mechanism of action of sinecatechins is unknown. In vitro, sinecatechins has anti-oxidant activity; the clinical significance of this finding is unknown.

FDA-approved indications: Topical treatment of external genital and perianal warts (condylomata acuminata) in immunocompetent patients 18 years of age and older.

Adverse reactions: Application site reactions, dysuria, skin ulcer, genital herpes simplex, and superinfection.

Drug interactions: Ointment should not be used until skin has healed from other treatments applied to the same area.

Monitoring parameters: Open sores, signs or symptoms of genital herpes simplex, and superinfection of warts.

Patient counseling: Do not wash off the ointment from the treated area before the next application. When you wash the treatment area or bathe, apply the ointment afterwards. The treatment area should not be bandaged.

Drug
Atralin™ (tretinoin)

Class: Retinoic acid derivative

New formulation: 0.05% gel in 45 g tubes

18. Chapter 28: Asthma and Chronic Obstructive Pulmonary Disease

Drug
Brovana™ (arformoterol tartrate)

Class: Long-acting beta$_2$-adrenergic agonist

Form: Aqueous solution

Formulations: Each vial contains 15 mcg/2 mL arformoterol tartrate aqueous solution.

Dose: Inhalation via nebulizer twice daily (morning and evening); daily dosage should not exceed one vial (15 mcg) by inhalation twice daily (30 mcg total daily dose).

Mechanism of action: Selective beta$_2$-adrenergic bronchodilator; stimulation of adenyl cyclase leads to relaxation of bronchial smooth muscle and inhibition of release of mediators of immediate hypersensitivity from cells, particularly mast cells.

FDA-approved indications: Long-term maintenance treatment of bronchoconstriction in patients with chronic obstructive pulmonary disease (COPD), including chronic bronchitis and emphysema. For use by nebulization only.

Adverse reactions: Fever, headache, palpitations, chest pain, rapid heart rate, tremor, and nervousness.

Drug interactions:
- Use additional adrenergic drugs with caution
- Dose adjustments are not necessary with concurrent administration of potent CYP2D6 inhibitors
- Concomitant administration of methylxanthines, steroids, or diuretics may potentiate hypokalemic effect; ECG changes and/or hypokalemia that may result from non-potassium-sparing diuretics can be worsened
- Administer with caution to patients treated with monoamine oxidase inhibitors, tricyclic antidepressants, or drugs known to prolong the QTc interval.

Monitoring parameters: Therapeutic response as indicated by peak expiratory flow rates and supplemental ipratropium and rescue albuterol use.

Patient counseling: Arformoterol is not indicated to relieve acute respiratory symptoms, and extra doses should not be used for that purpose. Patients should not inhale more than one dose at any one time. Use medication by nebulizer only and do not inject or swallow inhalation solution. Protect vials from light and excessive heat.

Drug
Alvesco® (ciclesonide)

Class: Inhaled corticosteroid

New formulation: 80 mcg and 160 mcg inhalers

Drug
Advair DISKUS® 250/50 (fluticasone propionate/salmeterol)

Class: Corticosteroid and long-acting beta$_2$-adrenergic agonist

New FDA-approved indication: Reduction of exacerbations of COPD in patients with a history of exacerbations.

Drug
Advair® HFA (fluticasone propionate/salmeterol)

Class: Anti-inflammatory/bronchodilator combination

New formulation: 45/21 mcg, 115/21 mcg, and 230/21 mcg HFA inhalation aerosol in metered-dose canisters containing 120 metered inhalations

Drug
Foradil® Certihaler® (formoterol fumarate)

Class: Long-acting beta$_2$-adrenergic agonist

Form: Inhalation powder

Formulations: Powder, metered-dose 10 mcg formoterol fumarate; inhaler device delivers 8.5 mcg per dose and contains 60 doses.

Dose: For adults and children 5 years of age and older, the usual dosage is 10 mcg inhalation every 12 hours.

Mechanism of action: Selective beta$_2$-adrenergic bronchodilator; stimulation of adenyl cyclase leads to relaxation of bronchial smooth muscle and inhibition of release of mediators of immediate hypersensitivity from cells, particularly mast cells.

FDA-approved indications: Long-term maintenance treatment of asthma; prevention of bronchospasm in adults and children 5 years of age and older with reversible obstructive airway disease.

Adverse reactions: Nasopharyngitis, headache, cough, nasal congestion, tremor, and rash.

Drug interactions:
- Use additional adrenergic drugs with caution
- Concomitant administration of methylxanthines, steroids, or diuretics may potentiate hypokalemic effect; ECG changes and/or hypokalemia that may result from non-potassium-sparing diuretics can be worsened
- Administer with caution to patients being treated with monoamine oxidase inhibitors, tricyclic antidepressants, or drugs known to prolong the QTc interval
- Administer cardioselective beta-blockers with caution.

Monitoring parameters: Proper inhalation technique, reduction in asthma symptoms, and pulmonary function tests.

Patient counseling: Formoterol is not indicated to relieve acute asthma symptoms, and extra doses should not be used for that purpose. Formoterol should not be used as a substitute for oral or inhaled corticosteroids. Never use a spacer with the device, and never exhale into the device. The device should never be washed and should be kept dry.

Drug
Perforomist™ (formoterol fumarate)

Class: Long-acting beta$_2$-adrenergic agonist

New formulation: 2 mL sterile solution for nebulization in 2.5 mL unit dose vials, carton of 60 vials

Drug
Singulair® (montelukast sodium)

Class: Leukotriene receptor antagonist

New FDA-approved indication: Prevention of exercise-induced bronchoconstriction/asthma in patients 15 years of age and older.

Drug
Flo-Pred® (prednisolone acetate)

Class: Corticosteroid

New formulation: Oral suspension, 5 mg per 5 mL (as 5.6 mg/5 mL of prednisolone acetate) and 15 mg per 5 mL (as 16.7 mg/5 mL of prednisolone acetate)

Drug
Orapred ODT™ (prednisolone sodium phosphate)

Class: Corticosteroid

New formulation: Orally disintegrating tablets available in strengths containing 13.4 mg, 20.2 mg, and 40.3 mg prednisolone sodium phosphate (equivalent to 10 mg, 15 mg, or 30 mg prednisolone base, respectively)

Drug
Zyflo CR™ (zileuton)

Class: Leukotriene synthesis inhibitor

New formulation: 600 mg extended-release tablet

19. Chapter 30: Anti-Infective Agents

Drug
Moxatag™ (amoxicillin extended release)

Class: Penicillin

New formulation: 775 mg extended-release tablet

Dose: 775 mg once daily for 10 days with a meal.

Drug
AzaSite™ (azithromycin)

Class: Macrolide antibiotic

Form: Ophthalmic solution

Formulations: 5 mL bottle containing 2.5 mL of a 1% sterile topical ophthalmic solution, containing a total of 25 mg azithromycin

Dose: Instill 1 drop in the affected eye(s) twice daily 8 to 12 hours apart for the first 2 days, and then instill 1 drop in the affected eye(s) once daily for the next 5 days.

Mechanism of action: Binds to the 50S ribosomal subunit of susceptible microorganisms and interferes with microbial protein synthesis.

FDA-approved indications: Treatment of bacterial conjunctivitis caused by susceptible isolates of CDC coryneform group G, *Haemophilus influenzae*, *Staphylococcus aureus*, *Streptococcus mitis* group, and *Streptococcus pneumoniae*.

Adverse reactions: Eye irritation.

Drug interactions: Drug interaction studies have not been conducted.

Monitoring parameters: Signs of superinfection or bacterial conjunctivitis.

Patient counseling: Thoroughly wash hands prior to use. Avoid contaminating the applicator tip by allowing it to touch the eye, fingers, or other sources. Patients should not wear contact lenses if they have signs or symptoms of bacterial conjunctivitis.

Drug
Doribax™ (doripenem)

Class: Carbapenem

Form: Intravenous infusion

Formulations: 500 mg single-use vial

Dose: 500 mg every 8 hours by intravenous infusion administered over 1 hour for patients ≥18 years of age.

Mechanism of action: Doripenem exerts its bactericidal activity by inhibiting bacterial cell wall biosynthesis.

FDA-approved indications: Treatment of complicated intraabdominal infections. Treatment of complicated urinary tract infections, including pyelonephritis.

Adverse reactions: Headache, nausea, diarrhea, rash, and phlebitis.

Drug interactions: Concomitant administration with probenecid results in increased plasma concentrations of doripenem. Doripenem may reduce serum valproic acid concentrations.

Monitoring parameters: Hypersensitivity reactions and serious skin reactions, and renal function because of extensive excretion via the kidneys.

Patient counseling: Allergic reactions could occur. Serious reactions require immediate treatment. Patients should report any previous hypersensitivity reactions to carbapenems, beta-lactams, or other allergens. The medication should be taken exactly as directed.

Drug
Doryx® (doxycycline hyclate delayed release)

Class: Tetracycline

New formulation: 150 mg delayed-release tablet

Drug
Mycamine® (micafungin sodium)

Class: Echinocandin antifungal

New FDA-approved indication: Treatment of candidemia, acute disseminated candidiasis, *Candida* peritonitis and abscesses.

Drug
Noxafil® (posaconazole)

Class: Triazole antifungal agent

Form: Oral suspension

Formulations: 105 mL cherry-flavored suspension containing 40 mg of posaconazole per milliliter in 4-ounce amber glass bottles with child-resistant closures

Dose: 200 mg (5 mL) three times daily. The duration of therapy is based on recovery from neutropenia or immunosuppression.

Mechanism of action: Blocks the synthesis of ergosterol, a key component of the fungal cell membrane, through the inhibition of the enzyme lanosterol 14α-demethylase and accumulation of methylated sterol precursors.

FDA-approved indications: Prophylaxis of invasive *Aspergillus* and *Candida* infections in severely immunocompromised patients 13 years of age and older; treatment of oropharyngeal candidiasis, including oropharyngeal candidiasis refractory to itraconazole and/or fluconazole.

Adverse reactions: Fever, headache, nausea, vomiting, diarrhea, fatigue, hypertension, anemia, neutropenia, bacteremia, bilirubinemia, hypokalemia, hypomagnesemia, hyperglycemia, thrombocytopenia, insomnia, cough, dyspnea, and rash.

Drug interactions:
- Concomitant administration of rifabutin, phenytoin, and cimetidine may result in lower plasma concentrations of posaconazole
- Posaconazole is an inhibitor primarily of CYP3A4. Plasma concentrations of drugs predominantly metabolized by CYP3A4 may be increased by posaconazole. Dose adjustments and/or monitoring may be necessary for cyclosporine, tacrolimus, rifabutin, midazolam, and phenytoin
- Avoid concomitant use with cimetidine, rifabutin, and phenytoin unless the benefits outweigh the risks.

Monitoring parameters: Liver function tests, electrolytes (potassium, magnesium, and calcium), and phenytoin and cyclosporine whole-blood trough concentrations.

Patient counseling: Take each dose with a full meal or liquid nutritional supplement in order to enhance absorption. Inform your physician if you develop severe diarrhea or vomiting, as these conditions may change blood levels of posaconazole.

Drug
Tyzeka™ (telbivudine)

Class: Synthetic thymidine nucleoside analogue

Form: Film-coated tablets

Formulations: 600 mg tablet

Dose: Recommended dose for adults and adolescents 16 years of age or older is 600 mg once daily. Adjustment of dose interval is required in patients with creatinine clearance <50 mL/min, including those with ESRD on hemodialysis. For patients with ESRD, telbivudine should be administered after hemodialysis.

Mechanism of action: Telbivudine inhibits HBV DNA polymerase (reverse transcriptase) by competing with the natural substrate, thymidine 5′-triphosphate. Incorporation of telbivudine 5′-triphosphate into viral DNA causes DNA chain termination, resulting in inhibition of HBV replication.

FDA-approved indication: Treatment of chronic hepatitis B in adult patients with evidence of viral replication and either evidence of persistent elevations in serum aminotransferases (ALT or AST) or histologically active disease.

Adverse reactions: Upper respiratory tract infection, fatigue, malaise, abdominal pain, nasopharyngitis, headache, increased blood CPK, cough, nausea, vomiting, lactic acidosis, and severe hepatomegaly with steatosis.

Drug interactions: Telbivudine is eliminated primarily by passive diffusion, so the potential for interactions between telbivudine and other drugs eliminated by renal excretion is low. However, because telbivudine is eliminated primary by renal excretion, co-administration of telbivudine with drugs that alter renal function may alter plasma concentrations of telbivudine. The potential for CYP450-mediated interactions involving telbivudine with other medicinal products is low.

Monitoring parameters: Liver function tests and creatinine clearance.

Patient counseling: Counsel patients about signs of lactic acidosis, hepatotoxicity, and muscle pain. Advise patients to contact their physician immediately if they experience any symptoms of lactic acidosis, hepatotoxicity, or muscle pain. If you miss a dose, take it as soon as you remember, and then take your next dose at its regular time. If it is almost time for your next dose, skip the missed dose. Do not take two doses at the same time.

Drug
Tindamax® (tinidazole)

Class: Antiprotozoal, antibacterial agent

New FDA-approved indications: Treatment of bacterial vaginosis in non-pregnant women. Other pathogens commonly associated with vulvovaginitis such as *Trichomonas vaginalis*, *Chlamydia trachomatis*, *Neisseria gonorrhoeae*, and *Candida albicans*. Herpes simplex virus should be ruled out prior to initiation of therapy.

20. Chapter 31: Human Immunodeficiency Virus and the Acquired Immunodeficiency Syndrome

Drug
Prezista™ (darunavir)

Class: Protease inhibitor/antiretroviral agent

Form: Tablet

Formulations: 300 mg tablet

Dose: Adults: 600 mg twice daily taken with ritonavir 100 mg twice daily.

Mechanism of action: Inhibition of the HIV-1 protease, which prevents the formation of mature virus particles.

FDA-approved indication: Treatment of HIV infection in antiretroviral treatment-experienced adult patients; co-administer with 100 mg ritonavir and with other antiretroviral agents.

Adverse reactions: Headache, rash, diarrhea, nausea, vomiting, and nasopharyngitis.

Drug interactions: Contraindicated with drugs that are highly dependent on CYP3A for clearance and have a narrow therapeutic index (anticonvulsants, antihistamines, rifampin, ergot derivatives, cisapride, St. John's wort, HMG-CoA reductase inhibitors, pimozide, and sedatives/hypnotics).

Monitoring parameters: Liver function tests, glucose, lipids, and pancreatic lipases.

Patient counseling: If you miss a dose by more than 6 hours, wait and take the next dose at the regularly scheduled time. If a dose is skipped, do not double the next dose. Always take with food.

Drug
Atripla™ (efavirenz, emtricitabine, and tenofovir disoproxil fumarate)

Class: Combination antiretroviral agent

Formulations: New combination: efavirenz 600 mg, emtricitabine 200 mg, and tenofovir disoproxil fumarate 300 mg tablet

Drug
Intelence™ (etravirine)

Class: Human immunodeficiency virus type 1 (HIV-1) specific, non-nucleoside reverse transcriptase inhibitor (NNRTI)

Form: Tablet

Formulations: 100 mg tablet

Dose: 200 mg twice daily following a meal.

Mechanism of action: Etravirine binds directly to reverse transcriptase and blocks the RNA-dependent and DNA-dependent DNA polymerase activities by causing disruption of the enzyme's catalytic site.

FDA-approved indication: In combination with other antiretroviral agents, treatment of HIV-1 infection in treatment-experienced adult patients who have evidence of viral replication and HIV-1 strains resistant to an NNRTI and other antiretroviral agents.

Adverse reactions: Rash, nausea, hypertension, abdominal pain, elevated liver enzymes, paresthesia, and peripheral neuropathy.

Drug interactions: Should not be coadministered with tipranavir/ritonavir, fosamprenavir/ritonavir, atazanavir/ritonavir, protease inhibitors administered without ritonavir, or NNRTIs. Inhibitors, inducers, and substrates of CYP3A4, CYP2C9, and/or CYP2C19 may alter the therapeutic effect or adverse reaction profile of etravirine.

Monitoring parameters: Virologic response, HIV RNA load, CD4 cell counts, severe rash, and signs and symptoms of immune reconstitution syndrome.

Patient counseling: Etravirine is not a cure for HIV infection, nor does the medication reduce the chance of passing HIV to others through sexual contact, sharing needles, or being exposed to blood. People taking etravirine may still get infections or other conditions common in people with HIV (opportunistic infections). The long-term effects of etravirine are not known at this time. It is very important to stay under a physician's care during treatment with etravirine. Take etravirine following a meal twice a day as prescribed. If unable to swallow the etravirine tablets whole, disperse the tablets in a glass of water, stir well, and drink immediately. Rinse the glass several times and completely swallow each rinse to ensure that the entire dose is consumed. Always use etravirine in combination with other antiretroviral drugs. If a dose is missed within 6 hours of the time the dose is usually taken, take etravirine following a meal as soon as possible, then take the next dose at the regularly scheduled time. Do not take the missed dose if it is missed by more than 6 hours from the time it is usually taken; resume usual dosing schedule.

Drug
Lexiva® (fosamprenavir calcium)

Class: HIV protease inhibitor

Forms: Tablet, oral suspension

Formulations: 700 mg tablet, 50 mg/mL oral suspension

Dose:
Therapy-naïve adults:
- 1400 mg twice daily
- 1400 mg once daily plus ritonavir 200 mg once daily
- 1400 mg once daily plus ritonavir 100 mg once daily
- 700 mg twice daily plus ritonavir 100 mg twice daily.

Protease inhibitor-experienced adults:
- 700 mg twice daily plus ritonavir 100 mg twice daily.

Pediatric patients (2 to 18 years of age):
- Dosage should be calculated on the basis of body weight (kg) and should not exceed adult dose.

Hepatic impairment:
- Dose adjustments are recommended in patients with mild, moderate, or severe hepatic impairment.

Mechanism of action: Fosamprenavir is a prodrug that is rapidly hydrolyzed to amprenavir by cellular phosphatases and inhibits HIV-1 protease.

FDA-approved indication: Indicated in combination with other antiretroviral agents for the treatment of HIV-1 infection.

Adverse reactions: Diarrhea, rash, nausea, vomiting, headache, and laboratory abnormalities.

Drug interactions:
- Drugs that induce CYP3A4 may decrease amprenavir (active metabolite) concentrations, leading to potential loss of virologic activity
- Coadministration with drugs that inhibit CYP3A4 may increase amprenavir concentrations

- Coadministration with ritonavir may result in clinically significant interactions with drugs metabolized by CYP2D6
- Drugs that should not be administered with fosamprenavir include antiarrhythmics (flecainide, propafenone), rifampin, ergot derivatives, cisapride, HMG CoA reductase inhibitors, pimozide, delavirdine, sedative/hypnotics (midazolam, triazolam), oral contraceptives, and St. John's wort.

Monitoring parameters: Liver function tests.

Patient counseling: If a dose is missed, patients should take the dose as soon as possible and then return to their normal schedule. However, if a dose is skipped, the patient should not double the next dose. For the oral suspension, shake the bottle vigorously before each use; refrigerate to improve taste. Adults should take the oral suspension form without food. Children should take the oral suspension with food.

Drug
Selzentry™ (maraviroc)

Class: CCR5 co-receptor antagonist

Form: Tablet

Formulations: 150 mg and 300 mg tablets

Dose:
- 150 mg twice daily when given with strong CYP3A4 inhibitors (with or without CYP3A inducers) including protease inhibitors (except tipranavir/ritonavir), delavirdine
- 300 mg twice daily when given with nucleoside reverse-transcriptase inhibitors, tipranavir/ritonavir, nevirapine, enfuvirtide, and other drugs that are not strong CYP3A inhibitors or CYP3A inducers
- 600 mg twice daily when given with CYP3A inducers, including efavirenz (without a strong CYP3A inhibitor).

Mechanism of action: Maraviroc selectively binds to the human chemokine receptor CCR5 present on the cell membrane, preventing the interaction of HIV-1 glycoprotein (gp) 120 and CCR5 necessary for CCR5-tropic HIV-1 to enter cells.

FDA-approved indication: In combination with antiretrovirals for treatment of adults infected with only CCR5-tropic HIV-1 who have evidence of viral replication and HIV-1 strains resistant to multiple antiretroviral agents.

Adverse reactions: Cough, pyrexia, upper respiratory tract infections, rash, musculoskeletal symptoms, abdominal pain, and dizziness.

Drug interactions:
- Coadministration with CYP3A inhibitors, including protease inhibitors (except tipranavir/ritonavir) and delavirdine, will increase the concentration of maraviroc
- Coadministration with CYP3A inducers, including efavirenz, may decrease the concentration of maraviroc.

Monitoring parameters: CD4 cell counts, plasma HIV-1 RNA, body weight, temperature, absence of AIDS-defining symptoms, quality of life, liver function test and viral hepatitis B or C screening prior to or during therapy when hepatitis is suspected, and signs and symptoms of hepatitis.

Patient counseling: Maraviroc is not a cure for HIV infection or AIDS, nor does the medication reduce the chance of passing HIV to others through sexual contact, sharing needles, or being exposed to blood. People taking maraviroc may still get infections or other conditions common in people with HIV (opportunistic infections). It is very important to stay under a physician's care during treatment with maraviroc. If a dose is missed, take the dose as soon as the missed dose is realized. Skip the missed dose if it is less than 6 hours before the next scheduled dose; resume the regular schedule. Do not take two tablets of maraviroc at the same time. Inform a health care provider if any unusual symptoms develop, or if any known symptoms persist or worsen.

Drug
Isentress® (raltegravir potassium) *integrase inhib*

Class: Human immunodeficiency virus integrase strand transfer inhibitor (HIV-1 INSTI)

Form: Tablet

Formulations: 400 mg tablets

Dose: 400 mg administered orally twice daily with or without food.

Mechanism of action: Raltegravir inhibits the catalytic activity of HIV-1 integrase, thereby preventing the covalent integration of unintegrated linear HIV-1 DNA into the host cell genome, preventing the formation of the HIV-1 provirus, ultimately preventing propagation of the viral infection.

FDA-approved indication: In combination with other antiretroviral agents for the treatment of HIV-1 infection in treatment-experienced adult patients who have evidence of viral replication and HIV-1 strains resistant to multiple antiretroviral agents.

Adverse reactions: Nausea, headache, diarrhea, pyrexia, creatine kinase elevations, myopathy, and rhabdomyolysis.

Drug interactions: Strong inducers of uridine diphosphate glucuronosyltransferase (UGT) 1A1 (e.g., rifampin) may reduce plasma concentrations of raltegravir.

Monitoring parameters: Virologic response, HIV RNA load, creatine kinase, routine blood chemistry, and signs and symptoms of immune reconstitution syndrome or inflammatory response to indolent or residual opportunistic infections, especially during the initial phase of treatment.

Patient counseling: Raltegravir is not a cure for HIV infection or AIDS, nor does the medication reduce the chance of passing HIV to others through sexual contact, sharing needles, or being exposed to blood. People taking raltegravir may still get infections or other conditions common in people with HIV (opportunistic infections). The long-term effects of raltegravir are not known at this time. It is very important to stay under a physician's care during treatment with raltegravir. If a dose is missed, take the dose as soon as the missed dose is realized. Skip the missed dose if it is not realized until it is time for the next scheduled dose; resume the regular schedule. Do not take two tablets of raltegravir at the same time. Inform a health care provider if any unusual symptoms develop, or if any known symptoms persist or worsen.

21. Chapter 32: Immunization

Drug
Kinrix™ (diphtheria and tetanus toxoids and acellular pertussis adsorbed and inactivated poliovirus vaccine)

Class: Inactivated vaccine

New formulations: Single-dose vial and prefilled syringe containing a 0.5 mL suspension for injection of diphtheria and tetanus toxoids, acellular pertussis antigens, and inactivated poliovirus types 1, 2, and 3

Dose: A single intramuscular injection (0.5 mL)

Drug
Pentacel® (diphtheria and tetanus toxoids and acellular pertussis adsorbed, inactivated poliovirus, and Haemophilus b conjugate [tetanus toxoid conjugate]) (DTaP-IPV/Hib)

Class: Inactivated vaccine

New formulation: Five-dose package containing 5 vials of DTaP-IPV component to be used to reconstitute 5 single-dose vials of lyophilized ActHIB vaccine component

Dose: The first dose may be administered as early as 6 weeks of age. The vaccine is approved for administration as a four-dose series at 2, 4, 6, and 15 to 18 months of age.

Drug
Gardasil® (quadrivalent human papillomavirus [Types 6, 11, 16, 18] recombinant vaccine)

Class: Vaccine

Form: Intramuscular injection

Formulations: 0.5 mL single-use vial or prefilled syringe

Dose: Shake well. Administer intramuscularly as three separate 0.5 mL doses. The second dose should be given 2 months after the first dose. The third dose should be given 6 months after the first dose. Administer in the deltoid region of the upper arm or in the higher anterolateral area of the thigh.

Mechanism of action: Development of humoral immune responses.

FDA-approved indications: Girls and women 9 to 26 years of age for the prevention of the following diseases caused by human papillomavirus (HPV) types 6, 11, 16, and 18: cervical cancer, genital warts (condylomata acuminata), and other precancerous or dysplastic lesions.

Adverse reactions: Fever, injection site pain, erythema, and swelling.

Drug interactions: Gardasil may be administered concomitantly (at a separate injection site) with hepatitis B vaccine (recombinant). Co-administration with other vaccines has not been studied. Immunosuppressive therapies may reduce the immune responses to vaccines.

Monitoring parameters: Monitor for adverse effects and anaphylaxis.

Patient counseling: Vaccination does not substitute for routine cervical cancer screening.

Drug
Influenza Virus Vaccine, H5N1

Class: Inactivated monovalent influenza virus vaccine

Form: Injection

Formulations: Each 1 mL dose contains 90 mcg influenza virus hemagglutinin of strain A/Vietnam/1203/2004 (H5N1, clade 1); suspension in a 5 mL multi-dose vial; contains thimerosal, a mercury derivative (50 mcg mercury/dose) added as a preservative.

Dose: Immunization consists of two 1 mL (90 mcg) intramuscular injections; the second 1 mL dose is given approximately 28 days after the first dose (window, 21 to 35 days).

Mechanism of action: Not well understood. Influenza vaccines induce antibodies against the viral hemagglutinin in the vaccine, thereby blocking viral attachment to human respiratory epithelial cells.

FDA-approved indication: Active immunization of persons 18 through 64 years of age at increased risk of exposure to the H5N1 influenza virus subtype contained in the vaccine.

Adverse reactions: Pain at injection site, headache, malaise, and myalgia.

Drug interactions: Do not mix with other vaccines in the same syringe or vial. Immunosuppressive therapies may reduce the immune response.

Monitoring parameters: Monitor for adverse effects and anaphylaxis.

Patient counseling: Inform patients of the benefits and risks of immunization. Influenza Virus Vaccine, H5N1, contains non-infectious particles. Instruct patients to report any serious adverse reaction to their physician.

Drug
Afluria® (influenza virus vaccine)

Class: Inactivated influenza virus vaccine

New formulations: 0.5 mL preservative-free, single-dose, pre-filled syringe; 5 mL multi-dose vial containing 10 doses.

New FDA-approved indication: Active immunization of persons ages 18 years and older against influenza disease caused by influenza virus subtypes A and type B present in the vaccine.

Drug
FluLaval™ (influenza virus vaccine)

Class: Influenza virus vaccine

Form: Intramuscular injection

Formulations: 5 mL multi-dose vial containing 10 doses. Each 0.5 mL dose contains 15 mcg influenza virus hemagglutinin of each of the following three strains: A/New Caledonia/20/99 (H1N1), A/Wisconsin/67/2005 (H3N2), and B/Malaysia/2506/2004. Thimerosal, a mercury derivative, is added as a preservative. Each 0.5 mL dose contains 25 mcg mercury.

Dose: A single 0.5 mL intramuscular injection.

Mechanism of action: Induces antibodies against the viral hemagglutinin in the vaccine, thereby blocking viral attachment to human respiratory epithelial cells.

FDA-approved indication: Active immunization of adults 18 years and older against influenza disease caused by influenza virus subtypes A and type B contained in the vaccine.

Adverse reactions: Pain, redness, and/or swelling at the injection site, headache, fatigue, myalgia, low-grade fever, and malaise.

Drug interactions: Do not mix with any other vaccine in the same syringe or vial. May increase blood levels of warfarin, theophylline, and phenytoin. Immuno-suppressive therapies may reduce immune response.

Monitoring parameters: Monitor for adverse effects and anaphylaxis.

Patient counseling: This vaccine is contraindicated for persons with known systemic hypersensitivity reactions to egg proteins. Safety and effectiveness have not been established in pregnant women and children. Antibody responses were lower in geriatric subjects than in younger subjects. Patients should report adverse reactions to their health care provider. Annual revaccination is recommended.

Drug
Rotarix® (rotavirus vaccine, live, oral)

Class: Live vaccine

New formulation: Vial of lyophilized vaccine to be reconstituted with a liquid diluent in a prefilled oral applicator. Each 1 mL dose contains a suspension of at least 10^6 median cell culture infective dose ($CCID_{50}$) of live, attenuated human G1P rotavirus after reconstitution.

Dose: Each dose is 1 mL administered orally. Administer first dose to infants beginning at 6 weeks of age. Administer second dose after an interval of at least 4 weeks and prior to 24 weeks of age.

Drug
Tetanus and Diphtheria Toxoids Adsorbed for Adult Use

Class: Tetanus diphtheria vaccine

New formulation: Unit dose preservative-free vial containing one dose

22. Chapter 33: Pediatrics

Drug
Orencia® (abatacept)

Class: Selective T cell co-stimulation modulator

New FDA-approved indication: Moderately to severely active polyarticular juvenile idiopathic arthritis in pediatric patients 6 years of age and older.

Dose: For patients 6 to 17 years of age weighing less than 75 kg, the recommended dose is 10 mg/kg. Pediatric patients weighing 75 kg or more should be administered abatacept according to the adult dosing regimen, not to exceed a maximum dose of 1000 mg.

Drug
Humira® (adalimumab)

Class: Tumor necrosis factor (TNF) blocker

New FDA-approved indication: Polyarticular juvenile idiopathic arthritis in patients 4 years of age and older.

Drug
Strattera® (atomoxetine hydrochloride)

Class: Selective serotonin norepinephrine reuptake inhibitor

New FDA-approved indication: Maintenance of attention-deficit/hyperactivity disorder in children and adolescents.

Drug
Nexium® (esomeprazole magnesium delayed release)

Class: Proton pump inhibitor

New FDA-approved indication: Short-term treatment of symptomatic gastroesophageal reflux disease in children 1 to 11 years of age.

Dose: 10 mg once daily for up to 8 weeks.

Drug
Flumist® (influenza virus vaccine live, intranasal)

Class: Influenza virus vaccine live intranasal

New FDA-approved indication: Active immunization of children 2 to 5 years of age against influenza virus subtypes A and type B contained in the vaccine.

Dose:

- Children 2 to 8 years of age not previously vaccinated with influenza vaccine: two doses (0.2 mL, administered as 0.1 mL per nostril, each, at least 1 month apart)
- Children 2 to 8 years of age previously vaccinated with influenza vaccine: one dose (0.2 mL administered as 0.1 mL per nostril).

Drug
Epivir® (lamivudine)

Class: Nucleoside reverse transcriptase inhibitor (NRTI)

New formulation: 150 mg scored tablet designed to facilitate dosing in pediatric patients with HIV-1

Drug
Kaletra® (lopinavir/ritonavir)

Class: HIV-1 protease inhibitor

New formulation: Film-coated tablets: 100 mg lopinavir and 25 mg ritonavir

Dose: Twice-daily dose in pediatric patients age 14 days and older is based on body weight. See prescribing information for additional information. Children >12 years of age or >40 kg should receive the adult dosage.

Drug
Menactra® (meningococcal [groups A, C, Y and W-135] polysaccharide diphtheria toxoid conjugate vaccine) for intramuscular injection

Class: Meningococcal vaccine

New FDA-approved indication: Active immunization of children age 2 to 10 years for the prevention of invasive meningococcal disease caused by *Neisseria meningitides* serogroups A, C, Y and W-135.

Drug
Asmanex® Twisthaler (mometasone furoate)

Class: Inhaled corticosteroid

New FDA-approved indication: Once-daily maintenance treatment of asthma in children 4 to 11 years of age.

Dose: The recommended starting dose is 110 mcg once daily in the evening.

Drug
Tamiflu® (oseltamivir phosphate)

Class: Neuraminidase inhibitor

New formulations: 30 mg and 45 mg capsules

Dose: For prophylaxis of influenza in pediatric patients, dosing is based on weight:

- ≤15 kg: 30 mg once daily for 10 days
- >15 kg to 23 kg: 45 mg once daily for 10 days
- >23 to 40 kg: 60 mg once daily for 10 days
- >40 kg: 75 mg once daily for 10 days.

Drug
Risperdal® (risperidone)

Class: Atypical antipsychotic

New FDA-approved indications: Treatment of adolescents age 13 to 17 years with schizophrenia. Short-term treatment of children and adolescents age 10 to 17 years with acute manic or mixed episodes of bipolar I disorder.

Dose:

- Schizophrenia in adolescents: initial dose 0.5 mg daily, titration 0.5 to 1 mg daily, target dose 3 mg daily, effective dose range 1 to 6 mg daily
- Bipolar mania in children and adolescents: initial dose 0.5 mg daily, titration dose 0.5 to 1 mg daily, target dose 2.5 mg daily, effective dose range 0.5 to 6 mg daily.

Drug
Accretropin™ (somatropin)

Class: Recombinant human growth hormone (r-hGH)

Form: Subcutaneous injection

Formulations: 5 mg/mL multi-dose vial

Dose: All doses should be divided into equal daily doses given 6 or 7 times per week subcutaneously.

- For growth hormone deficiency: 0.18 mg/kg body weight to 0.3 mg/kg (0.90 IU/kg) body weight weekly
- For Turner syndrome: 0.36 mg/kg body weight weekly.

Mechanism of action: Somatropin promotes skeletal, visceral, and general body growth, stimulates protein anabolism, and affects fat and mineral metabolism.

FDA-approved indications:
- Treatment of pediatric patients with growth hormone failure due to inadequate secretion of normal endogenous growth hormone
- Treatment of short stature associated with Turner syndrome in pediatric patients whose epiphyses are not closed.

Adverse reactions: Some patients may develop antibodies to the protein. Most frequently reported adverse reactions include injection site reactions, nausea, headache, fatigue, and scoliosis.

Drug interactions: Excessive glucocorticoid therapy may attenuate the growth-promoting effects of somatropin in children. Glucocorticoid therapy should be adjusted in children with concomitant growth hormone and glucocorticoid deficiency. Somatropin may alter the clearance of compounds metabolized by CP450 enzymes (e.g., corticosteroids, sex steroids, anticonvulsants, cyclosporine); careful monitoring is recommended. Treatment with somatropin may decrease insulin sensitivity; doses of antihyperglycemic agents may require adjustment.

Monitoring parameters: Urinary nitrogen excretion, serum urea nitrogen, insulin-like growth factor-1 (IGF-1), serum alkaline phosphatase, and centimeters of growth per year.

Patient counseling: Rotate injection sites to avoid localized tissue atrophy. A puncture-resistant container should be used for the disposal of used needles or syringes. Needles and syringes must not be reused. Seek prompt medical attention if an allergic reaction occurs. Contact a health care provider if adverse reactions or discomfort occur during therapy.

Drug
Norditropin® Cartridges (somatropin [rDNA origin] injection)

Class: Recombinant human growth hormone

New FDA-approved indication: Treatment of children with short stature associated with Turner syndrome

Dose: A dosage of up to 0.067 mg/kg/day is recommended.

Drug
Lamisil® (terbinafine hydrochloride)

Class: Allylamine antifungal

New FDA-approved indication: Treatment of tinea capitis in patients 4 years of age and older.

Dose: Take once a day with food for 6 weeks. Dosage is based on body weight:
- <25 kg: 125 mg/day
- 25 to 35 kg: 187.5 mg/day
- >35 kg: 250 mg/day.

Drug
Aptivus® (tipranavir)

Class: Protease inhibitor

New FDA-approved indication: Treatment of HIV-1 infected, treatment-experienced pediatric patients between the ages of 2 and 18 years.

Dose: Recommended dose is 14 mg/kg with 6 mg/kg ritonavir taken twice daily, not to exceed a maximum dose of tipranavir 500 mg coadministered with ritonavir 200 mg twice daily.

Drug
Diovan® (valsartan)

Class: Angiotensin II receptor blocker

New FDA-approved indication: Use in pediatric hypertension in patients 6 to 16 years of age.

Dose:
- Starting dose: 1.3 mg/kg once daily (up to 40 mg total)
- Dose range: 1.3 to 2.7 mg/kg once daily (up to 40 to 160 mg total).

23. Chapter 34: Geriatrics and Gerontology

Drug
Stalevo® (carbidopa/levodopa/entacapone)

Class: Antiparkinsonian agents: decarboxylase inhibitor, dopamine precursor, and catechol-O-methyl-transferase (COMT) antagonist

New formulation: 200 mg film-coated tablet containing 50 mg carbidopa, 200 mg levodopa, and 200 mg entacapone

Drug
Lucentis™ (ranibizumab)

Class: Recombinant humanized IgG1 kappa isotype monoclonal antibody fragment

Form: Ophthalmic intravitreal injection

Formulations: 10 mg/mL single-use vial

Dose: 0.5 mg (0.05 mL) is recommended to be administered by intravitreal injection once per month.

Mechanism of action: Binds to the receptor-binding site of active forms of VEGF-A (contributes to the progression of the neovascular form of age-related macular degeneration).

FDA-approved indication: Treatment of patients with neovascular (wet) age-related macular degeneration.

Adverse reactions: Conjunctival hemorrhage, eye pain, vitreous floaters, increased intraocular pressure, intraocular inflammation, eye irritation, increased lacrimation, headache, nausea, and hypertension.

Drug interactions: Drug interaction studies have not been conducted.

Monitoring parameters: Monitor patients during the week following the injection for increased intraocular pressure, endophthalmitis, and retinal detachments.

Patient counseling: If the eyes become red, sensitive to light, or painful, or a change in vision occurs, patients should seek immediate care from an ophthalmologist.

Drug
Exelon® Patch (rivastigmine)

Class: Acetylcholinesterase inhibitor

New formulation: Transdermal patch:
- 4.6 mg/24 hours: 5 cm^2 size containing 9 mg rivastigmine
- 9.5 mg/24 hours: 10 cm^2 size containing 18 mg rivastigmine.

Dose:
- Initial dose: one patch 4.6 mg/24 hours once daily
- Maintenance dose: one patch 9.5 mg/24 hours once daily.

Drug
Zelapar™ (selegiline hydrochloride)

Class: Monoamine oxidase type-B (MAO-B) inhibitor

Form: Orally disintegrating tablets

Formulations: 1.25 mg selegiline hydrochloride in a Zydis® formulation

Dose: Initiate treatment with 1.25 mg once daily for at least 6 weeks; the dose may be escalated to 2.5 mg given once daily if a desired benefit has not been achieved and the patient is tolerating treatment.

Mechanism of action: Inhibition of monoamine oxidase type B (MAO-B) activity; selegiline may act through other mechanisms to increase dopaminergic activity.

FDA-approved indication: Adjunctive treatment in the management of patients with Parkinson's disease treated with levodopa/carbidopa who exhibit deterioration in the quality of their treatment response.

Adverse reactions: Dizziness, chest pain, myasthenia, hypertension, nausea, and hypokalemia.

Drug interactions: CYP2B6 and CYP3A4 are involved in the metabolism of selegiline. CYP2A6 may have a minor role in the metabolism of selegiline. Concurrent use of meperidine, dextromethorphan, other selegiline products, sympathomimetic agents, tricyclic antidepressants, or selective serotonin reuptake inhibitors may lead to serious adverse events.

Monitoring parameters: Symptoms of parkinsonism, depression, and blood pressure.

Patient counseling: Selegiline should be taken in the morning before breakfast and without liquid. Patients should be cautioned about the possibility of developing hallucinations and instructed to report them to their health care provider. Patients should be advised of the possible need to reduce levodopa dosage.

24. Chapter 36: Anemias

Drug
Soliris™ (eculizumab)

Class: Monoclonal antibody

Form: Intravenous infusion

Formulations: 300 mg single-use vials each containing 30 mL of 10 mg/mL sterile, preservative-free eculizumab solution

Dose: Administer 600 mg every 7 days for the first 4 weeks, followed by 900 mg for the fifth dose 7 days later, then 900 mg every 14 days thereafter. Administer a meningococcal vaccine at least 2 weeks prior to initiation of treatment. Revaccinate according to current medical guidelines for vaccine use.

Mechanism of action: Eculizumab inhibits terminal complement-mediated intravascular hemolysis.

FDA-approved indication: Treatment of patients with paroxysmal nocturnal hemoglobinuria (PNH) to reduce hemolysis.

Adverse reactions: Headache, nasopharyngitis, nausea, fatigue, herpes simplex infections, influenza-like illness, anemia, infusion reactions, and increased risk of meningococcal infections.

Drug interactions: Drug interaction studies have not been conducted.

Monitoring parameters: Serum LDH levels, signs and symptoms of infusion reactions, and meningococcal infections.

Patient counseling: Eculizumab may lower the ability of the immune system to fight infections and may increase your chance of getting meningococcal infections.

25. Chapter 37: Venous Thromboembolic Disease

Drug
Plavix® (clopidogrel bisulfate)

Class: Antiplatelet agent

New formulation: 300 mg tablet to facilitate use of the FDA-approved loading dose for appropriate acute coronary syndrome patients as soon as possible after hospital admission

Drug
Fragmin® (dalteparin sodium)

Class: Low molecular weight heparin

New FDA-approved indication: Extended treatment of symptomatic venous thromboembolism (VTE) (proximal deep vein thrombosis [DVT] and/or pulmonary embolism [PE]) to reduce the recurrence of VTE in patients with cancer.

39. Appendices

Erin M. Timpe, PharmD, BCPS
Associate Professor and Director, Drug Information
Southern Illinois University, Edwardsville

Contents

Appendix 1

Normal Laboratory Values

Test	Conventional units	SI units
Albumin	3.5-5 g/dL	35-50 g/L
Alkaline phosphatase		
Adult	4.5-13 King-Armstrong U/dL	32-92 U/L
Infant	10-30 King-Armstrong U/dL	71-213 U/L
Amylase	60-160 Somogyi U/dL	25-125 U/L
Anion Gap	7-16 mEq/L	7-16 mmol/L
Arterial blood gases (ABG)		
HCO_3	21-28 mEq/L	21-28 mEq/L
O_2 saturation	94-100%	0.94-1
pH	7.35-7.45	7.35-7.45
Po_2	83-108 mmHg	11.04-14.36 kPa
Pco_2	35-45 mmHg	4.7-6 kPa
Basal metabolic panel (BMP)		
Bicarbonate	22-29 mEq/L	22-29 mmol/L
Blood urea nitrogen (BUN)	6-20 mg/dL	2.1-7.1 mmol/L
Chloride	98-107 mEq/L	98-107 mmol/L
Creatinine	0.6-1.3 mg/dL	53-115 micromol/L
Glucose	60-110 mg/dL	3.3-6.1 mmol/L
Potassium	3.5-5.1 mEq/L	3.5-5.1 mmol/L
Sodium	136-145 mEq/L	136-145 mmol/L
Blood pressure (mm Hg)		
Optimal	<120/<80	<120/<80
Normal	<130/<85	<130/<85
High normal	130-139/85-89	130-139/85-89
Hypertension		
Stage 1	140-159/90-99	140-159/90-99
Stage 2	160-179/100-109	160-179/100-109
Stage 3	>180/>110	>180/>110
Isolated systolic	>140/<90	>140/<90
Calcitonin	<150 pg/mL	<150 ng/L
Calcium	8.6-10 mg/dL	2.15-2.50 mmol/L
Carbon dioxide	22-29 mEq/L	22-29 mmol/L
Coagulation screen		
Activated partial thromboplastin time (aPTT)	<35 seconds	<35 seconds
Antithrombin III	21-30 mg/dL	210-300 mg/L
Bleeding time	1-<10 min	1-<10 min
Partial thromboplastin time (PTT)	22-37 seconds	22-37 seconds
Protein C	70-140%	0.70-1.40
Protein S	67-140%	0.67-1.40
Prothrombin time (PT)	11-15 seconds	11-15 seconds
Complete blood count (CBC)		
Hemoglobin (Hb)		
Male	13.1-18 g/dL	131-180 g/L
Female	11.7-16 g/dL	117-160 g/L
Hematocrit (Hct)		
Male	40-54%	0.40-0.54
Female	34-47%	0.34-0.47
Mean corpuscular volume (MCV)	80-96 micrometer^3	80-96 fL

(continued)

Appendix 1

Normal Laboratory Values (continued)

Test	Conventional units	SI units
CBC (continued)		
Mean corpuscular hemoglobin (MCH)	27-33 pg	27-33 pg
Mean corpuscular hemoglobin concentration (MCHC)	32-36%	0.32-0.36
Platelets	150-400 x 10^3/microliter	150-400 x 10^9/microliter
Red blood cells (RBC):		
Male	4.1-5.8 x 10^6 cells/microliter	4.1-5.8 x 10^{12} cells/L
Female	3.8-5.4 x 10^6 cells/microliter	3.8-5.4 x 10^{12} cells/L
White blood cells (WBC)	4.5-11 x 10^3 cells/microliter	4.5-11 x 10^9 cells/L
White blood cell differential:		
Band neutrophils	0.0-2.1 10^3 cells/microliter	0.0-2.1 10^9 cells/L
Basophils	0.0-0.19 10^3 cells/microliter	0.0-0.19 10^9 cells/L
Eosinophils	0.0-0.7 10^3 cells/microliter	0.0-0.7 10^9 cells/L
Lymphocytes	1.2-4.0 10^3 cells/microliter	1.2-4.0 10^9 cells/L
Monocytes	0.1-0.95 10^3 cells/microliter	0.1-0.95 10^9 cells/L
Segmented neutrophils	1.1-6.9 10^3 cells/microliter	1.1-6.9 10^9 cells/L
Corticotropin (ACTH) 08:00h	<120 pg/mL	<26 pmol/L
Cortisol 08:00h	5-23 mcg/dL	138-635 nmol/L
Creatinine kinase:		
Male	38-174 U/L	0.65-2.96 microKat/L
Female	26-140 U/L	0.46-2.38 microKat/L
Glucose tolerance test		
Baseline fasting blood glucose	70-105 mg/dL	3.9-5.8 mmol/L
30-Minute fasting blood glucose	110-170 mg/dL	6.1-9.4 mmol/L
60-Minute fasting blood glucose	120-170 mg/dL	6.7-9.4 mmol/L
90-Minute fasting blood glucose	100-140 mg/dL	5.6-7.8 mmol/L
120-minute fasting blood glucose	70-120 mg/dL	3.9-6.7 mmol/L
Hematologic tests		
Erythrocyte sedimentation rate (ESR)		
≥50 year old male	0-15 mm/h	0-15 mm/h
≥50 year old female	0-20 mm/h	0-20 mm/h
<50 year old male	0-20 mm/h	0-20 mm/h
<50 year old female	0-30 mm/h	0-30 mm/h
Ferritin		
Male	20-250 ng/mL	20-250 mcg/L
Female	10-120 ng/mL	10-120 mcg/L
Fibrinogen	200-400 mg/dL	2.00-4.00 g/L
Hemoglobin A1$_C$	4-6%	0.040-0.060
Reticulocytes	0.5-1.5%	0.005-0.015
Vitamin B$_{12}$	200-835 pg/mL	148-616 pmol/L
Iron		
Male	65-175 (g/dL)	11.6-31.3 (mol/L)
Female	50-170 (g/dL)	9.0-30.4 (mol/L)
Total iron binding capacity (TIBC)	250-425 (g/dL)	44.8-76.1 (mol/L)
Transferrin saturation	20-50%	0.20-0.50

(continued)

Appendix 1

Normal Laboratory Values (continued)

Test	Conventional units	SI units
Isoenzymes		
Creatine phosphokinase (MM)	5-70 U/L	5-70 U/L
Creatine phosphokinase (MB)	0-7 U/L	0-7 U/L
Creatine phosphokinase (BB)	0-3 U/L	0-3 U/L
Lipase	<200 U/L	<3.4 microKat/L
Lipids		
Total cholesterol		
Desirable	<200 mg/dL	<5.2 mmol/L
Borderline-high	200-239 mg/dL	<5.2-6.2 mmol/L
High	>239 mg/dL	>6.2 mmol/L
LDL		
Desirable	<130 mg/dL	<3.36 mmol/L
Borderline-high	130-159 mg/dL	3.36-4.11 mmol/L
High	>159 mg/dL	>4.11 mmol/L
HDL		
Low	<40 mg/dL	<1.04 mmol/L
High	>60 mg/dL	>1.55 mmol/L
Triglycerides		
Desirable	<150 mg/dL	<1.7 mmol/L
Borderline-high	150-199 mg/dL	1.7-2.25 mmol/L
High	200-499 mg/dL	2.26-5.64 mmol/L
Very high	>500 mg/dL	>5.65 mmol/L
Liver function tests (LFTs)		
Aspartate aminotransferase (AST, SGOT)	8-20 U/L	0.14-0.34 microKat/L
Alanine aminotransferase (ALT, SGPT)	10-40 U/L	0.17-0.68 microKat/L
Ammonia (NH_4^+)	15-45 mcg/dL	11-32 micromol/L
Bilirubin		
Conjugated	<2 mg/dL	<3.4 microMol/L
Total	0.2-1 mg/dL	3-19 microMol/L
Lactate dehydrogenase (LDH)	90-280 U/L	1.50-4.67 microKat/L
Magnesium	1.3-2.6 mg/dL	0.65-1.07 mmol/L
Phosphate	2.5-4.5 mg/dL	0.81-1.45 mmol/L
Prolactin		
Male	3-15 ng/mL	3-15 mcg/L
Female	3-23 ng/mL	3-23 mcg/L
Protein, total	6.4-8.3 g/dL	64-83 g/L
Thyroid hormone function tests		
Free thyroxine (Free T_4)	0.8-2.7 ng/dL	10-35 pmol/L
Thyroid-stimulating hormone (TSH)	0.4-8.9 microU/mL	0.4-8.9 mU/L
Thyroxine-binding globulin capacity	16-24 mcg/dL	206-309 nmol/L
Total triiodothyronine (T_3)	70-204 ng/dL	1.08-3.14 nmol/L
Total thyroxine by RIA (T_4)	4.6-11.0 mcg/dL	59-142 nmol/L
Uric acid	2.3-8.0 ng/dL	137-476 micromol/L

References

Malarkey LM, McMorrow ME. *Nurse's Manual of Laboratory Tests and Diagnostic Procedures.* Philadelphia: WB Saunders; 1996.

Tietz NW. *Clinical Guide to Laboratory Tests,* 3rd ed. Philadelphia: WB Saunders; 1995.

Appendix 2

Drugs in Renal Failure

Generic name (trade name)	Normal dose	CrCl 30-50 mL/min	CrCl 10-30 mL/min	CrCl <10 mL/min	Hemodialysis
Analgesics					
Acetaminophen	650 mg PO q4h	650 mg PO q6h	650 mg PO q6h	650 mg PO q6h	No supplementation required
Aspirin	650 mg PO q4h	650 mg PO q 4h	650 mg PO q6h	Avoid	Dose after HD
Codeine	30-60 mg PO q4-6h	20-45 mg PO q4-6h	20-45 mg PO q4-6h	15-30 mg PO q4-6h	No data
Fentanyl (Sublimaze®)	0.5 mcg/kg IV q1-2h	Same	0.375 mcg/kg IV q1-2h	0.25 mcg/kg IV q1-2h	0.25 mcg/kg IV q1-2h
Hydromorphone (Dilaudid®)	1-2 mg IV q4-6h	Same	Same	Same	Same
Meperidine (Demerol®)	50-100 mg IV or PO q3-4h	37.5-75 mg IV or PO q3-4h	37.5-75 mg IV or PO q3-4h	25-50 mg IV or PO q3-4h	Avoid
Morphine	20-25 mg PO q4h; 2-15 mg IV q2-4h	15-20 mg PO q4h; 1.5-12 mg IV q2-4h	15-20 mg PO q4h; 1.5-12 mg IV q2-4h	10 pg PO q4h; 1-8 mg IV q2-4h	No supplemental PO dose required; 1-8 mg IV q2-4
Propoxyphene (Darvon®)	65 mg PO q6-8h	Same	Same	Avoid	Avoid
Antiarrhythmics					
Adenosine (Adenocard®)	6 mg IV push over 1-2 s, may repeat second dose at 12 mg IV if necessary, may repeat 12 mg dose x 1	Same	Same	Same	Same
Atropine	0.5-1 mg IV push q 3-5 min, max 0.04 mg/kg	Same	Same	Same	Same
Class I					
Moricizine (Ethmozine®)	200-300 mg PO q8h	Same	Same	Same	Same
Propafenone (Rythmol®)	150-300 mg PO q8h	Same	Same	Same	Same
Class Ia					
Disopyramide (Norpace®)	300 mg IR LD, then 150-300 mg PO q6h	100 mg PO q6h	100 mg PO q12h	100 mg PO q24h	100 mg post-HD
Procainamide (Procan®, Pronestyl®)	500-1000 mg PO q4-6h; 50-100 mg/min IV until arrhythmia is suppressed or reach 500-1000 mg, then 2-6 mg/min	500 mg PO q6h	500 mg PO q12h	500 mg PO q12-24h	500 mg PO q24h post HD
Quinidine (Quinidex®, Quinaglute®)	Sulfate: 200-400 mg PO q4-6h; gluconate: 324-648 mg PO q8-12h; 200-300 mg IM q2-6h	Same	Same	Sulfate: 150-300 mg PO q4-6h	Sulfate: 100-200 mg post-HD

(continued)

Appendix 2

Drugs in Renal Failure (continued)

Generic name (trade name)	Normal dose	CrCl 30-50 mL/min	CrCl 10-30 mL/min	CrCl <10 mL/min	Hemodialysis
Antiarrhythmics (cont)					
Class Ib					
Lidocaine (Xylocaine®)	50-100 mg IV over 1-2 min bolus, then 1-4 mg/min IV	Same	Same	Same	Same
Mexilitine (Mexitil®)	200-400 mg PO q8h	Same	Same	Same	Same
Tocainide (Tonocard®)	200-400 mg PO q8h	Same	Same	Same	Same
Class Ic					
Encainide (Enkaid®)	25-50 mg PO q12h	25-50 mg PO q8h	25 mg PO q8h	25 mg PO q12-24h	Same
Flecainide (Tambocor®)	100-200 mg PO q12h	No change	50-100 mg PO q12h	50 mg PO q12h	Same
Class II (see β-blockers in antihypertensives					
Class III					
Amiodarone (Cordarone®)	800-1600 mg/d in divided doses for 1-2 weeks LD, then 100-600 mg/d	Same	Same	Same	Same
Bretylium (Bretyol®)	5 mg//kg IV bolus, may repeat at 10 mg/kg to max of 30 mg/kg	Same	Same	Same	Same
Class IV (see calcium channel blockers in antihypertensives)					
Antibiotics					
Aminoglycosides					
Amikacin (Amikin®)	7.5 mg/kg IV q12h	7.5 mg/kg IV q18-24h	7.5 mg/kg IV q24-48h	7.5 mg/kg IV q48h	7.5 mg/kg IV based on serum levels; redose if level <5 mcg/mL
Gentamicin (Garamycin®)	1.7 mg/kg q8h	0.5-1 mg/kg IV q12h or 1.7 mg/kg q24-48h	0.5-1 mg/kg IV q12h or 1.7 mg/kg q24-48h	0.35-0.5 mg/kg IV q24-48h or 1.7 mg/kg IV q48-72h	50% of dose post-HD
Tobramycin (Nebcin®)	1/7 mg/kg q8h	0.5-1 mg/kg IV q12h or 1.7 mg/kg q24-48h	0.5-1 mg/kg IV q12h or 1.7 mg/kg q24-48h	0.35-0.5 mg/kg IV q24-48h or 1.7 mg/kg IV q48-72h	50% of dose post-HD
Cephalosporins					
Cefaclor (Ceclor®)	250-500 mg PO tid	125-500 mg PO tid	125-500 mg PO tid	125-250 mg PO tid	250 mg PO post-HD
Cefadroxil (Duricef®)	0.5-1 g PO q12h	0.5-1 g PO q12-24h	0.5-1 g po q12-24h	0.5-1 g PO q24-48h	0.5-1 g PO post-HD
Cefazolin (Ancef®, Kexol®)	1-2 g IV q8h	1-2 g PO q8h	1-2 g IV q12h	1-2 g IV q24h	1-2 g IV q24h given post-HD
Cefepime (Maxipime®)	1-2 g IV q8-12h	1-2 g IV q12-24h	1-2 g IV q24h	0.5-1 g IV q24h	0.5-1 g IV q24h given post-HD

(continued)

Appendix 2

Drugs in Renal Failure (continued)

Generic name (trade name)	Normal dose	CrCl 30-50 mL/min	CrCl 10-30 mL/min	CrCl <10 mL/min	Hemodialysis
Cephalosporins (cont)					
Cefixime (Suprax®)	200 mg PO q12h	150-200 mg PO q12h	150 mg PO q12h	100 mg PO q12h	300 mg PO post-HD
Cefotaxime (Claforan®)	1-2 g IV q8h	1-2 g IV q8h	1-2 g IV q12h	1-2 g IV q24h	1-2 g IV q24h given post-HD
Cefotetan (Cefotan®)	1-2 g IV q12h	1-2 g IV q12h	1-2 g IV q24h	1-2 g IV q48h	1-2 g IV q48h given post-HD
Cefoxitin (Mefoxin®)	1-2 g IV q6-8h	1-2 g IV q8h	1-2 g IV q12h	1-2 g IV q24h	1-2 g IV q24h given post-HD
Cefpodoxime (Vantin®)	200 mg PO q12h	200 mg PO q16h	200 mg PO q16h	200 mg PO q24-48h	200 mg PO post-HD only
Cefprozil (Cefzil®)	500 mg PO q12h	250 mg PO q12-16h	250 mg PO q12-16h	250 mg PO q24h	250 mg PO post-HD
Ceftazidime (Ceptaz®, Fortaz®, Tazicef®, Tazidime®)	2 g IV q8h	2 g IV q12h	2 g IV, then 0.5-1 g IV q24h	2 g IV, then 1 g IV q48h	2 g IV, then 1 g IV q48h given post-HD
Ceftizoxime (Cefizox®)	1-2 g IV q8h	1-2 g IV q12h	1-2 g IV q12h	1-2 g IV q24h	1 g IV q48h given post-HD
Ceftriaxone (Rocephin®)	1-2 g IV q24h	Same	Same	Same	Same
Cefuroxime (Ceftin®, Kefurox®, Zinacef®)	0.75-1.5 g IV q8h	0.75-1.5 g IV q8h	0.75-1.4 g IV q12h	0.75-1.5 g IV q24h	0.75-1.5 g IV q24h given post-HD
Cephalexin (Keflex®)	250-500 mg PO q6h	250-500 mg PO q8-12h	240-500 mg PO q12h	250-500 mg PO q12h	Dose post-HD
Fluoroquinolones					
Ciprofloxacin (Cipro®)	500-750 mg PO; 400 mg IV q12h	250-500 mg PO; 400 mg IV q12h	250-500 mg PO q18h; 400 mg IV q24h	250-500 mg PO q18h; 400 mg IV q24h	250-500 mg PO q24h; 400 mg IV q24h given post-HD
Gatifloxacin (Tequin®)	400 mg PO or IV q24h	400 mg PO or IV x 1, then 200 mg PO or IV q24h	400 mg PO or IV x1, then 200 mg PO or IV q24h	400 mg IV or PO x 1, then 200 mg PO or IV q24h	400 mg PO or IV x 1, then 200 mg PO or IV q24h given post-HD
Levofloxacin (Levaquin®)	250-500 mg PO or IV q24h	500 mg PO or IV x 1, then 250 mg PO or IV q24h	500 mg PO or IV x 1, then 250 mg PO or IV q48h	500 mg PO or IV, x 1, then 250 mg PO or IV q48h	500 mg PO or IV x1, then 250 mg PO or IV q48h given post-HD
Miscellaneous					
Aztreonam (Azactam®)	1-2 g IV q6-8h	1-2 g IV q6-8h	1-2 g IV LD, then 1 g IV q6-8h	1-2 g IV LD, then 0.5 g IV q6-8h	1-2 g IV LD, then 0.5 g IV q6-8h given post-HD
Erythromycin (E-Mycin®)	250 mg PO q8h	Same	Same	Same	Same
Imipenem (Primaxin®)	500 mg IV q6h	500 mg IV q8h	500 mg IV q12h	250 mg IV q12h	250 mg IV q12h given post-HD
Linezolid (Zyvox®)	600 mg IV q12h	No data	No data	No data	Give post-HD

(continued)

Appendix 2

Drugs in Renal Failure (continued)

Generic name (trade name)	Normal dose	CrCl 30-50 mL/min	CrCl 10-30 mL/min	CrCl <10 mL/min	Hemodialysis
Misc. antibiotics (cont)					
Meropenem (Merrem®)	1 g IV q8h	1 g IV q12h	500 mg IV q12h	500 mg IV q24h	500 mg IV q24h given post-HD
Quinupristin-dalfopristin (Synercid®)	7.5 mg/kg IV q8h	Same	Same	Same	Same
Rifampin (Rifadin®)	600 mg PO q24h	300-600 mg PO q24-48h	300-600 mg PO q24-48h	300-600 mg PO q48h	300-600 mg PO q48h given post-HF
Trimethoprim-sulfamethoxazole (Bactrim®, Septra®)	8-20 mg/kg/d PO 6-12h; IV q12h	4-10 mg/kg/d PO or IV q12h	4-10 mg/kg/d PPO or IV q12h	2-5 mg/kg/d PO or IV q24h	2-5 mg/kg/d PO or IV q24h given post-HD
Vancomycin (Vancocin®)	500 mg IV q6h or 1 g q12h	1 g IV q24-96h	1 g IV q24-96g	1 g IV q4-7d	1 g IV q4-7d
Penicillins					
Amoxicillin-clavulanic acid (Augmentin®)	250-500 mg PO q8h 875 mg PO bid	Same	250-500 mg PO q12h; 875 mg PO bid	250-500 mg PO q24h; 875 mg PO q24h	Give post-HD
Ampicillin (Principen®, Omnipen®)	1-2 g IV q4-6g	1-2 g IV q6-8h	1-2 g IV q8-12h	1-2 g IV q12h	1-2 g IV q12h
Ampicillin-sulbactam (Unasyn®)	1.5-3 g IV q6h	1.5-3 g IV q8h	1.5-3 g IV q12h	1.5-3 g IV q24h	1.5-3 g IV q24h given post-HD
Methicillin (Staphcillin®)	1-2 g IV q4-6h	1-2 g IV q8h	1-2 g IV q6-8h	1-2 g IV q8-12h	1-2 g IV q8-12h
Nafcillin (Nafcin®, Unipen®)	1-2 g IV q4-6h	Same	Same	Same	Same
Oxacillin (Bactocil®)	1-2 g IV q4-6h	Same	Same	Same	Same
Penicillin G	1-4 MU IV q4-6h	1-4 MUIV q6-8h	1-4 MU IV q8-12h	1-4 MU IV q12-18h	1-4 MU IV q12-18h
Piperacillin (Pipracil®)	3 g IV q4-6h	3 g IV q6h	3 g IV q8h	3 g IV q12h	2 g IV q8h given post-HD
Piperacillin-tazobactam (Zosyn®)	3.375 g IV q4-6h	3.375 g IV q6h	3.375 g IV q8h	3.375 g IV q12h	2.25 g IV q8h given post-HD
Ticarcillin (Ticar®)	3 g IV q4h	1-2 g IV q4-8h	1-2 g IV 8h	1-2 g IV q12h	3 g IV post-HD
Ticarcillin-clavulanic acid (Timentin®)	3.1 g IV q4-6h	2 g IV q4h	2 g IV q12h	2 g IV q12h	2 g IV q12h given post-HD
Anticoagulants					
Enoxaparin (Lovenox®)	30 mg SC q12h 40 mg SC qd 1 mg/kg SC q12h	Same Same Same	30 mg SC qd 30 mg SC qd 1 mg/kg SC qd	30 mg SC qd 30 mg SC qd 1 mg/kg SC qd	No data
Anticonvulsants					
Carbamazepine (Tegretol®)	200 mg PO bid to 1200 mg PO q24h	Same	Same	Same	Same
Diazepam (Valium®)	2-10 mg PO q6-12h prn; 2-10 mg IV or IM q2-4h prn	Same	Same	Same	Same

(continued)

Appendix 2

Drugs in Renal Failure (continued)

Generic name (trade name)	Normal dose	CrCl 30-50 mL/min	CrCl 10-30 mL/min	CrCl <10 mL/min	Hemodialysis
Anticonvulsants (cont)					
Ethosuximide (Zarontin®)	500-1500 mg PO q24h	Same	Same	Same	Same
Gabapentin (Neurontin®)	300-600 mg PO tid	200-700 mg PO bid	300 mg PO q12-24h	300 mg PO qod	300 mg load, then 200-300 mg post-HD
Lamotrigine (Lamictal®)	15 mg PO q12-24h initially, then 100-500 mg PO q24h	Same	Same	Same	No data
Lorazepam (Ativan®)	0.5-10 mg PO q4-6h prn; 1-10 mg IV or IM q2-4h prn	Same	Same	Same	Same
Oxcarbazepine (Trileptal®)	200-400 mg PO tid	Same	Same	Same	No data
Phenobarbital (Luminal®, Solfoton®)	60-250 mg PO q24h; 10-20 mg/kg IV	Same	Same	60-100 mg PO q24h	Give dose post-HD
Phenytoin (Dilantin®)	15 mg/kg LD, then 200-400 mg/d PO or IV divided q8-12h	Same	Same	Same	Same
Primidone (Mysoline®)	250-500 mg PO qid	250-500 mg PO q8-12h	250-500 mg PO q8-12h	250-500 mg PO q12-24h	80-160 mg PO q12-24h
Sodium valproate (Depakene®, Depakote®)	15-60 mg/kg q24h	Same	Same	Same	Same
Topiramate (Topamax®)	100-400 mg PO q12-24h	50-400 mg PO q12-24h	50-200 mg PO q12-24h	25-100 mg PO q12-24h	No data
Antiemetics					
Metoclopramide (Reglan®)	10-20 mg IV q6h	7.5-15 mg IV q6h	7.5-15 mg IV 6h	5-10 mg IV q6h	7.5-15 mg IV q6h
Antifungals					
Amphotericin B nonlipid (Fungizone®)	0.4-1 mg/kg IV q24h	0.4-1 mg/kg IV q24h	0.4-1 mg/kg IV q24h	0.4-1 mg/kg IV q48h	0.4-1 mg/kg IV q48h
Am B lipid complex (Abelcet®)	5 mg/kg IV q24h	5 mg/kg IV q24h	5 mg/kg IV q24h	5 mg/kg IV q48h	5 mg/kg IV q48h
Am B cholecteryl sulfate complex (Amphotec®)	3-6 mg/kg/d IV q24h	3-6 mg/kg/d IV q24h	3-6 mg/kg/d IV q24h	3-6 mg/kg/d IV q48h	3-6 mg/kg/d IV q 48h
Am B liposome (Ambisome®)	3-5 mg/kg IV q24h	3-5 mg/lg IV q24h	3-5 mg/kg IV q24h	3-5 mg/kg IV q48h	3-5 mg/kg IV q48h
Fluconazole (Diflucan®)	100-400 mg PO or IV q24h	LD: 100-400 mg PO or IV, then 50-200 mg PO or IV q24h	LD: 100-400 mg PO or IV, then 50-200 mg PO Iv q24h	LD: 100-400 mg PO or IV, then 50-200 mg PO or IV q24h	100-400 mg PO or IV only after HD
Itraconazole (Sponanox®)	100-200 mg PO or IV q12h	100-200 mg PO or IV q12h	100-200 mg PO IV q12h	100-200 mg PO or IV q24h	100 mg PO q12-24h; 200 mg IV q24h post-HD
Ketoconazole (Nizoral®)	20 mg PO q24h	Same	Same	Same	Same

(continued)

Appendix 2

Drugs in Renal Failure (continued)

Generic name (trade name)	Normal dose	CrCl 30-50 mL/min	CrCl 10-30 mL/min	CrCl <10 mL/min	Hemodialysis
Antihistamines (cont)					
Cimetidine (Tagamet®)	400 mg PO bid; 300 mg IV q6h; 37.5-50 mg/h continuous infusion	200 mg PO bid; 300 mg IV q8h; 25-37.5 mg/h continuous infusion	200 mg PO bid; 200 mg IV q8h; 25-37.5 mg/h continuous infusion	100 mg PO bid; 300 mg IV q12h; 18-25 mg/h continuous infusion	No PO supplementation required; 300 mg IV q12h given post-HD
Famotidine (Pepcid®)	20-40 mg PO qhs; 20-40 mg IV q12h	5-20 mg PO qhs; 20 mg IV q12h	5-10 mg PO qhs; 20 mg IV q12h	2-4 mg PO qhs; 20 mg IV q24h, or 40 mg IV q48h	No PO supplementation required; 20 mg IV q24h given post-HD
Nizatidine (Axid®)	150 mg PO q12h or 300 mg PO hs	150 mg PO q24h	150 mg PO q24h	150 mg PO q48h	150 mg PO q48h
Ranitidine (Zantac®)	150-300 mg PO qhs; 50 mg IV q8h; 6.25 mg/h continuous infusion	75-150 mg PO qhs; 50 mg IV a12h	75-150 mg PO qhs; 50 mg IV q12h	75 mg PO qhs; 50 mg IV q24h	50% of PO dose post-HD; 50 mg IV q24h given post-HD
Antihypertensives					
ACE inhibitors					
Benazepril (Lotensin®)	10-40 mg PO q24h	5-20 PO q24h	5-20 mg PO q24h	5-20 mg PO q24h	5-20 PO q24h
Captopril (Capoten®)	25-200 mg PO q8h	18.75-75 mg PO q12-18h	18.75-75 mg PO q12-18h	12.5-50 mg PO q24h	Supplement 25-30% of dose after HD
Enalapril (Vasotec®)	5-10 mg PO q12h	2.5-7.5 mg PO q12h	2.5 mg PO q24h	2.5 mg PO q24h	2.5-7.5 PO q12h
Enalaprilat (Vasotec®)	1.25-5 mg IV q6h	1.25-2.5 mg IV q6h	0.625 mg IV x 1, then up to 1.25 mg q6h if inadequate response	0.625 mg IV x 1, then up to 1.25 me q6h if inadequate response	0.625 mg IV q6h
Fosinopril (Monopril®)	10-40 mg PO q24h	10-40 mg q24h	10-40 mg PO q24h	7.5-30 mg PO q24h	Same
Lisinopril (Zestril®)	10-40 mg PO q24h	5-30 mg PO q24h	5-30 mg PO q24h	2.5-20 mg PO q24h	2.5 mg initially, then 20% of patient's dose after HD if on a dosing regimen
Quinapril (Accupril®)	10-80 mg PO q24h	7.5-60 mg PO q24h	7.5-60 mg PO q24h	7.5-60 mg PO q24h	2.5 mg initially, then 25-35% of patient's dose after HD if on a dosing regimen
Ramipril (Altace®)	2.5-20 mg PO q24h	1.25-15 mg PO q24h	1.25-15 mg PO q24h	1.25-10 mg PO q24h	Supplement 20% of the patient's dose after HD
α-Blockers					
Doxazosin (Cardura®)	1-16 mg PO q24h	Same	Same	Same	Same
Prazosin (Minipress®)	1-15 mg PO q12h	Same	Same	Same	Same
Terazosin (Hytrin®)	1-20 mg/d PO	Same	Same	Same	Same

(continued)

Appendix 2

Drugs in Renal Failure (continued)

Generic name (trade name)	Normal dose	CrCl 30-50 mL/min	CrCl 10-30 mL/min	CrCl <10 mL/min	Hemodialysis
Angiotensin-receptor blockers					
Candesartan (Atacand®)	8-32 PO q24h	Same	Same	No data	Same
Losartan (Cozaar®)	25-100 mg PO q12-24h	Same	Same	Same	No data
Angiotensin-receptor blockers (cont)					
Irbesartan (Avapro®)	150-300 mg PO q24h	Same	Same		Same
Valsartan (Diovan®)	80-320 mg PO q24h	Same	Same	No data	No data
β-Blockers					
Atenolol (Ternormin®)	50-100 mg PO q24h	25-50 mg q48h	25-50 mg PO q24h	25-50 mg PO q96h	25-50 mg PO q96h; supplement 12.5-25 mg post-HD
Carvedilol (Coreg®)	6.25-50 mg PO q12h	Same	Same	Same	No data
Metoprolol (Lopressor®)	50-450 mg/d PO in 2-3 divided doses	Same	Same	Same	Supplement 50 mg PO post-HD
Labetalol (Normodyne®)	200-600 mg PO bid	Same	Same	Same	Same
Nadolol (Corgard®)	40-320 mg/d PO single or divided doses	20-160 mg/d PO q24-36h	20-160 mg/d PO q24-48h	10-80 mg/d PO q48h	Supplement 40 mg PO post-HD
Pindolol (Visken®)	10-40 mg PO q12h	Same	Same	Same	Same
Propranolol (Inderal®)	80-320 mg PO q6-12h	Same	Same	Same	Same
Sotalol (Betapace®)	80-320 mg PO q12h	80-320 mg PO q24h	80-320 mg PO q36-48h	10-100 mg PO according to clinical response	Same Supplement 80 mg post-HD
Calcium channel blockers					
Amlodipine (Norvasc®)	2.5-10 mg PO q24h	Same	Same	Same	Same
Diltiazem (Dilacor®, Cardizem®, Tiazac®)	30-90 mg PO q6-8h	Same	Same	Same	Same
Felodiopine (Plendil®)	5-15 mg PO q 8-24 h	Same	Same	Same	Same
Isradipine (Dynacirc®)	1.25-10 mg/d PO bid	Same	Same	Same	Same
Nicardipine (Cardene®)	20-40 mg PO tid	Same	Same	Same	Same
Nifedipine (Adalat®, Procardia®)	10-30 mg/d PO tid	Same	Same	Same	Same
Nimodipine (Nimotop®)	60 mg PO q4h	Same	Same	Same	Same
Verapamil (Calan®, Isoptin®, Verelan®)	40-120 mg PO q8h	Same	Same	20-60 mg PO q8h	20-60 mg PO q8h

(continued)

Appendix 2

Drugs in Renal Failure (continued)

Generic name (trade name)	Normal dose	CrCl 30-50 mL/min	CrCl 10-30 mL/min	CrCl <10 mL/min	Hemodialysis
Diuretics					
Bumetanide (Bumex®)	1-2 mg IV q8-12h	Same	Same	8-10 mg PO or IV single dose, or 12 mg infusion over 12h	Same
Furosemide (Lasix®)	40-80 mg IV q12h	Same	Same	Same	Not effective
Hydrochlorothiazide (Hydrodiuril®)	25-200 mg PO qd-tid	Same	Same	Not effective	Not effective
Spironloactone (Aldactone®)	25-200 mg/d PO in 2-4 divided doses	12.5-100 mg PO q12-24h	12.5-100 mg PO q24h	Not effective	Not effective
Triamterene (Dyrenium®)	50-100 mg PO bid	Same	Same	Not effective	Not effective
Antivirals					
Acyclovir (Zovirax®)	5-10 mg/kg PO or IV q8h	5-10 mg/kg PO or IV q12h	5-10 mg/kg PO or IV q24h	2.5 mg/kg PO or IV q24h	2.5-5 mg/kg PO or IV q24h given post-HD
Amantadine (Symmetrel®)	100 mg PO q12h	100 mg PO q24h	100 mg PO q48h	200 mg PO q7d	200 mg PO q7d
Didanosine (Videx®)	200 mg PO q12h	200 mg PO q12-24h	200 mg PO q24h	100 mg PO q24h	Dose after HD
Entecavir (Baraclude®)	0.5-1 mg qd	0.25-0.5 mg qd	0.15-0.3 mg qd	0.05-0.1 mg qd	Dose after HD
Famciclovir (Famvir®)	125 mg PO q12h, or 500 mg PO q8h	125 mg PO q12h, 500 mg PO q12h	125 mg PO q12-48h, 500 mg PO 12-48h	62.5 mg PO q48h, or 250 mg PO q48h	Dose after HD
Ganciclovir (Cytovene®)	1000 mg PO q8h, 5 mg/kg IV q12h, then 5 mg IV q24h	No data: 500-1000 mg PO q24h, 2.5 mg/kg IV q24h, then 1.24 mg/kg IV q24h	No data: 500-1000 mg PO q24h. 1.25 mg/kg IV q24h, then 0.625 mg/kg IV q24h	No data: 500 mg PO q48-96 h, 1.25 mg IV three times a week, then 0.625 mg/kg IV three times a week	No data: Dose PO after dialysis, 1.25 mg IV three times a week, then 0.625 mg/kg IV three times a week
Indinavir (Crixan®)	800 mg PO q8h	No data	No data	No data	No data
Lamivudine (Epivir®)	150 mg PO q12h	50-150 mg PO q24h	50-150 PO q24h	25-50 mg PO q25h	Dose after HD
Nelfinavir (Viracept®)	750 mg PO q8h	No data	No data	No data	No data
Nevirapine (Viramune®)	200 mg PO q24 h x 14 d, then q12h	No data	No data	No data	No data
Ribavirin (Rebetrol®)	200 mg PO 8h	200 mg PO q8h	200 mg PO q8h	100 mg PO q8h	Dose after HD
Ritonavir (Norvir®)	600 mg PO q12h	No data	No data	No data	No data
Saquinavir (Fortovase®, Invirase®)	600 mg PO q8h	No data	No data	No data	No data
Stavudine (Zerit®)	30-40 mg PO q12h	15-20 mg PO q12-24h	15-20 mg PO q12-24h	15-20 mg PO q24h	15-20 mg PO q24h
Valaciclovir (Valtrex®)	500 mg PO q12h to 1000 mg PO q8h	500-1000 mg PO q12-24h	500-1000 mg PO q12-24h	500 mg q24h	Dose after HD
Zalcitabine (Hivid®)	0.75 mg PO q8h	0.75 mg PO q8-12h	0.75 mg PO q12h	0.75 mg PO q24h	No data; dose after HD
Zidovudine (Retrovir®)	200 mg PO q8h; 300 mg PO q12h	200 mg PO q8h; 300 mg PO q12h	200 mg PO q8h; 300 mg PO q12h	100 mg PO q8h	100 mg PO q8h
Bisphosphonates					
Zoledronic acid (Zometa®)	4 mg IV	3-3.5 mg IV	No data	No data	No data

(continued)

Drugs in Renal Failure (continued)

Generic name (trade name)	Normal dose	CrCl 30-50 mL/min	CrCl 10-30 mL/min	CrCl <10 mL/min	Hemodialysis
Gout agents					
Allopurinol (Zyloprim®)	300 mg PO q24h	150-200 mg PO q24h	150 mg PO q24h	100 mg PO q48h	150 mg supplemental dose
Colchicine (Acetycol®, Colsalide®)	Acute: 2 mg, then 0.5 mg PO q6h; Chronic: 0.5-1 mg PO q24h	Decrease dose by 50% to no change	Decrease dose by 50%	Decrease dose by 25%	Same
Probenecid (Benemid®)	500 mg PO bid	Not effective	Not effective	Not effective	Not effective
Hypoglycemic agents					
Acarbose (Precose®)	50-200 mg PO tid	Avoid	Avoid	Avoid	No data
Acetohexamide (Dymelor®)	250-1500 mg PO q24h	Avoid	Avoid	Avoid	No data
Chlorpropamide (Diabinese®)	100-500 mg PO q24h	Avoid	Avoid	Avoid	Avoid
Exenatide (Byetta®)	5-10 mcg SC q bid	Same	Avoid	Avoid	Avoid
Glipizide (Glucotrol®)	2.5-15 mg PO q24h	1.25-7.5 mg Po q24h	1.25-7.5 mg PO q24h	1.24-7.5 mg PO q24h	No data
Glyburide (Diabeta®, Glynase®, PresTab®, Micronase®)	1.25-20 mg PO q24h	Avoid	Avoid	Avoid	No supplement necessary
Insulin	Variable	75% of usual dose	75% of usual dose	50% of usual dose	No supplement necessary
Metformin (Glucophage®)	500-850 mg PO bid	125-425 mg PO bid	125-212 mg PO bid	Avoid	No data
Tolazamide (Tolinase®)	100-250 mg PO q24h	Same	Same	Same	No data
Tolbutamide (Orinase®)	1-2 g q24h	Same	Same	Same	No supplement necessary
Nonsteroidal anti-inflammatory agents					
Diclofenac (Voltaren®)	25-75 mg PO bid	12.5-37.5 mg PO bid	6.25-37.5 mg PO bid	6.25-18.75 mg PO bid	No supplement necessary
Etodolac (Lodine®)	200 mg bid	Same	Same	Same	Same
Ibuprofen (Advil®, Motrin®)	200-800 mg PO q6h	Same	Same	Same	Same
Indomethacin (Indocin®)	25-50 mg PO q6-12h	Same	Same	Same	Same
Ketorolac (Toradol®)	60 mg IM LD, then 15-30 mg q6h; 30 mg IV LD, then 15 mg q6h	Same	Same	15 mg IM or IV q6h (no bolus dose)	15 mg IM or IV q6h (no bolus dose)
Nabumetone (Relafen®)	1-2 g PO q24h	Same	0.5-1 g PO q24h	0.5-1 g PO q24h	No supplement necessary
Naproxen (Naprosyn®)	250-500 mg PO 8-12h	Same	Same	Same	Same
Oxaprozin (Daypro®)	1200 mg PO q24h	Same	Same	Same	Same
Tolmetin (Tolectin®)	400 mg PO tid	Same	Same	Same	Same
Proton pump inhibitors					
Esomeprazole (Nexium®)	20-40 mg PO q24h	Same	Same	Same	Same
Lansoprazole (Prevacid®)	15-30 mg PO q12-24h	Same	Same	Same	Same
Omeprazole (Prilosec®)	20-40 mg PO q12-24h	Same	Same	Same	Same
Pantoprazole (Protonix®)	20-80 mg PO q24h; 80 mg IV q12h	Same	Same	Same	Same

Reference: Micromedex® Healthcare Series, (electronic version). Thomson Micromedex, Greenwood Village, CO.

Available at: http://www.thomsonhc.com (cited 8/3/2006)

Appendix 3

Drugs in Hepatic Failure

Drug	Dose
Amiodarone (Cordarone®, Pacerone®)	Dose adjustment may be necessary in patients with hepatic dysfunction
Amitriptyline (Elavil®)	Decrease dose in patients with cirrhosis
Aspirin	Avoid in severe hepatic dysfunction
Atomoxetine (Strattera®)	Decrease dose by 50% in moderate hepatic dysfunction; give 25% of normal dose in severe hepatic dysfunction
Azole antifungals	Consider decreased doses in patients with severe hepatic dysfunction
Azathioprine (Imuran®)	Monitor hepatic transaminases every 2 weeks for 4 weeks, then monthly thereafter
Benzodiazepines	No dose adjustments are necessary with oxazepam (Serax®), lorazepam (Ativan®), or temazepam (Restoril®) Alprazolam (Xanax®): dose 0.25 mg bid-tid in patients with hepatic dysfunction Chlordiazepoxide (Librium®): avoid or decrease dose in patients with cirrhosis or hepatitis Diazepam (Valium®): decrease dose by 50% in patients with cirrhosis Midazolam (Versed®): doses may need to be decreased by 50% Triazolam (Halcion®): doses may need to be decreased by 50%
Bicalutamide (Casodex®)	Use with caution in patients with moderate to severe hepatic dysfunction
Bisoprolol (Zebeta®)	Decrease initial dose to 2.5 mg in patients with hepatic insufficiency; do not exceed a dose of 10 mg daily
Bosentan (Tracleer®)	Liver function should be tested monthly
Buspirone (Buspar®)	Avoid in patients with severe hepatic dysfunction
Carbamazepine (Tegretol®)	Avoid in patients with hepatic disease
Celecoxib (Celebrex®)	Decrease dose by 50% in patients with moderate hepatic dysfunction; avoid in patients with severe hepatic dysfunction
Clindamycin (Cleocin®)	Decrease dose in patients with hepatic dysfunction
Cimetidine (Tagamet®)	Decrease dose (50%) in patients with severe hepatic dysfunction
Darunavir (Prezista®)	Monitor liver function tests at baseline, then periodically thereafter
Delavirdine (Rescriptor®)	Decrease dose in patients with moderate hepatic disease
Diazepam (Valium®)	Decrease dose by 50% in patients with cirrhosis
Diltiazem (Cardizem®, Cartia®, Dilacor®, Tiazac®)	Doses should not exceed 90 mg/d in patients with cirrhosis
Disulfram (Antabuse®)	Use with caution in patients with hepatic cirrhosis or hepatic insufficiency; avoid in patients with advanced or severe hepatic disease
Erythromycin (E-Mycin®)	Dose may need to be decreased in patients with severe hepatic dysfunction
Esomeprazole (Nexium®)	Do not exceed a dose of 20 mg in patients with severe hepatic dysfunction
Estrogens	Use with caution in patients with impaired liver function
HMG-CoA reductase inhibitors	Avoid in patients with elevated serum transaminases
Indinavir (Crixivan®)	Decrease dose to 600 mg q8h in patients with mild to moderate hepatic dysfunction
Interferon beta-1a (Avonex®)	Consider a dose reduction
Interferon beta-1b (Betaseron®)	Liver function should be tested at months 1, 3, and 6, then periodically thereafter
Isoniazid (Laniazid®, Nydrazid®)	Defer therapy for prevention of tuberculosis in patients with acute hepatic disease
Isotretinoin (Accutane®)	Monitor liver function tests at baseline, then at weekly or biweekly intervals until a response to the treatment is established
Lamivudine-zidovudine (Combivir®)	Decrease zidovudine dose by 50% in hepatic insufficiency
Lamotrigine (Lamictal®)	Reduce initial, escalation, and maintenance doses by 50% in patients with moderate hepatic dysfunction; decrease doses by 75% in patients with severe hepatic dysfunction
Lansoprazole (Prevacid®)	Decrease dose in patients with hepatic dysfunction
Leflunomide (Arava®)	Avoid in patients with moderate to severe hepatic dysfunction; decrease dose to 10 mg/d if liver enzymes are elevated to 2 times the upper limit of normal; discontinue if liver enzymes are elevated to 3 times the upper limit of normal
Losartan (Cozaar®)	Decrease initial dose to 25 mg; total daily dose should not exceed 100 mg
Methotrexate (Folex®, Rheumatrex®)	Decrease dose by 25% when the bilirubin is 3.1-5 mg% and the AST is >180 IU; avoid if the bilirubin is >5 mg%
Metoprolol (Lopressor®)	Dose adjustment may be necessary in patients with hepatic insufficiency
Nabumetone (Relafen®)	Use with caution in patients with severe hepatic insufficiency
Nefazodone (Serzone®)	Avoid in patients with elevated transaminases
Nelfinavir (Viracept®)	Use with caution in patients with hepatic impairment
Ofloxacin (Floxin®)	Do not exceed 400 mg/d in patients with severe liver dysfunction
Omeprazole (Prilosec®)	Decrease dose in patients with hepatic dysfunction
Ondansetron (Zofran®)	Do not exceed 8 mg/d in patients with severe hepatic insufficiency
Oxycodone (Oxycontin®)	Initiate dose at one third to one half the usual dose in patients with hepatic dysfunction; increase dose conservatively

(continued)

Appendix 3

Drugs in Hepatic Failure (continued)

Drug	Dose
Pantoprazole (Protonix®)	Consider every-other-day dosing in patients with severe hepatic dysfunction
Pioglitazone (Actos®)	Avoid in patients with hepatic disease or serum transaminases >2.5 times the upper limit of normal
Phenobarbital (Barbita®, Luminal®, Solfoton®)	Dose may need to be decreased in patients with hepatic dysfunction
Phenytoin (Dilantin®)	Monitor levels frequently as the dose may need to be decreased in hepatic failure
Procainamide (Procanbid®, Promine®, Pronestyl®, Rhythmin®)	Lower doses or longer dosing intervals may be required in patients with hepatic failure
Propranolol (Betachron®, Inderal®)	Monitor more frequently in patients with hepatic dysfunction
Quinidine (Cardioquin®, Quinaglute®, Quinalan®, Quinidex, Quinora®)	Maintenance doses may need to be decreased by 50% in patients with chronic hepatitis
Risperidone (Risperdal®)	Decrease dose in patients with hepatic dysfunction
Rofecoxib (Vioxx®)	Use the lowest dose possible in patients with moderate hepatic impairment
Rifampin (Rifadin®, Rimactane®)	Decrease dose in patients with a serum bilirubin >50 micromol/L; doses should not exceed 6-8 mg/kg biweekly in patients with severe hepatic dysfunction
Ritonavir (Norvir®)	Use with caution in patients with moderate to severe hepatic dysfunction
Saquinavir (Invirase®, Fortovase®)	Avoid in severe hepatic dysfunction

Selective serotonin reuptake inhibitors (SSRIs) and serotonin-norepinephrine reuptake inhibitors	The dose should be decreased or the dosing interval increased in patients with hepatic insufficiency
	    Citalopram (Celexa®): a dose of 20 mg is recommended for patients with decreased hepatic function
	    Fluoxetine (Prozac®): a 50% dose reduction is recommended in patients with cirrhosis
	    Fluvoxamine (Luvox®): decrease the dose and titrate slowly in patients with hepatic insufficiency
	    Paroxetine (Paxil®): dose initially at 10 mg daily or 12.5 mg daily of the controlled-release product; doses should not exceed 40 mg daily or 50 mg daily of the controlled-release product
	    Sertraline (Zoloft®): decrease the dose or increase the interval
	    Venlafaxine (Effexor®): decrease the dose by 50% in patients with moderate hepatic impairment

Sulfonylureas	Dose may need to be decreased in hepatic disease
Tacrolimus (Prograf®)	Dose at the low end of the dosing range in patients with hepatic insufficiency
Tetracyclines	Avoid in patients with hepatic dysfunction
Theophylline (Aerolate®, Aminophyllin®, Aquaphyllin®, Asmalix®, Bronkodyl®, Choledyl®, Duraphyl®, Respbid®, Slo-bid®, Slo-Phyllin®, Sustaire®, Theo-24®, Theo-bid®, Theochron®, Theo-clear®, Theo-Dur®, Theo-lair®, Theon®, Theospan®, Theovent®, Truphylline®)	Dose may need to be decreased and serum levels should be monitored frequently in patients with hepatic insufficiency
Tipranavir (Aptivus®)	Contraindicated in patients with moderate to severe hepatoxicity; monitor liver functions at baseline then periodically thereafter
Tramadol (Ultram®)	Dose 50 mg PO q12h in patients with cirrhosis
Tricyclic antidepressants: amitriptyline (Elavil®), clomipramine (Anafranil®), desipramine (Norpramin®), doxepin (Sinequan®), imipramine (Tofranil®), nortriptyline (Pamelor®), protriptyline (Vivactil®)	Dose should be decreased in patients with cirrhosis
Valdecoxib (Bextra®)	Do not exceed 10 mg/d in patients with moderate hepatic impairment; avoid in severe hepatic dysfunction
Valproic acid (Depakote®, Depakene®)	Avoid in patients with hepatic disease or significant hepatic insufficiency
Warfarin (Coumadin®)	Monitor INR more frequently
Zafirlukast (Accolate®)	Consider a decreased dose in patients with cirrhosis
Zalcitbine (Hivid®)	Avoid in patients with liver function tests >5 times the upper limit of normal
Zidovudine (Retrovir®)	Decrease dose by 50% in patients with cirrhosis

References: Micromedex® Healthcare Series (electronic version). Thomson Micromedex, Greenwood Village, CO.
Available at: http://www.thomsonhc.com (cited 8/3/2006).

Appendix 4

Top 200 Prescription Drugs

The following is a list of the top 200 prescriptions for 2005 by the number of U.S. prescriptions dispensed; obtained with permission from rxlist.com with data furnished by NDC Health.

	Brand name	Generic name		Brand name	Generic name
1.	Hydrocodone w/ APAP	hydrocodone w/ APAP	51.	Levaquin	levofloxacin
2.	Lipitor	atorvastatin	52.	Tramadol	tramadol
3.	Amoxicillin	amoxicillin	53.	Ciprofloxacin	ciprofloxacin
4.	Lisinopril	lisinopril	54.	Lotrel	amlodipine/benazepril
5.	Hydrochlorothiazide	hydrochlorothiazide	55.	Ranitidine	ranitidine
6.	Atenolol	atenolol	56.	Allegra	fexofenadine
7.	Zithromax	azithromycin	57.	Levoxyl	levothyroxine
8.	Furosemide	furosemide	58.	Diovan	valsartan
9.	Alprazolam	alprazolam	59.	Enalapril	enalapril
10.	Toprol XL	metoprolol XL	60.	Diazepam	diazepam
11.	Albuterol Aerosol	albuterol	61.	Naproxen	naproxen
12.	Norvasc	amlodipine	62.	Fluconazole	fluconazole
13.	Levothyroxine	levothyroxine	63.	Lisinopril/hydrochlorothiazide	lisinopril/hydrochlorothiazide
14.	Synthroid	levothyroxine	64.	Klor-Con	potassium chloride
15.	Metformin	metformin	65.	Altace	ramipril
16.	Zoloft	sertraline	66.	Wellbutrin XL	bupropion
17.	Lexapro	escitalopram	67.	Celebrex	Celecoxib
18.	Ibuprofen	ibuprofen	68.	Viagra	sildenafil citrate
19.	Cephalexin	cephalexin	69.	Doxycycline	doxycycline
20.	Ambien	zolpidem	70.	Zetia	ezetimibe
21.	Prednisone	prednisone	71.	Avandia	rosiglitazone maleate
22.	Nexium	esomeprazole	72.	Lovastatin	lovastatin
23.	Triamterene/ hydrochlorothiazide	triamterene/hydrochlorothiazide	73.	Diovan HCT	valsartan/hydrochlorothiazide
			74.	Carisoprodol	carisoprodol
24.	Propoxyphene N/APAP	propoxyphene N/APAP	75.	Yasmin 28	drospirenone/ethinyl estradiol
25.	Zocor	simvastatin	76.	Allopurinol	allopurinol
26.	Singulair	montelukast	77.	Clonidine	clonidine
27.	Prevacid	lansoprazole	78.	Methylprednisolone	methylprednisolone
28.	Metoprolol tartrate	metoprolol	79.	Actos	pioglitazone
29.	Fluoxetine	fluoxetine	80.	Pravachol	pravastatin
30.	Lorazepam	lorazepam	81.	Actonel	risedronate
31.	Plavix	clopidogrel	82.	Ortho Evra	norelgestromin/ethinyl estradiol
32.	Oxycodone/APAP	oxycodone/APAP	83.	Citalopram	citalopram
33.	Amoxicillin/clavulanate	amoxacillin/clavulanate	84.	Verapamil SR	verapamil
34.	Advair Diskus	salmeterol/fluticasone	85.	Isosorbide	isosorbide
35.	Fosamax	alendronate	86.	Penicillin VK	penicillin VK
36.	Effexor XR	venlafaxine	87.	Glyburide	glyburide
37.	Warfarin	warfarin	88.	Adderall XR	amphetamine mixed salts
38.	Paroxetine	paroxetine	89.	Nasonex	mometasone
39.	Clonazepam	clonazepam	90.	Folic acid	folic acid
40.	Zyrtec	cetirizine	91.	Seroquel	quetiapine
41.	Protonix	pantoprazole	92.	Cozaar	losartan
42.	Potassium chloride	potassium chloride	93.	Tricor	fenofibrate
43.	Acetaminophen/codeine	acetaminophen/codeine	94.	Coreg	carvedilol
44.	Trimethoprim/ sulfamethoxazole	trimethoprim/sulfamethoxazole	95.	Concerta	methylphenidate XR
			96.	Vytorin	ezetimibe/simvastatin
45.	Gabapentin	gabapentin	97.	Lantus	insulin glargine
46.	Premarin	conjugated estrogens	98.	Promethazine	promethazine
47.	Flonase	fluticasone	99.	Mobic	meloxicam
48.	Trazodone	trazodone	100.	Flomax	tamsulosin
49.	Cyclobenzaprine	cyclobenzaprine	101.	Crestor	rosuvastatin
50.	Amitriptyline	amitriptyline	102.	Glipizide ER	glipizide ER

(continued)

Appendix 4

Top 200 Prescription Drugs (continued)

Brand name	Generic name	Brand name	Generic name
103. Ortho Tri-Cyclen Lo	norgestimate/ethinyl estradiol	152. Zyprexa	olanzapine
104. Temazepam	temazepam	153. Lamictal	lamotrigine
105. Omeprazole	omeprazole	154. Zyrtec Syrup	cetirizine
106. Omnicef	cefdinir	155. Glycolax	polyethylene glycol 3350
107. Albuterol Nebulizer Solution	albuterol nebulizer solution	156. Acyclovir	acyclovir
108. Risperidal	risperidone	157. Propranolol	propranolol
109. Aciphex	rabeprazole	158. Nasacort AQ	triamcinolone acetonide
110. Digitek	digoxin	159. Aricept	donepezil
111. Sprionolactone	spironolactone	160. Butalbital/ acetaminophen/caffeine	butalbital/acetaminophen/caffeine
112. Valtrex	valacyclovir	161. Niaspan	niacin
113. Xalatan	latanoprost	162. Azithromycin	azithromycin
114. Metformin ER	metformin ER	163. Depakote	divalproex
115. Hyzaar	losartan/hydrochlorothiazide	164. Buspirone	buspirone
116. Quinapril	quinapril	165. Tri-Sprintec	norgestimate/ethinyl estradiol
117. Clindamycin	clindamycin	166. Methotrexate	methotrexate
118. Metronidazole Tabs	metronidazole	167. OxyContin	oxycodone
119. Triamcinolone	triamcinolone	168. Rhinocort Aqua	budesonide
120. Topamax	topiramate	169. Benicar HCT	olmesartan/hydrochlorothiazide
121. Combivent	ipratropium/albuterol	170. Terazosin	terazosin
122. Benazepril	benazepril	171. Skelaxin	metaxalone
123. Gemfibrozil	gemfibrozil	172. Clotrimazole/betamethasone	clotrimazole/betamethasone
124. Avapro	irbesartan	173. Cialis	tadalafil
125. Amaryl	glimepiride	174. Avalide	irbesartan/hydrochlorothiazide
126. Trinessa	norgestimate/ethinyl estradiol	175. Fexofenadine	fexofenadine
127. Estradiol	estradiol	176. Ortho Tri-Cyclen	norgestimate/ethinyl estradiol
128. Hydroxyzine	hydroxyzine	177. Bupropion SR	bupropion
129. Metoclopramide	metoclopramide	178. Benzonatate	benzonatate
130. Allegra-D 12 Hour	fexofenadine/pseudoephedrine	179. Patanol	olopatadine
131. Doxazosin	doxazosin	180. Quinine	quinine
132. Coumadin	warfarin	181. Cartia XT	diltiazem
133. Glipizide	glipizide	182. Humalog	insulin lispro
134. Diclofenac	diclofenac	183. Paxil CR	paroxetine
135. Evista	raloxifene	184. Aviane	levonorgestrel/ethinyl estradiol
136. Diltiazem CD	diltiazem	185. Lanoxin	digoxin
137. Detrol LA	tolterodine	186. Amphetamine mixed salts	amphetamine mixed salts
138. Meclizine	meclizine	187. Famotidine	famotidine
139. Glyburide/metformin	glyburide/metformin	188. Digoxin	digoxin
140. Strattera	atomoxetine	189. Levothroid	levothyroxine
141. Cymbalta	duloxetine	190. Nifedipine ER	nifedipine
142. Nitrofurantoin	nitrofurantoin	191. Nortriptyline	nortriptyline
143. Promethazine/codeine	promethazine/codeine	192. Tussionex	hydrocodone/chlorpheniramine
144. Benicar	olmesartan	193. Nitroquick	nitroglycerin
145. Mirtazapine	mirtazapine	194. Phenytoin	phenytoin
146. Bisoprolol/ hydrochlorothiazide	bisoprolol/hydrochlorothiazide	195. Endocet	oxycodone/acetaminophen
147. Clarinex	desloratadine	196. Etodolac	etodolac
148. Oxycodone	oxycodone	197. Atenolol/chlorthalidone	atenolol/chlorthalidone
149. Minocycline	minocycline	198. Phentermine	phentermine
150. Imitrex	sumatriptan	199. Tramadol/acetaminophen	tramadol/acetaminophen
151. Nabumetone	Nabumetone	200. Tizanidine	tizanidine

The Top 200 Prescriptions for 2005 by Number of U.S. Prescriptions Dispensed. RxList the internet drug index web site.
Available at: www.rxlist.com/top200.htm. Accessed on: August 4, 2006.

Appendix 5

Top 200 Over-the-Counter Products

The following is a list of over-the-counter (OTC) and health and beauty care brands based on dollar amount in 2004.

Rank	Product	Rank	Product
1.	Private-label internal analgesic tablets	51.	Trojan male contraceptives
2.	Private-label cold/allergy/sinus tablets/packets	52.	Metamucil laxative/stimulant liq/pwdr/oil
3	Private-label mineral supplements	53.	Osteo Bi Flex mineral supplements
4.	Advil internal analgesic tablets	54.	Boost weight control/nutritionals liq/pwd
5.	Tylenol internal analgesic tablets	55.	Private-label weight control/nutritionals liq/pwd
6.	Prilosec OTC antacid tablets	56.	Private-label cough syrup
7.	Depend adult incontinence products	57.	Tums EX antacid tablets
8.	Nicorette anti-smoking gum	58.	Ensure Plus weight control/nutritionals liq/pwd
9.	Private-label one- and two-letter vitamins	59.	Private-label nasal spray/drops/inhaler
10.	Private-label adult incontinence products	60.	Atkins Advantage weight control/nutritionals liq/pwd
11.	Private-label multivitamins	61.	Tylenol Arthritis internal analgesic tablets
12.	Aleve internal analgesic tablets	62.	Alavert cold/allergy/sinus tablets/packets
13.	Private-label first aid ointments/antiseptics	63.	Mucinex cold/allergy/sinus tablets/packets
14.	Ensure weight control/nutritionals liq/pwd	64.	Tylenol Sinus cold/allergy/sinus tablets/packets
15.	Private-label laxative tablets	65.	Sudafed cold/allergy/sinus tablets/packets
16.	Private-label antacid tablets	66.	Abreva lip balm/cold sore medication
17.	Slim Fast meal options weight control/nutritionals liq/pwd	67.	Imodium A-D diarrhea tablets
18.	Depend Poise adult incontinence products	68.	Private-label vaginal treatments
19.	Claritin D cold/allergy/sinus tablets/packets	69.	Private-label pregnancy test kits
20.	Private-label cold/allergy/sinus liquid/powder	70.	Commit anti-smoking tablets
21.	Benadryl cold/allergy/sinus tablets/packets	71.	Tylenol internal analgesic liquids
22.	Claritin cold/allergy/sinus tablets/packets	72.	Imodium Advanced diarrhea tablets
23.	Bayer internal analgesic tablets	73.	Children's Motrin internal analgesic liquids
24.	Tylenol PM internal analgesic tablets	74.	Neosporin Plus first aid ointments/antiseptics
25.	Nature Made one- and two-letter vitamins	75.	Tylenol Cold cold/allergy/sinus tablets/packets
26.	Centrum Silver multivitamins	76.	Private-label laxative/stimulant liq/pwdr/oil
27.	PediaSure weight control/nutritionals liq/pwd	77.	Futuro muscle/body support devices
28.	Private-label anti-smoking gum	78.	Monistat 3 vaginal treatments
29.	Private-label first aid – tape/bandage/gauze/cotton	79.	E P T pregnancy test kits
30.	Halls cough/sore throat drop	80.	Icy Hot external analgesics rubs
31.	Private-label eye/lens care solutions	81.	Tylenol Plus cold/allergy/sinus liquid/powder
32.	Pepcid AC antacid tablets	82.	Dulcolax laxative tablets
33.	Nicoderm CQ anti-smoking patch	83.	Theraflu cold/allergy/sinus tablets/packets
34.	Band-Aid first aid – tape/bandage/gauze cotton	84.	Private-label anti-smoking patch
35.	Dr. Scholl's foot care devices	85.	Alka-Seltzer plus cold/allergy/sinus tablets/packets
36.	Centrum multivitamins	86.	Breathe Right nasal strips
37.	Vicks Nyquil cold/allergy/sinus liquid/powder	87.	Bengay external analgesics rubs
38.	Nature Made mineral supplements	88.	Primatene Mist nasal spray/drops/inhaler
39.	Motrin IB internal analgesic tablets	89.	Pepcid Complete antacid tablets
40.	Bausch & Lomb ReNu Multiplus eye/lens care solutions	90.	Preparation H hemorrhoidal cream/ointment/spray
41.	Alcon Opti Free Express eye/lens care solutions	91.	Ensure Glucerna weight control/nutritionals liq/pwd
42.	Johnson & Johnson first aid – tape/bandage/gauze/cotton	92.	Private-label cough/sore throat drop
43.	Zantac 75 antacid tablets	93.	Zicam nasal spray/drops/inhaler
44.	Nature's Bounty mineral supplements	94.	Trim Spa weight control candy/tablets
45.	Ace muscle/body support devices	95.	First Response pregnancy test kits
46.	Robitussin DM cough syrup	96.	Excedrin Migraine internal analgesic tablets
47.	ThermaCare heat/ice packs	97.	Neosporin first aid ointments/antiseptics
48.	Private-label anti-itch treatments (inc. calamine)	98.	Advil cold & sinus cold/allergy/sinus tablets/packets
49.	Pepto-Bismol stomach remedy liquid/powder	99.	St. Joseph internal analgesic tablets
50.	Excedrin internal analgesic tablets	100.	Sundown mineral supplements

(continued)

Appendix 5

Top 200 Over-the-Counter Products (continued)

Rank	Product
101.	Gas X antacid tablets
102.	Tylenol 8 Hour internal analgesic tablets
103.	Rolaids antacid tablets
104.	One-A-Day multivitamins
105.	Monistat 1 vaginal treatments
106.	Trojan Enz male contraceptives
107.	Tylenol allergy sinus cold/allergy/sinus tablets/packets
108.	Vicks Dayquil cold/allergy/sinus tablets/packets
109.	Private-label internal analgesic liquids
110.	Afrin nasal spray/drops/inhaler
111.	Lamisil AT foot care/athletes foot medication
112.	Vicks VapoRub chest rubs
113.	Alka-Seltzer antacid/analgesic combo
114.	Phillips stomach remedy liquid/powder
115.	ChapStick lip balm/cold sore medication
116.	Serenity adult incontinence products
117.	Ricola cough/sore throat drop
118.	Metamucil laxative tablets
119.	Private-label sleeping aid tablets
120.	Triaminic cold/allergy/sinus liquid/powder
121.	Rogaine hair growth products
122.	Nature's Resource mineral supplements
123.	Delsym cough syrup
124.	Robitussin cough syrup
125.	Private-label foot care/athletes foot medication
126.	Ex-Lax laxative tablets
127.	Private-label diarrhea tablets
128.	Benadryl cold/allergy/sinus liquid/powder
129.	Viactiv mineral supplements
130.	Lotrimin A F foot care/athletes foot medication
131.	Midol feminine pain relievers
132.	Vicks Nyquil cold/allergy/sinus tablets/packets
133.	Ecotrin internal analgesic tablets
134.	Claritin Reditabs cold/allergy/sinus tablets/packets
135.	Dimetapp cold/allergy/sinus liquid/powder
136.	Robitussin CF cold/allergy/sinus liquid/powder
137.	Sundown one- and two-letter vitamins
138.	Preparation H hemorrhoidal remedies
139.	Private-label foot care devices
140.	Tinactin foot care/athletes foot medication
141.	Caltrate 600 mineral supplements
142.	Citracal mineral supplements
143.	Benadryl anti-itch treatments (inc. calamine)
144.	Os Cal mineral supplements
145.	Private-label stomach remedy liquid/powder
146.	Bausch & Lomb ReNu eye/lens care solutions
147.	Coricidin HBP cold/allergy/sinus tablets/packets
148.	Pediacare cold/allergy/sinus liquid/powder
149.	One-A-Day Weight Smart multivitamins
150.	Cold Eeze cough/sore throat drop
151.	Mylanta antacid liquid/powder
152.	Monistat 7 vaginal treatments
153.	Rid lice treatments
154.	Nature's Bounty one- and two-letter vitamins
155.	Cortizone 10 anti-itch treatments (inc. calamine)
156.	Private-label hair growth products
157.	Private-label Epsom salts
158.	Flintstones multivitamins
159.	Halls Fruit Breezers cough/sore throat drop
160.	Tums Ultra antacid tablets
161.	Citrucel laxative/stimulant liq/pwdr/oil
162.	3M Nexcare first aid – tape/bandage/gauze/cotton
163.	Infants' Motrin internal analgesic liquids
164.	Allergan Refresh Tears eye/lens care solutions
165.	Blistex lip balm/cold sore medication
166.	Centrum Performance multivitamins
167.	Ultra Slim-Fast weight control/nutritionals liq/pwd
168.	Zantrex 3 weight control candy/tablets
169.	Pepto-Bismol stomach remedy tablets
170.	Natrol mineral supplements
171.	Estroven mineral supplements
172.	Tylenol Flu cold/allergy/sinus tablets/packets
173.	Excedrin Tension Headache internal analgesic tablets
174.	Clearblue Easy pregnancy test kits
175.	Vicks Dayquil cold/allergy/sinus liquid/powder
176.	Robitussin cold/allergy/sinus liquid/powder
177.	Xenadrine EFX weight control candy/tablets
178.	Lifestyles male contraceptives
179.	Hydroxycut weight control candy/tablets
180.	Halls Defense cough/sore throat drop
181.	Private-label lice treatments
182.	Boost Plus weight control candy/tablets
183.	Ludens cough/sore throat drop
184.	Tums antacid tablets
185.	Excedrin PM internal analgesic tablets
186.	Sudafed Sinus cold/allergy/sinus tablets/packets
187.	Maalox Max antacid liquid/powder
188.	Summers Eve all other fem. Hygiene/med. treatments
189.	K-Y Warming Liquid personal lubricants
190.	Motrin cold/allergy/sinus liquid/powder
191.	Visine eye/lens care solutions
192.	Chloraseptic sore throat remedy liquids
193.	EAS Carb Control weight control/nutritionals liq/pwd
194.	Mederma first aid ointments/antiseptics
195.	Metabolife Ultra weight control candy/tablets
196.	Vicks Sinex nasal spray/drops/inhaler
197.	Benefiber laxative/stimulant liq/pwdr/oil
198.	AMO Complete Moisture Plus eye/lens care solutions
199.	Slim Fast Optima weight control/nutritionals liq/pwd
200.	Bausch & Lomb Ocuvite Presr Vision multivitamins

Top 200 OTC /HBC brands in 2004. *Drug Topics*.

Available at: http://www.drugtopics.com/drugtopics/data/articlestandard/drugtopics/162005/156502/article.pdf. Accessed on: August 4, 2006.

Appendix 6

Drugs Excreted in Breast Milk

The following is not comprehensive; generics and alternate brands of some products may exist. When recommending drugs to pregnant or nursing patients, always check product labeling for specific precautions.

Accolate	Compazine	Floxin	Meruvax II	Phenergan	Tegretol
Accuretic	Cordarone	Fluorescite	Methergine	Phenobarbital	Tenoretic
Achromycin	Corgard	Fortaz	Methotrexate	Phrenilin	Tenormin
Actiq	Cortisporin	Furosemide	MetroCream/Gel/Lotion	Pipracil	Tenuate
Activella	Corzide	Gabitril	Mexitil	Plan B	Testoderm
Adalat	Cosopt	Galzin	Mezlin	Platinol-AQ	Thalitone
Adderall	Coumadin	Garamycin	Micronor	Ponstel	Theo-24
Advicor	Covera-HS	Glucophage	Microzide	Pravachol	Theo-Dur
Aggrenox	Crinone	Glyset	Midamor	Premphase	Thorazine
Aldactazide	Cyclessa	Guaifed	Migranal	Prempro	Tiazac
Aldactone	Cystospaz	Halcion	Miltown	Prevacid	Timolide
Aldoclor	Cytomel	Haldol	Minizide	Preven	Timoptic
Aldomet	Cytotec	Helidac	Minocin	PREVPAC	Tobi
Aldoril	Cytoxan	Hydrocet	Mirapex	Prinzide	Tofranil
Alesse	Dapsone	Hydrocortone	Mircette	Procanbid	Tolectin
Allegra-D	Daraprim	HydroDIURIL	M-M-R II	Prograf	Tol-Tab
Alfenta	Darvon	Iberet-Folic	Modicon	Proloprim	Toprol-XL
Aloprim	Darvon-N	Ifex	Moduretic	Prometrium	Toradol
Altace	Decadron	Imitrex	Monodox	Pronestyl	Trandate
Ambien	Deconsal II	Imuran	Mono-Gesic	Propofol	Tranxene
Anaprox	Demerol	Inderal	Monopril	Prosed/DS	Trental
Ancef	Demulen	Inderide	Morphine	Provera	Trilafon
Androderm	Depacon	Indocin	MS Contin	Prozac	Trileptal
Apresoline	Depakene	INFeD	MSIR	Pseudoephedrine	Tri-Levlen
Aralen	Depakote	Invanz	Myambutol	Pulmicort	Trilisate
Arthrotec	Depo-Provera	Inversine	Mykrox	Pyrazinamide	Tri-Norinyl
Asacol	Desogen	Isoptin	Mysoline	Quibron	Triostat
Astramorph/PF	Desoxyn	Kadian	Naprelan	Quibron-T	Triphasil
Ativan	Desyrel	Keflex	Naprosyn	Quinidex	Trivora
A/T/S	Dexedrine	Keftab	Nascobal	Quinine	Trizivir
Augmentin	DextroStat	Kefurox	Necon	Reglan	Trovan
Avalide	D.H.E. 45	Kefzol	NegGram	Relpax	Tylenol
AVC	Diabinese	Keppra	Nembutal	Renese	Tylenol with Codeine
Axid	Diastat	Kerlone	Neoral	Requip	Ultram
Axocet	Diflucan	Klonopin	Niaspan	Reserpine	Unasyn
Azactam	Digitek	Kronofed-A	Nicotrol	Restoril	Uniphyl
Azathioprine	Dilacor	Kutrase	Nizoral	Retrovir	Uniretic
Azulfidine	Dilantin	Lamictal	Norco	Ridaura	Unithroid
Bactrim	Dilaudid	Lamisil	Nor-QD	Rifadin	Urimax
Benadryl	Diovan	Lamprene	Nordette	Rifamate	Uroqid-Acid
Bentyl	Diprivan	Lanoxicaps	Norinyl	Rifater	Valium
Betapace	Disalcid	Lanoxin	Noritate	Rimactane	Valtrex
Bexxar	Diuril	Lariam	Normodyne	Risperdal	Vanceril
Bicillin	Dolobid	Lescol	Norpace	RMS	Vancocin
Blocadren	Dolophine	Levbid	Norplant	Robaxisal	Vantin
Brethine	Doral	Levlen	Novantrone	Rocaltrol	Vascor
Brevicon	Doryx	Levlite	Nubain	Rocephin	Vaseretic
Brontex	Droxia	Levora	Nucofed	Roferon A	Vasotec
Cafergot	Duraclon	Levothroid	Nydrazid	Roxanol	Verelan
Calan	Duragesic	Levoxyl	Oramorph	Salflex	Vermox
Capoten	Duramorph	Levsin	Oretic	Sandimmune	Versed
Capozide	Duratuss	Levsinex	Ortho-Cept	Sansert	Vibramycin
Captopril	Duricef	Lexapro	Ortho-Cyclen	Sarafem	Vibra-Tabs
Carbatrol	Dyazide	Lexxel	Ortho-Novum	Seconal	Vicodin
Cardizem	Dyrenium	Lindane	Ortho Tri-Cyclen	Sectral	Viramune
Cataflam	E.E.S.	Lioresal	Orudis	Sedapap	Voltaren
Catapres	EC-Naprosyn	Lithium	Ovcon	Semprex-D	Wellbutrin
Ceclor	Ecotrin	Lithobid	Ovral	Septra	Xanax
Cefizox	Effexor	Lo/Ovral	Ovrette	Sinequan	Zagam
Cefobid	EMLA	Loestrin	Oxistat	Slo-bid	Zantac
Cefotan	Enduron	Lomotil	OxyContin	Solganal	Zarontin
Ceftin	ERYC	Loniten	OxyFast	Soma	Zaroxolyn
Celexa	EryPed	Lopressor	OxyIR	Sonata	Zestoretic
Ceptaz	Ery-Tab	Lortab	Pacerone	Sporanox	Ziac
Cerebyx	Erythrocin	Lotensin	Pamelor	Stadol	Zinacef
Ceredase	Erythromycin	Lotrel	Pancrease	Streptomycin	Zithromax
Cipro	Esgic-plus	Lufyllin	Panlor SS	Stromectol	Zoloft
Claforan	Eskalith	Lufyllin-GG	Paxil	Symmetrel	Zonalon
Clarinex	Estrostep	Luminal	PCE	Syn-Rx	Zonegran
Claritin	Ethmozine	Luvox	Pediapred	Synthroid	Zosyn
Claritin-D	Felbatol	Macrobid	Pediazole	Tagamet	Zovia
Cleocin	Feldene	Macrodantin	Pediotic	Tambocor	Zovirax
Clozaril	femhrt	Mandol	Pentasa	Tapazole	Zyban
Codeine	Fero-Folic	Marinol	Pepcid	Tarka	Zydone
CombiPatch	Fiorinal	Maxipime	Periostat	Tavist	Zyloprim
Combipres	Flagyl	Maxzide	Persantine	Tazicef	Zyrtec
Combivir	Florinef	Mefoxin	Pfizerpen	Tazidime	

From Fleming T., ed. *Drug Topics Red Book*. Montvale, NJ: Thompson PDR, 2004.

Appendix 7

Drugs That May Cause Photosensitivity

The drugs in this table are known to cause photosensitivity in some individuals. Effects can range from itching, scaling, rash, and swelling to skin cancer, premature skin aging, skin and eye burns, cataracts, reduced immunity, blood vessel damage, and allergic reactions.

The list is not all-inclusive, and shows only representative brands of each generic. When in doubt, always check specific product labeling. Individuals should be advised to wear protective clothing and to apply sunscreens while taking the medications listed below.

Generic	Brand
Acetazolamide	Diamox
Acitretin	Soriatane
Alatrofloxacin	Trovan I.V.
Alendronate	Fosamax
Alitretinoin	Panretin
Almotriptan	Axert
Amiloride/hydrochlorothiazide	Moduretic
Aminolevulinic acid	Levulan Kerastick
Amiodarone	Cordarone, Pacerone
Amitriptyline	Elavil
Amitriptyline/chlordiazepoxide	Limbitrol
Amitriptyline/perphenazine	Triavil
Amoxapine	
Anagrelide	Agrylin
Aripiprazole	Abilify
Atazanavir	Reyataz
Atenolol/chlorthalidone	Tenoretic
Atorvastatin	Lipitor
Aurothioglucose	Solganal
Azatadine/pseudoephedrine	Rynatan, Trinalin
Azithromycin	Zithromax
Benazepril	Lotensin
Benazepril/hydrochlorothiazide	Lotensin HCT
Bendroflumethiazide/nadolol	Corzide
Bexarotene	Targretin
Bismuth/metronidazole/ tetracycline	Helidac
Bisoprolol/hydrochlorothiazide	Ziac
Brompheniramine/ dextromethorphan/ phenylephrine	Alacol DM
Brompheniramine/ dextromethorphan/ pseudoephedrine	Bromfed-DM
Buffered aspirin/ pravastatin	Pravigard PAC
Bupropion	Wellbutrin, Zyban
Candesartan/ hydrochlorothiazide	Atacand HCT
Capecitabine	Xeloda
Captopril	Capoten
Captopril/hydrochlorothiazide	Capozide
Carbamazepine	Carbatrol, Tegretol, Tegretol-XR
Carbinoxamine/ pseudoephedrine	Palgic-D, Palgic-DS, Pediatex-D
Carvedilol	Coreg
Celecoxib	Celebrex
Cetirizine	Zyrtec
Cetirizine/pseudoephedrine	Zyrtec-D
Cevimeline	Evoxac
Chlorhexidine gluconate	Hibistat
Chloroquine	Aralen
Chlorothiazide	Diuril
Chlorpheniramine/ hydrocodone/ pseudoephedrine	Tussend
Chlorpheniramine/ phenylephrine/pyrilamine	Rynatan
Chlorpromazine	Thorazine
Chlorpropamide	Diabinese
Chlorthalidone	Thalitone
Chlorthalidone/clonidine	Clorpres

Generic	Brand
Cidofovir	Vistide
Ciprofloxacin	Cipro
Citalopram	Celexa
Clemastine	Tavist
Clozapine	Clozaril
Cromolyn sodium	Gastrocrom
Cyclobenzaprine	Flexeril
Cyproheptadine	Periactin
Dacarbazine	DTIC-Dome
Dantrolene	Dantrium
Demeclocycline	Declomycin
Desipramine	Norpramin
Diclofenac potassium	Cataflam
Diclofenac sodium	Voltaren
Diclofenac sodium/ misoprostol	Arthrotec
Diflunisal	Dolobid
Dihydroergotamine	D.H.E. 45
Diltiazem	Cardizem, Tiazac
Diphenhydramine	Benadryl
Divalproex	Depakote
Doxepin	Sinequan
Doxycycline hyclate	Doryx, Periostat, Vibra-Tabs, Vibramycin
Doxycycline monohydrate	Monodox
Enalapril	Vasotec
Enalapril/felodipine	Lexxel
Enalapril/hydrochlorothiazide	Vaseretic
Enalaprilat	Vasotec I.V.
Epirubicin	Ellence
Eprosartan mesylate/ hydrochlorothiazide	Teveten HCT
Erythromycin/sulfisoxazole	Pediazole
Estazolam	ProSom
Estradiol	Gynodiol
Ethionamide	Trecator-SC
Etodolac	Lodine
Felbamate	Felbatol
Fenofibrate	Tricor, Lofibra
Floxuridine	Sterile FUDR
Flucytosine	Ancobon
Fluorouracil	Efudex
Fluoxetine	Prozac, Sarafem
Fluphenazine	Prolixin
Flutamide	Eulexin
Fluvastatin	Lescol
Fluvoxamine	Luvox
Focinopril	Monopril
Fosphenytoin	Cerebyx
Furosemide	Lasix
Gabapentin	Neurontin
Gatifloxacin	Tequin
Gemfibrozil	Lopid
Gemifloxacin mesylate	Factive
Gentamicin	Garamycin
Glatiramer	Copaxone
Glimepiride	Amaryl
Glipizide	Glucotrol
Glyburide	DiaBeta, Glynase, Micronase
Glyburide/metformin HCl	Glucovance
Griseofulvin	Fulvicin P/G, Grifulvin, Gris-PEG

Generic	Brand
Haloperidol	Haldol
Hexachlorophene	pHisoHex
Hydralazine/ hydrochlorothiazide	Apresazide
Hydrochlorothiazide	HydroDIURIL, Microzide, Oretic
Hydrochlorothiazide/fosinopril	Monopril HCT
Hydrochlorothiazide/irbesartan	Avalide
Hydrochlorothiazide/lisinopril	Prinzide, Zestoretic
Hydrochlorothiazide/ losartan potassium	Hyzaar
Hydrochlorothiazide/ methyldopa	Aldoril
Hydrochlorothiazide/ moexipril	Uniretic
Hydrochlorothiazide/ propranolol	Inderide
Hydrochlorothiazide/ quinapril	Accuretic
Hydrochlorothiazide/ spironolactone	Aldactazide
Hydrochlorothiazide/telmisartan	Micardis HCT
Hydrochlorothiazide/timolol	Timolide
Hydrochlorothiazide/triamterene	Dyazide, Maxzide
Hydrochlorothiazide/valsartan	Diovan HCT
Hydroflumethiazide	Diucardin
Hydroxychloroquine	Plaquenil
Hypericum	Kira, St. John's Wort
Hypericum/vitamin B₁/ vitamin C/kava-kava	One-A-Day Tension & Mood
Ibuprofen	Motrin
Imatinib Mesylate	Gleevec
Imipramine	Tofranil
Indapamide	Lozol
Interferon alfa-2b, recombinant	Intron A
Interferon alfa-n3 (human leukocyte derived)	Alferon-N
Interferon beta-1a	Avonex
Interferon beta-1b	Betaseron
Irbesartan/ hydrochlorothiazide	Avalide
Isoniazid/pyrazinamide/ rifampin	Rifater
Isotretinoin	Accutane, Amnesteem
Ketoprofen	Orudis, Oruvail
Lamotrigine	Lamictal
Leuprolide	Lupron
Levamisole	Ergamisol
Lisinopril	Prinivil, Zestril
Lomefloxacin	Maxaquin
Loratadine	Claritin
Loratadine/pseudoephedrine	Claritin-D
Losartan	Cozaar
Lovastatin	Mevacor, Altocor
Lovastatin/niacin	Advicor
Maprotiline	Ludiomil
Mefenamic acid	Ponstel
Meloxicam	Mobic
Meperidine/promethazine	Mepergan
Mesalamine	Pentasa

(continued)

Appendix 7

Drugs That May Cause Photosensitivity (continued)

Generic	Brand	Generic	Brand	Generic	Brand
Methazolamide		Pentosan polysulfate	Elmiron	Somatropin	Serostim
Methotrexate	Trexall	Pentostatin	Nipent	Sotalol	Betapace, Betapace AF
Methoxsalen	Uvadex, Oxsoralen, 8-MOP	Perphenazine	Trilafon	Sparfloxacin	Zagam
		Phenazopyridine/ sulfamethizole	Urobiotic-250	Sulfamethoxazole/ trimethoprim	Bactrim, Septra
Methyclothiazide	Enduron	Pilocarpine	Salagen		
Methyldopa/ Chlorothiazide	Aldoclor	Pimpinella major	Burnet	Sulfasalazine	Azulfidine
Metolazone	Mykrox, Zaroxolyn	Piroxicam	Feldene	Sulfisoxazole	Gantrisin Pediatric
Minocycline	Dynacin, Minocin	Polythiazide	Renese	Sulindac	Clinoril
Mirtazapine	Remeron	Polythiazide/prazosin	Minizide	Sumatriptan	Imitrex
Moexipril	Univasc	Porfimer sodium	Photofrin	Tacrolimus	Prograf, Protopic
Moxifloxacin	Avelox	Pravastatin	Pravachol	Tazarotene	Tazorac
Nabumetone	Relafen	Prochlorperazine	Compazine, Compro	Tetracycline	Sumycin
Nalidixic acid	NegGram	Promethazine	Phenergan	Thalidomide	Thalomid
Naproxen	Naprosyn, EC-Naprosyn	Protriptyline	Vivactil	Thioridazine hydrochloride	Mellaril
		Pyrazinamide	Pyrazinamide	Thiothixene	Navane
Naproxen sodium	Anaprox, Naprelan	Quetiapine	Seroquel	Tiagabine	Gabitril
Naratriptan	Amerge	Quinapril	Accupril	Topiramate	Topamax
Nefazodone	Serzone	Quinidine gluconate	Quinidine	Triamcinolone	Azmacort
Nifedipine	Procardia	Quinidine sulfate	Quinidex	Triamterene	Dyrenium
Nisoldipine	Sular	Rabeprazole sodium	Aciphex	Trifluoperazine	Stelazine
Norfloxacin	Noroxin	Ramipril	Altace	Trimipramine	Surmontil
Nortriptyline	Pamelor	Riluzole	Rilutek	Trovafloxacin	Trovan Tablets
Ofloxacin	Floxin	Risperidone	Risperdal	Valacyclovir	Valtrex
Olanzapine	Zyprexa	Ritonavir	Norvir	Valdecoxib	Bextra
Olmesartan medoxomil/ hydrochlorothiazide	Benicar HCT	Rizatriptan	Maxalt	Valproate	Depacon
		Ropinirole	Requip	Valproic acid	Depakene
Olsalazine	Dipentum	Ruta graveolens	Rue	Venlafaxine	Effexor
Oxaprozin	Daypro	Saquinavir	Fortovase	Verteporfin	Visudyne
Oxcarbazepine	Trileptal	Saquinavir mesylate	Invirase	Vinblastine	
Oxycodone	Roxicodone	Selegiline	Eldepryl	Voriconazole	Vfend
Oxytetracycline	Terramycin	Sertraline	Zoloft	Zalcitabine	Hivid
Pantoprazole	Protonix	Sibutramine	Meridia	Zaleplon	Sonata
Paroxetine	Paxil	Sildenafil	Viagra	Ziprasidone	Geodon
Pastinaca sativa	Parsnip	Simvastatin	Zocor	Zolmitriptan	Zomig
				Zolpidem	Ambien

From Fleming T., ed. *Drug Topics Red Book.* Montvale. NJ: Thompson PDR, 2004.

Appendix 8

Drug Information Resources by Category

Adverse drug reactions/side effects

AHFS Drug Information
Drug Facts & Comparisons
Drug Information Handbook
Martindale: The Complete Drug Reference
Meyler's Side Effects of Drugs
Micromedex DRUGDEX
Physician's Desk Reference
Side Effects of Drugs Annual
Textbook of Adverse Drug Reactions
EMBASE
International Pharmaceutical Abstracts
Medline
TOXLINE (NLM Database)
ClinAlert (www.nlm.nih.gov/databases/
    alerts/clinical_alerts.html)
FDA Medwatch Program
    (http://www.fda.gov/medwatch/safety.htm)
Institute for Safe Medication Practices
    (http://www.ismp.org/)
Vaccine Adverse Event Reporting System
    (http://www.vaers.org/)

Alternative medicine/herbals/natural products

Herbs of Choice
Honest Herbal
Natural Medicines Comprehensive Database
PDR for Nonprescription Drugs and Dietary
    Supplements
Review of Natural Products
The Complete German Commission E
    Monographs
FDA CFSAN Dietary Supplements
    (http://vm.cfsan.fda.gov)
National Center for Alternative and
    Complimentary Medicine
    (http://nccam.nih.gov)
NIH Office of Dietary Supplements
    (http://dietary-supplements.info.nih.gov)

Drug dosing in renal dysfunction

AHFS Drug Information
Drug Facts & Comparisons
Drug Information Handbook
Drug Prescribing in Renal Failure
Handbook of Dialysis
Physician's Desk Reference
Sanford Guide to Antimicrobial Therapy
    (Antimicrobials Only)

EMBASE
International Pharmaceutical Abstracts
Medline
Global Pharmacist Renal Dosing
    (http://www.globalrph.com/renaldosing.htm &
    http://www.globalrph.com/crcl.htm)
John Hopkins Aids Service
    (http://www.hopkins-aids.edu/publications/
    book/ch4_agents_tab0428.html#tab0428)
Nephrology Pharmacy Associates (http://www.
    nephrologypharmacy.com/pub_dialysis.html)
University of Louisville, Kidney Disease
    Program (http://www.kdp-baptist.
    louisville.edu/renalfailure/)

Drug interactions

AHFS Drug Information
Drug Facts & Comparisons
Drug Interaction Facts
Drug Therapy Screening System (DTSS)
Evaluation of Drug Interactions
Hansten & Horn's Analysis and Management of
    Drug Interactions
Micromedex DRUG-REAX
EMBASE
International Pharmaceutical Abstracts
Medline
Drug Store (http://www.drugstore.com/
    pharmacy/drugchecker/)
Facts & Comparisons (www.
    factsandcomparisons.com/NewsArticle.asp?I
    D=91)
Liverpool Pharmacology HIV group (http://
    www.hiv-druginteractions.org/)
University of Indiana (http://medicine.
    iupui.edu/flockhart/)

Drug therapy/therapeutics

Applied Therapeutics: The Clinical Use of
    Drugs
Cecil Textbook of Medicine
Harrison's Principles of Internal Medicine
Medical Letter
Pharmacist's Letter
Pharmacotherapy: A Pathophysiologic
    Approach
Textbook of Therapeutics: Drug and Disease
    Management
Washington Manual of Medical Therapeutics
EMBASE

International Pharmaceutical Abstracts (IPA)
Medline
Global Pharmacist (http://www.globalrph.com)
Merck Manual Diagnosis and Therapy Text
    (http://www.merck.com/pubs/mmanual_hom
    e/contents.htm)
Mdchoice (http://www.mdchoice.
    com/calculators.asp)
Excipient/Inactive Ingredient Information
Drug Manufacturer/Company
Handbook of Pharmaceutical Additives
Micromedex POISINDEX
Physician's Desk Reference/ Package
    Insert/Product Label

Legal and regulatory

Guide to Federal Pharmacy Law
Pharmacy Law Digest
USPDI Volume III: Approved Drugs and Legal
    Requirements
USP/NF
Code of Federal Regulations (Title 21)
    (www.gpo.gov)
FDA website (www.fda.gov)
Joint Commission on Accreditation of
    Healthcare Organizations
    (www.jcaho.org)
National Association of Boards of Pharmacy
    (http://www.nabp.net)
US Drug Enforcement Administration
    (http://www.usdoj.gov/dea/)
World Health Organization
    (http://www.who.int/en/)

Monographs/medication use evaluation (MUE, DUE)

AHFS Drug Information
Drug Usage Evaluations (ASHP)
Formulary Monograph Service (F & C)
International Pharmaceutical Abstracts (IPA)
ASHP Practices (http://www.ashp.org/
    bestpractices/index.cfm
The FIX System (www.theformulary.com)

News/new drug approvals

FAXStat
Medical Letter
Pharmacist's Letter
The Pink Sheet
CenterWatch (http://www.centerwatch.
    com/patient/drugs/druglist.html)

(continued)

Appendix 8

Drug Information Resources by Category (continued)

FDA Website (http://www.fda.gov/cder/
approval/index.htm)
Lexi-Comp (http://www.lexi.com/web/
newdrugs.jsp)
Reuters News Service (www.reutershealth.
com)

Nonprescription drugs/ OTC information
American Drug Index
Drug Facts & Comparisons
Drug Topics Redbook
Handbook of Nonprescription Drugs
Micromedex DRUGDEX, POISINDEX
PDR for Nonprescription Drugs and Dietary
Supplements
DrugStore.com (www.drugstore.com)

Off-label/unlabeled/non-FDA approved
uses
AHFS Drug Information
Drug Fact and Comparisons
Martindale
Micromedex DRUGDEX
Mosby's GenRX
USPDI Volume I
EMBASE
International Pharmaceutical Abstracts
Medline

Patient counseling/education
AHFS Drug Information
Drug Facts and Comparisons
Handbook of Nonprescription Drugs
Medication Teaching Manual (ASHP)
Micromedex DRUGDEX
Patient counseling handbook
Patient Drug Facts
USPDI Volume II: Advice for the Patient

Pediatric dosing and therapeutics
AHFS Drug Information
Drug Facts & Comparisons
Harriet Lane Handbook
Micromedex DRUGDEX
Nelson Textbook of Pediatrics
Neofax
Pediatric Dosage Handbook
Physician's Desk Reference
Principles and Practice of Pediatrics
EMBASE

International Pharmaceutical Abstracts
Medline

Pharmaceutics/compounding/
manufacturing
Allen's Compounded Formulations
Extemporaneous Ophthalmic Preparations
Handbook on Extemporaneous Formulations
International Journal of Pharmaceutical
Compounding
Stability of Compounded Formulations
US Pharmacist Contemporary Compounding
Compendium
EMBASE
International Pharmaceutical Abstracts
Medline
Center for Drug Evaluation and Research
(http://www.fda.gov/cder/pharmcomp/)
International Journal of Pharmaceutical
Compounding (www.ijpc.com)

Pharmacokinetics
AHFS Drug Information
Applied Pharmacokinetics
Basic Clinical Pharmacokinetics
Clinical Pharmacokinetics
Drug Facts & Comparisons
Martindale
Micromedex DRUGDEX
Physician's Desk Reference
Principles of Therapeutic Drug Monitoring
USPDI Volume 1
EMBASE
International Pharmaceutical Abstracts
Medline

Foreign drug identification
Drugs Available Abroad
Drug Facts & Comparisons (Canadian Trade
Name Index)
European Drug Index
Martindale
Merck Index
Diccionario de Especialidades
Micromedex Index Nominum
Mosby's GenRX (International Drug Name
Index)
The British Pharmacopoeia
USP Dictionary
World Pharmaceuticals Directory

EMBASE
International Pharmaceutical Abstracts
Medline
British National Formulary
(http://bnf.vhn.net/home/)
Electronics Medicines Compendium
(http://emc.vhn.net/)
Royal Pharmaceutical Society of Great
Britain http://www.pharmj.com/
noticeboard/info/pip/foreignmedicines.
html

General drug information resources
(compendia)
AHFS Drug Information
Drug Facts & Comparisons
Martindale's
Micromedex DRUGDEX
Mosby's GenRX
Physician's Desk Reference
USPDI Volume I: Drug Information for
Health Care Provider

Geriatrics
AHFS Drug Information
Consultant Pharmacist Journal
Drug Facts & Comparisons
Drug Therapy and the Elderly
Geriatric Dosage Handbook
Geriatric Pharmacology
Micromedex DRUGDEX
Physician's Desk Reference
Therapeutics in the Elderly
USPDI Volume I
EMBASE
International Pharmaceutical Abstracts
Medline
American Society of Consultant
Pharmacists (http://www.ascp.com/)
Geriatrics and Aging (http://www.
geriatricsandaging.com/ga_links.htm)

Immunology/biotechnology/vaccines
Concepts in Immunology and
Immunotherapeutics
ImmunoFacts
Center for Disease Control (CDC) website
(www.cdc.gov/nip)
Immunize Action Coalition (http://www.
immunize.org/)

(continued)

Appendix 8

Drug Information Resources by Category (continued)

US Health and Human Services
(http://www.hrsa.gov/osp/vicp/)
Vaccine Adverse Event Reporting System
(http://www.vaers.org/)

Intravenous stability/compatibility
AHFS Drug Information
Guide to Parenteral Admixtures
Handbook on Injectable Drugs
Micromedex DRUGDEX
Trissel's Tables of Physical Compatibility
EMBASE
International Pharmaceutical Abstracts
Medline
Handbook of Parenteral Drug Administration
(http://members.ozemail.com.au/~jamesbc/
frames.htm)

Investigational drug identification
Drug Facts & Comparisons
Index Nominum
Martindale
Merck Index
Micromedex DRUGDEX, POISINDEX
NDA Pipeline
Unlisted Drugs
World Pharmaceuticals Directory
EMBASE
International Pharmaceutical Abstracts
Medline
Aids Clinical Trials (http://www.actis.org/)
CenterWatch (http://www.centerwatch.
com/patient/trials.html)
NIH Clinical Trials Database (www.
clinicaltrials.gov)
Pharmaceutical Research and Manufacturers
of America (http://www.newmedicines.org/)
Reuters News Service
(www.reutershealth.com)

Laboratory Tests and Microbiology
Basic Skills in Interpreting Laboratory Data
Clinical Guide to Laboratory Tests
Laboratory Tests and Diagnostic Procedures
Laboratory Test Handbook

Pregnancy and lactation information
Breastfeeding: A Guide for the Medical
Profession
Drugs in Pregnancy and Lactation
Micromedex REPRORISK

Focus Information Technology (http://www.
perinatology.com/exposures/druglist.htm)
Safety of Drugs in Pregnancy and Lactation
(http://www.accp.com/pod/p3b11pre01.pdf)
UK's Drugs in Lactation Advisory Service
(http://www.ukmicentral.nhs.uk/drugpreg/
guide.htm)

Pharmacology
AHFS Drug Information
Basic Concepts & Clinical Applications
Clinical Pharmacology
Drug Facts & Comparisons
Goodman & Gilman's Pharmacological Basic
of Therapeutics
Principles of Pharmacology
Textbook of Pharmacology

Phone numbers and addresses
American Drug Index
Drug Facts & Comparisons
Drug Topics Redbook
Martindale
Micromedex DRUGDEX, POISINDEX
Mosby's GenRX
NDA Pipeline
PDR
Manufacturer websites (various)

Chemical/physical properties
CRC Handbook of Chemistry and Physics
Merck Index
Textbook of Organic, Medicinal, and
Pharmaceutical Chemistry
USP-Dictionary
USP/NF

Product availability/shortages
American Drug Index
Drug Topics Red Book
Handbook of Nonprescription Drugs
ASHP Drug Shortage Center (http://www.
ashp.org/shortage/)
Drug Wholesaler websites (various)
FDA Drug Shortage site (http://www.fda.gov/
cder/drug/shortages/default.htm)

Product identification
American Drug Index
AHFS Drug Information
Diccionario de Especialidades Farmaceuticas
Drug Facts & Comparisons

Drug Topics Redbook
Drugs Available Abroad
European Drug Index
Index Nominum
Martindale
Merck Index
Micromedex POISINDEX
NDA Pipeline
Pharmacist's Letter
Unlisted Drugs
USP Dictionary
World Pharmaceuticals Directory
EMBASE
International Pharmaceutical Abstracts
Medline
FDA website (www.fda.gov)
Internet (various search engines, websites)
Reuters News Service (www.
reutershealth.com)

Tablet/capsule identification
Drug Facts & Comparisons
Ident-A-Drug
Micromedex IDENTIDEX
Mosby's GenRX
Physician's Desk Reference (PDR)
RX-List website (www.rxlist.com)

Toxicology/poisoning
Clinical Management of Poisoning and Drug
Overdose
Clinical Toxicology of Drugs
Handbook of Poisoning
Micromedex DRUGDEX, POISINDEX
Poisoning and Toxicology Compendium
Principles of Clinical Toxicology
Toxicologic Emergencies
EMBASE
International Pharmaceutical Abstracts
Medline
ToxNet
American Association of Poison Control
Centers (http://www.aapcc.org/)
Environmental Protection Agency
(http://www.epa.gov/iris/)
Merck Manual (http://www.merck.com/
pubs/mmanual/section23/chapter307/307a.
htm)
Oxford University
(http://physchem.ox.ac.uk/MSDS/)

Appendix 9

Drugs That Should Not Be Crushed

Pharmacists may sometimes encounter patients who cannot swallow tablets or capsules. When an alternative liquid formulation is not available, pulverizing the solid dosage form before administration can serve as a quick, safe solution to the problem.

However, not all pharmaceutical products may be crushed before administration. A variety of slow-release formulations can deliver dangerous immediate doses of their active ingredients if the integrity of the delivery system is destroyed, and enteric-coated products must remain intact in order to prevent their dissolution in the stomach.

Listed below are various slow-release as well as enteric-coated products that should not be crushed or chewed. Slow-release (sr) represents products that are controlled-release, extended-release, long-acting, or timed-release. Enteric-coated (ec) represents products that are delayed-release.

In general, capsules containing slow-release or enteric-coated particles may be opened and their contents administered on a spoonful of soft food. Instruct patients not to chew the particles, though. (Patients should, in fact, be discouraged from chewing any medication unless it is specifically formulated for that purpose.)

This list should not be considered all-inclusive. Generic and alternate brands of some products may exist. Tablets intended for sublingual or buccal administration (not included in this list) should also be administered only as intended, in an intact form.

Drug	Manufacturer	Form	Drug	Manufacturer	Form
Accuhist LA	Pediamed	sr	Bromfenex	Ethex	sr
Aciphex	Janssen	ec	Bromfenex PD	Ethex	sr
Adalat CC	Bayer	sr	Bromfenex PE	Ethex	sr
Adderall XR	Shire US	sr	Bromfenex PE Pediatric	Ethex	sr
Advicor	KOS	sr	Caffedrine	Blairex	sr
Aerohist	Aero	sr	Calan SR	Pharmacia	sr
Aerohist Plus	Aero	sr	Carbatrol	Shire US	sr
Afeditab CR	Watson	sr	Cardene SR	Roche	sr
Aggrenox	Boehringer Ingelheim	sr	Cardizem CD	Biovail	sr
Aldex	Zyber	sr	Cardizem LA	Biovail	sr
Aleve Cold & Sinus	Bayer Consumer	sr	Cardizem SR	Biovail	sr
Aleve Sinus & Headache	Bayer Consumer	sr	Carox Plus	Seneca	sr
Allegra-D	Aventis	sr	Cartia XT	Andrx	sr
Allerx	Adams	sr	Catemine	Tyson Neutraceuticals	ec
Allerx-D	Adams	sr	Cemill 1000	Miller	sr
Allfen	MCR American	sr	Cemill 500	Miller	sr
Allfen-DM	MCR American	sr	Certuss-D	Capellon	sr
Alophen	Numark	ec	Cevi-Bid	Lee	sr
Altex-PSE	Alphagen	sr	Chlorex-A	Cypress	sr
Altocor	Andrx	sr	Chlor-Phen	Truxton	sr
Ambifed-G	MCR American	sr	Chlor-Trimeton Allergy	Schering Plough	sr
Ambifed-G DM	MCR American	sr	Chlor-Trimeton Allergy Decongestant	Schering Plough	sr
Amdry-C	PrasCo	sr			
Amdry-D	PrasCo	sr	Cipro XR	Bayer	sr
Amibid DM	Amide	sr	Claritin-D	Schering Plough	sr
Amibid LA	Amide	sr	Claritin-D 24-Hour	Schering Plough	sr
Amidal	Amide	sr	Coldamine	Breckenridge	sr
Aminoxin	Tyson Neutraceuticals	ec	Coldec D	Breckenridge	sr
Ami-Tex PSE	Amide	sr	Coldec TR	Breckenridge	sr
Aquabid-DM	Alphagen	sr	Coldex-A	United Research	sr
Aquatab C	Adams	sr	Coldmist DM	Breckenridge	sr
Aquatab D	Adams	sr	Coldmist Jr.	Breckenridge	sr
Aquatab DM	Adams	sr	Coldmist LA	Breckenridge	sr
Arthrotec	Pharmacia	ec	Colfed-A	Breckenridge	sr
Asacol	Procter & Gamble	ec	Concerta	McNeil Consumer	sr
Ascocid-1000	Key	sr	Contac 12-hour	GlaxoSmithKline Consumer	sr
Ascocid-500-D	Key	sr			
Ascriptin Enteric	Novartis Consumer	ec	Correctol	Schering Plough	ec
ATP	Tyson Neutraceuticals	ec	Cotazym-S	Organon	ec
Atrohist Pediatric	Celltech	sr	Covera-HS	Pharmacia	sr
Augmentin XR	GlaxoSmithKline	sr	Crantex ER	Breckenridge	sr
Avinza	Ligand	sr	Crantex LA	Breckenridge	sr
Azulfidine Entabs	Pharmacia	ec	Creon 10	Solvay	ec
Bayer Aspirin Regimen	Bayer Consumer	ec	Creon 20	Solvay	ec
Bellahist-D LA	Cypress	sr	Creon 5	Solvay	ec
Biaxin XL	Abbott	sr	C-Tym	Emrex/Economed	sr
Bidex-DM	Stewart-Jackson	sr	Dairycare	Plainview	ec
Biohist LA	Ivax	sr	Dallergy	Laser	sr
Bisac-Evac	G & W	ec	Dallergy- Jr.	Laser	sr
Biscolax	Global Source	ec	D-amine-SR	Alphagen	sr
Bontril Slow-Release	Amarin	sr	Deconamine SR	Kenwood	sr
Bromfed	Muro	sr	Deconex	Poly	sr
Bromfed-PD	Muro	sr	Decongest II	Qualitest	sr

| Enteric-coated = ec | Slow-release = sr |

(continued)

Appendix 9

Drugs That Should Not Be Crushed (continued)

Drug	Manufacturer	Form	Drug	Manufacturer	Form
De-Congestine	Qualitest	sr	Fero-Folic 500	Abbott	sr
Deconsal II	Carolina	sr	Fero-Grad-500	Abbott	sr
Depakote	Abbott	ec	Ferro-Sequels	Inverness	sr
Depakote ER	Abbott	sr	Ferro-Time	Time-Cap	sr
Depakote Sprinkles	Abbott	ec	Ferrous Fumarate DS	Vita-Rx	sr
Despec SR	Int'l Ethical Labs	sr	Fetrin	LunsCo	sr
Detrol LA	Pharmacia	sr	Flagyl ER	Pharmacia	sr
Dex GG TR	Boca	sr	Fleet Bisacodyl	C.B. Fleet	ec
Dexaphen SA	Major	sr	Folitab 500	Rising	sr
Dexedrine Spansules	GlaxoSmithKline	sr	Fumatinic	Laser	sr
D-Feda II	WE Pharm	sr	G/P 1200/75	Cypress	sr
Diamox Sequels	Duramed	sr	Genacote	Ivax	ec
Dilacor XR	Watson	sr	Gentlax	Purdue Frederick	ec
Dilantin Kapseals	Pfizer	sr	GFN 1000/DM 50	Cypress	sr
Dilatrate-SR	Schwarz	sr	GFN 1200/DM 20/PE 40	Cypress	sr
Diltia XT	Andrx	sr	GFN 1200/DM 60/PSE 60	Cypress	sr
Dimetane Extentabs	Wyeth Consumer	sr	GFN 1200/Phenylephrine 40	Cypress	sr
Disophrol Chronotab	Schering Plough	sr	GFN 1200/PSE 50	Cypress	sr
Ditropan XL	Ortho-McNeil	sr	GFN 500/DM 30	Cypress	sr
Donnatal Extentabs	PBM	sr	GFN 550/PSE 60	Cypress	sr
Doryx	Warner Chilcott	ec	GFN 550/PSE 60/DM 30	Cypress	sr
Drexophed SR	Qualitest	sr	GFN 595/PSE 48	Cypress	sr
Drihist SR	PrasCo	sr	GFN 595-PSE 48-DM 32	Cypress	sr
Drituss GP	Qualitest	sr	GFN 795-PSE 85	Cypress	sr
Drixomed	IoPharm	sr	GFN 800/DM 30	Cypress	sr
Drixoral	Schering Plough	sr	GFN 800/PSE 60	Cypress	sr
Drixoral Plus	Schering Plough	sr	Giltuss TR	Gil	sr
Drixoral Sinus	Schering Plough	sr	Glucophage XR	Bristol-Myers Squibb	sr
Drize-R	Monarch	sr	Glucotrol XL	Pfizer	sr
Drysec	A.G. Marin	sr	GP-1200	IoPharm	sr
Dulcolax	Boehringer Ingelheim Consumer	ec	G-Phed	Alphagen	sr
			Guaifed	Verum	sr
Duradryl Jr.	Breckenridge	sr	Guaifed-PD	Verum	sr
Durahist	Proethic	sr	Guaifenex DM	Ethex	sr
Durahist PE	Proethic	sr	Guaifenex G	Ethex	sr
Duraphen DM	Proethic	sr	Guaifenex GP	Ethex	sr
Duraphen II	Proethic	sr	Guaifenex LA	Ethex	sr
Durasal II	PrasCo	sr	Guaifenex PSE 120	Ethex	sr
Dynabac	Muro	ec	Guaifenex PSE 60	Ethex	sr
Dynabac D5-Pak	Muro	ec	Guaifenex PSE 80	Ethex	sr
Dynacirc CR	Reliant	sr	Guaifenex-Rx	Ethex	sr
Dynahist-ER Pediatric	Breckenridge	sr	Guaifenex-Rx DM	Ethex	sr
Dynex	Athlon	sr	Guaimax-D	Schwarz	sr
Easprin	New River	ec	Gua-SR	Seatrace	sr
EC Naprosyn	Roche	ec	Guiadex D	Breckenridge	sr
Ecotrin	GlaxoSmithKline Consumer	ec	Guiadex PD	Breckenridge	sr
			Guiadrine DM	Breckenridge	sr
Ecotrin Adult, Low-Strength	GlaxoSmithKline Consumer	ec	Guiadrine G-1200	Breckenridge	sr
			Guiadrine GP	Breckenridge	sr
Ecotrin Maximum-Strength	GlaxoSmithKline Consumer	ec	Guiadrine PSE	Breckenridge	sr
			H 9600 SR	Hawthorn	sr
Ecpirin	Prime Marketing	ec	Halfprin	Kramer	ec
Ed-A-Hist	Edwards	sr	Hematron-AF	Seyer Pharmatec	sr
Effexor-XR	Wyeth-Ayerst	sr	Hemax	Pronova	sr
Efidac 24 Chlorpheniramine	Novartis Consumer	sr	Histaclear D	Ethex	sr
Efidac 24 Pseudoephedrine	Novartis Consumer	sr	Histade	Breckenridge	er
Endal	Pediamed	sr	Histade MX	Breckenridge	sr
Entab-DM	Rising	sr	Hista-Vent DA	Ethex	sr
Entercote	Global Source	ec	Hista-Vent PSE	Ethex	sr
Entex ER	Andrx	sr	Histex CT	TEAMM	sr
Entex LA	Andrx	sr	Histex I/E	TEAMM	sr
Entex PSE	Andrx	sr	Histex SR	TEAMM	sr
Entocort EC	Astra Zeneca	ec	Humavent LA	WE Pharm	sr
Eryc	Warner Chilcott	ec	Humibid DM	Carolina	sr
Ery-Tab	Abbott	ec	Humibid LA	Carolina	sr
Eskalith-CR	GlaxoSmithKline	sr	Hydro Pro DM SR	Breckenridge	sr
Eudal SR	Forest	sr	Hyoscyamine TR	Breckenridge	sr
Extendryl Jr.	Fleming	sr	Iberet-500	Abbott	sr
Extendryl SR	Fleming	sr	Iberet-Folic-500	Abbott	sr
Feen-A-Mint	Schering Plough	ec	Icaps TR	AlCon	sr
Femilax	G & W	ec	Icar-C Plus SR	Hawthorn	sr

Enteric-coated = ec	Slow-release = sr

Appendix 9

Drugs That Should Not Be Crushed (continued)

Drug	Manufacturer	Form	Drug	Manufacturer	Form
Imdur	Key	sr	Mintab D	Breckenridge	sr
Inderal LA	Wyeth-Ayerst	sr	Mintab DM	Breckenridge	sr
Indocin SR	Forte	sr	Miraphen PSE	CaraCo	sr
Innopran XL	Reliant	sr	Modane	Savage	ec
Iobid DM	IoPharm	sr	MS Contin	Purdue Frederick	sr
Ionamin	Celltech	sr	MSP-BLU	Cypress	ec
Iosal II	IoPharm	sr	Mucinex	Adams	sr
Iotex PSE	IoPharm	sr	Muco-Fen DM	Ivax	sr
Isochron	Forest	sr	Multi-Ferrous Folic	United Research	sr
Isoptin SR	Abbott	sr	Multiret Folic-500	Amide	sr
K-10	Alra	sr	Nalex-A	Blansett	sr
K-8	Alra	sr	Naprelan	Elan	sr
Kadian	Faulding	sr	Nasatab LA	ECR	sr
Kaon-CL 10	Savage	sr	ND Clear	Seatrace	sr
K-Dur 10	Key	sr	New Ami-Tex LA	Amide	sr
K-Dur 20	Key	sr	Nexium	Astra Zeneca	ec
Klor-Con 10	Upsher-Smith	sr	Niaspan	KOS	sr
Klor-Con 8	Upsher-Smith	sr	Nicomide	Sirius	sr
Klor-Con M10	Upsher-Smith	sr	Nifedical XL	Teva	sr
Klor-Con M15	Upsher-Smith	sr	Nitrocot	Truxton	sr
Klor-Con M20	Upsher-Smith	sr	Nitro-Time	Time-Cap	sr
Klotrix	Bristol-Myers Squibb	sr	Norflex	3M	sr
Kronofed-A	Ferndale	sr	Norpace CR	Pharmacia	sr
Kronofed-A-Jr.	Ferndale	sr	Omnihist LA	WE Pharm.	sr
K-Tab	Abbott	sr	Oramorph SR	AAI Pharma	sr
Lescol XL	Novartis	sr	Oruvail	Wyeth-Ayerst	sr
Levall G	Athlon	sr	Oxycontin	Purdue	sr
Levbid	Schwarz	sr	Palgic-D	Pamlab	sr
Levsinex	Schwarz	sr	Pancrease	Ortho-McNeil	ec
Lexxel	Astra Zeneca	sr	Pancrease MT 10	Ortho-McNeil	ec
Lipram 4500	Global	ec	Pancrease MT 16	Ortho-McNeil	ec
Lipram-CR10	Global	ec	Pancrease MT 20	Ortho-McNeil	ec
Lipram-CR20	Global	ec	Pancrecarb MS-4	Digestive Care	ec
Lipram-CR5	Global	ec	Pancrecarb MS-8	Digestive Care	ec
Lipram-PN10	Global	ec	Pancrelipase 20,000	United Research	ec
Lipram-PN16	Global	ec	Pangestyme CN-10	Ethex	ec
Lipram-PN20	Global	ec	Pangestyme CN-20	Ethex	ec
Lipram-UL12	Global	ec	Pangestyme EC	Ethex	ec
Lipram-UL18	Global	ec	Pangestyme MT16	Ethex	ec
Lipram-UL20	Global	ec	Pangestyme UL12	Ethex	ec
Liquibid-D	Capellon	sr	Pangestyme UL18	Ethex	ec
Liquibid-D 1200	Capellon	sr	Pangestyme UL20	Ethex	ec
Liquibid-PD	Capellon	sr	Panmist DM	Pamlab	sr
Lithobid	Solvay	sr	Panmist Jr.	Pamlab	sr
Lodine XL	Wyeth-Ayerst	sr	Panmist LA	Pamlab	sr
Lodrane 12D	ECR	sr	Pannaz	Pamlab	sr
Lodrane 12-hour	ECR	sr	Papacon	Consolidated Midland	sr
Lodrane LD	ECR	sr	Para-Time SR	Time-Cap	sr
Lusonex	Wraser	sr	Paser	Jacobus	sr
Mag Delay	Major	ec	Pavacot	Truxton	sr
Mag64	Rising	ec	Paxil CR	GlaxoSmithKline	sr
Mag-SR	Cypress	sr	PCE Dispertab	Abbott	ec
Mag-SR Plus Calcium	Cypress	sr	PCM Allergy	Boca	sr
Mag-Tab SR	Niche	sr	PCM LA	Cypress	sr
Maxifed	MCR American	sr	Pentasa	Shire US	sr
Maxifed DM	MCR American	sr	Pentopak	Zoetica	sr
Maxifed-G	MCR American	sr	Pentoxil	Upsher-Smith	sr
Maxovite	Tyson Neutraceuticals	sr	Pharmadrine	Breckenridge	sr
Medent DM	Stewart-Jackson	sr	Phendiet-105	Truxton	sr
Medent LD	Stewart-Jackson	sr	Phenyleph 20/CPM 8/	United Research	sr
Mega-C	Merit	sr	Methscop 2.5 LA		
Melfiat	Numark	sr			
Mescolor	First Horizon	sr	Phenytek	Bertek	sr
Mestinon Timespan	ICN	sr	Plendil	Astra Zeneca	sr
Metadate CD	Celltech	sr	Poly Hist Forte	Poly	sr
Metadate ER	Celltech	sr	Poly-Vent	Poly	sr
Methylin ER	Mallinckrodt	sr	Poly-Vent Jr.	Poly	sr
Micro-K	Ther-Rx	sr	Prehist D	Marnel	sr
Micro-K 10	Ther-Rx	sr	Prelu-2	Roxane	sr
Mindal	Breckenridge	sr	Prevacid	Tap	ec
Mindal DM	Breckenridge	sr	Prilosec	Astra Zeneca	ec
Mintab C	Breckenridge	sr	Prilosec OTC	Procter & Gamble	ec
			Procanbid	Monarch	sr

Enteric-coated = ec   Slow-release = sr

Appendix 9

Drugs That Should Not Be Crushed (continued)

Drug	Manufacturer	Form	Drug	Manufacturer	Form
Procardia XL	Pfizer	sr	Sular	First Horizon	sr
Profen Forte	Ivax	sr	Sulfazine EC	Qualitest	ec
Profen Forte DM	Ivax	sr	Symax-SR	Capellon	sr
Profen II	Ivax	sr	Tarka	Abbott	sr
Profen II DM	Ivax	sr	Taztia XT	Andrx	sr
Prohist-8	Emrex/Economed	sr	Tegretol-XR	Novartis	sr
Prolex PD	Blansett	sr	Tenuate Dospan	Aventis	sr
Prolex-D	Blansett	sr	Theo-24	UCB	sr
Pronestyl-SR	Bristol-Myers Squibb	sr	Theocap	Forest	sr
Protid	LunsCo	sr	Theochron	Forest	sr
Protonix	Wyeth-Ayerst	ec	Theo-Time	Major	sr
Prozac Weekly	Eli Lilly	ec	Thiamilate	Tyson Neutraceuticals	ec
Pseubrom	Alphagen	sr	Tiazac	Forest	sr
Pseubrom-PD	Alphagen	sr	Time-Hist	MCR American	sr
Pseudo CM TR	Boca	sr	Toprol XL	Astra Zeneca	sr
Pseudo GG TR	Boca	sr	TotalDay	National Vitamin	sr
Pseudocot-C	Truxton	sr	Touro Allergy	Dartmouth	sr
Pseudocot-G	Truxton	sr	Touro CC	Dartmouth	sr
Pseudovent	Ethex	sr	Touro DM	Dartmouth	sr
Pseudovent DM	Ethex	sr	Touro EX	Dartmouth	sr
Pseudovent PED	Ethex	sr	Touro LA	Dartmouth	sr
P-tuss DM	PrasCo	sr	Tranxene SD	Ovation	sr
Q-bid DM	Qualitest	sr	Tranxene-SD	Ovation	sr
Qdall	Atley	sr	Trental	Aventis	sr
Quadra-Hist D	Ethex	sr	Trikof-D	Respa	sr
Quadra-Hist D Ped	Ethex	sr	Trinalin Repetabs	Key	sr
Quibron-T/SR	Monarch	sr	Trituss-ER	Everett	sr
Quindal	Qualitest	sr	Tussafed-LA	Everett	sr
Reliable Gentle Laxative	Ivax	ec	Tussall-ER	Everett	sr
Rescon Jr.	Capellon	sr	Tussi-BID	Capellon	sr
Rescon MX	Capellon	sr	Tylenol Arthritis	McNeil Consumer	sr
Respa-1st	Respa	sr	Ultrabrom	WE Pharm	sr
Respa-AR	Respa	sr	Ultrabrom PD	WE Pharm	sr
Respa-DM	Respa	sr	Ultrase	Axcan ScandiPharm	ec
Respa-GF	Respa	sr	Ultrase MT12	Axcan ScandiPharm	ec
Respa-PE	Respa	sr	Ultrase MT18	Axcan ScandiPharm	ec
Respahist	Respa	sr	Ultrase MT20	Axcan ScandiPharm	ec
Respaire-120 SR	Laser	sr	Uniphyl	Purdue Frederick	sr
Respaire-60 SR	Laser	sr	Urimax	Integrity	ec
Rhinacon A	Breckenridge	sr	Urocit-K 10	Mission	sr
Ribo-2	Tyson Neutraceuticals	ec	Urocit-K 5	Mission	sr
Rinade-BID	Emrex/Economed	sr	Uroxatral	Sanofi-Synthelabo	sr
Risperdal Consta	Janssen	sr	Vanex Forte-D	Monarch	sr
Ritalin LA	Novartis	sr	V-Dec-M	Seatrace	sr
Ritalin SR	Novartis	sr	Veracolate	Numark	ec
Rodex Forte	Legere	sr	Verelan	Schwarz	sr
Rondamine	Major	sr	Verelan PM	Schwarz	sr
Rondec-TR	Biovail	sr	Versacaps	Seatrace	sr
Ru-Tuss 800	Sage	sr	Videx EC	Bristol-Myers Squibb	ec
Ru-Tuss 800 DM	Sage	sr	Vitamin C/Rose Hips	ADH Health	sr
Ru-Tuss Jr.	Sage	sr	Vivotif Berna	Berna	ec
Sam-E	Pharmavite	ec	Voltaren	Novartis	ec
Sinemet CR	Bristol-Myers Squibb	sr	Voltaren-XR	Novartis	sr
Sinutuss DM	WE Pharm	sr	Vospire ER	Odyssey	sr
Sinuvent PE	WE Pharm	sr	WE Mist II LA	WE Pharm	sr
Slo-Niacin	Upsher Smith	sr	WE Mist LA	WE Pharm	sr
Slow FE	Novartis Consumer	sr	Wellbutrin SR	GlaxoSmithKline	sr
Slow FE With Folic Acid	Novartis Consumer	sr	Wellbutrin XL	GlaxoSmithKline	sr
Slow-Mag	Purdue	ec	Wobenzym N	Marlyn	ec
Spacol T/S	Dayton	sr	Xanax XR	Pharmacia	sr
St. Joseph Pain Reliever	McNeil Consumer	ec	Xiral	Hawthorn	sr
Sta-D	Magna	sr	Zaptec PSE	American Generics	sr
Stahist	Magna	sr	Z-Cof LA	Zyber	sr
Stamoist E	Magna	sr	Zephrex LA	Sanofi-Synthelabo	sr
Sudafed 12-Hour	Pfizer Consumer	sr	Zorprin	Par	sr
Sudafed 24-Hour	Pfizer Consumer	sr	Zyban	GlaxoSmithKline	sr
Sudal 60/500	Atley	sr	Zymase	Organon	ec
Sudal DM	Atley	sr	Zyrtec-D	Pfizer	sr
Sudal SR	Atley	sr			

Enteric-coated = ec   Slow-release = sr

From Fleming T., ed. *Drug Topics Red Book*. Montvale. NJ: Thompson PDR, 2004.

Appendix 10

Use-in-Pregnancy Ratings

The U.S. Food and Drug Administration's Use-in-Pregnancy rating system weighs the degree to which available information has ruled out risk to the fetus against the drug's potential benefit to the patient. Below is a listing of drugs (by generic name) for which ratings are available.

CONTRAINDICATED IN PREGNANCY

Studies in animals or humans, or investigational or post-marketing reports, have demonstrated fetal risk which clearly outweighs any possible benefit to the patient.

Acitretin
Anisindione
Atorvastatin Calcium
Bicalutamide
Clomiphene Citrate
Danazol
Demecarium Bromide
Desogestrel/Ethinyl Estradiol
Diclofenac Sodium/Misoprostol
Dienestrol
Dihydroergotamine Mesylate
Estazolam
Estradiol
Estrogens, Conjugated
Estrogens, Conjugated/
    Medroxyprogesterone
    Acetate
Estrogens, Esterified
Estrogens, Esterified/
    Methyltestosterone
Estropipate
Ethinyl Estradiol
Ethinyl Estradiol/Ethynodiol
    Diacetate
Ethinyl Estradiol/Levonorgestrel
Ethinyl Estradiol/Norethindrone
Ethinyl Estradiol/Norethindrone
    Acetate
Ethinyl Estradiol/Norgestimate
Ethinyl Estradiol/Norgestrel
Finasteride
Fluorouracil
Fluvastatin Sodium
Follitropin Alpha
Follitropin Beta
Gonadotropin, Chorionic
    (Profasi)
Goserelin Acetate
Interferon Alfa-2B/Ribavirin
Isotretinoin
Leflunomide
Leuprolide Acetate
Levonorgestrel
Lovastatin
Medroxyprogesterone Acetate

Megestrol Acetate
    (Megace Suspension)
Menotropins
Mestranol/Norethindrone
Methyltestosterone
Misoprostol
Nafarelin Acetate
Norethindrone
Norethindrone Acetate
Norgestrel
Oxandrolone
Oxymetholone
Plicamycin
Pravastatin Sodium
Raloxifene Hydrochloride
Ribavirin
Rosuvastatin Calcium
Simvastatin
Stanozolol
Tazarotene
Testosterone
Testosterone Enanthate
Thalidomide
Tositumomab/Iodine I 131
    Tositumomab
Triazolam
Urofollitropin
Warfarin Sodium
Yohimbine Hydrochloride

POSITIVE EVIDENCE OF RISK

Investigational or postmarketing data show risk to the fetus. Nevertheless, potential benefits may outweigh the potential risk.

Alitretinoin
Alprazolam
Altretamine
Amiodarone Hydrochloride
Amlodipine Besylate/Benazepril
    Hydrochloride*
Anastrozole
Atenolol
Atenolol/Chlorthalidone
Azathioprine
Azathioprine Sodium
Benazepril Hydrochloride*
Benazepril Hydrochloride/
    Hydrochlorothiazide*
Bortezomib
Busulfan
Candesartan Cilexetil*

Capecitabine
Captopril*
Carbamazepine
Carboplatin
Carmustine
Chlorambucil
Cladribine
Clonazepam
Cytarabine Liposome
Dactinomycin
Daunorubicin Citrate Liposome
Daunorubicin Hydrochloride
Demeclocycline Hydrochloride
Divalproex Sodium
Docetaxel
Doxorubicin Hydrochloride
Doxorubicin Hydrochloride
    Liposome
Doxycycline Calcium
Doxycycline Hyclate
Doxycycline Monohydrate
Enalapril Maleate*
Enalapril Maleate/Felodipine*
Enalapril Maleate/
    Hydrochlorothiazide*
Enalaprilat*
Floxuridine
Fludarabine Phosphate
Flutamide
Fosinopril Sodium*
Fosphenytoin Sodium
Gemcitabine Hydrochloride
Gentamicin Sulfate
Goserelin Acetate
Hydrochlorothiazide/Irbesartan*
Hydrochlorothiazide/Lisinopril*
Hydrochlorothiazide/Losartan
    Potassium*
Hydrochlorothiazide/Moexipril
    Hydrochloride*
Hydrochlorothiazide/Valsartan*
Idarubicin Hydrochloride
Ifosfamide
Imatinib Mesylate
Irbesartan*
Letrozole
Lisinopril*
Lithium Carbonate
Lithium Citrate
Lorazepam
Losartan Potassium*
Mechlorethamine Hydrochloride
Megestrol Acetate
    (Megace Tablets)
Melphalan
Mephobarbital
Mercaptopurine
Methimazole

Midazolam Hydrochloride
Minocycline Hydrochloride
Mitoxantrone Hydrochloride
Moexipril Hydrochloride*
Neomycin Sulfate/Polymyxin B
    Sulfate
Nicotine
Paclitaxel
Pamidronate Disodium
Pentobarbital Sodium
Pentostatin
Perindopril Erbumine*
Potassium Iodide
Procarbazine Hydrochloride
Quinapril Hydrochloride*
Ramipril*
Streptomycin Sulfate
Tamoxifen Citrate
Telmisartan
Thioguanine
Thiotepa
Tobramycin (Inhalation)
Tobramycin Sulfate
Topotecan Hydrochloride
Toremifene Citrate
Trandolapril*
Trandolapril/Verapamil
    Hydrochloride*
Tretinoin (Oral)
Valproate Sodium
Valproic Acid
Valsartan*
Vinblastine Sulfate
Vincristine Sulfate
Vinorelbine Tartrate
Voriconazole

C

RISK CANNOT BE RULED OUT

Human studies are lacking, and animal studies are either positive for risk or are lacking as well. However, potential benefits may outweigh the potential risk.

Abacavir Sulfate
Abciximab
Acetaminophen/Butalbital
Acetaminophen/Butalbital/
    Caffeine
Acetaminophen/Caffeine/
    Chlorpheniramine
    Maleate/Hydrocodone
    Bitartrate/Phenylephrine
    Hydrochloride
Acetaminophen/Codeine

Phosphate
Acetaminophen/Hydrocodone
    Bitartrate
Acetaminophen/Oxycodone
    Hydrochloride
Acetaminophen/Pentazocine
    Hydrochloride
Acetazolamide
Acetic Acid/Oxyquinoline
    Sulfate/Ricinoleic Acid
Adapalene
Adenosine
Alatrofloxacin Mesylate
Albendazole
Albumin, Human
Albuterol
Albuterol Sulfate
Albuterol Sulfate/Ipratropium
    Bromide
Alclometasone Dipropionate
Aldesleukin
Alendronate Sodium
Allopurinol Sodium
Alprostadil
Alteplase, Recombinant
Amantadine Hydrochloride
Amifostine
Aminohippurate Sodium
Aminosalicylic Acid
Amlodipine Besylate
Amlodipine Besylate/Benazepril
    Hydrochloride*
Amoxicillin/Clarithromycin/
    Lansoprazole
Amphetamine &
    Dextroamphetamine Mixture
Amprenavir
Amylase/Cellulase/Hyoscyamine
    Sulfate/Lipase/Phenyl-
    toloxamine Citrate/Protease
Amylase/Cellulase/Lipase/
    Protease
Amylase/Lipase/Protease
Anagrelide Hydrochloride
Antihemophilic Factor IX
    Complex (Human)
Antihemophilic Factor IX
    Complex (Recombinant)
Antihemophilic Factor VIIa
    (Recombinant)
Antihemophilic Factor VIII
    (Human)
Antihemophilic Factor VIII
    (Human)/Von Willebrand
    Factor Complex (Human)
Antihemophilic Factor VIII
    (Recombinant)
Antihemophilic Factor VIII:C

* Category C or D depending on the trimester the drug is given.

From Fleming T., ed. *Drug Topics Red Book*. Montvale. NJ: Thompson PDR; 2004.

(continued)

Appendix 10

Use-in-Pregnancy Ratings (continued)

(Human)
Anti-Inhibitor Coagulant
  Complex
Antipyrine/Benzocaine
Anti-Thymocyte Globulin
Antivenin (Latrodectus
  Mactans)
Apraclonidine Hydrochloride
Aripiprazole
Asparaginase
Aspirin/Carisoprodol
Aspirin/Carisoprodol/Codeine
  Phosphate
Aspirin/Methocarbamol
Atovaquone
Atropine Sulfate/Benzoic
  Acid/Hyoscyamine
  Sulfate/Methenamine/Methyl-
  ene Blue/Phenyl Salicylate
Atropine Sulfate/Difenoxin
  Hydrochloride
Atropine Sulfate/Diphenoxylate
  Hydrochloride
Atropine Sulfate/Hyoscyamine
  Sulfate/Phenobarbital/
  Scopolamine Hydrobromide
Azelastine Hydrochloride
Bacillus of Calmette & Guerin,
  Live (BCG Live)
Becaplermin
Beclomethasone Dipropionate
Beclomethasone Dipropionate
  Monohydrate
Benazepril Hydrochloride*
Benazepril Hydrochloride/
  Hydrochlorothiazide*
Bendroflumethiazide/Nadolol
Benoxinate Hydrochloride/
  Fluorescein Sodium
Benzocaine
Benzonatate
Benzoyl Peroxide
Benzoyl Peroxide/Erythromycin
Bepridil Hydrochloride
Betamethasone Dipropionate,
  Augmented
Betamethasone
  Dipropionate/Clotrimazole
Betaxolol Hydrochloride
Bethanechol Chloride
Bisoprolol Fumarate
Bisoprolol Fumarate/
  Hydrochlorothiazide
Botulinum Toxin Type A
Brinzolamide
Budesonide
Bupivacaine Hydrochloride
Bupivacaine Hydrochloride/
  Epinephrine Bitartrate
Buprenorphine Hydrochloride
Butabarbital/Hyoscyamine
  Hydrobromide/
  Phenazopyridine
  Hydrochloride
Butorphanol Tartrate
Calcitonin, Salmon
Calcitriol

Calcium Acetate
Candesartan Cilexetil*
Captopril*
Carbachol
Carbetapentane
  Tannate/Chlorpheniramine
  Tannate/Ephedrine
  Tannate/Phenylephrine
  Tannate
Carbetapentane
  Tannate/Chlorpheniramine
  Tannate/Phenylephrine
  Tannate
Carbidopa/Levodopa
Carbinoxamine Maleate
Carvedilol
Celecoxib
Chloramphenicol
Chloroprocaine Hydrochloride
Chlorothiazide
Chlorothiazide Sodium
Chlorothiazide/Methyldopa
Chloroxine
Chlorpheniramine
  Maleate/Methscopolamine
  Nitrate/Phenylephrine
  Hydrochloride
Chlorpheniramine
  Maleate/Pseudoephedrine
  Hydrochloride
Chlorpheniramine
  Polistirex/Hydrocodone
  Polistirex
Chlorpheniramine
  Tannate/Phenylephrine
  Tannate/Pyrilamine Tannate
Chlorpropamide
Chlorthalidone/Clonidine
  Hydrochloride
Choline Magnesium Trisalicylate
Cidofovir
Cilastatin Sodium/Imipenem
Cilostazol
Ciprofloxacin
Ciprofloxacin Hydrochloride
Ciprofloxacin Hydrochloride/
  Hydrocortisone
Citalopram Hydrobromide
Clarithromycin
Clobetasol Propionate
Clofibrate
Clonidine
Clonidine Hydrochloride
Clotrimazole (Oral)
Codeine Phosphate/Guaifenesin
Codeine Phosphate/
  Phenylephrine Hydrochloride/
  Promethazine Hydrochloride
Codeine Phosphate/
  Promethazine Hydrochloride
Colistimethate Sodium
Corticorelin Ovine Triflutate
Corticotropin, Repository
Cosyntropin
Crotamiton
Cyanocobalamin (Nascobal)
Cyclosporine

Cytomegalovirus Immune
  Globulin Intravenous, Human
Dacarbazine
Daclizumab
Dantrolene Sodium
Dapsone
Deferoxamine Mesylate
Delavirdine Mesylate
Denileukin Diftitox
Desonide
Desoximetasone
Dexamethasone Sodium
  Phosphate
Dexamethasone Sodium
  Phosphate/Neomycin Sulfate
Dexamethasone/Neomycin
  Sulfate/Polymyxin B Sulfate
Dexamethasone/Tobramycin
Dexrazoxane
Dextroamphetamine Sulfate
Dextromethorphan
  Hydrobromide/Guaifenesin
Dextromethorphan
  Hydrobromide/Promethazine
  Hydrochloride
Dichlorphenamide
Diflorasone Diacetate
Diflunisal
Digoxin
Digoxin Immune Fab (Ovine)
Diltiazem Hydrochloride
Dinoprostone
Diphtheria Toxoid/Haemophilus
  B Conjugate Vaccine/
  Pertussis Vaccine/Tetanus
  Toxoid
Diphtheria Toxoid/Pertussis
  Vaccine, Acellular/Tetanus
  Toxoid
Diphtheria Toxoid/Tetanus
  Toxoid
Dirithromycin
Disopyramide Phosphate
Donepezil Hydrochloride
Dopamine Hydrochloride
Dorzolamide Hydrochloride
Dorzolamide Hydrochloride/
  Timolol Maleate
Doxazosin Mesylate
Dronabinol
Dyphylline
Dyphylline/Guaifenesin
Echothiophate Iodide
Efalizumab
Efavirenz
Enalapril Maleate*
Enalapril Maleate/Felodipine*
Enalapril Maleate/
  Hydrochlorothiazide*
Enalaprilat*
Epinephrine
Epinephrine Hydrochloride
Epoetin Alfa
Ergocalciferol
Erythromycin, Solution (A/T/S)

Erythromycin Ethylsuccinate/
  Sulfisoxazole Acetyl
Escitalopram Oxalate
Esmolol Hydrochloride
Ethiodized Oil
Ethionamide
Etidronate Disodium
Etodolac
Etomidate
Felbamate
Felodipine
Fenofibrate
Fentanyl
Fentanyl Citrate
Ferrous Fumarate/Folic Acid/
  Intrinsic Factor/Vitamin B12/
  Vitamin C
Ferrous Fumarate/Folic Acid/
  Vitamins, Multi
Fexofenadine Hydrochloride
Fexofenadine Hydrochloride/
  Pseudoephedrine
  Hydrochloride
Filgrastim (G-CSF)
Flecainide Acetate
Fluconazole
Flucytosine
Flumazenil
Flunisolide
Fluocinolone Acetonide
Fluocinonide
Fluorometholone
Fluorometholone Acetate
Fluorometholone/Sulfacetamide
  Sodium
Flurandrenolide
Fluticasone Propionate
Fluvoxamine Maleate
Formoterol Fumarate
Fosamprenavir Calcium
Foscarnet Sodium
Fosinopril Sodium*
Furosemide
Gabapentin
Gallium Nitrate
Ganciclovir
Ganciclovir Sodium
Gemfibrozil
Gentamicin Sulfate
Glimepiride
Glipizide
Globulin, Immune
Glyburide
Gonadotropin, Chorionic
  (Novarel)
Guaifenesin
Guaifenesin/Hydrocodone
  Bitartrate
Guaifenesin/Hydrocodone
  Bitartrate/Pseudoephedrine
  Hydrochloride
Guaifenesin/Pseudoephedrine
  Hydrochloride (Duratuss,
  Zephrex)
Haemophilus B Conjugate
  Vaccine
Haemophilus B Conjugate

Vaccine/Hepatitis B,
  Recombinant Vaccine
Halcinonide
Haloperidol Decanoate
Halothane
Hemin
Heparin Sodium
Hepatitis A Vaccine, Inactivated
Hepatitis B Immune Globulin
Hepatitis B Vaccine-
  Recombinant
Hexachlorophene
Homatropine Methylbromide/
  Hydrocodone Bitartrate
Hydrochlorothiazide/Irbesartan*
Hydrochlorothiazide/Lisinopril*
Hydrochlorothiazide/Losartan
  Potassium*
Hydrochlorothiazide/
  Methyldopa
Hydrochlorothiazide/Metoprolol
  Tartrate
Hydrochlorothiazide/Moexipril
  Hydrochloride*
Hydrochlorothiazide/
  Propranolol Hydrochloride
Hydrochlorothiazide/
  Spironolactone
Hydrochlorothiazide/Timolol
  Maleate
Hydrochlorothiazide/Triamterene
Hydrochlorothiazide/Valsartan*
Hydrocodone Bitartrate/
  Ibuprofen
Hydrocortisone
Hydrocortisone Acetate
Hydrocortisone Acetate/
  Neomycin Sulfate/
  Polymyxin B Sulfate
Hydrocortisone Acetate/
  Pramoxine Hydrochloride
Hydrocortisone Butyrate
Hydrocortisone Probutate
Hydrocortisone Valerate
Hydrocortisone/Iodoquinol
Hydrocortisone/Neomycin
  Sulfate/Polymyxin B Sulfate
Hydromorphone Hydrochloride
Hydroquinone
Hyoscyamine
Hyoscyamine Sulfate
Ibutilide Fumarate
Imiglucerase
Indinavir Sulfate
Indocyanine Green
Influenza Virus Vaccine
  (Subvirion)
Influenza Virus Vaccine
  (Whole-Virus)
Interferon Alfa-2A
Interferon Alfa-2B
Interferon Alfacon-1
Interferon Alfa-N3
Interferon Beta-1A
Interferon Beta-1B
Interferon Gamma-1B
Irbesartan*

* Category C or D depending on the trimester the drug is given.

(continued)

Appendix 10

Use-in-Pregnancy Ratings (continued)

Iron Dextran
Isoniazid/Pyrazinamide/
   Rifampin
Isosorbide Dinitrate
Isosorbide Mononitrate (Ismo)
Isradipine
Itraconazole
Ivermectin
Japanese Encephalitis Virus
   Vaccine
Ketoconazole
Ketorolac Tromethamine
Labetalol Hydrochloride
Lamivudine
Lamivudine/Zidovudine
Lamotrigine
Latanoprost
Levalbuterol Hydrochloride
Levamisole Hydrochloride
Levetiracetam
Levofloxacin
Levorphanol Tartrate
Linezolid
Lisinopril*
Losartan Potassium*
Mafenide Acetate
Measles/Mumps/Rubella
   Vaccine
Mebendazole
Mefenamic Acid
Mefloquine Hydrochloride
Meningitis Vaccine
Mepivacaine Hydrochloride
Metaproterenol Sulfate
Metaraminol Bitartrate
Methamphetamine
   Hydrochloride
Methenamine
   Mandelate/Sodium Acid
   Phosphate
Methocarbamol
Methoxsalen
Metoprolol Succinate
Metoprolol Tartrate
Metyrosine
Mexiletine Hydrochloride
Midodrine Hydrochloride
Milrinone Lactate
Mirtazapine
Modafinil
Moexipril Hydrochloride*
Mometasone Furoate
Monobenzone
Morphine Sulfate
Moxifloxacin Hydrochloride
Mumps Virus Vaccine
Muromonab-Cd3
Mycophenolate Mofetil
Mycophenolate Mofetil
   Hydrochloride
Nabumetone
Nadolol
Nalidixic Acid
Naloxone Hydrochloride/
   Pentazocine Hydrochloride
Naphazoline Hydrochloride

Naratriptan Hydrochloride
Natamycin
Nateglinide
Nefazodone Hydrochloride
Neostigmine Methylsulfate
Niacin
Nicardipine Hydrochloride
Nifedipine
Nilutamide
Nimodipine
Nisoldipine
Nitroglycerin
Norfloxacin
Nystatin
Ofloxacin
Olanzapine
Olopatadine Hydrochloride
Olsalazine Sodium
Omeprazole
Oprelvekin
Orphenadrine Citrate
Oxaprozin
Oxcarbazepine
Oxymorphone Hydrochloride
Palivizumab
Pancrelipase
Paricalcitol
Paroxetine Hydrochloride
Pegademase Bovine
Pegaspargase
Peginterferon Alpha-2A
Penbutolol Sulfate
Pentoxifylline
Perindopril Erbumine*
Phentermine Hydrochloride
Phenylephrine Hydrochloride
Phenylephrine Hydrochloride/
   Promethazine Hydrochloride
Phytonadione
Pilocarpine Hydrochloride
Pimozide
Pioglitazone Hydrochloride
Pirbuterol Acetate
Piroxicam
Plasma Protein Fraction
Pneumococcal Vaccine
Podofilox
Polio Vaccine, Inactivated
Polyethylene Glycol
Polyethylene Glycol/Potassium
   Chloride/Sodium
   Bicarbonate/Sodium Chloride
Polyethylene Glycol/Potassium
   Chloride/Sodium
   Bicarbonate/Sodium
   Chloride/Sodium Sulfate
Polymyxin B
   Sulfate/Trimethoprim Sulfate
Polythiazide/Prazosin
   Hydrochloride
Potassium Acid Phosphate
Potassium Chloride
Potassium Citrate
Potassium Phosphate/Dibasic

Sodium Phosphate/
   Monobasic Sodium
   Phosphate
Potassium Phosphate/Sodium
   Phosphate
Pralidoxime Chloride
Pramipexole Dihydrochloride
Prazosin Hydrochloride
Prednicarbate
Prednisolone Acetate
Prednisolone Acetate/
   Sulfacetamide Sodium
Prednisolone Sodium
   Phosphate
Procainamide Hydrochloride
Promethazine Hydrochloride
Propafenone Hydrochloride
Proparacaine Hydrochloride
Propranolol Hydrochloride
Protamine Sulfate
Proteinase Inhibitor (Human),
   Alpha 1
Protirelin
Pyrazinamide
Pyrimethamine
Quetiapine Fumarate
Quinapril Hydrochloride*
Quinidine Gluconate
Quinidine Sulfate
Rabies Immune Globulin
Rabies Vaccine
Ramipril*
Repaglinide
Reteplase, Recombinant
Rho (D) Immune Globulin
Rifampin
Rifapentine
Riluzole
Rimantadine Hydrochloride
Rimexolone
Risedronate Sodium
Risperidone
Rituximab
Rizatriptan Benzoate
Rocuronium Bromide
Rofecoxib
Ropinirole Hydrochloride
Rosiglitazone Maleate
Rubella Virus Vaccine
Rubeola Virus Vaccine
Salicylsalicylic Acid
Salmeterol Xinafoate
Sargramostim
Scopolamine
Selegiline Hydrochloride
Sermorelin Acetate
Sertraline Hydrochloride
Sevelamer Hydrochloride
Sibutramine Hydrochloride
Sodium Polystyrene Sulfonate
Somatrem
Somatropin, E-Coli Derived
Spiriva
Spironolactone
Stavudine
Streptokinase

Succimer
Succinylcholine Chloride
Sulconazole Nitrate
Sulfabenzamide/Sulfacetamide/
   Sulfathiazole
Sulfacetamide Sodium
Sulfacetamide Sodium/Sulfur
Sulfamethoxazole/Trimethoprim
Sulfanilamide
Sumatriptan
Sumatriptan Succinate
Tacrine Hydrochloride
Tacrolimus
Telmisartan*
Terazosin Hydrochloride
Terconazole
Testolactone
Tetanus Immune Globulin
Tetanus Toxoid
Theophylline
Thiabendazole
Thrombin
Thyrotropin Alfa
Tiagabine Hydrochloride
Tiludronate Disodium
Timolol Maleate
Tizanidine Hydrochloride
Tocainide Hydrochloride
Tolcapone
Tolmetin Sodium
Tolterodine Tartrate
Topiramate
Tramadol Hydrochloride
Trandolapril*
Trandolapril/Verapamil
   Hydrochloride*
Tretinoin (Topical)
Triamcinolone Acetonide
Triamterene
Trientine Hydrochloride
Triethanolamine Polypeptide
   Oleate
Trifluridine
Trimethoprim
Trimipramine Maleate
Trovafloxacin Mesylate
Tuberculin
Typhoid Vaccine
Typhoid Vi Polysaccharide
   Vaccine
Valrubicin
Valsartan*
Vancomycin Hydrochloride
   (Injection, Suspension)
Varicella Virus Vaccine
Vecuronium Bromide
Venlafaxine Hydrochloride
Verapamil Hydrochloride
Vitamin B12 (Injection)
Yellow Fever Vaccine
Zalcitabine
Zaleplon
Zidovudine
Zileuton
Zolmitriptan
Zonisamide

B

NO EVIDENCE OF RISK IN HUMANS

Either animal findings show risk while human findings do not, or, if no adequate human studies have been done, animal findings are negative.

Acarbose
Acebutolol Hydrochloride
Acetylcysteine
Acrivastine/Pseudoephedrine
   Hydrochloride
Acyclovir
Acyclovir Sodium
Alfuzosin Hydrochloride
Amiloride Hydrochloride
Amiloride Hydrochloride/
   Hydrochlorothiazide
Amlexanox
Amoxicillin
Amoxicillin/Clavulanate
   Potassium
Amphotericin B Lipid Complex
Amphotericin B Liposome
Ampicillin Sodium/Sulbactam
   Sodium
Amylase/Lipase/Protease
   (Pancrease)
Antithrombin III (Human)
Aprotinin
Atazanavir Sulfate
Azelaic Acid
Azithromycin Dihydrate
Aztreonam
Basiliximab
Brimonidine Tartrate
Budesonide
   (Pulmicort Turbuhaler)
Bupropion Hydrochloride
Butenafine Hydrochloride
Cabergoline
Carbenicillin Indanyl Sodium
Cefaclor
Cefadroxil
Cefamandole Nafate
Cefazolin Sodium
Cefdinir
Cefepime Hydrochloride
Cefixime
Cefoperazone Sodium
Cefotaxime Sodium
Cefotetan Disodium
Cefoxitin Sodium
Cefpodoxime Proxetil
Cefprozil
Ceftazidime
Ceftazidime Sodium
Ceftibuten
Ceftizoxime Sodium
Ceftriaxone Sodium
Cefuroxime Axetil

---

* Category C or D depending on the trimester the drug is given.

Use-in-Pregnancy Ratings (continued)

Cefuroxime Sodium	Enoxaparin Sodium	Lidocaine	Ondansetron	Sulfasalazine
Cephalexin	Epinephrine/Lidocaine	Lidocaine Hydrochloride	Ondansetron Hydrochloride	Tadalafil
Cetirizine Hydrochloride	Hydrochloride	Lidocaine/Prilocaine	Orlistat	Tamsulosin Hydrochloride
Chlorhexidine Gluconate	Epoprostenol Sodium	Lindane	Oxiconazole Nitrate	Terbinafine Hydrochloride
Ciclopirox Olamine	Eptifibatide	Lodoxamide Tromethamine	Oxybutynin Chloride	Terbutaline Sulfate
Cimetidine	Erythromycin	Loracarbef	Oxycodone Hydrochloride	Ticlopidine Hydrochloride
Cimetidine Hydrochloride	Erythromycin Ethylsuccinate	Loratadine	Palonosetron Hydrochloride	Tirofiban Hydrochloride
Clavulanate	Erythromycin Stearate	Loratadine/Pseudoephedrine	Pemoline	Tobramycin (Ophthalmic)
Potassium/Ticarcillin	Etanercept	Sulfate	Penicillin G Benzathine	Torsemide
Disodium	Ethacrynate Sodium	Malathion	Penicillin G Benzathine/	Trastuzumab
Clindamycin Hydrochloride	Ethacrynic Acid	Meclizine Hydrochloride	Penicillin G Procaine	Urokinase
Clindamycin Phosphate	Famotidine	Memantine Hydrochloride	Penicillin G Potassium	Ursodiol
Clopidogrel Bisulfate	Fenoldopam Mesylate	Meropenem	Pentosan Polysulfate Sodium	Valacyclovir Hydrochloride
Clotrimazole (Topical)	Ferric Sodium Gluconate	Mesalamine	Pergolide Mesylate	Vancomycin Hydrochloride
Clozapine	Flavoxate Hydrochloride	Metformin Hydrochloride	Permethrin	(Capsules)
Cromolyn Sodium	Fondaparinux Sodium	Methohexital Sodium	Piperacillin Sodium	Vardenafil Hydrochloride
Cyclobenzaprine Hydrochloride	Fosfomycin Tromethamine	Methyldopa	Piperacillin Sodium/Tazobactam	Zafirlukast
Cyproheptadine Hydrochloride	Glatiramer Acetate	Metoclopramide Hydrochloride	Sodium	Zolpidem Tartrate
Dalteparin Sodium	Glucagon Hydrochloride	Metolazone	Praziquantel	
Danaparoid Sodium	Glycopyrrolate	Metronidazole	Progesterone	
Daptomycin	Gonadorelin Hydrochloride	Metronidazole Hydrochloride	Propofol	
Desflurane	Guaifenesin/Pseudoephedrine	Miglitol	Psyllium	
Desmopressin Acetate	Hydrochloride (Guaifed)	Montelukast Sodium	Quinupristin/Dalfopristin	
Diclofenac Potassium	Guanfacine Hydrochloride	Mupirocin	Ranitidine Hydrochloride	
Diclofenac Sodium	Hydrochlorothiazide	Mupirocin Calcium	Rifabutin	
Didanosine	Ibuprofen	Naftifine Hydrochloride	Ritonavir	
Diphenhydramine	Imiquimod	Nalbuphine Hydrochloride	Ropivacaine Hydrochloride	
Hydrochloride	Indapamide	Nalmefene Hydrochloride	Saquinavir	
Dipyridamole	Infliximab	Naloxone Hydrochloride	Saquinavir Mesylate	
Dobutamine Hydrochloride	Insulin Lispro, Human	Naproxen	Sildenafil Citrate	
Dolasetron Mesylate	Ipratropium Bromide	Naproxen Sodium	Silver Sulfadiazine	
Dornase Alpha	Isosorbide Mononitrate	Nelfinavir Mesylate	Sodium Fluoride	
Doxapram Hydrochloride	(Monoket, Imdur)	Nitrofurantoin, Macrocrystals	Somatropin, E-Coli Derived	
Doxepin Hydrochloride	Ketoprofen	Nitrofurantoin, Macrocrystals/	(Genotropin)	
(Zonalon)	Lactulose	Nitrofurantoin Monohydrate	Somatropin, Mammalian	
Edetate Calcium Disodium	Lansoprazole	Nizatidine	Derived (Serostim)	
Emedastine Difumarate	Lepirudin	Octreotide Acetate	Sotalol Hydrochloride	
Emtricitabine	Levocarnitine	Omalizumab	Sucralfate	

**CONTROLLED STUDIES
SHOW NO RISK**

*Adequate, well-controlled
studies in pregnant women
have failed to demonstrate
risk to the fetus.*

Levothyroxine Sodium
Liothyronine Sodium

* Category C or D depending on the trimester the drug is given.

From Fleming T, ed. *Drug Topics Red Book.* Montvale. NJ: Thompson PDR; 2004.

Appendix 11

Sugar-Free Products

Listed below, by therapeutic category, is a selection of drug products that contain no sugar. When recommending these products to diabetic patients, keep in mind that many may contain sorbitol, alcohol, or other sources of carbohydrates. This list should not be considered all-inclusive. Generics and alternate brands of some products may be available. Check product labeling for a current listing of inactive ingredients.

Analgesics

Actamin Maximum Strength Liquid	Cypress
Addaprin Tablet	Dover
Aminofen Tablet	Dover
Aminofen Max Tablet	Dover
Aspirtab Tablet	Dover
Back Pain-Off Tablet	Textilease Medique
Backprin Tablet	Hart Health and Safety
Buffasal Tablet	Dover
Dyspel Tablet	Dover
Febrol Liquid	Scot-Tussin
I-Prin Tablet	Textilease Medique
Medi-Seltzer Effervescent Tablet	Textilease Medique
Ms.-Aid Tablet	Textilease Medique
PMS Relief Tablet	Textilease Medique
Silapap Children's Elixir	Silarx

Antacids/Antiflatulents

Almag Chewable Tablet	Textilease Medique
Alcalak Chewable Tablet	Textilease Medique
Aldroxicon I Suspension	Textilease Medique
Aldroxicon II Suspension	Textilease Medique
Baby Gasz Drops	Lee
Dimacid Chewable Tablet	Otis Clapp & Son
Diotame Chewable Tablet	Textilease Medique
Diotame Suspension	Textilease Medique
Gas-Ban Chewable Tablet	Textilease Medique
Mallamint Chewable Tablet	Textilease Medique
Mylanta Gelcaplet	Johnson & Johnson/Merck
Neutralin Tablet	Dover
Tums E-X Chewable Tablet	GlaxoSmithKline Consumer

Antiasthmatic/Respiratory Agents

Jay-Phyl Syrup	Pharmakon

Antidiarrheals

Diarrest Tablet	Dover
Di-Gon II Tablet	Textilease Medique
Imogen Liquid	Pharmaceutical Generic

Blood Modifiers/Iron Preparations

I.L.X. B-12 Elixir	Kenwood
Irofel Liquid	Dayton
Nephro-Fer Tablet	R & D

Corticosteroids

Pediapred Solution	Celltech

Cough/Cold/Allergy Preparations

Accuhist DM Pediatric Drops	Pediamed
Accuhist LA Tablets	Pediamed
Accuhist Pediatric Drops	Pediamed
Alacol DM Syrup	Ballay
Anaplex DM Syrup	ECR
Anaplex HD Syrup	ECR
Atuss EX Liquid	Atley
Benadryl Allergy/ Sinus Children's Solution	Warner-Lambert Consumer
Biodec DM Drops	Bio-Pharm
Biodec DM Syrup	Bio-Pharm
Bromdec Solution	Scientific Laboratories
Bromdec DM Solution	Scientific Laboratories
Bromhist-DM Solution	Cypress
Bromhist Pediatric Solution	Cypress
Bromophed DX Syrup	Qualitest
B-Tuss Liquid	Blansett
Carbofed DM Syrup	Hi-Tech
Carbofed DM Drops	Hi-Tech
Cardec Syrup	Qualitest
Cardec DM Syrup	Qualitest
Cetafen Cold Tablet	Hart Health and Safety
Cheratussin DAC Liquid	Qualitest
Codal-DM Syrup	Cypress
Coldmist DM Syrup	Breckenridge
Coldonyl Tablet	Dover
Co-Tussin Liquid	American Generics
Cotuss-V Syrup	Alphagen
Cytuss HC Syrup	Cypress
Decorel Forte Tablet	Textilease Medique
Despec Liquid	International Ethical
Despec-SF Liquid	International Ethical
Diabetic Tussin Allergy Relief Liquid	Health Care Products
Diabetic Tussin Allergy Relief Gelcaplet	Health Care Products
Diabetic Tussin C Expectorant Liquid	Health Care Products
Diabetic Tussin Cold & Flu Gelcaplet	Health Care Products
Diabetic Tussin DM Liquid	Health Care Products
Diabetic Tussin DM Maximum Strength Liquid	Health Care Products
Diabetic Tussin EX Liquid	Health Care Products
Dimetapp Allergy Children's Elixir	Wyeth Consumer
Diphen Capsule	Textilease Medique
Double-Tussin DM Liquid	Reese
Dynatuss Syrup	Breckenridge
Dynatuss HC Solution	Breckenridge
Dynatuss HCG Solution	Breckenridge
Echotuss-HC Syrup	Superior
Endal HD Liquid	Pediamed

(continued)

Appendix 11

Sugar-Free Products (continued)

Endal HD Plus Liquid	Pediamed	Hydro-Tussin HD Liquid	Ethex	Phanasin Syrup	Pharmakon
Endotuss-HD Syrup	American Generics	Hyphen-HD Syrup	Alphagen	Phanasin Diabetic Choice Syrup	Pharmakon
Enplus-HD Syrup	Alphagen	Hytuss Tablet	Hyrex	Phanatuss Syrup	Pharmakon
Entex Syrup	Andrx	Hytuss 2X Capsule	Hyrex	Phenydryl Solution	Scientific Laboratories
Entex HC Syrup	Andrx	Iofen-C NF Liquid	Superior		
Exo-Tuss Syrup	American Generics	Iofen-DM NF Liquid	Superior	Pneumotussin 2.5 Syrup	ECR
		Iofen-NF Liquid	Superior	Poly-Tussin Syrup	Poly
Gani-Tuss NR Liquid	Cypress	Jaycof Expectorant Syrup	Pharmakon	Poly-Tussin DM Syrup	Poly
Gani-Tuss-DM NR Liquid	Cypress			Poly-Tussin HD Syrup	Poly
Genecof-HC Liquid	Pharmaceutical Generic	Jaycof-HC Liquid	Pharmakon	Poly-Tussin XP Syrup	Poly
		Jaycof-XP Liquid	Pharmakon	Pro-Cof Liquid	Qualitest
Genecof-XP Liquid	Pharmaceutical Generic	Kita LA Tos Liquid	R.I.D.	Pro-Cof D Liquid	Qualitest
		Levall 5.0 Liquid	Athlon	Prolex DH Liquid	Blansett
Genedel Syrup	Pharmaceutical Generic	Lodrane Liquid	ECR	Prolex DM Liquid	Blansett
		Lortuss DM Solution	Proethic Laboratories	Protex Solution	Scientific Laboratories
Genedotuss-DM Liquid	Pharmaceutical Generic				
		Lortuss HC Solution	Proethic Laboratories	Protex D Solution	Scientific Laboratories
Genexpect DM Liquid	Pharmaceutical Generic				
		Marcof Expectorant Syrup	Marnel	Protuss Liquid	First Horizon
Genexpect-PE Liquid	Pharmaceutical Generic	Maxi-Tuss HCX Solution	MCR American	Protuss-D Liquid	First Horizon
		M-Clear Syrup	McNeil, R.A.	Quintex Syrup	Qualitest
Genexpect-SF Liquid	Pharmaceutical Generic	Mytussin AC Cough Syrup	Morton Grove	Quintex HC Syrup	Qualitest
				Romilar AC Liquid	Scot-Tussin
Giltuss Liquid	Gil	Mytussin DAC Syrup	Morton Grove	Romilar DM Liquid	Scot-Tussin
Giltuss HC Syrup	Gil	Nalex DH Liquid	Blansett	Rondec Syrup	Biovail
Giltuss Pediatric Liquid	Gil	Nalex-A Liquid	Blansett	Rondec DM Syrup	Biovail
Giltuss TR Tablet	Gil	Nalspan Senior DX Liquid	Morton Grove	Rondec DM Drops	Biovail
Guai-Co Liquid	Alphagen			Scot-Tussin Allergy Relief Formula Liquid	Scot-Tussin
Guaicon DMS Liquid	Textilease Medique	Neotuss S/F Liquid	A.G. Marin		
		Neotuss-D Liquid	A.G. Marin	Scot-Tussin DM Liquid	Scot-Tussin
Guai-DEX Liquid	Alphagen	Norel DM Liquid	U.S. Corp	Scot-Tussin DM Cough Chasers Lozenge	Scot-Tussin
Guaitussin AC Solution	Scientific Laboratories	Norel SD Solution	U.S. Corp		
		Nycoff Tablet	Dover	Scot-Tussin Expectorant Liquid	Scot-Tussin
Guaitussin DAC Solution	Scientific Laboratories	Onset Forte Tablet	Textilease Medique		
				Scot-Tussin Original Liquid	Scot-Tussin
Guiatuss AC Syrup	Alpharma	Orgadin Liquid	American Generics		
Guiatuss AC Syrup	Ivax			Scot-Tussin Senior Liquid	Scot-Tussin
Guiatuss DAC Syrup	Alpharma	Orgadin-Tuss Liquid	American Generics		
Halotussin AC Liquid	Watson			Siladryl Allergy Liquid	Silarx
Halotussin DAC Liquid	Watson	Orgadin-Tuss DM Liquid	American Generics	Siladryl DAS Liquid	Silarx
Hayfebrol Liquid	Scot-Tussin			Sildec Syrup	Silarx
H-C Tussive Syrup	Vintage	Organidin NR Liquid	Wallace	Sildec Drops	Silarx
Histex PD Liquid	TEAMM	Organidin NR Tablet	Wallace	Sildec-DM Syrup	Silarx
Histinex HC Syrup	Ethex	Palgic-DS Syrup	Pamlab	Sildec-DM Liquid	Silarx
Histinex PV Syrup	Ethex	Pancof Syrup	Pamlab	Silexin Syrup	Otis Clapp & Son
Histuss HC Solution	Scientific Laboratories	Pancof EXP Syrup	Pamlab	Silexin Tablet	Otis Clapp & Son
		Pancof HC Liquid	Pamlab	Siltussin DAS Liquid	Silarx
Hydro PC Syrup	Cypress	Pancof XP Liquid	Pamlab	Siltussin DM DAS Cough Syrup Formula	Silarx
Hydron KGS Liquid	Cypress	Pediatex DM Liquid	Zyber		
Hydro-Tussin DM Elixir	Ethex	Pediatex D	Zyber	Siltussin SA Syrup	Silarx
Hydro-Tussin HC Syrup	Ethex				

(continued)

Appendix 11

Sugar-Free Products (continued)

S-T Forte 2 Liquid	Scot-Tussin	Metamucil Smooth Texture Powder	Procter & Gamble	Vademecum Mouthwash & Gargle Concentrate	Dermatone
Sudodrin Tablet	Textilease Medique	Reguloid Powder	Rugby	**Potassium Supplements**	
Supress DX Pediatric Drops	Kramer-Novis	**Miscellaneous**		Cena K Liquid	Century
Suttar-SF Syrup	Gil	Acidoll Capsule	Key	Kaon Elixir	Savage
Tricodene Syrup	Pfeiffer	Alka-Gest Tablet	Key	Kaon-Cl 20% Liquid	Savage
Trispec-PE Liquid	Deliz	Bicitra Solution	Ortho-McNeil	Rum-K Liquid	Fleming
Tussafed Syrup	Everett	Colidrops Pediatric Drops	A.G. Marin	**Vitamins/Minerals/Supplements**	
Tussafed-EX Pediatric Drops	Everett	Cytra-2 Solution	Cypress	Action-Tabs Made For Men	Action Labs
Tussafed-HC Syrup	Everett	Cytra-K Solution	Cypress	Adaptosode For Stress Liquid	HVS
Tuss-DM Liquid	Seatrace	Cytra-K Crystals	Cypress	Adaptosode R+R For Acute Stress Liquid	HVS
Tuss-ES Syrup	Seatrace	Melatin Tablet	Mason Vitamins	Aminoplex Powder	Tyson
Tussi-Organidin DM NR Liquid	Wallace	Methadose Solution	Mallinckrodt	Aminostasis Powder	Tyson
Tussi-Organidin DM-S NR Liquid	Wallace	Neutra-Phos Powder	Ortho-McNeil	Aminotate Powder	Tyson
Tussi-Organidin NR Liquid	Wallace	Neutra-Phos-K Powder	Ortho-McNeil	Apetigen Elixir	Kramer-Novis
Tussi-Organidin-S NR Liquid	Wallace	Polycitra-K Solution	Ortho-McNeil	Apptrim Capsules	Physician Therapeutics
Tussi-Pres Liquid	Kramer-Novis	Polycitra-LC Solution	Ortho-McNeil	B-C-Bid Caplet	Lee
Tussirex Liquid	Scot-Tussin	Questran Light Powder	Par	Bevitamel Tablet	Westlake
Vi-Q-Tuss Syrup	Vintage	**Mouth/Throat Preparations**		Biosode Liquid	HVS
Vitussin Expectorant Syrup	Cypress	Aquafresh Triple Protection Gum GlaxoSmithKline		Biotect Plus Caplet	Gil
Vortex Syrup	Superior		Consumer	C & M Caps-375 Capsule	Key
Z-Cof DM Syrup	Zyber	Cepacol Maximum Strength Spray	J.B. Williams	Calbon Tablet	Emrex/Economed
Z-Cof HC Syrup	Zyber	Cepacol Sore Throat Lozenges	J.B. Williams	Cal-Cee Tablet	Key
Zyrtec Syrup	Pfizer	Cheracol Sore Throat Spray	Lee	Calcimin-300 Tablet	Key
Fluoride Preparations		Cylex Lozenges	Pharmakon	Cal-Mint Chewable Tablet	Freeda Vitamins
Ethedent Chewable Tablet	Ethex	Diabetic Tussin Cough Drops	Health Care Products	Carox Plus Tablet	Seneca
Fluor-A-Day Tablet	Pharmascience	Fisherman's Friend Lozenges	Mentholatum	Cerefolin Tablet	Pamlab
Fluor-A-Day Lozenge	Pharmascience	Fresh N Free Liquid	Geritrex	Cevi-Bid Tablet	Lee
Flura-Loz Tablet	Kirkman	Isodettes Sore Throat Spray	GlaxoSmithKline Consumer	Cholestratin Tablet	Key
Lozi-Flur Lozenge	Dreir	Larynex Lozenges	Dover	Chromacaps Tablet	Key
Sensodyne w/Fluoride Gel	GlaxoSmithKline Consumer	Listerine Pocketpaks Film	Pfizer Consumer	Chromium K6 Tablet	Rexall Consumer
Sensodyne w/Fluoride Tartar Control Toothpaste	GlaxoSmithKline Consumer	Medikoff Drops	Textilease Medique	Combi-Cart Tablet	Atrium Bio-Tech
Sensodyne w/Fluoride Toothpaste	GlaxoSmithKline Consumer	N'Ice Lozenges	Heritage Brand/Insight	Daily Herbs Formulas	Mason Vitamins
Laxatives		Oragesic Solution	Parnell	Delta D3 Tablet	Freeda Vitamins
Citrucel Powder	GlaxoSmithKline Consumer	Orasept Mouthwash/Gargle Liquid	Pharmakon	Detoxosode Liquids	HVS
Fiber Ease Liquid	Plainview	Robitussin Lozenges	Wyeth Consumer	DHEA Capsule	ADH Health Products
Fibro-XL Capsule	Key	Sepasoothe Lozenges	Textilease Medique	Diabeze Tablet	Key
Genfiber Powder	Ivax			Diatx Tablet	Pamlab
Konsyl Easy Mix Formula Powder	Konsyl	Thorets Maximum Strength Lozenges	Otis Clapp & Son	Diet System 6 Gum	Applied Nutrition
Konsyl-Orange Powder	Konsyl	Throto–Ceptic Spray	S.S.S.	Diucaps Capsule	Legere
				Dl-Phen-500 Capsule	Key

(continued)

Appendix 11

Sugar-Free Products (continued)

Product	Manufacturer
Electrotab Tablet	Hart Health And Safety
Endorphenyl Capsule	Tyson
Ensure Nutra Shake Pudding	Ross Products
Enterex Diabetic Liquid	Victus
Essential Nutrients Plus Silica Tablet	Action Labs
Evening Primrose Oil Capsule	National Vitamin
Evolve Softgel	Bionutrics Health Products
Ex-L Tablet	Key
Extress Tablet	Key
Eyetamins Tablet	Rexall Consumer
Fem-Cal Tablet	Freeda Vitamins
Fem-Cal Plus Tablet	Freeda Vitamins
Folacin-800 Tablet	Key
Foltx Tablet	Pamlab
Gram-O-Leci Tablet	Freeda Vitamins
Hemovit Tablet	Dayton
Herbal Slim Complex Capsule	ADH Health Products
Legatrin GCM Formula Tablet	Columbia
Lynae Calcium/Vitamin C Chewable Tablet	Boscogen
Lynae Chondroitin/ Glucosamine Capsule	Boscogen
Lynae Ginse-Cool Chewable Tablet	Boscogen
Mag-Caps Capsule	Rising
Mag-Ox 400 Tablet	Blaine
Mag-SR Tablet	Cypress
Medi-Lyte Tablet	Textilease Medique
New Life Hair Tablet	Rexall Consumer
Nutrisure OTC Tablet	Westlake
O-Cal Fa Tablet	Pharmics
Plenamins Plus Tablet	Rexall Consumer
Powermate Tablet	Green Turtle Bay Vitamin
Prostaplex Herbal Complex Capsule	ADH Health Products
Prostatonin Capsule	Pharmaton Natural Health
Protect Plus Liquid	Gil
Protect Plus NR Softgel	Gil
Quintabs-M Tablet	Freeda Vitamins
Re/Neph Liquid	Ross Products
Replace Capsule	Key
Replace w/o Iron Capsule	Key
Resource Arginaid Powder	Novartis Nutrition
Ribo-100 T.D. Capsule	Key
Samolinic Softgel	Key
Boscogen	
Sea Omega 30 Softgel	Rugby
Sea Omega 50 Softgel	Rugby
Soy Care for Bone Health	Inverness Medical Tablet
Soy Care for Menopause	Inverness Medical Capsule
Strovite Forte Syrup	Everett
Sunnie Tablet	Green Turtle Bay Vitamin
Sunvite Tablet	Rexall Consumer
Sunvite Platinum Tablet	Rexall Consumer
Supervite Liquid	Seyer Pharmatec
Suplevit Liquid	Gil
Triamin Tablet	Key
Triamino Tablet	Freeda Vitamins
Ultramino Powder	Freeda Vitamins
Uro-Mag Capsule	Blaine
Vitalize Liquid	Scot-Tussin
Vitamin C/Rose Hips Tablet	ADH Health Products
Vitrum Jr Chewable Tablet	Mason Vitamins
Xtramins Tablet	Key
Yohimbe Power Max 1500 For Women Tablet	Action Labs
Yohimbized 1000 Capsule	Action Labs
Ze-Plus Softgel	Everett

From Fleming T., ed. *Drug Topics Red Book*. Montvale. NJ: Thompson PDR, 2004.

Appendix 12

Alcohol-Free Products

The following is a selection of alcohol-free products grouped by therapeutic category. The list is not comprehensive. Generic and alternate brands may exist. Always check product labeling for definitive information on specific ingredients.

Analgesics

Product	Manufacturer
Acetaminophen Infants Drops	Ivax
Actamin Maximum Strength Liquid	Cypress
Addaprin Tablet	Dover
Advil Children's Suspension	Wyeth Consumer
Aminofen Tablet	Dover
Aminofen Max Tablet	Dover
APAP Elixir	Bio-Pharm
Aspirtab Tablet	Dover
Buffasal Tablet	Dover
Demerol Hydrochloride Syrup	Sanofi-Synthelabo
Dolono Elixir	R.I.D.
Dyspel Tablet	Dover
Genapap Children Elixir	Ivax
Genapap Infant's Drops	Ivax
Motrin Children's Suspension	McNeil Consumer
Motrin Infants' Suspension	McNeil Consumer
Silapap Children's Elixir	Silarx
Silapap Infant's Drops	Silarx
Tylenol Children's Suspension	McNeil Consumer
Tylenol Extra Strength Solution	McNeil Consumer
Tylenol Infant's Drops	McNeil Consumer
Tylenol Infant's Suspension	McNeil Consumer

Antiasthmatic Agents

Product	Manufacturer
Dilor-G Liquid	Savage
Dy-G Liquid	Cypress
Elixophyllin-GG Liquid	Forest

Anticonvulsants

Product	Manufacturer
Zarontin Syrup	Pfizer

Antiviral Agents

Product	Manufacturer
Epivir Oral Solution	GlaxoSmithKline

Cough/Cold/Allergy Preparations

Product	Manufacturer
Accuhist Pediatric Drops	Propst
Alacol DM Syrup	Ballay
Allergy Relief Medicine Children's Elixir	Hi-Tech Pharmacal
Anaplex DM Syrup	ECR
Anaplex HD Syrup	ECR
Andehist DM Drops	Cypress
Andehist DM Syrup	Cypress
Andehist DM NR Liquid	Cypress
Andehist DM NR Syrup	Cypress
Andehist NR Syrup	Cypress
Atuss DR Syrup	Atley
Atuss EX Liquid	Atley
Atuss G Liquid	Atley
Atuss HC Syrup	Atley
Atuss MS Syrup	Atley
Benadryl Allergy Solution	Pfizer Consumer
Biodec DM Drops	Bio-Pharm
Biodec DM Syrup	Bio-Pharm
Bromaline Solution	Rugby
Bromaline DM Elixir	Rugby
Bromanate Elixir	Alpharma USPD
Bromaxefed DM RF Syrup	Morton Grove
Bromaxefed RF Syrup	Morton Grove
Broncotron Liquid	Seyer Pharmatec
Bromdec Solution	Scientific Laboratories
Bromdec DM Solution	Scientific Laboratories
Bromhist Pediatric Solution	Cypress
Bromhist-DM Pediatric Syrup	Cypress
Bromhist-DM Solution	Cypress
Bron-Tuss Liquid	American Generics
B-Tuss Liquid	Blansett
Carbatuss Liquid	GM
Carbofed DM Drops	Hi-Tech Pharmacal
Carbofed DM Syrup	Hi-Tech Pharmacal
Cardec Syrup	Qualitest
Cardec DM Syrup	Qualitest .
Cepacol Sore Throat Liquid	J.B. Williams
Chlordex GP Syrup	Cypress
Chlor-Trimeton Allergy Syrup	Schering Plough
Codal-DH Syrup	Cypress
Codal-DM Syrup	Cypress
Codotuss Liquid	Major
Coldonyl Tablet	Dover
Complete Allergy Elixir	Cardinal Health
Co-Tussin Liquid	American Generics
Cotuss-V Syrup	Alphagen
Creomulsion Complete Syrup	Summit Industries
Creomulsion Cough Syrup	Summit Industries
Creomulsion For Children Syrup	Summit Industries
Creomulsion Pediatric Syrup	Summit Industries
Cytuss HC Syrup	Cypress
Dehistine Syrup	Cypress
Deltuss Liquid	Deliz
Despec Liquid Labs	International Ethical
Diabetic Tussin Allergy Relief Liquid	Healthcare Products
Diabetic Tussin C Expectorant Liquid	Healthcare Products
Diabetic Tussin Cold & Flu Tablet	Healthcare Products
Diabetic Tussin DM Liquid	Healthcare Products
Diabetic Tussin DM Maximum Strength Liquid	Healthcare Products
Diabetic Tussin DM Maximum Strength Capsule	Healthcare Products
Diabetic Tussin EX Liquid	Healthcare Products
Dimetapp Allergy Children's Elixir	Whitehall-Robins
Dimetapp Cold & Fever Children's Suspension	Wyeth Consumer
Dimetapp Decongestant Pediatric Drops	Wyeth Consumer
Double-Tussin DM Liquid	Reese
Dynatuss Syrup	Breckenridge
Dynatuss EX Syrup	Breckenridge
Dynatuss HC Solution	Breckenridge
Dynatuss HCG Solution	Breckenridge
Echotuss-HC Syrup	Superior
Endagen-HD Syrup	Monarch
Endal HD Solution	Pediamed
Endal HD Syrup	Propst
Endal HD Plus Syrup	Propst
Endotuss-HD Syrup	American Generics
Enplus-HD Syrup	Alphagen
Entex Syrup	Andrx
Entex HC Syrup	Andrx
Exo-Tuss	American Generics
Father John's Medicine Plus Drops	Oakhurst
Friallergia DM Liquid	R.I.D.
Friallergia Liquid	R.I.D.
Gani-Tuss NR Liquid	Cypress
Gani-Tuss-DM NR Liquid	Cypress
Genahist Elixir	Ivax
Giltuss HC Syrup	Gil
Giltuss Liquid	Gil
Giltuss Pediatric Liquid	Gil
Guai-Co Liquid	Alphagen
Guaicon DMS Liquid	Textilease Medique
Guai-Dex Liquid	Alphagen
Guaifed Syrup	Muro
Guaitussin AC Solution	Scientific Laboratories
Guaitussin DAC Solution	Scientific Laboratories
Halotussin AC Liquid	Watson Pharma
Hayfebrol Liquid	Scot-Tussin
H-C Tussive Syrup	Vintage
Histex HC Syrup	TEAMM
Histex Liquid	TEAMM
Histex PD Drops	TEAMM
Histex PD Liquid	TEAMM
Histinex HC Syrup	Ethex
Histinex PV Syrup	Ethex
Histuss HC Solution	Scientific Laboratories
Hycomal DH Liquid	Alphagen
Hydone Liquid	Hyrex
Hydramine Elixir	Ivax
Hydro-Tussin DM Elixir	Ethex
Hydro-Tussin HC Syrup	Ethex
Hydro-Tussin HD Liquid	Ethex
Hydro-Tussin XP Syrup	Ethex
Hyphen-HD Syrup	Alphagen
Iofen-C NF Liquid	Superior
Iofen-DM NF Liquid	Superior
Iofen-NF Liquid	Superior
Jaycof Expectorant Syrup	Pharmakon
Jaycof-HC Liquid	Pharmakon
Jaycof-XP Liquid	Pharmakon
Kita La Tos Liquid	R.I.D.
Levall Liquid	Andrx
Levall 5.0 Liquid	Andrx
Lodrane Liquid	ECR
Marcof Expectorant Syrup	Marnel
M-Clear Syrup	McNeil, R.A.
Medi-Brom Elixir	Medicine Shoppe
Motrin Cold Children's Suspension	McNeil Consumer
Mytussin-PE Liquid	Morton Grove
Nalex DH Liquid	Blansett Pharmacal
Nalex-A Liquid	Blansett Pharmacal
Nalspan Senior DX Liquid	Morton Grove
Neotuss S/F Liquid	A.G. Marin
Neotuss-D Liquid	A.G. Marin
Norel DM Liquid	U.S. Pharmaceutical
Nucofed Syrup	Monarch
Nycoff Tablet	Dover
Orgadin Liquid	American Generics
Orgadin-Tuss Liquid	American Generics
Orgadin-Tuss DM Liquid	American Generics
Organidin NR Liquid	Wallace
Palgic-DS Syrup	Pamlab
Pancof Syrup	Pamlab
Pancof EXP Syrup	Pamlab
Pancof HC Liquid	Pamlab
Pancof XP Liquid	Pamlab
Panmist DM Syrup	Pamlab
Panmist-S Syrup	Pamlab
PediaCare Cold + Allergy Children's Liquid	Pharmacia
PediaCare Cough + Cold Children's Liquid	Pharmacia
PediaCare Decongestant Infants Drops	Pharmacia

Appendix 12

Alcohol-Free Products (continued)

PediaCare Decongestant Plus Cough Drops	Pharmacia
PediaCare Multi-Symptom Liquid	Pharmacia
PediaCare Nightrest Liquid	Pharmacia
Pediahist DM Syrup	Boca
Pedia-Relief Liquid	Major
Pediatex Liquid	Zyber
Pediatex-D Liquid	Zyber
Pediox Liquid	Atley
Phanasin Syrup	Pharmakon
Phanatuss Syrup	Pharmakon
Phena-S Liquid	GM
Pneumotussin 2.5 Syrup	ECR
Poly-Tussin Syrup	Poly
Poly-Tussin DM Syrup	Poly
Poly-Tussin HD Syrup	Poly
Poly-Tussin XP Syrup	Poly
Primsol Solution	Medicis
Pro-Cof Liquid	Qualitest
Prolex DH Liquid	Blansett Pharmacal
Prolex DM Liquid	Blansett Pharmacal
Protuss Liquid	First Horizon
Protuss-D Liquid	First Horizon
Q-Tussin PE Liquid	Qualitest
Quintex Syrup	Qualitest
Robitussin Cough & Congestion Liquid	Wyeth Consumer
Robitussin DM Syrup	Wyeth Consumer
Robitussin PE Syrup	Wyeth Consumer
Robitussin Pediatric Drops	Wyeth Consumer
Robitussin Pediatric Cough Syrup	Wyeth Consumer
Robitussin Pediatric Night Relief Liquid	Wyeth Consumer
Romilar AC Liquid	Scot-Tussin
Romilar DM Liquid	Scot-Tussin
Rondec Syrup	Biovail
Rondec DM Drops	Biovail
Rondec DM Syrup	Biovail
Scot-Tussin Allergy Relief Formula Liquid	Scot-Tussin
Scot-Tussin DM Liquid	Scot-Tussin
Scot-Tussin Expectorant Liquid	Scot-Tussin
Scot-Tussin Original Syrup	Scot-Tussin
Scot-Tussin Senior Liquid	Scot-Tussin
Siladryl Allergy Liquid	Silarx
Siladryl DAS Liquid	Silarx
Sildec Liquid	Silarx
Sildec Syrup	Silarx
Sildec-DM Drops	Silarx
Sildec-DM Syrup	Silarx
Siltussin DAS Liquid	Silarx
Siltussin DM Syrup	Silarx
Siltussin DM DAS Cough Formula Syrup	Silarx
Siltussin SA Syrup	Silarx
Simply Cough Liquid	McNeil Consumer
Simply Stuffy Liquid	McNeil Consumer
S-T Forte 2 Liquid	Scot-Tussin
Sudatuss DM Syrup	Pharmaceutical Generic
Sudatuss-2 Liquid	Pharmaceutical Generic
Sudatuss-SF Liquid	Pharmaceutical Generic
Triaminic Infant Decongestant Drops	Novartis Consumer
Trispec-PE Liquid	Deliz
Tussafed Syrup	Everett
Tussafed-EX Syrup	Everett
Tussafed-EX Pediatric Liquid	Everett
Tussafed-HC Syrup	Everett
Tuss-DM Liquid	Seatrace
Tuss-ES Syrup	Seatrace
Tussi-Organidin DM NR Liquid	Wallace
Tussi-Organidin DM-S NR Liquid	Wallace
Tussi-Organidin NR Liquid	Wallace
Tussi-Organidin-S NR Liquid	Wallace
Tussi-Pres Liquid	Kramer-Novis
Tussirex Liquid	Scot-Tussin
Tussirex Syrup	Scot-Tussin
Tylenol Allergy-D Children's Liquid	McNeil Consumer
Tylenol Cold Children's Liquid	McNeil Consumer
Tylenol Cold Children's Suspension	McNeil Consumer
Tylenol Cold Infants' Drops	McNeil Consumer
Tylenol Cold Plus Cough Children's Liquid	McNeil Consumer
Tylenol Cold Plus Cough Infants' Suspension	McNeil Consumer
Tylenol Flu Children's Suspension	McNeil Consumer
Tylenol Flu Night Time Max Strength Liquid	McNeil Consumer
Tylenol Sinus Children's Liquid	McNeil Consumer
Vanex-HD Syrup	Monarch
Vicks 44E Pediatric Liquid	Procter & Gamble
Vicks 44M Pediatric Liquid	Procter & Gamble
Vicks Dayquil Multi-Symptom Liquicap	Procter & Gamble
Vicks Dayquil Multi-Symptom Liquid	Procter & Gamble
Vicks Nyquil Children's Liquid	Procter & Gamble
Vi-Q-Tuss Syrup	Vintage
Vitussin Expectorant Syrup	Cypress
Vortex Syrup	Superior
Z-Cof DM Syrup	Zyber
Z-Cof HC Syrup	Zyber

Ear/Nose/Throat Products

4-Way Saline Moisturizing Mist Spray	Bristol-Myers
Ayr Baby Saline Spray	Ascher, B.F.
Bucalcide Solution	Seyer Pharmatec
Bucalcide Spray	Seyer Pharmatec
Bucalsep Solution	Gil
Bucalsep Spray	Gil
Cepacol Sore Throat Liquid	Combe
Cheracol Sore Throat Spray	Lee
Fresh N Free Liquid	Geritrex
Gly-Oxide Liquid	GlaxoSmithKline Consumer
Isodettes Sore Throat Spray	GlaxoSmithKline Consumer
Lacrosse Mouthwash Liquid	Aplicare
Larynex Lozenges	Dover
Listermint Liquid	Pfizer Consumer
Nasal Moist Gel	Blairex
Orajel Baby Liquid	Del
Orajel Baby Nighttime Gel	Del
Oramagic Oral Wound Rinse Powder for Suspension	MPM Medical
Orasept Mouthwash/ Gargle Liquid	Pharmakon Labs
Tanac Liquid	Del
Tech 2000 Dental Rinse Liquid	Care-Tech Laboratories
Throto-Ceptic Spray	S.S.S.
Zilactin Baby Extra Strength Gel	Zila Consumer

Gastrointestinal Agents

Baby Gasz Drops	Lee
Colidrops Pediatric Drops	A.G. Marin
Diarrest Tablet	Dover
Imogen Liquid	Pharmaceutical Generic
Kaodene NN Suspension	Pfeiffer
Kaopectate Advanced Formula Suspension	Pharmacia Consumer
Kaopectate Children's Liquid Suspension	Pharmacia Consumer
Liqui-Doss Liquid	Ferndale
Mylicon Infants' Suspension	J&J–Merck
Neoloid Liquid	Kenwood Therapeutics
Neutralin Tablet	Dover
Senokot Children's Syrup	Purdue Frederick

Hematinics

Irofol Liquid	Dayton

Miscellaneous

Cytra-2 Solution	Cypress
Cytra-K Solution	Cypress
Emetrol Solution	Pharmacia Consumer
Fluorinse Solution	Oral B
Rum-K Liquid	Fleming

Psychotropics

Thorazine Syrup	GlaxoSmithKline

Topical Products

Aloe Vesta 2-N-1 Antifungal Ointment	Convatec
Fleet Pain Relief Pads	Fleet
Fresh & Pure Douche Solution	Unico
Handclens Solution	Woodward
Joint-Ritis Maximum Strength Ointment	Naturopathic
Klenz Kloth Pads	Geritrex
Neutrogena Acne Wash Liquid	Neutrogena
Neutrogena Antiseptic Liquid	Neutrogena
Neutrogena Clear Pore Gel	Neutrogena
Neutrogena T/Derm Liquid	Neutrogena
Neutrogena Toner Liquid	Neutrogena
Podiclens Spray	Woodward
Propa pH Foaming Face Wash Liquid	Del
Sea Breeze Foaming Face Wash Gel	Clairol
Stri-Dex Pad	Blistex
Stri-Dex Maximum Strength Pad	Blistex
Stri-Dex Sensitive Skin Pad	Blistex
Stri-Dex Super Scrub Pad	Blistex
Therasoft Anti-Acne Cream	SFC/Solvent Free
Therasoft Skin Protectant Cream	SFC/Solvent Free

Vitamins/Minerals/Supplements

Adaptosode For Stress Liquid	HVS
Adaptosode R+R For Acute Stress Liquid	HVS
Apetigen Elixir	Kramer-Novis
Biosode Liquid	HVS
Detoxosode Products Liquid	HVS
Genesupp-500 Liquid	Pharmaceutical Generic
Genetect Plus Liquid	Pharmaceutical Generic
Multi-Delyn w/Iron Liquid	Silarx
Poly-Vi-Sol Drops	Mead Johnson
Poly-Vi-Sol w/Iron Drops	Mead Johnson
Protect Plus Liquid	Gil
Soluvite-F Drops	Pharmics
Strovite Forte Syrup	Everett
Supervite Liquid	Seyer Pharmatec
Suplevit Liquid	Gil
Tri-Vi-Sol Drops	Mead Johnson
Tri-Vi-Sol w/Iron Drops	Mead Johnson
Vitafol Syrup	Everett
Vitalize Liquid	Scot-Tussin
Vitamin C/Rose Hips Tablet, Extended Release	ADH Health Products

From Fleming T., ed. *Drug Topics Red Book.* Montvale. NJ: Thompson PDR, 2004.

Appendix 13

Common Drug Interactions

Pharmacodynamic interactions

Object drug (trade name)	Precipitant drug (trade name)	Mechanism of Interaction
Antiarrhythmics	Antipsychotics, cisapride (Propulsid®), erythromycin (E-Mycin®), fluoroquinolones, fluoxetine (Prozac®), 5HT-3 antagonists, tricyclic antidepressants	Additive effects cause prolonged QT interval
Anticholinergic agents	Antihistamines, phenothiazine derivatives	Increased anticholinergic side effects
Aspirin, clopidogrel (Plavix®), heparin, low molecular weight heparins, ticlopidine (Ticlid®), warfarin (Coumadin®)	Garlic, gingko	Increased bleeding due to displacement of platelet-activating factor from its binding site
Clopidogrel (Plavix®), heparin, low molecular weight heparins, ticlopidine (Ticlid®), warfarin (Coumadin®)	Aspirin, NSAIDs	Increased bleeding due to inhibition of platelet aggregation
Benzodiazepines	Flumazenil (Romazicon®)	Antagonistic activity
β-Blockers	β-Agonists	Antagonistic activity
Naloxone (Narcan®)	Opiates	Antagonistic activity

Pharmacokinetic interactions

Digoxin (Lanoxin®), phenytoin (Dilantin®), quinolones, tetracyclines, warfarin (Coumadin®)	Antacids, cholestyramine (Questran®, Prevalite®, LoCHOLEST®), didanosine (Videx®), divalent cations (Ca^{2+}, Co^{2+}, Cu^{2+}, Fe^{2+}, Mg^{2+}, Mn^{2+}), sucralfate (Carafate®)	Decreased efficacy of object drug due to complexation and chelation
Dapsone, itraconazole (Sporanox®), ketoconazole (Nizoral®)	Antacids, H$_2$-receptor antagonists, proton pump inhibitors	Decreased efficacy of object drug due to increased pH of GI fluids
Oral contraceptives, warfarin (Coumadin®)	Antibiotics	Decreased efficacy of object drug due to change in bacterial flora of GI tract
Phenytoin (Dilantin®), valproic acid (Depakene®, Depakote®), warfarin (Coumadin®)	Chloral hydrate, (Aquachloral®, Supprettes®), salicylates, valproic acid (Depakene®, Depakote®)	Increased fraction of object drug due to drug displacement with multiple highly protein-bound drugs
Digoxin (Lanoxin®)	Aminoglycosides, amphotericin B (Amphotec®, Amphocin®, Fungizone®, Abelcet®, Ambisome®)	Nephrotoxicity due to decreased glomerular filtration rate
Lithium (Eskalith®, Lithobid®)	NSAIDs, thiazides	Decreased clearance of lithium
Cephalosporins, penicillins, quinolones	Probenecid (Benemid®)	Decreased antibiotic excretion due to competition for renal tubular secretion
Aspirin	Acetazolamide (Diamox®), sodium bicarbonate	Increased elimination of aspirin due to increased urinary pH

Cytochrome P450 interactions
CYP1A2

Substrates (trade name)	Inhibitors (trade name)	Inducers (trade name)
Amitriptyline (Elavil®)	Cimetidine (Tagamet®)	Cigarette smoke
Clomipramine (Anafranil®)	Ciprofloxacin (Cipro®)	Phenobarbital (Luminal sodium®)
Clozapine (Clozaril®)	Clarithromycin (Biaxin®)	Phenytoin (Dilantin®)
Cyclobenzaprine (Flexeril®)	Erythromycin (E-Mycin®)	Rifampin (Rifadin®, Rimactane®)
Desipramine (Norpramin®)	Fluvoxamine (Luvox®)	Ritonavir (Norvir®)
Diazepam (Valium®)	Grapefruit juice	
Fluvoxamine (Luvox®)	Isoniazid (Nydrazid®)	
Gingko	Ketoconazole (Nizoral®)	

(continued)

Appendix 13

Common Drug Interactions (continued)

CYP1A2 (cont)

Substrates (trade name)	Inhibitors (trade name)	Inducers (trade name)
Haloperidol (Haldol®)	Levofloxacin (Levaquin®)	
Imipramine (Tofranil®)	Norfloxacin (Chibroxin®, Noroxin®)	
Mexiletine (Mexitil®)		
Propranolol (Inderal®)	Ofloxacin (Floxin®)	
Theophylline, aminophylline (Aerolate®, Aquaphyllin®, Asmalix®, Bronkodyl®, Choledyl®, Constant-T®, Duraphyl®, Elixophyllin®, Phyllocontin®, Quibron®, Respbid®, Slo-bid®, Slo-Phyllin®, Sustaire®, Theo-24®, Theobid®, Theochron®, Theoclear®, Theo-Dur®, Theolair®, Theon®, Theospan®, Theovent®, Truphylline®), R-warfarin (Coumadin®)	Paroxetine (Paxil®), ticlopidine (Ticlid®)	

CYP2C9

Substrates (trade name)	Inhibitors (trade name)	Inducers (trade name)
Celecoxib (Celebrex®)	Amiodarone (Cordarone®, Pacerone®)	Phenobarbital (Luminal sodium®)
Diclofenac (Cataflam®, Voltaren®)	Cimetidine (Tagamet®)	Phenytoin (Dilantin®)
Flurbiprofen (Ansaid®)	Fluconazole (Diflucan®)	Rifampin (Rifadin®, Rimactane®)
Ibuprofen (Advil®, Motrin®)	Fluoxetine (Prozac®)	
Leflunomide (Arava®)	Fluvastatin (Lescol®)	
Losartan (Cozaar®)	Isoniazid (Nydrazid®)	
Montelukast (Singulair®)	Paroxetine (Paxil®)	
Naproxen (Aleve®, Naprosyn®)	Sertraline (Zoloft®)	
Phenytoin (Dilantin®)	Sulfamethoxazole (Bactrim®, Gantanol®, Septra®, Sulfatrim®)	
Piroxicam (Feldene®)	Ticlopidine (Ticlid®)	
Rosiglitazone (Avandia®)	Trimethoprim (Bactrim®, Primsol®, Proloprim®, Septra®, Sulfatrim®, Trimpex®)	
Sulfamethoxazole (Bactrim®, Gantanol®, Septra®, Sulfatrim®)	Zafirlukast (Accolate®)	
Tolbutamide (Orinase®)		
S-Warfarin (Coumadin®)		

CYP2C19

Substrates (trade name)	Inhibitors (trade name)	Inducers (trade name)
Amitriptyline (Elavil®)	Cimetidine (Tagamet®)	Carbamazepine (Tegretol®)
Citalopram (Celexa®)	Fluoxetine (Prozac®)	Norethindrone
Clomipramine (Anafranil®)	Fluvastatin (Lescol®)	
Cyclophosphamide (Cytoxan®, Neosar®)	Fluvoxamine (Luvox®)	
Diazepam (Valium®)	Ketoconazole (Nizoral®)	
Imipramine (Tofranil®)	Lansoprazole (Prevacid®)	
Lansoprazole (Prevacid®)	Omeprazole (Prilosec®)	
Nelfinavir (Viracept®)	Paroxetine (Paxil®)	
Omeprazole (Prilosec®)	Sertraline (Zoloft®)	
Pantoprazole (Protonix®)	Ticlopidine (Ticlid®)	
Phenytoin (Dilantin®)		

CYP2D6

Substrates (trade name)	Inhibitors (trade name)	Inducers (trade name)
Amitriptyline (Elavil®)	Amiodarone (Cordarone®, Pacerone®)	Carbamazepine (Tegretol®)
Bisoprolol (Zebeta®)		Phenobarbital (Luminal sodium®)
Chlorpromazine (Thorazine®)	Celecoxib (Celebrex®)	Phenytoin (Dilantin®)

(continued)

Appendix 13

Common Drug Interactions (continued)

CYP2D6 (cont)

Substrates (trade name)	Inhibitors (trade name)	Inducers (trade name)
Clomipramine (Anafranil®)	Cimetidine (Tagamet®)	Rifampin (Rifadin®, Rimactane®)
Clozapine (Clozaril®)	Clomipramine (Anafranil®)	Ritonavir (Norvir®)
Codeine	Desipramine (Norpramin®)	
Cyclobenzaprine (Flexeril®)	Fluoxetine (Prozac®)	
Desipramine (Norpramin®)	Haloperidol (Haldol®)	
Dextromethorphan	Indinavir (Crixivan®)	
Doxepin (Sinequan®)	Paroxetine (Paxil®)	
Fluoxetine (Prozac®)	Propafenone (Rhythmol®)	
Gingko	Quinidine (Cardioquin®, Quinaglute®, Dura-	
Haloperidol (Haldol®)	Tabs®, Quinidex®)	
Hydrocodone		
Imipramine (Tofranil®)	Ritonavir (Norvir®)	
Metoprolol (Lopressor®)	Sertraline (Zoloft®)	
Nortriptyline (Aventyl®, Pamelor®)	Thioridazine (Mellaril®)	
Oxycodone (Endocodone®, OxyContin®, OxyIR®, Percolone®, Roxicodone®)		
Paroxetine (Paxil®)		
Perfenazine (Trilafon®)		
Propafenone (Rhythmol®)		
Propranolol (Inderal®)		
Risperidone (Risperdal®)		
Thioridazine (Mellaril®)		
Timolol (Betimol®, Blocadrin®, Timoptic®)		
Tramadol (Ultram®)		
Trazodone (Desyrel®)		
Venlafaxine (Effexor®)		

CYP2E1

Acetaminophen (Tylenol®)	Disulfram (Antabuse®)	Chronic ethanol
Chlorzoxazone (Parafon Forte®)		Isoniazid (Nydrazid®)
Ethanol, enflurane, halothane, isoflurane		

CYP3A

Alprazolam (Xanax®)	Amiodarone (Cordarone®, Pacerone®)	Carbamazepine (Tegretol®)
Astemizole (Hismanal®)	Cimetidine (Tagamet®)	Glucocorticoids
Atorvastatin (Lipitor®)	Clarithromycin (Biaxin®)	Phenobarbital (Luminal sodium®)
Buspirone (Buspar®)	Erythromycin (E-Mycin®)	Phenytoin (Dilantin®)
Calcium channel blockers	Fluconazole (Diflucan®)	Primidone (Mysoline®)
Carbamazepine (Tegretol®)	Fluoxetine (Prozac®)	Rifampin (Rifadin®, Rimactane®)
Cilostazol (Pletal®)	Fluvoxamine (Luvox®)	Ritonavir (Norvir®)
Cisapride (Propulsid®)	Grapefruit juice	St. John's wort
Citalopram (Celexa®)	Indinavir (Crixivan®)	
Clindamycin (Cleocin®)	Itraconazole (Sporanox®)	
Clomipramine (Anafranil®)	Ketoconazole (Nizoral®)	
Clonazepam (Klonopin®)	Metronidazole (Flagyl®)	
Cyclosporine (Gengraf®, Neoral®, Sandimmune®)	Miconazole (Monistat®)	

(continued)

Appendix 13

Common Drug Interactions (continued)

CYP3A (cont)

Substrates (trade name)	Inhibitors (trade name)	Inducers (trade name)
Dapsone	Nefazodone (Serzone®)	
Erythromycin (E-Mycin®)	Nelfinavir (Viracept®)	
Estrogens	Norfloxacin (Chibroxin®, Noroxin®)	
Garlic	Ritonavir (Norvir®)	
Gingko	Saquinavir (Fortovase®, Invirase®)	
Imipramine (Tofranil®)	Sertraline (Zoloft®)	
Protease inhibitors	Valerian	
Ketoconazole (Nizoral®)	Zafirlukast (Accolate®)	
Losartan (Cozaar®)		
Lovastatin (Mevacor®)		
Miconazole (Monistat®)		
Midazolam (Versed®)		
Montelukast (Singulair®)		
Nefazodone (Serzone®)		
Ondansetron (Zofran®)		
Prednisone (Deltasone®, Meticorten®, Orasone®)		
Quinidine (Cardioquin®, Quinaglute®, Quinidex®)		
Rifampin (Rifadin®, Rimactane®)		
Sertraline (Zoloft®)		
Simvastatin (Zocor®)		
Tacrolimus (Prograf®)		
Tamoxifen (Nolvadex®)		
Temazepam (Restoril®)		
Triazolam (Halcion®)		
R-Warfarin (Coumadin®)		

References

Goshman L, Fish J, Roller K. Clinically significant cytochrome P450 drug interactions. *J Pharmacy Soc Wisc.* 1999;May/June:23-38.

Michalets EL. Update: Clinically significant cytochrome P450 drug interactions. *Pharmacotherapy.* 1998;18:84-112.

MICROMEDEX" Healthcare Series: MICROMEDEX, Greenwood Village, CO (edition expires 3/2003).

Woosley RL. Drugs that prolong the QT interval and/or induce torsades de pointes. Available at www.qtdrugs.org/medical-pros/drug-lists/printable-drug-list.cfm. Accessed February 20, 2003.

From the American Pharmacists Association

The Leader in Providing the Most Comprehensive Line of Resources to Pharmacists and Health Professionals

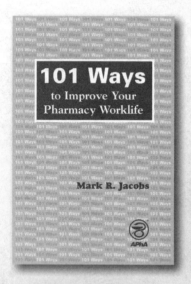

101 Ways to Improve Your Pharmacy Worklife

Mark R. Jacobs

In pharmacies across the country, pharmacists are busier, more stressed, and, some would say, unhappier than ever before, resulting from an increasing volume of prescriptions being written today, chronic delays in securing reimbursement from third-party payers, pharmacist shortages, and unprofessional working conditions.

Written by a frontline community pharmacist who has refused to passively accept the status quo during his many years in practice, *101 Ways to Improve Your Pharmacy Worklife* is the first book to offer pharmacists practical ways to reduce stress and improve their professional well-being.

ISBN: 978-1-58212-014-0 • 2001 • 165 pp • Softbound

APhA Member	$36.00
Nonmember	$40.00

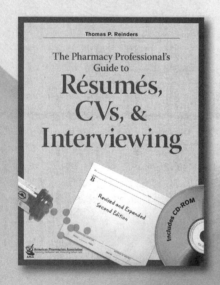

The Pharmacy Professional's Guide to Résumés, CVs, & Interviewing

Thomas P. Reinders

The latest edition of this popular resource geared specifically for job-seeking pharmacy professionals gives step-by-step instructions for developing written materials, such as résumés, CVs, and cover letters that get results, and prepares you for interviews that distinguish you from the crowd. New sections help you build a professional image by developing portfolios, business cards, and personal statements as well as putting e-mail to work in your favor. It contains 15 sample résumés, 6 sample CVs, and 20 sample letters for pharmacists and technicians in a variety of settings, including community pharmacy, hospitals, academia, and industry.

2nd Edition
ISBN: 978-1-58212-076-8 • 2006 • 164 pp • Softbound with CD-ROM

APhA Member	$41.00
Nonmember	$45.00

08

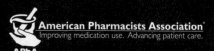